Motor Disorders

Motor Disorders

Editor

David S. Younger, M.D.
Associate Clinical Professor of Neurology
Director of Clinical Neuromuscular Disorders, and
Co-Director, Jerry Lewis Muscular Dystrophy Association Clinic at Rusk Institute
New York University Medical Center
Chief, Neuromuscular Diseases, and
Director of the Electromyography Laboratory
Lenox Hill Hospital
New York, New York

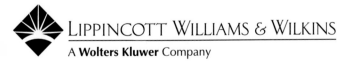

LIPPINCOTT WILLIAMS & WILKINS
A **Wolters Kluwer** Company
Philadelphia · Baltimore · New York · London
Buenos Aires · Hong Kong · Sydney · Tokyo

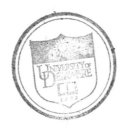

Acquisitions Editor: Anne M. Sydor
Developmental Editor: Mildred G. Ramos
Manufacturing Manager: Tim Reynolds
Production Manager: Liane Carita
Production Editor: Tony DeGeorge
Cover Designer: Jeane Norton
Indexer: Michael Ferreira
Compositor: Lippincott Williams & Wilkins Desktop Division
Printer: Edwards Brothers

Printed in the United States of America

9 8 7 6 5 4 3 2 1

Library of Congress Cataloging-in-Publication Data
Motor disorders / editor, David S. Younger.
    p. cm.
    Includes bibliographical references and index.
    ISBN 0-316-97600-8 (alk. paper)
    1. Neuromuscular diseases.   I. Younger, David S.
    [DNLM: 1. Neuromuscular Diseases. WE 550 M9185 1999]
  RC925.M65   1999
  616.7′44—dc21
  DNLM/DLC   98-32461
  For Library of Congress   CIP

This book is dedicated to the spouses, children, and significant others of all of the contributors. In that regard, personal appreciation and dedication goes to my wife Holly, our two sons Adam and Seth, and our dog Armand, who all sat by patiently and were often displaced while the process of editing and writing took place.

Contents

Part III: Spinal Cord Diseases

Part IV: The Neuronal Degenerations

Part V: Neurorehabilitation

Contributors

Editor for Neurorehabilitation

Stanley J. Myers, M.D.
Corning Professor of Rehabilitation Medicine
Columbia University and
New York Presbyterian Hospital
710 West 168th Street
New York, New York 10032

Steven M. Albert, Ph.D., MSc.
Assistant Professor of Neuropsychology
* and Public Health*
Gertrude H. Sergievsky Center
Columbia University
630 West 168th Street, P&S Box 16
New York, New York 10032

Anthony A. Amato, M.D.
Assistant Professor of Medicine/Neurology
Co-Director of Neuromuscular Service
University of Texas Health Science Center
* at San Antonio*
7703 Floyd Curl Drive
San Antonio, Texas 78284-7883

John R. Bach, M.D.
Vice Chair
Department of Physical Medicine and
* Rehabilitation*
UMDNJ-The New Jersey Medical School
110 Bergen Street, University Heights
Newark, New Jersey 07103

George D. Baquis, M.D.
Assistant Professor
Department of Neurology
Tufts University School of Medicine
145 Harrison Avenue
Boston, Massachusetts 02111, and
Director
Electromyography Laboratory
Division of Neurology
Baystate Medical Center
Springfield, Massachusetts 01199

Richard J. Barohn, M.D.
Professor of Neurology
Lois C. A. and Darwin E. Smith Distinguished
* Chair in Neurological Mobility Research*
Acting Chair
Department of Neurology
University of Texas Southwestern
* Medical Center at Dallas*
5323 Harry Hines Boulevard
Dallas, Texas 75235-8897

Andrew Blitzer, D.D.S.
New York Center for
* Voice and Swallowing Disorders at*
* Saint Luke's/Roosevelt Hospital Center*
Head and Neck Surgical Group
425 West 59th Street, Suite 4E
New York, New York 10019

Charles F. Bolton, M.D., F.R.C.P.(C)
Professor
Department of Clinical Neurological Sciences
University of Western Ontario, and
Consultant
Department of Clinical Neurological Sciences
London Health Sciences Centre
800 Commissioners Road East
London, Ontario N6A 4G5, Canada

Eduardo Bonilla, M.D.
Professor of Neurology and Pathology
Department of Neurology
Columbia University
* College of Physicians and Surgeons*
630 West 168th Street
New York, New York 10032

Thomas H. Brannagan III, M.D.
Department of Neurology
MCP-Hahnemann University
Broad and Vine, Mail Stop 308
Philadelphia, Pennsylvania 19102-1192

Susan Bressman, M.D.
Professor and Chair
Department of Neurology
Beth Israel Medical Center
Phillips Ambulatory Care Center
10 Union Square East
New York, New York 10003

Mitchell F. Brin, M.D.
Backman-Straus Professor of Neurology
Associate Professor
Director, Movement Disorders Program
Department of Neurology
Mount Sinai Medical Center
One Gustave Levy Place, Box 1052
New York, New York 10029

Mark B. Bromberg, M.D., Ph.D.
Associate Professor
Director
Neuromuscular Program
Department of Neurology
University of Utah School of Medicine
50 North Medical Drive
Salt Lake City, Utah 84132

Robert H. Brown, Jr., M.D., Ph.D., D.Phil.
Professor
Department of Neurology
Harvard Medical School
25 Shattuck Street
Boston, Massachusetts 02115, and
Associate
Department of Neurology
Massachusetts General Hospital
Building 149, 13th Street, Room 6627
Charlestown, Massachusetts 02129

Peter A. Calabresi, M.D.
Assistant Professor
Department of Clinical Neurosciences
Brown University, and
Director, Multiple Sclerosis Program
Rhode Island Hospital
110 Lockwood Street, Suite 342
Providence, Rhode Island 02903

Michael P. Collins, M.D.
Assistant Professor
Department of Neurology
Ohio State University School of Medicine
Means Hall, 4th Floor
Columbus, Ohio 43210

Marinos C. Dalakas, M.D.
Neuromuscular Diseases Section
National Institute of
*   Neurological Disorders and Stroke*
National Institutes of Health
Building 10 Room 4N248
9000 Rockville Pike
Bethesda, Maryland 20892

Josep Dalmau, M.D.
Assistant Attending Neurologist
Department of Neurology
Memorial Sloan-Kettering Cancer Center
1275 York Avenue
New York, New York 10021

Maura L. Del Bene, R.N., B.S.N.
Co-Director
The Eleanor and Lou Gehrig
*   Muscular Dystrophy Association/*
*   Amyotrophic Lateral Sclerosis Center*
Neurological Institute, and
Research Nurse Clinician
Department of Education Research
*   and Standards*
New York Presbyterian Hospital
710 West 168th Street
New York, New York 10032

Darryl C. De Vivo, M.D.
Sidney Carter Professor of Neurology and
*   Professor of Pediatrics*
Columbia University
*   College of Physicians and Surgeons, and*
Director of Pediatric Neurology
Neurological Institute and Babies Hospital
New York Presbyterian Hospital
710 West 168th Street
New York, New York 10032

Salvatore DiMauro, M.D.
Lucy G. Moses Professor of Neurology
Director
H. Houston Meritt Clinical Research Center for
*   Muscular Dystrophy and Related Diseases*
Columbia University
*   College of Physicians and Surgeons*
630 West 168th Street
New York, New York 10032

Judy Drucker, R.N., A.N.P.-C
Adult Nurse Practitioner
Department of Neurology
State University of New York
    Health Science Center at Syracuse
750 East Adams Street
Syracuse, New York 13210

Mark A. Ferrante, M.D.,
    Major, U.S.A.F., M.C.
Director, Electromyography Laboratory
Staff Neurologist,
    Department of Neurology
Keesler Medical Center
301 Fisher Street
Biloxi, Mississipi 39534

Amory J. Fiore, M.D.
Department of Neurosurgery
Neurological Institute
New York Presbyterian Hospital
710 West 168th Street
New York, New York 10032

Andrew D. Goodman, M.D.
Associate Professor
Department of Neurology
University of Rochester, and
Director
Multiple Sclerosis Center
Strong Memorial Hospital
601 Elmwood Avenue
Rochester, New York 14642

Robert C. Griggs, M.D., Ph.D.
Edward A. and Alma Vollertsen Rykenboer
    Professor of Neurophysiology
Professor and Chair
Editor-in-Chief
Department of Neurology
University of Rochester
601 Elmwood Avenue, Box 673
Rochester, New York 14642

John J. Halperin, M.D.
Professor
Department of Neurology
New York University School of Medicine
New York, New York 10016, and
Chairman
Department of Neurology
North Shore University Hospital
300 Community Drive
Manhassett, New York 11030

Asao Hirano, M.D.
Division of Neuropathology
Department of Pathology,
Montefiore Medical Center
111 East 210th Street
Bronx, New York 10467

Michio Hirano, M.D.
Florence Irving Assistant Professor
Department of Neurology
Columbia University School of Medicine, and
Assistant Attending Physician
New York Presbyterian Hospital
630 West 168th Street
New York, New York 10032

Robert N. N. Holtzman, M.D.
Assistant Clinical Professor
Department of Neurological Surgery
Columbia University School of Medicine, and
Associate Attending Physician
Department of Neurological Surgery
Neurological Institute
New York Presbyterian Hospital
710 West 168th Street
New York, New York 10032

Gerald W. Honch M.D.
Department of Neurology
University of Rochester, and
Rochester General Hospital
1425 Portland Avenue
Rochester, New York 14621

Susan T. Iannaccone, M.D.
Professor
Department of Neurology
University of Texas Southwestern
Medical Center at Dallas
5323 Harry Hines Boulevard
Dallas, Texas 75235, and
Director
Neuromuscular Diseases and
    Neurorehabilitation
Department of Neurology
Texas Scottish Rite Hospital for Children
222 Welborn Street
Dallas, Texas 75219

Burk Jubelt, M.D.
Department of Neurology
State University of New York
    Health Science Center at Syracuse
750 East Adams Street
Syracuse, New York 13210

Michael G. Kaiser, M.D.
Neurological Institute
New York Presbyterian Hospital
710 West 168th Street
New York, New York 10032

Dennis D. J. Kim, M.D.
Department of Rehabilitation Medicine
Albert Einstein College of Medicine, and
Department of Rehabilitation Medicine
Montefiore Medical Center
111 East 210th Street
Bronx, New York 10467

Heakyung Kim, M.D.
Vice Chairman and Fellow
Department of Physical Medicine
  and Rehabilitation
UMDNJ-The New Jersey
  Medical School, and
Department of Rehabilitation Medicine
University Hospital B403
150 Bergen Street
Newark, New Jersey 07103

John T. Kissel, M.D.
Professor
Department of Neurology
Ohio State University Hospital
1654 Upham Drive
Columbus, Ohio 43210

Christian Krarup, M.D., Ph.D.
Professor
Faculty of Medicine
University of Copenhagen
Blegdamsvej 3
2200 Copenhagen, Denmark and
Director
Department of
  Clinical Neurophysiology
Rigshospitalet
Blegdamsvej 9
2100 Copenhagen, Denmark

William E. Krauss, M.D.
Department of Neurology
Neurological Institute
New York Presbyterian Hospital
710 West 168th Street
New York, New York 10032

Hirofumi Kusaka, M.D.
Professor and Chairman
Department of Neurology
Kansai Medical University, and
Director
Department of Neurology
Kansai Medical University Hospital
10-15 Fumizonocho
Moriguchishi, Osaka 570-8506, Japan

Dale J. Lange, M.D.
Neurological Institute
New York Presbyterian Hospital
710 West 168th Street
New York, New York 10032

Andrew B. Lassman, M.D.
Columbia University
  College of Physicians and Surgeons, and
Department of Neurology
New York Presbyterian Hospital
710 West 168th Street
New York, New York 10032

Norman Latov, M.D., Ph.D.
Professor
Department of Neurology
Columbia University, and
Director
Peripheral Neuropathy Center
Department of Neurology
New York Presbyterian Hospital
710 West 168th Street
New York, New York 10032

Elan D. Louis, M.D.
Assistant Professor
Department of Neurology
Gertrude H. Sergievsky Center
Columbia University
  College of Physicians and Surgeons
710 West 168th Street
New York, New York 10032

Robert E. Lovelace, M.D., F.R.C.P.
Columbia University
  College of Physicians and Surgeons, and
Neurological Institute
New York Presbyterian Hospital
710 West 168th Street
New York, New York 10032

Timothy Lynch, M.D.
Assistant Professor of Neurology
Department of Neurology
Neurological Institute
New York Presbyterian Hospital
710 West 168th Street
New York, New York 10032

Daniel J. L. MacGowan, M.R.C.P.I.
Neuro-AIDS Research Program
Departments of Neurology and
*   Clinical Neurophysiology*
Mount Sinai Medical Center
One Gustave Levy Place, Box 1052
New York, New York 10029

Thornton B. Alex Mason II, M.D.
Assistant Professor
Department of Neurology
Columbia University, and
Assistant Attending Physician
New York Presbyterian Hospital
710 West 168th Street
New York, New York 10032

Paul C. McCormick, M.D.
Associate Professor of
*   Clinical Neurosurgery*
Department of Neurosurgery
Columbia University College of
*   Physicians and Surgeons, and*
Associate Attending Physician
New York Presbyterian Hospital
710 West 168th Street
New York, New York 10032

Jerry R. Mendell, M.D.
Professor and Chair
Department of Neurology
Ohio State University
473 Means Hall, Room 445
Columbus, Ohio 43210

Carlo Minetti, M.D.
Department of Pediatrics
University of Genova
Istituto G. Gaslini
Largo G. Gaslini 5
16147 Genova, Italy

Hugo W. Moser, M.D.
University Professor
Department of Neurology
*   and Pediatrics*
Johns Hopkins University, and
Director
Neurogenetics Research
Kennedy Krieger Institute
707 North Broadway
Baltimore, Maryland 21205

Peregrine L. Murphy, MSc, M.D.IV
The Eleanor and Lou Gehrig Muscular
*   Dystrophy Association/Amyotrophic*
*   Lateral Sclerosis Research Center*
Neurological Institute
New York Presbyterian Hospital
710 West 168th Street
New York, New York 10032

Mile Nikolic, M.Sc.
Clinical Assistant
Faculty of Medicine
University of Cophenhagen, and
Civil Engineer
Department of Clinical Neurophysiology
Rigshospitalet
Blegsdamsvej 9
2100 Copenhagen, Denmark

Gareth J. Parry, M.D.
Professor and Head
Department of Neurology
Fairview-University Medical Center
University of Minnesota
420 Delaware Street SE
Minneapolis, Minnesota 55455

James M. Powers, M.D.
Professor
Department of Pathology and
*   Laboratory Medicine*
University of Rochester
601 Elmwood Avenue
Rochester, New York 14642

Seth L. Pullman, M.D.
Neurological Institute
New York Presbyterian Hospital
710 West 168th Street
New York, New York 10032

Barry Rodstein, M.D.
Assistant Professor
Department of Rehabilitation Medicine
Albert Einstein College of Medicine, and
Attending Physician
Department of Rehabilitation Medicine
Montefiore Medical Center
111 East 210th Street
Bronx, New York 10467

Gustavo C. Román, M.D.
Department of Neurology
University of Texas
*   Health Sciences Center*
San Antonio, Texas 78284-7883

Michael Rose, M.D.
Honorary Senior Lecturer
Department of Neurology
Guys, Kings, and St. Thomas's
*   Medical School, and*
Consultant Neurologist
Kings College Hospital
Denmark Hill
London SE5 8A2, United Kingdom

Myrna R. Rosenfeld, M.D., Ph.D.
Assistant Professor
Department of Neurology
*   and Neuroscience*
New York Hospital–
*   Cornell Medical Center, and*
Assistant Attending Neurologist
Memorial Sloan-Kettering
*   Cancer Center*
1275 York Avenue
New York, New York 10021

Saud A. Sadiq, M.D.
Assistant Professor
Department of Neurology
Albert Einstein College of Medicine, and
Chief
Department of Neurology
St. Luke's-Roosevelt Hospital
425 West 59th Street, Suite 7C
New York, New York 10019

David S. Saperstein, M.D.
Chief
Neuromuscular Disease Service
Department of Neurology
Wilford Hall Medical Center
2200 Bergquist Drive, Suite 1
San Antonio, Texas 78236

Steven R. Schwid, M.D.
Assistant Professor of Neurology
University of Rochester
*   Medical Center*
601 Elmwood Avenue
Rochester, New York 14642

Stefano Simonetti, M.D.
Division of Neurology
E. O. Ospedali Galliera
Mura delle Cappuccine, 14
16128 Genova, Italy

David M. Simpson, M.D.
Associate Professor
Department of Neurology, and
Director
Clinical Neurophysiology Laboratories and
*   Neuro-AIDS Research Program*
Mount Sinai Medical Center
1 Gustave Levy Place, Box 1052
New York, New York 10029

Celia F. Stewart, M.D.
Department of Speech-Language
*   Pathology and Audiology*
New York University
719 Broadway, Room 237
New York, New York 10003, and
Department of Neurology
Movement Disorders Center
Mount Sinai School of Medicine and
the Mount Sinai Hospital
One Gustave Levy Place
New York, New York 10029

Samer D. Tabbal, M.D.
Movement Disorders Fellow
Columbia University
*   College of Physicians and Surgeons, and*
Department of Neurology
Neurological Institute
New York Presbyterian Hospital
710 West 168th Street
New York, New York 10032

Kurenai Tanji, M.D.
Associate Research Scientist
Department of Neurology
Columbia University
*   College of Physicians and Surgeons*
630 West 168th Street
New York, New York 10032

Chang-Yong Tsao, M.D.
Departments of Neurology and Pediatrics
Ohio State University and
*   Children's Hospital*
700 Children's Drive
Columbus, Ohio 43205

Louis H. Weimer, M.D.
Neurological Institute
Columbia University
*   College of Physicians and Surgeons, and*
Department of Neurology
New York Presbyterian Hospital
710 West 168th Street
New York, New York 10032

Asa J. Wilbourn, M.D.
Associate Clinical Professor
Department of Neurology
Case Western Reserve
*   School of Medicine, and*
Director
Electromyography Laboratory
Department of Neurology
Cleveland Clinic Foundation
9500 Euclid Avenue
Cleveland, Ohio 44195

David S. Younger, M.D.
Associate Clinical Professor
Department of Neurology
Director of
*   Clinical Neuromuscular Disorders, and*
Co-Director, Jerry Lewis Muscular Dystrophy
*   Association Clinic at Rusk Institute*
New York University Medical Center
550 First Avenue
New York, New York 10016
Chief, Neuromuscular Diseases, and
Director of the Electromyography Laboratory
Lenox Hill Hospital
100 East 77th Street
New York, New York 10021

Douglas W. Zochodne, M.D.
Associate Professor
Department of Clinical Neurosciences
Neurosciences Research Group
University of Calgary, and
Consultant Neurologist
Department of Clinical Neurosciences
Foothills Hospital
3330 Hospital Drive NW
182A Heritage Medical Research Building
Calgary, Alberta T2N 4N1, Canada

Preface

A striking aspect of the history of motor disorders has been the persistence of generations of neuroscientists and clinicians to search for a more cohesive understanding of the motor system in health and disease. Remarkable progress has been achieved over the past decade in the classification, diagnosis, etiopathogenesis, and treatment of many peripheral and central nervous system motor disorders. This has occurred along the diverse lines of electrophysiology, immunology, molecular genetics, ultrastructural analysis, as well as technical advances in neurosurgical and rehabilitative care. These advances have in turn fostered more effective and innovative treatments in many of the debilitating neuromuscular disorders, leading to sustained remissions, and at the least, improved outcomes and enhanced independence.

When first considering the outline of this book, it was clear that the proposed content differed from available standard textbooks of general neurology, myology, peripheral neuropathy, and rehabilitation medicine. The project most closely resembled Michael Brooke's monograph, *A Clinician's Guide to Neuromuscular Disease*, first published two decades ago, and still exerting influence on current generations of students of neuromuscular disease for the quality of its teaching and the ease of reading. In tribute to his contributions over the many years in the field of motor disorders, we were fortunate that Dr. Brooke agreed to write the Foreword.

The content of the book is divided into five sections. Part One encompasses general aspects of the clinical laboratory investigation of motor disorders. Parts Two through Four contain chapters on the most important motor disorders of the peripheral and central nervous system, working from the muscle and nerve, to the spinal cord, and brain. Part Five was coedited with Dr. Stanley Myers, Corning Professor of Rehabilitation Medicine at Columbia University. It covers the theory and practice of neurorehabilitation, topics not ordinarily found in a neurology textbook, as well as all the essential aspects of physiotherapy, bracing, respiratory therapy, management of spasticity and dystonia, speech and swallowing, bladder, bowel, and sexual disorders, and importantly, interdisciplinary palliative and psychosocial care.

The invited authors, all experts in their fields, were drawn from all parts of the United States and abroad. They demonstrated extreme tolerance in allowing their work to be carefully edited and blended together toward the larger goal of a single volume applicable to health professionals from different backgrounds. Many authors were drawn from the Columbia-Presbyterian Medical Center of the New York Presbyterian Hospital. That was where my clinical and academic career was launched, impassioned by mentors and contemporary colleagues who encouraged me to edit this book.

Mark Placito, Senior Editor initiated the process. It was ably continued by Anne Sydor, Associate Editor, Mildred Ramos, Editorial Assistant, and Tony DeGeorge, Associate Production Editor.

Foreword

I was delighted to be asked to compose a foreword for Dr. Younger's book on muscle diseases. Man is a self-centered creature and the request was pleasing, even though I remember the wry musings of a former Dean as to his selection for the post. The Faculty was scrutinized to see whose research was impoverished, and the choice was obvious. I researched the subject of forewords at some length and was fascinated to discover that they generally begin with a cliché and end with a homily. So be it.

Our generation is probably as entitled to the conceit that we live in momentous times as any of our forebears. When one considers that a textbook of medicine in the Renaissance was valid for centuries and that the practices of medicine in the time of Avicenna continued through the Middle Ages, it is amazing to witness in one lifetime the new renaissance. Even more remarkable that the one subspecialty, neuromuscular diseases, has been so much in the forefront of these developments. Merely forty years ago the clinician's responsibility ended with the diagnosis, more or less accurate. Muscle biopsy was in its infancy and the standard textbooks, written by Adams, Denny, Brown, and Pearson did not mention muscle histochemistry. There were no neuromuscular conditions whose fundamental cause was apparent, although myasthenia was becoming clearer. Treatment was based on not-so-benign neglect and even simple rehabilitative techniques were shunned. The scientific method had not yet been blossomed and clinical trials were based on whimsy.

In many ways, the progress in medicine has mirrored the general human lot. It is trite to note that we have come from the first powered flight to the boundaries of space in less than a century, but this is to overlook the real progress. The invention of the ballpoint pen and the adhesive note, both of which appeared within the last fifty years, have probably had more influence on the ordinary person. When it became possible to build higher than three stories, larger groups of people could work and live together and it spelled the end of isolation as surely as the Industrial Revolution spelled the end of the cottage industry. The significant development was not, however, the skyscraper, but the elevator, that made this space useful, an item which would hardly be credited today with the development of the Western world. Marconi is remembered because he and his predecessors showed that information could be sent without wires, but it was the invention of Lee de Forest's vacuum tube and of Armstrong's regenerative receivers that made wireless communication more than an atmospheric freak and provoked the radio boom of the 1920s.

Similarly, it is easy to recall the breakthroughs in neuromuscular disease such as the Lennon's animal model of myasthenia in 1975, which established the autoimmune basis of the disease. In the same decade, changes in the design of wheelchairs and the use of orthotics changed the lives of more people but did not provoke the same discussion over coffee. The revelation of the abnormal superoxide dismutase gene in amyotrophic lateral sclerosis (ALS) by the group at the Massachusetts General Hospital was and is an exciting piece of research with major implications in the illness, but the ALS patient is equally impressed by percutaneous gastrostomy. It is really the difference between the basic research which fascinates all of us in the field and applied research which impacts the lives of our patients.

Medicine, like many aspects of civilization, is dependent upon the spread of information; among researchers, practitioners, and out into the general public. In the 1400s Gutenberg and Caxton developed the printed page, and for the next 500 years the world learned to read. Medicine developed slowly and the best work was the careful observational studies from the great physicians such as Willis and Harvey. The physician was still the scholar, the seer. The abbreviation and the acronym had not yet displaced the elegance of writing that is so characteristic of the medical journals a century ago.

In the 1950s the photo typesetter appeared and the printed paperback, bringing an abundance of books within the reach of all. Communication vaulted into the airwaves where the equivalent of the paperback, the pocket radio, appeared following the invention of the transistor by Shockley and colleagues in 1947. Television replaced the hearth as a focal point. The generation brought up without TV is dying out. So is the musical evening, the quilting bee, and the reading club. The computer, which had its beginnings in the mammoth Electronic Numerical Integrator and Computer developed by Eckert and Mauchly in the 1940s, was slower to develop until the integrated circuit reduced the physical size and costs to practical levels. Once that happened, the development and application of the device has been astonishing. The printing press made it possible for everyone to read and liberated mankind from superstition and ignorance. The computer has enabled the individual to publish effortlessly to the far corners of the world, no matter how ignorant or superstitious the publication. Indeed we now live under the computer's dominance. Gutenberg could probably have foreseen the long-range effect of his invention. Marconi, deForest, and Armstrong could not.

Medicine has been profoundly affected by these changes at two levels. The first is the ease of communication within the profession. A myriad of journals assail our libraries with more information in a month than was available during the entire eighteenth century. Computers have made this information overload accessible as they process and search from everything from DNA sequences to the number of right-handed plumbers with carpal tunnel syndrome.

The second is probably far more reaching. The public now has access to medical information in a way that has never been possible. The paperback started it with a series of handbooks on medical matters ranging from Dr. Spock to Dr. Ruth. With the coming of the Internet, public access has broadened and we have all experienced patients who have researched their illness extensively on the Internet. Unfortunately, the information available electronically varies from the orthodox to the outlandish. It would be interesting to calculate the ratio of information to misinformation on the Internet. It may not reach parity. The result of all this is that the public is more critical and demanding, and, correspondingly, the physician must now be more informed than ever.

Neuromuscular disease has developed into a recognizable subspecialty in about the same time period that the computer has matured. Three decades ago, our knowledge of neuromuscular disease was based on the clinical descriptions pioneered by Duchenne, Erb, and others in the 1800s, akin to the demonstration of wireless telegraphy by Marconi. The pathophysiology of disease was debated but theories lacked proof and speculation often took us far afield. The topic of neuromuscular disease occurred rarely in the medical curriculum. Specialists in the area were unknown with the notable exceptions of the group at Columbia, the University of California, Los Angeles, the National Institutes of Health, and the University of Pennsylvania in the U.S. and Newcastle in England. The 1960s saw the spread of the specialty to other centers and the growing awareness that there was more to neuromuscular disease than limb girdle dystrophy and Duchenne dystrophy. Neurology appointed itself the guardian of the entire clinical discipline. This was not surprising, for the clinical care of patients and electromyography were traditional neuroscientific endeavors, but it was unusual in the realm of pathology. Before long, under the leadership of King Engel and others, muscle histochemistry became an essential part of the pathological diagnosis and was an area of which the general pathologist knew little. Universities across North America, Europe, and the rest of the world pressed recruitment in the area and the muscle doctors fanned out into the hinterlands. So active was the recruitment that soon it appeared that there were more people making a living from muscle disease than there were dying from it.

The Muscular Dystrophy Association (MDA), in the U.S. and Canada, raised large amounts of money to add to the government funds and the specialty became a popular one for the investigative scientist. The 1970s were associated with an upsurge of research in immunology, spurred by the identification of the immune attack on the end plate in myasthenia gravis. Much of the research was concentrated on the muscular dystrophies, probably due to the influence of the MDA. Observational research and case descriptions gave way to careful biochemical and electrophysiological characterization of disease. One of the problems in medical research arose from one of its early successes. When penicillin was discovered, its effect on infectious disease was so dramatic that there was no doubt about its efficacy. The patient with a fulminating pneumonia who was returned to immediate good health by the injection of the new penicillin was testimony enough to its effect. This lulled us into the belief that any agent which might be useful in the treatment of disease could be tested on one or at most a handful of patients. Vignos and colleagues had quietly changed the rehabilitative approach and made an enormous difference in the lives of patients with muscle disease, but the real search was for The Cure. There was a belief that if enough therapeutic agents were tried one of them would have this Lazarus effect. There was not felt to be any need for the large clinical trial upon which our sister specialty of cardiology, that other muscle specialty, was then embarking. Clinical trials in the 1970s were thus rare and usually case controls.

At the end of the 1970s it seemed as if the most promising line of approach in the muscular dystrophies was to be from the unraveling of the biochemical and physiological puzzles. Research often went far afield from the muscle and varied from looking at abnormalities in the structure, function, and proteins in lymphocytes and red blood cells in Duchenne dystrophy to speculation that an abnormality in the blood supply might be its cause.

Neuropathies remained an area for the descriptive scientist. The pathological findings and detailed clinical examinations carried out by Dyck and colleagues characterized the disease but did not reveal the cause. In ALS, research chased the causative agent, a virus, a toxin in the blood, one of the heavy metals, all to no avail.

The watershed came in the 1980s and did so in an area which few anticipated, except in hindsight. Molecular genetics had been making spectacular progress in other areas but it revolutionized the field of neuromuscular disease. Kunkel, Worton, Davies, and others whose omission here is not intended to offend, showed that it was possible to find and characterize the abnormal gene. Within a surprisingly short space of time, its product, dystrophin, was identified and tracked down to the sarcolemma. Duchenne dystrophy was the crucible for work which was extended by Campbell's group in Iowa and Tome and Fardeau in Paris among others. Today, the classification of muscular dystrophies, particularly the limb girdle and childhood groups, has been shattered by the discovery of the function and genetic basis of many of the errant proteins.

Parallel with the molecular biology of the dystrophies, the small group of diseases characterized by periodic paralysis yielded up their secrets. The abnormal structure of the malfunctioning ion channels in these illnesses has been characterized and their blueprints provide real hope that drugs may be tailor-made to correct the defects.

Another development of the 1980s was the recognition that the clinical trial was a scientific experiment and not simply an art form. The randomized controlled trial and the attendant rigorous diagnostic and selection criteria were recognized as essential as was the need for proper statistical analysis. Therapeutic agents were tested based on animal experiments and not simply on speculation. Leading the way in this area were the large ALS trials spurred on by the pharmaceutical companies to evaluate the newly synthesized neurotrophic factors. The results of several of these trials have stirred further debate over the difference between clinical significance and statistical significance and which one of these twins we should be pursuing.

Genetically engineered animals provide models of human disease and the possibility of treatment. The integration of the person with disability in the community has been reflected in building codes requiring wheelchair accessibility and by a change in the public's attitude.

The present decade has also seen challenges that have more to do with the environment of research than research itself. Traditionally research, medical and otherwise, has depended upon the backing and support of powerful sponsors. The church in the early years, the industrialists in the late part of the nineteenth and first half of the twentieth centuries, and governments after the Second World War. Each have supported research for their own aims and in each of these environments there have been penalties for stepping too far from the fold. In this way the direction of research was guided into areas that were considered meaningful.

The great contribution of the universities, other than teaching, was to provide a haven for academic researchers to pursue their own lines of investigation without the immediate possibility of losing their job when things were not going well. In the three decades after the 1940s, government believed that research in all areas was vital to the future well-being of their populations. It was an atmosphere in which the ills of mankind seemed to be on the brink of solution, death itself could be avoided if only enough funds were poured into the problem.

Setting aside military research, the governments did not attempt to force research into one channel or another and, since resources were ample, particularly in the United States, a multitude of projects blossomed. As always, some were good, some bad and some indifferent. As always, some of the good ones were disappointing and occasionally some of the most spectacular results came from unexpected sources. An awareness grew that to develop one good line of investigation, it was necessary to support a hundred less good.

Not only did research flourish, but the universities themselves grew with the influx of new scientists. Money is time and because salaries were available, junior medical faculty had the time to devote to their laboratory activities.

In the 1980s and in the current decade, the climate changed again. Countries and their governments were unable to devote the resources necessary to sustain the exponential growth of the medical system, both in health care and in medical research. Of the two it was easier to trim the research budget, but the health care budget posed a bigger threat by an order of several magnitudes. The well ran relatively dry. It was still possible to obtain funding for a top-notch research endeavor, but the merely ordinary were left to shrivel on the vine. Worse, medical faculty, particularly the young faculty members so essential to continuing research, spent most of their time having to generate their own income instead of being able to develop their research laboratory skills and become the next generation of productive researchers.

Into this void stepped the pharmaceutical industry. On the surface it looked like an ideal alliance. The companies responsible for the development and manufacturing of new drugs teaming up with the academic researchers whose laboratory research help discover these drugs. Indeed, it is an ideal system when it works well and there are many instances of collaborative research sponsored by the pharmaceutical firms, governments and universities.

There are potential problems and some have surfaced. In simplistic fashion, the goal of the researcher is to follow the research wherever it leads, even if the initial aim is the cure of an illness. The ultimate goal of the pharmaceutical company is to run a profitable company, be responsible to the stockholders and to market useful drugs to patients with illness.

Regulatory agencies play an important role in the lives of the pharmaceutical companies. Their function is an important one. The public cannot evaluate for themselves the effectiveness of a medication. There has always been a brisk market in nostrums and potions in neuromuscular diseases. As long as they are cheap and safe, little harm is done. With the increasing cost of medicines to society and the possibility of serious complications from the drugs, it was necessary to have some agency to evaluate the usefulness and safety of any new drug. The regulations are strict and the scrutiny intense. The ultimate proof of the drug is the controlled clinical trial. No new drug reaches the population without adequate demonstration of safety and efficacy by this means. The 1990s might be known as the decade of the clinical trial in neuromuscular disease. Not that the results were as spectacular as in molecular genetics. Far from it, but more energy and money was probably poured into this activity than most others and it was a major area of collaboration between the pharmaceutical industry and the research clinician. Drug testing developed a different connotation for the neuromuscular specialist than for the general public.

Industry had excellent research facilities and they were able to hire the brightest minds. Their own resources as well as venture capital provided the fuel. The components of the clinical trial included patients with a secure diagnosis, an illness which could be accurately measured and the likelihood that the measurements would change during the time of the trial.

Industry needed the research clinician in the academic setting for two reasons. First, access to the patients. Second, the clinical expertise of the specialist in the particular disease. The rules of the market place then took over. In the academic institutions, collaborative research with drug companies was not considered a suitable activity for the researcher. It just was not respectable. Further, the population of suitable patients was small and was concentrated in university centers. Drug companies found that they had to pay rather dearly to obtain access to these patients and there was no neighboring shop to go for competitive pricing.

Within a few years many departments were using the money from clinical trials to support their junior faculty and to give them the freedom for research that they had formerly enjoyed with federal funding. The pharmaceutical industry did not always get what they paid for. The regulatory agencies demanded, quite properly, meticulous record keeping, flawless case report forms and a host of other checks including on-site inspections. The clinical research team is not always sympathetic to such demands. A flawed clinical trial wastes a huge amount of money and some trials were less than perfect. More and more the pharmaceutical and biotechnology companies took control of all aspects of the clinical trials from the decision as to what drugs to test to data storage and analysis. Although the individual academic investigators were still able to provide input, the industry sponsored trial became the norm. It might be debated that there has been no loss of academic freedom in this process, but the danger is there. A pharmaceutical company certainly does not have to supply the resources for a project which might show its product in an unfavorable light. The company is also reluctant to make data from such studies freely available to any researcher that wants it, in fear that they might find their way to a competitor. Neither of these two are hypothetical examples. There is a further danger that has to be considered. Consider an active neuromuscular researcher, maintaining a laboratory and clinic staff with funds derived from clinical trials, who is approached to consider a clinical trial by two separate companies, each with a similar drug, say X and Y. Drug X is relatively free of known side effects and the per patient reimbursement will be $700 per patient. Drug Y has the same physiological effect but there is a small chance of liver or renal failure. The per patient reimbursement offered for this drug is $6,000 per patient. Who will choose which trial to accept, the investigator or the patient? If it be the patient, who will present him with the facts?

There is no malevolence on the part of the pharmaceutical industry. The people involved are as ethical, scrupulous and concerned as any in academic medicine. As an industry, however, their aim is different and each company has to explain itself to the annual general meeting. To have such a master might alter the concept of academic freedom and substitute the balance sheet for the curriculum vitae.

This may be especially relevant since the next step in neuromuscular diseases is about to be taken, akin to the invention of the integrated circuit for the computer. Within four years of the discovery of the abnormal gene in Duchenne dystrophy a technique to replace the missing protein was being discussed. The proposal was to infuse the abnormal muscle with normal myoblasts which would fuse with the regenerating muscle and carry the normal gene to the cell. The disappointment should probably have been anticipated in view of the efficiency with which the body rejects such interference.

Currently a more sophisticated delivery system is being tested in a logical and sequential fashion. This involves the insertion of a tailored gene into a viral carrier which has been gutted of its native genes. The virus is used to infect the animal and the genetic apparatus turned on in the muscle using a suitable promoter. With appropriate immunosuppression in animals the process is efficient enough to give hope that it might be used in human disease. Whether or not this particular model will work, it seems likely that within less than a decade some form of gene therapy will be available. When that happens it will light up the field of neuromuscular diseases as never before. Like all lights it will cast some shadows.

We will not only alter human disease we will alter human evolution. Ethics committees are already dealing with the ramifications of whether employers, insurance companies or children should be provided with the results of DNA testing. These problems will be nothing compared to whether one should be allowed to alter the intelligence, appearance or disease susceptibility of an individual. If so, will there be an ideal type to which the population will wish to conform? Science is poised on the brink of a change which may be as final as Armageddon if not as obvious.

In this maelstrom of change it is difficult to know when and where to place a book so that it doesn't get swept away. Dr. Younger has chosen a propitious moment and an excellent group of writers. There is a small hiatus as our knowledge of the pathophysiology of neuromuscular disease is refined. The community is gathering itself for the next leap forward. This will last until gene therapy becomes a reality and the next set of problems presents itself for the next generation to solve. In this pause it is useful to summarize the art and science of neuromuscular diseases. Dr. Younger and his colleagues are to be congratulated on seizing the day and producing a volume which will be useful to those of us trying to provide sensible advice to people with neuromuscular disease.

Michael Brooke
University of Alberta, Edmonton
Alberta, Canada

PART I

General Considerations

Motor Disorders,
edited by David S. Younger.
Lippincott Williams & Wilkins, Philadelphia © 1999.

CHAPTER 1

Overview of Motor Disorders

David S. Younger

The diagnosis of muscle weakness is an art that depends on experience and logical clinical reasoning because it encompasses much of clinical neurology. In this chapter we review aspects of the clinical and laboratory diagnosis of motor disorders, including recent achievements in electrophysiology, neuroimaging, molecular genetics, muscle and nerve biopsy analysis, and therapy, to serve as an introduction and background for the chapters and sections that follow.

HISTORY AND EXAMINATION

The history and neurologic examination are the important first steps in the diagnosis of motor disorders of the peripheral nervous system and central nervous system (CNS). The goal is to establish the neurologic symptoms and signs and their temporal progression and associated findings, and to formulate a categoric diagnosis and localize the disease process in the nervous system (1,2).

Patients should be asked about specific motor symptoms. Some patients may not use the term "weakness" but will instead give an equivalent history of difficulty in combing hair, brushing teeth, rising out of a chair, or going upstairs, indicative of proximal weakness; problems in buttoning a shirt or stepping over a curb point to predominant distal involvement. Progressive proximal weakness is the presenting symptom of polymyositis, dermatomyositis; mitochondrial, glycolytic, or lipid storage myopathy; and the Lambert-Eaton myasthenic syndrome (LEMS). Proximal weakness and prominent wasting is seen in facioscapulohumeral (FSH) and limb girdle muscular dystrophy (LGMD) and Duchenne and Becker muscular dystrophy (DMD and BMD, respectively), further separable by the distribution of weakness, inheritance pat-

D. S. Younger: Department of Clinical Neuromuscular Disorders and Jerry Lewis Muscular Dystrophy Association Clinic at Rusk Institute, New York University Medical Center and Department of Neuromuscular Disease and Electromyography Laboratory, Lenox Hill Hospital, New York, New York 10021.

tern, genetic studies, and distinctive findings on electomyography (EMG) and muscle biopsy. Myotonic dystrophy, scapuloperoneal dystrophy, distal myopathy, amyotrophic lateral sclerosis (ALS), and spinal muscular atrophy (SMA) are all associated with predominant distal weakness.

Patients should also be asked about specific sensory symptoms, because if there is sensory loss, there must be more than a myopathy, and the cause should be sought in a lesion in the peripheral nerves, dorsal root ganglia (DRG), or dorsal columns of the spinal cord. The symptoms should be recorded in the patients own words, such as various types of numbness, clumsiness, unsteadiness, pain, inability to recognize objects in the hand with eyes closed or in a pants pocket, and difficulty walking in the dark because of impaired proprioception.

Autonomic insufficiency may accompany motor disorders associated with diabetic, amyloid, or alcoholic neuropathy; acute intermittent porphyria; Guillain-Barré syndrome (GBS); botulism; tabes; Parkinson disease; and multiple system atrophy (MSA), and with the use of neuroleptic tranquilizers, antidepressant, and cardiovascular drugs. An early symptom of autonomic insufficiency is erectile failure in men because of a combination of autonomic and vascular disease that increases with age, duration of the underlying disorder, and vascular disease of the internal pudendal artery. Autonomic cardiovascular involvement in either gender leads to orthostatic lightheadedness and resting tachycardia. Gastric autonomic neuropathy leads to nausea, vomiting, early satiety, postprandial bloating, diffuse epigastric discomfort, and pancreatic exocrine insufficiency. Lower gastrointestinal motility disturbances can lead to diarrhea or constipation, bacterial overgrowth, intestinal mucosal insufficiency, and fecal incontinence. Genitourinary involvement is heralded by incomplete bladder emptying, overflow incontinence, frequent bladder infections, and retrograde ejaculation in men. Autonomic vasomotor insufficiency can lead to anhidrosis or hyperhidrosis, venous congestion, reflex pain, purplish discoloration of the feet, and facial gustatory sweating.

The tempo of the symptoms may provide a clue to the exact cause of weakness. The development of limb weakness and sensory loss over several weeks in the intensive care unit strongly suggests critical illness polyneuropathy. Fluctuation and variability over the course of a day, months, or years, leading to exacerbations and remissions in an otherwise healthy patient, is likely to be due to myasthenia gravis (MG). The distribution of weakness in MG is characteristic, affecting ocular, facial, limb, oropharyngeal, and respiratory muscles, and is confirmed by unequivocal and reproducible improvement after the intravenous injection of 10 mg edrophonium chloride (Tensilon), a rapidly acting acetylcholinesterase (AChE) inhibitor (3). Precipitous weakness may be due to myoglobinuria, so suggested by dark coloration of the urine, transient worsening over days, and a high creatine kinase (CK) in the serum, which often proves to be the first clue to a heritable enzymatic defect in muscle glycogenolysis, glycolysis, or mitochondrial metabolism (4). Recurrent attacks of slight to severe weakness lasting a few hours upon awakening, sparing oropharyngeal and respiratory muscles, are usually due to periodic paralysis. Weakness of the legs that evolves over years and progresses from the thighs to the rest of the legs is likely due to DMD in boys and inclusion body myositis (IBM) in older adults of either gender. The cause of an acute disorder such as GBS or polymyositis may lie in forgotten viral illness, immunization, new medication, potentially toxic exposure, or an underlying systemic illness.

The rule that proximal or girdle weakness equals myopathy and distal weakness implies neuropathy is useful when the latter is accompanied by sensory loss and early loss of tendon reflexes. Selective weakness of extensor neck muscles defines the "floppy" or "drooped" head syndrome that most often proves to be due to FSH and myotonic dystrophy, sclerodermatomyositis, ALS, or severe cervical spondylosis. Facial weakness may be so slowly progressive and symmetric as to escape notice in FSH and myotonic dystrophy and myotubular myopathy. Focal wasting or enlargement of muscles dramatic enough to be noticed by the patient are important clinical clues of an underlying neuromuscular disorder, whereas generalized wasting is also a feature of malnutrition and severe systemic disease. Painless wasting of the hand is often the first clue to ALS or syringomyelia, but the addition of radiating pain should then lead to consideration of peripheral nerve entrapment or cervical root compression. Although frank enlargement of calf muscles in DMD is due to replacement of muscle by fat and connective tissue, the diffuse hypertrophy in myotonia congenita results from continuous muscle contraction. A painful mass of muscle is usually due to rupture of a tendon or muscle but is frequently due to focal muscle infarction in a diabetic patient (5).

It is useful to ask about fatigue, cramps, myalgia, fasciculation, stiffness, and spasms. Fatigue and myalgia in the absence of specific weakness often signifies possible depression or systemic illness. Athough it is often stated that fatigue is never the solitary finding of MG, it can accompany true weakness and worsen with repetitive contraction. Frequent cramping with myalgia is seen in myoadenylate deaminase deficiency. There is a syndrome of benign fasciculation and cramps (6). Muscle contractures are separated from true cramps and dystonic postures or spasms by the absence, in the former, of electrical activity in the EMG. Stiffness is exquisitely painful in stiff-person syndrome and painless due to rigidity or spasticity alone in lesions of the extrapyramidal pathways or corticospinal tracts.

Clues to the cause of muscular weakness may be obtained in a pedigree. It should include the names, sex, age, and specific symptoms and physical characteristics of similarly affected family members. The pedigree will usually indicate the pattern of inheritance in an affected cohort but may not be informative if the patient is an index case or when failure of expressivity of the gene defect leads to a phenotypically normal heterozygote. The possible modes of single-gene inheritance include autosomal dominant (AD), autosomal recessive (AR), and X-linked dominant transmission. DNA analysis has revealed new insights into single-gene disorders and allowed more precise diagnosis and genetic counseling through improved carrier detection and prenatal screening. Possibly affected relatives should be examined and photographed, and the records of deceased family members with neurologic illnesses should be reviewed closely.

The distinctive biology of mitochondrial DNA (mtDNA) has added new concepts and terminology to classic Mendelian genetics (7). The human mitochondrial genome is contained in a tiny molecule of 16,569 base pairs. Thirteen of 37 genes encode structural proteins, including subunits of complexes I, III, IV, or cytochrome-c-oxidase and subunits of complex V. The remaining 24 mtDNA genes are required for protein translation; 22 encode transfer RNA, and 2 encode ribosomal RNA. Several biologic factors explain the heterogeneity of human mitochondria disease. First, each cell has multiple mitochondrial genomes, the absolute number depending on the requirement for oxidative energy; some organs such as the brain, heart, and skeletal muscle have lower thresholds for mitochondrial dysfunction. Second, a mutation can affect some or all of the mtDNA, leading to varying proportions of mutant mtDNA among tissues over the lifetime of the patient, explaining the appearance of particular syndromes of different ages. Third, virtually all mtDNA derives from the ooctye, so a mother transmits mutant mtDNA to all of her children, both boys and girls, but only the latter pass it on to their offspring.

A detailed neurologic examination is the next step in the elucidation of a motor disorder, discussed in detail elsewhere (8–10). It generally begins with an assessment of mental status for memory loss or frank dementia. The examination of cranial motor function includes assessment of ocular motility; strength in facial and neck muscles; and tests for audition, vestibular function, and patterns of speech. There are two useful signs for MG: the lid-twitch sign, elicited by asking the patient to gaze fully downward and then slowing bringing the eyes upward to a straight-ahead position, and the Hering's sign, in which ptosis is accentuated by passive opening of the contralateral lid. There are likewise several unmistakable signs of bulbar motor neuron disease (MND), usually seen in combination with dysarthria: mentalis muscle twitching, scalloping and twitching of the tongue, and copious pharyngeal secretions. Individual limb muscles should be examined and graded on a scale of 0 to 5 according to criteria of the Medical Research Council (10). It is useful to observe the patient rising from a low chair or deep squat, with arms folded on the chest, a maneuver described by Gowers (11) and named in his honor. Children with DMD are asked to stand from a seated position, characterized first by pushing with one arm, and bend forward and climb up the legs with both arms. The patient should be observed erect with both eyes open and closed, and gait should be assessed while on toes, heels, and walking tandem. Hopping on either foot tests strength, and coordination is tested by rapid successive movements and finger-to-nose pointing. Proprioceptive and vibratory sensation should be tested in the feet and hands. Thermal, pinprick, and light touch sensation by moving the stimulus proximally along the leg and arms should be rated by the patient. Tendon reflexes are best tested in the seated position with the hands folded in the lap and the legs dangling; knee jerks are considered absent only after reinforcement, and similarly ankle reflexes in the kneeling position.

The pattern of neurologic signs may be crucial to the diagnosis and may direct further evaluation toward the likeliest causes. Focal weakness, wasting, fasciculation, and tendon areflexia, sparing sensation, are classic lower motor neuron (LMN) signs, indicating either a primary or secondary lesion of anterior horn cells (AHC) due to MND or motor axons as in motor neuropathy (12), further separable by laboratory studies. Overly brisk reflexes in limbs with LMN signs, accompanied by Hoffman and Babinski signs and clonus, are unequivocal upper motor neuron signs indicative of a lesion in the corticospinal tracts (12). The combination of LMN and upper motor neuron signs in a suspected patient makes the clinical diagnosis of ALS "inescapable" (12). Upper motor neuron signs alone are the presenting feature of spastic paraplegia that is most often due to multiple sclerosis (MS), compressive tumor, vascular malformation of the spinal cord, foramen magnum, cervical spondylotic myelopathy, herniated thoracic nucleus pulposus, hereditary spastic paraplegia (HSP), spinocerebellar ataxia, MSA, vacuolar myelopathy due to infection with human immunodeficiency virus (HIV) type 1 or HIV-3–associated tropical spastic paraparesis, syringomyelia, or primary lateral sclerosis (PLS) (13).

An acquired or inherited cerebellar syndrome is unmistakable when signs and symptoms are accurately catalogued. Ataxia is the presenting feature of spinocerebellar ataxia further separable by age at onset, pattern of inheritance, and associated neurologic and nonneurologic features. The signs of vestibulocerebellar involvement, in addition, include rotated postures of the head and spontaneous nystagmus. Corticopontocerebellar involvement is further suggested by disturbances of speech, station, the rate and composition of voluntary movements, with dysmetria, hypotonia, and pendulous tendon reflexes. Likewise, the symptoms and signs of an extrapyramidal disorder such as Parkinson disease or parkinsonism are tremor at rest, rigidity, bradykinesia, flexed posture, loss of postural reflexes, and freezing phenomena. Patients with MSA, in addition, have dementia, motor neuron involvement, progressive supranuclear palsy, and primary autonomic failure. The combination of glove-and-stocking sensory loss, ataxia, and areflexia, indicative of DRG involvement, makes the clinical diagnosis of paraneoplastic encephalomyelitis and sensory neuronopathy likely; confirmation by anti-Hu serology subsequently directs the search for occult small cell lung cancer (SCLC) (14).

The clinical symptoms and signs of spinal cord lesions relate to four essential characteristics of the offending lesion (15): the *level,* because the higher the lesion, the greater the loss of motor, sensory, and autonomic function; the *extent of damage in the transverse plane* leading to expected incomplete or complete transverse cord syndromes; the *extent of the lesion in the longitudinal plane* and therefore the number of spinal segments involved; and the *duration of the lesion.* Whereas acute traumatic disruption of the spinal cord can irreversibly injure nerve cells, axons, synaptic connections, and their anatomic arrangement, making later recovery obsolete, the gradual compression by a tumor, spondylosis, or vascular malformation is generally amenable to surgery with the expectation of partial functional recovery. In transverse spinal cord syndromes, muscles innervated by the affected segments at the level of a spinal lesion show signs of flaccid paralysis due to injury of AHC; over time, spasticity ensues. *Selective AHC* involvement is usually due to poliomyelitis, the postpolio syndrome, or SMA. *Combined AHC and anterolateral tract* involvement leads to segmental paralysis, spasticity, and sensory loss, whereas alteration of bladder, bowel, and sexual function most often results from anterior spinal artery thrombosis or compression by an extramedullary tumor. The most frequent etiologies of a combined posterior column and lateral corticospinal tract involvement resulting in progressive ataxia and spasticity are B_{12} deficiency; hereditary ataxia; posterior spinal artery insufficiency; and posterior compression by cervical spondylosis, spinal tumor, or vascular malformation. Syringomyelia is the classic example of a *central spinal cord* syndrome with resulting pathology along a transverse and longitudinal plane. The common presenting findings of syringomyelia are weakness and wasting of small hand muscles due to AHC involvement and dissociated sensory loss due to damage of decussating pain and temperature fibers by the enlarging cavity, with relative preservation of the dorsal tracts. Spastic paraparesis with disturbances of bladder, bowel, and sexual function and sweating occur late in the course.

Motor syndromes that have historically defied easy interpretation on a clinical basis have also had ambiguous nosology. The terms LGMD and "limb girdle syndromes" describe patients with predominant shoulder-girdle and pelvic muscle weakness. The limits of LGMD have narrowed considerably through the application of molecular genetic analysis and histochemical studies to muscle biopsy specimens. Most affected patients prove to have chronic polymyositis, glycolytic or lipid storage myopathy, mitochondrial encephalomyopathy, DMD, BMD, or SMA. Nevertheless, a certain diagnosis of LGMD can be made with assurance when linkage analysis demonstrates association with one of the known chromosomal loci. Nosology has also proved inadequate in syndromes of progressive proximal weakness associated with diabetes mellitus. Charcot (16) coined the term "diabetic paraplegia" and "pseudotabes" in patients with pronounced leg weakness accompanied by pain and sensory loss. Bruns (17), and later Garland and Tavener (18), described a predominantly motor disorder characterized by painful asymmetric weakness of the thighs without sensory loss, so termed "diabetic myelopathy" because of the frequent association of Babinski signs. Garland (19) later called the same condition "diabetic amyotrophy" because of the profound weakness and wasting and acute spontaneous activity found on EMG. A variety of other descriptive terms have been used interchangeably: ischemic mononeuropathy multiplex (20), diabetic proximal amyotrophy (21), subacute proximal diabetic neuropathy (22), and painful lumbosacral plexopathy (23).

LABORATORY EVALUATION

The choice of laboratory studies in a patient with a motor disorder depends on the presumed etiologic or differential diagnosis and may include one or more of the following studies: EMG and nerve conduction studies (NCS), neuroradiologic studies of the brain and spinal cord, blood tests, lumbar cerebrospinal fluid (CSF) analysis, genetic analysis, and muscle and nerve biopsy.

Neurophysiologic Studies

Electrodiagnostic studies are necessary in the investigation of suspected myopathy, disorders of the neuromuscular junction (NMJ), peripheral neuropathy and entrapment neuropathy, plexus and root disorders, and MND. The electromyographic features of myopathy include normal NCS and short-duration low-amplitude motor unit potentials (MUPs) with excessive polyphasia and a full recruitment pattern at the onset of a forceful contraction in clinically weak muscles, also termed early recruitment. In myopathy, motor units are reduced in duration due to loss of slow initial and terminal components and a reduction in the temporal dispersion of surviving muscle fibers along the end-plate region. These findings correlate with the diffuse distribution of myofiber loss seen in a muscle biopsy of myopathies of various clinicopathologic types. The reduction in mean MUP duration is more pronounced in proximal than in distal muscles and in those with more weakness and advanced disease.

Demyelinating peripheral neuropathy is distinguished by significant slowing of nerve conductions velocities, prolongation of distal and F-wave latencies, motor conduction block, and absence of spontaneous activity in affected muscles. A drop of 50% or more of the proximal compound muscle action potential (CMAP) at sites not prone to compression is diagnostic of motor conduction block. A reduction of 20% is strongly suggestive of a block in the absence of abnormal temporal dispersion. Although motor conduction block and focal amplitude, waveform, and velocity changes of the CMAP are all potentially indicative of focal demyelination, only motor conduction block results in focal weakness. By comparison, axonal neuropathy is recognized by normal or mildly slow nerve conduction velocities, reduced CMAP and sensory nerve action potential amplitudes, normal distal latencies, and mildly prolonged F-wave latencies. In addition, there is variable active and chronic distal spontaneous activity, long-duration MUPs, and a reduced recruitment pattern in weak muscles.

The NMJ disorders are clinically, electrophysiologically, and pathogenically heterogenous. They have in common loss of the safety factor for NMJ transmission, with an abnormal response to repetitive nerve stimulation. A decremental response of 12% to 15% or more of successive CMAPs after 3-Hz stimulation, with aggravation of the block for several minutes after brief exercise, are indicative of a postsynaptic defect typical of MG. Maximal exercise for 15 seconds causes transient improvement of the decrement termed "postactivation facilitation," as does an injection of edrophonium chloride. Prolonged exercise for 1 minute, followed by repetitive trains of nerve stimulation at 1-minute intervals, worsens the block, termed "postactivation exhaustion." Exposure of the toxin of *Clostridium botulinum* in contaminated food leads to binding of a receptors along the terminal axon and the clinical and electrophysiologic syndrome of botulism. LEMS is instead due to the action of antibodies directed against presynaptic P/Q-type voltage gated calcium channels. Both botulism and LEMS show low amplitude CMAPs on conventional NCS, which increase by 100% to 200% after 20 Hz or more of repetitive nerve stimulation, indicative of the underlying presynaptic defect.

Single-fiber EMG supplements repetitive nerve stimulation by quantifying transmission at individual endplates while the patient voluntarily activates the muscle fiber under examination. However, it requires strict patient cooperation and examiner proficiency. Action potentials are recorded from two muscle fibers in the same motor unit near the single-fiber electrode. The variability in the time between consecutively recorded potentials is termed "jitter." Blocking is recognized by consecutive impulses that that do follow one another. The expected finding in MG is normal jitter in some potential pairs and increased jitter in others. As a rule, 20 potential pairs are studied in each muscle. Up to 85% of patients with generalized MG have abnormal decrement in a hand or shoulder muscle with repetitive nerve stimulation, whereas 86% of patients with generalized myasthenia and 65% of those with ocular involvement reveal abnormalities on single-fiber EMG studies. With the addition of a second muscle, jitter is seen in 99% of patients with generalized MG, making it a more sensitive method of analysis.

Electrodiagnostic studies can provide more accurate information than the clinical examination in the differentiation of a plexus lesion from a proximal mononeuritis or nerve root lesion, such as in the differentiation of axillary, suprascapular, and musculocutaneous neuropathies from C-5 root or upper trunk lesions; radial neuropathy from C-7 root, middle trunk, or posterior cord lesions; and combined median and ulnar neuropathies from C-8 root, lower trunk, or medial cord lesions. Most plexopathies are accompanied by axon loss, especially in those due to infiltrating carcinoma, radiation, hematomas, and gunshot wounds. In idiopathic brachial neuritis, pain, weakness, and wasting typically occur in an upper trunk distribution, and NCS show a reduction in CMAP and sensory nerve action potential amplitudes that parallel the severity of the illness, often in association with active spontaneous activity in muscles innervated by proximal and distal nerve branches.

Radiculopathy or a root lesion leads to peripheral motor deficits in a myotomal distribution. They most often occur in association with acute or chronic disc disease and degenerative arthritis with narrowing of the lateral recess or nerve root foramina. The resulting impingement leads to neuropraxic or axonopathic nerve injury. Because root lesions occur proximal to DRG, the sensory nerve action potential (SNAP) of the corresponding spinal segment remains normal. The one exception is herpes zoster virus infection because of concomitant involvement of the DRG. Motor NCS are generally normal because the studied segments are distal to the site of involvement; however, there may be slowing of veloci-

ties, a reduction in the amplitude, and prolongation of the duration of the CMAP in severe axon loss lesions. F-wave latencies along named nerves with a known root innervation may show a latency delay, abnormal impersistence, amplitude changes, duration, or asymmetry with side-to-side comparisons. However, F waves are of limited usefulness because they can only be recorded from a limited number of muscles with restricted myotomal distributions. H responses are more sensitive but are generally restricted to abnormality of the S-1 segment. EMG is performed in muscles sharing the same or different peripheral innervation and myotomal segments to establish the pattern of involvement. Fibrillations, positive sharp waves, fasciculation, and complex repetitive discharges may be delayed for weeks in the legs but are usually evident in paraspinal muscles 10 days after the initial injury and are clear evidence of a lesion proximal to the DRG. Fibrillation may be absent in chronic lesions if reinnervation has kept pace with denervation; then excessive polyphasia of MUPs will be present. Some muscles are useful to evaluate by needle EMG because they derive their innervation from single roots, including the rhomboids from the C-5, the pronator teres from the C-6, and the triceps from the C-7 roots. Examination of the extensor carpi ulnaris, a C-8 root-innervated muscle, is especially useful to avoid confusion with combined lesions of the median and ulnar nerves. The distinction of an L-5 root lesion from a peroneal or sciatic neuropathy requires examination of the tibialis posterior, tensor fascia lata, and gluteus medius muscles. The gluteus maximus is abnormal in an S-1 radiculopathy but is typically spared in high sciatic nerve lesions.

Electrodiagnostic studies are also imperative in the diagnosis and prognosis of ALS. The loss of spinal and brainstem motor neurons pathologically leads to the anticipated electrophysiologic findings of a widespread neurogenic disorder of AHCs and motor axons. NCS should be performed in all patients to demonstrate normality of SNAPs, to search for motor conduction block, and to estimate the degree of motor axon loss. Motor velocities may be slightly slowed and F-wave and distal motor latencies mildly prolonged because of loss of the fastest conducting fibers, usually in proportion to the reduction in CMAP amplitude. Even before muscle fibers fibrillate electrically, the degeneration of a portion of motor neurons leads to loss of innervation of muscle fibers in the respective motor units, whereas remaining ones sprout collateral fibers. The reinnervated fibers generate motor units, first with a variation in their configuration because of blocking of conduction and reduced synchrony of nerve terminal conduction. The inclusion of other fibers into the motor unit leads to motor units of longer duration, higher amplitude, and increased fiber density. The reduction in the number of motor neurons that can be activated leads to reduced recruitment upon voluntary contraction and with increasing effort, an abnormally high firing rate of individual motor units, and an increased ratio of the number of motor units to the firing rate. Although many parameters correlate with prognosis, the following bestow a poor prognosis: more severe disease, older age, the presence of widespread low CMAP amplitudes with reduced velocities, abnormalities on fiber density, single-fiber MG, and repetitive nerve stimulation.

A battery of autonomic studies can add useful information in selected patients with motor disorders to assist in management and prognosis (24). Autonomic neuropathy contributes to the risk of malignant ventricular arrhythmia due to prolongation of the QT interval of the resting electrocardiogram and to sudden cardiorespiratory arrest after general anesthesia or the use of medications that suppress baroreceptor responses. Noninvasive quantitative autonomic tests include studies of cardiovagal function such as heart rate response to deep breathing, Valsalva maneuver, and standing upright; sympathetic tests of blood pressure control to standing, tilting, or sustained handgrip; sudomotor control to thermally and chemically induced sweating; and the assessment of sphincter and erectile dysfunction.

Other neurophysiologic methods have a role in the evaluation of patients with spastic paraparesis and subtle or sublinical sensory symptoms. They include recordings of visual, brainstem auditory, and somatosensory evoked responses. An excessive interocular difference of 12 msec in the P100 latency of the visual evoked response reflects pathologic involvement of the anterior visual pathways due to optic neuropathy because each eye projects to both occipital hemispheres. The most commonly used pattern stimulus is a checkerboard of light and dark squares that reverses or shifts without a change in luminance. The cerebral response is recorded from the Oz electrode of the international 10-20 system, with reference to Cz, and linked to the mastoids. Brainstem auditory evoked responses are perfomed by monaural stimulation with refraction clicks of 60 to 70 decibels above the hearing threshold. For clinical purposes, calculations are made of the wave I to III, I to V, and the III to V interpeak latencies, reflecting central conduction time. Somatosensory evoked responses are elicited by stimulation of any accessible sensory or mixed nerve, but the median and posterior tibial are the most common ones chosen. The responses are generated by impulse traffic along proximal peripheral nerve pathways from the popliteal fossa and clavicle, to the dorsal horn, and along the posterior columns to the contralateral thalamus and cortex. Their respective waveforms are displayed by electrode montages or combinations, placed at various locations over the lumbar and cervical enlargements of the cord, and on the scalp. They correspond to local synaptic activity or near-field potentials or synchronous depolarizations along advancing white matter fiber tracts at a distance

from the recording electrodes or far-field potentials. Although the diagnostic yield of evoked responses is greatest when all three types of evoked response studies are performed together, their individual selection should be determined by the clinical situation. For example, an abnormal visual evoked response makes the diagnosis of MS essentially certain in the setting of progressive myelopathy, especially when there are high intensity subcortical T-2 lesions on brain magnetic resonance imaging (MRI), intrathecal synthesis of IgG, and oligoclonal bands.

Transcranial magnetic stimulation is potentially useful in motor disorders associated with primary degeneration of corticospinal tract pathways, such as ALS and PLS (25). In this test, circular high power coils are positioned on the scalp with its center over the vertex to record CMAPs and distal latencies in the arms and over Fz for the legs. The motor roots are stimulated with the cathode positioned over C-7 and L-1. The central motor conduction time is calculated by subtracting the distal motor latencies obtained after nerve root stimulation from those obtained by cortical stimulation. The CMAP amplitudes recorded after cortical stimulation are expressed as a percentage of those obtained from root stimulation. An abnormally prolonged central motor conduction time and reduced CMAP amplitude correlates with the presence of corticospinal tract involvement in patients with ALS and probably PLS. It also has a potential role in the evaluation of patients with ALS and PLS but less well in patients with bulbar palsy and MS.

Neuroimaging Studies

Radiologic studies are an important part of the laboratory evaluation of patients with motor disorders. MRI is the most widely used neuroimaging study for CNS disorders. The intravenous contrast agent gadopentetate dimeglumine crosses the blood–brain barrier and is associated with few side effects. It shortens T1 and T2 relaxation times of spin echo images and accumulates in lesions as areas of increased signal intensity compared with precontrast images. MRI of the spine has supplanted myelography in the evaluation of patients with spinal cord disorders due to compressive cervical spondylosis, Chiari and vascular malformations, extramedullary tumors, syringomyelia, MS, and acquired and hereditary anomalies of the craniocervical junction. It can be used to image the cross-sectional planes of individual limbs at sites of focal muscle wasting due to active myopathy and along selected nerves enlarged by lymphomatous infiltrates. MR spectroscopy supplements exercycle ergometry and treadmill protocols in patients with defects of muscle oxidative metabolism (26). Positron emission tomography compliments MRI in the CNS evaluation of mitochondrial encephalomyopathy, Parkinson disease, MSA, vasculitis, and other degenerative CNS disorders (27).

Blood Tests, Antibody Assays, and Cerebrospianl Fluid

Blood and CSF can be processed for a variety of studies depending on the presumptive diagnosis. An elevated serum CK is usually the first laboratory abnormality in myopathy and is almost always accompanied by increased levels of serum glutamic-oxaoacetic acid, glutamic-pyruvic transaminase, and lactate dehydrogenase. A CK level in the thousands of units is characteristic of DMD and in the tens to hundreds of thousands of units are found in attacks of myoglobulinuria. Lesser elevations of up to three times normal are seen in chronic myopathy and diverse neurogenic disorders. A forearm-ischemic test with simultaneous measurements of serum CK, venous lactate, and ammonia can help differentiate among the heritable enzymatic defects in glycogenolysis and glycolysis.

Autoimmune serology plays a pivotal role in the diagnosis of NMJ disorders (28). Binding, blocking, and modulating acetylcholine receptor (AChR) antibodies together assay the most important postulated disturbances of AChR function in MG, namely accelerated degradation and endocytosis (binding antibody), cross-linking of AChR antibodies (modulating antibody), and functional blockade (blocking antibody). The binding assay, expressed in nmol/L of bound AChR, is positive in up to 90% of patients with generalized MG and is the preferred screening test. Striational antibodies are found in 80% of patients with MG and a thymoma and in a quarter of those with thymoma without clinically apparent MG (29). However, many of them will have electrophysiologic evidence of MG when studied and can develop frank signs of MG later in their course, sometimes even after thymectomy. Patients with the LEMS should be studied in addition for antibodies to P/Q and N-type voltage gated calcium channels. The P/Q channels initiate the presynaptic release of ACh and are target antigens in LEMS. N-type channels are widely distributed in the CNS and may be a target antigen in rubrocortical, spinal, and autonomic syndromes in association with LEMS. High titers of either type should raise suspicion of a primary lung cancer. Fewer than 5% of patients with MG have voltage gated calcium channel antibodies, making them a useful assay to distinguish LEMS from MG, because even though the serologic profile of the two disorders may occasionally overlap, the two rarely do so clinically.

The specific blood studies that should be performed in patients with peripheral neuropathy should be guided by the clinical presentation and the postulated etiologic diagnosis. Tests for diabetes; renal and hepatic disease; B_{12} deficiency; thyroid and parathyroid dysfunction; monoclonal paraproteinemia; infectious hepatitis B and C; quantitative IgG, IgA, and IgM elevations; and peripheral T-cell studies are all relatively inexpensive and may reveal important information at the outset of the evaluation. HIV serology should be obtained in high-risk patients. Serum monoclonal paraproteins are best revealed by immunofixation electrophoresis. The neuropathies associated with monoclonal paraproteinemia are clinically and pathogenically heterogenous. They result from malignant and nonmalignant B-cell proliferation and may be the first clue to possible underlying multiple myeloma, cryoglobulinemia, amyloidosis, chronic lymphocytic leukemia, and lymphocytic lymphoma, often associated with IgG and IgA paraproteins. The nonmalignant IgM monoclonal paraproteins, once called "gammopathies of unknown significance" (30), are now better understood for their potential autoreactive specificities to peripheral nerve, although only a small number have been well characterized. The monoclonal IgM antibody directed against anti–myelin-associated glycoprotein (MAG) is one of the best understood autoantibody syndromes, satisfying five essential criteria (31). First, the autoantigen anti-MAG is known. Second, there is a specific antibody response, namely the anti-MAG glycoprotein antibody. Third, the disease can be transferred to laboratory animals with the sera of affected patients. Fourth, binding of the antibody at the site of the antigen leads to local destruction and alteration of myelin function, resulting in demyelinating neuropathy. Fifth, removal or suppression of the antibody response is associated with clinical benefit.

The emergence of several neurogenic disorders associated with polyclonal IgM and IgG antibodies directed against the peripheral nerve gangliosides and glycolipid antigens have transformed our concepts of motor nerve disorders and MND over the past decade. They in turn led to commercially available serologic testing for practicing neurologists. Between 1986 and 1988, Latov and colleagues (32,33) reported a single patient with a motor neuropathy that simulated MND clinically and electrophysiologically but differed in the presence of very high titers of a serum IgM GM1 antibody that cross-reacted with GD1b. At the same time, in 1988, Parry and Clarke (34) described similar patients with an LMN disorder that simulated MND but differed in the presence of multifocal conduction block. Pestronk et al. (35) ascribed the pathogenesis of multifocal motor neuropathy (MMN), so named, to the activity of GM1 antibodies and proposed therapy with the immunosuppressive agent cyclophosphamide. In 1993 there were three additional contributions: Chaudhry et al. (36) demonstrated the effectiveness of intravenous immune globulin (IVIg) in MMN; Yuki et al. (37) described acute axonal neuropathy with polyclonal IgM anti-GM1 that cross-reacted with GD1a and preceding *Campylobacter* enteritis; and Chiba et al. (38) showed increased titers of a polyclonal IgG GM1 ganglioside with a unique specificity to GQ1b in patients with the Miller Fisher variant of GBS, characterized clinically by areflexia, ataxia, and ophthalmoplegia. The accumulated evidence from experimental laboratory animal studies and the analysis of postmortem and peripheral nerve biopsies of affected patients suggests the importance of anti-ganglioside antibody studies in patients with motor neuropathy with or without conduction block, motor axonal forms of GBS, and in selected cases of neuronopathy, wherein the primary pathologic insult often cannot be ascribed with assurance to the motor axon or perikarya.

Although the anti-Hu or anti-neuronal nuclear antibody type 1-associated paraneoplastic encephalomyelitis and sensory neuronopathy (PEM-SN) is primarily a sensory disorder, up to 40% of patients can show frank spinal cord and brainstem motor neuron involvement (39). The anti-Hu antibody is a polyclonal IgG antibody that reacts with closely spaced protein antigens of molecular mass 35 to 40 kDa on immunoblots of human neuronal extracts and nuclei of SCLC cells (40). Direct immunoperoxidase studies of postmortem brain tissue show intranuclear deposits of anti-Hu IgG in a pattern similar to that seen when the sera of affected patients is applied to normal sections of brain (41). Three protein autoantigens, designated HuD, HuC, and Hel-N1, share sequence homologies (42). The expression of Hu antigens is a nearly universal feature of SCLC; however, paraneoplastic neurologic disease is seen with only the highest titers on Western blot (43).

Properly performed, a lumbar puncture is a safe and informative procedure in a variety of motor disorders. Acellular CSF with a raised protein content, of 100 mg/dL or more, supports the diagnosis of Kearns-Sayre syndrome (KSS) and both GBS and chronic inflammatory polyradiculoneuropathy (CIDP). Pleocytosis and a mild protein elevation that varies with the severity of the paralysis occurs in poliomyelitis, with a shift from polymorphonuclear to mononuclear cells over several days. It is useful to analyze CSF in patients with suspected spinal cord tumors for cytology and tumor markers and in patients with HIV infection and multicentric white matter lesions to differentiate progressive multifocal leukoencephalopathy from toxoplasmosis, because pleocytosis and a raised protein content are frequent in toxoplasmosis. Intrathecal synthesis of myelin basic protein and oligoclonal bands support the diagnosis of MS in clinically suspected cases. Virtually all patients with Lyme neuroborreliosis and acute meningitis, cranial neuritis, or radiculitis show evidence of CSF lymphocytosis, intrathecal production of *Borrelia burgdorferi*-specific antibody, and, in some, demonstration of the organism by culture or polymerase chain reaction (44). In such patients, the presence of CSF inflammation is only one element of a more disseminated process affecting the peripheral nerve, subarachnoid space, and corresponding levels of the spinal cord.

Genetic Analysis

The genetic analysis of motor disorders has witnessed unprecedented progress in the past two decades. Table 1 lists motor disorders of known genetic cause. The DNA analysis of primary myopathies, congenital MG, hereditary neuropathies, and inherited MND has revealed new insights into single-gene disorders and allowed more precise diagnosis and genetic counseling through improved carrier detection and prenatal screening. The defective gene in DMD was accomplished along several independent lines of investigation using restriction fragment length polymorphisms and the process of "reverse genetics" as follows. DNA analysis revealed deletions or duplications in a band near the middle of the short arm of the X chromosome, designated Xp21, in two clusters or "hot spots." Complementary DNA probes identified a messenger RNA that predicted the skeletal muscle protein that was named dystrophin (45,46). Antibodies against the dystrophin fusion peptide revealed its membrane-bound location (47). Out-of-frame deletions resulted in DMD, whereas in-frame deletions result in BMD (48). In the latter, the related dystrophin protein is altered in size or reduced in quantity but not altogether lost from the muscle (49). The recent application of DNA probes and anti-dystrophin antibodies to muscle biopsy specimens in turn resulted in a refinement in the diagnosis and expansion of the recognized Xp21 myopathies or dystrophinopathies. They include BMD variants such as those with atypical distribution like quadriceps or distal myopathies and others with minimal weakness or idiopathic elevations of the CK level.

Mitochondrial disorders can now be classified as to whether the gene defect lies in nuclear DNA, mtDNA, or in the faulty communication between the two genomes (50). The term "mitochondrial myopathy" has been replaced by "mitochondrial encephalomyopathy" to emphasize the more common widespread systemic and CNS involvement. Deletions and point mutations of mtDNA lead to two distinctive neurologic syndromes, progressive external ophthalmoplegia (PEO) and KSS. In purely clinical terms, PEO is characterized by the slow steady progression of ptosis and ophthalmoparesis beginning in childhood or young adulthood. Strictly defined, KSS includes PEO with onset before age 20 years and pigmentary retinopathy, with at least one of the following: heart block, a cerebellar syndrome, or CSF protein content above 100 mg/dL. In addition, there may be dementia, sensorineural hearing loss, short stature, diabetes mellitus, or hypothyroidism. Skeletal muscle biopsy in mitochondrial encephalomyopathy shows ragged red fibers, so named for their characteristic appearance with a modification of Gomori trichrome histochemical stain due to the accumulation of mitochondria along the borders of myofibers (51). Mitochondrial proliferation is believed to be a compensatory mechanism for the imbalance between energy requirements and the oxidative-phosphorylation capabilities of affected myofibers. Ultrastructural analysis when performed shows densely packed cristae with rodlike inclu-

TABLE 1. *Neuromuscular diseases of known transmission*

Disease	MIM	Mode of inheritance	Gene location	Gene product
Muscular dystrophies				
DMD	310200	XR	Xp21.2	Dystrophin
BMD	310200	XR	Xp21.2	Dystrophin
EDMD	310300	XR	Xq28	Emerin
FSH	158900	AD	4q35	
LGMD	253600	AR	15q	LGMD2
	253600	AR	2p	LGMD3
	159000	AD	5q	LGMD1
Severe childhood	253700	AR	13q12	SCARMD1
DM	160900	AD	19q13	Protein kinase
Congenital myopathies				
Myotubular	310400	XR	Xq28	MTM1
Central core	117000	AD	19q13.1	Ryanodine receptor
Nemaine	161800	AD	1q21-q23	NEM1
Fukuyama	253800	AR	9q31-q33	FCMD
Merosin deficiency		AR	6q2	Merosin
Other myotonic disorders				
Hyperkalemic period paralysis	170500	AD	17q13.1-13.3	Sodium channel
Paramyotonic congenita	168300	AD	17q13.1-q13.2	Sodium channel
Hypokalemic period paralysis	170400	AD	1q31-q32	Calcium channel (dihydropyridine receptor)
Metabolic myopathies				
Glycogenoses				
Type II-Pompe	232300	AR	17q23	GAA
Type IV-McArdle	232600	AR	11q13	Muscle phosphorylase
Type VII-Tarui	232800	AR	1ccnq32	Muscle phosphofructokinase
Type IX	311800	XR	Xq13	Phosphoglycerate kinase
Abnormal ACh-AChR interaction				
Slow channel				
Fast channel				
HSMN				
Type 1a	118220	AD	17p12-p11.2	PMP22
Type 1b	159440	AD	1q21.1-q23.3	Po
Type 11a	118210	AD	1p35-p36	
Type 11b			3q	
Type 111	145900	AD	17p11.2	PMP22
		AD	1q21-q23	Phytanic acid d-hydroxylase
Type IV	214400	AR	8q13-q21.1	TTR
CMT X$_1$	302800	XD	Xq13.1	GKB1 encoding connexin-32
CMT X$_2$	382801	XR	Xp22.2;Xq2	
HNPP	162500	AD	17p11.2	PMP22
Refsum disease	266500	AR		Phytanic acid α-hydroxylase
FAP	176300	AD	18q11.2-q12.1	TTR
Friedrich ataxia	229300	AR	9q13-q21.1	
Acute intermittent porphyria	176000	AD	11q24.1-q24.2	PGB deaminase
Familial dysautonomia	223900	AR	9q31-q33	
Tangier disease	205400	AR		
MLD	250100	AR	22q1331-qter	Arylsulfatase A
ALD	300100	XR	Xq28	ALD protein (peroxisomal transporter protein)
Fabry disease	301500	X-linked	X chromosome	α-Galactosidase
Multiple sulfatase deficiency	272200	AR		Arylsulfatase A, B, and C
Krabbe disease	245200	AR	12q21-q31	Galactocerebrosidase
Type X	261670	AR	7p12-p13	Phosphoglycerate mutase
Type XI	150000	AR	11p15.4	Lactate dehydrogenase
Lipidoses				
Carnitine palmitoyltransferase deficiency	255110	AR	11p11-p13	Carnitine palmitoyltransferase
Congenital myasthenic syndromes				
Familial infantile	259210	AR		
Paucity of synaptic vesicles		AR		
AChE deficiency		AR		
AChR deficiency		AR		
Paucity of synaptic folds		AR		

TABLE 1. *Continued.*

Disease	MIM	Mode of inheritance	Gene location	Gene product
Motor neuron diseases				
Wernig-Hoffman syndrome	253300	AR	5q11-q13	SMA
Kugelberg-Welander syndrome	253400	AR	5q11-q13	SMA
Familial ALS	105400	AD	21q22	SOD
	205100	AR	2q33-q35	ALS2
Kennedy syndrome	313200	XR	Xq21-22	Androgen receptor
Late-onset Tay-Sachs disease	278000		15q23-24	Hexosaminidase A deficiency
Sandhoff's disease	268800		5q11.2-13.6	Hexosaminidase A and B deficiency
AB variant disease	272750		5q	GM2 activator protein deficiency

Disease	MtDNA mutation	Mode of inheritance	DNA defect
Mitochondrial encephalomyopathies			
KSS	Deletion	Sporadic	
PEO	Deletion	Sporadic	
	Point mutation	Maternal	tRNA$^{Leu\ (UUR)}$
			tRNA^{Asn}
	Multiple deletions	AD	tRNA^{Leu}
PEO, myopathy, sudden death	Point mutation	Maternal	tRNA^{Leu}
MELAS	Point mutation	Maternal	tRNA^{Lys}
MERRF	Point mutation	Maternal	tRNA^{Lys}
MERRF/MELAS	Point mutation	Maternal	ATPase6
NARP	Point mutation	Maternal	ATPase6
MILS	Point mutation	Maternal	tRNA^{Leu}
Myopathy			
	Duplication	Sporadic	tRNA^{Pro}
	Multiple deletions	AR, AD	
MIMyCa	Point mutation A-G	Maternal	tRNA^{Leu}
Multisystem cardiomyopathy	Point mutation	Maternal	tRNA^{Ile}
Fatal congenital multisystem	Point mutation	Maternal	tRNA^{Thr}
LHON	Point mutation T-C, G-A, A-G	Maternal	ND1, ND2, III, ND4, ND5, ND6, Cytb Cox1, Cox
DAD	Point mutation A-G	Maternal	tRNA^{Leu}
	Duplication	Maternal	
Progressive encephalomyopathy	Multiple deletions	AD	
Familial recurrent myoglobinuria	Multiple deletions	AR	
MEPOP or MNGIE	Multiple deletions	AR	
Fatal infantile myopathy	Severe depletion		
Myopathy of childhood	Partial depletion		

MIM, McKusick "Mendelian inheritance in man"; DMD, Duchenne muscular dystrophy; BMD, Becker muscular dystrophy; EDMD, Emery Dreifuss muscular dystrophy; FSH, fascioscapulohumeral; LGMD, limb girdle muscular dystrophy; DM, dystrophica myotonica or myotonic muscular dystrophy; ACh, acetylcholine; AChE, ACh esterase; AChR, ACh receptor; HSMN, hereditary sensorimotor neuropathy; PMP, peripheral myelin protein; P, peripheral nerve protein; CMT, Charcot-Marie-Tooth disease; *GKB1,* gene of uncertain function; HNPP, hereditary neuropathy with pressure palsies; FAP, familial amyloid polyneuropathy; TTR, transthyretin; PBG, porphobilinogen; MLD, metachromatic leukodystrophy; ALD, adrenoleukodystrophy; ALS, amyotrophic lateral sclerosis; SMA, spinal muscular atrophy; SOD, superoxide dismutase; Hex, hexosaminidase; ALS, amyotrophic lateral sclerosis; AD, autosomal dominant; AR, autosomal recessive; XR, X-linked recessive; PEO, progressive external ophthalmoplegia; MELAS, mitochondrial myopathy with lactic acidosis and strokelike episodes; MERRF, myoclonic epilepsy with ragged-red fibers; NARP, neuropathy, ataxia, retinitis pigmentosa; MILS, maternally inherited Leigh syndrome; MIMyCa, maternally inherited myopathy and cardiomyopathy; LHON, Leber hereditary optic neuropathy; MEPOP, mitochondrial encephalomyopathy, polyneuropathy, ophthalmoplegia, and pseudoobstruction; MNGIE, mitochondrial neuropathy, gastrointestinal disorder, and encephalopathy; DAD, diabetes and deafness; KSS, Kearns-Sayre syndrome.

sions. The demonstration of the characteristic gene deletion (52) in KSS has assisted in classification of overlapping cases, such as those with KSS and strokelike episodes or, conversely, patients with progressive external ophthalmoplegia plus a few, but not all, of the features required for KSS. Two other multisystem mitochondrial disorders include myoclonic epilepsy with ragged red fibers (MERRF) and mitochondrial myopathy with encephalopathy, lactic acidosis, and strokelike episodes (MELAS), with additional distinctive features of seizures, exercise intolerance, dementia, retardation with normal early development, and onset before age 40 years. The last category of mitochondrial gene defects are those caused by faulty communication between nuclear DNA and mtDNA. These disorders are transmitted by Mendelian inheritance because the primary genetic error often resides in nuclear DNA.

Current understanding of the congenital myasthenic syndromes and ion channel abnormalities has been achieved by the application of molecular genetics to the detection of mutations in AChR subunit genes, accompanied by sophisticated morphologic and electrophysiologic studies of the NMJ (53). Clinical clues of a possible congenital myasthenic syndrome include a suggestive family history of onset in either the neonatal period, infancy, or childhood with progression into adolescence or adulthood; lack of a significant response to AChE drugs; and absent AChR antibodies. Symptomatic congenital myasthenia results from the loss of the safety factor for normal NMJ transmission and can be divided into presynpatic, synaptic, and postsynaptic disorders. Two presynaptic disorders are due to defects in ACh resynthesis or to a paucity of synaptic vesicles with reduced quantal release of ACh. End-plate AChE deficiency causes a synaptically mediated disorder. The postsynaptic form of congenital MG is generally associated with a kinetic abnormality of AChR, with or without receptor deficiency, or AChR deficiency without a primary kinetic abnormality. Those with AChR and a kinetic abnormality include ion channel disorders due to short open time, a slow channel syndrome associated with prolonged open time due to delayed channel closure, a slow channel syndrome due to increased affinity of the receptor for Ach causing repeated openings during prolonged acetylcholine occupancy, and another syndrome in which the nature of the kinetic abnormality is not yet elucidated. Those with ACh deficiency include the low-affinity fast-channel syndrome and the high-conductance fast-channel syndrome. Those with ACh deficiency without a primary kinetic abnormality are caused by nonsense mutations in the ε subunit gene of the receptor complex. Motor point biopsy adds precision to the diagnosis of congenital myasthenia in suspected patients but should be performed at centers with a genuine interest in the disorder because of the necessary detailed studies. The muscle tissue should first be processed for routine studies and then for cytochemical localization of AChE and immune deposits at end-plates. Electron microscopic and immunocytochemical studies are necessary to determine the size and density of synaptic vesicles and the morphology of nerve terminals and postsynaptic membranes. Quantitative assessment of AChR binding can be performed using peroxidase labeled α-bungarotoxin toxin. In vitro microelectrode studies including noise analysis and patch-clamp recordings provide additional information about the kinetic properties of abnormal AChR channels.

New insights gained through molecular genetics have also had an impact on the classification of the Charcot-Marie-Tooth (CMT) neuropathies (54). They were first categorized phenotypically by common clinical, electrophysiologic, histopathologic nerve findings and patterns of inheritance. Three genes have since been identified, peripheral myelin protein 22 (PMP22), peripheral nerve protein (Po), and connexin 32, located on chromosomes 17, 1, and the X chromosome, respectively. Other gene loci have yet to be defined on chromosomes 3 and 8. The most common phenotype, CMT1, presents as demyelinating neuropathy with slow conduction velocities, histologic evidence of remyelination in the form of onion bulbs in a nerve biopsy, and an AD inheritance. Locus heterogeneity results from defects in the PMP22 and Po gene, leading to phenotypic differences due to the involvement of different gene products. Different point mutations in the PMP22 gene leads to phenotypic heterogeneity in CMT-1A, as does the dose of the gene. For example, two copies of PMP22 result in the normal state, but a triple dose leads to expression of the abnormal phenotype. Sporadic cases of either CMT1A or 1B often prove to be new mutations in the specific genes.

A decade of intense research in molecular genetics has also begun to unravel the nature of the clinical diversity of familial MND, inherited ataxias, and hereditary spastic paraplegia (HSP). There are several types of progressive SMA. Three of them, infantile SMA type 1a and 1b or Wernig-Hoffman syndrome, SMA type 2, and SMA type 3 or Kugelberg-Welander syndrome, are transmitted with AD inheritance and demonstrate linkage to chromosome 5q (55). Differences in age at onset and distribution of weakness are examples of allelic heterogeneity. Three forms of adult-onset GM2 gangliosidoses can produce a clinical phenotype similar to that of SMA–late-onset Tay Sachs disease, caused by deficiency of the alpha subunit of Hex A. Sandhoff disease is caused by deficiency of the Hex A and B beta subunits. The AB variant syndrome is caused by deficiency of GM2 protein activation. Two disorders, one in childhood, Fazio-Lone syndrome, and the other in midlife, X-linked recessive bulbospinal muscular atrophy or Kennedy disease, are associated with prominent bulbar weakness. About 10% of cases of ALS demonstrate autosomal dominant inheritance. Familial autosomal dominant ALS (FALS) is indistinguishable clinically from sporadic ALS (56). However, it can differ from sporadic ALS in the subclinical involvement of the posterior columns, Clarke's column, and spinocerebellar tracts and in the presence of hyaline intraneuronal inclusions resembling Lewy bodies in the cytoplasm of surviving motor neurons (57,58). The gene locus for FALS has been identified, and several mutations have been reported in the gene for copper (Cu) zinc (Zn) superoxide dismutase (SOD) that are coinherited with FALS in large cohorts (59). Cu/ZnSOD1 is a metalloenzyme of 32 kilobases encoded by five exons with the SOD1 locus. It primary function is to detoxify free oxygen radicals that have the potential to interact adversely with cellular constituents of motor neurons. Given the clinical and pathologic similarities to familial ALS, it is a reasonable premise that some cases of sporadic ALS also may be mediated by free radical injury.

Historically, the inherited ataxias also defied easy interpretation, and this was reflected in ambiguous clinical nosology that was modified by the elucidation of separate ataxia gene loci among large kindreds of a common phenotype, genotype, identifiable mutant protein, and biochemical defect. A current classification recognizes a group with onset before age 20 years and AR inheritance, represented most commonly by Friedrich ataxia. A later onset group, the spinocerebellar ataxias, has AD inheritance and is divided into seven subgroups labeled spinocerebellar ataxia 1 to 7, all without a known biochemical defect. A third group of diverse ataxias has identifiable biochemical defects. The HSP syndromes are also clinically, genetically, and pathologically heterogeneous. A common pure form has slow progression in the legs and AD inheritance. These, in turn, are divided into two groups based on the age at onset (<35 years in type 1) and in the association of muscle weakness, urinary symptoms, and impaired sensation (in type 2). There are complicated forms of HSP, so termed because of the association with a variety of other neurologic and nonneurologic abnormalities. Adrenomyeloneuropathy (AMN) is an X-linked peroxisomal disorder and a cause of pure HSP in men and hemizygote women. It shares a common genetic origin with adrenoleukodystrophy (ALD) at the Xq28 gene locus. Patients with AMN and ALD accumulate abnormally high levels of saturated very-long-chain fatty acids that forms the basis for the diagnostic assay.

Muscle and Nerve Biopsy

The indications for muscle and nerve biopsy continue to broaden as the evaluative process improves (60). Properly handled, muscle biopsy is clinically useful in the evaluation of suspected inflammatory myopathy, glycolytic lipid-storage myopathy, progressive muscular dystrophy, mitochondrial encephalomyopathy, and congenital myasthenia.

The inflammatory myopathies include polymyositis, IBM, and dermatomyositis, further separable from one another by distinct clinical, morophologic, and immunohistochemical features (61). Polymyositis occurs alone or in association with systemic autoimmune or connective tissue diseases and viral or bacterial infections. The essential clinical features are myalgia, cranial and proximal limb weakness, and an elevated serum CK level. Biopsy of an affected muscle shows myofiber necrosis, regeneration, lymphocytic infiltration, and variable fibrosis. Cytotoxic CD8+ cells surround healthy endomysial myofibers, leading to phagocytosis and necrosis. IBM is distinguished by finger flexor and extensor leg weakness, onset usually after age 50, variable distal sensory loss, a

mildly elevated or normal serum CK level, and the finding of rimmed vacuoles and eosinophilic inclusions that strongly react with ubiquitin, Congo red, and crystal violet histochemistry. Patients with dermatomyositis have a characteristic violacious shiny rash of the upper eyelids, face, neck, trunk, elbows, knuckles, and nail beds and variable proximal weakness. B cells and CD4+ cells invade the endomysium and surround blood vessels, without significant lymphocytic invasion of non-necrotic muscle fibers. The disorder frequently overlaps with systemic sclerosis, mixed connective tissue disease, and systemic malignancy. It is not known whether patients with dermatomyositis are a greater risk for occult malignancy; nevertheless, it is reasonable to include CT of the chest, abdomen, and pelvis and manual rectal and pelvic examination, mammogram, and tumor markers in older patients who may be at greater risk.

Muscle histochemistry coupled with genetic analysis of muscle homogenates has revealed the molecular basis of the metabolic myopathies in which symptoms are presumably caused by the abnormal accumulation of a metabolic product resulting from a block in glycogenolysis, glycolysis, or lipid metabolism (62). Affected patients have slowly progressive, fluctuating, or fixed limb weakness. They include deficiencies of myophosphorylase, phosphofructokinase, carnitine palmityltranferase, phosphoglycerate mutase, phosphoglycerate kinase, and lactate dehydrogenase. Virtually all can be associated with recurrent myoglobinuria, and all but one, carnitine palmityltranferase, are due to a defect in glycogenolysis or glycolysis. With the exception of phosphoglycerate kinase, which is X linked, the others are generally inherited in an AR fashion.

Nerve biopsy may provide the necessary histologic proof of certain motor disorders such as peripheral nerve vasculitis, neurolymphomatosis, polyglucosan body disease, and amyloidosis. It also adds precision to the diagnosis of CIDP, diabetic neuropathy, MMN, metachromatic leukodystrophy, Krabbe disease, AMN, and ceroid lipofuscinosis when noninvasive tests of the blood, urine, skin, or conjunctiva are uninformative. Among several reported series of patients with histologically confirmed peripheral nerve vasculitis (63), about a third were of the nonsystemic type after intensive evaluation and two-thirds showed evidence of systemic involvement due to underlying polyarteritis nodosa, Wegener granulomatosis, rheumatoid arthritis, Sjögren syndrome, or systemic lupus erythematosus. The premise of an isolated peripheral nerve vasculitis defined by nerve biopsy alone has been questioned due to the frequent finding of necrotizing arteritis in a muscle biopsy specimen and the absence of long-term follow-up in most cases. Only one patient so studied at autopsy showed evidence of isolated peripheral nerve vasculitis (64); conversely, two others diagnosed by nerve biopsy in life failed to show vasculitis at postmortem examination (65).

Even though a motor biopsy is preferable in a patient with a purely motor syndrome, it entails a deeper dissection with potentially more serious operative risks. Nonetheless, one patient with the clinical and electrophysiologic syndrome of MMN and very high titers of serum IgM anti-GM1 antibodies had granular deposits of IgM at adjacent internodes and along the paranodal surface of myelin sheaths in a sural nerve specimen (66). Injection of that patient's serum into rat sciatic nerve resulted in similar pathologic findings and that binding activity was removed with GM1 (67).

TREATMENT

The medical treatment of motor disorders should be guided by the postulated or known mechanism of the underlying disease. The hope of gene therapy in DMD motivated a generation of neuromuscular scientists to isolate the gene and deficient protein, but in the end it could not be practically implemented. Dietary therapies to replace or supplement deficient nutrients or enzymes has been tried with limited success in the mitochondrial encephalomyopathies. Patients with ALD and AMN can be given a supplemental diet enriched in unsaturated fats to offset the abnormal accumulation of saturated very-long-chain fatty acids.

Immunosuppressive and immunomodulating therapies have had profound results in several disorders known to be caused by altered humoral or cell-mediated immunity, but there are few guiding principles and even experts disagree in the starting dose, duration of therapy, and sequence or combination of available agents. Prednisone is the mainstay of therapy in polymyositis to suppress the infiltrating cytotoxic T cells that recognize main histocompatibility type 1 antigens and, along with macrophages, assemble in a trimolecular complex to initiate the attack on healthy myofibers. Generalized MG is a prototypical autoimmune disorder that nearly always warrants treatment with immunosuppressant and immunomodulating therapies to achieve sustained remission. The pathogenesis of the disease begins with sensitized thymic T and B cells that stimulate the production of polyclonal antibodies that recognize highly conserved antigens in the AChR of skeletal muscle, resulting in their ultimate destruction. In the end, the treating neurologists must decide the sequence and combination of pyridostigmine, thymectomy, various corticosteroid preparations, azathioprine, plasmapheresis, and IVIg, sadly without the benefit of clinical trials.

IVIg is a rational initial therapy in dermatomyositis based on its ability to inhibit lymphocyte function, pathogenic cytokines, and the binding and activation of complement proteins, especially the terminal component C5b-9 membrane attack complex (MAC). However, it does not confer long-term benefit; therefore, most patients are treated with a second immunosuppressant. IVIg is accepted monotherapy for MMN, with or without elevated GM1 antibody titers, but beyond its presumed action at sites of reversible motor conduction block, its exact mode of benefit in MMN is not well understood. In some progressively fatal disorders of unknown cause such as ALS, potent immunosuppressive therapy should be offered and never purposely withheld when there is a concurrent lymphoproliferative disease or when the neurologic syndrome is the first manifestation of occult SCLC or breast cancer, because aggressive therapy might theoretically halt or slow progression of the neurologic illness by suppressing the systemic immune response to the tumor.

Neurotrophic and other growth factors are important in the treatment of motor disorders. They include nerve growth factor, brain-derived neurotrophic factor (BDNF), neurotrophin-3, neurotrophin-4/5, ciliary neurotrophic factor, glial-derived neurotrophic factor, and insulin growth factor. BDNF, neurotrophin-3, neurotrophin-4/5, and ciliary neurotrophic factor are potent mediators of motor neuron survival and presumably rescue neonatal spinal and cranial motor neurons from death after axonopathy; they also block apoptotic cell death. Collateral, and not regenerative, sprouting is neurotrophin factor dependent. Collateral sprouts emerge from intact rather than injured axons and can slow the apparent progression of the disease. Both BDNF and neurotrophin-3 prevented axotomy-induced death of adult rat corticospinal tract (68). Motor neuron degeneration in the wobbler mouse, a model of human MND, is slowed by BDNF (69). Insulin growth fator type 1 (Myotrophin) had equivocal benefit in a multicenter trial of ALS; however, multicenter phase III trials of ciliary neurotrophic factor and BDNF are underway. A possible important role for neurotrophins and non-neurotrophin growth factors has also been suggested in the treatment of muscular dystrophy, diabetic neuropathy, leprosy, traumatic nerve injury, Parkinson disease, and Alzheimer disease (70,71).

Rehabilitative therapy of patients with motor disorders should be tailored to the diagnosis and the specific motor deficits. The comprehensive management of patients with a potentially disabling motor disorder requires the commitment of a multidisciplinary team of health professionals and caregivers. A physiatrist, physical therapist, and occupational therapist should identify necessary adaptive aids; teach the proper use of a cane, orthoses, or walker; and recommend low-impact aerobic exercises to decrease fatigue and depression and increase muscle efficiency. If there is dysarthria and dysphagia, a speech and swallowing evaluation should be arranged with an otolaryngologist and speech therapist to recommend proper positioning and breathing techniques to maximize speech volume and articulation and, depending on the seriousness of the bulbar findings, educate the patient and family in airway care and augmentative communication devices. If there is weight loss due to dysphagia and a calorie count by a nutritionist reveals suboptimal caloric intake, then a gastroenterologist should be consulted to implement supplemental oral feedings, preferably through a percutaneous endoscopic gastrostomy (PEG) tube.

Spasticity should be treated first with oral baclofen and tizanidine, increasing the dose until side effects occur; severe symptoms can be treated with intrathecal baclofen delivered by a pump. Botulinum toxin injections have an important role in the management of dystonia and in refractory spasticity. Pain that accompanies spasticity, joint contractures, pressure sores, and spinal strains should be treated aggressively with pharmacologic and physical therapy. Bladder, bowel, and sexual disorders accompany a wide variety of peripheral nervous system and CNS motor disorders and require the involvement of a neurologist and gynecologist and other necessary subspecialists. Untreated or ineffectively treated, they can be a source of risk for further illness as, for example, when chronic urinary tract infections or antibiotic-associated diarrhea supervenes. At the least, these symptoms lead to heightened depression and isolation. The management of respiratory failure due to muscle weakness can be especially challenging and necessitates a thorough evaluation by a pulmonologist experienced in neuromuscular disorders. There are new assistive breathing devices that prolong the time to require endotracheal intubation while improving the quality and duration of life at home or in a hospice.

REFERENCES

1. Younger DS. The diagnosis of progressive flaccid weakness. *Semin Neurol* 1993;13:241–246.
2. Younger DS. The diagnosis of progressive spastic paraparesis. *Semin Neurol* 1993;13:319–321.
3. Younger DS, Hays AP, Uncini A, DiMauro S. Recurrent myoglobinuria and HIV seropositivity: incidental or pathogenic association? *Muscle Nerve* 1989;12:842–843.
4. Younger DS, Worrall BB, Penn AS. Myasthenia gravis: historical perspective and overview. *Neurology* 1997;48[Suppl 5]:S1–S7.
5. Bodner R, Younger DS. Diabetic muscle infarction. *Muscle Nerve* 1994;17:949–950.
6. Blexrud MD, Windebank AJ, Daube JR. Long-term followup of 121 patients with benign fasciculations. *Ann Neurol* 1993;34:622–625.
7. DiMauro S, Wallace DC, eds. *Mitochondrial DNA in human pathology.* New York: Raven Press, 1993.
8. Younger DS, Gordon PH. Diagnosis in neuromuscular diseases. *Neurol Clin* 1996;14:135–168.
9. Members of the Mayo Clinic Department of Neurology. *Clinical examination in neurology.* St Louis: Mosby, 1998:87–285.
10. Medical Research Council. *Aids to the examination of the peripheral nervous system.* Memorandum 45. London: Her Majesty's Stationary Office, 1982.
11. Gowers WR. *Pseudohypertrophic muscular paralysis: a clinical lecture.* London: Churchill, 1879.
12. Younger DS, Rowland LP, Latov N, et al. Motor neuron disease and ALS: relation of high CSF protein to paraproteinemia and clinical syndrome. *Neurology* 1990;40:595–599.
13. Younger DS, Chou S, Hays AP, et al. Primary lateral sclerosis: a clinical diagnosis reemerges. *Arch Neurol* 1988;45:1304–1307.
14. Younger DS, Dalmau J, Inghirami G, Sherman W, Hays AP. Anti-Hu-associated peripheral nerve and muscle microvasculitis. *Neurology* 1994;44:181–183.
15. Guttmann L. Clinical symptomatology of spinal cord lesions. In: Vinken PJ, Bruyn GW, eds. *Handbook of clinical neurology.* Vol. 2. Amsterdam: Elsevier, 1978:178–216.
16. Charcot M. Sur un cas de paraplegie diabetique. Lecon du 13 Decembre 1889. In: Guinon G, ed. *Clinique des maladies du system nerveu.* Paris: Progres Medical, 1891:257–284.
17. Bruns L. Ueber neuritische lahmungen beim diabetes mellitus. *Berl Klin Wochenschr* 1890;27:509–515.
18. Garland H, Tavener D. Diabetic myelopathy. *Br Med J* 1953;1:1405–1408.
19. Garland H. Diabetic amyotrophy. *Br Med J* 1955;2:1287–1290.
20. Raff MC, Sangalang V, Asbury AK, et al. Ischemic mononeuropathy multiplex associated with diabetes mellitus. *Arch Neurol* 1968;18:487–499.
21. Chokroverty S. Proximal nerve dysfunction in diabetic proximal amyotrophy. *Arch Neurol* 1982;39:403–407.
22. Williams IR, Mayer RF. Subacute proximal diabetic neuropathy. *Neurology* 1976;26:108–116.
23. Bradley WG, Chad D, Verghese JP, et al. Painful lumbosacral plexopathy with elevated erythrocyte sedimentation rate: a treatable inflammatory syndrome. *Ann Neurol* 1984;15:457–464.
24. Report of the therapeutics and technology assessment subcommittee of the American Academy of Neurology. Clinical autonomic testing. *Neurology* 1996;46:873–880.
25. Claus D, Brunholzl C, Kerling FP, Henschel S. Transcranial magnetic stimulation as a diagnostic and prognostic test in amyotrophic lateral sclerosis. *J Neurol Sci* 1995;129[Suppl]:30–34.
26. Argov Z, Bank WJ. Phosphorous magnetic resonance spectroscopy (31pMRS) in neuromuscular disorders. *Ann Neurol* 1991;30:90–97.
27. Eidelberg D. Functional brain networks in movement disorders. *Curr Opin Neurol* 1998;11:319–326.
28. Lennon VA. Serologic profile of myasthenia gravis and distinction from the Lambert-Eaton myasthenic syndrome. *Neurology* 1997;48[Suppl 5]:S23–S27.
29. Lovelace RE, Younger DS. Myasthenia gravis with thymoma. *Neurology* 1997;48[Suppl 5]:S76–S81.
30. Kyle RA. Monoclonal gammopathy of undetermined significance—natural history in 24 cases. *Am J Med* 1978;64:814–826.
31. Dalakas MC. Basic aspects of neuroimmunology as they relate to immunotherapeutic targets: present and future prospects. *Ann Neurol* 1995;37[Suppl 1]:S2–S14.
32. Freddo L, Yu RK, Latov N, et al. Ganglioside GM1 and GD1b are antigens for IgM M-protein in a patient with human motor neuron disease. *Neurology* 1986;36:454–458.
33. Latov N, Hays AP, Donofrio PD. Monoclonal IgM with unique specificity to gangliosides GM1 and GD1b and to lacto-*N*-tetraose associated with human motor neuron disease. *Neurology* 1988;38:763–768.
34. Parry GJ, Clarke S. Multifocal acquired demyelinating neuropathy masquerading as motor neuron disease. *Muscle Nerve* 1988;11:103–107.
35. Pestronk A, Cornblath DR, Ilyas AA, et al. A treatable multifocal motor neuropathy with antibodies to GM1 gangliosides. *Ann Neurol* 1988;24:73–78.
36. Chaudhry V, Corse AM, Cornblath DR, et al. Multifocal motor neuropathy: response to human immune globulin. *Ann Neurol* 1993;33:237–242.
37. Yuki N, Sato S, Tsuji S, et al. Frequent presence of anti-GQ1b antibody in Fisher's syndrome. *Ann Neurol* 1993;43:414–417.
38. Chiba A, Kusunoki S, Obata H, Machinami R, Kanazawa I. Serum anti-GQ1b IgG antibody is associated with ophthalmoplegia in Miller Fisher syndrome and Guillain-Barré syndrome: clinical and immunohistochemical studies. *Neurology* 1993;43:1911–1917.
39. Dalmau J, Graus F, Rosenblum MK, Posner JB. Anti-Hu-associated paraneoplastic encephalomyelitis/sensory neuronopathy: a clinical study of 71 patients. *Medicine* 1992;71:59–72.
40. Dalmau J, Furneaux HM, Cordon-Cardo C, Posner JB. The expression of the HU (paraneoplastic encephalomyelitis/sensory neuronopathy) antigen in human normal and tumor tissue. *Am J Pathol* 1992;141:881–886.
41. Dalmau J, Furneaux HM, Rosenblum MK, Graus F, Posner JB. Detection of the anti-Hu antibody in regions of the nervous system and tumor from patients with paraneoplastic encephalomyelitis/sensory neuronopathy. *Neurology* 1991;41:1757–1764.
42. Dropcho EJ. Autoimmune central nervous system paraneoplastic dis-

orders: mechanisms, diagnosis, and therapeutic options. *Ann Neurol* 1995;37[Suppl 1]:S102–113.

43. Dalmau J, Furneaux HM, Gralla RJ, Kris MG, Posner JB. Detection of the anti-Hu antibody in the serum of patients with small cell lung cancer: a quantitative Western blot analysis. *Ann Neurol* 1990;27:544–552.

44. Halperin JJ. Neuroborreliosis: central nervous system involvement. *Semin Neurol* 1997;17:19–24.

45. Koenig M, Monaco AP, Kunkel LM. The complete sequence of dystrophin predicts a rod-shaped cytoskeletal protein. *Cell* 1988;53:219–228.

46. Monaco AP, Bertelson CJ, Liechti-Gialata H, Mosner H, Kunkel LM. An explanation for the phenotypic differences between patients bearing deletions of the DMD locus. *Genomics* 1988;2:90–95.

47. Zubrzycka-Gaarn EE, Bulman DE, Karpati G, et al. The Duchenne muscular dystrophy gene product is localized in the sarcolemma of human skeletal muscle. *Nature* 1988;333:466–469.

48. Monaco AP, Neve RL, Colletti-Feener CJ, et al. Isolation of candidate cDNAs for portions of the Duchenne muscular dystrophy gene. *Nature* 1986;323:646–650.

49. Hoffman EP, Fischbeck RH, Brown RH, et al. Characterization of dystrophin in muscle biopsy specimens from patients with Duchenne's or Becker muscular dystrophy. *N Engl J Med* 1988;38:1363–1368.

50. DiMauro S, Moraes CT. Mitochondrial encephalomyopathies. *Arch Neurol* 1993;50:1197–1208.

51. Engel WK, Cunningham GC. Rapid examination of muscle tissue: an improved trichrome method for fresh-frozen biopsy sections. *Neurology* 1963;13:919–923.

52. Moraes CT, DiMauro S, Zeviani M, et al. Mitochondrial DNA deletions in progressive external ophthalmoplegia and Kearns-Sayre syndrome. *N Engl J Med* 1989;320:1293–1299.

53. Engel AG, Ohno K, Milone M, Sine SM. Congenital myasthenic syndromes caused by mutations in acetylcholine receptor genes. *Neurology* 1997;48[Suppl 5]:S28–S35.

54. Mendell JR. Charcot-Marie-Tooth neuropathies and related disorders. *Semin Neurol* 1998;18:41–47.

55. Kleyn PW, Gilliam TC. Progress toward cloning of the gene responsible for childhood spinal muscular atrophy. *Semin Neurol* 1993;13:276–282.

56. Mulder DW, Kurland LT, Offord KP, Beard CM. Familial adult motor neuron disease: amyotrophic lateral sclerosis. *Neurology* 1986;36:511–517.

57. Brownell B, Oppenheimer DR, Hughes JT. The central nervous system in motor neuron disease. *J Neurol Neurosurg Psychiatry* 1970;33:338–357.

58. Tanaka J, Nakamura H, Tabuchi Y, Takahishi K. Familial amyotrophic lateral sclerosis: features of multisystem degeneration. *Acta Neuropathol* 1984;64:22–29.

59. Rosen DR, Siddique T, Patterson D, et al. Mutations in Cu/Zn superoxide dismutase gene are associated with familial amyotrophic lateral sclerosis. *Nature* 1993;362:59–62.

60. Hays AP, Younger DS. Muscle and nerve biopsy. In: Rowland LP, ed. *Merritt's textbook of neurology*. Baltimore: Williams and Wilkins, 1995:97–100.

61. Dalakas MC. Polymyositis, dermatomyositis, and inclusion body myositis. *N Engl J Med* 1991;325:1487–1498.

62. DiMauro S, Tonin P, Servidei S. Metabolic myopathies. In: Rowland LP, DiMauro S, eds. *Handbook of clinical neurology*. Amsterdam: Elsevier, 1992:479–526.

63. Younger DS, Kass R. Vasculitis of the nervous system. Historical perspective and overview. *Neurol Clin* 1997;15:737–758.

64. Kernohan JW, Woltman HW. Periarteritis nodosa: a clinicopathologic study with specific reference to the nervous system. *Arch Neurol Psychiatry* 1938;39:655–686.

65. Younger DS, Rosoklija G, Hays AP. Diabetic peripheral neuropathy. *Semin Neurol* 1998;18:95–104.

66. Santoro M, Thomas FP, Fink ME, et al. IgM deposits at nodes of Ranvier in a patient with amyotrophic lateral sclerosis, anti-GM1 antibodies, and multifocal conduction block. *Ann Neurol* 1990;28:373–377.

67. Santoro M, Uncini A, Corbo M, et al. Experimental autoimmune block induced by serum from a patient with anti-GM1 antibodies. *Ann Neurol* 1992;31:385–390.

68. Giehl KM, Tetzlaff W. BDNF and NT-3, but not NGF, prevent axotomy-induced death of rat corticospinal neurons in vivo. *Eur J Neurosci* 1996;8:1167–1175.

69. Ikeda K, Klikosz B, Green T, et al. Effects of brain-derived neurotrophic factor (BDNF) on motor dysfunction in wobbler mouse motor neuron disease. *Ann Neurol* 1995;37:505–511.

70. Slonim AE, Rosenthal H, Manzione D, Goldberg T. Clinical trial of recombinant human insulin-like growth factor-1 in myotonic dystrophy. *Ann Neurol* 1995;38:334(abst).

71. Ebendal T, Lonnerberg P, Pei G, Kylberg A, Kullander K, Persson H. Engineering cells to secrete growth factors. *J Neurol* 1994;242[Suppl 1]:S5–S7

72. McKusick VA. *Mendelian inheritance in man*, 10th ed. Baltimore: Johns Hopkins University Press, 1992.

Motor Disorders,
edited by David S. Younger.
Lippincott Williams & Wilkins, Philadelphia © 1999.

CHAPTER 2

Basic Principles and Practice of Electromyography

Mark A. Ferrante and Asa J. Wilbourn

The electrodiagnostic examination[1] is an extension of the clinical neurologic examination and provides important information about the peripheral nervous system (PNS) that usually cannot be obtained in any other manner. It includes nerve conduction studies (NCS), the needle examination, and a variety of special studies including F waves, H responses, and repetitive nerve stimulation. Motor NCS and the needle examination assess the motor system from the lower motor neuron (LMN) in the brainstem and spinal cord to the muscle fibers they innervate; needle electromyography (EMG) also provides some information about the central nervous system. Sensory NCS assess sensory axons from the dorsal root ganglia to the recording or stimulating site, whichever is more distal. This chapter reviews aspects of PNS anatomy, physiology, and pathology; the technical and diagnostic features of NCS and the needle examination; and the electrophysiologic manifestations of specific disorders of the motor unit.

ANATOMIC CONSIDERATIONS

Cortical motor neurons, the upper motor neurons (UMNs), give rise to corticospinal and corticobulbar tract fibers that in turn synapse with brainstem and spinal cord LMNs. The smallest element of movement is the product of an individual motor unit, which consists of a single LMN, its axon, and all muscle fibers it innervates across the intervening neuromuscular junctions (NMJs). Motor axons of the same spinal segment exit the spinal cord and fuse to form a single ventral root, which subsequently joins sensory axons of the respective dorsal root to form a mixed spinal nerve. The latter exits the intervertebral foramen and gives off a posterior branch, the posterior primary ramus, which is the source of paraspinal muscle innervation and sensation to the dorsal aspect of the neck and trunk. The remaining sensory and motor axons, termed the "anterior primary ramus" (APR), subsequently intermingle to form the somatic plexuses of the body (i.e., cervical, brachial, lumbar, and sacral), except in the thoracic and abdominal regions, where they remain independent. These fibers supply muscle innervation and sensation to the ventral and lateral aspects of the trunk and all parts of the limbs (Fig. 1) (1).

Distally, the mixed nerves segregate into motor and sensory components. Motor axons derived from LMNs of the same spinal cord segment innervate muscles belonging to the same myotome, whereas sensory axons derived from the same level innervate sensory receptors of a common dermatome. An understanding of the pathways traversed by the motor and sensory axons studied during the electrodiagnostic examination is important for students of neurology and mandatory for electromyographers. Knowing the muscle domain of each PNS segment permits competent performance of the study and accurate localization of any identified abnormalities. For example, because the upper trunk is formed by the joining of the C-5 and C-6 APR, its muscle domain is equal to the sum of the C-5 and C-6 muscle domains *minus* the muscle domains of the long thoracic and dorsal scapular nerves, because these two nerves receive axons derived from the C-5 and C-6 APR before upper trunk formation. This approach permits deduction of the muscle domain of any PNS element. Frequently exam-

M. A. Ferrante: Electromyography Laboratory and Department of Neurology, Keesler Medical Center, Biloxi, Mississippi 39534.

A. J. Wilbourn: Department of Neurology, Case Western Reserve School of Medicine and Electromyography Laboratory and Department of Neurology, Cleveland Clinic Foundation, Cleveland, Ohio 44195.

[1]The opinions and assertions contained herein are the private views of the authors and are not to be construed as the official policy or position of the U.S. Government, the Department of Defense, or the Department of the Air Force.

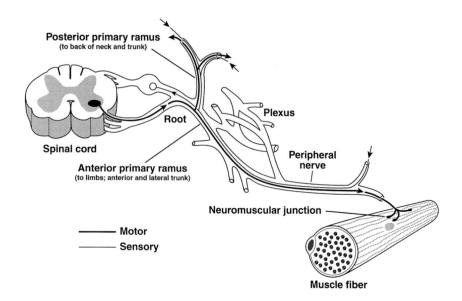

FIG. 1. Portions of the peripheral neuro-muscular system. (From Wilbourn A. How can electromyography help you? Postgrad Med 1983;6:188, with permission.)

ined muscles belonging to the muscle domains of the cervical and lumbosacral roots and the trunk and cord elements of the brachial plexus are provided, respectively, in Tables 1 through 4 (2–7). The sensory nerve domains of the PNS elements are equally important. Sensory nerve domains of the brachial plexus elements were recently reviewed and are provided in Table 5 (8). In addition, illustrations of the dermatomes (Figs. 2 through 5) and cutaneous nerve distributions (Figs. 6 through 9) of the body and the course and muscle domain for the median, ulnar, radial, femoral, sciatic, superficial peroneal, and deep peroneal nerves (Figs. 10 through 16) are provided.

TABLE 1. *Muscle domains of the cervical root elements*

C-5:	Rhomboideus major and minor, **supraspinatus, infraspinatus, deltoid, biceps, brachioradialis**
C-6:	Supraspinatus, infraspinatus, **deltoid, biceps,** triceps, anconeus, **brachioradialis,** extensor carpi radialis, **pronator teres, flexor carpi radialis**
C-7:	**Triceps, anconeus,** extensor carpi radialis, extensor digitorum communis, extensor carpi ulnaris, **pronator teres, flexor carpi radialis**
C-8:	Extensor digitorum communis, extensor carpi ulnaris, **extensor pollicis brevis, extensor indicis proprius, flexor pollicis longus, pronator quadratus, abductor pollicis brevis, flexor carpi ulnaris, flexor digitorum profundus, abductor digiti minimi, adductor pollicis, first dorsal interosseous**
T-1:	Flexor pollicis longus, **pronator quadratus, abductor pollicis brevis,** flexor carpi ulnaris, **flexor digitorum profundus, abductor digiti minimi, adductor pollicis, first dorsal interosseous**

Only our own muscle preferences are shown. Paraspinal muscles belong to all root elements and therefore are not listed. Muscles shown in bold type are more likely to be involved with disease of the listed root element.

TABLE 2. *Muscle domains of the lumbosacral root elements*

L-2:	**Iliacus**
L-3:	**Iliacus, adductor longus, vastus lateralis, vastus medialis, rectus femoris**
L-4:	**Adductor longus, vastus lateralis, vastus medialis, rectus femoris, tibialis anterior,** extensor hallucis
L-5:	**Tensor fascia lata, gluteus medius,** gluteus maximus, **semimembranosus, semitendinosus, tibialis anterior, extensor hallucis, peroneus longus, extensor digitorum brevis, tibialis posterior, flexor digitorum longus,** gastrocnemius (lateral head)
S-1:	Tensor fascia lata, gluteus medius, **gluteus maximus, biceps femoris (short head), biceps femoris (long head), extensor digitorum brevis,** tibialis posterior, flexor digitorum longus, **gastrocnemius (lateral head), gastrocnemius (medial head), soleus, abductor hallucis, abductor digiti quinti pedis**
S-2:	Biceps femoris (short head), biceps femoris (long head), gastrocnemius (medial head), **soleus, abductor hallucis, abductor digiti quinti pedis**

Only our own muscle preferences are shown. Paraspinal muscles belong to all root elements and therefore are not listed. Muscles shown in bold type are more likely to be involved with disease of the listed root element.

TABLE 3. *Muscle domains of the trunk elements*

Upper trunk	Middle trunk	Lower trunk
Supraspinatus	Pronator teres	Flexor pollicis longus
Infraspinatus	Flexor carpi radialis	Abductor pollicis brevis
Biceps	Triceps	Extensor carpi ulnaris
Deltoid	Anconeus	Extensor digitorum communis
Teres minor	Extensor carpi radialis	Extensor pollicis brevis
Triceps	Extensor carpi ulnaris	Extensor indicis proprius
Pronator teres	Extensor digitorum communis	Flexor carpi ulnaris
Flexor carpi radialis	Extensor indicis proprius	Flexor digitorum profundus- 3,4
Brachioradialis		Abductor digiti minimi
Extensor carpi radialis		First dorsal interosseous

TABLE 4. *Muscle domains of the cord elements*

Lateral cord	Posterior cord	Medial cord
Biceps	Deltoid	Flexor pollicis longus
Pronator teres	Teres minor	Abductor pollicis brevis
Flexor carpi radialis	Triceps	Flexor carpi ulnaris
	Anconeus	Flexor digitorum profundus- 3,4
	Brachioradialis	Abductor digiti minimi
	Extensor pollicis brevis	First dorsal interosseous
	Extensor carpi radialis	
	Extensor indicis proprius	
	Extensor digitorum communis	
	Extensor carpi ulnaris	

TABLE 5. *SNAP domains of the brachial plexus elements*
(and their involvement incidence)

Upper trunk: LABC (96%); Med-D1 (96%); radial (58%); Med-D2 (20%); Med-D3 (8%)
Middle trunk: Med-D2 (80%); Med-D3 (79%); radial (42%)
Lower trunk: Uln-D5 (96%); DUC (96%); MABC (100%); Med-D3 (13%)
Lateral cord: LABC (100%); Med-D1 (100%); Med-D2 (100%); Med-D3 (87%)
Posterior cord: radial (100%)
Medial cord: Uln-D5 (100%); DUC (100%); MABC (100%); Med-D3 (13%)

Values in parentheses indicate the incidence of involvement for the various brachial plexus elements (8).

SNAP, sensory nerve action potential; LABC, lateral antebrachial cutaneous digit; Med-D1, median, recording first digit; Med-D2, median, recording second digit; Med-D3, median, recording third digit; Uln-D5, ulnar, recording fifth digit; DUC, dorsal ulnar cutaneous; MABC, medial antebrachial cutaneous.

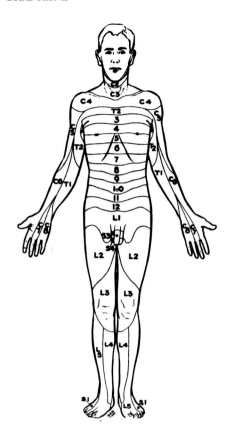

FIG. 2. Anterior view of the dermatomes of the body. The C-2 dermatome adjoins the cutaneous nerve distribution of the mandibular division of the fifth cranial nerve. The arrows indicate the lateral extensions of the T-3 dermatome. (From Haymaker W, Woodhall B. *Peripheral nerve injuries: principles of diagnosis.* Philadelphia: WB Saunders, 1953:28, with permission.)

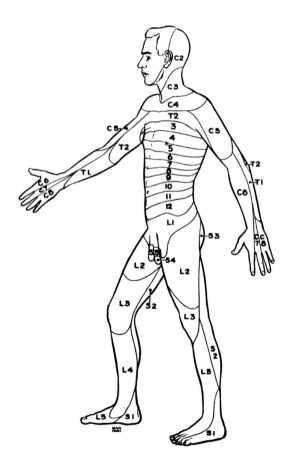

FIG. 3. Anterolateral view of the dermatomes of the body. (From Haymaker W, Woodhall B. *Peripheral nerve injuries: principles of diagnosis.* Philadelphia: WB Saunders, 1953:28, with permission.)

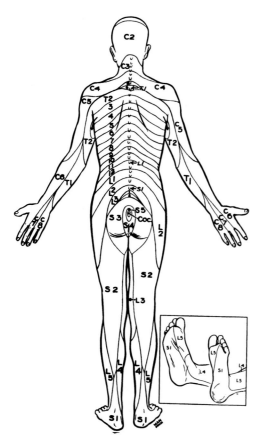

FIG. 4. Posterior view of the dermatomes of the body. Note the absence of a C-1 dermatome. The arrows in the region of the vertebral column identify the T-1, L-1, and S-1 vertebral processes, whereas those in the axillary regions indicate the lateral extent of the T-3 dermatome. The inset shows the dermatomes of the plantar aspects of the feet. (From Haymaker W, Woodhall B. *Peripheral nerve injuries: principles of diagnosis.* Philadelphia: WB Saunders, 1953:28, with permission.)

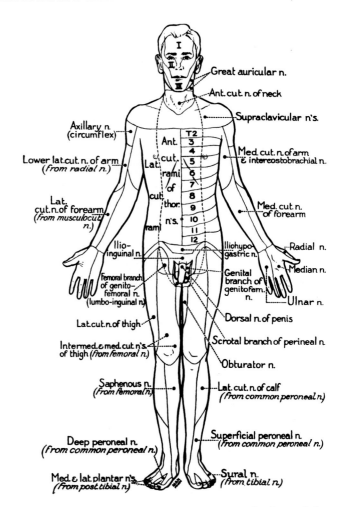

FIG. 6. Anterior view of the cutaneous distributions of the peripheral nerves of the body. The intercostal nerves are indicated on the left side of the trunk by numbers, the cutaneous distributions of the branches of the anterior primary rami are shown on the right side of the trunk, and the asterisk just below the scrotum lies within the field of the posterior cutaneous nerve of the thigh. (From Haymaker W, Woodhall B. *Peripheral nerve injuries: principles of diagnosis.* Philadelphia: WB Saunders, 1953:28, with permission.)

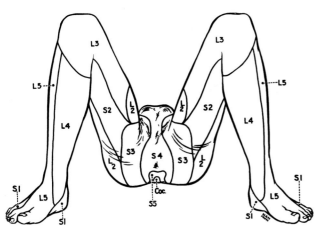

FIG. 5. The dermatomes of the perineum and lower extremities. (From Haymaker W, Woodhall B. *Peripheral nerve injuries: principles of diagnosis.* Philadelphia: WB Saunders, 1953:28, with permission.)

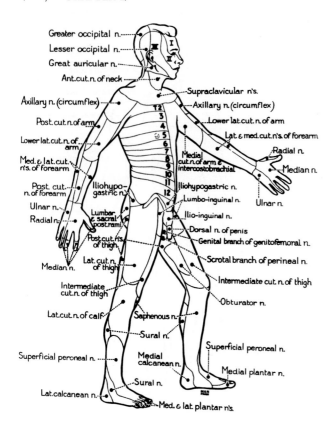

FIG. 7. Anterolateral view of the cutaneous distributions of the peripheral nerves of the body. The roman numerals indicate the ophthalmic (I), maxillary (II), and mandibular (III) divisions of the fifth cranial nerve. (From Haymaker W, Woodhall B. *Peripheral nerve injuries: principles of diagnosis.* Philadelphia: WB Saunders, 1953:28, with permission.)

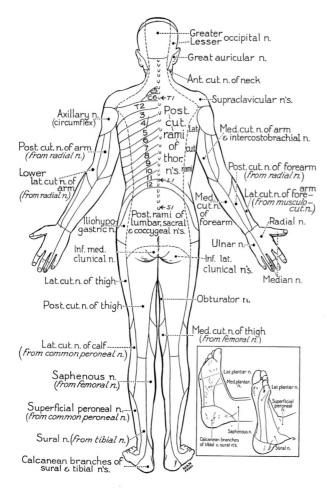

FIG. 8. Posterior view of the cutaneous distributions of the peripheral nerves of the body. The broken lines indicate the boundaries of the cutaneous supply of the posterior primary rami. (From Haymaker W, Woodhall B. *Peripheral nerve injuries: principles of diagnosis.* Philadelphia: WB Saunders, 1953:28, with permission.)

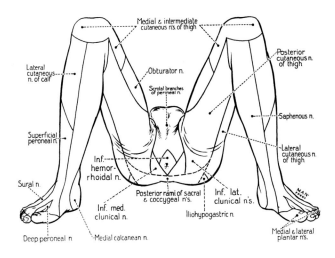

FIG. 9. The cutaneous distributions of the peripheral nerves of the perineum and lower extremities. (From Haymaker W, Woodhall B. *Peripheral nerve injuries: principles of diagnosis.* Philadelphia: WB Saunders, 1953:28, with permission.)

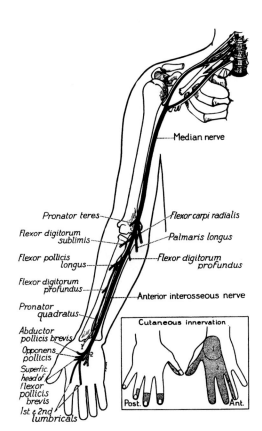

FIG. 10. The course and distribution of the median nerve and the muscles it supplies. The inset shows the cutaneous boundaries of the palmar cutaneous (1) and the palmar digital (2) nerve branches. (From Haymaker W, Woodhall B. *Peripheral nerve injuries: principles of diagnosis.* Philadelphia: WB Saunders, 1953:28, with permission.)

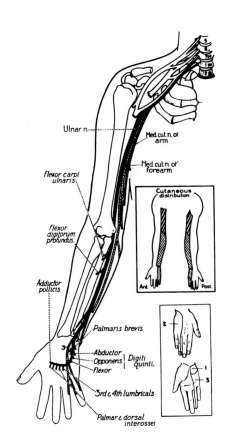

FIG. 11. The course and distribution of the medial cutaneous nerves of the arm and forearm and the ulnar nerve and the muscles supplied by the latter. The patterns of the three nerves are duplicated in the upper inset. The lower inset shows the cutaneous boundaries of the palmar (1), dorsal (2), and superficial terminal (3) branches of the ulnar nerve. (From Haymaker W, Woodhall B. *Peripheral nerve injuries: principles of diagnosis.* Philadelphia: WB Saunders, 1953:28, with permission.)

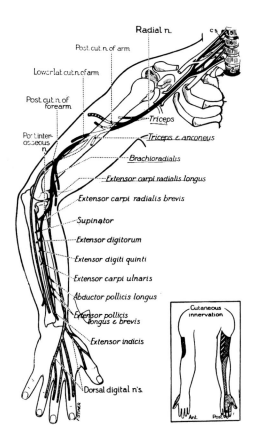

FIG. 12. The course and distribution of the radial nerve and the muscles it supplies. The patterns of the cutaneous nerves are duplicated in the inset. (From Haymaker W, Woodhall B. *Peripheral nerve injuries: principles of diagnosis.* Philadelphia: WB Saunders, 1953:28, with permission.)

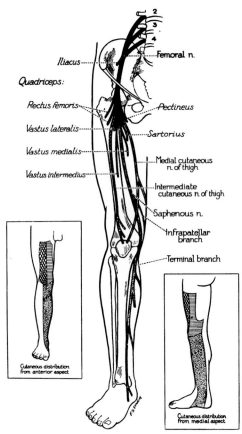

FIG. 13. The course and distribution of the femoral nerve and the muscles it supplies. The patterns of the cutaneous nerves are duplicated in the inset. The broken line indicates the boundaries between the infrapatellar and terminal branches of the saphenous nerve. (From Haymaker W, Woodhall B. *Peripheral nerve injuries: principles of diagnosis.* Philadelphia: WB Saunders, 1953:28, with permission.)

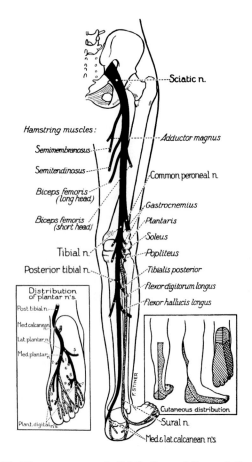

FIG. 14. The course and distribution of the sciatic, tibial, posterior tibial, and plantar nerves and the muscles they supply. The patterns of the cutaneous nerves are duplicated in the inset. (From Haymaker W, Woodhall B. *Peripheral nerve injuries: principles of diagnosis.* Philadelphia: WB Saunders, 1953:28, with permission.)

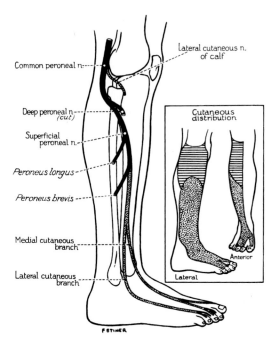

FIG. 15. The course and distribution of the superficial peroneal nerve and the muscles it supplies. The patterns of the cutaneous nerves are duplicated in the inset. (From Haymaker W, Woodhall B. *Peripheral nerve injuries: principles of diagnosis.* Philadelphia: WB Saunders, 1953:28, with permission.)

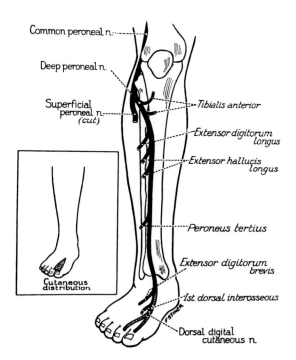

FIG. 16. The course and distribution of the deep peroneal nerve and the muscles it supplies. Its cutaneous distribution is shown in the inset. (From Haymaker W, Woodhall B. *Peripheral nerve injuries: principles of diagnosis.* Philadelphia: WB Saunders, 1953:28, with permission.)

ELECTRODIAGNOSTIC EXAMINATION

Introduction to Nerve Conduction Studies

Standard NCS assess large myelinated nerve fibers of named sensory, motor, and mixed nerves depending on the axon type(s) under study; thinly myelinated and unmyelinated fibers, for example, those that transmit pain and temperature, are not amenable to evaluation by standard NCS. When a peripheral nerve is electrically depolarized by negative charge accumulation beneath the cathode of the stimulator, bidirectionally propagating nerve fiber action potentials are generated. Two electrodes positioned away from the stimulation site record the summation of these potentials, termed the evoked response. The electrode closest to the stimulation site is the active, or G1 electrode, and the more distant one is termed the reference, or G2 electrode. The electrical activity recorded by these two electrodes is amplified differentially and displayed on the oscilloscope screen.

The actual performance of NCS is deceptively simple. The G1 and G2 electrodes are positioned over the nerve being studied when sensory or mixed NCS are being performed and along the motor point of the muscle belly and the tendon (for G1 and G2 electrodes, respectively) when motor NCS are performed. A ground electrode is affixed between the stimulating and recording sites to reduce shock artifact. The nerve is then stimulated, beginning with a low stimulus intensity which is progressively increased until a response is evoked. The stimulus intensity is continually increased until the size of the response ceases to increase. At this point, the response is called, incorrectly, a *supramaximal* response. In fact, it is obviously a *maximal* response; the stimulus that ultimately elicited it was supramaximal. Whenever NCS are performed, various components of the response are evaluated. These provide information concerning the conduction status of the nerve fibers being assessed, information that often is unobtainable from clinical examination and other laboratory studies.

Sensory Nerve Conduction Studies

The recorded sensory nerve action potential (SNAP) is the summation of many evoked nerve fiber action potentials. These recordings are generally made with surface recording electrodes placed proximal or distal to the stimulating electrodes by orthodromic or antidromic techniques, respectively. We prefer the antidromic technique because it produces higher SNAP amplitudes and less patient discomfort. Measurable waveform parameters include the nerve response amplitude, duration, morphology, and, depending on the NCS technique preferred, a latency or conduction velocity (CV). The response components for a sensory NCS are illustrated in Fig. 17. Waveform morphology may be biphasic or triphasic, depending on the particular sensory NCS being per-

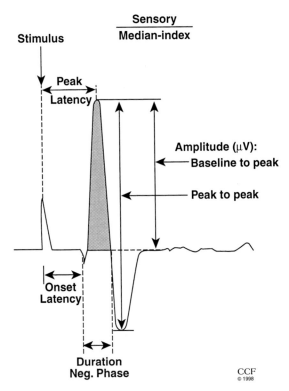

FIG. 17. The various components of the sensory nerve conduction response. (From Levin KH, Shields RW Jr, Wilbourn AJ. Electromyography/electrodiagnosis. In: Isley MR, Krauss GL, Levin KH, et al., eds. *Electromyography/electroencephalography.* Redmond, WA: SpaceLabs Medical, Inc., 1993, with permission.)

formed. The amplitude of the SNAP, in microvolts, is measured from the trough of the initial positive component to the peak of the subsequent negative component when the response is triphasic or from the baseline to the initial negative component when the response is biphasic. The amplitude varies with the number of functioning axons, their relative conduction rates, and the distance between the stimulation and recording sites. A longer distance decreases the amplitude by increasing temporal dispersion among the recorded impulses. The amplitude is considered abnormal when it falls below published or individual laboratory control values. In addition, when the amplitude is 50% or less of the contralateral homologous response, it is considered to be *relatively* abnormal. The duration, in milliseconds, is the time between the onset and termination of the first negative phase of the SNAP. The latency and CV reflect the rate of conduction along the stimulated axons. One or both can be reported, depending on whether the distance between the stimulating and recording electrodes is predefined or variable.

We prefer to use constant distances between the stimulating and recording electrodes for two reasons. First, the need to calculate a CV is eliminated, thereby permitting the elapsed time or latency, in milliseconds, to be directly reported without manipulation. Second, it removes the

effect that temporal dispersion has on the amplitude of the recorded responses. The *onset* latency reflects the conduction rate along the *fastest* conducting fibers, whereas the *peak* latency corresponds to the *average* conduction rate of the fastest conducting fibers. There are theoretical reasons why onset latencies are more sensitive. Nonetheless, we use peak latencies because they are easier to identify and because there are no published studies showing onset latencies to be of greater diagnostic value. The CV, in meters per second, is calculated by dividing the distance between the stimulating and recording sites, in millimeters, by the time required, in milliseconds, for some portion of the SNAP to appear after the nerve is stimulated. Whenever a distal sensory CV is reported, it usually reflects the preference of the person performing the NCS for using anatomic landmarks to define the stimulation and recording sites. With this approach, the distance between the stimulation and recording sites varies among individuals. Thus, both the time and the distance are variable and, for that reason, must be measured. Although infrequently performed, sensory nerves can also be stimulated at more proximal sites. By dividing the surface distance in millimeters by the latency difference in milliseconds, between the peak latencies of the two recorded responses, a CV along more proximal segments of the sensory nerve can be calculated. This can be especially helpful in the assessment of patients with suspected polyneuropathy.

Although sensory NCS do not assess components of the motor system, they are important in its evaluation for several reasons. First, they may be a clue to the localization of the lesion, as, for example, in patients with paraneoplastic sensory neuronopathy due to circulating anti-Hu antibodies directed against dorsal root ganglia and central nervous system neurons. Second, sensory NCS are more sensitive than motor NCS in detecting axon loss or focal demyelinating lesions and may be the only NCS abnormality identified. For example, the peak latency of the median SNAP in the carpal tunnel syndrome (CTS), a disorder that produces focal demyelination, precedes abnormality of the distal motor latency. SNAP amplitudes are also reduced to a greater extent than those of the motor responses in axon-loss lesions. Third, sensory NCS are the only component of the basic electrodiagnostic study that assesses any portion of the peripheral sensory system. A significant drawback of sensory NCS, however, is their greater vulnerability to physiologic, physical, and pathologic factors. The small size of the SNAP makes it much more vulnerable to obesity, edema, physiologic temporal dispersion, temperature, and pathologic influences. Thus, even among normal individuals, their procurement is technically more demanding. Of the controllable factors, temperature is by far the most problematic. Cooling of the studied extremity increases the amplitude and duration, prolongs the latency, and decreases the CV of the recorded sensory response.

Therefore, whenever a prolonged latency and decreased CV are encountered and the amplitude is not reduced, warming is required; otherwise, these changes may be wrongly ascribed to a demyelinating disorder. Aging also interferes with NCS interpretation. For example, normal individuals over the age of 60 years can have bilaterally unelicitable sural and superficial peroneal SNAPs.

Although many different sensory NCS have been reported throughout the years, the frequency with which they are used varies among EMG laboratories. Most consider the median (recording index finger), ulnar (recording fifth finger), and the sural NCS as the standard sensory NCS. In our EMG laboratories, we also include the radial (recording thumb base) and the superficial peroneal (recording dorsum of ankle) NCS in this category. Several nonstandard studies [e.g., the median (recording thumb and middle finger), the lateral and medial antebrachial cutaneous, and the dorsal ulnar cutaneous studies] are used in certain situations. In our EMG laboratories, for example, they are used primarily to localize axon loss brachial plexus lesions (8). The saphenous and the lateral femoral cutaneous nerves are not reliable enough for routine clinical use. Consequently, we have no means of assessing the sensory fibers traversing the lumbar plexus. Details concerning the assessment of individual sensory NCS are outside the scope of this chapter but are available to the interested reader (9).

Motor NCS

In the case of motor NCS, only orthodromic studies, using the belly-tendon method, can be performed. The recorded activity represents the summation of the muscle fiber action potentials generated by activated motor axons and is termed a compound muscle action potential (CMAP). The innervation ratio, or number of muscle fibers innervated by a single motor axon, explains why CMAP amplitudes, measured in millivolts, are so much larger than SNAPs (measured in microvolts). This *magnification effect* significantly reduces CMAP vulnerability to physiologic, physical, and pathologic factors.

Measured waveform parameters include amplitude, duration, latency, CV, and morphology. The CMAP morphology is biphasic because placement of the G1 electrode over the motor point of the muscle results in a CMAP response recorded at its inception; therefore, an initial positive phase is not present, as it often is with SNAPs, and the amplitude is measured from baseline to peak. Because the negative phase duration of a CMAP is so much greater than that of a SNAP, CMAPs are quite resistant to physiologic temporal dispersion (10). This allows the distance between the stimulating and recording electrodes to be much greater, thereby permitting the assessment of a much longer nerve segment. As a result, motor NCS are the best means for identifying focal demyelinating conduction blocks. Although spinal root

level stimulation can be performed, it is seldom necessary to stimulate proximal to the supraclavicular level, with upper extremity assessment, or to the popliteal fossa level with lower extremity evaluations. As with sensory NCS, when constant distances are used between the stimulating and recording sites, latencies can be obtained and compared among individuals. However, the distal latency alone cannot be used to calculate a motor nerve CV because the motor response, unlike the sensory one, is not generated directly by the motor nerve fibers but rather by their innervated muscle fibers. For that reason, the calculated CV reflects NMJ transmission and muscle fiber conduction times, in addition to motor nerve conduction times. Consequently, to independently assess the conduction rate of the motor nerve fibers, the nerve must be stimulated at two separate sites; this results in distal and proximally evoked responses. Each provides an amplitude and a latency measurement. Because the time required for NMJ transmission and muscle fiber conduction is the same for both responses, the latency difference (i.e., the proximal latency minus the distal latency) reflects the time required for the impulses to travel between the two sites. The motor nerve CV (in milliseconds) between the two stimulation sites equals the distance between them (in millimeters) divided by their latency difference (in milliseconds). Figure 18 illustrates the response components for motor NCS.

In most EMG laboratories, the median, ulnar, peroneal, and posterior tibial responses, recording from the abductor pollicis brevis, abductor digiti minimi, extensor digitorum

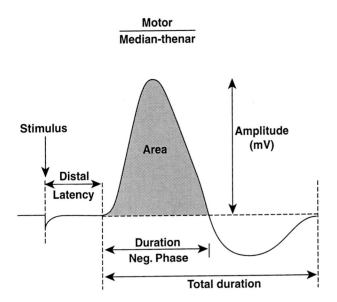

FIG. 18. The various components of the motor nerve conduction response. (From Levin KH, Shields RW Jr, Wilbourn AJ. Electromyography/electrodiagnosis. In: Isley MR, Krauss GL, Levin KH, et al., eds. *Electromyography/electroencephalography*. Redmond, WA: SpaceLabs Medical, Inc., 1993, with permission.)

brevis, and abductor hallucis muscles, respectively, comprise *standard* motor NCS. Other limb and cranial motor nerves can also be assessed provided that recording and stimulating sites are accessible. When only a single stimulation site is available, as for example along the axillary nerve recording from the deltoid muscle and the spinal accessory nerve recording from the trapezius muscle, only distal motor latencies and amplitudes are analyzed.

Mixed Nerve Conduction Studies

In such studies, the nerve is stimulated distally, whereas the response is recorded proximally along the nerve. These evoked responses are typically triphasic but may be biphasic when a limited amount of tissue lies between the recording electrodes and the axons (e.g., in thin individuals) or absent when a significant amount of intervening tissue is present (e.g., in obesity). Their amplitudes and latencies are measured as for SNAPs. Mixed NCS technically are difficult to perform in large-limbed individuals and, except for the palmar and plantar nerves, offer little additional information over conventional sensory NCS.

Electrophysiologic Manifestations of Various Nerve Lesions

Nerve Conduction Studies

The pathologic responses to nerve injury are limited as are their corresponding electrophysiologic manifestations. Pathologically, axon loss, focal demyelination, or some combination of the two is ultimately produced. Axon disruption causes the distal stump of the involved axon to undergo degeneration (termed Wallerian degeneration), thereby making it incapable of conducting evoked impulses to the recording site. Thus, the pathophysiologic counterpart of axon loss is conduction failure. The number of nerve fibers that contribute action potentials to the compound response is the major determinant of the SNAP and CMAP amplitudes. Consequently, the amplitude of the evoked response is often the only parameter affected by disorders that produce axon loss. Because focal axon disruption causes Wallerian degeneration of the entire distal stump, its effects do not remain focal. As a result, axon-loss lesions produce decreased response amplitudes regardless of whether the nerve is stimulated above, at, or below the site of the original lesion. For this reason, axon-loss lesions related to LMN or dorsal root ganglia insults are identifiable by electrodiagnostic studies. As the number of disrupted axons increases, the amplitude of the recorded response decreases. Once most or all fibers undergo axon loss, the responses become unelicitable. For unknown reasons, the SNAP amplitude is more sensitive to a given degree of axon loss than the CMAP amplitude. Lesions resulting in the loss of approximately 50% of the axons of a mixed nerve often lead to unelicitable SNAPs, whereas the CMAP amplitudes remain about one-half normal.

With two exceptions, the latency and CV measurements tend to be normal in partial axon-loss lesions because of ample conduction along uninjured nerve fibers. First, when all or most of the fastest conducting fibers are affected, there can be mild prolongation of distal latencies and mild slowing of CVs; however, this generally requires a severe amount of axon loss, and the degree of amplitude reduction is then much more pronounced than the decline in velocity. Second, substantial slowing can be seen when there is a severe axon-loss lesion and subsequent regeneration. This reflects the smaller diameter (higher impedance) and thinner myelin sheaths (increased capacitance) of the regenerating axons.

The observed alterations in demyelinating lesions depend on its degree. Overall, processes producing demyelination tend to affect the largest fibers and, hence, the fastest conducting ones. Mild demyelinating lesions cause widening of the nodal gap and slow the rate of propagation of nerve fiber action potentials; thus, distal latencies are prolonged and CVs are decreased. When more pronounced demyelination occurs, the propagating impulses are blocked across the lesioned site and, as in the case of axon loss-associated conduction failure, the amplitude of the recorded response is decreased on stimulation proximal to the lesion. Thus, with demyelinating conduction block, the NCS response amplitude again becomes the most important NCS parameter, with the degree of amplitude reduction dependent on the number of nerve fibers affected. Importantly, unlike axon-loss processes in which the recorded response amplitudes are low or unobtainable regardless of the site of stimulation, focal demyelinating conduction block lesions are truly focal because they do not affect conduction along more proximal and distal nerve segments. Thus, unless the site of demyelinating conduction block lies between the stimulating and recording sites, it will go undetected by NCS. Whenever two separate stimulation sites yield CMAPs with significantly different amplitudes and various technical and anatomic factors can be excluded, a focal demyelinating conduction block lesion is present somewhere between the two sites. The single exception to this rule is in axon-loss processes before the development of Wallerian degeneration, when the distal nerve segment is still capable of conducting responses. In addition to focal demyelinating lesions, multifocal and generalized distributions can also be identified.

After the fourth to seventh day from the onset of weakness and before reinnervation occurs, the amount of accompanying axon loss can be estimated by comparing the percentage loss of the CMAP amplitude between the distally recorded abnormal response and its normal contralateral counterpart. For example, when the distal CMAP amplitude is 5 mV and the proximal CMAP amplitude is 2.5 mV along an affected nerve compared with a normal contralateral distal CMAP amplitude of 10 mV, then 50% of the affected nerve fibers are affected by axon loss, 25% by demyelinating conduction block, and 25% conduct normally.

When a focal demyelinating conduction block lesion is suspected, further evaluation along more proximal stimulation sites (e.g., at the elbow, spiral groove, axilla, and supraclavicular fossa) can be undertaken. Further localization can be determined using the *inching* technique (11). With this technique, stimulation is applied at progressively more distal sites until the proximally identified amplitude reduction normalizes.

The clinical correlation of these various pathophysiologies is straightforward. Concerning motor axons, clinical weakness occurs when propagating nerve fiber action potentials do not reach their muscle fiber pool, an outcome that occurs only with axon-loss–induced conduction failure or demyelinating conduction block. Because all nerve fiber action potentials traverse the lesion site, weakness does not occur secondary to lesions producing demyelinating conduction slowing. Regarding sensory axons, fixed sensory deficits only occur with dropout of propagating sensory nerve fiber action potentials, again reflecting either axon-loss–induced conduction failure or demyelinating conduction block but not demyelinating conduction slowing. Hence, regardless of fiber type, demyelinating conduction slowing has essentially no clinical accompaniment; it is an electrodiagnostic phenomenon (Table 6).

Needle Examination

This is the most sensitive test for axon-loss lesions and the only one capable of identifying disorders involving the UMN system and, for practical purposes, the muscle fibers themselves. Either concentric or monopolar needle electrodes are used. Concentric needles are hollow with a central small metal wire surrounded by an insulating resin. The tip of the wire is exposed distally and functions as the G1 electrode, whereas the intramuscular portion of the cannula functions as the G2 electrode. Monopolar needles are composed of a metal shaft coated with Teflon, except at the tip, which functions as the G1 recording electrode in conjunction with a separate electrode, typically a surface one, used as the G2 recording electrode. The electrical activity recorded by the G1 and G2 leads of the needle electrode passes through a differential amplifier and the voltage difference between them is displayed on the oscilloscope. The sound characteristics of the recorded responses are fed into an audio system. The standard needle examination includes a sampling of distal, middle, and proximal limb muscles of different root, plexus, and nerve origins, and paraspinal muscles; several muscle domains are indicated in Tables 1 to 4. When a myopathy is suspected, this approach is modified (12). The three phases of the needle examination include needle insertion, rest, and activation.

TABLE 6. *EDX abnormalities of the motor neuraxis*

1. Upper motor neuron
   Normal sensory NCS
   Decreased spatial recruitment
   Decreased temporal recruitment
2. Intraspinal canal lesion
   Normal sensory NCS
   Abnormal motor NCS—uncommon
   Fibrillation potentials
   MUAP configuration changes
   Decreased spatial recruitment
   Increased temporal recruitment
3. Postganglionic lesions
   Abnormal sensory NCS
   Abnormal motor NCS
   Fibrillation potentials
   Increased MUAP duration
   Decreased spatial recruitment
   Increased temporal recruitment
4. *Pure* motor axon lesion
   Normal sensory NCS
   Abnormal motor NCS (+/-)
   Fibrillation potentials
   Increased MUAP duration
   Decreased spatial recruitment
   Increased temporal recruitment
5. Terminal nerve branch(es)
   Disintegration of the motor unit
      Normal sensory NCS
      Abnormal motor NCS (+/-)
      Fibrillation potentials
      Decreased MUAP duration and amplitude
      Polyphasic potentials
      Increased recruitment
6. NMJ disorders
   Disintegration of the motor unit
      As listed in no. 5
      Also, abnormal RSS
7. Muscle disorders
   Disintegration of the motor unit
      As listed in no. 5

None, some, or all of the above-listed EDX abnormalities may be observed, depending on the degree of severity of the underlying disorder.

EDX, electrodiagnostic; NCS, nerve conduction studies; MUAP, motor unit action potentials; RSS, repetitive nerve stimulation studies.

Insertion Phase

This includes needle insertion below the skin with small advances in different directions. *Insertional activity* is derived from needle-induced mechanical excitation of muscle fibers that typically lasts less than a third of a second. When fat or connective tissue replaces muscle, insertional activity decreases and ultimately disappears. Increased insertional activity is said to be present when various types of electrical potentials follow the needle insertion. The latter may be normal (e.g., *snap-crackle-pop*) or abnormal, such as when brief trains of insertional positive sharp waves follow needle insertion. (13).

Rest Phase

Both normal and abnormal spontaneous activity may be observed during this period between needle advancements, when the needle is held motionless in a relaxed muscle. End-plate *noise*, a type of normal spontaneous activity, occurs when the needle electrode records activity from the nearby end-plate region, a location typically painful for the patient. It consists of two distinct types of electrical activity, miniature end-plate potentials and end-plate spikes. Miniature end-plate potentials are irregular, short duration, low amplitude, monophasic, negative waveforms that reflect the spontaneous release of quanta of acetylcholine (ACh), which have a sound reminiscent of seashell noise. End-plate spikes are irregular, longer duration, higher amplitude, biphasic waveforms with an initial negative phase and a sound likened to sputtering fat in a frying pan. During the rest phase, several types of abnormal spontaneous activity may be observed.

Fibrillation potentials are regularly firing potentials that result from spontaneous repetitive activation of muscle fibers that have lost their innervation for 3 or more weeks. Generally, they fire with metronomic regularity at 1 to 15 Hz and are the most common type of abnormal spontaneous activity encountered. They are the *sine qua non* of motor axon loss and have two presentations, either biphasic spikes or positive sharp waves. The two simply reflect the relationship between the needle electrode and the muscle fiber membrane (9) and, for that reason, are referred to by the single term fibrillation potentials. A muscle fiber unable to generate spontaneous fibrillation potentials may be abnormal enough to generate brief trains of insertional positive sharp wave activity when injured by the needle tip. Compared with end-plate spikes, the initial phases of fibrillation potentials are positive. After muscle fiber denervation, ion channel changes develop that produce 0.5- to 15-Hz autonomous muscle fiber depolarizations. Although these potentials are best characterized by their metronomic regularity, irregularity may be noted in the acute setting. The high innervation ratio of most limb muscles accounts for the extreme sensitivity of the needle examination for the detection of motor axon loss. When a *single* motor axon is disrupted, fibrillation potentials occur in all muscle fibers of that motor unit, a degree of insult not discernible by motor NCS or clinical examination. Fibrillation potentials are also commonly seen in primary muscle disorders such as polymyositis due to the separation of a portion of the muscle fiber from its end-plate because of segmental muscle necrosis. Myopathic fibrillation potentials are identical to neurogenic ones but, unlike the latter, may fire at very slow rates (14). Although fibrillation potentials themselves are nonspecific, their distribution has a strong localizing role, and their size and density yields information on disease duration and severity. For example, large amplitude potentials are observed in acute dis-

orders and in greater density with more severe disorders. They persist until reinnervation occurs or degeneration of the muscle fibers is complete (9,15).

Fasciculation potentials fire irregularly with the configuration of motor unit action potentials (MUAPs). They represent the spontaneous activation of individual or portions of motor units. They signify irritability rather than denervation. Their firing frequency varies from a few per minute to one per second. Their significance is determined by the company they keep. They are of little importance in isolation, such as in the clinical syndrome of benign fasciculation, whereas they are quite important if accompanied by fibrillation potentials and prolonged duration MUAPs, as with anterior horn cell disease. They may also be seen in chronic demyelinating processes (e.g., radiation plexopathy), and thyrotoxicosis.

Complex repetitive discharges derive from the near-synchronous firing of multiple muscle fibers, with one fiber ephaptically pacing the others. They typically have a bizarre appearance, usually continuously disrupt the baseline, and have an abrupt onset and cessation. Although the amplitude, duration, configuration, and frequency vary among different complex repetitive discharges, these aspects are essentially constant for an individual complex repetitive discharge. These nonspecific discharges, which are observed in both neuropathic and myopathic disorders, are a sign of chronicity, typically indicating the lesion is of at least 6 months duration.

Myotonic discharges are action potentials of single muscle fibers that also occur in trains. They occur as spikes or positive sharp waves. Their firing frequency and amplitude continuously change, a feature that produces a characteristic pitch variation like that of a diving airplane. These potentials most often reflect muscle membrane disorders. Their recognition has important clinical consequences because their occurrence with clinical myotonia is suggestive of either myotonic dystrophy, myotonia congenita, or paramyotonia congenita. Importantly, they are also seen without accompanying clinical myotonia as in polymyositis, acid maltase deficiency, hypothyroidism, hyperkalemic periodic paralysis, and with use of diazo-cholesterols and monocarboxylate drugs.

Grouped repetitive discharges are the repeated firing of groups of several potentials that display a simple waveform. The time period between individual potentials of the group is termed the intrapotential interval, whereas the time period separating each group is termed the interpotential interval; the latter is usually silent, unlike the case with complex repetitive discharges. They can vary in the number of potentials composing a group and their firing frequency. When two or more grouped repetitive discharges fire concurrently and asynchronously, it is termed myokymia. Facial myokymia is seen commonly with multiple sclerosis and pontine gliomas, limb myokymia with radiation-induced plexopathy and multifocal motor neuropathy, and generalized myokymia with chronic inflammatory demyelinating polyradiculoneu-ropathies (CIDP) and gold intoxication (16).

Cramp potentials, like fasciculation activity, are abnormal MUAPs. Two characteristic features of the observed MUAPs are their rapid firing rate and their synchronicity. Normally, motor unit recruitment proceeds one at a time, from the smallest to the largest. Normally, single MUAPs can only be studied while they are firing at the lower end of their normal range; further MUAP recruitment limits individual MUAP differentiation and, consequently, the ability to observe MUAPs while they are firing at the upper end of their normal range. With a cramp, MUAPs recruit synchronously and individually fire at frequencies well above 40 Hz. This accounts for the accompanying pain, a likely reflection of cramp-induced ischemia. Cramp potentials have a strong association with fasciculation activity and, like them, reflect irritability. Among patients with abundant fasciculations, cramping is a frequent complaint. Conversely, among those referred with cramps, fasciculations are frequently observed. Cramp potentials can be benign or associated with a serious disorder such as motor neuron disease.

Activation Phase

During this phase the patient voluntarily contracts the muscle under study, with the needle electrode held stationary, while the recruitment, firing pattern, and morphology of the evoked MUAPs are examined. Much has been learned over the past several decades in this area. Individual muscle fiber action potentials of a particular motor unit do not contribute equally to the observed MUAP. Whereas all of its muscle fiber action potentials contribute to the motor unit potential duration, only the muscle fiber action potentials nearest to the recording electrode significantly contribute to its amplitude and to the time that elapses between the positive trough and the negative peak of its main spike component, termed the "rise time." The study of single MUAPs requires a gentle contraction. At a basal firing rate of 5 to 10 Hz, MUAPs fire almost regularly and exhibit a stable waveform morphology. As the force of the muscle contraction progressively increases, more MUAPs appear on the oscilloscope screen signifying spatial recruitment; those previously recruited increase their firing rate, termed temporal recruitment. Together, spatial and temporal recruitment lead to smooth increments in muscle contraction force. Eventually, individual MUAPs are no longer discernible and a full interference pattern is said to be present.

Recruitment is abnormal when it is reduced or early. *Reduced recruitment* refers to decreased spatial recruitment, a reflection of motor unit dropout. The latter occurs in LMN and motor axon disorders that result in Wallerian degeneration and therefore axon-loss conduction failure and also in demyelinating conduction block lesions due to inactivation of the involved motor units. An advanced stage of MUAP dropout results in a *discrete interference pattern*. Normally, individual MUAPs cannot be discernible at the upper end of their normal firing range because as spatial recruitment increases, it becomes impossible to detect the firing characteristics of the individual MUAPs. However, with impaired spatial recruitment, MUAPs of the functioning motor units can still be detected and, for that reason, they can be distinguished while they are firing at the upper end of their firing range. Both spatial and temporal recruitment are normal in lesions that produce demyelinating conduction slowing because they do not produce motor unit dropout.

Early recruitment refers to the increase in spatial recruitment for a given degree of force. It occurs in disorders that produce disintegration of the motor unit (e.g., in lesions that affect the terminal axon branch(es), the NMJ, or the muscle fibers). Because the number of muscle fibers per activated LMN is less, the amount of force an affected motor unit is capable of generating decreases and the result is that more motor units are required to produce a given amount of contractile force. Otherwise stated, motor unit recruitment proceeds at a faster rate, and the number of motor units firing is out of proportion to the effort. The result is a full interference pattern with a submaximal effort.

Another type of abnormal recruitment is a UMN firing pattern due to disorders of the corticospinal tracts. Both spatial and temporal recruitment are decreased and, for that reason, the interference pattern is incomplete. A similar MUAP firing pattern is seen with incomplete voluntary effort. Unlike the faster firing frequency observed with reduced recruitment, the discernible MUAPs fire at their basal rate.

The morphology of the observed MUAP can be described in terms of its external and internal configuration. The *external configuration* refers to the duration and amplitude. With UMN lesions, because the disorder is proximal to the LMN, the motor unit territory and fiber density are unchanged and hence the duration and amplitude of the MUAP are unaltered. Incomplete LMN and motor axon loss disorders produce motor unit dropout and hence denervation throughout the entire motor unit. Unaffected motor units supplying a partially denervated muscle may subsequently adopt some of the denervated muscle fibers, via collateral sprouting, thereby increasing their muscle fiber territories and muscle fiber densities and hence their duration. An increase in their amplitude may also be noted, especially in the setting of static (e.g., remote poliomyelitis) or very slowly progressive (e.g., Kugelberg-Welander disease) LMN disorders because muscle fiber reinnervation is able to keep pace with muscle fiber denervation. These MUAP changes are referred to as chronic neurogenic MUAP changes. When motor unit dropout follows demyelinating conduction block, the MUAP configuration is not affected because the motor axons remain in continuity. The motor unit territory and muscle fiber density are decreased in disorders that produce disintegration of the motor unit, and therefore MUAPs with a shorter duration and lower amplitude are observed.

The *internal configuration* of an MUAP refers to its phases (i.e., area under the curve between any two baseline crossings) and its turns (i.e., directional changes not crossing the baseline). UMN lesions do not effect the muscle fiber territory or density of the motor units and hence do not lead to configurational changes in their MUAPs. LMN and motor axon loss lesions may increase the number of MUAP phases and turns by collateral sprouting. Demyelinating conduction block of motor axons leads to motor unit dropout, but the internal configurations of the remaining MUAPs are unaffected. However, when demyelinating conduction block affects individual terminal nerve branches, alterations may be observed. Disorders that produce disintegration of the motor unit tend to produce an increased number of turns and phases. Polyphasic MUAPs have more than four phases. Only when an excessive number of them are observed is it considered an abnormality because about 10% of the MUAPs of any normal muscle are polyphasic. Chronic neurogenic MUAPs are usually polyphasic.

The primary diagnostic value of polyphasic MUAPs is with disorders producing disintegration of the motor unit (e.g., myopathies). They are also useful in the identification of early proximodistal reinnervation, because initially there are less muscle fibers per regenerating motor axon, and therefore an MUAP appearance similar to that of motor unit disintegration is observed. Because the conduction rate along recently regenerated terminal axons is quite slow, the duration of the MUAP may be markedly prolonged.

Timing of the Electrodiagnostic Examination

An understanding of the temporal pathophysiologic changes that accompany various neuromuscular disorders is of importance in the proper timing of electrodiagnostic studies. At their onsets, focal axon-loss and demyelinating conduction block lesions produce motor unit dropout and, for that reason, display similar electrical features. SNAP and CMAP responses from stimulation distal to the causative lesion are always of normal amplitude, whereas those obtained with stimulation proximal to the lesion are low in amplitude or unelicitable. Needle EMG reveals a reduced recruitment pattern or an absence of voluntary MUAPs in muscles innervated by affected nerves.

From day 2 to day 10, motor and sensory amplitudes decrease. Concerning motor axons, Wallerian degeneration, when present, appears by about 3 days and reaches a nadir at about 1 week. Importantly, axon-loss lesions reduce CMAP amplitudes with stimulation above, at, or below the lesion (i.e., the response amplitudes are uniformly reduced); when substantial, the responses may be unelicitable. With demyelinating conduction block, abnormal responses are only observed with stimulation at or above the lesion; normal responses are observed with stimulation below the lesion. Hence, the electrical differentiation of these two pathophysiologic processes requires a period of at least 5 to 7 days from the onset of the clinical weakness. Similar changes are observed in sensory NCS, but with axon-loss lesions the abnormalities manifest at about day 6 and peak around day 11. During this period, the needle examination remains unchanged from its day 1 appearance.

From day 15 to day 20, *insertional positive sharp waves* begin to appear in denervated muscles just distal to the lesion site and, subsequently, throughout the entire muscle domain of the affected nerve. These potentials remain for approximately 1 week and are then replaced by fibrillation potentials. Demyelinating conduction block lesions are frequently accompanied by at least some fibrillation potentials, especially when the process is severe or acute. During this time period, the NCS are unchanged.

Muscle fibers affected by axon-loss lesions undergo reinnervation or complete degeneration. There are two mechanisms available for reinnervation. The first and fastest is collateral sprouting, in which normal unaffected motor axons branch out to adopt denervated muscle fibers. Collateral sprouting occurs best with incomplete lesions, because unaffected fibers are required for the collateral sprout. Thus, the greater the percentage of affected motor axons, the less likely are the chances that collateral sprouting will successfully take place. The second mechanism of reinnervation is by regrowth of the proximal axon stump, a process that proceeds slowly at a rate of about an inch per month. Proximal-to-distal regeneration occurs best when the distance between the site of the lesion and the denervated muscles is short. Without reinnervation, muscle fiber degeneration occurs around 20 to 24 months. Consequently, when the affected muscles are separated by more than 20 to 24 inches from the lesion site, proximal-to-distal regeneration will be relatively ineffective. For these reasons, muscle fibers affected by complete lesions can only be reinnervated through proximal-to-distal regeneration, whereas those more than 2 feet from the lesion can only be reinnervated by collateral sprouting. In conclusion, the completeness of the lesion and the distance between the lesion site and the affected muscles are important in prognostication.

Special Studies

H Responses

These responses are elicited by stimulating the tibial nerve in the popliteal fossa, with the cathode oriented proximally, while recording from the gastrocnemius-soleus complex. Low stimulus intensities activate large Ia sensory fibers because of their lower threshold compared with motor fibers. The evoked action potentials reach the S-1 segment of the spinal cord and, in turn, activate S-1 motor fibers, producing an H-wave response at the recording site. As the stimulus intensity is increased, the H-wave amplitude increases, but when the stimulus intensity exceeds the threshold for activation of the motor nerve fiber, bidirectionally propagating action potentials are generated. The distally propagated action potential results in an early motor response or M wave, whereas the proximally propagated action potential negates, through collision, some of the S-1 motor fiber potential, producing the H wave. As the stimulus intensity is increased further, the H-wave amplitude diminishes and eventually disappears. Conversely, the M-wave amplitude increases with increasing stimulus intensity and eventually becomes maximal. The H response is used in the evaluation of generalized polyneuropathies and S-1 radiculopathies. Not unexpectedly, the amplitude of the response, and not the latency, is usually the most sensitive parameter. H responses are consistently elicited from the gastrocnemius-soleus muscle complex in adults, but a drawback is the tendency of their amplitude to decrease with aging. In fact, bilaterally absent H responses are frequently encountered among normal individuals over the age of 60 years. Also, they frequently become permanently unelicitable after S-1 radiculopathies and lumbar laminectomies.

F Waves

These are elicited by the supramaximal stimulation of a motor nerve, which induces bidirectionally propagating action potentials. Those traveling distally produce the M wave, whereas those traveling proximally reach spinal cord LMNs. Depending on the state of excitation of the latter, backfiring may occur among some (about 5% to 10%) of the LMNs, thereby resulting in centrifugally propagating motor nerve fiber action potentials. These in turn are recorded distally as an F-wave response. Unlike H responses, F waves can be elicited from any motor nerve. Theoretically, these responses should be quite useful in the detection of proximal nerve lesions. However, they are insensitive to motor axon loss and, regarding demyelination, are usually only abnormal when severe demyelinating lesions, affecting all or nearly all motor axons of an individual nerve, are encountered. Consequently, they typically do not identify processes already detected during the basic electrodiagnostic study. Probably their main usefulness is with early Guillain-Barré syndrome.

Repetitive Nerve Stimulation Studies

Repetitive nerve stimulation studies (RSS) are performed in patients with suspected NMJ disorders. The safety factors for NMJ transmission are the overabundance of ACh release from axon terminals, the abundant number of postsynaptic receptors, and the breadth of the cleft separating the presynaptic and postsynaptic membranes. These features ensure muscle fiber depolarization and, consequently, the generation of a muscle fiber action potential. Disorders that lower the safety factor can be identified by RSS. RSS, when performed at low stimula-

tion rates such as 2 to 3 Hz, identify postsynaptic disorders such as acquired autoimmune myasthenia gravis (MG), whereas rates of 40 Hz or more identify presynaptic disorders, such as Lambert-Eaton myasthenic syndrome (LEMS). The stimulation and recording techniques are identical to those of individual motor NCS except that trains of motor responses are collected. In 2- to 3-Hz RSS, a baseline CMAP train is initially recorded and followed by an exercise period of 30 to 120 seconds. Subsequently, several more CMAP trains are recorded. The length of the exercise period is determined by the baseline recording. When the baseline CMAP train shows a decremental response, a 30-second exercise period is used; otherwise, an exercise period of 120 seconds is used.

ELECTRODIAGNOSTIC FEATURES OF NEUROMUSCULAR DISORDERS

Incomplete Voluntary Effort

Incomplete voluntary effort occurs principally with pain, hysteria-conversion reactions, and malingering, but because none of these produce structural damage to the central nervous system or PNS, all parts of the electrophysiologic examination are normal, including the sensory and motor NCS, the late responses, and the various phases of the needle examination. Although the activation phase of the needle examination discloses decreased MUAP recruitment, it is not abnormal because the degree of recruitment is appropriate for the degree of effort. When weak muscles yield normal CMAP amplitudes and needle EMG shows only reduced MUAP recruitment, there are two possibilities, either incomplete voluntary effort or a UMN disorder. Pain-related incomplete voluntary effort displays normal MUAP recruitment up to the point at which the patient stops muscle activation due to pain. With hysteria-conversion disorders and malingering, variations in the MUAP firing pattern can often be disclosed by an experienced examiner (17). The significance of MUAP firing pattern variation during the activation phase of the needle examination in hysteria conversion is similar to that of variable resistance during the assessment of muscle strength on clinical examination and suggests a functional process. In addition, the electrodiagnostic features of give-away weakness and alternating agonist-antagonist contraction patterns may be observed, namely the sudden disappearance of MUAP activation and poorly synchronized MUAPs firing in bursts, respectively. A functional disorder may be superimposed upon actual organic disease, in which case more extensive electrodiagnostic studies are necessary to confirm that the degree of disability far exceeds the boundaries of the actual organic process.

Upper Motor Neuron Disorders

Sensory and motor NCS, late responses, and the insertion and rest phases of the needle examination are normal in UMN disorders. However, because UMN disorders cause impaired spatial and temporal MUAP recruitment, the activation phase of the needle examination, during maximal effort, reveals a less than expected number of MUAPs firing at the lower end of their normal range or below it, depending on the threshold of the individual motor unit generating the MUAP (18). The effect of UMN lesions on the motor unit firing rate and on the contractile and myosin isoform composition properties of single muscle fibers has been reviewed elsewhere (18). Regardless of the degree of coaxing, affected patients cannot recruit more MUAPs or increase their firing rate. Because the muscle fiber densities and territories of these motor units are not affected, their MUAP configurations remain normal. Occasionally, in patients with marked UMN lesions, the amount of MUAP activity generated by a stimulus-induced involuntary response (e.g., stroking the sole while a needle electrode records from the tibialis anterior muscle) far exceeds that observed with voluntary activation. Unfortunately, when the underlying central process also produces tremor, the ability to evaluate the rest and activation phases of the needle examination may be severely hampered, rendering the electrodiagnostic study inconclusive. The electrical features of incomplete voluntary effort and UMN disorders are very similar. A possible hint to a UMN disorder is a continuous tremulous MUAP firing pattern that fires in poorly synchronized bursts (19). With hysteria conversion and malingering it notoriously tends to appear intermittently.

Spinal Canal and Spinal Cord Disorders

The intraspinal canal houses the spinal cord (including the anterior horn cells and their exiting motor axons), the primary ventral rootlets and the centrally directed preganglionic sensory axons.

Intrinsic spinal cord disorders may affect motor element(s), such as the corticospinal tract, anterior horn cells, the intraparenchymal component of the peripherally directed motor axons, or some combination of motor and sensory elements (i.e., preganglionic sensory axons). Because preganglionic sensory axon involvement does not affect either the dorsal root ganglia or the postganglionic sensory axons, their involvement is not recognized by sensory NCS (i.e., the sensory NCS are normal). Because the H response assesses the S-1 preganglionic sensory fibers, it may be abnormal. Anterior horn cell injury results in Wallerian degeneration of the affected motor axons, thereby causing muscle fiber denervation throughout the territories of the affected motor units. The affected motor units do not produce MUAPs and hence are unable to contribute to the generation of muscle contraction force. The expected electrical findings are normal SNAPs, normal, low amplitude, or unelicitable CMAPs, and an abnormal needle examination; motor

latencies and CVs generally remain normal until very severe axon loss has occurred. On needle examination, the insertion phase shows positive sharp waves, usually from day 15 to day 20 after muscle fiber denervation; these are replaced by fibrillation potentials, usually between day 21 and day 35. Fasciculation potentials are a common finding in anterior horn cell disorders, particularly amyotrophic lateral sclerosis (ALS). Spatial recruitment is impaired due to a dropout of whole motor units that leads to reduced MUAPs firing at the upper end of the normal range. Later, collateral sprouting from unaffected motor axons increases the muscle fiber territory and density of these motor units, and consequently their MUAPs become increased in duration and possibly amplitude. During the activation phase, cramp potentials may be induced. At rapid rates of progressive injury, reinnervation fails to keep pace with denervation, and insertional positive waves and fibrillation potentials are continually noted. Depending on the severity of anterior horn cell loss along the S-1 spinal segment, the H- and M-wave responses may be reduced in amplitude. F waves are generally not affected by axon loss lesions; however, the number recorded may be decreased, termed F-wave impersistence.

Poliomyelitis

Acute poliomyelitis is now infrequent in developed countries, due to widespread vaccination beginning around the middle of the twentieth century. Two features are specific to acute poliomyelitis: asymmetric distribution and the absence of chronic MUAP changes. Fasciculation and cramp potentials may or may not be present. In *remote* poliomyelitis, muscle fiber reinnervation is already present. Therefore, CMAPs sometimes have a normal amplitude and needle examination shows alterations in MUAP firing rate and configuration more so than the extent of spontaneous activity. When abnormal needle examination features are observed in muscles with reportedly near-normal strength clinically and near-normal CMAP amplitudes, it indicates that the muscle was previously affected, that reinnervation was nearly complete, and that the muscle fiber territories and densities of the surviving motor units are significantly increased (because the CMAP amplitude normalized).

Amyotrophic Lateral Sclerosis

There are five distinguishing electrophysiologic features of ALS. First, the distribution of abnormalities is asymmetric. Second, routine motor NCS are frequently abnormal, a reflection of distal muscle wasting. Third, fasciculation activity is usually widespread. Less-affected muscles tend to disclose more fasciculation potentials, whereas more affected musculature reveals a greater extent of fibrillation potentials and MUAP loss. Fourth, in contrast to poliomyelitis, the rate of denervation with ALS far exceeds the capacity for reinnervation; in other words, it is rapidly progressive. For that reason, the duration and amplitude of the MUAPs do not have the opportunity to increase to the magnitude that they do in poliomyelitis. Hence, the extent of insertional positive waves and fibrillation potentials is much more pronounced than are the changes in MUAP configuration. Fifth, a UMN firing pattern is usually encountered along with a LMN one. The presence of a UMN firing pattern is inconsistent with a pure LMN lesion. Like other diffuse motor neuron disorders, needle examination abnormalities are sought in muscles of three limbs with differing nerve and root innervations, and in bulbar and thoracic paraspinal muscles.

Spinal Muscular Atrophy

Of the several disorders in this category, only Werdnig-Hoffman disease [spinal muscular atrophy (SMA) type 1 (SMA-1)] and Wohlfart-Kugelberg-Welander disease (SMA-3) are mentioned here. In both, the distribution of electrical abnormalities is symmetric, proximally predominant, and fasciculation potentials may or may not be observed. The degree of chronic neurogenic MUAP changes differs between the two disorders. SMA-1 is widespread (i.e., involves the brainstem LMNs, in addition to the somatic LMNs) and rapidly progressive. Consequently, reinnervation is outpaced by denervation. For that reason, the CMAP amplitudes are reduced or unelicitable and the spectrum of needle examination abnormalities is similar to that encountered in patients with rapidly evolving ALS. Conversely, the slower progression of SMA-3 permits reinnervation to keep pace with denervation and hence produces a spectrum of needle examination abnormalities similar to remote poliomyelitis. The brainstem LMNs are involved in only about one-third of these patients.

Kennedy Disease

Also known as bulbospinal neuronopathy, this is an X-linked recessive disorder involving both sensory and motor neurons (20,21). A recent report described the electrical findings in 19 patients with this disease (22). Low amplitude of unelicitable SNAPs are usually observed. Interestingly, the lack of uniformity among the SNAP abnormalities suggests an *acquired*, rather than a hereditary, process. Low amplitude CMAPs are less frequently observed. These NCS findings suggest an acquired "pure" sensory neuropathy. However, the needle examination reveals sparse fibrillation potentials and pronounced chronic neurogenic MUAP changes, features consistent with the very slowly progressive nature of this disorder. Although the distribution of these electrical abnormalities is often generalized, they may be more pro-

nounced at, or even restricted to, the onset segment. In our experience, this particular pattern of electrical abnormalities is essentially unique to Kennedy disease.

Primary Root Disorders

A root disorder, or *radiculopathy,* is one of the most common referral diagnoses to EMG laboratories. The dorsal and ventral roots consist of sensory and motor axons, respectively. With the exception of the S-1 preganglionic sensory fibers, which are assessed by the H-response test, the sensory axons of most roots are unavailable for study with conventional NCS and EMG; consequently, sensory NCS are normal. This is unfortunate because isolated sensory root involvement is the most frequent clinical type of radiculopathy (23). The results of motor NCS are variable, depending on the particular root(s) affected, the underlying pathophysiology, the severity of the lesion, and the timing of the study. Significant CMAP amplitude reduction is infrequent, even in muscles of the affected myotome. Two reasons account for this. First, most lesions affect a minority of motor axons in a root, a feature that facilitates collateral sprouting; and second, most muscles are innervated by more than one spinal segment.

The basic motor NCS can be used to study the C-8, T-1, L-5, and S-1 roots, whereas nonroutine motor NCS are required to assess disorders affecting other roots, for example, the phrenic CMAP for the third to fifth cervical roots. Hence, the distribution of the radicular disease influences the likelihood of identifying motor NCS abnormalities. When the cause is demyelinating conduction block, it may go unnoticed because the needle examination is less sensitive to this pathophysiology. Axon loss is a more common associated finding in radiculopathy and is more easily discernible on needle examination. The latter is likely to be abnormal in the acute phase, from 3 weeks to 3 months after the lesion and before collateral sprouting, when hundreds of muscle fibers for each involved motor axon are denervated. The insertion and rest phases of the needle examination reveals insertional positive sharp waves and fibrillation potentials. It is uncommon for a muscle to be so severely denervated that an abnormal MUAP firing pattern is detected. Once collateral sprouting occurs, chronic neurogenic MUAP changes become apparent.

Acute radiculopathy is classically diagnosed by the finding of fibrillation potentials in myotomal limb and adjacent paraspinal muscles patterns. Reinnervation proceeds in a proximal-to-distal direction; accordingly, the needle abnormalities can be limited to the most distally located muscles of an involved root. As reinnervation proceeds, fibrillation activity becomes more sparse, making it more difficult to recognize this process. The H-response amplitude, more than the latency, is a sensitive marker of S-1 radiculopathy, whereas F-wave responses are usually normal. With affliction of multiple contiguous roots (e.g., cauda equina syndrome), the sensitivity of the electrical study markedly increases due to substantive muscle denervation. This produces low amplitude or unelicitable CMAPs and abundant fibrillation activity.

Electrodiagnostic studies in well-defined root lesions can show false-negative findings due to involvement of sensory fibers alone or roots that cannot be adequately assessed, such as the L-2 root. Often, the study is performed before fibrillation potentials have had time to develop or after they have disappeared because the muscle fibers generating them may be reinnervated. There are four reasons to pursue electrical studies in the diagnosis of radiculopathy. First, the EMG can often localize the process and correctly identify the predominant pathophysiology. Second, unlike neuroimaging studies that can often yield false-positive information, electrical testing rarely provides false-positive results in the hands of experienced electromyographers. Third, serial electrical assessment can be used to follow the course of the neurologic disorder. Fourth, when the clinical diagnosis is in error, the electrodiagnostic study may redirect the evaluation. For example, when an ALS patient presents with a foot drop and weakness in an L-5 distribution, suggesting an L-5 radiculopathy, the extreme sensitivity of the needle examination in detecting motor axon loss and fasciculation potentials results in the easy recognition of needle examination abnormalities outside of the L-5 myotome, thereby identifying a more generalized intraspinal canal process such as ALS.

Plexus Disorders

Together, the NCS and needle examination are helpful in the electrodiagnosis of plexopathies. They show motor abnormalities similar to axon-loss radiculopathies of the same magnitude, including fibrillation potentials in mild lesions and decreased CMAP amplitudes and MUAP loss with more severe lesions. The difference in plexopathies is the involvement of sensory NCS, as manifested by SNAP amplitude reduction out of proportion to the degree of axon loss. Another distinctive finding of a plexopathy is the lack of fibrillation activity in paraspinal muscles, although this is also frequently observed with radiculopathies. The cervical plexus is made up of the C-1 through C-4 APR, lies in the lateral neck, and except for its phrenic nerve derivative, is the most difficult of the plexuses to assess in the EMG laboratory. The phrenic nerve represents an exception because phrenic nerve conduction (i.e., phrenic CMAP) and needle examination of the diaphragm can be performed and may be of assistance in identifying the nature and site of respiratory insufficiency (24).

The brachial plexus extends from the lower cervical vertebrae to the axilla. Because the neck and shoulder are highly mobile, the brachial plexus is quite vulnerable to traumatic injury. It is for this reason that the brachial plexus is the most frequently injured of the plexuses (25). Anatomically, the brachial plexus is composed of five APR, three trunks, six divisions, three cords, and several named nerves. The C-5 through T-1 APR combine to form the three trunks of the brachial plexus in the following manner: the C-5 and C-6 roots combine to form the upper trunk, C-8 and T-1 join to form the lower trunk, and C-7 continues as the middle trunk. Each trunk in turn divides into anterior and posterior divisions, the latter of which combine to form the posterior cord, whereas the anterior divisions of the upper and middle trunk form the lateral cord and the anterior division of the lower trunk continues as the medial cord. Five named nerves of the brachial plexus enter the arm (e.g., median, ulnar, radial, musculocutaneous, and axillary). The suprascapular, dorsal scapular, and long thoracic nerves exit more proximally. The divisions of the brachial plexus are situated behind the clavicle. This permits its disorders to be grouped as *supra*clavicular and *infra*clavicular, a system that has both diagnostic and prognostic utility. For example, disorders affecting the supraclavicular portion are often due to severe traction and carry a poor prognosis (25), whereas infraclavicular lesions, which are also most often traumatic in nature, are more frequently associated with a better outcome. As would be expected from its anatomic organization, supraclavicular element lesions are easily confused with radiculopathies, whereas infraclavicular element lesions are frequently mistaken for single or multiple mononeuropathies.

Because most brachial plexus lesions cause some degree of axon-loss–induced conduction failure and because the SNAP and the muscle domains of each brachial plexus element are known, the investigation of axon-loss brachial plexopathy is usually straightforward, as shown in Tables 3 to 5. Disorders that produce demyelinating conduction block along plexus fibers distal to the midtrunk level can be identified by comparing the CMAP amplitudes after proximal and distal stimulation. A clue to the presence of proximal demyelinating conduction block is the relative preservation of CMAP amplitudes despite a significant reduction in MUAP recruitment. Because the basic electrodiagnostic study does not assess all brachial plexus elements, additional NCS and needle examinations of additional muscles, as well as contralateral comparison studies, are usually required, the precise studies being determined by the referral diagnosis and the electrodiagnostic findings noted as the study unfolds (Table 5). Of note is that the median SNAPs cannot be used for comparison in the presence of CTS involving either side if the latter has caused decreased median SNAP amplitudes. As expected, the late responses generally are not helpful with these disorders. Certain patterns of abnormality indicate not only the localization of the underlying disorder but also its likely etiology (e.g., true neurogenic thoracic outlet syndrome, postmedian sternotomy, and radiation-induced plexopathies) (26,27).

Lumbar and sacral plexopathies are encountered much less frequently than brachial plexopathies because their location makes them less vulnerable to trauma. Also, the limited number of sensory and motor NCS available for assessment makes them more difficult to identify. Femoral motor NCS assess many of the L-2– to L-4–derived motor axons that traverse the lumbar plexus. However, without a reliable corresponding sensory NCS, their postganglionic localization cannot be confirmed. Fibrillation potentials in femoral- and obturator-innervated muscles, but not among lumbar paraspinal muscles, justifies the tentative diagnosis of a lumbar plexopathy. Needle examination differentiates lumbar plexopathies from peripheral nerve lesions. For example, in the setting of a lumbar plexus lesion involving the L-3 and L-4 motor axons, a clinically suspected femoral mononeuropathy can be excluded when needle abnormalities are noted also in obturator-innervated muscles. Theoretically, sacral plexopathy should be readily diagnosed, at least those causing moderate or severe axon loss, because reliable sensory NCS exist to assess L-5 and S-1 sensory fibers. Unfortunately, sacral plexopathy occurs most often among the elderly, in whom the SNAPs of the lower extremities are often absent bilaterally. Unilateral abnormalities, however, are always indicative of a postganglionic lesion, regardless of age. Another problem with the diagnosis of sacral plexopathy is the tendency for bilateral occurrence. In these situations, side-to-side SNAP amplitude comparisons are of limited value. Routine motor NCS assess the L-5 to S-2 nerve fibers. Unfortunately, because of the sensory and motor axon overlap between the sciatic nerve and the sacral plexus, it is frequently impossible to differentiate these two entities. Their NCS findings are virtually identical. Needle examination abnormalities in the glutei and tensor fascia lata muscles helps localize the lesion to the sacral plexus. Although abnormalities in paraspinal muscles indicate a problem at the spinal root level, their absence does not exclude a root-level lesion. H-response abnormalities occur in radicular, plexus, and sciatic nerve lesions when the S-1 sensory or motor fibers are affected and, consequently, cannot be used to discriminate between these two entities.

Peripheral Nerve Disorders

PNS disease processes can be grouped as focal (i.e., mononeuropathies), multifocal (i.e., multiple mononeuropathies), or generalized (i.e., polyneuropathies). Pathologically, these disorders may be due to demyelination, axon loss, or both. Therefore, electrodiagnostic assessment may reveal evidence of demyelinating conduction slowing, demyelinating conduction block, axon-loss–induced conduction failure, or some combination of these. Neuropathies produce quite variable electrical findings, depending on their rapidity of onset, underlying pathophysiology, distribution, severity, and duration (e.g., acute or chronic) and the particular fiber types (e.g., sensory, motor) affected. By identifying the pathophysiology and severity of an underlying mononeuropathy, the electrodiagnostic study can offer prognostic information, guide subsequent management (e.g., surgical exploration versus watchful waiting), and, through serial examinations, follow the status of reinnervation.

Focal mononeuropathies can develop abruptly or gradually. Regarding demyelination, in general, abruptly developing disorders are associated with demyelinating conduction block, whereas those developing more gradually are associated with demyelinating conduction slowing. Axon-loss–induced conduction failure is associated with both abruptly and gradually developing disorders. Thus, the underlying pathophysiology of slowly progressive focal PNS lesions (e.g., entrapment and compression neuropathies) usually is demyelinating conduction slowing (e.g., CTS, some ulnar neuropathies about the elbow) or axon-loss–induced conduction failure (e.g., neoplasm-induced neuropathies). Both types of pathophysiology are seen with some slow-onset mononeuropathies, the exact blend reflecting the severity and rate of progression of the lesion, and the temporal relationship between symptom onset and the electrodiagnostic study.

With sudden onset focal lesions, the underlying pathophysiology generally is either demyelinating conduction block, axon-loss–induced conduction failure, or both. Examples include common peroneal neuropathies at the fibular head, most radial neuropathies at the spiral groove, and some ulnar neuropathies at the elbow. Noteworthy is that of these, the first two characteristically present with weakness (i.e., foot drop and wrist drop, respectively), so the underlying pathology must be preventing impulses from reaching the muscle fibers; therefore, it must be causing either demyelinating conduction block or axon-loss–induced conduction failure and not demyelinating conduction slowing. Demyelinating processes due to abrupt trauma typically resolve over a 6- to 8-week period. As a result, electrodiagnostic studies performed more than 8 weeks postinjury typically disclose only axon loss, even if some demyelinating conduction block (i.e., clinical neurapraxia) was present earlier. An important exception to this statement is tourniquet paralysis, which may show prolonged conduction block lasting up to 10 months. Also, demyelinating conduction block lesions continue to accrue when the precipitating practice persists, such as elbow leaning (ulnar neuropathies at the elbow) and leg crossing (common peroneal lesions at the fibular head). In contrast to the short-lived focal demyelinating lesions resulting from acute trauma, demyelinating conduction blocks along axons can persist indefinitely with certain nontraumatic conditions such as radiation-induced brachial plexopathy and multifocal motor neuropathy.

The amount of clinical weakness that accompanies both demyelinating conduction block and axon-loss–induced conduction failure can be approximated by comparing the distal CMAP amplitude recorded from the affected muscle with the response recorded from the contralateral normal side and with the ipsilateral proximally generated response. The difference between the distal CMAP amplitudes in the two limbs reflects the amount of axon loss, whereas the difference between the proximal and distal CMAP amplitudes in the involved limb indicates the amount of demyelinating conduction block. In this regard, it is possible to estimate the percentage of fibers affected by demyelinating conduction block and, consequently, the amount of early recovery. The pathologies and pathophysiologies of the most frequently encountered mononeuropathies are provided in Table 7.

Acquired polyneuropathies are generally due to either demyelination or axonal loss, whereas many, but not all, genetic neuropathies are demyelinating. Two exceptions are Charcot-Marie-Tooth neuropathy type II and porphyria, which are hereditary disorders producing axon loss. Most toxic and metabolic disorders are also caused by axon loss. Chronic sensorimotor axon-loss polyneuropathy has a typical electrical and temporal progression, which generally parallels the clinical course. The pathologic process starts distally with a stocking distribution and evolves to a stocking-glove pattern. In its mildest form, initial findings are seen distally in intrinsic foot muscles on needle examination in the form of fibrillation potentials. Sensory and mixed NCS, including the sural, superficial peroneal, and plantar nerves and the H responses, are more sensitive to axon loss than the motor NCS and are affected next. When needle examination abnormalities appear in the foreleg, the H response and lower extremity SNAP amplitudes will already have begun to diminish, even

before upper extremity sensory responses are affected. Next, denervation of intrinsic foot muscles produces markedly diminished motor NCS responses and MUAP dropout on needle examination. When H responses and lower extremity SNAP responses are unelicitable, SNAP amplitudes in the upper extremity begin to decrease. In addition, intrinsic hand muscles show features of axon loss on needle examination and, still later, diminished motor NCS responses appear. In the course of an axon-loss polyneuropathy, distal changes remain more pronounced than proximal ones. When the CMAP amplitudes are very low, the motor conduction velocities may be modestly reduced due to loss of the fastest conducting fibers.

With hereditary demyelinating polyneuropathies (e.g., Charcot-Marie-Tooth type I), the most prominent NCS parameter abnormality is conduction slowing. Thus, prolonged peak (SNAP) and onset (CMAP) latencies and decreased CVs are observed. In general, the sensory NCS are more affected than the motor NCS. Usually, the lower extremity SNAPs are unelicitable and the upper extremity SNAPs reveal decreased amplitude and increased duration, in addition to prolonged peak latencies. Because of the hereditary nature of the pathologic insult, the involved nerves are uniformly affected, and consequently, the degree of conduction slowing is quite uniform. This uniformity of involvement tends to preserve the synchrony of impulse conduction along individual nerve fibers. Hence, the morphology of the recorded motor waveforms, including their amplitudes, is less distorted over distance than those seen in acquired demyelinating polyneuropathies. Although some dispersion of responses typically occurs, it is generally distal. A mild amount of fibrillation activity is present in the distal leg muscles, along with prominent chronic neurogenic MUAP changes.

TABLE 7. *Characteristic pathologies and pathophysiologies of various mononeuropathies*

Disorder	Pathology/pathophysiology
Long thoracic neuropathy	Axon loss/ALICF
Suprascapular neuropathy	Axon loss/ALICF
Axillary neuropathy	Axon loss/ALICF
Radial neuropathy—spiral groove	Axon loss and demyelination/ALICF and DCB
Posterior interosseous neuropathy	Axon loss/ALICF
Ulnar neuropathy	
Across the elbow	Axon loss and demyelination/ALICF, DCB, DCS
At the wrist	Axon loss (demyelination)/ALICF (DCB)
Anterior interosseous neuropathy	Axon loss/ALICF
Carpal tunnel syndrome	Demyelination/DCS[a]
Femoral neuropathy	Axon loss (demyelination)/ALICF (DCB)
Sciatic neuropathy	Axon loss/ALICF
Peroneal neuropathy—fibular head	Axon loss and demyelination/ALICF and DCB
Tarsal tunnel syndrome	Axon loss (demyelination)/ALICF (DCS)

The pathologies and pathophysiologies shown in parentheses occur less frequently.
[a]Axon loss and ALICF appear later in the course of carpal tunnel syndrome.
ALICF, axon-loss–induced conduction failure; DCB, demyelinating conduction block; DCS, demyelinating conduction slowing.

Acquired demyelinating polyneuropathy (i.e., polyradiculoneuropathy) shows various combinations of low amplitude or unelicitable CMAPs and SNAPs, prolongation of latencies, decreased CVs, and prolonged durations. If slowing is present but not uniform along the individual nerve fibers, the reduced synchrony results in an increase in the negative phase duration and a reduction in the CMAP amplitude. One of the principal features identifying the process as acquired is the variability among the different studied nerve segments. Moreover, because these disorders, particularly those of rapid onset, also tend to produce some axon loss, fibrillation potentials may also be observed. There may be rapid or gradual clinical onset. In Guillain-Barré syndrome, demyelinating conduction block is the major pathophysiologic process, although some axon loss is typically seen. The proximal, middle, or distal segments of the peripheral nerves may be disproportionately affected. With midsegment lesions, conduction block can sometimes be demonstrated on motor NCS. Conduction blocks that are situated distal to the supraclavicular stimulation site can be detected on motor NCS, whereas those in the lower extremity must be located distal to the popliteal fossa to be detectable. Whenever MUAPs firing in decreased numbers at faster than their basal firing rate are seen during the activation phase of the needle examination in a muscle from which a normal motor NCS response amplitude was previously obtained, a proximally situated block is likely. With significant demyelinating conduction blocks distal to the wrist and ankle, both the proximal and distal CMAPs are low in amplitude, a pattern suggestive of axon-loss–induced conduction failure. Unfortunately, this pattern of uniformly decreased CMAP amplitudes may yield an erroneous impression of early axon loss when a distal demyelinating block is not considered. The SNAP amplitudes may be decreased but often not to the extent of the CMAPs; F waves and H responses may also show abnormalities. When terminal nerve branches are affected by demyelinating conduction block, only a fraction of the muscle fibers belong to the affected motor unit dropout, leading to disintegration of the motor unit. This produces early recruitment with an apparent *myopathic* appearance, that is, short duration, low amplitude, and perhaps polyphasic MUAPs.

In CIDP, low amplitude or unelicitable SNAPs and CMAPs, prominent sensory and motor nerve slowing, and prolonged latencies are observed and, much less often, demyelinating conduction blocks. In CIDP, the SNAP abnormalities and the degree of demyelinating conduction slowing tend to be more pronounced compared with Guillain-Barré syndrome, whereas the extent of fibrillation potentials is less pronounced. Some patients show no abnormalities on needle examination, despite an extensive evaluation. The electrical features of CIDP may be similar to a hereditary demyelinating process. Low amplitude or unelicitable sensory NCS responses in the upper extremities, with normal lower extremity responses, is virtually never encountered in hereditary demyelinating neuropathies. *Mixed* polyneuropathies show features of both axon loss and demyelination. Diabetic polyneuropathy is often placed in this category. It is mainly an axon-loss process but is often accompanied by mild motor slowing, although not in the definite demyelinating range. It is the most commonly encountered polyneuropathy in the United States and other developed countries; CTS and ulnar neuropathies about the elbow are frequently superimposed (28).

Polyneuropathies variably involve sensory, motor, and autonomic axons; however, some affect only one type of fiber. The most common is a *pure* sensory polyneuropathy, a term that includes sensory neuronopathies because the exact site of the lesion cannot often be determined electrically. These disorders can also be divided into acquired and hereditary forms. The electrical abnormalities noted in the hereditary forms are usually most pronounced in the lower extremities and uniform among the affected axons, whereas those associated with the acquired forms may not show a lower extremity predominance and often are nonuniform in nature. An exception is the sensory neuronopathy observed with Kennedy disease that has an acquired appearance. Again, the H responses are very sensitive, diagnostically, to the presence of a demyelinating polyneuropathy because they are usually unelicitable.

Neuromuscular Junction Disorders

These can be divided into presynaptic and postsynaptic types, classic examples of which are LEMS and MG, respectively. MG is an autoimmune disorder that results in postsynaptic ACh receptor destruction and postsynaptic membrane reduction and synaptic cleft widening. Each of these three changes lowers the safety factor of NMJ transmission and either produces or predisposes to NMJ transmission failure. Weakness, when present, typically has a proximal predominance. Consequently, a thorough assessment of the proximal muscles with slow RSS and needle examination is needed because these muscles are more likely to show abnormalities. In some patients, symptoms are restricted to the ocular and bulbar muscles. Because the clinical hallmark of the weakness associated with MG is fatigability, sustained effort and exercise are used to enhance the electrical abnormalities. Sensory NCS are unaffected in MG. Because single motor nerve stimulation does not induce fatigue, the motor NCS and late responses are usually normal. Needle examination is normal as well, unless moment-to-moment amplitude variation of single firing MUAPs is specifically sought during the activation phase of the needle examination or unless the disorder has advanced enough to cause disintegration of the motor unit, in which case *myopathic*-appearing MUAPs are observed. Moreover, even when moment-to-moment amplitude variation is noted during the needle examination, it is not specific for MG. For that reason, further studies are required. The major procedure used is 2- to 3-Hz RSS. At this rate, repetitive stimulation decreases the size of the immediately releasable ACh pool, thereby reducing the number of ACh-containing vesicles released with each subsequent stimulus. In normal individuals, the safety factor ensures a maximum CMAP response to each motor nerve stimulation, and therefore the train of evoked CMAPs is uniform in appearance. With MG, when 2- to 3-Hz RSS is applied and the ACh pool is reduced, progressively greater numbers of NMJ transmission failures occur among the synapses within the motor units of the stimulated motor nerve. Thus, fewer and fewer muscle fibers are activated, and for that reason progressively smaller MUAPs are generated; this in turn produces progressively smaller CMAPs—the decremental response of MG. This physiologic explanation also accounts for the needle observations mentioned above. Because the subset of failing NMJs varies each time a given motor unit is activated, the individual muscle fiber action potentials that contribute to the MUAP must also vary. Myopathic-appearing MUAPs reflect less than complete activation of all muscle fibers composing the motor unit. Sustained effort or exercise enhances the degree of CMAP decrement by facilitating ACh utilization, so explaining the rationale for combining exercise with RSS. Because exercise further worsens the already reduced safety factor, it further worsens the degree of CMAP decrement. Consequently, it may bring out a decremental CMAP response when the baseline CMAP train is normal.

With unsuspected mild generalized MG, the electrodiagnostic examination may appear normal. Moreover, when the basic NCS are normal, the needle examination in patients with MG may suggest a nonnecrotizing myopathic process. Consequently, whenever the latter is considered, it is important to perform slow RSS to exclude the possibility of MG. These studies are performed at two or more sites, especially proximal ones (e.g., spinal accessory nerve, recording upper trapezius; facial nerve, recording various facial muscles; peroneal nerve, recording tibialis anterior). RSS may be flawed by artifacts such as electrode movement. Cold temperature may normalize NMJ transmission and the abnormal decremental response induced by slow RSS. When slow RSS is normal and MG is still the most likely diagnosis, single fiber EMG should be performed because of its higher yield.

LEMS is an autoimmune disorder in which antibodies bind to calcium channels of the presynaptic membrane, thereby producing a decrease in the number of active zone particles and presynaptic membrane disorganization. An increase in intracellular calcium concentration at the nerve terminal increases the number of ACh-containing vesicles released with depolarization. Consequently, the result of active zone particle destruction is that less ACh is released with nerve fiber depolarization. This decrease is substan-

tial and severely lessens the number of muscle fiber action potentials generated by nerve fiber activation. Because NMJ disorders have no effect on the sensory NCS, the latter are normal. However, the motor NCS are nearly always abnormal. Unlike with MG, the routine CMAPs usually are very low in amplitude, often less than 10% of their expected value. The needle examination reveals moment-to-moment amplitude variation and MUAPs with a *myopathic* appearance. Because slow RSS further decreases the amount of ACh released with repetitive stimulation, CMAP decrement occurs. However, when the initial CMAP is extremely small, this decremental pattern may not be discernible. By increasing the intracellular calcium concentration of the nerve branch terminal, fast RSS at 40 to 50 Hz significantly increases the amount of ACh released. For that reason, with fast RSS an increase in CMAP size occurs, the so-called incremental response. Often, the amplitude increases severalfold in magnitude compared with baseline. Fast RSS is painful, and the same outcome can be generated by exercise. For that reason, most electromyographers do not perform fast RSS as a screening test for a presynaptic disorder. Instead, when low CMAP amplitudes are noted during the routine motor NCS, the studied muscle is exercised for 10 seconds and a single motor stimulation is repeated, the so-called Lambert-Eaton test. If this causes an increment in CMAP amplitude of 100% or more, fast RSS can be performed to confirm the presynaptic disorder. Some patients are so weak that they are unable to perform the requested 10 seconds of exercise. In these instances fast RSS is mandatory. No differences are noted in the electrical features of LEMS secondary to cancer versus those due to primary immunologic disorders.

Myopathic Disorders

Myopathy refers to a heterogeneous group of muscle disorders. The heterogeneity of electrical manifestations of myopathies reflects the differences in underlying physiology, pathology, stage of the disease, and the effect of treatment. NCS are generally normal in myopathy, although the CMAP amplitudes may be significantly reduced when the recorded muscles are severely affected. All myopathic features sought during the needle examination of a patient with myopathy are nonspecific and can be seen with both terminal peripheral nerve and NMJ disorders. Nonetheless, when these nonspecific features are present in certain patterns and combinations, the likelihood of a myopathy increases. Several modifications of the electrodiagnostic study are required whenever a myopathy is suspected. Given that a generalized process is suspected, an upper and a lower extremity should be assessed, including at least one sensory and one motor NCS per studied limb. This would typically include the peroneal and median motor NCS and sural and median sensory NCS. Because myopathic processes

Motor Disorders,
edited by David S. Younger.
Lippincott Williams & Wilkins, Philadelphia © 1999.

CHAPTER 3

Electrophysiology of the Motor Unit

Stefano Simonetti, Mile Nikolic, and Christian Krarup

The motor unit is the smallest functional unit of skeletal muscle, and its electrophysiologic characteristics are central in the diagnosis of neuromuscular disorders associated with partial denervation and myopathy. Since the introduction of electromyography (EMG), it has been apparent that the interpretation of the electrical activity of muscle is influenced by both technical and biologic factors and that the variability of the individual muscle requires quantitation for proper evaluation. With the introduction of computer technology, this quantitative evaluation has become less time consuming; however, the methods themselves influence the results of the interpretation.

In this chapter we review aspects of the different methods used to record the motor unit action potential (MUAP) and discuss the parameters for the interpretation of the EMG and the principal pathophysiologic alterations.

DEFINITION AND CLASSIFICATION OF THE MOTOR UNIT

The concept of the motor unit was developed by Liddell and Sherrington (1) and Sherrington (2) over 70 years ago; it is defined as the motoneuron, its axon, and the muscle fibers that it innervates. The basic organization of motor units is similar in most mammals (3). Multilead electrode studies reveal that the territory of the motor unit is usually circular or elliptical, with a diameter, for example, in the brachial biceps muscle of 15 mm with space for 15 to 30 motor units (4,5). In animals, glycogen-depletion experiments have shown that the relative territory of the motor unit varies considerably (6,7) from 8% to 76% of the whole cross-section of the muscle

with large areas in the soleus (41% to 76%) and smaller ones in anterior tibial muscle (8% to 22%) (8). The muscle fibers of one motor unit are intermingled with fibers of others; rarely, two to four muscle fibers from the same motor unit are adjacent to one another (6,9,10). The likelihood in human muscle that a fiber is placed within 300 μm from another fiber of the same motor unit is about 50% (11). With single-fiber recording, about 1.5 fibers belong to the same motor unit (12), indicating that the pickup area comprises about six motor units. There is a larger concentration of fibers at the center of the motor unit than at its periphery (5,7).

Muscle fibers have different physiologic, biochemical, and mechanical properties, and the motor unit composition, size, and number vary greatly in individual muscles (13–17). This is of particular importance because involvement of motor units in a given disease may be determined by their properties. The recruitment of motor units during the development of force is nonrandom; with weak efforts it is possible to examine the characteristics of individual units.

Classification of Motor Units

All muscle fibers in the same motor unit are of a similar histochemical type (7). Different criteria have been used to classify motor units (17–21). Three groups of motor units emerge when physiologic, mechanical, biochemical, and histochemical criteria are used (22,23) (Table 1), although in fact they probably fall into a continuum (17). In experimental animals, fast-twitch motor unit fibers are characteristically larger, the twitch tension is increased, the twitch:tetanus ratio is higher, the conduction velocity along the motor axon is faster, and the motoneuron diameter is larger; however, the input resistance of the motoneuron is lower.

The number of muscle fibers in each motor unit or the innervation ratio, defined as the number of muscle fibers innervated by a single a-motor neuron, varies in individual

S. Simonetti: Division of Neurology, E.O. Ospedali Galliera, 16128 Genova, Italy.

M. Nikolic: Faculty of Medicine, University of Copenhagen and Department of Clinical Neurophysiology, Rigshospitalet, 2100 Copenhagen, Denmark.

C. Krarup: Faculty of Medicine, University of Copenhagen and University Hospital, Rigshospitalet, Copenhagen, Denmark.

TABLE 1. *Classification of motor units*

Motor unit type	Muscle fiber type		
	Mitochondrial enzyme	ATPase activity (pH 9.4)	Physiologic classification + oxidative metabolism
Slow fatigue resistant	Type C (high mitochondrial staining)	Type 1 muscle fibers (low activity)	Slow oxidative
Fast fatigue resistant	Type B (intermediate mitochondrial staining)	Type 2a muscle fibers (high activity)	Fast-twitch oxidative glycolytic
Fast fatiguing	Type A (low mitochondrial staining)	Type 2b muscle fibers (high activity)	Fast-fatigued glycolytic

muscles from 5 to 20 fibers in extraocular eye muscles (24,25) to more than 2,000 in large extremity muscles (gastrocnemius) (26). The innervation ratio is the main determinant in the force each motor unit can produce (27); the force per unit area in most studies is similar among different fiber types (28,29). The innervation area is subject to influence by both biologic factors and pathologic lesions; increasing age is associated with a reduction in motor neuron number and an increase in the innervation ratio due to collateral sprouting (30–35). The innervation ratio is subject to change in pathologic processes that cause Wallerian, axonal, or neuronal degeneration. Collateral sprouting in these conditions has a marked influence on the physiologic parameters of the motor unit and is of major importance as a compensatory mechanism to delay or reduce the degree of weakness (36–40).

Gradation of Force

Muscle may increase force output by recruitment of additional motor units and by modulation of the discharge frequency of different motor units. Additional mechanisms may influence the force output (41) such as potentiation, fatigue, and change in stiffness, related to prior activity. At low levels of force there is a recruitment of additional motor units before changes in firing rate. In most muscles, the increase in force amounts to about 80% of the maximum, whereas 20% derive from an increase in discharge frequency (42–44). In some muscles, motor units may be recruited at a force level of 50%, and the remaining force level is determined by rate coding that ensures more precise gradation (42,45). In reflex movement and during gradual and rapidly increasing force production, the sequence of recruitment of motor units follows the size principle (46–48): Small, low force, slow-twitch, fatigue-resistant motor units are recruited at low levels of force, whereas the largest fatigable motor units are recruited at maximal levels. The input–output relationship of the motoneuron is, however, under additional suprasegmental control such that the order of recruitment may be changed according to the specific task (49–52). The order of recruitment may also be changed by altering afferent input (43,53,54) disease states and injury (55,56). The rise times of MUAPs in fast

muscles is faster than in slowly contracting muscle, without appreciable differences in the shape, amplitude, or duration of the MUAPs (17).

It is believed that with steady isometric contraction, motor units active at the beginning of the contraction remain active (43,57,58) with a time-dependent replacement of active motor units by different motor units believed to delay fatigue (49–60), although this has not been confirmed in other studies (61,62).

In human muscles during slow ramp contractions, motor units fire at 2 to 3 Hz and with slight effort reach a stable regular firing rate of 5 to 7 Hz (17,63–67). At maximum effort, discharge frequencies vary somewhat in different muscles but rarely increase above 30 to 40 Hz (42,44,68–70); however, at brisk brief contractions, discharge rates of 150 Hz have been recorded (71). The firing rates of motor units with different recruitment thresholds suggest that at moderate force, the low-threshold motor units have higher maximal firing rates than high-threshold motor units (42,68,69); however, the high-threshold motor units seem to have higher and phasic discharge rates at high force (68,72).

Number of Motor Units

The number of functioning motor units in the muscle is of considerable interest both to distinguish neurogenic from myopathic processes as causes of muscle weakness and to follow the loss of motor units in neurogenic disorders. Considerable efforts have been made to develop methods of motor unit number estimation (MUNE) by recording single MUAPs evoked by electrical stimulation and during voluntary contractions (Table 2). These methods include manual incremental stimulation (73–77), computer-assisted incremental stimulation (78), multiple-point threshold stimulation (79,80), analysis of F waves (81–83), and spike-triggered averaging of MUAPs (84–86).

The basic principle of all these methods is the determination of the size of the physiologic response of a representative motor unit that is then divided into the size of the maximal compound muscle response considered to be a sum of individual motor unit responses. A number of assumptions are made to determine the representative quantal motor unit response whether obtained as the force

TABLE 2. *Motor unit number estimates using different methods*

Muscle	Mean ± SD	Subjects	Age (yr)	Method	Authors	Reference
Thenar group	253 ± 34	61	<40	Manual incremental stimulation	Brown, 1972	74
	340 ± 87	67	<60	Manual incremental stimulation	Sica et al., 1974	75
	83 ± 46	12	>60	Manual incremental stimulation	Sica et al., 1974	75
	261 ± 116	14		Alternation corrected incremental stimulation	Milner-Brown and Brown, 1976	77
	228 ± 93	33	21–56	Computer-assisted incremental stimulation	Galea et al., 1991	78
	288 ± 95	17	20–40	Multiple point stimulation	Doherty and Brown, 1993	80
	139 ± 68	20	63–81	Multiple point stimulation	Doherty and Brown, 1993	80
	170 ± 62	10	26–49	Manual incremental stimulation	Stein and Yang, 1990	86
	135 ± 27	10	26–49	STA/EMG	Stein and Yang, 1990	86
	130 ± 39	10	26–49	STA/force	Stein and Yang, 1990	86
	116 ± 45	10	26–49	STA (microstimulation)/force	Stein and Yang, 1990	86
	122 ± 38	10	26–49	STA (microstimulation)/EMG	Stein and Yang, 1990	86
	287 ± 103	18	31 ± 11	F response (automated)	Stashuk et al., 1994	82
	195 ± 34	15	68 ± 3	F response (automated)	Stashuk et al., 1994	82
	234/95*	30		Statistical	Daube, 1995	88
Extensor digitorum brevis	199 ± 60	41	4–58	Manual incremental stimulation	McComas et al., 1971	73
	197 ± 49	39	35 ± 14	Manual incremental stimulation	Ballantyne and Hansen, 1974	76
	163 ± 84	10		Alternation corrected incremental stimulation	Milner-Brown and Brown, 1976	77
	131 ± 45	33	21–56	Computer-assisted incremental stimulation	Galea et al., 1991	78
	158/58	30		Statistical	Daube, 1995	88
Hypothenar group	380 ± 79	77	<60	Manual incremental stimulation	Sica et al., 1974	75

STA, spike-triggered averaging; EMG, electromyography. *indicates mean/ lower limit.

of the motor unit or the MUAP. These assumptions pertain to activation of individual α-motor axons at low levels of stimulation and may be influenced by fluctuating activation of several axons with similar thresholds (alternation).

Such alternation has been minimized by multiple point stimulation, wherein the nerve is stimulated at several points along its length and the very first all-or-nothing response used to measure the MUAP. In this method, the stimulation at different sites along the length of the nerve does not take into consideration branching of the α-motor axon that increases distally and takes place at considerable distances from the nerve (87). Analysis of F waves to extract MUAP information also claims to reduce alternation, although the firing of α-motor neurons may be influenced by central nervous system disorders, such as amyotrophic lateral sclerosis (ALS), associated with an increased motor neuron excitability due to corticospinal degeneration. The alternation due to overlapping axon thresholds has been used statistically in the Poisson distribution of discrete events. The average size of MUAPs at different levels of stimulation is then assessed from the variance of a series of 30 measurements (88).

Rather than using electrical stimulation of single motor axons, MUNE may be carried out during voluntary contractions: Individual MUAPs are recorded with a concentric needle, and using spike-triggered averaging, the surface recordings of associated MUAPs are then recorded. This method avoids the possibility of alternation, but at slight effort, small motor units may be preferentially recruited and the number of motor units therefore overestimated. The resolution of MUAPs at higher degrees of effort may be improved by computer-assisted decomposition of the EMG interference pattern (89). In all methods of MUNE it is required that the motor unit response, whether it is an MUAP or a mechanical twitch response, remains stable during repeated stimulations and that the motor unit responses add arithmetically to yield the maximal compound response. Surface electrodes are placed over the end-plate region to yield biphasic MUAPs with a negative onset. In the intrinsic hand muscles with a wide distribution of end-plates, some MUAPs may have a positive onset, and cancellation of phases thus influences the compound response. The MUAPs must have an amplitude sufficient to allow them to be distinguished from noise. In large muscles, deeper placed motor units may not be detected at the surface recording. Similarly, in myopathic disorders where the number of motor units remain normal while muscle fibers are affected, the MUAP amplitude may decrease below detectable levels, and the calculated number of motor units may therefore be misleading (90,91).

Despite these potential sources of error, MUNE using different methods in the same muscles yielded comparable results of both the number of motor units (e.g., 300 in median innervated hand muscles and about 200 in the extensor digitorum brevis muscle) and the distribution of MUAP sizes (86,92) (Table 2). Repeated measures have shown the results to be reasonably stable over time (80,93) in normal subjects and in patients with ALS. Direct anatomic assessment of motor unit counts are only to some extent comparable with physiologic measures of MUNE. In counts of large myelinated fibers of a motor nerve to assess the number of α-motor axons, sensory fibers comprise 40% to 60% of the total number of large myelinated fibers of diameter greater than 6 to 7 μm (94). These studies are therefore subject to error in the distinction between large and small motor and sensory fibers.

At maximal stimulation of the median nerve at the wrist, all of its innervated muscles in the hand contribute to the compound muscle action potential. In the monkey (*Macaca fascicularis*), the number of motor units using manual incremental stimulation and recording through a subcutaneous electrode over the abductor pollicis brevis was about 150 (S. Archibald, R. Lacin, L. Wrage, R. Madison, and C. Krarup, unpublished data). Acute sectioning of individual nerve branches in the baboon showed that the recorded compound muscle action potential was derived from all thenar and median innervated lumbrical muscles, in accordance with a count of 40 to 50 motor units in anatomic measurements of the abductor pollicis brevis (87).

PARAMETERS OF THE MOTOR UNIT POTENTIAL

In most laboratories, the needle EMG examination is carried out by a concentric needle electrode referenced to the cannula or a monopolar electrode referenced to a surface electrode at a frequency interval of 2 to 10k Hz. The recording area of the concentric needle is 0.07 mm², whereas the monopolar needle is insulated with Teflon except for a bared recording area of 0.17 mm². Because of the different properties of the electrodes, the MUAP parameters are not directly comparable (95,96). The control values used in Copenhagen were obtained using concentric needle electrodes (97).

The EMG examination usually falls into three parts: recording at rest to ascertain the presence of diverse forms of spontaneous activity resulting from denervation activity such as fibrillation potentials or positive sharp waves, fasciculations, myotonic bursts, complex repetitive discharges, miniature end-plate potentials, and end-plate spikes; recording during low levels of voluntary effort to obtain individual MUAPs without interference from other MUAPs; and recording during maximal voluntary effort to evaluate interference patterns.

The MUAP is a compound signal reflecting the summation and cancellation of phases of the action potentials from individual muscle fibers in the motor unit. With intracellular recordings, the action potential is a monophasic waveform of about 100 mV, whereas the extracellular potential is a volume-conducted derivative of the rate of membrane depolarization. The MUAP represents the spatial and temporal summation of these bi(tri)phasic spikes, wherein the negative spike in the normal muscle is obtained from two to three fibers within 0.5 to 1 mm of the electrode. The contribution of activity from fibers at a slightly longer distance is negligible because of the steep spatial decay of the high-frequency spike. In contrast, the slow initial and terminal positive phases represent activity from fibers at greater distances because the decay of these slow components is much smaller (25). The amplitude of the spike is determined by the proximity of the closest active fibers as indicated by the fact that fibrillation potentials that originate from single fibers may have as high an amplitude as the MUAP.

The shape and duration of the MUAP reflects the architecture of the motor unit. Recorded outside the end-plate region, the MUAP typically has three phases: an initial positive phase, a negative spike, and a terminal positive phase. A negative afterpotential is sometimes recorded and is enhanced when the lower limiting amplifier frequency is set above 2 Hz (98). At the end-plate region the MUAP is biphasic in shape with a sharp negative onset. In some instances, the MUAP may be split up into four or more phases, reflecting a greater asynchrony of discharges. In normal humans, the number of polyphasic MUAPs, that is, with five or more phases, comprises about 3% of a large number of control subjects, and when 20 to 25 MUAPs are recorded, less than 12% of the total number of potentials are polyphasic. In the deltoid and facial muscles, less than 25% are polyphasic, and similarly it is less than 20% in the vastus lateralis and the anterior tibial muscles (99,100). An

MUAP may contain a spike component separate from the main spike. These so-called satellite potentials represent action potentials of a single or a few fibers temporally dispersed from the main bulk of the fibers in the motor unit in disease states and contributes up to 3% of MAUPs of healthy muscle (101–105). A stationary far-field positive potential is sometimes recorded during the positive terminal phase of the MUAP with monopolar needle electrodes; it represents extinction of the action potential at the myotendinous transition (106,107).

Three MUAP parameters are of clinical importance: the MUAP duration, peak-to-peak amplitude, and the phasicity (Fig. 1).

Duration of the Motor Unit Action Potential

The duration of the MUAP reflects the temporal dispersion of activity of fibers constituting the motor unit and is primarily due to the spatial distribution of endplates along muscle fibers measuring 20 to 30 mm, with a conduction velocity of 3 to 5 m/sec (4,5,108). The duration is also related to the number of muscle fibers present in a semicircle 2.5 mm from the active recording surface (109,110) and the diameter of muscle fibers in the motor unit (111,112). It is measured from the first deflection of

the MUAP from baseline to the return of the terminal positive phase (Fig. 1). The duration is highly dependent on amplifier settings. Normal values from the Clinical Neurophysiology Laboratory at Rigshospitalet were obtained at a gain of 100 µV/cm; the measured duration was shorter at lower gain settings and longer at higher gains. In modern equipment with digitalized signals, the deviation and return to baseline is usually determined by amplitude or slope criteria (113) and the normal values developed for the manual measurements may therefore not be applicable.

In a given muscle, the normal duration of individual MUAPs can vary by a factor of 3 to 5 and in the brachial biceps range from 5 to 15 msec. This variability is mainly due to the variability in fiber content of the motor units. It is therefore necessary to record several MUAPs (20 to 30) at different sites in the muscle to obtain a representative sample. The duration of simple units, defined by the presence of four or less phases, and polyphasic MUAPs are averaged separately and together and the values compared with age-matched control subjects. The normal range is defined as the normal mean ± 20% (Table 3). MUAP duration is the most important parameter in the separation of myopathic disorders in which there is a loss of muscle fibers from chronic neurogenic disorders in which there is an increased number of muscle fibers due to collateral sprouting (114–116).

Amplitude of the Motor Unit Action Potential

MUAP amplitude is measured peak-to-peak from the most positive to the sequentially most negative peak (Fig. 1). Because of cancellation between phases, the MUAP amplitude is less than the sum of individual fiber potentials and may even be smaller than the amplitude of single fiber potentials. It depends on the proximity of the closest 2 to 15 fibers of the motor unit within about a 0.5-mm diameter (109,110,112,117) and is propor-

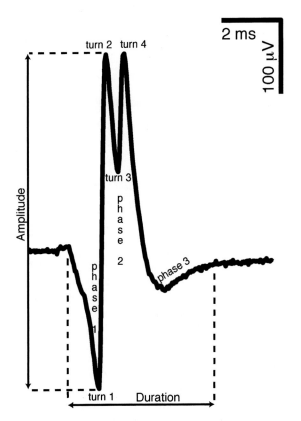

FIG. 1. Motor unit potential from normal muscle recorded with concentric needle electrodes. The measured parameters and the different components are indicated.

TABLE 3. EMG limits in normal muscle (95% confidence limits)

Voluntary activity	
Weak effort (%)	
Duration of the motor unit potential	±20[a]
Amplitude of motor unit potential	±50[a]
Incidence of polyphasic potentials	12[b]
Full effort	
Pattern	Full recruitment
Amplitude of envelope curves (mV)	>2, <4
Spontaneous activity	
Upper limit, number of sites outside end-plate region with fibrillation potentials or positive sharp waves	2

[a]Mean of 25 or more motor unit action potentials.
[b]In the deltoid and facial muscles 25%, in the anterior tibial and lateral vastus muscles, 20%.
From Ref. 186.

tional to the number and density of fibers in the motor unit. Because of the large effect of distance between the active fibers and the recording surface, the amplitudes of the MUAPs are markedly variable. The amplitude also depends on the type of electrode used. The amplitude is larger when using monopolar than concentric needle electrodes (118,119). It is important to hear the crisp sound of discharging MUAPs, indicating that the electrode is placed close to active motor units. Manipulating the electrode should be avoided because this can yield larger amplitude MUAPs. The recordings that form the basis for the control material at Rigshospitalet were obtained without manipulating the needle to obtain larger amplitudes; however, the variability of the amplitude is such that we require it to be more than 100% above controls to be clearly abnormal.

Better standardization of recording MUAPs has been attempted by adhering to rules on the rise time of the MUAP, as measured from the maximum positive to the maximum negative peak (120). A general recommendation is to accept a rise time of no more than 0.5 msec (121); however, this also depends on the number of fibers that summate to generate the MUAP. It tends to increase in chronic partial denervation with reinnervation of muscle fibers, whereas it is shorter in myopathy due to loss of muscle fibers. In practice, we exclude potentials with slow rise times and amplitudes of less than 50 μV. The rise time is negatively correlated to the amplitude of the MUAP but, if less than 2 msec, has little influence on the duration of the MUAP that is determined by the slow initial and terminal phases of the MUAP (122).

Shape of the Motor Unit Action Potential

MUAPs can be simple in shape or polyphasic. The latter are of long or short duration in myopathy depending on the degree of muscle fiber regeneration. It is important to calculate amplitudes and durations of simple and polyphasic potentials separately and to collect more MUAPs than necessary in case additional ones are needed (123). Irregularities of the MUAP that do not result in baseline crossings are termed "turns" if they have an amplitude of more than 100 μV (Fig. 1). Studies of MUAPs have shown variability in the shape in successive discharges or jiggle (124) not due to electrode displacement. This is more pronounced in myasthenia gravis and in early collateral sprouting with immature axonal sprouts.

Firing Rates of the Motor Unit Action Potential

The firing rates of MUAPs are not usually considered in routine EMG studies. Deafferentiation has been shown to reduce the firing rate, emphasizing the important contribution of proprioceptors (67,125). Increased firing rates were reported in some cases of neuropathy (126), but this was not confirmed in other studies (127,128). Abnormalities in

firing rates have also been reported in patients with various central nervous system disorders (129–131).

Biologic and Physical Factors that Influence the Motor Unit Action Potential

Age

The duration of the MUAP increases from 20 to 80 years, although the amount varies in different muscles (132–134), and there is disagreement as to the age when an increase in duration occurs (135). It may be due to remodeling of the motor units with collateral sprouting (31,32,136) that presumably starts in the third decade due to progressive loss of anterior horn cells (137). The increase in MUAP duration at ages less than 20 years is probably due to growth. Single-fiber EMG (SFEMG) studies have shown an increase in fiber density with age older than 60 years (138) that may be partly due to a reduction in muscle mass and fiber diameter (139). An increase in fiber density could cause an increase in the amplitude of initial and terminal phases and consequently a longer duration of the MUAP. The amplitude of the MUAP does not change significantly with age.

Temperature

A reduction in muscle fiber and axon conduction velocities occurs at low temperatures, and MUAP duration increases with a reduction of the intramuscular temperature (132,140). The mean duration of MUAPs increases by 6%/°C between 30 and 36°C and by 9%/°C between 22 and 30°C. At normal intramuscular temperatures, the MUAP does not change enough to cause errors in diagnosis; however, at temperatures lower than 32°C, considerable errors may occur. MUAP polyphasia increases from about 3% at 37°C to 25% at 29°C (100). The amplitude of the MUAP may increase or decrease at low temperature due to variable phase cancellations (132). At ADEMG the MUAP duration is prolonged at low temperature, although amplitudes and turns remain unchanged (141).

Special Electrodes

Concentric electrodes record a somewhat distorted signal from the MUAP. This has led to considerable efforts in developing other electrode types to examine the architectural and spatial extent of the MUAP.

Multilead Electrodes

It has long been recognized that the shape and duration of the MUAP recorded with a concentric electrode depends on its location within the motor unit. Buchthal et al. (5,142) developed a multielectrode with up to 14 recording areas placed 1 mm apart and each corresponding to that of a concentric needle to determine the spatial distribution of individual spikes and hence delineate the shape and territory of the motor unit in normal and diseased muscle. By placing two multielectrodes perpendicularly to each other, the motor unit in normal muscle was found to be usually circular in shape and with a larger concentration of muscle fibers at the center of the motor unit than at the periphery (5) in agreement with earlier histochemical findings (6,143). In myopathy (144), the size of the motor unit was found to be decreased, whereas it was increased in neurogenic lesions (145). However, an enlarged territory of the motor unit as indicated by the electrical activity could be due to an increased fiber density that would cause the spike activity to be seen at a longer distance, leading to an interpretation of a spatially larger motor unit.

Stålberg et al. (146) studied the extent of the motor unit by using a multilead single-fiber electrode. The SFEMG recording electrode is 25 μm in length (0.005 mm²), and the uptake area is about 300 μm. Normal muscles spikes of at least 200 μV are recorded from one to two muscle fibers from the same motor unit, and the average number of spikes at 20 sites is used to calculate the fiber density (average 1.5 in normal muscle). Studies with multilead SFEMG showed that the density of fibers within the motor unit increased in neurogenic lesions but that the territory of the motor unit remains unchanged.

Scanning Electromyography

To evaluate the spatial distribution of the electrical activity within the motor unit, a concentric needle electrode was pulled through the motor unit and the MUAP recorded at 50-μm-space intervals and averaged by means of a trigger-potential obtained from an SFEMG needle placed within the same motor unit (147). The spatial profile showed that in about one half of control patients, a single major negative peak was present, but some had up to four peaks. The scan of patients with myopathy may show increased fractionation of the motor unit with a larger number of spikes, whereas the number of silent areas with an activity of less than 50 μV was decreased in neurogenic lesions due to reinnervation within the motor unit area. The relatively normal scan length supports the view of newly incorporated muscle fibers originating within the original motor unit territory and that collateral branches do not cross fascicular borders. In most cases, the technique does not distinguish between neurogenic lesions and myopathy (148), possibly because of the contribution of regeneration in the latter.

Macro Electromyography

The MUAP recorded with a concentric needle is a relatively poor indicator of the total activity contained in the motor unit. Recording with an electrode of a surface area 15 mm in length improves the evaluation of the size of the motor unit by sampling a larger portion of the motor unit (149,150). The motor unit activity is then averaged to reduce the contribution of activity from other motor units and recorded by means of a trigger potential recorded from an SFEMG lead incorporated in the same electrode. The MUAP is the compound of a large number of muscle fibers in the cylindrical recording area surrounding the exposed tip with a radius of about 2 mm and a length of 15 mm (151–153). The area and amplitude of the MUAP are correlated with the number and size of muscle fibers in the entire motor unit (149), whereas the duration is difficult to measure accurately. A variant of the method has been developed by Jabre (154), where the macroelectrode has been combined with a concentric needle. The amplitude of the macro MUAP increases with age due to reinnervation after motor neuron loss. Such changes are also found in progressive neuropathy. In patients with ALS and the postpolio syndrome, the size of the MUAP decreases as the disease progresses, suggesting loss of large motor units. In myopathy, the mean amplitude of the MUAPs has been found to be normal or slightly decreased (155). This could be due to increased density of muscle fibers in the motor unit, as also indicated by SFEMG.

Surface Recording of the Electromyography

Surface recordings, by means of elaborate electrode arrays and spike triggering, may be useful to assess endplate distribution, muscle tendon transition, motor unit depth and firing rate, and MUAP propagation along muscle fibers (156–159).

Bipolar Needle Electrodes

In these electrodes, two concentric leads are placed together in the cannula and the electrical activity is recorded between them (119). The pickup area is restricted and the electrode is therefore not suitable for MUAP evaluation. The electrode is useful to ascertain whether the electrical activity is volume conducted from a distance.

METHODS OF ANALYZING MOTOR UNIT ACTIVITY

Recording the Motor Unit Action Potential in Clinical Practice

Sampling of a representative number of motor units is necessary because of the large variability in innervation ratios and therefore the duration and amplitude of MUAPs of individual muscles. Reliance on a visual impression of MUAP characteristics is inaccurate (Fig. 2). We therefore require a mean MUAP duration or amplitude outside the 95% confidence limits to establish abnormality. In instances of mild disease or heterogeneous affection of the muscle by myositis or monoradic-

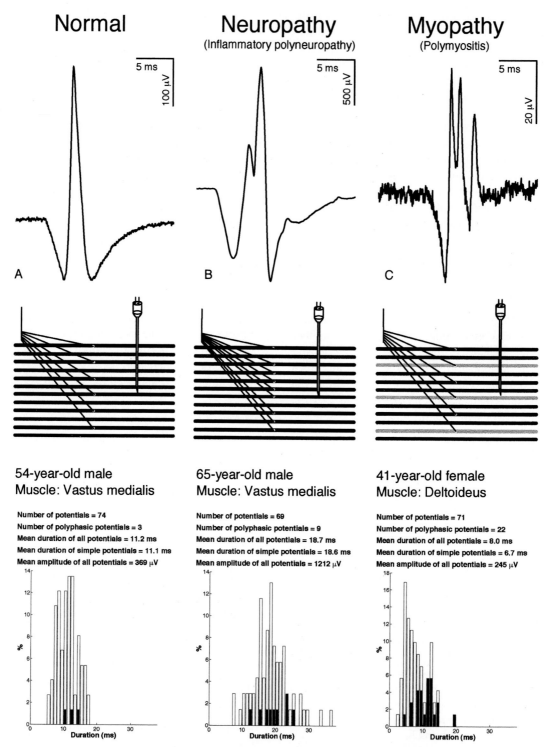

Normal

Neuropathy
(Inflammatory polyneuropathy)

Myopathy
(Polymyositis)

A

B

C

54-year-old male
Muscle: Vastus medialis

65-year-old male
Muscle: Vastus medialis

41-year-old female
Muscle: Deltoideus

Number of potentials = 74
Number of polyphasic potentials = 3
Mean duration of all potentials = 11.2 ms
Mean duration of simple potentials = 11.1 ms
Mean amplitude of all potentials = 369 μV

Number of potentials = 69
Number of polyphasic potentials = 9
Mean duration of all potentials = 18.7 ms
Mean duration of simple potentials = 18.6 ms
Mean amplitude of all potentials = 1212 μV

Number of potentials = 71
Number of polyphasic potentials = 22
Mean duration of all potentials = 8.0 ms
Mean duration of simple potentials = 6.7 ms
Mean amplitude of all potentials = 245 μV

FIG. 2. Motor unit action potentials (MUAPs) recorded with concentric needle electrodes. The MUAPs were extracted using the EMGPAD system. **(A)** Normal subject; **(B)** patient with polyneuropathy; **(C)** patient with myopathy. The topmost traces are examples of MUAPs from each muscle. The middle drawing is a schematic interpretation of distribution of muscle fibers. Black bars **(A–C)** indicate muscle fibers from the active motor unit; dark gray bars **(A–C)** indicate muscle fibers from another nonactive motor unit; light gray bars **(C)** indicate degenerated muscle fibers belonging to the active motor unit. The lowermost histograms show the distribution of durations of MUAPs in the muscles. The white bars indicate simple potentials and the black bars indicate polyphasic potentials (4% in **A**, 13% in **B**, 31% in **C**). The mean values of parameters are indicated above the histograms. In **B**, the duration of the MUAPs was 51% prolonged and the amplitude was 427% increased; in **C**, the duration of simple potentials was 41% shortened and of all potentials 29% shortened, and the amplitude was normal.

ular disease, the mean duration and amplitude may not deviate from normal, and the determination of outliers has been suggested as a supplementary criterion of abnormality (160).

In the recording of activity from single motor units, it is important to obtain signals that are not contaminated by activity from adjacent motor units. At low effort, MUAPs are recorded by the use of a trigger circuit and a delay that allows the whole MUAP to be included on the oscilloscope to measure its total duration and amplitude. To ensure that the signal is derived from a single motor unit, undisturbed by activity from others, three to five similar signals are recorded. This "template" method has the inherent bias of recording large MUAPs, and it is therefore important to ensure that all MUAPs at each needle position are included in the analysis. At low effort it is usually possible to record two to three MUAPs at each site. The sampling should include recordings from about 10 recording sites. To ensure that the sampling is well distributed over the entire muscle, we record from three sites at distances of not less than 0.5 cm each at three to four needle positions. Even though modern integrated EMG machines allow the recording, storing, and analysis of MUAPs to proceed faster and easier, the bias of the sampling may be greater because only those MUAPs that are triggered are captured at times to the exclusion of smaller MUAPs.

The reliability of MUAP analysis depends on the expertise of the examiner. For this reason we find it necessary to keep hard copies or computer data files of all recordings to ensure that the mean and SD of amplitudes and durations are obtained from different and undisturbed MUAPs. The parameters are calculated for the simple and the polyphasic MUAPs separately if the incidence of polyphasic potentials is increased.

Automatic Decomposition of Motor Unit Action Potentials During Voluntary Effort

A number of automatic EMG analysis systems have been developed over the last 15 years to extract MUAPs from the EMG signal. This reduces the sampling bias inherent in the selection of MUAPs captured by a trigger function. They can measure the duration, amplitude,

turns, and phases of the MUAPs. Whereas some methods are designed primarily for analysis of individual MUAPs, others have had the primary goal of analyzing the firing pattern during different degrees of voluntary effort. More recently developed systems allow both measurements of MUAP parameters at a partial or a full firing pattern.

Five features are desirable in an automated system of MUAP analysis (Table 4): a short on- or off-line response time; analysis of firing frequency, firing variability, and recruitment time; a decomposition algorithm to segregate signals from the individual motor units, especially to measure duration, amplitude, number of phases, and turns; use of a concentric needle electrode, especially for decomposition of the EMG signal; and special needle electrodes for decomposition of the interference pattern at higher levels of force.

In all systems, MUAP identification is a multistep task that includes recording, amplification, filtering, and sampling of the EMG signal; segmentation of the signal into time intervals that contain EMG activity, either an MUAP or superimposed MUAPs; clustering of signals into MUAPs according to whether criteria of similarity are fulfilled, followed in some systems by resolution of superimposed MUAPs; and display of identified MUAPs, with measurements of necessary parameters and, in some systems, presentation of partial or complete firing patterns.

Template matching is a method used by different systems to detect MUAPs. In the system designed by Andreassen (161), sequential signals are assigned to templates according to whether the power of the signal differs by less than 12% of the power of the template; a MUAP is assigned when four matching potentials are accepted. Up to four templates are accepted at each recording site.

In the "Multi-MUP" analysis system, a 4.8-second signal is analyzed (162–164) and parametric measurements of the potential shape are used to assign potentials to matching classes. A maximum of six MUAPs can be recorded from each site. The resolved MUAPs are averaged for measurements of parameters. Superimposed MUAPs are not resolved, and only a partial firing pattern is produced.

In the ADEMG system developed by McGill and Dorfman (165), a 10-second signal is initially high-pass fil-

TABLE 4. *Comparison of five automatic EMG analysis systems*

	On-line/ off-line	Firing pattern	MUAP shape parameters	Type of needle electrode	Contractile force
Andreassen	On-line	No	Yes	Conventional	Low
Stålberg et al. (multi-MUP)	On-line	Partial	Yes	Conventional	Low
McGill and Dorfman (ADEMG)	On-line	Partial	Yes	Conventional	Low
Hass and Meyer (ARTMUP)	Off-line	Full	Yes	Conventional	Low
Nikolic et al. (EMGPAD)	Off-line	Full	Yes	Conventional	Low
LeFever and DeLuca	Off-line	Full	No	Special	High

EMG, electromyography; MUAP, motor unit action potentials; MUP, motor unit potential; ADEMG, automatic decomposition electromyography; ARTMUP, automatic recognition and tracking of motor unit potentials; EMGPAD, EMG precision automatic decomposition.

tered using a first- or a second-order differentiating filter to enhance spikes with a fast rise time. The spikes are detected according to a preset threshold and subsequently transformed to a frequency domain and classified using template matching. The identified MUAPs are averaged for measurements. Superimposed MUAPs are not resolved, and only a partial firing pattern, used to confirm the MUAP assignment, is obtained.

The system developed by Hass and Meyer (166) has a selectable degree of decomposition so that a fast extraction of the MUAP parameters for a routine clinical examination or a more time-consuming complete decomposition for research can be chosen. First, a 10-second EMG signal is segmented into time intervals containing MUAP activity using a slope criterion. Similar segments are then clustered by a minimal spanning tree method. The minimal spanning tree is constructed by comparing all segments pairwise using nonparametric distance measure. The user can stop at this point and can be presented with the MUAPs and their parameters or continue with a multistep resolution of up to three superimposed MUAPs. After the resolution stage, the firing patterns are produced for each identified motor unit.

By using both the MUAP shape and an estimate of the interpotential intervals (167–169), similar looking potentials from different motor units and variability in the MUAP shape can be detected by inconsistency or consistency in the interpotential intervals, respectively.

We have developed a decomposition system for the detailed analysis of MUAP shape parameters, firing patterns, and MUAP shape variability (EMG precision automatic decomposition (PAP) (170)). The electrical activity is sampled by a concentric needle electrode at a frequency of 23.5 kHz. The EMG signal is first separated into segments containing MUAP activity and then clustered by a minimum spanning tree method. This analysis leads to a partition consisting of clusters containing isolated MUAPs and clusters composed of superimposed MUAPs. The number of segments in a cluster is used to detect potentials from one motor unit. From each of these clusters, a template is selected. The clusters containing superimposed MUAPs are analyzed by a recursive algorithm. The cross-correlation between superimposed MUAPs and a template are computed and timeshifts with high correlation are detected. The template is subtracted for each of these timeshifts, and a subsequent pass through the algorithm processes the residual segments. The output of the decomposition algorithm is the MUAP parameters, plots of the MUAPs, and their firing patterns. We have found the firing patterns useful for detecting and discriminating between needle movement and MUAP shape variability and studying central nervous system motor unit control.

Whereas the above systems are aimed at decomposing EMG signals at relatively low force, the decomposition system developed by LeFever and DeLuca (171) was primarily designed to separate the EMG signal into its constituent MUAP trains at high contractile force. The recording is carried out using a quadripolar needle electrode that allows each motor unit to be defined by three different MUAPs and hence to give a unique description of the MUAP at even high contractile force.

Analysis of the Electromyography Signal at Higher Levels of Voluntary Effort

To ascertain pathophysiologic changes at higher levels of effort, different methods have been developed to analyze the interference pattern when individual MUAPs cannot be distinguished. This has the advantage of activating motor units at other than low levels of effort.

Turns-Amplitude Analysis

In this analysis, the number of turns in the interference pattern and the mean amplitude difference between turns are measured within an epoch of fixed duration (172,173). A turn was defined as a change in voltage of 100 μV and may arise as a peak in a MUAP or interaction between MUAPs, and the number of turns reflects the number of active motor units, the proportion of polyphasic MUAPs, and the firing rate. The mean amplitude increases with increased force output and with the amplitudes of recruited MUAPs.

Fuglsang-Frederiksen et al. (174–176) counted the number of turns at a given absolute force equal to 30% of the maximal voluntary force. Measurements during a relative force output better discriminated between myopathy, neurogenic lesions, and controls than during 2- or 5-kg fixed force output, respectively, in the brachial biceps and medial vastus muscles (177). The number of turns increases in patients with myopathy, as does the mean amplitude between turns in patients with neurogenic lesions. An increase in the ratio of turns:mean amplitude was found to be a sensitive indicator of myopathy, and a reduced ratio was an indicator of neurogenic disorders (173,174,178–181). In patients with myopathy, the number of small intervals between turns is increased, and decreased in neurogenic disorders (173,174,182). The use of turns-amplitude analysis of the interference pattern at 30% of maximal effort was found to have the same diagnostic yield as analysis of MUAPs at low effort but the two methods supplemented rather than replaced each other (172,173). The diagnostic yield was not further improved by analysis at forces greater than 30% of maximum (183–185).

In an effort to reduce the cooperation required by the patient, the turns-amplitude analysis has been modified in various ways to obtain measurements independent of measured force. These include measurements of the number of turns as a function of the mean amplitude at three to five force levels from minimum to maximum. The scatter plot in control patients forms a cloud wherein the borders include 90% of normal values. Studies in myopathy and neurogenic lesions deviate in opposite directions (186). The peak ratio method uses the ratio of turns:mean amplitude as a function of increasing force. It is measured every 100 msec during gradually increasing force over a period of 10 seconds and at peak ratio; at maximum force the intervals between turns are indicated (187–189). Patients with myopathy have a higher peak ratio or an increased number of intervals of less than 1.5 msec or both, whereas patients with neurogenic lesions deviate in the opposite directions.

In addition to the turns-amplitude analysis, the interference pattern has been studied by *power spectral analysis* in patients with neuromuscular disorders and in the study of muscle fatigue, which lead to a shift of the interference pattern spectrum toward lower frequencies (190,191).

PATHOPHYSIOLOGIC CHANGES IN THE MOTOR UNIT ACTION POTENTIAL

The primary aim of the EMG examination is to determine whether weakness is due to a myopathic or neurogenic lesion. Proximal and distal weak muscles are generally studied. Spontaneous muscle fiber activity during rest may be recorded in normal muscle and in myopathy and chronic partial denervation. In control and affected muscle, the end-plate zone shows miniature end-plate potentials and spontaneous muscle fiber discharges that have a sharp

negative onset. Outside the end-plate zone, propagated action potentials are rarely recorded in normal muscle. In myopathy fibrillation, activity is abundant in conditions with muscle fiber necrosis such as myositis and some types of muscular dystrophy, whereas they are rare, for example, in mitochondrial myopathy or thyrotoxicosis. In neurogenic disorders, denervation activity indicates failure of reinnervation but may be seen for several years after the insult has occurred, as for example in poliomyelitis. An increased incidence of fibrillation potentials and positive sharp waves is a nonspecific criterion of pathologic changes in the muscle, as are complex repetitive discharges that usually arise from groups of muscle fibers and may be seen in both myopathy and neurogenic lesions. Abundant waxing and waning complex repetitive discharges are characteristically seen in radiation-induced peripheral nerve damage. Fasciculations are defined as irregular discharges in groups of muscle fibers and may occur in normal muscle and in myositis and neurogenic lesions. They tend to have long discharge intervals of more than 3 seconds and most often arise from groups of muscle fibers that are not under voluntary control. Analysis of the MUAPs at weak effort has a central position in the EMG examination because the duration, amplitude, and shape of the MUAPs recorded with a concentric or a monopolar needle electrode reflects the architecture of the motor unit.

The basic pathophysiologic change in myopathy (Table 5) is an inability to propagate action potentials, the degen-

TABLE 5. *EMG criteria of neuromuscular disease*

Specific criteria	Nonspecific criteria
Criteria of myopathy	
MUAP during weak effort	MUAP during weak effort
Decrease in duration	Increased incidence of polyphasic potentials
	Decreased amplitude
Recruitment pattern	
Full recruitment in a weak and wasted muscle	Recruitment pattern
Decreased amplitude of full recruitment pattern	Reduced recruitment pattern
	Activity at rest
Criteria of peripheral nerve and root disease	Fibrillation activity and positive sharp waves
MUAP during weak effort	
Increase in duration	MUAP during weak effort
Increase in amplitude	Increased incidence of polyphasic potentials
Recruitment pattern	
Discrete activity	Recruitment pattern
Increased amplitude	Reduced recruitment pattern
	Activity at rest
Criteria of anterior horn cell disease	Fibrillation activity and positive sharp waves (4–10 sites)
MUAP during weak effort	
Increase in duration	MUAP during weak effort
Increase in amplitude (>500% increased)	Increase in amplitude of individual
Recruitment pattern	MUAPs (200%)
Discrete activity	
Increased amplitude (>6 mV)	
Activity at rest	Activity at rest
Fasciculations (malignant, intervals of >3 sec)	Fasciculations (benign, intervals < 1 sec)

EMG, electromyography; MUAP, motor unit action potentials. For normal limits, see Table 3.

eration of muscle fibers, and a loss of muscle fibers in the individual motor unit. Whether these abnormalities are reflected in the EMG depends on the stage of the disease and whether compensatory regeneration mechanisms have already occurred. At early stages of the disorder, muscle contraction may be affected primarily at the level of excitation-contraction coupling, in which case MUAP analysis may show only mild or unspecific changes. The incidence of polyphasic potentials is increased in patients with myopathy for two reasons. First, muscle fibers of the motor units are lost and hence summation of muscle fiber action potentials in the MUAP is reduced. Because of the loss of muscle fibers, the duration of the MUAP is reduced (Fig. 2). Second, there is regeneration of muscle fibers from satellite cells, and this is associated with polyphasic potentials due to increased dispersion caused by a reduced conduction velocity along the regenerated muscle fibers or along collateral nerve sprouts. The incidence of polyphasic potentials is related to the duration of the MUAPs and to the number of regenerating basophilic fibers at muscle biopsy. At an early stage of myopathy, the incidence of long duration polyphasic potentials is increased, whereas they decrease with advancing severity (115). The presence of long polyphasic potentials may lead to the erroneous conclusion of a neurogenic disorder. To avoid this error, we also measure the duration of simple MUAPs separately (Fig. 2).

In chronic partial denervation, reinnervation due to collateral sprouting enlarges the motor unit territory (Table 5). In reinnervation due to axonal regeneration, nascent motor units may be polyphasic and of short duration. However, even in such cases the mean MUAP duration of 20 to 30 MUAPs is usually prolonged, although amplitudes of the severely polyphasic MUAPs may be small. In chronic neuropathies, the duration, amplitude, and incidence of polyphasic MUAPs are increased (Fig. 2). Polyphasic potentials arise from dispersion of muscle fiber action potentials in the motor unit due to low conduction velocity of reinnervated atrophic muscle fibers and axonal sprouts. In early reinnervation, conduction along immature sprouts is insecure, and the MUAP may show pronounced variability (jiggle) with intermittent dropout of segments of the MUAP. In long-standing neurogenic lesions, such as remote poliomyelitis, polyphasic potentials may be near normal due to maturation of the collateral sprouts. It has been suggested that in the postpolio syndrome, the extended sprout tree may show regressive changes with degeneration of sprouts; however, it is also possible that the whole motor neuron degenerates, leaving motor units with a smaller innervation ratio and hence a smaller metabolic load on the motoneuron. In patients with ALS, simple and polyphasic potentials are enlarged, due to either long-standing reinnervation or coupled-discharges of more than one motor unit.

In cases where the findings of MUAP analysis are uncertain, it is often helpful to supplement the study with turns-amplitude analysis of the interference pattern. This aspect of muscle function allows examination at higher degrees of muscle force than the slight effort required to study individual MUAPs. Evaluation of the interference pattern at maximal voluntary effort is an integral part of the EMG examination and gives a semiquantitative measure of the presence of motor unit loss. Normally, maximal voluntary contraction in cooperative subjects is associated with a full interference pattern where individual MUAPs cannot be discerned. The amplitude of the envelope curve of the interference pattern is measured, and at maximal effort, the amplitude recorded with a concentric needle is in most muscles 2 to 4 mV (192). In myopathy, the interference pattern is generally full and of lower amplitude than in normal muscle. It starts abruptly even at lower levels of effort than in controls. In severe myopathy with extensive muscle fiber loss, the interference pattern may be reduced and may show less pronounced summation than in normal muscle. In neurogenic lesions, the interference pattern is reduced in moderate cases with loss of motor units, whereas it is discrete in severe cases wherein individual MUAPs stand out with a flat baseline between successive discharges. In chronic motor neuron disorders with reinnervation due to collateral sprouting, the amplitude of the reduced or discrete interference pattern is increased and may reach values of 8 to 10 mV (Table 5).

The distribution, type, and degree of abnormalities at the EMG examination are important in the specific diagnosis of neuromuscular disorders. Although the EMG examination should include clinically affected muscles, it may be crucial to study muscles not overtly affected. For example, in patients with suspected motor neuron disease, the initial weakness and atrophy may have a segmental distribution, raising suspicion of either radicular affection or mononeuropathy. However, EMG examination of muscles with normal force and bulk often shows that the involvement is distributed more widely than suggested by the clinical examination and therefore indicate a generalized disorder. These aspects of the clinical neurophysiology examination are covered in chapters 2 and 32.

SUMMARY

The interpretation of the EMG is based on the combination of clinical findings and the abnormalities during rest, at weak effort to analyze individual MUAPs, and with maximal effort for the interpretation of the interference pattern. The individual changes are interpreted as signs of myopathy or of neurogenic involvement, but the individual criteria are in some instances nonspecific for the diagnosis. There are specific and nonspecific signs of myopathic and neurogenic lesions (Table 5).

ACKNOWLEDGMENT

Supported by the Danish Medical Research Council.

REFERENCES

1. Liddell EGT, Sherrington CS. Recruitment and some other factor on reflex inhibition. *Proc R Soc Lond* 1925;B97:488–518.
2. Sherrington CS. Remarks on some aspects of reflex inhibition. *Proc R Soc Lond* 1925;B97:519–545.
3. Burke RE. Physiology of motor units. In: Engel AG, Franzini-Armstrong C, eds. *Myology*, 2nd ed. New York: McGraw-Hill, 1994:464–483.
4. Buchthal F, Guld C, Rosenfalck P. Volume conduction of the spike of the motor unit potential investigated with a new type of multielectrode. *Acta Physiol Scand* 1957;38:331–354.
5. Buchthal F, Guld C, Rosenfalck P. Multielectrode study of the territory of a motor unit. *Acta Physiol Scand* 1957;39:83–104.
6. Edström L, Kugelberg E. Histochemical composition, distribution of fibres and fatiguability of single motor units. Anterior tibial muscle of the rat. *J Neurol Neurosurg Psychiatry* 1968;31:424–433.
7. Kugelberg E. Properties of the rat hindlimb motor units. In: Desmedt JE, ed. *New developments in electromyography and clinical neurophysiology*. Vol. 1. Basel: Karger, 1973:2–13.
8. Bodine-Fowler SC, Garfinkel A, Roy RR, Edgerton VR. Spatial distribution of muscle fibers within the territory of a motor unit. *Muscle Nerve* 1990;13:1133–1145.
9. Doyle AM, Mayer RF. Studies of the motor unit in the cat. *Bull Univ MD School Med* 1969;54:11–17.
10. Brandstater ME, Lambert EH. Motor unit anatomy. Type and spatial arrangement of muscle fibers. In: Desmedt JE, ed. *New developments in electromyography and clinical neurophysiology*. Vol. 1. Basel: Karger, 1973:14–22.
11. Stålberg E, Trontelj JV. *Single fiber electromyography in healthy and diseased muscle*, 2nd ed. New York: Raven Press, 1994.
12. Stålberg E, Ekstedt J. Single fiber electromyography and microphysiology of the motor unit in normal and diseased human muscle. In: Desmedt JE, ed. *New developments in electromyography and clinical neurophysiology*. Vol. 1. Basel: Karger, 1973:113–129.
13. Guth L, Samaha FJ. Qualitative differences between actomyosin ATPase of slow and fast mammalian muscle. *Exp Neurol* 1969;25:138–163.
14. Brooke MH, Kaiser KK. Muscle fibre types. How many and what kind? *Arch Neurol* 1970;23:369–379.
15. Peter JB, Barnard RJ, Edgerton VR, Gillespie GA, Stempel KE. Metabolic profiles of three fibre types of skeletal muscle in guinea pigs and rabbits. *Biochemistry* 1972;11:2627–2633.
16. Khan MA. Histochemical characteristic of vertebrate striated muscle: a review. *Prog Histochem Cytochem* 1976;8:1–48.
17. Buchthal F, Schmalbruch H. Motor unit of mammalian muscle. *Physiol Rev* 1980;60:90–142.
18. Burke RE, Levine DN, Tsairis P, Zajac FE. Physiological types and histochemical profiles in motor units of the cat gastrocnemius. *J Physiol (Lond)* 1973;234:749–765.
19. Close RI. Dynamic properties of mammalian skeletal muscles. *Physiol Rev* 1972;52:129–197.
20. Spurway NC. Interrelationship between myosin-based and metabolism-based classification of skeletal muscle fibers. *J Histochem Cytochem* 1981;29:87–90.
21. Spurway NC. Objective characterization of cells in terms of microscopical parameters: an example from muscle histochemistry. *Histochem J* 1981;13:269–317.
22. Hamm TM, Nemeth PM, Solanki L, Gordon DA, Reinking RM, Stuart DG. Association between biochemical and physiological properties in single motor units. *Muscle Nerve* 1988;11:245–254.
23. Dahl HA, Roald L. How equivocal is the muscle fiber type concept? *Anat Embryol* 1991;184:269–273.
24. Torre M. Nombre et dimensions des unites dans les muscles extrinseques de l'oeil et, en general, dans les muscles squelettiques relies a des organes de sens. *Arch Suisses Neurol Psychiatry* 1953;72:362–376.
25. Buchthal F. The general concept of the motor unit. *Res Publs Assoc Res Nerv Ment Dis* 1961;38:1–30.
26. Feinstein B, Lindegard B, Nyman E, Wohlfart G. Morphologic studies of motor units in normal human muscle. *Acta Anat* 1955;23:127–142.
27. Tötösy de Zepetnek J, Zung HV, Erdebil S, Gordon T. Innervation ratio is an important determinant of force in normal and reinnervated rat tibialis anterior muscles. *J Neurophysiol* 1992;67:1385–1403.
28. Lucas SM, Ruff RL, Binder MD. Specific tension measurements in single soleus and medial gastrocnemius muscle fibers of the cat. *Exp Neurol* 1987;95:142–154.
29. Brooks SV, Faulkner JA. Contractile properties of skeletal muscles from young, adult and aged mice. *J Physiol (Lond)* 1988;404:71–82.
30. Galganski ME, Fuglevand AJ, Enoka RM. Reduced control of motor output in a human hand muscle of elderly subjects during submaximal contractions. *J Neurophysiol* 1993;69:2108–2115.
31. Rosenheimer JL. Ultraterminal sprouting in innervated and partially denervated adult and aged rat muscle. *Neuroscience* 1990;38:763–770.
32. Desypris G, Parry DJ. Relative efficacy of slow and fast motoneurons to reinnervate mouse soleus muscle. *Am J Physiol* 1990;258:C62–C70.
33. Kanda K, Hashizume K. Factors causing differences in force output among motor units in the rat medial gastrocnemius muscle. *J Neurophysiol* 1989;448:677–695.
34. Ishihara A, Araki H. Effects of age on the number and histochemical properties of muscle fibers and motoneurons in the rat extensor digitorum longus muscle. *Mech Ageing Dev* 1988;45:213–221.
35. Faulkner JA, Brooks SA. Muscle fatigue in old animals: unique aspects of fatigue in elderly human beings. In: Gandevia SC, Enoka RM, McComas AJ, Stuart DG, Thomas CK, eds. *Fatigue: neural and muscular mechanisms*. New York: Plenum, 1995.
36. Rafuse VF, Gordon T, Orozco R. Proportional enlargement of motor units after partial denervation of cat triceps surae muscles. *J Neurophysiol* 1992;68:1261–1276.
37. Gordon T, Yang JF, Ayer K, Tyreman N. Recovery potential of muscle after partial denervation: a comparison between rats and humans. *Brain Res Bull* 1993;30:477–482.
38. Dantes M, McComas J. The extent and time course of motoneuron involvement in amyotrophic lateral sclerosis. *Muscle Nerve* 1991;14:416–421.
39. Bromberg MB, Forshew DA, Nau KL, Bromberg J, Simmons Z, Fries TJ. Motor unit number estimation, isometric strength and electromyographic measures in amyotrophic lateral sclerosis. *Muscle Nerve* 1993;16:1213–1219.
40. Einarsson G, Grimby G, Stålberg E. Electromyographic and morphological functional compensation in late poliomyelitis. *Muscle Nerve* 1990;13:165–171.
41. Sinkjær T. Muscle, reflex and central components in the control of the ankle joint in healthy and spastic man. *Acta Neurol Scand* 1997;96 [Suppl 170]:3–28.
42. De Luca CJ, LeFever RS, McCue MP, Xenakis AP. Behaviour of human motor units in different muscles during linearly varying contractions. *J Physiol (Lond)* 1982;329:13–28.
43. Grimby L, Hannerz J. Firing rate and recruitment order of toe extensor motor units in different modes of voluntary contractions. *J Physiol (Lond)* 1977;264:865–879.
44. Kukulka CG, Clamann HP. Comparison of the recruitment and discharge properties of motor units in human brachial biceps and adductor pollicis during isometric contractions. *Brain Res* 1981;219:45–55.
45. Milner-Brown HS, Stein RB, Yemm R. Changes in firing rate of human motor units during linearly changing voluntary contractions. *J Physiol (Lond)* 1973;230:371–390.
46. Henneman E, Mendell LM. Functional organizations of motoneuronal pool and its input. In: Brooks VB, ed. *Handbook of physiology. Section 1. The nervous system. Vol. 2. Motor control*. Bethesda, MD: American Physiological Society, 1981:423–507.
47. Burke RE. Motor units: anatomy, physiology, and functional organization. In: Brooks VB, ed. *Handbook of physiology. Section 1. The nervous system. Vol. 2. Motor control*. Bethesda, MD: American Physiological Society, 1981:345–422.
48. Buchthal F, Schmalbruch H. Contraction times of twitches evoked by H-reflexes. *Acta Physiol Scand* 1970;80:378–382.
49. Person RS. Rhythmic activity of a group of human motoneurones during voluntary contraction of a muscle. *Electroencephalogr Clin Neurophysiol* 1974;36:585–595.
50. Thomas JS, Schmidt EM, Hambrecht FT. Facility of motor unit control during tasks defined in terms of unit behaviours. *Exp Neurol* 1978;59:384–395.
51. Desmedt JE, Godaux E. Ballistic contractions in man. Characteristic recruitment pattern of single motor units of the tibialis anterior muscle. *J Physiol (Lond)* 1977;264:673–693.
52. Desmedt JE, Godaux E. Spinal motoneuron recruitment in man. Rank deordering with direction but not with speed of voluntary movement. *Science* 1981;214:933–936.
53. Hannerz J. Discharge properties of motor units in relation to recruitment order in voluntary contraction. *Acta Physiol Scand* 1974;91:374–384.

54. Kanda K, Burke RE, Walmsley B. Differential control of fast and slow twitch motor units in the decerebrate cat. *Exp Brain Res* 1977;29:57–74.

55. Powers RK, Rymer WZ. Effects of acute dorsal spinal hemisection on motoneuron discharge in the medial gastrocnemius of the decerebrate cat. *J Neurophysiol* 1988;59:1540–1556.

56. Glendinning DS, Enoka RM. Motor unit behaviour in Parkinson's disease. *Phys Ther* 1994;74:61–70.

57. Gilson AS, Mills WB. Activities of single motor units in man during slight voluntary efforts. *Am J Physiol* 1941;133:658–669.

58. Masland WS, Sheldon D, Hershey CD. The stochastic properties of individual motor unit interspike intervals. *Am J Physiol* 1969;217:1384–1388.

59. Edwards RG, Lippold OC. The relation between force and integrated electrical activity in fatigued muscle. *J Physiol (Lond)* 1956;132:677–681.

60. Vredenbregt J, Rau G. Surface electromyography in relation to force, muscle length and endurance. In: Desmedt JE, ed. *New developments in electromyography and clinical neurophysiology.* Vol. 1. Basel: Karger, 1973:607–622.

61. De Luca CJ, Forrest WJ. Probability distribution function of the inter-pulse intervals of single motor unit action potential during isometric contraction. In: Desmedt JE, ed. *New developments in electromyography and clinical neurophysiology.* Vol. 1. Basel: Karger, 1973:638–647.

62. De Luca CJ, Forrest WJ. Some properties of motor unit action potential trains recorded during constant force isometric contractions in man. *Kybernetik* 1973;12:160–168.

63. Petajan JH, Phillip BA. Frequency control of motor unit action potentials. *Electroencephalogr Clin Neurophysiol* 1969;27:66–72.

64. Petajan JH. Clinical electromyographic studies of diseases of the motor unit. *Electroencephalogr Clin Neurophysiol* 1974;36:395–401.

65. Petajan JH. Motor unit frequency control in normal man. In: Desmedt JE, ed. *Motor unit types, recruitment and plasticity in health and disease. Progress in clinics neurophysiology.* Vol. 9. Basel: Karger, 1981:184–200.

66. Kudina LP, Alexeeva NP. After-potential and control of repetitive firing in human motoneurones. *Electroencephalogr Clin Neurophysiol* 1992;85:345–353.

67. Macefield VG, Gandevia SC, Bigland-Ritchie B, Gorman RB, Burke D. The firing rates of human motoneurones voluntarily activated in the absence of muscle afferents feedback. *J Physiol (Lond)* 1993;471:429–443.

68. Monster AW, Chan H. Isometric force production by motor units of extensor digitorum communis muscle in man. *J Neurophysiol* 1977;40:1432–1443.

69. Tanji J, Kato M. Firing rate of individual motor units in voluntary contraction of abductor digiti minimi muscle in man. *Exp Neurol* 1973;40:771–783.

70. Freund HJ, Budingen HJ, Dietz V. Activity of single motor units from human forearm muscles during voluntary isometric contractions. *J Neurophysiol* 1975;38:933–946.

71. Marsden CD, Meadows JC, Merton PA. Isolated single motor units in human muscle and their rate of discharge during maximal voluntary effort. *J Physiol (Lond)* 1971;217:12–13.

72. Gydikov A, Kosarov D. Some features of different motor units in human biceps brachii. *Pflugers Arch* 1974;347:75–88.

73. McComas AJ, Fawcett PRW, Campbell MJ, Sica REP. Electrophysiological estimation of the number of motor units within a human muscle. *J Neurol Neurosurg Psychiatry* 1971;34:121–131.

74. Brown WF. A method for estimating the number of motor units in thenar muscles and the change in motor unit count with aging. *J Neurol Neurosurg Psychiatry* 1972;35:845–852.

75. Sica REP, McComas AJ, Upton ARM. Motor unit estimation in small muscles of the hand. *J Neurol Neurosurg Psychiatry* 1974;37:55–67.

76. Ballantyne JP, Hansen S. Computer method for the analysis of evoked motor unit potential. *J Neurol Neurosurg Psychiatry* 1974;37:1187–1194.

77. Milner-Brown HS, Brown WF. New methods of estimating the number of motor units in a muscle. *J Neurol Neurosurg Psychiatry* 1976;39:258–265.

78. Galea V, deBruin H, Cavasin R, McComas AJ. The numbers and relative sizes of motor unit estimated by computer. *Muscle Nerve* 1991;14:1123–1130.

79. Kadrie HA, Yates SK, Milner-Brown HS, Brown WF. Multiple point electrical stimulation of ulnar and median nerves. *J Neurol Neurosurg Psychiatry* 1976;39:973–985.

80. Doherty TJ, Brown WF. The estimated numbers and relative sizes of thenar motor units as selected by multiple point stimulation in young and older adults. *Muscle Nerve* 1993;16:355–366.

81. Stashuk DW, Doherty TJ, Brown WF. Automatic analysis of F-responses. New methods for deriving motor unit estimates and analyzing relative latencies and conduction velocities in single motor fibres. *Muscle Nerve* 1992;15:1204–1205.

82. Stashuk DW, Doherty TJ, Kassam A, Brown WF. Motor unit estimates based on automated analysis of F responses. *Muscle Nerve* 1994;17:881–890.

83. Doherty TJ. Physiological properties of single thenar motor units in the F response of younger and older adults. *Muscle Nerve* 1994;17:860–872.

84. Lee RG, Ashby P, White DG, Aguayo A. Analysis of motor conduction velocity in the human median nerve by computer simulation of compound muscle action potentials. *Electroencephalogr Clin Neurophysiol* 1975;39:225–237.

85. Brown WF, Strong MJ, Snow RS. Methods for estimating numbers of motor units in biceps-brachialis muscles and losses of motor unit with aging. *Muscle Nerve* 1988;11:423–432.

86. Stein RB, Yang JF. Methods for estimating the number of motor units in human muscles. *Ann Neurol* 1990;28:487–495.

87. Wray SH. Innervation ratios for large and small limb muscles in the baboon. *J Comp Neurol* 1969;137:227–250.

88. Daube JR. Estimating the number of motor units in a muscle. *J Clin Neurophysiol* 1995;12:585–594.

89. Stashuk D, Brown WF. Decomposition enhanced spiked triggered averaging: an improved method for estimating motor unit numbers in proximal muscle. *Muscle Nerve* 1994;17:1098(abst).

90. Scarpalezos S, Panayiotopoulos CP. Myopathy or neuropathy in thyrotoxicosis. *N Engl J Med* 1973;289:918–919.

91. McComas AJ, Sica REP, Brandstater ME. Further motor unit studies in Duchenne muscular dystrophy. *J Neurol Neurosurg Psychiatry* 1977;40:1147–1151.

92. Doherty TJ, Simmons Z et al. Methods for estimating the numbers of motor units in human muscles. *J Clin Neurophysiol* 1995;12:565–584.

93. Felice KJ. Thenar motor unit number estimates using the multiple point stimulation technique: reproducibility studies in ALS patients and normal subjects. *Muscle Nerve* 1995;18:1412–1416.

94. Boyd IA, Davey MR. *Composition of peripheral nerves.* Edinburgh: Churchill Livingstone, 1968.

95. Guld C. On the influence of measuring electrodes duration and amplitude of muscle action potentials. *Acta Physiol Scand* 1951;25:30–32.

96. Buchthal F, Pinelli P. Muscle action potentials in polymyositis. *Neurology* 1953;3:424–436.

97. Rosenfalck P, Rosenfalck A. *Electromyography-sensory and motor conduction. Findings in normal subjects.* Copenhagen: Laboratory of Clinical Neurophysiology, Rigshospitalet, 1975:1–49.

98. Lang AH, Vaahtoranta K. The baseline, the time characteristics and the slow afterwaves of the motor unit potential. *Electroencephalogr Clin Neurophysiol* 1973;35:387–394.

99. Thage O. Quadriceps weakness and wasting. Copenhagen FADLs forlag, 1974:1–132.

100. Buchthal F. Electromyography in the evaluation of muscle diseases. *Methods Clin Neurophysiol* 1991;2:25–45.

101. Denny-Brown D. Interpretation of the electromyogram. *Arch Neurol Psychiatry* 1949;61:99–128.

102. Takahashi K. The coupling discharge in neurogenic muscular atrophy. *Arch Neurol* 1966;14:617–623.

103. Desmedt JE, Borenstein S. Collateral reinnervation of muscle fibre by motor axons of dystrophic motor units. *Nature* 1973;246:500–501.

104. Buchthal F, Rosenfalck P. On the structure of motor units. In: Desmedt J, ed. *New developments in electromyography and clinical neurophysiology.* Vol. 1. Basel: Karger, 1973:71–85.

105. Lang AH, Partanen I. Satellite potentials and the duration of potentials in normal, neuropathic and myopathic muscles. *J Neurol Sci* 1976;27:513–525.

106. Kosarov D, Gydikov A. The influence of volume conduction on the shape of action potentials recorded by various types of needle electrodes in normal human muscles. *Electromyogr Clin Neurophysiol* 1970;333:319–325.

107. Gydikov A, Kosarov D. Extraterritorial potential field of impulses

from separate motor units in human muscles. *Electromyogr Clin Neurophysiol* 1972;12:283–305.

108. Buchthal F, Rosenfalck P. Action potential parameters in different human muscles. *Acta Physiol Scand* 1955;30:125–131.

109. Nandedkar S, Sanders D, Stålberg E. Selectivity of the EMG recording techniques: a simulation study. *Med Biol Eng Comput* 1985;23:536–540.

110. Nandedkar S, Stålberg E, Sanders D. Simulation techniques in electromyography. *IEEE Trans Biomed Eng* 1985;32:775–785.

111. Andreassen S, Jørgensen N. A model for the motor unit potential. *Electroencephalogr Clin Neurophysiol* 1981;52:1163.

112. Nandedkar S, Sanders D, Stålberg E, Andreassen S. Simulation of concentric needle EMG motor unit action potential. *Muscle Nerve* 1988;2:151–159.

113. Stålberg E, Andreassen A, Falck B, Lang H, Rosenfalck A, Trojaborg W. Quantitative analysis of individual motor unit potentials—a proposition for standardized terminology and criteria for measurements. *J Clin Neurophysiol* 1986;3:313–348.

114. Buchthal F. Electromyography. In: Remond A, ed. *Handbook of electroencephalography and clinical neurophysiology*. Amsterdam: Elsevier, 1976.

115. Buchthal F. Electrophysiological signs of myopathy as related with muscle biopsy. *Acta Neurol* 1977;32:1–29.

116. Buchthal F. Electromyography in evaluation of muscle diseases. In: Aminoff MJ, ed. *Neurologic clinics*. Philadelphia: W.B. Saunders, 1985:573–598.

117. Buchthal F. *An introduction to electromyography*. Copenhagen: Gyldendal, 1957:1–43.

118. Kohara N, Kaji R, Kimura J. Comparison of recording characteristics of monopolar and concentric needle electrodes. *Electroencephalogr Clin Neurophysiol* 1993;89:242–246.

119. Buchthal F, Guld C, Rosenfalck P. Action potential parameters in normal muscle and their dependence on physical variables. *Acta Physiol Scand* 1954;32:200–218.

120. AAEM glossary. *Muscle Nerve* 1987;10:8S.

121. International Federation of Societies for Electroencephalography and Clinical Neurophysiology. *Recommendations for the practice of clinical neurophysiology*. Amsterdam: Elsevier, 1983:143.

122. Barkhaus P, Nandedkar S. On the selection of concentric needle electromyogram motor unit action potentials: is the rise time criterion too restrictive? *Muscle Nerve* 1996;19:1554–1560.

123. Trojaborg W. Quantitative electromyography in polymyositis: a reappraisal. *Muscle Nerve* 1990;13:964–971.

124. Stålberg E, Sonoo M. Assessment of variability in the shape of the motor unit action potential, the "jiggle", at consecutive discharges. *Muscle Nerve* 1994;17:1135–1144.

125. Young RR, Hagbarth KE. Physiological tremor enhanced by manoeuvres affecting the segmental stretch reflex. *J Neurol Neurosurg Psychiatry* 1980;43:248–256.

126. Halonen JP, Falck B, Kalimo H. The firing rate of motor units in neuromuscular disorders. *J Neurol* 1981;225:269–276.

127. Dietz V, Freund HJ. Entladungsverhalten einzelner motorischer Einheiten bei uramischen Patienten. Ein Beitrag zur Frühdiagnose demyelinisierender Polyneuropathien. *J Neurol* 1974;207:255–269.

128. Miller RG, Sherrat M. Firing rates of human motor units in partially denervated muscle. *Neurology* 1978;28:1241–1248.

129. Freund HJ, Dietz V, Wita CW, Kapp H. Discharge characteristics of single motor units in normal subjects and patients with supraspinal motor disturbances. In: Desmedt JE, ed. *New developments in electromyography and clinical neurophysiology*. Vol. 1. Basel: Karger, 1973:242–250.

130. Rosenfalck A, Andreassen S. Impaired regulation of force and firing pattern of single motor units in patients with spasticity. *J Neurol Neurosurg Psychiatry* 1980;43:907–916.

131. Young RR, Shahani BT. A clinical neurophysiological analysis of single motor unit discharge patterns in spasticity. In: Feldman RG, Young RR, Koella WP, eds. *Spasticity: disordered motor control*. Chicago: Year Book Medical Publishers, 1980:219–231.

132. Buchthal F, Pinelli P, Rosenfalck P. Action potentials parameters in normal human muscles and their physiological determinants. *Acta Physiol Scand* 1954;32:219–229.

133. Sacco G, Buchthal P, Rosenfalck P. Motor unit potentials at different ages. *Arch Neurol* 1962;6:44–51.

134. Howard J, McGill C, Dorfman L. Age effects on properties of motor unit action potentials: ADEMG analysis. *Ann Neurol* 1988;24:207–213.

135. Bischoff C, Machetanz J, Conrad B. Is there an age-dependent continuous increase in the duration of the motor unit action potentials? *Electroencephalogr Clin Neurophysiol* 1991;81:304–311.

136. Barker D, Ip MC. Sprouting and degeneration of mammalian motor axons in normal and deafferentated skeletal muscle. *Proc R Soc B* 1966;163:538–554.

137. Tomlinson BE, Irving D. The numbers of limb motor neurons in the human lumbosacral cord throughout the life. *J Neurol Sci* 1977;34:213–219.

138. Stålberg E, Thiele B. Motor units fibre density in the extensor digitorum communis muscle. *J Neurol Neurosurg Psychiatry* 1975;38:874–880.

139. Roos MR, Rice CL, Vandervoort AA. Age-related changes in motor unit function. *Muscle Nerve* 1997;20:679–690.

140. Tackmann W, Vogel P. Zur Abhangigkeit der Muskelaktionspotentialdauer von der intramuskularen Temperatur. *Z EEG-EMG* 1987;8:72–75.

141. Bertram M, Nishida T, Minieka M, Janssen I, Levy C. Effects of temperature on motor unit action potentials during isometric contraction. *Muscle Nerve* 1995;18:1443–1446.

142. Buchthal F, Erminio F, Rosenfalck P. Motor unit territory in different human muscles. *Acta Physiol Scand* 1959;45:72–87.

143. Kugelberg E, Edström L, Abbruzzese M. Mapping of motor units in experimentally reinnervated rat muscle. *J Neurol Neurosurg Psychiatry* 1970;33:319–329.

144. Buchthal F, Rosenfalck G, Erminio F. Motor unit and fiber density in myopathies. *Neurology* 1960;10:389–408.

145. Erminio F, Buchthal F, Rosenfalck P. Motor unit territory and muscle fiber concentration in paresis due to peripheral nerve injury and anterior horn cell involvement. *Neurology* 1959;9:657–671.

146. Stålberg E, Schwartz MS, Thiele B, Schiller HH. The normal motor unit in man. A single fiber EMG multielectrode investigation. *J Neurol Sci* 1976;27:291–301.

147. Stålberg E, Antoni L. Electrophysiological cross-section of the motor unit. *J Neurol Neurosurg Psychiatry* 1980;43:469–474.

148. Stålberg E, Dioszeghy P. Scanning EMG in normal muscle and in neuromuscular disorders. *Electroencephalogr Clin Neurophysiol* 1991;81:403–416.

149. Stålberg E. Macro EMG, a new recording technique. *J Neurol Neurosurg Psychiatry* 1980;43:475–482.

150. Stålberg E, Fawcett PR. Macro EMG in healthy subjects of different ages. *J Neurol Neurosurg Psychiatry* 1982;45:870–878.

151. Nandedkar SD, Stålberg E. Simulation of macro EMG motor unit potentials. *Electroencephalogr Clin Neurophysiol* 1983;56:52–62.

152. Nandedkar SD, Stålberg E, Kim YI, et al. Use of signal representation to identify abnormal motor unit potentials in macro EMG. *IEEE Trans Biomed Eng* 1984;31:220–227.

153. Hilton-Brown P, Nandedkar SD, Stålberg E. Simulation of fibre density in single-fiber electromyography and its relationship to macro-EMG. *Med Biol Eng Comp* 1985;23:541–546.

154. Jabre JF. Concentric macro electromyography. *Muscle Nerve* 1991;14:820–825.

155. Hilton-Brown P, Stålberg E. Motor unit size in muscular dystrophy, a macro EMG and scanning EMG study. *J Neurol Neurosurg Psychiatry* 1983;46:996–1005.

156. Masuda T, Sadoyama T. The propagation of single motor unit potential detected by a surface electrode array. *Electroencephalogr Clin Neurophysiol* 1986;63:590–598.

157. Schneider J, Rau G, Silny J. A noninvasive EMG technique for investigating the excitation propagation in single motor units. *Electromyogr Clin Neurophysiol* 1989;22:385–400.

158. Merletti R, De Luca CJ. New techniques in surface electromyography. In: Desmedt JE, ed. *Computer-aided electromyography and expert systems*. Amsterdam: Elsevier, 1989:115–124.

159. Blok J, Stegeman D, van Dijk H, Drost G, Zwarts M. Single motor unit analysis from surface EMG topography. *Electroencephalogr Clin Neurophysiol* 1997;103:220(abst).

160. Stålberg E, Bischoff C, Falck B. Outliers, a way to detect abnormality in quantitative EMG. *Muscle Nerve* 1994;17:392–399.

161. Andreassen S. Methods for computer-aided measurement of motor unit parameters. In: Ellington RJ, Murray NMF, Halliday AM, eds. *The London symposia* (EEG Suppl 39). New York: Elsevier, 1987:13–20.

162. Stålberg E, Falck B, Sonoo M, Åström M. Multi-MUP EMG analysis—a two year experience with a quantitative method in daily routine. *Electroencephalogr Clin Neurophysiol* 1994;97:145–154.

163. Nandedkar S, Barkhaus P, Charles A. Multi-motor unit action potential analysis (MMA). *Muscle Nerve* 1995;18:1155–1166.
164. Bischoff C, Stålberg E, Falck B, Edebol Eeg-Olofsson K. Reference values of motor unit action potentials obtained with multi-MUAP analysis. *Muscle Nerve* 1994;17:842–851.
165. McGill KC, Dorfman L. Automatic EMG decomposition in brachial biceps. *Electroencephalogr Clin Neurophysiol* 1985;61:1453–1461.
166. Haas WF, Mayer M. An automatic EMG decomposition system for routine clinical examinations and clinical research (ARTMUP). In: Desmedt JE, ed. *Computer-aided electromyography and expert systems*. Amsterdam: Elsevier, 1989:67–81.
167. Stashuk D, Qu Y. Adaptive motor unit action potential clustering using shape and temporal information. *Med Biol Eng Comput* 1996;34:41–49.
168. Etawil H, Stashuk D. Resolving superimposed motor unit action potentials. *Med Biol Eng Comput* 1996;34:33–40.
169. Stashuk D, Qu Y. Robust method for estimating motor unit firing-pattern statistics. *Med Biol Eng Comput* 1996;34:50–57.
170. Nikolic M, Sørensen AJ, Dahl K, Krarup C. Detailed analysis of motor unit activity. 19th Annual International Conference of the IEEE Engineering in Medicine and Biology Society, Chicago, 1997:123.
171. LeFever RS, DeLuca CJ. A procedure for decomposing myoelectric signal into its constituent action potentials. *IEEE Trans BME* 1982;29: 149–162.
172. Willison RG. Analysis of electrical activity in healthy and dystrophic muscle in man. *J Neurol Neurosurg Psychiatry* 1964;27:386–394.
173. Fitch P. An analyser for use in human electromyography. *Electron Eng* 1967;39:240–243.
174. Fuglsang-Frederiksen A, Månsson A. Analysis of electrical activity of normal muscle in man at different degrees of voluntary effort. *J Neurol Neurosurg Psychiatry* 1975;38:683–694.
175. Fuglsang-Frederiksen A, Scheel U, Buchthal F. Diagnostic yield of analysis of the pattern of electrical activity and of individual motor unit potentials in myopathy. *J Neurol Neurosurg Psychiatry* 1976;39: 742–750.
176. Fuglsang-Frederiksen A, Scheel U, Buchthal F. Diagnostic yield of analysis of the pattern of electrical activity of muscle and individual motor unit potentials in neurogenic involvement. *J Neurol Neurosurg Psychiatry* 1977;40:544–554.
177. Fuglsang-Frederiksen A, Månsson A. Pattern of electrical activity during moderate effort and properties of motor unit potentials sampled during weak effort in progressive muscular dystrophy. *Electroencephalogr Clin Neurophysiol* 1974;36:576.
178. Serra C, Rossi A, Mozzillo A, Ruocco A, Facciolla D, Biondi A. Quantitative EMG and EEG findings in patients exposed to chronic intoxication from industrial adhesives. *Acta Neurol (Napoli)* 1980;35: 276–284.
179. Smyth DPL. Quantitative electromyography in babies and young children with primary muscle disease and neurogenic lesions. *J Neurol Sci* 1982;56:199–207.
180. Cruz Martinez A, Ferrer MT, Perez Conde MC. Automatic analysis of the electromyogram. 2. Studies in patients with primary muscle disease and neurogenic involvement. Comparison of diagnostic yields versus individual motor unit parameters. *Electromyogr Clin Neurophysiol* 1984;24:17–38.
181. Gilchrist JM, Nandedkar SD, Stewart CS, Massey JM, Sanders DB, Barkhaus PE. Automatic analysis of the electromyographic interference pattern using the turns:amplitude ratio. *Electroencephalogr Clin Neurophysiol* 1988;70:534–540.
182. Dowling MH, Fitch P, Willison RG. A special purpose digital computer (Biomac 500) used in the analysis of the human electromyogram. *Electroencephalogr Clin Neurophysiol* 1968;25:570–573.
183. Fuglsang-Frederiksen A. Electrical activity and force during voluntary contraction of normal and diseased muscles. *Acta Neurol Scand* 1981; 63[Suppl 83]:1–60.
184. Fuglsang-Frederiksen A, Dahl K, Lo Monaco M. Electrical muscle activity during a gradual increase in force in patients with neuromuscular diseases. *Electroencephalogr Clin Neurophysiol* 1984;57:320–329.
185. Fuglsang-Frederiksen A, Lo Monaco M, Dahl K. Integrated electrical activity and number of zero crossing during a gradual increase in muscle force in patients with neuromuscular diseases. *Electroencephalogr Clin Neurophysiol* 1984;58:211–219.
186. Stålberg E, Chu J, Bril V, Nandedkar S, Stålberg S, Ericsson M. Automatic analysis of the EMG interference pattern. *Electroencephalogr Clin Neurophysiol* 1983;56:672–681.
187. Liguori R, Dahl K, Vingtoft S, Fuglsang-Frederiksen A. Determination of peak-ratio by digital turns-amplitude analysis on line. *Electromyogr Clin Neurophysiol* 1990;30:371–378.
188. Liguori R, Dahl K, Fuglsang-Frederiksen A. Turns-amplitude analysis of the electromyographic recruitment pattern disregarding force measurement. I. Method and reference values in healthy subjects. *Muscle Nerve* 1992;15:1314–1318.
189. Liguori R, Dahl K, Fuglsang-Frederiksen A, Trojaborg W. Turns-amplitude analysis of the electromyographic recruitment pattern disregarding force measurement. II. Findings in patients with neuromuscular disorders. *Muscle Nerve* 1992;15:1319–1324.
190. Rønager J, Christensen H, Fuglsang-Frederiksen A. Power spectrum of the EMG pattern in normal and diseased muscles. *J Neurol Sci* 1989;94:283–294.
191. Fuglsang-Frederiksen A, Rønager J. EMG power spectrum, turns-amplitude analysis and motor unit potential duration in neuromuscular disorders. 1990;97:81–91.
192. Buchthal F, Kamieniecka Z. The diagnostic yield of quantified electromyography and quantified muscle biopsy in neuromuscular disorders. *Muscle Nerve* 1982;5:265–280.

Motor Disorders,
edited by David S. Younger.
Lippincott Williams & Wilkins, Philadelphia © 1999.

CHAPTER 4

Neurophysiology of Clinical Motor Control

Samer D. Tabbal and Seth L. Pullman

In this chapter we present an overview of clinically relevant issues in the physiology of motor control. Anatomic structures and pathways, pathophysiology, and clinical phenomenology are described within the context of motor control and behavior in a select number of representative movement disorders. This is not intended to be exhaustive but rather a delineation of the basic principles and current understanding of motor disorders. We specifically provide an overview of key anatomic pathways, Parkinson disease (PD) and the theories underlying current surgical approaches to treatment, some hyperkinetic syndromes, dystonia, tremor, myoclonus, and gait and postural abnormalities.

ANATOMY OF KEY PATHWAYS INVOLVED IN MOTOR CONTROL

The cortex, basal ganglia, thalamus, cerebellum, and brainstem function together to influence directly and indirectly the behavior of the motor unit, the final common pathway from the spinal cord (Fig. 1). Motor control is achieved through the integration and modulation of these interconnecting pathways on the thousands of motor neurons and interneurons at each level of the spinal cord. The motor unit and all its associated muscle fibers, tendon, bones, and joints ultimately work together to produce movement or isometric force. What follows is a brief description of the critical pathways involved in motor control.

The *corticospinal tract* originates from the motor cortex (Brodmann area 4), the premotor cortex (Brodmann area 6), and the parietal cortex (somatic sensory areas 3, 1, and 2) at a ratio of about 3:3:4, respectively. These glut-

aminergic fibers travel through the posterior internal capsule into the brainstem, forming the pyramids. They adopt a somatotopic arrangement in the spinal cord with ventromedial subdivisions projecting onto spinal motor neurons and interneurons to innervate axial and proximal muscles; dorsolateral subdivisions project onto the dorsolateral motor neuron and interneuron pools that innervate limb muscles. Corticospinal tract fibers originating from the primary somatic sensory of the parietal cortex project primarily onto the dorsal horn of the spinal cord. Corticobulbar fibers originating in a similar somatotopic pattern project to nuclei of the brainstem, dorsal columns, and pons that project in turn to the cerebellum.

The *basal ganglia* play a major role in motor control through dozens of parallel and interconnected pathways. In particular, they impart upon the ventrolateral (VL) and ventroanterior (VA) nuclei of the thalamus. The internal globus pallidus (GPi) and the substantia nigra pars reticulata (SNr) are the major basal ganglia output relay stations ultimately influencing primary motor and premotor areas and the brainstem. Complex models of corticobasal ganglia thalamocortical circuits have been proposed (Fig. 2), and several have proven to be useful in predicting clinical syndromes and therapeutic outcomes (Fig. 3) (1,2). Two GABAergic striatonigral circuits converge on the Gpi/SNr in one model to inhibit the VL/VA nuclei of the thalamus, which in turn facilitate the generation of forces or movement.

The first is a direct pathway in which cortically initiated stimulation of a subset of putaminal GABAergic neurons carrying D1 receptors inhibit the GPi/SNr. This relieves the VL/VA from the GPi/SNr-generated inhibition, consequently promoting movement and contributing a positive feedback loop. An indirect pathway is a multisynaptic circuit that begins with cortically initiated stimulation of other putaminal GABAergic neurons carrying D2 receptors that inhibit the external globus pallidus (GPe). This reduces GABAergic GPe-generated inhibition on the subthalamic nuclei (STN). Unopposed,

S.D. Tabbal: Columbia University College of Physicians and Surgeons and Department of Neurology, Neurological Institute, New York Presbyterian Hospital, New York, New York 10032.

S.L. Pullman: Neurological Institute, New York Presbyterian Hospital, New York, New York 10032.

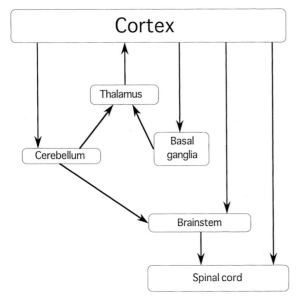

FIG. 1. The parallel projections of the cortex to multiple levels of the motor system, including two parallel reentrant systems (cortex-cerebellum thalamus cortex and cortex-basal ganglia-thalamus-cortex).

the STN stimulates the GPi/SNr, which consequently inhibit the VL/VA nuclei of the thalamus. The GPe has a direct inhibitory connection to the Gpi/SNr, and when the GPe is inhibited by the activation of the indirect pathway, the GPi/SNr is also relieved from the GPe-generated inhibition, so promoting further inhibition of the VL/VA. The inhibition of the thalamic nuclei by the two arms of the indirect pathway suppresses the genera-

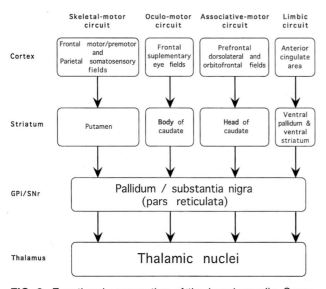

FIG. 2. Functional segregation of the basal ganglia. Somatotopy is maintained in the GPi/SNr and in the thalamus; the later projects back to the cortex.

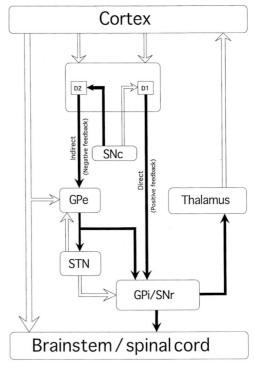

FIG. 3. Functional basal ganglia anatomy of movement disorders. The white arrows indicate glutaminergic excitatory effects, whereas the black arrows indicate GABAergic inhibitory effects. Cortically initiated activation of both pathways results in a net inhibition of the GPi/SNr through the direct pathway and a net facilitation of the GPi/SNr through the indirect pathway. The former results in increased movement (positive feedback to the cortex due to inhibition of inhibitory influences) and the latter results in decreased movement (negative feedback to the cortex). SNc stimulation, however, facilitates movements through its effect on both pathways, namely, the activation of the direct (positive feedback) pathway and the inhibition of the indirect (negative feedback) pathway. Conversely, the decreased SNc influences, as occurs in Parkinson disease, and inhibits the generation of movement.

tion of movement by the cortex that can be considered a negative feedback loop.

Preponderance of the activity of the direct positive feedback pathway predisposes to a *hyperkinetic* state, whereas greater activity of the indirect negative feedback pathway predisposes to a *hypokinetic* state. Under normal conditions, the direct and the indirect pathways are in balance ensuring normal motor control. This balance is consolidated further by multiple feedback circuits, in particular cortical excitatory input to the STN and STN excitatory feedback inputs into the GPe and putamen. In contrast to cortically initiated stimulation of the two striatonigral pathways, nigral (SNc) stimulation promotes activation of the direct pathway via D1 receptors carrying putaminal neurons and inhibition of the indirect pathway via the D2 receptor carrying putaminal neurons, both of which enhance increased force generation or movement.

D1 and D2 receptors are located along the dendritic spines and shafts of medium-sized spiny putaminal neurons (MSN), whereas corticostriatal glutaminergic synapses are located almost exclusively on the head of the dendritic spines, so allowing for the modulation of corticostriatal transmission. Putaminal MSN have been the subject of extensive investigation given their critical location in the basal ganglia circuit. They represent 80% to 90% of putaminal neurons and have an extrinsic dopaminergic innervation (from the SNc). Two populations of putaminal dopaminergic neurons have been recently identified (3): abundant 5-μm neurons that lack dendritic spines and 10- to 12-μm neurons with numerous dendritic spines. These neurons are dramatically unregulated in 1-methyl-4-phenyl-1-1,2,3,6-tetrahydropyridine (MPTP) induced parkinsonian monkeys. The clinical significance of these neurons remains uncertain, although it has been speculated that their degeneration may have a role in the delayed development of dyskinesia and motor fluctuations, one of the common complications of chronic L-dopa treatment in PD. Another observation of unclear clinical significance is the exclusive presence of substance P in D1 receptor containing MSN and of Met-enkephalin in the D2 receptor containing MSN. N-methyl-D-aspartate (NMDA) receptors also have been implicated in the activity-dependent synaptic plasticity of the basal ganglia (4).

Efferent pathways of the *cerebellum* indirectly affect the motor output through the VL thalamus and the red nucleus before modulating higher cortical activity. Afferent cerebellar pathways influence motor control through the dorsal spinocerebellar tract along the inferior cerebellar peduncle from pontine nuclei and the middle cerebellar peduncle. They convey information about ongoing movements and are processed in a local synaptic relays that eventuates on the Purkinje cells. It communicates with a burst of excitation in deep cerebellar nuclei followed by Purkinje cell-mediated inhibition. The output of the deep cerebellar nuclei along the superior cerebellar peduncle influences the VL and the red nucleus, generating a complex pattern of muscle activation devoid of motor overshoot. The cerebellum also plays important roles in planning, motor learning, and as a comparator of actual with intended movements.

Descending pathways from the brainstem are the most primitive phylogenic motor pathways. Critical descending pathways in motor control belong to the ventromedial and dorsolateral pathway groups. The ventromedial pathway includes the reticulospinal tract originating from the reticular formation in the medulla and pons, the lateral and medial vestibulospinal tracts originating from the lateral and medial vestibular nucle, and the tectospinal tract originating from the tectum and superior colliculi. The fibers of these pathways project bilaterally and widely over disparate segments of the spinal cord and synapse on motor neurons and interneurons, including long priospinal neurons that control proximal and axial muscles. These tracts provide gross postural adjustments, especially by the reticulospinal tract, and head control and eye movement coordination, particularly by the tectospinal tract. The reticulospinal pathways have been shown to be critical in the generation of the startle response to sudden and intense acoustic stimuli (5). The ventromedial pathways receive multiple input from the interstitial nucleus of Cajal, the serotonergic raphe, and the noradrenergic locus ceruleus nuclei.

Dorsolateral pathways include the rubrospinal and rubrobulbar fibers. The former originates from the magnocellular red nucleus and projects onto dorsolateral motor neurons and interneurons of a small number of spinal segments. These neurons innervate the muscle of the limbs in parallel to the dorsolateral division of the corticospinal tract. Similarly, the rubrobulbar fibers project to the facial nuclei, the sensory trigeminal nuclei, and the cuneate and gracile dorsal column nuclei.

The *spinal cord* has interconnected segmental circuits consisting of motor and sensory neurons, and hundreds of thousands of interneurons at each level that mediate virtually all reflexes below the neck and establish the fundamental network that initiates the synergy of basic movement. Injections of spinal cord axons with anatomic tracers show that corticospinal neurons and spinal motor neurons have a connection pattern that is somatotopically both convergent and divergent; namely, a corticospinal neuron synapses on several motor neurons and an individual motor neuron receives projections from several corticospinal neurons (6). This arrangement ensures synchrony and balance between neighboring motor neurons that innervate muscle fibers of functionally related muscles.

CLINICAL DISORDERS OF MOTOR CONTROL

Parkinson Disease and Related Syndromes

In 1957, Carlsson et al. (7) demonstrated that reserpine caused an akinetic-rigid parkinsonian syndrome that could be reversed by dopamine. Three years later, Ehringer and Hornykiewicz (8) discovered that PD was a state of profound dopamine deficiency in the brain and later attributed it to degeneration of the substantia nigra (SNc). The reduction in striatal dopamine results in a preponderance of indirect D2 receptor-mediated pathway activity (Fig. 4) and partly explains the bradykinesia and rigidity seen in PD and experimentally lesioned animals and humans (9–12), including electrophysiologic studies performed on patients with PD during therapeutic stereotactic lesioning of basal ganglia output structures. These studies confirm that the neuronal discharge rates in GPi are increased compared with the GPe (13). The clinical improvement achieved after a GPi lesion (14–16) and after the presumed inactivation of STN by high-frequency stimulation (17) lends credence to this model. Stereotactic pallidotomy partly reverses the

A

B

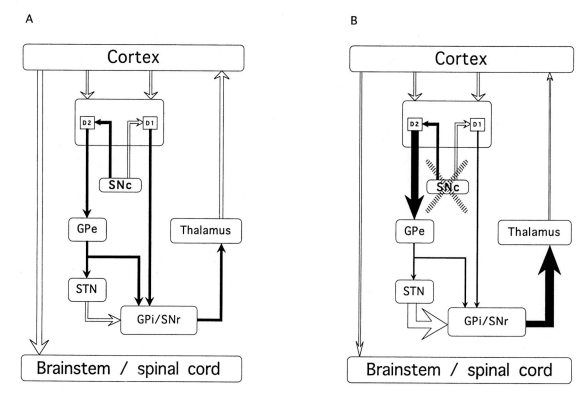

FIG. 4. Changes in basal ganglia circuitry in **(A)** the normal state compared with **(B)** Parkinson disease.

lack of cortical activation attributed to excessive GPi/SNr outflow demonstrated by positron emission tomography studies in PD patients (17–19).

The hypokinetic state model presented in Fig. 4 may be overly simplistic to explain other observations. For instance, inhibition of the thalamocortical neurons via GPi/SNr feedback inhibition causes akinesia, whereas lesions at the area where the VL/VA thalamic nuclei receive their input from the basal ganglia do not (20). This suggests that lesions in other parts of the circuit also contribute to the pathophysiology of akinesia. It is not clear whether parkinsonian symptoms are due to the absolute increase in firing rate or to an abnormal firing pattern of the GPi/SNr (21). The latter explanation would explain how a lesion in the GPi could cause both amelioration of dyskinesia or excessive movement associated with reduced activity of the GPi and bradykinesia/rigidity in PD or a paucity of movement associated with increased activity of the GPi. It is likely that dyskinesia and bradykinesia are worsened by an abnormal firing pattern of the GPi/SNr rather than by an abnormal firing rate because pallidotomy improves both. Indeed, there is no doubt that PD affects multiple cortical and subcortical structures (22–24) that are critical in motor control, including those in the cortex and the brainstem. The supplementary motor area has been shown to be critical in the generation of self-initiated movements. Its dysfunction in positron emission tomography studies in PD patients (25) and in single-unit studies in MPTP-treated

monkeys (26) accounts for the difficulty in performing self-initiated movements in patients with relative sparing of their ability to perform sensory cue-triggered movements. There are many studies showing abnormal cortical activity, including prolonged cognitive reaction times and homonymous hemispiral abnormalities in PD patients (27–30). Attributing the phenomenology of parkinsonism to the basal ganglia alone would be unreasonable.

Therapeutic modulation of glutaminergic pathways has been considered in PD. It is possible that a blockade of glutaminergic receptors in the striatum or the GPi/SNr could ameliorate PD in a manner similar to pallidotomy. Indeed, this pharmacologic alternative to pallidotomy has been confirmed in rodents and nonhuman primates by stereotactic injections (31,32) and by the systemic administration of selective glutamate-receptor antagonists. For example, alpha-amino-3-hydroxy-5-methyl-4-isoxazole proportionate (AMPA) receptors are abundant in the Gpi/SNr; an anti-parkinsonian effect was achieved in MPTP-treated monkeys by systemic administration of NBQX (a highly specific AMPA-receptor antagonist) at doses that did not produce behavioral side effects in normal monkeys. On the other hand, NMDA receptors are widespread in the basal ganglia but are exceptionally concentrated in the striatum. Remacemide, an NMDA receptor antagonist, potentiates subthreshold doses of L-dopa when given orally to MPTP-treated monkeys. Clinical studies with remacemide in PD are in progress.

Tremor in PD has been attributed to unmasking of the oscillatory activity of thalamic nuclei mediated by the inhibitory or hyperpolarizing influence of increased basal ganglia output (33,34). This rhythmic oscillation can be further enhanced by periodic bursts of the reticular thalamus that is known to occur during moments of immobility, accounting for the typical parkinsonian tremors at rest. Another theory states that it is the unmasking of pacemaker-like properties of the basal ganglia themselves (35) due to the loss of their dopaminergic modulation. Indeed, rhythmic bursts of spikes synchronous to the parkinsonian tremor have been recorded in STN and GPi during pallidotomy (13,36,37). Opposing these central hypotheses, a peripheral theory suggests that the tremor in PD is due to oscillation of unstable long loop reflexes that involve muscle stretch receptors, dorsal columns, the thalamus, and the cortex. Long loop reflexes may affect the firing of pyramidal motor neurons and the resulting muscle contraction in response to a muscle stretch (38). These reflexes are increased in magnitude in PD (39,40) proportionally to the degree of increase in tone (41), implying a role in the pathophysiology of the rigidity and tremors in PD.

Hyperkinetic Movement Syndromes

Hemiballism occurs secondary to lesion of the STN in most cases (42–44). The interrupted indirect pathways with an STN lesion leaves the direct pathway unopposed, promoting excessive involuntary movement (Fig. 5A). The selective degeneration of striatal projections to the GPe results in decreased indirect pathway activity (Fig. 5B) and chorea seen early in the course of Huntington disease. With progression of the degeneration of striatal projections, output of the direct pathway is also compro-

mised, resulting in increased GPi activity and a corresponding reduction in chorea and the development of parkinsonian signs late in the disease (Fig. 5C). This model, however, does not explain other observations, for example, how a lesion in the pallidum promotes involuntary movements or why GPi lesions in normal monkeys and in humans do not cause long-term involuntary movements and hyperkinesia or hemiballism after lesioning of the STN (15,45).

Drug-induced dyskinesia is also difficult to explain. It has been postulated that chronic administration of L-dopa in PD, intended to replace the dopaminergic stimulation of putaminal neurons normally provided by the SNc, favors the direct pathway promoting excessive movements; a change in dopamine receptor number or binding properties likely also plays a role (46). The beneficial effect of pallidotomy in dyskinesia is likely to be due to changes in the abnormal GPi/SNr pattern of firing as described above.

Dystonia

Dystonia is characterized by sustained muscle contractions that cause twisting, repetitive movements, and abnormal postures (47). They are classified according to the distribution of the involved muscles and named by their genetic inheritance patterns for the most affected body part or region. Hereditary childhood dystonia is due to an abnormal gene on chromosome 9q (DYT1) (48) that encodes for an ATP-binding heat shock protein, the function of which is still unknown (49). In most instances of secondary dystonia, there are lesions in the contralateral basal ganglia and occasionally in the cerebral cortex, diencephalon, and brainstem (50).

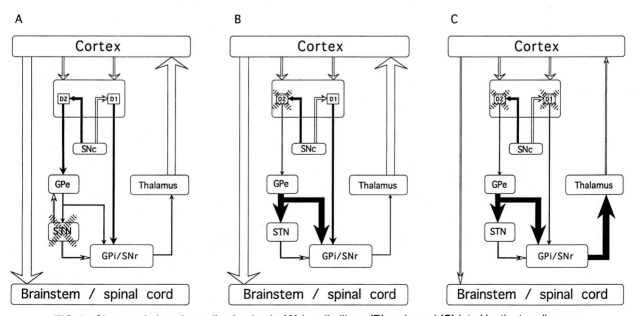

FIG. 5. Changes in basal ganglia circuitry in **(A)** hemiballism, **(B)** early, and **(C)** late Huntington disease.

The theory that dystonia is a hyperkinetic disorder is supported by its appearance at peak (L-dopa) doses in PD and its relief with thalamotomy. Paradoxically, dystonia occurs spontaneously in patients with PD treated during their "off" periods, when they are most hypokinetic. Preliminary studies suggest a loss of putaminal D2 receptors in some forms of idiopathic focal dystonia (51); accordingly, dystonia cannot be classified strictly as either a hypokinetic or a hyperkinetic disorder. It has been suggested that dystonia is primarily a sensory disorder (52) and not simply a motor disturbance. A current useful model for dystonia is based on the theory that dystonia results from a reduction or imbalance in cortical, brainstem, and spinal inhibitory and aberrant sensory influences (53,54). Repetitive tasks, which in addition cause changes in brain representation of movements, could lead to the development of dystonia through overflow of muscle activity on attempted action. Several lines of reasoning support this. First, sensory symptoms may precede the development of dystonia (55). Second, the response of the brain to somatosensory stimuli is abnormal in dystonia (56–59). Dystonic symptoms may result from a mismatch between central motor output and sensory input from muscles to the central nervous system, thus leading to the muscle spasms and cocontractions. Third, in contrast to PD patients, the sensory defects in dystonia involve long loop reflexes that are known to be increased in *duration* but not in magnitude (40,60). Accordingly, the peripheral electromyography (EMG) silent period is significantly more prolonged in focal dystonia (61). Fourth, the stimulation of the ventralis intermedius nucleus of the thalamus produces cocontraction of muscles like dystonia, and this nucleus has been shown to contain more sensory cells in patients with dystonia compared with controls. Mexiletine, an oral derivative of lidocaine, ameliorates a small group of patients with idiopathic spasmodic torticollis and blepharospasm (59).

Tremor

Tremors are rhythmic oscillations of part of the body around one or more joints (62,63). There are many different types and numerous underlying causes, so it is important to characterize the specific tremor type to establish a correct diagnosis and offer the most appropriate treatment. They are classified according to whether they occur at rest, while maintaining a posture, with generalized activity, or during the performance of a specific task. There is still no universally accepted method of measurement (62). The clinical evaluation and rating scales are usually too subjective and imprecise to discern subtle changes over time or too objective to determine significant responses to therapy. Graphic evidence of tremor activity can be obtained by performing certain tasks, such as writing or drawing the Archimedes spiral, but they are not easily standardizable across subjects.

Physiologic tremor (PT) is generated and mediated both peripherally and centrally. The peripheral component of PT contributes irregular very low amplitude and variable oscillations, usually 8 to 12 Hz depending on the physiologic characteristics of mass, stiffness, and other properties of the tremorous body part. The central component of PT, often referred to as the "central oscillator," also contributes weak 8- to 12-Hz oscillations and probably many higher frequencies and low-amplitude oscillations. Exaggerated physiologic tremor (EPT) has the same peripheral and central components as PT, but there is greater participation of the stretch reflex and the 8- to 12-Hz central oscillator. When EPT becomes constant and clinically symptomatic with posture or movement, without provoking factors, it can be termed essential tremor (ET). The results of activation positron emission tomography (64) suggest that the cerebellum, thalamus, and cortex together mediate ET. Inertial loading identifies PT when there is absence of EMG activity corresponding to the mechanical-reflex component. The clear separation of EPT from ET is more difficult, but there should be greater relative power of the mechanical-reflex component, more involvement of peripheral reflexes, and lower amplitudes in EPT. In older subjects, EPT can be distinguished from ET based on higher EPT and lower ET frequencies as well.

ET, PD, cerebellar, dystonic, and other pathologic tremors have different central generators resulting in a variety of tremors of 1 to 20 Hz. EMG-to-movement and side-to-side frequency coherences, EMG topography, reflex responses, tremor amplitude ratios during different clinical tasks, and others are diagnostically useful quantitative methods in tremor analysis. Computerized tremor analysis using electronic transducing devices are highly sensitive, objective, and reproducible. Tremors are amenable to quantitative mathematical analysis because they are quasi-sinusoidal movements, with two measurable parameters, frequency (measured in Hz) and amplitude (measured in mm). Other waveform characteristics are useful in the physiologic research of central and peripheral aspects of motor control (63), such as side-to-side differences in PD and ET (66), and in the differentiation of dystonia and ET (67).

There are several different techniques to measure tremor. The most commonly used is the electronic detection of motion by accelerometry. Miniature accelerometers can be attached to the tremorous part of the body and do not interfere with voluntary or involuntary movements. High-speed microcomputers are capable of acquiring, processing, and analyzing accelerometric data quickly and efficiently to analyze the accelerometric signals. Simultaneous EMG can provide information about motor unit recruitment and synchronization with the tremor activity (62,68) and the relationship of the synergistic muscles. In tremor analysis, the EMG signal is often processed by rectification, integration, or smoothing to place its frequency profile into the tremor range (62).

The tremor activity, accelerometric, EMG, and other data are generally acquired through an analog-to-digital board, processed, digitized, and analyzed off-line. With faster computers and digital signal processing boards, however, they can be analyzed in real time. If the number of sampled points is N over a period of time T sec, then the sampling rate is N/T, the frequency resolution is $1/T$ Hz and the maximum recordable frequency is $N/2T$ Hz (also known as the Nyquist frequency) (69). Thus, if the highest frequency of concern is 25 Hz, the sampling rate of the recording device must be at least 50 Hz and preferably several times that for better signal processing. Low-pass filtering and other techniques can be used to improve further signal-to-noise ratios.

The objective and detailed findings of a tremor analysis test are most helpful when the clinical picture is unclear or very complicated. Depending on the recording circumstances, tremor frequencies can be reliably calculated to within 0.1 Hz and tremor displacement amplitudes can be determined accurately to less than 0.1 mm. For example, parkinsonian and ET are often difficult to separate but obviously important to distinguish for prognosis and treatment (63,70). Both conditions occur with increasing age and both may occur at rest or with actions. There are, however, objective physiologic characteristics that can be used to separate the clinical phenomenology of these conditions. Typically, parkinsonian rest tremors have characteristic waveforms and identical side-to-side peak frequency spectra, despite very asymmetric displacement amplitudes in each hand. ET, however, has been shown to have much less side-to-side frequency correlation but more similar side-to-side amplitudes (67). Other diagnostically challenging disorders such as orthostatic tremor, dystonic tremor, primary writing, and voice tremors can also be effectively evaluated and quantified with physiologic techniques (66,71,72).

Myoclonus

Myoclonus results from brief involuntary muscle contractions leading to quick body movements or limb jerks. A remarkable number of different pathologic conditions result in similar-appearing jerks yet no single biochemical or physiologic mechanism is common to all of them. Myoclonus occurs in more pathologic and normal physiologic conditions than any other movement disorder. It may be focal, multifocal, or generalized; symmetric or asymmetric; periodic or aperiodic. It can be generated cortically, subcortically, in the brainstem, spinal cord, or more peripherally and is not associated with loss or change in consciousness (73,74). Cortical and subcortical myoclonic jerks characteristically are bursts of muscle activity, irregular in timing, separated by distinct pauses, and irregular in amplitude and force. Brief lapses in muscle tone, or asterixis, is a form of "negative" myoclonus because it phenomenologically appears as quick limb movements and physiologically may be caused by similar cerebral mechanisms as muscle jerks (75). Brainstem, spinal, and peripheral myoclonus represent different forms of myoclonus from the more typical quick irregular jerks. These types of myoclonus are comprised of longer duration, more rhythmic muscle activity in segmental axial or limb myotomes and may be generated by discrete spinal lesions or more diffusely in the propriospinal interneurons (76).

The various presentations of myoclonus can be differentiated from other movement disorders and epilepsy; in particular, it can be distinguished from hemiballism dystonia, chorea, tics, clonus, tremor, startle, and fasciculations for proper treatment and management. Some types of myoclonus differ from epilepsy only in degree of motor involvement. Although a long-standing controversy, animal models and hippocampal slice preparations have shown that the same pathophysiologic mechanism occurs in both myoclonus originating from the cerebral cortex or brainstem and epilepsy (77). Epilepsia partialis continua, therefore, is a form of continuous or repetitive focal myoclonus (78). Clinically, many patients with myoclonus have an underlying epileptic disorder, and there are many reports of patients having myoclonus along with several different types of motor epilepsies (73).

Distinguishing myoclonus from other movement disorders may be difficult and requires both clinical examination and specialized physiologic tests to resolve the problem. Hemiballism is generally unilateral, irregular in timing and scaling, with long duration muscle bursts (>500 msec) that are typically very proximal, characteristics that, together, are different from myoclonus of cortical or subcortical origin. Dystonia is usually quite different phenomenologically from myoclonus, but some forms can be so quick as to be called myoclonic dystonia (79) with an associated alcohol-responsive autosomal dominant syndrome (80). Myoclonus never has the fluidity and proximal-to-distal randomness of chorea or the stereotypy and partial voluntary control of tics. Myoclonus is different from clonus in that it is never sustained after tendon stretch (73) and differs from tremor in that it is usually not sinusoidal without discrete intervals between jerks. Some forms of brainstem or spinal myoclonus such as palatal myoclonus, however, can appear very rhythmic and sinusoidal. Myoclonus differs from normal startle in that it is often asymmetric and does not habituate. More complex pathologic startle syndromes, however, share similar elements with myoclonus and require special testing for diagnosis (81). Fasciculations originate from single motor units either in the anterior horn cell or its axons, and although myoclonus may originate in the spinal cord or peripheral nervous system, it always involves the synchronous firing of more than single motor units (73).

There are many classifications of myoclonus, but the most helpful distinguishes it from other hyperkinetic involuntary movements and provides methods for its evaluation. Stimulus sensitivity is probably the most useful classification clinically and physiologically. Stimulus sensitivity occurs over a continuum from epilepsia partialis continua in which cortical motor neurons fire regularly and continuously, to spontaneous myoclonus that discharges without afferent input but not regularly or continually, to reflex myoclonus in which afferent input is needed to evoke a myoclonic jerk (82), to the stimulus-insensitive forms of myoclonus. Stimulus-sensitive myoclonia is also referred to as reflex or action myoclonus depending on whether external or internal afferent information triggers a jerk. These are either cortical or reticular in origin and can be distinguished clinically and with physiologic tests. The nonstimulus sensitive myoclonia are comprised of the more rhythmic jerking of palatal or spinal myoclonus, the slower and more periodic discharges found in some acquired disorders such as Creutzfeldt-Jacob disease, and the faster but nonrepetitive irregular nonstimulus sensitive jerks of benign essential and physiologic myoclonus (74,82,83).

The physiologic investigation of myclonus includes direct and intercorrelation of EMG recordings of jerks, electroencephalographic measurement of cortical activity, and sensory evoked potentials to monitor sensory processing (74). The EMG alone is useful for determining the burst durations of myoclonic jerks and the patterns of antagonist actions and activation orders up or down the brainstem or spinal cord. Although there are no set burst durations diagnostic of myoclonus, as a general rule, irregular cocontracting antagonists 10 to 50 msec in duration are characteristic of cortical myoclonus, whereas EMG bursts of up to 300 msec characterize brainstem and spinal segmental myoclonus. The EMG in hemiballism would be of long duration but not rhythmic and would not spread up or down the spinal cord. Normal voluntary activity usually takes the form of triphasic agonist-antagonist-agonist ballistic activity; however, certain actions can trigger a form of subcortical myoclonus that results in ballistic overflow myoclonus, a variant of essential myoclonus (84).

Gait and Posture Control

Normal walking is achieved through a repeating series of leg and hip flexion and extension movements with concomitant hip and trunk stabilization procedures. The step cycle in locomotion is divided into the swing phase, when the foot is swinging forward as in stepping, and the stand phase, when the foot is planted with the leg moving backward. The rhythmic alternation between flexion and extension during walking is mediated in the spinal cord even in the absence afferent input (85–87). This rudimentary spinal pattern generator has multiple connections with virtually all supraspinal motor centers (Fig. 6). The interplay between all these structures generates various

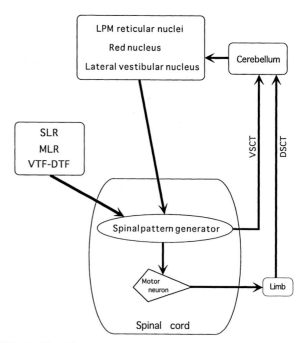

FIG. 6. Simplified connections between the "spinal pattern generator" and multiple supraspinal motor levels involved in gait and posture control. LPM, lateral pontomedullary (reticular nuclei); VSCT, DSCT, ventral, dorsal spinocerebellar tracts; SLR, subthalamic locomotor region; MLR, mesencephalic locomotor region; VTF, DTF, ventral, dorsal tegmental fields.

locomotion patterns and posture control. The vestibulospinal tract from the lateral vestibular nucleus shares antigravity muscle tone control with the nuclei gigantocellularis and the pontis caudalis. The latter are modulated by the anterior lobe of the cerebellum and the fastigial nuclei during the swing or stepping phase of the gait cycle. Indeed, lesions of the anterior cerebellum result in truncal ataxia such as in the anterior vermis syndrome of alcohol intoxication and lesions of the fastigium that cause truncal dysequilibrium with a tendency to fall to the side of the lesion (88). The lateral and paravermal cerebellar cortices and the globose-emboliform nuclei affect the rhythmicity of the spinal generator of locomotion and coordination via connections with the rubrospinal, the lateral pontomedullary reticulospinal, and the vestibulospinal pathways (89,90). In cats (88), the brainstem and diencephalon contain four vaguely defined areas that are critical in gait initiation and posture control. The first is the subthalamic locomotor region (SLR), which is located in the lateral hypothalamus. When stimulated, the SLR causes the stealth gait pattern as seen in the pursuit of prey. Second is the mesencephalic locomotor region (MLR), which is located in the pedunculopontine nucleus of the dorsolateral midbrain and has extensive bilateral connections with the basal ganglia and the cerebellum. When stimulated briefly, it produces rapid walking followed by running. Inhibition of the MLR by the GPi/SNr, as in PD, suppresses locomotion (91,92), whereas its excitation by the STN and motor cortex promote locomotion. Third is the ventral tegmental field (VTF) within the rostral nucleus raphe magnus of the caudal midline pons, which when stimulated increases antigravity muscle tone. Fourth, is the dorsal tegmental field in the caudal nucleus raphe centralis superior in the caudal midline pons that when stimulated decreases antigravity muscle tone.

The VTF and dorsal tegmental field control postural tone during locomotion along with reticulospinal and vestibulospinal pathway modulation (90). These nuclei also connect with the MLR and SLR (88), enhancing the integration of locomotion patterns to appropriate tone changes. Purposeful modification and initiation of locomotion are functions of the frontal cortex via connections with the MLR, SLR, basal ganglia, and spinal networks (89,93). Precise foot placement (e.g., in walking on a grid or a horizontal ladder) requires an intact frontal lobe (89,94). Limbic structures are also involved in the control of locomotion. When stimulated pharmacologically or by the VTF, the nucleus accumbens promotes prolonged locomotion activity in rats (95). It has connections to the dorsal medial thalamus nuclei that project to the medial prefrontal cortex within the limbic system.

Balance Control Against Postural Perturbation

The vertical line passing through the center of gravity of the body, known as the line of gravity, is 3 to 8 cm anterior to the ankles (96). Its fluctuation within a narrow limit is called postural sway. This is achieved by continuous feedback to the central nervous system provided by muscle, joint, cutaneous receptors, vestibular, and visual inputs. A loss of sensory inputs from one system can be compensated to some degree by the inputs of the other systems. For example, in the absence of visual input, balance is effectively maintained by the somatosensory and vestibular information. The impairment of two sensory modalities, however, causes postural instability, and the loss of all three invariably results in falls (97,98). The extent of the compromise of postural stability is also proportional to the age and to the extent of central nervous system damage of the patient (99). Several maneuvers can be used to counteract destabilizing perturbations. The ankle strategy consists of a set of muscle contractions of the legs and torso that produces opposing torques about the ankles. The *hip strategy* combines hip flexion or extension with appropriate arm movements to prevent a fall. Both are mediated by the monosynaptic stretch reflex of latency 45 to 50 msec and by longer latency somatosensory reflexes of about 100 msec, known as functional stretch reflexes. The latter are mediated through transcortical neural loops. Their amplitude and latency are dictated by a prior experience acquired in a previous similar context of somatosensory, vestibular,

and visual information (100–102). Severe destabilizing perturbations require more complex body movements to assume a new base of support, as for example, using three limbs to prevent injury or grabbing a fixed object for support. These are called rescue responses and require input from the frontal lobes and adequate strength and agility. When a destabilizing disturbance is expected by an individual, the central nervous system is able to perform a stabilizing anticipatory postural activity (103). This is achieved by activating a set of stabilizing muscles before the body is challenged by the postural perturbation. Lesions of the anterior lobe of the cerebellum and the frontal cortex interfere with this preparatory program (104,105), which is also abnormal in PD patients (106).

REFERENCES

1. Albin RL, Young AB, Penney JB. The functional anatomy of basal ganglia disorders. *Trends Neurosci* 1989;12:366–375.
2. DeLong MR. Primate models of movement disorders of basal ganglia origin. *Trends Neurosci* 1990;13:281–285.
3. Betarbet R, Turner R, Chockkan V, et al. Dopaminergic neurons intrinsic to the primate striatum. *J Neurosci* 1997;17:6761–6768.
4. Rauschecker JP. Mechanisms of visual plasticity: Hebb synapses, NMDA receptors, and beyond. *Physiol Rev* 1991;71:587–615.
5. Wu M, Suzuki SS, Siegel JM. Autonomical distribution and response patterns of reticular neurons active in relation to acoustic startle. *Brain Res* 1988;457:399–406.
6. Dum RP, Strick PL. Premotor areas: nodal points for parallel efferent systems involved in the central control of movement. In: Humphrey DR, Freund H-J, eds. *Motor control: concepts and issues.* New York: John Wiley & Sons, 1991:383–397.
7. Carlsson A, Lindquist M, Magnusson T. 3-4-Dihydroxyphenylalanine and 5-hydroxytryptophan as reserpine antagonists. *Nature* 1957;180:1200.
8. Ehringer H, Hornykiewicz O. Verteilung von Noradrenalin und Dopamin (3-hydroxytyramin) im Gehirn des Menschen und ihr Verhalten bei Erkrankungen des extrapyramidalen systems. *Klin Wochenschr* 1960;38:1236–1239.
9. Mink JW, Thach WT. Basal ganglia motor control. III. Pallidal ablation: normal reaction time, muscle co-contraction, and slow movement. *J Neurophysiol* 1991;65:330–351.
10. Strub RL. Frontal lobe syndrome in a patient with bilateral globus pallidus lesions. *Arch Neurol* 1986;46:1024–1027.
11. Kato M, Kimura M. Effects of reversible blockade of basal ganglia on a voluntary arm movement. *J Neurophysiol* 1992;68:1516–1534.
12. DeLong MR, Coyle JT. Globus pallidus lesions in the monkey produced by kainic acid: histologic and behavioral effects. *Appl Neurophysiol* 1979;42:95–97.
13. Vitek JL, Kaneoke Y, Turner R. Neuronal activity in the internal (GPi) and external (GPe) segments of the globus pallidus (GP) of parkinsonian patients is similar to that in the MPTP-treated primate model of parkinsonism. *Soc Neurosci Abstr* 1993;19:1584.
14. Dogali M, Fazzini E, Kolodny E, et al. Stereotactic ventral pallidotomy for Parkinson's disease. *Neurology* 1995;45:753–761.
15. Laitinen LV, Bergenheim AT, Hariz MI. Leksell's posteroventral pallidotomy in the treatment of Parkinson's disease. *J Neurosurg* 1992;76:53–61.
16. Sutton JP, Couldwell W, Lew MF, et al. Ventroposterior medial pallidotomy in patients with advanced Parkinson's disease. *Neurosurgery* 1995;36:1116–1125.
17. Pollak B, Benabrid AL, Gross C, et al. Effects de la stimulation du noyau sous-thalamique dans la maladie de Parkinson. *Rev Neurol (Paris)* 1994;149:175–176.
18. Obeso JA, Rothwell JC, Ceballos-Bauman AO, et al. The mechanism of action of pallidotomy in Parkinson's disease: physiological and imaging studies. *Soc Neurosci Abstr* 1982;21:1995.
19. Ceballos-Bauman AO, Obeso JA, Vitek JL, et al. Restoration of thal-

amocortical activity after posterventrolateral pallidotomy in Parkinson's disease. *Lancet* 1994;344:814.

20. Narabayashi H, Maeda T, Yokochi F. Long term follow up study of nucleus ventralis intermedius and ventrolateralis thalamotomy using microelectrode technique in parkinsonism. *Appl Neurophysiol* 1987; 50:330–337.

21. Greenamyre JT. Pharmacological pallidotomy with glutamate antagonists [editorial]? *Ann Neurol* 1996;39:557–558.

22. Forno LS, De Lanney LE, Irwin I, Langston JW. Similarities and differences between MPTP-induced parkinsonian and Parkinson's disease. *Adv Neurol* 1993;60:600–608.

23. Gibb WR. Neuropathology of Parkinson's disease and related syndromes. *Neurol Clin* 1992;10:361–376.

24. Jellinger KA. Pathology of Parkinson's disease changes other than the nigrarostriatal pathway. *Mol Chem Neuropath* 1991;14:153–197.

25. Jahanshahi M, Jenkins IH, Brown RG, Marsden CD, Passingham RE, Brooks DJ. Self-initiated versus externally triggered movements I. An investigation using measurement of regional cerebral blood flow with PET and movement-related potentials in normal and Parkinson's disease. *Brain* 1995;118:913–933.

26. Watts RL, Mandir AS, Montgomery EB. Abnormalities of supplementary motor area (SMA) neuronal activity in MPTP parkinsonism. *Soc Neurosci Abstr* 1989;15:787.

27. Dick JPR, Rothwell JC, Day BL, et al. The Bereitschafts potential is abnormal in Parkinson's disease. *Brain* 1989;112:233–244.

28. Pullman SL, Watts RL, Juncos JL, Chase TN, Sanes JN. Dopaminergic effects on simple and choice reaction times performance in Parkinson's disease. *Neurology* 1988;38:249–254.

29. Pullman SL, Watts RL, Juncos JL, Sanes JN. Movement amplitude choice reaction time performance in Parkinson's disease may be independent of dopaminergic status. *J Neurol Neurosurg Psychiatry* 1990; 53:279–283.

30. Yu QP, Pullman SL, Fahn S, Pedersen SF. Homonymous hemispiral abnormalities in patients with Parkinson's disease. *Soc Neurosci Abstr* 1997;23:1898.

31. Starr MS. Glutamate/dopamine/D1/D2 balance in the basal ganglia and its relevance to Parkinson's disease. *Synapse* 1995;19:264–293.

32. Klockgether T, Turki L, Honoré T, et al. The AMPA receptor antagonist in NBQX has antiparkinsonian effects on monoamine-depleted rats and MPTP-treated monkeys. *Ann Neurol* 1991;30:717–723.

33. Buzsaki G, Smith A, Berger S, Fisher LJ, Gage FH. Petit mal epilepsy and parkinsonian termor: hypothesis of a common pacemaker. *Neuroscience* 1990;36:1–14.

34. Lenz FA, Tasker RR, Kwan MC, et al. Single unit analysis of the human ventral thalamic nuclear group: correlation of the thalamic "tremor cells" with the 3–6 Hz component of parkinsonian tremor. *J Neurosci* 1988;8:754–764.

35. Nambu A, Llinas R. Electrophysiology of the globus pallidus neurons: an in vitro study in guinea pig brain slices. *Soc Neurosci Abstr* 1990; 16:428.

36. Bergman H, Wichman T, Karmon B, DeLong MR. The primate subthalamic nucleus. Neuronal activity in the MPTP model of parkinsonism. *J Neurophysiol* 1994;7:507–520.

37. Vitek JT, Wichman T, DeLong MR. Current concepts of basal ganglia neurophysiology with respect to tremorogenesis. In: Findley LJ, Koller W, eds. *Handbook of tremor disorders*. New York: Marcel Dekker, 1994:37–50.

38. Evarts EV, Fromm C. The pyramidal tract neuron as summing point in a closed-loop control system in monkey. In: Desmedt JE, ed. *Cerebral Motor Control in Man: Long Loop Mechanisms. Progress in Clinical Neurophysiology.* Base, New York: Karger, 1978:56–69.

39. Struppler F, Lehmann-Horn F, Klein W, Luching CM, Deuschl G. Effects of stereoencephalotomy on long-latency EMG responses and motor control of arm movement in Parkinson syndrome. *Adv Neurol* 1984;40:437–445.

40. Tatton WG, Bedingham W, Verrier MC, Blair RDG. Characteristic alterations in responses to imposed wrist displacements in parkinsonian rigidity and dystonia musculorum deformans. *Can J Neurol Sci* 1984;11:281–287.

41. Tatton WG, Lee RG. Evidence of abnormal long-loop reflexes in rigid parkinsonian patients. *Brain Res* 1975;100:671–676.

42. Carpenter MB, Whittier JR, Mettler FA. Analysis of choreoid hyperkinesia in the rhesus monkey. Surgical and pharmacological analysis of hyperkinesia resulting from lesions in the subthalamic nucleus of Luys. *J Comp Neurol* 1950;92:293–332.

43. Kase CS, Mauslsby GO, Dejuan E, Mohr JP. Hemichorea hemiballism and lacunar infarctions in the basal ganglia. *Neurology* 1981;31: 452–455.

44. Hamada I, DeLong MR. Excitotoxic acid lesions of the primate subthalamic nucleus result in transient dyskinesia of the contralateral limb. *J Neurophysiol* 1992;68:1859–1866.

45. Wichman T, Bergman H, DeLong MR. The primate subthalamic nucleus. III. Changes in motor behavior and neuronal activity in the internal pallidus induced by subthalamic inactivation in the MPTP model of parkinsonism. *J Neurophysiol* 1994;58:14–21.

46. Gerfen CR. Dopamine receptor function in the basal ganglia. *Clin Neuropharmacol* 1995;18:5162–5177.

47. Fahn S. Concept and classification of dystonia. In: Fahn S, Marsden CD, Caln DB, eds. *Advances in neurology: dystonia 2.* New York: Raven Press, 1988:1–8.

48. Bressman SB, de Leon D, Kramer PL, et al. Dystonia in Ashkenazi Jews: clinical characterization of a founder mutation. *Ann Neurol* 1994;36:771–777.

49. Ozelius LJ, Hewett JW, Page CE, et al. The early onset torsion dystonia gene (DYT1) encodes an ATP-binding protein. *Nat Genet* 1997; 17:40–48.

50. Calne DB, Lang AE. Secondary dystonia. In: Fahn S, Marsden CD, Calne DB, eds. *Advances in neurology: dystonia 2.* New York: Raven Press, 1988:9–33.

51. Perlmutter JS, Stambuck M, Markham J, Moerlein S. Quantified binding of [F18]spiperone in focal dystonia. *Mov Disord* 1996;11:217.

52. Hallett M. Is dystonia a sensory disorder? *Ann Neurol* 1995;38: 139–140.

53. Alexander GE, Crutcher MD. Functional architecture of basal ganglia circuits: neural substrates of parallel processing. *Trends Neurosci* 1990;13:266–271.

54. Mink JW. Focused selection and inhibition of competing motor programs. *Prog Neurobiol* 1996;50:381–425.

55. Ghika J, Regli F, Growdon JH. Sensory symptoms in cranial dystonia: a potential role in the etiology? *J Neurol Sci* 1993;116:142–147.

56. Lenz FA, Seike SE, Jaeger CJ, et al. Single neuron analysis of thalamic activity in patients with dystonia. *J Neurophysiol* (in press).

57. Tempel LW, Perlmutter JS. Abnormal cortical responses in patients with writer's cramp. *Neurology* 1993;43:2252–2257.

58. Grissom J, Toro C, Trettau J, Hallett M. The N30 and N140-P190 median somatosensory evoked potential waveforms in dystonia involving the upper extremity. *Neurology* 1995;45[Suppl 4]:A458.

59. Ohara S, Miki J, Momoi H, Unno H, Shindo M, Yanagisawa N. Treatment of spasmodic torticollis with mexiletine: a case report. *Mov Disord* 1997;12:466–468.

60. Rothwell JC, Obeso JA, Day BL, Marsden CD. Pathophysiology of dystonias. In: Desmedt JE, ed. *Advances in neurology: motor control mechanisms in health and disease.* New York: Raven Press, 1983: 851–863.

61. Pullman SL, Ford B, Elibol B, Uncini A, Su PC, Fahn S. Cutaneous electromyographic silent period findings in brachial dystonia. *Neurology* 1996;46:503–508.

62. Elble RJ, Koller WC. *Tremor*. Baltimore: The Johns Hopkins University Press, 1990:143–157.

63. Marsden CD. Origins of normal and pathological tremor. In: Findley LJ, Capildeo R, eds. *Movement Disorders: Tremor*. New York: Oxford University Press, 1984:37–84.

64. Brooks DJ, Jenkins IH, Bain P, et al. A comparison of the abnormal patterns of cerebral activation associated with neuropathic and essential tremor. *Neurology* 1992;42:423.

65. Reference deleted in proofs.

66. Pullman SL, Fahn S, Rueda J. Physiologic characterization of dystonic and essential tremors. *Neurology* 1992;42:471.

67. Pullman SL, Mirski DF, Vira J. Physiologic analysis of side-to-side variability in parkinsonian and essential tremors. *Mov Disord* 1992; 7:299.

68. Elble RJ. Physiologic and essential tremor. *Neurology* 1986;36: 225–231.

69. Glaser EM, Ruchkin DS. *Principles of neurobiological signal analysis*. New York: Academic Press, 1976:9–17.

70. Hubble JP, Busenbark KL, Koller WC. Essential tremor. *Clin Neuropharmacol* 1989;12:453–482.

71. Kachi T, Rothwell JC, Cowan JMA, Marsden CD. Writing tremor: its relationship to benign essential tremor. *J Neurol Neurosurg Psychiatry* 1985;45:545–550.

72. Rivest J, Marsden CD. Trunk and head tremor as isolated manifestations of dystonia. *Mov Disord* 1990;5:60–65.

73. Snodgrass SR. Myoclonus: analysis of monoamine, GABA, and other systems. *FASEB J* 1990;4:2775–2788.

74. Shibasaki H. Electrophysiologic studies of myoclonus. *Muscle Nerve* 1988;11:899–907.

75. Artieda J, Muruzabal J, Larumbe R, Garcia de Casasola C, Obeso J. Cortical mechanisms mediating asterixis. *Mov Disord* 1992;7:209–216.

76. Chokroverty S, Walters A, Zimmerman T, Picone M. Propriospinal myoclonus. *Neurology* 1992;42:1591–1595.

77. Halliday AM. Evolving ideas on the neurophysiology of myoclonus. In: Fahn S, Marsden CD, Van Woert MH, eds. *Advances in neurology: myoclonus*. New York: Raven Press, 1986:339–355.

78. Watanabe K, Kuroiwa Y, Toyokura Y. Epilepsia partialis continua: epileptogenic focus in motor cortex and its participation in transcortical reflexes. *Arch Neurol* 1984;41:1040–1044.

79. Ravits J, Hallett M, Baker M, Wilkins D. Primary writing tremor and myoclonic writer's cramp. *Neurology* 1985;35:1387–1391.

80. Gasser T, Bereznai B, Muller B, et al. Linkage studies in alcohol-responsive myoclonic dystonia. *Mov Disord* 1996;11:363–370.

81. Wilkins DE, Hallett M, Wess M. Audiogenic startle reflex of man and its relationship to startle syndromes. A review. *Brain* 1986;3:561–573.

82. Marsden CD, Hallett M, Fahn S. The nosology and pathology of myoclonus. In: Marsden CD, Fahn S, eds. *Movement disorders*. London: Butterworth, 1982:196–248.

83. Obeso JA, Rothwell JC, Marsden CD. The spectrum of cortical myoclonus. *Brain* 1985;108:193–224.

84. Hallett M, Chadwick D, Marsden CD. Ballistic movement overflow myoclonus. A form of essential myoclonus. *Brain* 1977;100:299–312.

85. Brown TG. On the nature of the fundamental activity of the nervous centers, together with an analysis of the conditioning of rhythmic activity in progression, and a theory of evolution of function in the nervous system. *J Physiol (Lond)* 1914;48:18–46.

86. Dietz V, Columbo DM, Jensen L, Baumgartner L. Locomotor capacity of spinal cord in paraplegic patients. *Ann Neurol* 1995;37:574–582.

87. Bussel B, Roby-Brami A, Néris OR, Yakovleff A. Evidence for a spinal stepping generator in man. Electrophysiological study. *Acta Neurobiol* 1996;56:465–468.

88. Mori S. Integration of posture and locomotion in acute decerebrate cats in awake, freely moving cats. *Prog Neurol* 1987;28:161–195.

89. Armstrong DM. The supraspinal control of mammalian locomotion. *J Physiol (Lond)* 1988;405:1–37.

90. Kawahara K, Moris S, Tamiyama T, Kanaya T. Discharges in neurons in the midpontine dorsal tegmentum of mesencephalic cat during locomotion. *Brain Res* 1985;341:377–380.

91. Garcia-Rill E, Kinjo N, Atsuta Y, Ishikawa Y, Webber M, Shinner RD. Posterior midbrain-induced locomotion. *Brain Res Bull* 1990;24:499–508.

92. DeLong MR, Wichmann T. Basal ganglia-thalamocortical circuits in parkinsonian signs. *Clin Neurosci* 1993;1:18–26.

93. Drew T. Motor cortical cell discharge during voluntary gait modification. *Brain Res* 1988;457:181–187.

94. Henneman E. Motor functions of the brainstem and basal ganglia. In: Mountcastle VB, ed. *Medical physiology*. St Louis: CV Mosby Co., 1974:678–721.

95. Wu M, Brudzynski SM. Mesolimbic dopamine terminals and locomotor activity induced from the subiculum. *NeuroReport* 1995;6:1602–1604.

96. Elble RJ, Moody C, Leffler K, Sinha R. The initiation of normal walking. *Mov Disord* 1994;9:139–146.

97. Horak FB, Nashner LM, Diener NC. Postural strategies associated with somatosensory and vestibular loss. *Exp Brain Res* 1990;82:167–177.

98. Lestienne F, Soechting J, Berthoz A. Postural readjustments induced by linear motion of visual scenes. *Exp Brain Res* 1977;28:363–384.

99. Gatev P, Thomas S, Lou JS, Lim M, Hallett M. Effects of diminished and conflicting sensory information on balance in patients with cerebral deficits. *Mov Disord* 1996;11:654–664.

100. Nashner LM, McCollum G. The organization of human postural movement: a formal basis and experimental synthesis. *Behav Brain Sci* 1985;8:135–172.

101. Aniss AM, Diener MC, Hore J, Gandevia SC, Burke D. Behavior of human muscle receptors when reliant on proprioceptive feedback during standing. *J Neurophysiol* 1990;64:661–670.

102. Timmann D, Belting C, Schwartz M, Diener MC. Influence of visual and somatosensory input on leg EMG responses in dynamic posturography in normals. *EEG Clin Neurophysiol* 1994;93:7–14.

103. Belen'kii UY, Gurfinkel VS, Pal'tsev YI. Elements of control of voluntary movements. *Biofizika* 1967;12:135–141.

104. Traub MM, Rothwell JC, Marsden CD. Anticipatory postural reflexes in Parkinson's disease and other akinetic-rigid syndromes and in cerebellar ataxia. *Brain* 1980;103:393–412.

105. Diener MC, Dichgans J, Guschlbauer B, Backer M, Rapp H, Klockgether T. The coordination of posture and voluntary movement in patients with cerebral dysfunction. *Mov Disord* 1992;7:14–22.

106. Dick JPR, Rothwell JC, Berardelli A, et al. Associated postural adjustments in Parkinson's disease. *J Neurol Neurosurg Psychiatry* 1986;49:1378–1385.

Motor Disorders,
edited by David S. Younger.
Lippincott Williams & Wilkins, Philadelphia © 1999.

CHAPTER 5

Muscle Pathology

Eduardo Bonilla, Kurenai Tanji, and Carlo Minetti

During the past decade, advances in molecular genetics have revealed the cause of the most common forms of hereditary myopathies, including Duchenne and Becker muscular dystrophy (DMD and BMD) and myotonic dystrophy. Similar studies are being conducted for other forms of muscular dystrophy, and rapid progress is to be expected in our understanding of the pathogenesis of these disorders. Concomitant advances in muscle morphology have been applied to the investigation of muscle biopsies. This has led to important observations of the cellular localization of normal and mutated gene products, contributed to a better understanding of the pathogenesis of muscle cell dysfunction, and provided new approaches for the diagnosis of muscular dystrophy.

This chapter is a signpost for the new directions that have been taken in the evaluation of muscle pathology, emphasizing the application of immunologic probes for the diagnosis of muscular dystrophy. The metabolic disorders, including the mitochondrial myopathies and distal myopathies, inflammatory myopathies, and other acquired myopathies, are discussed in Chapters 9, 10, and 12 of this book.

MUSCULAR DYSTROPHIES

The muscular dystrophies comprise a group of hereditary myopathies characterized by progressive muscle weakness and wasting. The muscle pathology shows signs of degeneration, regenerative changes, and proliferation of connective tissue but no distinctive morphologic abnormalities.

E. Bonilla and K. Tanji: Department of Neurology, Columbia University College of Physicians and Surgeons, New York, New York 10032.

C. Minetti: Department of Pediatrics, University of Genova, Istituto G. Gaslini, 16147 Genova, Italy.

Duchenne Muscular Dystrophy

DMD is the most common childhood dystrophy, affecting approximately 1 male in 3,500. It is inherited as an X-linked recessive trait, and about one third of cases are due to new mutations (1). It begins in early childhood, usually before the age of 4 years. Muscle biopsy shows various degrees of the following changes, depending on the stage of the disease: increased variation in fiber size, large hyper-contracted fibers, focal areas of degenerating and regenerating fibers, increased numbers of internal nuclei, and infiltration of fat and connective tissue. The diagnosis is based on clinical features, muscle biopsy, analysis of serum creatine kinase (CK) levels, and evidence of a mutation in the DMD gene, which can be based either on the analysis of DNA or the gene product, dystrophin. Mutations in the DMD gene cause a shift in the translational reading frame of the dystrophin messenger RNA, a nonsense mutation, and therefore a failure of protein synthesis (2).

Dystrophin is a large (427 kDa) cytoskeletal protein localized to the plasma membrane of the muscle fibers. The protein is tightly associated through its cysteine-rich and C-terminal domains to a large group of dystrophin-associated proteins. These proteins have been divided into three complexes: dystroglycan, syntrophin, and sarcoglycan complexes. The dystroglycan complex consists of α-dystroglycan and β-dystroglycan. The syntrophin complex consists of α_1-syntrophin and β_1-syntrophin. The sarcoglycan complex consists of at least four proteins: α-sarcoglycan, β-sarcoglycan, δ-sarcoglycan, and τ-sarcoglycan. In muscle fibers, interactions between cytoskeletal actin filaments and dystrophin and between α-dystroglycan and the α_2-chain of laminin have been identified, suggesting that one function of the dystrophin-glycoprotein complex is to provide a link between the cytoskeleton and the extracellular matrix (2–5). Also, it should be noted that mutations in at least five components of the dystrophin-based membrane cytoskeleton (dystrophin, α-sarcoglycan, β-sarcoglycan, τ-sarcoglycan, and δ-sarcoglycan) each cause an inherited muscular dystrophy with very similar histopathologic features (6).

DNA analysis detects about 65% of patients with DMD, whereas immunologic analysis of the protein allows the detection of all patients. Immunohistochemistry of frozen muscle sections using antibodies against dystrophin shows no staining in DMD patients, whereas in sections of normal muscle, dystrophin is localized at the sarcolemma (Fig. 1). Similarly, immunoblot analysis of muscle extracts shows a severe defect of dystrophin with concentrations less than 3% of normal (Fig. 1).

Because of the lack of specific therapy, female carriers must be detected to prevent new occurrences. Identification of some, but not all, carriers can be achieved by direct DNA analysis, the analysis of polymorphic DNA sequences linked to the DMD gene, or dystrophin immunohistochemistry of muscle biopsies (7). Prenatal diagnosis is carried out by direct DNA analysis of amniocytes or chorionic villi.

Becker Muscular Dystrophy

This is an allelic form of DMD that is about ten times less common than DMD. The clinical manifestations and distribution of weakness are similar to those of DMD, but the onset is usually after age 5 years. Most patients are still able to walk beyond the age of 12 years. As in DMD, the serum CK concentration is greatly increased even before weakness becomes manifest. Muscle biopsy shows fiber splitting, occasional hypercontracted fibers, segmental myonecrosis, and proliferartion of connective tissue.

BMD is due to mutations in the dystrophin gene, but mutations in this disorder do not cause a frame-shift of the coding sequence. The result is synthesis of shorter dystrophin molecules, which may be only partially functional and more susceptible to degradation (5). In agreement with these molecular defects, the immunohistochemical stain for dystrophin in muscle biopsies is present but shows low intensity and appears discontinuous (Fig. 1). Immunoblot shows qualitative and quantitative alterations of the protein with dystrophin molecules that are smaller than normal (Fig. 1).

Familial X-linked Myalgia and Cramps

This disorder is considered a variant or milder form of BMD. Onset varies, and the cramps, which are usually exercise induced, may begin in early childhood or adoles-

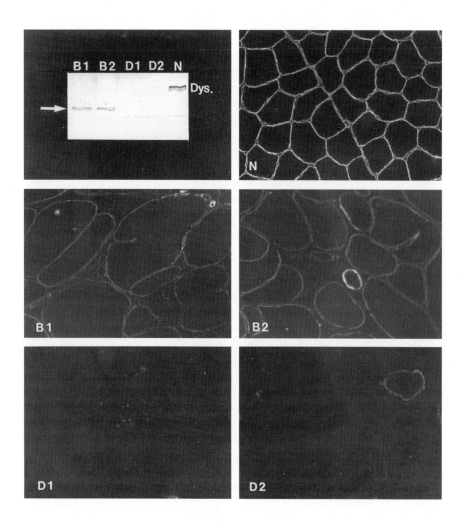

FIG. 1. Dystrophin analysis in Duchenne/Becker muscular dystophies (DMD/BMD). **Top, left:** Western blot containing a sample from a normal control (*N*), two brothers with BMD (*B1* and *B2*), and samples from two brothers with DMD (*D1* and *D2*). The control shows a normal dystrophin (Dys.); the protein is absent in the brothers with DMD, and in the brothers with BMD a mutated protein is seen migrating at a lower position. The corresponding immunostains on frozen sections show a normal pattern in the control (*N*, **top right**), low intensity immunostain in the brothers with BMD (*B1* and *B2*, **middle**), and a markedly reduced immunoreaction in the DMD brothers (*D1* and *D2*, **bottom**). ×110.

cence. Affected patients show elevated resting serum CK levels, calf hypertrophy, and no muscle weakness. There is no history of progressive deterioration of muscle function, and muscle biopsy findings do not show changes consistent with a dystrophic process (7).

Demonstration of a mutation or in-frame deletion in the dystrophin gene is provided by DNA analysis or by direct study of the protein by immunoblotting that shows a smaller dystrophin band (Fig. 2).

Emery-Dreifuss Dystrophy

This rare form of X-linked childhood muscular dystrophy is distinguished from BMD by the presence of contractures of the elbow, ankle, and neck and by cardiomyopathy that causes conduction block. The muscle disorder is slowly progressive and rarely disabling, but sudden death attributable to heart conduction disturbances is not uncommon. The serum CK concentration is only mildly elevated, and the electrocardiogram shows various degrees of atrioventricular block. The muscle biopsy usually shows nonspecific myopathic features, including variation in fiber size, muscle fiber necrosis, and endomysial and perimysial fibrosis. The gene for Emery-Dreifuss dystrophy is located on the distal end of the long arm of the X chromosome. The protein encoded by the gene has been called emerin and has been localized to the nuclear membrane of the muscle fibers (9,10). The diagnosis is based on clinical features, evidence of a mutation in the Emery-Dreifuss dystrophy gene, or the immunologic and immunohistochemical analysis of the gene product, emerin (Fig. 3).

Congenital Muscular Dystrophy

Congenital muscular dystrophy (CMD) is a heterogeneous group characterized by floppiness and profound muscle weakness at birth. In addition, contractures or joint deformities and a variable involvement of the central nervous system (CNS) are usually present. Four autosomal recessive forms have been identified on the basis of differential involvement of the CNS. Fukuyama type CMD, muscle-eye-brain disease, and Walker-Warburg type CMD are dominated by signs of CNS involvement. The last form, occidental CMD, is characterized by skeletal muscle involvement in the absence of clinically evident CNS manifestations.

The morphologic hallmark of these clinically heterogeneous syndromes is a marked increase in connective tissue, so suggesting that abnormalities of components of the extracellular matrix might be involved in the pathogenesis of these disorders. The demonstration that laminin, a component of the basal lamina, was a ligand for α-dystroglycan later prompted studies of whether one of the laminin subunits could be involved in CMD. Laminin is a heterotrimer of one heavy chain and two light chains, and the α_2-chain (merosin) is a 400-kDa isoform found in muscle, in some regions of the CNS, and in Schwann cells of the peripheral nervous system (11). In 1994, a systematic study of several French patients with typical CMD showed that the laminin α_2-chain was deficient in about half of the patients (12). Other studies supported this observation in muscle of patients with CMD from other Western countries (Fig. 4) (13). Because the chromosomal location of the laminin α_2-chain was known (chromosome 6q2), genetic studes confirmed the localization of the CMD gene to the 6q2 locus (14). Later, mutations (splice site and nonsense) in the laminin α_2-chain gene were reported in patients with the Occidental form of CMD (11,15). The gene for Fukuyama type CMD has been localized to chromosome 9q31-33 (16).

Facioscapulohumeral Dystrophy

This autosomal dominant (AD) disorder becomes apparent in adolescence and progresses slowly. The expression of the disease varies greatly among different patients and in

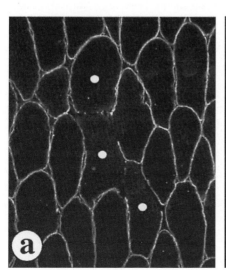 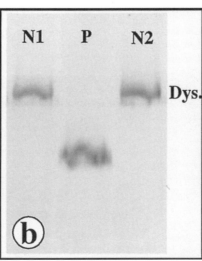

FIG. 2. Dystrophin analysis in familial X-linked myalgia and cramps. **a:** Dystrophin immunohistochemistry shows a few fibers with discontinuous dystrophin stain at the sarcolemma (white circles). ×200. **b:** Western blot shows a normal dystrophin (Dys.) in two controls (*N1* and *N2*) and a mutated protein migrating at a lower position in the patient (*P*) with myalgia and cramps.

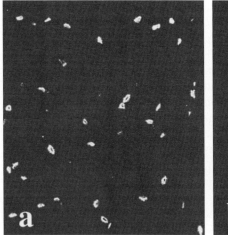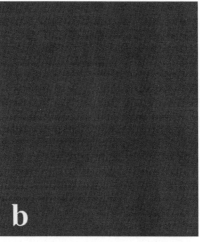

FIG. 3. Emerin immunohistochemistry. **a:** The normal control shows immunoreaction at the nuclear membrane (white arrows) of the muscle nuclei. **b:** A patient with Emery-Dreifuss dystrophy shows lack of emerin in the membrane of the muscle nuclei. ×220.

subsequent generations, from a virtually asymptomatic condition to a severe, although rarely disabling, weakness. The serum CK concentration is only slightly increased, and muscle biopsy abnormalities are not very remarkable, often consisting of scattered atrophic fibers. In some families, however, muscle biopsy shows striking inflammatory changes. The gene for facioscapulohumeral dystrophy has been localized on the long arm of chromosome 4. Available genetic markers can be used for genetic counseling and prenatal diagnosis; however, until flanking markers are found, the accuracy of diagnostic testing is limited (17).

Limb Girdle Muscular Dystrophy (LGMD)

This is the least well-defined of all muscular dystrophies, and it probably includes different diseases, which may explain the variation in age at onset and severity in different patients. Typically, it begins in the second or third decade, with slowly progressive weakness, generally affecting one limb girdle first and then spreading to the other. Serum CK concentrations vary widely from normal to grossly increased. Electromyography (EMG) and muscle biopsy are helpful to rule out more specific disorders that may be clinically indistinguishable from LGMD: structurally defined congenital myopathies, metabolic myopathies, and spinal muscular atrophy.

Recently, genetic linkage studies and molecular mutation investigations of candidate genes have begun to elucidate the underlying cause of some forms of LGMD. In a new nomenclature, the dominantly inherirted LGMDs have been labeled LGMD 1, with the letters indicating the specific loci: LGMD 1A has been mapped to chromosome 5q and LGMD 1B has been localized to chromosome 1q11-21. All recessively inherited LGMDs have been labeled LGMD 2 and the following loci have been assigned: LGMD 2A (chromosome 15q), LGMD 2B (chromosome 2p), LGMD 2C (chromosome 13q12), LGMD 2D (chromosome 17q21), LGMD 2E (chromosome 4q12), and LGMD 2F (chromosome 5q33).

Mutation studies of candidate genes in recessively inherited LGMD have identified the proteins that, when mutated, are responsible for five of these disorders: LGMD 2A is caused by calpain 3 deficiency, LGMD 2C by δ-sarcoglycan deficiency, LGMD 2D by α-sarcoglycan deficiency, LGMD 2E by β-sarcoglycan deficiency, and LGMD 2F by τ-sarcoglycan deficiency (5,18).

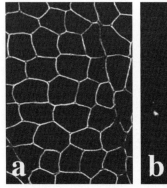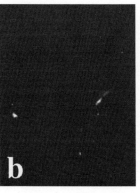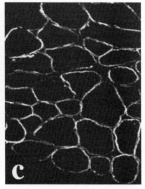

FIG. 4. Congenital muscular dystrophy (CMD) with laminin α_2-chain deficiency. **a:** A normal control shows immunoreaction for laminin α_2-chain at the sarcolemma of all fibers. **b:** A patient with CMD shows lack of laminin α_2-chain at the sarcolemma of all fibers. **c:** The same patient shows immunoreaction for dystrophin at the cell surface of the muscle fibers. ×110.

Oculopharyngeal Muscular Dystrophy

This is a late-onset AD disorder typically of the fourth to fifth decade and is manifested by progressive ptosis, dysphagia, and limb weakness. Linkage of oculopharyngeal muscular dystrophy to 14q11.2-q13 has been reported in several French Canadian families (19). This disorder has been ultrastructurally characterized by the presence of filamentous inclusions in muscle nuclei (20).

MYOTONIC DISORDERS

Myotonia is an alteration of muscle relaxation characterized electromyographically by repetitive high-frequency discharges that wax and wane in frequency and amplitude and are not abolished by curarization or peripheral nerve block.

Myotonic Dystrophy

This is the most common form of adult muscular dystrophy, with an estimated incidence of 1 per 7,500. It is a multisystem disorder characterized by muscle weakness, wasting and myotonia, cardiomyopathy, cataract, baldness, and endocrine dysfunctions. The onset is usually in adolescence, and the course is slowly progressive, but one of the striking features of this disorder is the variability of phenotype both within and between families. EMG shows a combination of myotonic and myopathic features.

The inheritance pattern is AD with the affected gene locus on the long arm of chromosome 19. The disease is due to a variable trinucleotide repeat insert in the myotonic dystrophy gene consisting of 50 to several thousand CTG repeats (21). This mutation interrupts the 3′ untranslated region of a protein kinase gene that has been named myotonin protein kinase. The measurement of the $(CTG)_n$ repeat is considered an accurate diagnostic test (22). The muscle pathology is relatively distinct and consist of numerous central nuclei, sarcoplasmic masses, ring fibers, and variable type I fiber atrophy (23).

Congenital Myotonic Dystrophy

Affected infants manifest a clinical picture very different from that in adolescents; they show severe hypotonia, bilateral facial weakness with difficulty in sucking, and respiratory distress. The almost exclusively maternal transmission of congenital myotonic dystrophy has been attributed to genetic imprinting. An important negative feature is the absence of clinical and often electrical evidence of myotonia in these infants; however, clinical or electrical evidence of myotonia in the mother is a useful diagnostic clue. The most significant pathologic abnormatity in the muscle biopsy is immaturity of muscle fibers. The fibers are of small caliber and have basophilic cytoplasm with internally placed nuclei, showing the histologic features of myotubes.

Myotonia Congenita

Myotonia congenita is an AD disorder due to mutations of the gene coding for the voltage-sensitive chloride channel of skeletal muscle (24). The symptoms are limited to myotonia, and muscle hypertrophy is common. Becker described an autosomal recessive (AR) form of congenital myotonia in which muscle hypertrophy is more pronounced than in the dominant form and weakness is often present. This form is also due to mutations of the voltage-sensitive chloride channel. Serum CK concentrations are normal in both forms of myotonia congenita, and EMG shows myotonic discharges but no myopathic features. Muscle biopsy findings are usually normal, except for lack of type IIB fibers.

Paramyotonia Congenita

The clinical hallmarks of this disorder are the temperature-sensitive nature of the myotonia and episodic paralysis. Transmission is AD, and the disorder is due to mutations of the gene coding for the voltage-sensitive sodium channel of the muscle fibers. Muscle biopsy shows no particular pathologic features (25).

Hypokalemic Periodic Paralysis

This condition is characterized by attacks of flaccid paralysis involving trunk and limb muscles, typically sparing respiratory and ocular muscles. Transmission is autosomal dominant, with a striking predominance of affected males, and the disorder is due to mutations in the voltage-dependent calcium channel of the muscle fibers (25). During attacks, muscle is inexcitable, and EMG shows electrical silence. Serum potassium concentrations are characteristically decreased, probably because of a shift of potassium into the muscle. Muscle biopsy taken during and between attacks show numerous vacuoles that may be empty or may contain granular or hyaline material. Another characteristic alteration that may be seen in period paralysis is the collection of structures referred to as tubular aggregates (Fig. 5).

Hyperkalemic Periodic Paralysis

Hyperkalemic periodic paralysis is transmitted as an AD trait. As in paramyotonia congenita, the disorder is due to a mutation resulting in a single amino acid change of voltage-sensitive sodium channels that alters the gating properties of the channel (25). Attacks are shorter than in the hypokalemic disorder and may be precipitated by rest after heavy exercise and by cold or fasting. Clinical or electrical evidence of myotonia is present in most

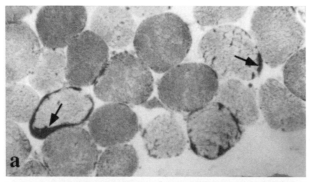

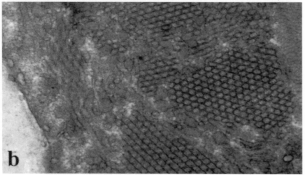

FIG. 5. Hypokalemic periodic paralysis. **a:** Nicotinamide dehydrogenase tetrazolium reductase **(NADH-TR)** histochemistry shows several collections of tubular aggregates (*black arrows*) confined to type II fibers. ×260. **b:** Electron microscopy shows that the aggregates are in a hexagonal array and contain a moderately electron-dense core. ×70,000.

affected families, but weakness, not myotonia, is the main clinical complaint. Serum potassium concentrations are variably increased during the attacks, and attacks may be induced by administration of potassium. The most frequent changes in muscle biopsies are the presence of vacuoles and tubular aggregates, which have features identical to those observed in the hypokalemic form, but they are usually less numerous.

MORPHOLOGICALLY DEFINED CONGENITAL MYOPATHIES

Congenital myopathies are defined as nonprogressive myopathies of the neonatal period with weakness and hypotonia of varying severity. They have been classified according to the pathologic features on histochemical study of frozen sections of muscle tissue. The following are brief descriptions of the most common congenital myopathies with incorporation of recent molecular pathology data when available.

Central Core Disease

In this disorder, well-circumscribed central areas or cores, usually extending along the entire length of the muscle fibers, show decreased staining with reactions for oxidative enzymes and phosphorylase (Fig. 6). The lesions are usually limited to type I fibers, and in most patients there is marked type I fiber predominance. By electron microscopy, the central cores can be divided into two types: structured cores, in which the architecture of the sarcomeres is preserved, and unstructured cores, in which the organization of the sarcomeres is lost. The ultrastructure of the cores shows streaming of the Z-disc, decreased numbers of mitochondria, and few glycogen granules within the core (Fig. 6). It is transmitted in an AD fashion, and the gene for both central core disease and malignant hyperthermia has been localized on chromosome 19q12-13. The protein encoded by this gene is the calcium release channel of the sarcoplasmic reticulum, and mutations of the gene have been found in families with malignant hyperthermia and central core disease (26).

Multicore (Minicore) Disease

This was originally described in two children with nonprogressive weakness at birth and delayed motor milestones. There were multiple small cores in each affected fiber, with abnormalities resembling those of unstruc-

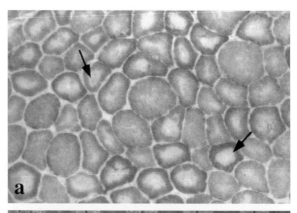

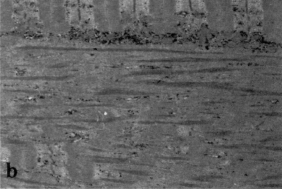

FIG. 6. Central core disease. **a:** Cytochrome *c* oxidase histochemistry shows areas lacking oxidative activity (*arrows*) in several muscle fibers. ×240. **b:** Electron microscopy shows a region of a core with streamimg of Z-disc material and lack of mitochondria. ×12,000.

tured central cores. The cores, however, did not extend along the entire length of the fiber.

Nemaline (Rod) Myopathy

This disorder is characterized by multiple "rod" structures in muscle fibers that are best revealed with the modified Gomori trichrome stain (Fig. 7). Both fiber types may be affected, but rods tend to be more abundant in type I fibers, and type I fiber predominance is common. The electron microscopy of the rods is similar to that of the Z-disks, from which they appear to originate (Fig. 7). The patients usually have dysmorphic features such as an elongated face, high arched palate, club foot, and kyphosis. It is usually transmitted as an AD trait, but AR cases have also been reported. Linkage studies assigned the gene for autosomal dominant nemaline myopathy to 1p13-25. When the gene for α-tropomyosin was assigned to the same region, it became a good candidate for nemaline myopathy, and Laing et al. (27) showed a point mutation in exon 1 of the gene that segregated with the expression of the disease in one family. Similar studies in other families with AD nemaline myopathy showed no mutation in different exons of the α-tropomyosin gene, suggesting the presence of genetic heterogeneity in the disease. In addition, AR nemaline myopathy did not show

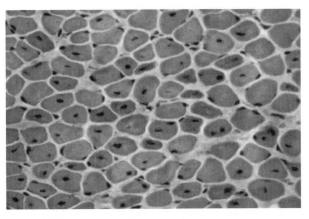

FIG. 8. Myotubular myopathy. Modified Gomori trichrome stain shows several centrally placed myonuclei. ×220.

linkage to the α-tropomyosin locus, and linkage analysis mapped this form to chromosome 2q21 (28).

Myotubular (Centronuclear) Myopathy

The morphologic hallmark of this disorder is the presence of rows of central nuclei in both fiber types but predominantly in type I fibers (Fig. 8). Type I fiber preponderance and hypotrophy have also been described. The central nuclei are surrounded by areas of cytoplasm devoid of myofibrils and containing variably increased oxidative enzymes and decreased ATPase activity, a picture reminiscent of myotubes. Because of the similarity of these fibers to myotubes, it has been proposed that this disorder may be due to an arrest of normal muscle development. When type I hypotrophy is the predominant feature of the biopsy, the disorder is called type I fiber hypotrophy with central nuclei.

The most common mode of transmission is AR, but X-linked recessive transmission has been described in several families. Linkage studies of families with the X-linked form mapped the locus to Xq28, and recently, mutations in a gene coding for a tyrosine phosphatase have been reported in 12% of patients with myotubular myopathy. The putative protein, myotubularin, may play a role in the control of cell growth, proliferation, and differentiation (29).

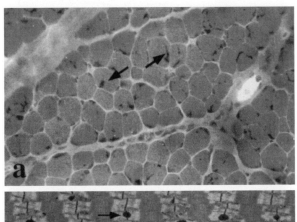
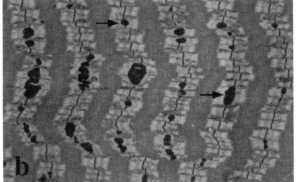

FIG. 7. Nemaline myopathy. **a:** Modified Gomori trichrome shows rods (*arrows*) in several muscle fibers. ×180. **b:** Electron microscopy shows that the rods (*arrows*) originated from the Z-disc. ×5,400.

REFERENCES

1. Moser H. Duchenne muscular dystrophy: pathogenetic aspects and genetic prevention. *Hum Genet* 1984;66:17–40.
2. Hoffman EP, Brown RH, Kunkel LM. Dystrophin: the protein product of the Duchenne muscular dystrophy locus. *Cell* 1987;51:919–928.
3. Koenig M, Monaco AP, Kunkel LM. The complete sequence of dystrophin predicts a rod-shaped cytoskeletal protein. *Cell* 1988;53:219–228.
4. Bonilla E, Samitt CE, Miranda AF, et al. Duchenne muscular dystrophy: deficiency of dystrophin at the muscle cell surface. *Cell* 1988;54:447–452.
5. Hoffman EP. The muscular dystrophies. In: Rosenberg RN, Prusiner

SB, DiMauro S, Barchi RL, eds. *The molecular and genetic basis of neurological disease.* Boston: Butterworth-Heinemann, 1996:877–930.

6. Campbell KP. Three muscular dystrophies: loss of cytoskeleton-extracellular matrix linkage. *Cell* 1995;80:675–679.

7. Bonilla E, Schmidt B, Samitt CE, et al. Normal and dystrophin-deficient muscle fibers in carriers of the gene for Duchenne muscular dystrophy. *Am J Pathol* 1988;133:440–445.

8. Gospe SM, Lazaro RP, Lava NS, Grootscholten PM, Scott MO, Fischbeck KH. Familial X-linked myalgia and cramps: a nonprogressive myopathy associated with a deletion in the dystrophin gene. *Neurology* 1989;39:1277–1280.

9. Bione S, Tamanini F, Rivella S, et al. Identification of a novel X-linked gene responsible for Emery-Dreifuss muscular dystrophy. *Nat Genet* 1994;8:323–327.

10. Nagano A, Koga R, Ogawa M, et al. Emerin deficiency at the nuclear membrane in patients with Emery-Dreifuss muscular dystrophy. *Nat Genet* 1996;12:254–259.

11. Pegoraro E, Mancias P, Swerdlow SH, et al. Congenital muscular dystrophy with primary laminin α2 (merosin) deficiency presenting as inflammatory myopathy. *Ann Neurol* 1996;40:782–791.

12. Tome FMS, Evangelista T, Leclerc A, et al. Congenital muscular dystrophy with merosin deficiency. *CR Acad Sci Paris* 1994;317:351–357.

13. Minetti C, Bado M, Morreale G, Pedemente M, Cordone G. Disruption of basal lamina in congenital muscular dystrophy with merosin deficiency. *Neurology* 1996;46:1354–1358.

14. Hillaire D, Leclerc A, Faure S, et al. Localization of merosin-negative congenital muscular dystrophy to chromosome 6q2 by homozygosity mapping. *Hum Mol Genet* 1994;3:1657–1661.

15. Helbling-Leclerc A, Zhang X, Topaloglu H, et al. Mutations in the laminin α2-chain gene (LAMA2) cause merosin-deficient congenital muscular dystrophy. *Nat Genet* 1995;11:216–218.

16. Toda T, Segawa M, Nomura Y, et al. Localization of the gene for Fukuyama type congenital muscular dystrophy to chromosome 9q31-33. *Nat Genet* 1993;5:283–286.

17. Tawil R, Griggs RC. Facioscapulohumeral muscular dystrophy. In: Rosenberg RN, Prusiner SB, DiMauro S, Barchi RL, eds. *The molecular and genetic basis of neurological disease.* Boston: Butterworth-Heinemann, 1996:931–937.

18. Nigro V, de Sa Moreira E, Piluso G, et al. Autosomal recessive limb-girdle muscular dystrophy, LGMD 2F, is caused by a mutation in the τ-sarcoglycan gene. *Nat Genet* 1996;14:195–198.

19. Brais B, Xie Y-G, Sanson M, et al. The oculopharyngeal muscular dystrophy locus maps to the region of the cardiac α and β myosin heavy chain genes on chromosome 14q11.2-q13. *Hum Mol Genet* 1995;4:429–434.

20. Tome FMS, Fardeau M. Oculopharyngeal muscular dystrophy. In: Engel AG, Franzini-Armstrong C, eds. *Myology.* New York: McGraw-Hill, 1994:1233–1245.

21. Brook JD, McCurrach ME, Harley HG, et al. Molecular basis of myotonic dystrophy: expansion of a trinucleotide (CTG) repeat at the 3' end of a transcript encoding a protein kinase family member. *Cell* 1992;68:799–808.

22. Roses AD. Myotonic dystrophy. In: Rosenberg RN, Prusiner SB, DiMauro S, Barchi RL, eds. *The molecular and genetic basis of neurological disease.* Boston: Butterworth-Heinemann, 1996:913–930.

23. Engel AG. Diseases of muscle (myopathies) and neuromuscular junction. In: Wyngaarden JB, Smith LH, Bennett JC, eds. *Cecil textbook of medicine.* Philadelphia: W.B. Saunders Company, 1992:2250–2268.

24. Jentsch TJ. Myotonia congenita. In: Rosenberg RN, Prusiner SB, DiMauro S, Barchi RL, eds. *The molecular and genetic basis of neurological disease.* Boston: Butterworth-Heinemann, 1996:715–721.

25. Barchi RL. Molecular pathology of the period paralysis. In: Rosenberg RN, Prusiner SB, DiMauro S, Barchi RL, eds. *The molecular and genetic basis of neurological disease.* Boston: Butterworth-Heinemann, 1996:723–731.

26. MacLennan DH, Phillips MS, Britt BA. The molecular and genetic basis for malignant hyperthermia and central core disease. In: Rosenberg RN, Prusiner SB, DiMauro S, Barchi RL, eds. *The molecular and genetic basis of neurological disease.* Boston: Butterworth-Heinemann, 1996:733–748.

27. Laing NG, Wilton SD, Akkari PA, et al. A mutation in the α-tropomyosin gene TPM3 associated with autosomal dominant nemaline myopathy. *Nat Genet* 1995;9:75–79.

28. Wallgren-Pettersson C, Avela K, Marchand S, et al. A gene for autosomal recessive nemaline myopathy assigned to chromosome 2q by linkage analysis. *Neuromusc Disord* 1995;5:441–449.

29. Laporte J, Hu LJ, Kretz et al. A gene mutated in X-linked myotubular myopathy defines a new puutative tyrosine phosphatase family conserved in yeast. *Nat Genet* 1996;13:175–181.

Motor Disorders,
edited by David S. Younger.
Lippincott Williams & Wilkins, Philadelphia © 1999.

CHAPTER 6

Peripheral Nerve Pathology

David S. Younger

Spectacular progress has been made in the application of immunohistochemical and immunocytochemical techniques, molecular genetics, ultrastructural and morphometric studies, and teased nerve analysis to nerve biopsies in the evaluation of patients with peripheral neuropathy and related disorders. The has resulted in greater accuracy in the assignment of specimens, for diagnostic purposes, to more certain proposed mechanisms of injury, and the more rational selection of immunomodulating and immunosuppressive therapies. This chapter reviews aspects of peripheral nerve microscopic anatomy, morphologic and immunopathologic alterations in peripheral nervous system disorders, and the contribution of nerve biopsy to neuropathic motor disorders.

GENERAL CONSIDERATIONS

Exclusive of the pathologic alterations of individual nerve axons, disease processes that affect the peripheral nerve often lead to specific alterations of the epineurial, perineurial, and endoneurial compartments described in more detail below.

Epineurium

The fibrous adipose tissue of the epineurium invests the whole nerve trunk and space between the individual fascicles and is the site of entry of the vasa nervorum (Fig. 1). The vascular anatomy of the nerves of the limbs has been recognized for over 50 years since the detailed studies of Sunderland (1,2). The nutrient vessels ramify within the nerve trunk, anastomosing longitudinally and penetrating the perineurium, ending in an unbroken network of endoneurial microvessels (Fig. 2A and B). The

D. S. Younger: Department of Clinical Neuromuscular Disorders and Jerry Lewis Muscular Dystrophy Association Clinic at Rusk Institute, New York University Medical Center and Department of Neuromuscular Disease and Electromyography Laboratory, Lenox Hill Hospital, New York, New York 10021.

proximal circulation of named nerves of the arm and leg may be sustained by long stretches of a single arterial vessel, such as in the axilla-to-elbow and knee-to-elbow segments (Fig. 3) (1–4), most often located peripherally in the nerve trunk, but this does not generally translate into watershed zones unless there is associated vasculitis or abrupt thrombosis of large named vessels (5).

The epineurium provides mechanical support, cushioning nerve trunks as they pass by bony prominences. Focal nerve compression is enhanced when there is a reduction in the epineurial fat cushion due to chronic disease or malnutrition with accompanying weight loss in association with syndromes of severe generalized weakness and chronic bedridden or immobile states and prolonged stays in the intensive care unit. The sites most prone to compression are the ulnar nerve at the elbow, the sciatic nerve in the buttock and thigh, and the peroneal nerve at the fibular head.

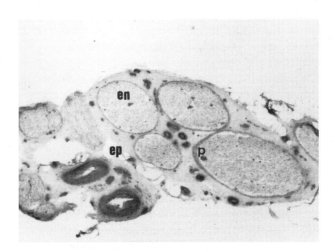

FIG. 1. The distribution of blood vessels in the peripheral nerve trunk. A cross-section of sural nerve is shown in low magnification stained with hematoxylin and eosin and counterstained with anti-actin smooth muscle antibody. *ep*, epineurium; *en*, endoneurium; *p*, perineurium.

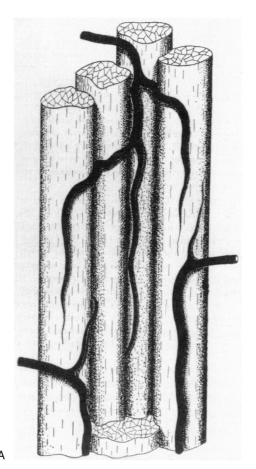
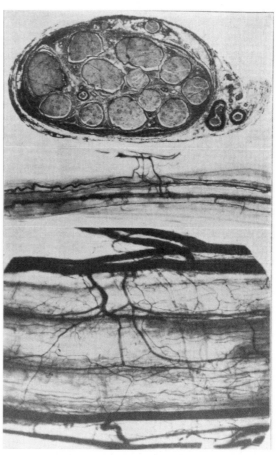

FIG. 2. The vascular supply of the peripheral nerves of the limbs. **A:** An artists view of the intraneural supply. **B:** The injection of india ink shows the actual internal architecture of the vascular supply. Reproduced by permission of The American Medical Association.

Perineurium

Individual nerve fascicles are surrounded by alternating layers of specialized densely packed cells, the pericytes, and longitudinally oriented collagen fibers. The perineurium is subject to nonspecific morphologic alterations such as thickening of the basal lamina as a consequence of a variety of disorders and normal aging. There is a primary inflammatory syndrome of the perineurium, termed perineuritis (6), which classically presents with sensory loss; however, one reported patient had prominent motor involvement (7).

Endoneurium

The endoneurium is the supporting matrix for myelinated and unmyelinated nerve fibers contained within a single fascicle. This compartment reacts to a vast number of nonspecific processes with a limited number of alterations. Collectively, the observed pathologic findings generally point toward either segmental demyelination or axonopathy as the primary pathologic process. Segmental

demyelination is generally attributable to a primary disturbance of Schwann cell function or immune-mediated injury of internodal myelin segments; however, in both instances, the axon is left essentially intact. Standard cryostat- and paraffin-stained sections do not adequately demonstrate the histologic features of demyelination and remyelination in a given nerve specimen. However, plastic embedded, 1-μm, semithin sections can show demyelinated axons and thinly myelinated fibers because of the production of a new myelin sheath. Teased nerve fiber studies are ideally suited to show the segmental character of the lesions. Repeated episodes of demyelination and remyelination lead to onion bulb formations, visible by electron microscopy as concentrically laminated Schwann cell processes.

Active axonal degeneration due to nerve ischemia, compression, trauma, infection, and primary or secondary degeneration of motor axons is suggested by the presence of myelin ovoids, myelin debris, and macrophage recruitment along the course of degenerated fibers, best seen in longitudinally stained sections. The signs of chronic axonopathy are a marked depletion of

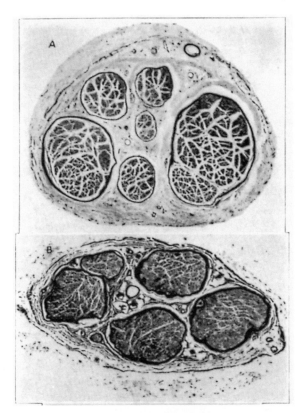

FIG. 3. The relation of blood vessels to the components of the nerve in the upper arm. The major arteriole is situated peripherally in the median **(A)** and ulnar **(B)** nerve. Reproduced by permission of The American Medical Association.

myelinated and unmyelinated nerve fibers and endoneurial fibrosis.

IMMUNOPATHOLOGY

Significant advances have been made in the basic understanding of immune reactions of the peripheral nerves (8), and these in turn have had wide-ranging impacts on the immunopathologic evaluation of nerve tissue. Under normal circumstances, the peripheral nervous system is protected from immune reactions by the blood–nerve barrier that consists of perineurial and endoneurial vascular tight junctions. In the early phases of inflammation, there is enhancement of vascular permeability by vasoactive substances, complement activation, and cytokine secretion. These alterations lead to leakage of inflammatory mediators and the immigration of lymphocytes and macrophages in the endoneurial compartment. Much has been learned about each of these constituents in the past decade.

Local immune activation requires the interaction of a specific autoantigen, a main histocompatibility (MHC) Class II antigen-presenting cell and antigen-specific T cells in the trimolecular complex. This interaction leads to the proliferation of specific helper (CD4+) and cytotoxic (CD8+) T cells, with expression of human leukocyte antigen-DR, interleukin-2 receptor, and the secretion of tumor necrosis factor-α and other interleukins. Macrophages are the primary antigen-presenting cell of the peripheral nervous system (9). They appear as immunoreactive CD68+ cells with elongated or cylindrical cell bodies, scattered in the endoneurium, often in proximity to blood vessels. Intensely stained MHC Class II-positive macrophages appear in excessive numbers at foci of acute axonal degeneration and in other primary immune-mediated neuropathies. They also have a role in the initiation of myelinated nerve fiber regeneration (10). The complement system also contributes to vascular and neural injury. Activation of the classic or alternative pathways leads to cleavage of C3 to C3d that then results in activation of the terminal lytic sequence C5b-9 or membrane attack complex (MAC).

Commercially available monoclonal and polyclonal antibodies directed against T-cell subsets, B cells, macrophages, immunoglobulins, complement proteins, cytokines and other inflammatory mediators, and MHC class antigens can be easily applied to clinical and research protocols for the evaluation of patients with various immune-mediated neuropathies (11).

NERVE BIOPSY: GENERAL CONSIDERATIONS

Over the past decade, the demand for nerve biopsy has increased along with advances in the assessable process and treatment of diverse neuropathic disorders, and the availability of outpatient biopsy surgery has allowed far easier and less expensive access of the procedure to patients. The nerve chosen for biopsy should be clinically and electrophysiologically involved. A segment of the sural, superficial peroneal, and femoral intermedius nerves can be surgically removed, depending on the clinical circumstances, without incurring a serious deficit; each has the advantage of allowing biopsy of underlying muscle, respectively, from the soleus, peroneus brevis, and rectus femoris (Fig. 4A–D). The estimated risk of residual pain, paresthesia, analgesia, or anesthesia from a sural nerve biopsy is about 5% (12). There is a technique for the biopsy of the gracilis motor nerve in the medial thigh that does not lead to a noticeable deficit (13); however, it entails a deeper dissection. Examination of a specimen of muscle tissue is useful to exclude unsuspected myopathy. It also increases the yield of vasculitic lesions and provides useful information about the severity of an underlying neuropathy. Full-thickness nerve biopsy is preferable to a fascicular biopsy; however, some still prefer the latter technique to minimize dermatomal sensory loss and afford regeneration across the gap.

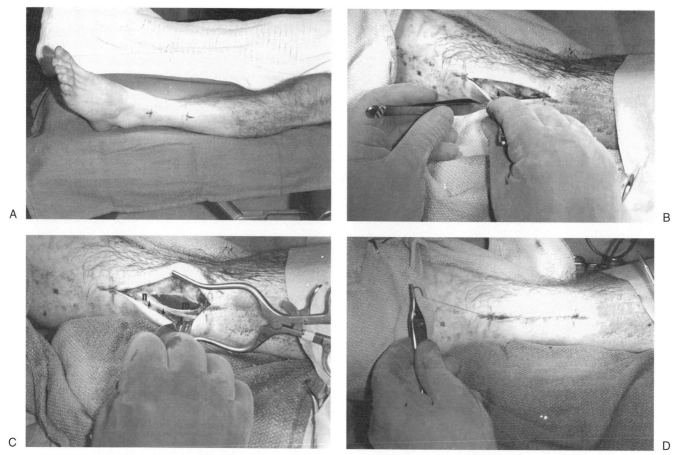

FIG. 4. Superficial peroneal sensory nerve and peroneus brevis muscle biopsy procedure. **A:** The nerve is palpated laterally along the distal third of the leg along a line between the fibular head and lateral malleolus providing the markings for the incision. **B:** Under monitored anesthesia care, an incision is made and the area is dissected revealing the nerve (n) obliquely traversing the field (arrow). **C:** Incising the aponeurosis reveals underlying muscle tissue (m) in addition to nerve (n, and arrows) available for biopsy. **D:** After the specimens are removed and the site irrigated, a subcuticular closure is performed using absorbable sutures.

SPECIFIC NEUROPATHIC MOTOR DISORDERS

Nerve biopsy is useful in the diagnosis of several neuropathic motor disorders, discussed in more detail below.

Peripheral Nerve Vasculitis

In 1938, Harry Lee Parker recommended biopsy of a peripheral nerve to diagnose cases of polyarteritis nodosa (14). Coers and Woolf (15) later described the suitability of the superficial peroneal musculocutaneous nerve and peroneus brevis muscle that was later implemented in the diagnosis of other similar patients with mononeuritis multiplex (16,17). A quarter century later, Dyck et al. (18), Kissel et al. (19), and Said et al. (20) established an important role for sural nerve biopsy in the definition of peripheral nerve vasculitis.

Necrotizing arteritis affects small- and medium-sized epineurial vessels of the range found in the vasa nervorum leading to narrowing, occlusion, and recanalization of vessel lumina in individual nerves (Fig. 5). The resulting lesions interrupt nutritional and oxygen support, leading to ischemia and infarction of a portion of the nerve fascicle, usually in a centrofascicular or wedge-shaped area and best seen in cross-section of the nerve trunk. Nerve biopsy is essential in the proper management of peripheral nerve vasculitis because unrecognized and therefore untreated, the outcome is often fatal (21). Conversely, the risk of potentially fatal medication side effects in histologically unproved cases outweighs the potential benefits of empiric immunosuppressive therapy (22).

Cholesterol Emboli Syndrome

Nerve biopsy is essential in the antemortem diagnosis of cholesterol emboli syndrome (23). The neurologic disorder includes myalgia, livedo reticularis, mononeuritis multiplex or distal symmetrical polyneuropathy, increased erythrocyte sedimentation rate, and weight loss. Vascular

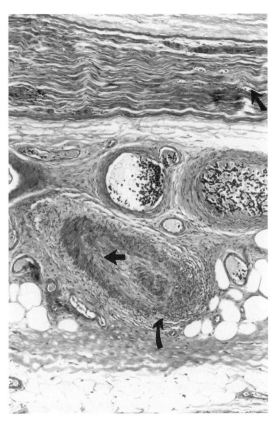

FIG. 5. Peripheral nerve vasculitis. A superficial peroneal sensory nerve in longitudinal section stained with hematoxylin and eosin shows necrotizing arteritis in the epineurium with resultant invasion and destruction of the vessel wall (*curved arrow*), proliferation, and narrowing of the lumen (*horizontal arrow*). There is a moderate loss of myelinated nerve fibers with foci of myelin debris (*diagonal arrow*). Reproduced by permission of Thieme Medical Publishers.

catheter procedures and severe aortic atherosclerosis are probably the most important risk factors in susceptible patients. Biopsy of an affected nerve and muscle shows cholesterol crystals in the lumina of epineurial and epimysial vessels accompanied by necrotizing arteritis and foreign body giant cell reaction (Fig. 6). It can be argued that intraluminal deposition of cholesterol leads to arteritis rather than a coincidence of two separate disorders. Cholesterol clefts are not seen in other arteritic processes that result in the entrapment of cholesterol crystals. Similar pathologic findings in animals occur after injection of human atheromata. Necrotizing arteritis was noted at other sites of the peripheral nervous system in patients with cholesterol emboli neuropathy, including the lumbar plexus and skeletal muscles, and in other organs at postmortem examination.

Familial Amyloid Polyneuropathy and Primary Systemic Amyloidosis

Familial amyloid polyneuropathy is a group of autosomal dominant disorders characterized by deposits of amy-

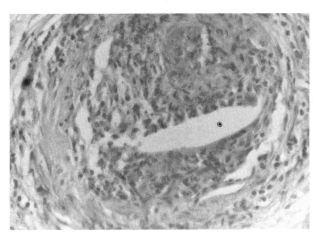

FIG. 6. Cholesterol emboli syndrome. A cross-section of gastrocnemius muscle stained with hematoxylin and eosin demonstrates active and healed arteritis in the vicinity of a cholesterol cleft (*circle*).

loid fibrils in the peripheral nerve (24,25). The amyloid fibrils are derived from mutant forms of a plasma protein transthyretin or prealbumin (26). The various familial amyloid polyneuropathy phenotypes differ in the clinical presentation of neuropathy, age at onset from the third to seventh decade, and the pattern of systemic involvement variably affecting skin, liver, heart, vitreous, and other organs. Although the polyneuropathy is mainly sensory, one reported patient with an Asp 70 mutation presented with carpal tunnel syndrome followed by generalized weakness, wasting, and fasciculation, suggesting prominent motor nerve involvement (27). Sural nerve biopsy in that patient revealed axonopathy with homogenous masses of hyaline, deeply eosinophilic material deposited in the endoneurium and epineurium, typical tinctorial and optical properties of amyloid, and immunoreactivity to transthyretin antisera (Fig. 7). By electron microscopy, the

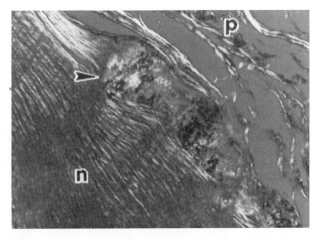

FIG. 7. Familial amyloidotic polyneuropathy. A longitudinal section of sural nerve stained with Congo red and viewed under crossed polarized lenses demonstrates endoneurial (*n*) amyloid deposition immediately subjacent to the perineurium (*p*).

amyloid deposits appeared as fine, haphazard, non-branched filaments with a diameter of 8 to 10 nm.

Painful small-fiber neuropathy with progressive autonomic involvement is a common presenting feature of primary systemic amyloidosis. It results from the excessive production of immunoglobulin light chains due to plasma cell dyscrasia and is detectable by immunohistochemical analysis of a nerve biopsy specimen. In one patient with generalized weakness and wasting, laboratory studies suggested a neuropathic cause; however, electrodiagnostic studies were more compatible with a myopathic process, and muscle biopsy instead showed amyloid deposits in myofibers (Fig. 8A and B).

Adult Polyglucosan Body Disease

Adult polyglucosan body disease is a rare neurologic disorder characterized clinically by peripheral neuropathy with motor and sensory loss, corticospinal tract signs, urinary incontinence, and dementia and pathologically by polyglucosan bodies distributed in the peripheral and central nervous system of affected patients. One patient with autopsy proven adult polyglucosan body disease simulated amyotrophic lateral sclerosis (ALS) clinically and pathologically (28). At postmortem examination, polyglucosan bodies were found extensively in neuronal and astrocytic processes, nerve roots, and peripheral nerves. A second similar patient had polyglucosan bodies in myelinated axons in a sural nerve biopsy (Fig. 9A and B).

Neurolymphomatosis

Neurolymphomatosis is defined histologically by lymphomatous infiltration of the nerve in a biopsy specimen or at postmortem examination. Virtually all patients present with signs of peripheral neuropathy. Of 41 histolog-

ically proven cases, 16 were diagnosed antemortem by nerve biopsy and the remainder at postmortem examination; all but one had non-Hodgkin's lymphoma (29,30). Less than one half of patients have known lymphoma; therefore, nerve biopsy is crucial in establishing the diagnosis and prompting effective therapy. One recently studied patient with progressive leg weakness was found to have B-cell non-Hodgkin's lymphoma in a superficial peroneal nerve biopsy (Fig. 10A and B). He improved neurologically with intravenous cyclophosphamide therapy, but a higher grade of lymphoma appeared 6 months later as an isolated neck mass prompting further therapy.

Charcot-Marie-Tooth Neuropathies

Prominent motor involvement is the cause of the common foot deformity, pes cavus, and the "inverted champagne bottle" appearance of the leg in long-standing cases of Charcot-Marie-Tooth (CMT) neuropathy. The classification of the CMT neuropathies historically relied on the concordance of the clinical aspects, inheritance patterns, and electrophysiologic and nerve biopsy findings. However, modern genetic analysis added a fifth criterion, demonstration of the responsible gene defect. These include point mutations, duplications, overexpressions, and other alterations in the responsible gene loci for peripheral myelin protein 22, Po, and connexin 32 situated, respectively, on chromosomes 17, 1, and the X chromosome; other gene defects have been reported on chromosome 3 and 8 (31). There is generally little difficulty in establishing the diagnosis of CMT in index cases of well-studied families. However, several clinical situations might constitute diagnostic dilemmas warranting nerve biopsy to provide clinicopathologic correlation, for example, index cases of CMT1A with de novo duplications at the 17p11.2-12; families with hereditary neu-

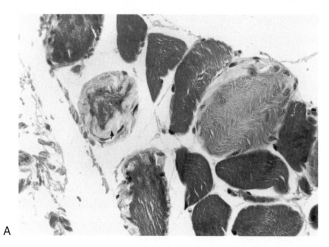
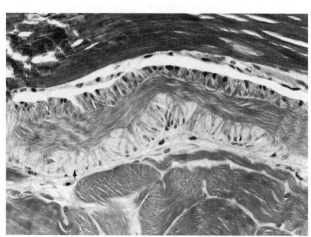

A   B

FIG. 8. Amyloid myopathy. Vastus lateralis muscle viewed in cross-section **(A)** and in longitudinal section **(B)** shows amyloid deposition at the peripheral of myofibers stained with Masson trichrome (*arrows*).

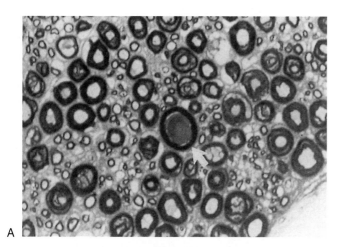
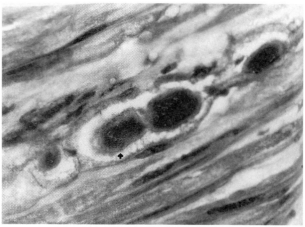

A

B

FIG. 9. Adult polyglucosan body disease. **A:** A polyglucosan body is seen within a large myelinated axon from a ventral root in a semithin section stained with toluidine blue (*arrow*). **B:** Several polyglucosan bodies are seen within a myelinated axon stained with hematoxylin and eosin (*arrow*).

ropathy with liability to pressure palsy (HNPP) or so-called tomaculous neuropathy, in which linkage to chromosome 17p may be lacking; or patients with CMT2C that resemble hereditary juvenile hereditary spinal muscular atrophy clinically.

Chronic Inflammatory Demyelinating Polyneuropathy

Chronic inflammatory demyelinating polyneuropathy (CIDP) is probably the most common cause of undiagnosed demyelinating neuropathy. The disorder is characterized clinically by slow or stepwise progressive or relapsing symmetric sensorimotor neuropathy with loss of tendon reflexes, elevation of the cerebrospinal fluid protein content, widespread slowing of nerve conduction velocities, and morphologic evidence of primary demyelination in a nerve biopsy. Several factors may contribute to the occurrence of prominent motor involvement

in some affected patients (32). First, a relatively larger proportion of large myelinated motor fibers contained in mixed nerves could lead to a greater devastation of motor function. Second, motor fibers in the ventral roots may be selectively involved pathologically by inflammatory demyelinating lesions and axon loss. Third, demyelinated motor fibers might be selectively impaired due to their lower safety factor for impulse propagation. Fourth, depending on the fascicular arrangement of motor fibers in a given nerve trunk, inflammatory-demyelinating lesions might be relatively restricted to motor fascicles, leaving sensory fibers intact.

There is no general consensus as to the appropriateness of nerve biopsy in all patients with CIDP. However, most authorities would probably advocate biopsy of an affected nerve to confirm the diagnosis pathologically and to exclude other etiologies before commencing therapy. Nonetheless, nerve biopsy findings can be quite variable. Among 60 patients with CIDP (33), 48% had

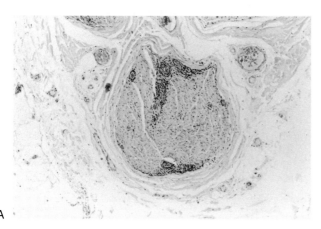
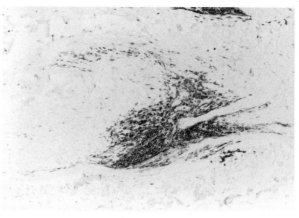

A

B

FIG. 10. Neurolymphomatosis. **A:** Superficial peroneal sensory nerve demonstrates an intense lymphocytic invasion stained with H&E, which in **B** stains positively for leukocyte common antigen (LCA). Further evaluation showed gene rearrangement indicative of a malignant non-Hodgkin lymphoma.

evidence of demyelination and remyelination, 21% had axonopathy, 13% had features of both myelinopathy and axonopathy, and 18% were normal; only 11% had inflammation; however, lymphocyte marker immunohistochemistry was not performed.

Motor Neuropathy and Motor Neuron Disease

Our present concepts of motor neuropathy have evolved over the past two decades, influenced by the delineation of several lower motor neuron (LMN) syndromes separable from classic CIDP and motor neuron disease (MND). In 1982, Lewis and Sumner (34) described 5 patients from among 40 cases of CIDP with a primarily motor form of mononeuritis multiplex especially involving the arms, with multifocal conduction block of mixed nerves severe enough to account for the observed weakness. This syndrome, termed multifocal demyelinating motor neuropathy, was considered a variant of CIDP. Sural nerve biopsies in three patients so studied showed primarily demyelination and remyelination with varying axon loss. Treatment with immunosuppressant medication led to neurologic improvement. In the same volume of the journal *Neurology*, Lewis and Sumner (35) demonstrated that conduction block was specific for acquired immune demyelination and rarely if ever occurred in inherited neuropathy.

Several years later, Parry and Clarke (36), Pestronk et al. (37), Bradley et al. (38), and Krarup et al. (39) described other patients with focal weakness, wasting, and fasciculation without sensory involvement that

resembled progressive spinal muscular atrophy. The defining feature of so-called multifocal motor neuropathy (MMN) was conduction block restricted to motor axons with normal conduction in uninvolved nerves. Other laboratory findings have included high serum titers of GM1 antibodies in many, but not all, patients and demyelination and remyelination leading to large caliber axons with thinly myelinated fibers, minor onion bulbs, and variable axon loss in sural and mixed nerve biopsy specimens (Fig. 11A and B). The distinction between MMN and MND has been important because motor neuropathy is treatable with immunomodulating and immunosuppressant medications, whereas MND is irreversibly fatal.

In the same period, morphometric and later immunohistochemical studies were undertaken in the nerves of patients with ALS, and these in turn led to improved understanding of motor neuropathy. The concept that weakness and wasting resulted from neuronal degeneration or neuronopathy initially stemmed from neuropathologic studies of patients with ALS. However, there was lingering uncertainty as to contribution of focal proximal axonopathy and distal "dying back" degeneration of peripheral motor axons, an issue that was addressed during a symposium sponsored by the Muscular Dystrophy Association in 1981 in Scottsdale, Arizona. Dyck (40) presented morphometric data showing selective loss of motor neurons in ALS spinal cords, with evidence of acute axonal degeneration in peripheral motor axons. In a discussion of that article, Bradley et al. (41) commented that an equal proportion of acute axonal degeneration was observed along proximal and distal segments of the phrenic nerve of patients with

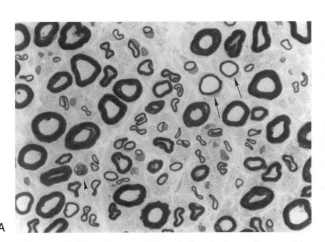

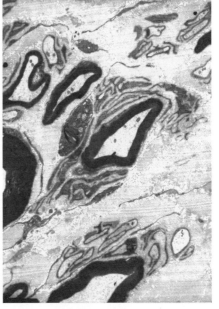

A   B

FIG. 11. Multifocal motor neuropathy. **A:** A sural nerve biopsy in semithin section stained with toluidine blue shows increased numbers of thinly myelinated large caliber fibers (*arrows*) and a single degenerating axon (*arrowhead*). **B:** Electron microscopy of the sural nerve shows thinly myelinated large fibers and minor onion bulbs.

ALS at autopsy, with only a 16% loss of distal large myelinated fibers. Corbo et al. (13) later showed statistically more frequent regenerative clusters of small myelinated fibers in motor nerve biopsy specimens of patients with motor neuropathy than in those with MND in which few or no regenerative clusters were found (Fig. 12A–C).

Direct immunofluorescence staining of sural nerve cryosections in over 50 cases of ALS generally showed no morphologic differences compared with normal control subjects (42); however, two reported patients had exceptional findings. The first was a 73-year-old woman with typical ALS, before breast cancer, and a monoclonal IgA serum paraprotein. Sural nerve biopsy showed deposits of IgA and light chains along axons. At postmortem examination, indirect immunofluorescence revealed binding of IgA to axons and the perikarya of nerve cells and specificity for the high-molecular-weight subunit of neurofilament protein and a neuronal surface antigen (43,44). The second patient was a 38-year-old woman with atypical ALS because of progressive paraplegia in association with multifocal motor conduction block and a high serum IgM GM1 antibody titer (45). Sural nerve biopsy showed granular IgM deposits at nodal and paranodal regions of myelinated nerve fibers. When the patient's serum was injected into rat sciatic nerve, the serum IgM bound to the nodes of Ranvier, and this binding activity was removed by preincubation with GM1 (46).

LMN syndromes associated with lymphoma presented additional challenges to nomenclature and etiopathogenesis of motor disorders. First described in 1963 by Rowland and Schneck (47), and then named by Schold et al. (48), so called subacute motor neuronopathy presents with progressive painless asymmetric limb weakness, with few or no signs of sensory involvement, reminiscent of motor neuropathy. Altogether, LMN disease accounts for some patients with MND and lymphoma (49) and includes patients that differ clinically and pathologically from sporadic forms of MND. Among 26 reported patients with MND and lymphoma seen over the past two decades at Columbia Presbyterian Medical Center in New York (50), all 3 with pure LMN disease improved with treatment of the underlying malignancy. One patient had multifocal motor conduction block and chronic lymphocytic leukemia (49). A second patient had IgM paraproteinemia with reactivity to GM1 and GD1b gangliosides (51); sural nerve biopsy in that patient showed axon loss, focal demyelination, and increased numbers of regenerative clusters. A third patient had progressive paraplegia with

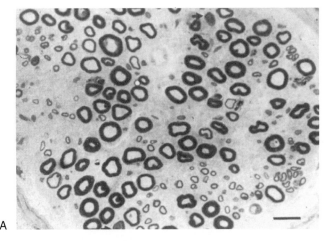

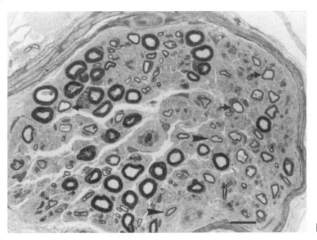

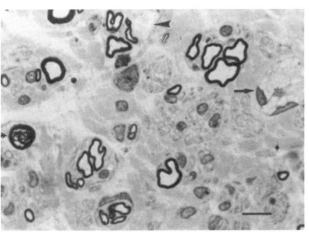

FIG. 12. Motor nerve biopsy studies in motor neuropathy and motor neuron disease. Semithin sections of a motor nerve in a patient with motor neuron disease (A), showing a reduction of myelinated fibers and a few foci of myelin debris (arrows). (B and C) Motor nerve fascicle from a patient with motor neuropathy demonstrates in addition many thinly myelinated fibers (arrows) and small onion bulbs (arrowheads). At higher power, a motor fascicle shows four regenerative clusters of myelinated fibers, a band of Bungner (arrow), a demyelinated axon (arrowhead), and myelin ovoid (curved arrow). Reproduced by permission of John Wiley and Sons Publishers.

IgA monoclonal paraproteinemia (61). Whereas the postmortem examination of patients with ALS and lymphoma differs little from sporadic ALS, those with subacute motor neuronopathy demonstrate, in addition, mild inflammatory cell infiltration and degeneration of the posterior columns sparing the corticospinal tracts, with patchy demyelination in peripheral nerves (47,48,52,53).

Diabetic Neuropathy

There are several recognizable clinicopathologic neuropathic syndromes associated with diabetes mellitus and different methods of classification; significant motor involvement is not uncommon (54). Progressive painful pelvifemoral weakness is the predominant manifestation of proximal diabetic neuropathy, lumbosacral plexitis, and diabetic amyotrophy, further separable by electrodiagnostic studies. Distal weakness parallels the severity of sensory involvement in distal polyneuropathy. Weakness occurs in the arms in the distribution of mixed or motor nerve trunks in mononeuritis multiplex and simplex.

Although early investigations of diabetic neuropathy used nerve trunks from amputated limbs or postmortem specimens (55–57), the modern analysis of peripheral nerve biopsies has played an important role in elucidating the pathology of peripheral nerve injury in this disorder. Although it can still be debated how much ischemia, metabolic alterations, and immunologic mechanisms of nerve injury each contribute to diabetic microangiopathy or to a particular form of neuropathy, one fact is clear: Nerve biopsy is an important tool in appreciating the type and extent of pathologic alterations in a given patient (54).

Diabetic microangiopathy refers to the collective morphologic and biochemical alterations of nerve microvessels and is the major determinant of neuropathy. Under the influence of microangiopathy and accelerated arteriosclerosis, a range of ischemic events occur in a given patient, ranging from a mild reduction in the delivery of oxygen and essential nutrients to frank infarction of one or more fascicles, depending on the severity of the vascular alterations, acuteness of the injury, and the efficiency of the collateral circulation. Microscopically, there is thickening of microvessels due to reduplication of basal lamina, pericyte degeneration, and deposition of polysaccharide in vessel walls, recognized by positive periodic acid-Schiff staining (58). Although early ultrastructural studies found abnormal closure of endoneurial capillaries and intraluminal platelet thrombi in sural nerve microvessels (59), these findings were not confirmed in later analyses (60). Using immunohistochemical studies, we noted an increased density of microvessels in diabetes compared with normal control subjects.

Chronic sustained hyperglycemia leads to diverse metabolic sequela in peripheral nerve fibers including increased flux in the polyol pathway, nonenzymatic glycation of protein elements, an accumulation of vasoactive substances, alterations in lipid metabolism, and abnormal neurotropism (10). It is proposed that these, in turn, lead to alterations in basement membrane structure, impaired axon transport mechanisms, and further perturbation of neuropathy.

Humoral and cellular autoimmunity also contribute to the development of diabetic microangiopathy and neuropathy. Direct counting of immunoperoxidase stained T cells in peripheral nerve sections of patients with severe proximal diabetic neuropathy, distal polyneuropathy, and mononeuritis multiplex revealed significant vascular and endoneurial infiltrates compared with normal control subjects and other patients with IgM antibodies to antimyelin associated glycoprotein (54). Up to 60% of severely affected cases overall had evidence of epineurial T-cell microvasculitis in a sural nerve biopsy and the remainder had variable perivascular lymphocytic infiltrates (Fig. 13A and B). Most T cells expressed the acti-

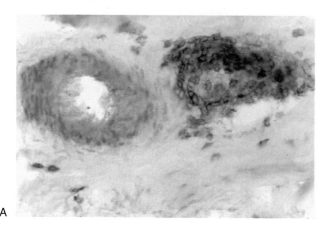
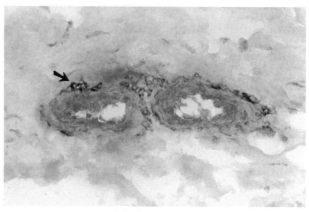

A   B

FIG. 13. T-cell infiltrates in diabetic neuropathy. Microvasculitis **(A)** with frank invasion of an endoneurial vessel wall, and perivascular infiltration **(B)** are seen in the sural nerves of patients with distal diabetic neuropathy using an immunoperoxidase staining procedure of monoclonal antibodies that recognize CD3+ T cells and smooth muscle actin in vessel walls (*arrow*). Reproduced by permission of Thieme Medical Publishers.

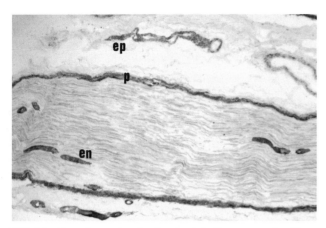

FIG. 14. Complement activation in diabetic neuropathy. Complement immunofluorescence studies in longitudinal section of the sural nerve in a patient with distal diabetic neuropathy demonstrates C5b-9 membrane attack complex activation along the walls of endoneurial (*en*) and epineurial (*ep*) blood vessels and nonspecifically along the perineurium (*p*).

vation marker interleukin-2 receptor (CD25) and MHC Class II antigen. The significance of the T-cell infiltrates in diabetic nerves is not well understood; however, they might be directed against antigens specific for the peripheral nerve or shared by pancreas and nerve. T-cell clones might become sensitized early in the course of the illness by superantigens expressed in pancreatic islets or they might be induced by the metabolic stress of diabetes.

Complement mediated injury of microvessels also contributes to microangiopathy by the deposition of MAC along peripheral nerve microvessels detectable by immunofluorescence staining methods (Fig. 14) (11). The initiating factor in the abnormal activation of complement in diabetic nerves is still speculative, but one possibility is a defect in the expression of certain regulatory membrane proteins that normally protects cells by limiting activation of MAC.

ACKNOWLEDGMENT

I am grateful to Arthur P. Hays, M.D., and Gorazd Rosoklija, M.D., Ph.D. (Department of Pathology, Division of Neuropathology, Columbia Presbyterian Medical Center, NY) for providing Fig. 14.

REFERENCES

1. Sunderland S. Blood supply of the nerves of the upper limb in man. *Arch Neurol Psychiatry* 1945;53:91–115.
2. Sunderland S. Blood supply of the sciatic nerve and its popliteal divisions in man. *Arch Neurol Psychiatry* 1945;53:283–289.
3. Dyck PJ, Conn DL, Okazaki H. Necrotizing angiopathic neuropathy. Three dimensional morphology of fiber degeneration related to sites of occluded vessels. *Mayo Clin Proc* 1972;47:461–475.
4. Moore PM, Fauci AS. Neurologic manifestations of systemic vasculitis. A retrospective and prospective study of the clinicopathologic features and response to therapy in 25 patients. *Am J Med* 1981;71:517–524.
5. Younger DS. Nerve models, role models, reminiscences, and a tribute to Robert E. Lovelace, MD, FRCP. *Semin Neurol* 1998;18:145–149.
6. Asbury AK, Picard EH, Barringer JR. Sensory perineuritis. *Arch Neurol* 1972;26:302–312.
7. Younger DS, Quan D. Nonvasculitic neuritis. *Neurology* 1994;44:194.
8. Dalakas MC. Basic aspects of neuroimmunology as they relate to immunotherapeutic targets: present and future prospects. *Ann Neurol* 1995;37[Suppl 1]:S2–13.
9. Griffin JW, George R, Ho T. Macrophage systems in peripheral nerve. A review. *J Neuropathol Exp Neurol* 1993;52:553–560.
10. Sima AAF. Metabolic alterations of peripheral nerve in diabetes. *Semin Neurol* 1996;16:129–137.
11. Younger DS, Rosoklija G, Hays AP. Peripheral nerve immunohistochemistry in diabetic neuropathy. *Semin Neurol* 1996;16:139–142.
12. Hays AP, Younger DS. Muscle and nerve biopsy. In: Rowland LP, ed. *Merritt's textbook of neurology.* Baltimore: Williams & Wilkins, 1995:97–100.
13. Corbo M, Abouzhahr MK, Latov N, et al. Motor nerve biopsy studies in motor neuropathy and motor neuron disease. *Muscle Nerve* 1997;20:15–21.
14. Kernohan JW, Woltman HW. Periarteritis nodosa: a clinicopathologic study with special reference to the nervous system. *Arch Neurol Psychiatry* 1938;39:655–686.
15. Coers C, Woolf AL. *The innervation of muscle: a biopsy study.* Oxford: Oxford University Press, 1943:2–3.
16. Bleehan SS, Lovelace RE, Cotton RE. Mononeuritis multiplex in polyarteritis nodosa. *Q J Med* 1962;32:193–209.
17. Lovelace RE. Mononeuritis multiplex in polyarteritis nodosa. *Neurology* 1964;14:434–442.
18. Dyck PJ, Benstead TJ, Conn DL, Stevens JC, Windebank AJ, Low PA. Nonsystemic vasculitic neuropathy. *Brain* 1987;110:843–854.
19. Kissel JT, Slivka AP, Warmolts JR, Mendell JR. The clinical spectrum of necrotizing angiopathy of the peripheral nervous system. *Ann Neurol* 1985;18:251–257.
20. Said G, Lacroix-Ciaudo C, Fujimura H, Blas C, Faux N. The peripheral neuropathy of necrotizing arteritis: a clinicopathologic study. *Ann Neurol* 1988;23:461–465.
21. Hawke SHB, Davies L, Pamphlett R, Guo Y-P, Pollard JD, McLeod JG. Vasculitic neuropathy: a clinical and pathologic study. *Brain* 1991;114:2175–2190.
22. Younger DS, Kass RM. Vasculitis and the nervous system: historical perspective and overview. *Neurol Clin* 1997;15:737–758.
23. Bendixen BM, Younger DS, Hair LS, Gutierrez C, Meyers ML, Homma S, Jaffe IA. Cholesterol emboli syndrome. *Neurology* 1992;42:428–430.
24. Andrade C. Amyloid neuropathy. In: Vinken PJ, Bruyn GW, Myrianthropolous NC, eds. *Handbook of clinical neurology. Vol. 42. Neurogenetic directory. I.* Amsterdam: Elsevier, 1981:518–524.
25. Benson MD, Wallace MR. Amyloidosis. In: Scriver CR, Beaudet AL, Sly WS, Volle D, eds. *The metabolic basis of inherited disease,* 6th ed. Vol. 2. New York: McGraw-Hill, 1989:2439–2460.
26. Costa PP, Figuerira AS, Bravo FR. Amyloid fibril protein related to prealbumin in familial amyloidotic polyneuropathy. *Proc Natl Acad Sci USA* 1978;75:4499–4503.
27. Izumoto S, Younger DS, Hays AP, Mantone RL, Smith RT, Herbert J. Familial amyloidotic polyneuropathy presenting with carpal tunnel syndrome and a new transthyretin mutation, asparagine 70. *Neurology* 1992;42:2094–2102.
28. McDonald TD, Fault PL, Bruno C, DiMauro S, Goldman JE. Polyglucosan body disease simulating amyotrophic lateral sclerosis. *Neurology* 1993;43:785–790.
29. Diaz-Arrastia R, Younger DS, Hair L, et al. Neurolymphomatosis: a clinicopathologic syndrome re-emerges. *Neurology* 1992;42:1136–1141.
30. Gordon PH, Younger DS. Neurolymphomatosis [letter]. *Neurology* 1996;46:1191–1192.
31. Mendell JR. Charcot-Marie-Tooth neuropathies and related disorders. *Semin Neurol* 1998;18:41–47.
32. Sumner AJ. Separating motor neuron disease from pure motor neuropathy. Multifocal motor neuropathy with persistent conduction block. *Adv Neurol* 1991;56:399–403.
33. Matusmmuro K, Izumo S, Umehara F, Osam M. Chronic inflammatory demyelinating polyneuropathy: histological and immunpathological studies in biopsied sural nerves. *J Neurol Sci* 1994;127:170–178.
34. Lewis RA, Sumner AJ, Brown MJ, Asbury AK. Multifocal demyelinating neuropathy with persistent conduction block. *Neurology* 1982;32:958–964.

35. Lewis RA, Sumner AJ. The electrodiagnostic distinctions between chronic familial and acquired demyelinative neuropathies. *Neurology* 1982;32:592–596.

36. Parry GJ, Clarke S. Multifocal acquired demyelinating neuropathy masquerading as motor neuron disease. *Muscle Nerve* 1988;11: 103–107.

37. Pestronk A, Cornblath DR, Ilyas AA, et al. A treatable multifocal motor neuropathy with antibodies to GM1 ganglioside. *Ann Neurol* 1988;24: 73–78.

38. Bradley WG, Bennett RK, Good P, Little B. Multifocal chronic inflammatory polyneuropathy with multifocal conduction block. *Arch Neurol* 1988;45:451–455.

39. Krarup C, Stewart JD, Sumner AJ, Pestronk A, Lipton SA. A syndrome of asymmetric limb weakness with motor conduction block. *Neurology* 1990;40:118–127.

40. Dyck PJ. Are motor neuropathies and motor neuron diseases separable? *Adv Neurol* 1982;36:105–114.

41. Bradley WG, Good P, Rasool CG, Adelman LS. Morphometric and biochemical studies of peripheral nerves in amyotrophic lateral sclerosis. *Ann Neurol* 1983;14:267–277.

42. Hays AP. Separation of motor neuron diseases from pure motor neuropathies: pathology. *Adv Neurol* 1991;56:385–398.

43. Sadiq SA, van den Berg LH, Kilidireas K, Hays AP, Latov N. Human monoclonal antineurofilament antibody cross-reacts with a neuronal surface protein. *J Neurosci Res* 1991;29:319–325.

44. Hays AP, Roxas A, Sadiq SA, et al. A monoclonal IgA in a patient with amyotrophic lateral sclerosis reacts with neurofilaments and surface antigen on neuroblastoma cells. *J Neuropath Exp Neurol* 1990;49:383–398.

45. Santoro M, Thomas FP, Fink ME, et al. IgM deposits at nodes of Ranvier in a patient with amyotrophic lateral sclerosis, anti-GM1 antibodies and multifocal motor conduction block. *Ann Neurol* 1990;28:373–377.

46. Santoro M, Uncini A, Corbo M, Lugaresi A, Latov N. Conduction abnormalities induced by sera of patients with multifocal motor neuropathy and anti-GM1 antibodies. *Muscle Nerve* 1993;16:610–615.

47. Rowland LP, Schneck SA. Neuromuscular diseases associated with malignant neoplastic diseases. *J Chronic Dis* 1963;16:777–795.

48. Schold SC, Eun-Sook C, Somasundaram M, Posner JB. Subacute motor neuronopathy: a remote effect of lymphoma. *Ann Neurol* 1979;5: 271–287.

49. Younger DS, Rowland LP, Hays AP, et al. Lymphoma, motor neuron disease, and amyotrophic lateral sclerosis. *Ann Neurol* 1991;29:78–86.

50. Gordon PH, Rowland LP, Younger DS, et al. Lymphoproliferative disorders and motor neuron disease: an update. *Neurology* 1997;48: 1671–1678.

51. Latov N, Hays AP, Donofrio PD, et al. Monoclonal IgM with unique specificity to gangliosides GM1 and to lactose-*N*-tetrose associated with human motor neuron disease. *Neurology* 1988;38:763–768.

52. Rosenfeld MR, Posner JB. Paraneoplastic motor neuron disease. *Adv Neurol* 1991;56:445–449.

53. Forsyth PA, Dalmau J, Graus F, Cwik V, Rosenblum MK, Posner JB. Motor neuron syndromes in cancer patients. *Ann Neurol* 1997;41: 722–730.

54. Younger DS, Rosoklija G, Hays AP, Latov N. Diabetic peripheral neuropathy: a clinicopathologic and immunohistochemical analysis of sural nerve biopsies. *Muscle Nerve* 1996;19:722–727.

55. Dolman CL. The morbid anatomy of diabetic neuropathy. *Neurology* 1963;13:135–142.

56. Raff MC, Sangalang V, Asbury AK. Ischemic mononeuropathy multiplex associated with diabetes mellitus. *Arch Neurol* 1968;18:487–499.

57. Woltman HW, Wilder RM. Diabetes mellitus: pathological changes in the spinal cord and peripheral nerves. *Arch Intern Med* 1929;44:576–605.

58. Fagerberg SE. Diabetic neuropathy—a clinical and histological study of the significance of vascular affections. *Acta Med Scand* 1959;164 [Suppl 345]:1–97.

59. Yasuda H, Dyck PJ. Abnormalities of endoneurial microvessels and sural nerve pathology in diabetic neuropathy. *Neurology* 1987;37:20–28.

60. Giannini C, Dyck PJ. Ultrastructural morphometric abnormalities of sural nerve endoneurial microvessels in diabetes mellitus. *Ann Neurol* 1994;36:408–415.

Motor Disorders,
edited by David S. Younger.
Lippincott Williams & Wilkins, Philadelphia © 1999.

CHAPTER 7

Cytopathology of the Motor Neuron

Hirofumi Kusaka and Asao Hirano

Large neurons in the anterior horn of the spinal cord are well-known targets of the neuropathology of various diseases (1). Among these, amyotrophic lateral sclerosis (ALS) is an age-associated neurodegenerative disease primarily affecting the motor neuron system and characterized by loss of motor neurons. Degenerative processes have only recently been studied in detail with the aid of immunohistochemical and electron microscopic techniques. An overview of some of the new findings associated with lower motor neuron (LMN) alterations is presented here.

PHOSPHORYLATED NEUROFILAMENTS

Round argyrophilic structures were originally described by Wohlfart (2) in the anterior horn of ALS patients in 1959. Then, in 1968, Carpenter (3) delineated light and electron microscopic features of accumulation of neurofilaments within the proximal axons of the anterior horn cells. He distinguished larger, over 20 μm in diameter, spheroids and globules and smaller argyrophilic structures. Globules are limited to the ventral medial portion of the anterior horns in various conditions, including normal control subjects. On the other hand, spheroids are also found in control subjects (4), but their incidence is high in sporadic ALS patients. The discovery of numerous spheroids and chromatolytic neurons in one patient with a short clinical course suggested accumulation of neurofilaments as early alteration of anterior horn cell degeneration (5,6) and led to extensive studies thereafter (7).

Spheroids are faintly eosinophilic or occasionally hematoxylinophilic by hemotoxylin and eosin (H&E) staining (Fig. 1A) and markedly argyrophilic. They have round contours with crumpled margins and whorled con-

tents. They are seen in the anterior horns of the spinal cord and cranial motor nuclei and are common in areas with many remaining neurons, like lumbar anterior horns. They are rarely found in the motor cortex (8) or in the corticospinal tract of the midbrain and upper pons (9). Immunohistochemically, phosphorylated neurofilaments and peripherin are strongly expressed in spheroids (10).

Under the electron microscope, spheroids appear as a large collection of bundles of 10-nm neurofilaments. Each bundle interlaces the other, resulting in a characteristic complicated pattern (Fig. 1B). Despite this intermingled pattern of bundles, each neurofilament stands apart from the other because of its side arms. Among the bundles, a small number of mitochondria, vesicles, smooth endoplasmic reticulum, and other organelles are sometimes mixed (6,11).

Some spheroids are found in the proximal axon of morphologically unremarkable neurons, specifically between the distal portion of the initial segment and the first internode of the axon (12). But continuity of spheroids with the cell body is generally difficult to confirm (5).

The cytoplasm of anterior horn cells in normal control subjects is usually negative for phosphorylated high- and medium-molecular-weight neurofilament proteins. However, in sporadic ALS, Guamanian ALS, and especially in a subset of familial ALS with posterior column and spinocerebellar tract degeneration, considerable amounts of phosphorylated neurofilaments are accumulated within the soma of the anterior horn cells (13,14). Although phosphorylated neurofilaments accumulate focally in the cytoplasm in sporadic and familial ALS (13), in the latter (14) they take distinctly different forms and occur in much larger amounts than in those with sporadic ALS. Some of these accumulations are associated with Lewy body-like hyaline inclusion (LBHI) bodies that are described later. Neurofilamentous accumulations within the axon in familial ALS are also different from those seen in sporadic cases. They take cordlike or more irregular forms and ultrastructurally consist of neurofilaments

H. Kusaka: Department of Neurology, Kansai Medical University and Kansai Medical University Hospital, Morguchishi, Osaka 570-8507, Japan.

A. Hirano: Division of Neuropathology, Department of Pathology, Montefiore Medical Center, Bronx, New York 10467.

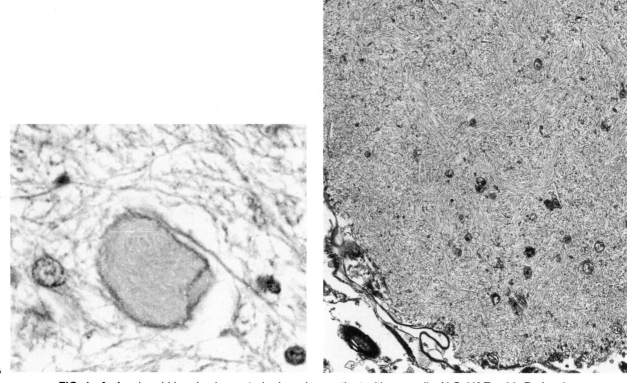

A

B

FIG. 1. A: A spheroid in a lumbar anterior horn in a patient with sporadic ALS. H&E × 80. **B:** A spheroid is composed of interwoven bundles of neurofilaments. From the same patient. ×12,000.

arranged parallel to the long axis of the axon (15), different from the interwoven pattern of the spheroid as seen in sporadic ALS (11).

Several lines of evidence from studies of transgenic mice overexpressing neurofilaments suggest that abnormal neurofilamentous accumulations play a leading role in motor neuron degeneration (16,17). Recent reports of neurofilamentous accumulation in patients with familial ALS caused by a mutation in the gene for Cu/Zn superoxide dismutase (*SOD1*) supports this view (18,19).

UBIQUITIN

Discovery of ubiquitinated proteins in neurodegenerative diseases markedly advanced our understanding of cell degeneration in motor neuron disease (MND) (20,21). At least three types of ubiquitinated structures are recognized in MND: LBHI in a subgroup of familial ALS, round hyaline inclusions in sporadic ALS or LMN syndromes, and skeinlike inclusions (SLI).

Lewy Body-like Hyalin Inclusions

LBHI was originally described as hyaline inclusion in an American "C" family of ALS (22,23). It is a faintly eosinophilic or hematoxylinophilic round structure, a core,

surrounded by a halo. As implied in its name, LBHI resembles the Lewy body of Parkinson disease but lacks the concentric pattern in its core and stains blue, not red, with Masson trichrome. It is usually located within the cytoplasm but occasionally is found in the cordlike swollen axon and dendrite. LBHI occurs mainly in the LMN but also develops in the brainstem reticular formation, Clarke's column, lateral cuneatus nucleus (15,23,24), and rarely in the motor cortex (25), in line with the degeneration of multiple systems in familial ALS. LBHI is considered characteristic for a subset of familial ALS with posterior column and spinocerebellar tract involvement (22).

Immunohistochemically, some LBHIs show diffuse staining patterns but most display characteristic intense expression of both ubiquitin and phosphorylated neurofilaments in their halos, suggesting colocalization of ubiquitin and phosphorylated neurofilament proteins (26). Cores are occasionally stained with anti-ubiquitin antibody (27). In addition to ubiquitin and phosphorylate neurofilaments, the expression of Cu/Zn *SOD1* was confirmed in LBHI from the original "C" family that showed a point mutation at the second position of codon 4 (Ala 4 Val) in exon 1 of the *SOD1* gene, the most frequent mutation, accounting for 50% of *SOD1*-linked familial ALS (28).

Under the electron microscope, LBHI appears to be composed of an accumulation of randomly oriented neu-

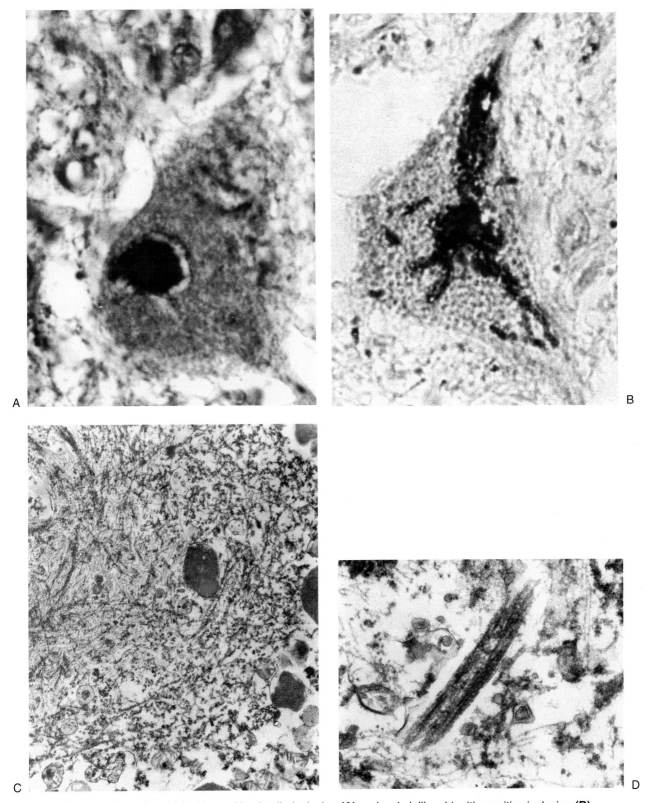

FIG. 2. A round antiubiquitin-positive hyalin inclusion **(A)** and a skeinlike ubiquitin-positive inclusion **(B)** in large anterior horn cells from the same patient shown in Fig. 1A and B. Electron microscopically, the inclusion consists of collections of thick filaments studded with granules and neurofilaments **(C)**. Occasionally, bundles of thick filaments are located close to the inclusion **(D)**. (**A** and **B**) Anti-ubiquitin antibody counterstained with hematoxylin and eosin. ×900. **(C)** ×22,000. **(D)** ×44,000.

rofilaments that are intermingled with thick linear structures associated with granular material. The core has denser collections of thick linear structures and neurofilaments, whereas the halo contains mainly neurofilaments (15,27,29).

Round Hyaline Inclusions

In sporadic ALS or MND, particularly with shorter clinical courses (30), round hyaline inclusions are observed along with other characteristic pathologic findings like spheroids and Bunina bodies (31). Some have a halo and a core and are almost indistinguishable from LBHI. However, some lack halos, and their cores have small vacuolar parts inside or irregular margins attached with filamentous materials. Despite several discrepancies, it appears homogeneously and densely stained with anti-ubiquitin antibody (Fig. 2A) (32,33) and negatively or weakly stained with anti-phosphorylated neurofilament antibodies (31,33–35). *SOD1* is only weakly expressed in round hyaline inclusion (36, 37). Ultrastructurally, bundles of 15- to 20-nm-thick filaments with granules and bundles of 10-nm neurofilaments are intermingled in various proportion forming, as a whole, a round collection without limiting membrane (Fig. 2C) (38). Within or around the inclusion, SLIs are occasionally found (33), and Bunina bodies are situated close to the inclusion (33,39). Round hyaline inclusions are usually observed in the LMN of patients with sporadic ALS, lower MND (31) with LBHI, and sporadic ALS with dementia (37). It is also reported in Betz cells, small neurons of the motor cortex (40), and rarely in the Onufrowicz's nucleus (41) in patients with sporadic ALS.

Skeinlike Inclusions

SLI is a filamentous structure virtually and clearly recognizable with anti-ubiquitin antibodies (Fig. 2B) (21). It takes various patterns from a single filament or a coarse meshwork of filaments to a rather dense collection of filaments. Ultrastructurally, it appears to consist of a small bundle of thick filaments of 15 to 25 nm in diameter, with a hollow space in the center (Fig. 2D) (42). Electron-dense granules are seen freely and attached to thick filaments, which are indistinguishable from those found in round hyaline inclusions (38).

SLI is characteristically seen in the LMN, motor cortex (8), and inferior olivary nucleus (25) of patients with MND. SLI is common in sporadic ALS (21,33,34), lower MND (32), ALS with dementia (37), Guamanian ALS (43), and familial ALS with posterior column involvement (42) but not in Werdnig-Hoffmann disease, longstanding poliomyelitis, and juvenile or adult ALS with basophilic inclusions (BIs) (44). However, it should be noted that SLI has been found in patients with parkinsonism (34), Machado-Joseph disease (45), and dentatorubropallidoluisian atrophy (25).

BUNINA BODY

This cytoplasmic inclusion was originally described by the Russian pathologist Bunina in 1962 in two patients with familial ALS (46). The inclusion was considered a neurovirus, and her group allegedly succeeded in transmitting it to a monkey. It is now known to occur in cases of sporadic ALS (47), ALS with dementia (48), and Guamanian ALS (47) and considered highly characteristic of LMN degeneration in MND. Under the light microscope, the Bunina body is a brightly eosinophilic inclusion of several microns in diameter and round to oval in shape. It develops singularly among the lipofuscin granules or Nissl substance in the cytoplasm, but sometimes multiple inclusions make a cluster or chainlike formation. A larger inclusion may have a lucid part within. It stains bright red by H&E, deep blue by phosphotangustic acid hematoxylin, and blue by Luxol fast blue. It is not argyrophilic or autofluorescent and is negative for periodic acid-Schiff, Sudan Black B, and Congo red.

Immunocytochemically, the Bunina body remains an enigma because of its inert reactivity to many antibodies such as neurofilaments, tau, amyloid precursor protein, synaptophysin, glial fibrillary acidic protein (GFAP), microtubule-associated proteins (MAPs), alpha- and beta-tubulins, actin, desmin, or Golgi. Ubiquitin immunoreactivity seems to be negative despite several contradictory results (34,49). Recently, Okamoto et al. (50) reported the expression of cystatin C protein in Bunina bodies (Fig. 3A).

The ultrastructure of the Bunina body was first reported by Hart et al. in 1977 (51) and confirmed by several other authors (52). It consisted of an electron-dense amorphous substance margined with tubules or vesicles (Fig. 3B). The amorphous substance occasionally includes a cytoplasmic island containing neurofilaments and other organella. Tubules or vesicles are shown to be reactive with anti-cystatin C antibody, a property similar to that of tubular structure of the Golgi apparatus in the anterior horn cells of a cat (50).

Bunina bodies are usually seen within the cytoplasm or dendrites of degenerated LMNs but sometimes in normal-looking large neurons as well. Bunina bodies tend to appear in the lumbar anterior horn because this segment contains more remaining large neurons in sporadic ALS patients. Bunina bodies have also been seen to develop in a patient with a shorter clinical course. However, so far, no Bunina body has been found within the axoplasm.

Although Bunina bodies are found in sporadic ALS and Guamanian ALS, they are particularly common in a so-called Mitsuyama type of ALS with dementia (48,53). Therefore, it is considered a pathologic hallmark of ALS. However, it should be noted that Bunina bodies are not observed in a subset of familial ALS with posterior col-

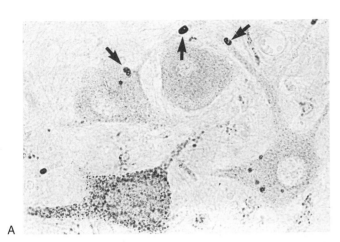 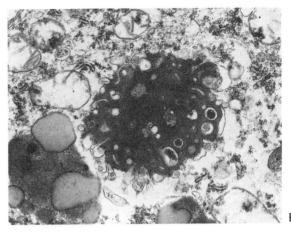

FIG. 3. A: Bunina bodies (*arrows*) are strongly stained with anti-cystatin C antibody. A normal-looking neuron contains no Bunina bodies but displays diffusely small granules stained with anti-cystatin C antibody. A lumbar anterior horn from a patient with sporadic amyotrophic lateral sclerosis. ×430. **B:** A Bunina body is composed of electron-dense amorphous substances and attached vacuoles and vesicles. A large anterior horn cell in a patient with sporadic amyotrophic lateral sclerosis. ×24,000.

umn and spinocerebellar tract involvement or juvenile or adult-onset MND with BI (54,55). They are mainly distributed in LMNs of the spinal cord and brainstem. A single report described them in Betz cells (8). Furthermore, several recent studies have revealed the occurrence of Bunina bodies in several neurons that are so far considered to be exempt from the pathology of ALS, such as the oculomotor nucleus (56), Onufrowicz's nucleus (35), Clarke's nucleus (57), reticular formation of the brainstem (58), and subthalamic nucleus (59,60).

Despite its bright eosinophilia, distinct expression of cystatin C, and conspicuous ultrastructure, the origin of Bunina bodies remains unknown. Several fascinating hypotheses have been proposed but none have been proven. Hart et al. (51) suggested the derivation of Bunina bodies from autophagic vacuoles or from degenerated mitochondria. Tomonaga et al. (52) proposed a link to laminated cytoplasmic bodies. A relationship with hyaline inclusion or SLIs has also been suggested (33). Recently, Nakano et al. (58) and Okamoto et al. (50) independently proposed the origin of Bunina bodies from the Golgi apparatus. In addition to the occurrence in neurons other than motor neurons in some ALS patients, ultrastructurally similar or identical inclusions are reported in neurons of aged rats (61), the olfactory bulb of aged humans (62), the spinal cord of a patient without ALS (4), and gangliocytoma (63). It probably represents a facet of the degenerating process of a neuron. A high incidence in ALS, particularly in LMNs, seems to lend a diagnostic priority to the presence of Bunina bodies.

SYNAPTOPHYSIN

Synaptophysin is a 38-kDa glycoprotein, an integral constituent of the membrane of presynaptic vesicles. It serves as a useful marker for the study of synaptic pathology, heretofore a virtually unexplored field in MND. Kawanami et al. (64) first reported a profound decrease in levels of synaptophysin expression in the anterior horns of ALS patients. The reduction was more marked in the neuropil and corresponded to the severity of neuronal loss. However, the soma and proximal dendrites of the remaining neurons are frequently reactive or hyperreactive with anti-synaptophysin antibodies (64). Confirmed by subsequent studies (65,66), these observations correlate with the loss and atrophy of distal dendrites, previously demonstrated by Kato et al. (67) in Golgi preparations. Therefore, there is a loss of presynaptic terminals in the anterior horns of ALS patients. The increased immunoreactivity around the perikarya and dendrites of some remaining neurons could reflect cell shrinkage or a synaptic rearrangement associated with degeneration of the dendritic tree.

However, Matsumoto et al. (68) found no reduction of reaction products in lumbar cords after transection of the pyramidal tract, indicating no apparent effect on synaptophysin expression from the upper motor neuron pathology.

GOLGI APPARATUS

Applying an antiserum against MG-160, an intrinsic membrane sialoglycoprotein of medial cisterna of the Golgi apparatus, Gonatas et al. (69) disclosed fragmentation and dispersion of the apparatus in approximately 30% of the LMNs of ALS patients, whereas only 1% of the cells of patients with other neurologic diseases or age-matched control subjects showed similar changes. They proposed that fragmentation of the Golgi apparatus was an early event in the pathogenesis of the neuronal degeneration in ALS. Interestingly, neurons with ubiquitin-positive SLIs in

Guamanian ALS and non-Guamanian ALS had fragmented Golgi apparatus (70), indicating the relationship between the Golgi apparatus fragmentation and SLI formation. Bunina bodies, another pathologic hallmark of ALS, represent an abnormal accumulation of a still unknown proteinaceous material associated with the Golgi apparatus (50). In addition, spinal cord neurons from transgenic mice expressing a mutant form of Cu/Zn *SOD1* also showed fragmentation of the Golgi apparatus (71). However, this alteration is not unique to sporadic ALS or Guamanian ALS. It is observed in patients with Werdnig-Hoffmann's disease, infantile neuronal degeneration, adult-type familial bulbospinal atrophy, and mitochondrial myopathy with cytochrome *c* oxidase deficiency. Similar changes are found in patients with lymphoma or leukemia with leptomeningeal involvement and multiple myeloma associated with a chronic inflammatory demyelinating polyneuropathy as well. Furthermore, it is inducible by colchicine, brefeldin A, microtubule-depolymerizing agents, and infection with herpes simplex virus 1 (70,72).

SUPEROXIDE DISMUTASE

A 15-kb gene, comprised of five exons on chromosome 21, encodes a free radical scavenger enzyme, Cu/Z *SOD1*, composed of 153 amino acids. The discovery by Rosen et al. (73) of missense mutations at exons 2 and 4 of the *SOD1* gene in a subgroup of familial ALS is a notable landmark in ALS research. More than 45 mutations within exons 1, 2, 4, and 5 of the Cu/Zn *SOD1* gene have been reported as the proven primary cause of ALS (74). Furthermore, development of motor neuron dysfunction and degeneration of anterior horn cells in several lines of transgenic mice expressing *SOD1* mutations (G93A, G37R) lends further support to a central role played by *SOD1* gene mutations in the pathogenesis of MND (75–77). In one of these models, the earliest pathology is fragmentation of Golgi apparatus (71). In several days, there is microvesiculation of anterior horn cells with many of the vacuoles originating from dilatation of the rough endoplasmic reticulum and from degenerating mitochondria (75). In some of the surviving neurons, interestingly, filamentous hyaline inclusions are formed (78) that currently await the immunohistochemical and ultrastructural comparison with LBHIs seen in familial ALS. The reexamination of the "C" family (A4V) failed to disclose the characteristic mitochondrial pathology (79).

Recently, a transgenic mouse model expressing the mutant human *SOD1*, G85R, was reported to show a different pathology consisting of striking astroglial alteration without vacuoles. This suggests the heterogeneity of pathology in these transgenic mice expressing mutant *SOD1* genes (80). Similar heterogeneity also begins to appear among familial ALS, whereas the clinicopathologic features are analyzed in terms of *SOD1* gene muta-

tion. An I113T substitution in exon 4 seems to correlate with marked neurofilamentous pathology in the motor neuron and other neurons (18,19). A4T (28) and A4V mutation (81) in exon 1 and E100G in exon 4 (82) and two base pair deletions in exon 5 (83) seem to relate to the classic pathology of familial ALS with posterior column and spinocerebellar degeneration and LBHI. However, one patient with familial ALS displayed multisystem degeneration similar to the "C" family but without LBHIs or *SOD1* gene abnormalities (84). Another patient with familial ALS lacked a gene abnormality but showed multisystem involvement and accumulation of phosphorylated neurofilaments (85). Although only 5% to 10% of ALS belongs to the familial type and 20% of the familial type might be related to *SOD1* gene abnormality, further studies of a correlation between clinicopathologic phenotype and genotype would afford valuable insight into the pathomechanism of motor neurons, even in sporadic ALS and related conditions.

BASOPHILIC INCLUSIONS

BIs were first described by Wohlfart and Swank (86) in large anterior horn cells of a 14-year-old patient and thereafter found in a subset of juvenile or young adult patients with MND or juvenile ALS (87). The clinical course was 11 to 18 months, but some had autonomic dysfunction or eye movement disorders. BIs, generally larger than Bunina bodies, have various forms like clovers, horseshoes, or globules. They are faintly basophilic on H&E stain and anilinophilic (Fig. 4A). Their argyrophilia is not so distinct. The distribution is not limited to the motor neurons but also found in thalamus, globus pallidus, substantia nigra, red nucleus, reticular formation, Clarke's column, posterior horn, and other areas. The ultrastructure consists of interwoven aggregation of 13- to 17-nm-thick filaments studded with granules (Fig. 4B). They are vaguely or partly reactive to ubiquitin but negative for antineurofilament or tau proteins. No Bunina bodies or SLIs were observed in these cases; therefore, juvenile ALS is different from classic ALS both clinically and pathologically.

BIs have not been observed in classic ALS by several systematic studies (33,88). However, recently, three adult ALS patients with ages at onset of 36, 38, and 53 years (54,55,89) showed widespread BIs at postmortem examination, associated clinically with ophthalmoplegia and artificial respirator (89) or gaze palsy and dysuria before the start of artificial respiration (55). Bunina bodies, ubiquitin-positive SLI, or LBHI were not found. Spheroids were rare. One patient, in addition, had Alzheimer's neurofibrillary tangles in Betz cells, which is usually devoid of tangles even in patients with Alzheimer's disease (54). Although clinical manifestation is prominently expressed in the motor neuron system, it seems that the juvenile and adult patients with BIs constitute a multisys-

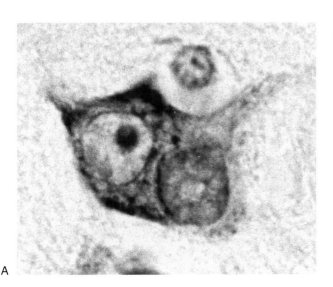
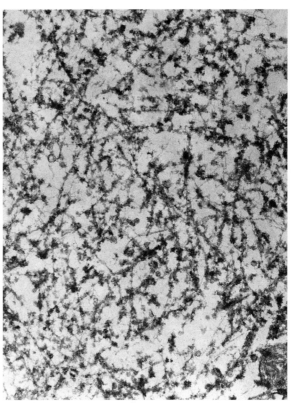

A   B

FIG. 4. A: A large basophilic inclusion seen in a neuron of the motor cortex. Nissl × 720. **B:** A basophilic inclusion consists of a collection of thick filaments and granules in a neuron of the motor cortex from a patient with an adult-onset motor neuron disease with basophilic inclusions. ×22,000.

tem degeneration distinct from classic or familial ALS, with posterior column and spinocerebellar tract involvement. The neurochemical architecture of the striatum is also different between patients with BIs and sporadic classic ALS (90), providing additional evidence for the heterogeneity of MND.

REFERENCES

1. Hirano A. *A guide to neuropathology.* 1st ed. New York: Igaku-Shoin Medical Publishers, Inc., 1981.
2. Wohlfart G. Degenerative and regenerative axonal changes in the ventral horns, brainstem and cerebral cortex in amyotrophic lateral sclerosis. *Acta Univ Lund* 1959;50:1–24.
3. Carpenter S. Proximal axonal enlargement in motor neuron disease. *Neurology* 1968;18:842–851.
4. Kusaka H, Hirano A. Fine structure of anterior horns in patients without amyotrophic lateral sclerosis. *J Neuropathol Exp Neurol* 1985;44:430–438.
5. Inoue K, Hirano A. Early pathological changes of amyotrophic lateral sclerosis. Autopsy findings of a case of 10 months duration. *Neurol Med (Tokyo)* 1979;11:448–453.
6. Hirano A, Inoue K. Early pathological changes of amyotrophic lateral sclerosis. Electron microscopic study of chromatolysis, spheroids and Bunina bodies. *Neurol Med (Tokyo)* 1980;13:148–160.
7. Gambetti P, Shecket G, Ghetti B, Hirano A, Dahl D. Neurofibrillary changes in human brain. An immunocytochemical study with neurofilaments antisera. *J Neuropathol Exp Neurol* 1983;42:69–79.
8. Sasaki S, Maruyama S. Immunocytochemical and ultrastructural studies of the motor cortex in amyotrophic lateral sclerosis. *Acta Neuropathol* 1994;87:578–585.
9. Okamoto K, Hirai S, Shoji M, Senoh Y, Yamazaki T. Axonal swellings in the corticospinal tracts in amyotrophic lateral sclerosis. *Acta Neuropathol* 1990;80:222–226.
10. Corbo M, Hays A. Peripherin and neurofilament protein coexist in spinal spheroids of motor-neuron disease. *J Neuropathol Exp Neurol* 1992;51:531–537.
11. Hirano A, Donnenfeld H, Sasaki S, Nakano I. Fine structural observations of neurofilamentous changes in amyotrophic lateral sclerosis. *J Neuropathol Exp Neurol* 1984;43:461–470.
12. Sasaki S, Maruyama S. Increase in diameter of the axonal initial segment is an early change in amyotrophic lateral sclerosis. *J Neurol Sci* 1992;110:114–120.
13. Matsumoto S, Mizusawa H, Yen S-H, Hirano A. Immunocytochemical study of phosphorylated neurofilaments in the anterior horn cells of amyotrophic lateral sclerosis. *Neurol Med (Tokyo)* 1989;30:370–377.
14. Mizusawa H, Hirano A, Yen S, Matsumoto S, Rojas-Corona R, Donnenfeld H. Focal accumulation of phosphorylated neurofilaments within anterior horn cell in familial amyotrophic lateral sclerosis. *Acta Neuropathol* 1989;79:37–43.
15. Hirano A, Nakano I, Kurland L, Mulder D, Holley P, Saccomanno G. Fine structural study of neurofibrillary tangles in a family with amyotrophic lateral sclerosis. *J Neuropathol Exp Neurol* 1984;43:471–480.
16. Lee M, Marszalek J, Cleveland D. A mutant neurofilament subunit causes massive, selective motor-neuron death—implications for the pathogenesis of human motor-neuron disease. *Neuron* 1994;13:975–988.
17. Julien JP, Cote F, Collard JF. Mice overexpressing the human neurofilament heavy gene as a model of ALS. *Neurobiol Aging* 1995;16:487–490.
18. Orrell RW, King AW, Hilton DA, Campbell MJ, Lane RJ, de Belleroche JS. Familial amyotrophic lateral sclerosis with a point mutation of SOD-1: intrafamilial heterogeneity of disease duration associated with neurofibrillary tangles. *J Neurol Neurosurg Psychiatry* 1995;59:266–270.
19. Rouleau G, Clark A, Rooke K, et al. SOD1 mutation is associated with accumulation of neurofilaments in amyotrophic lateral sclerosis. *Ann Neurol* 1996;38:128–131.

20. Leigh P, Anderton B, Dodson A, Gallo J, Swash M, Power D. Ubiquitin deposits in anterior horn cells in motor neuron diseases. *Neurosci Lett* 1988;93:197–203.

21. Lowe J, Lennox G, Jefferson D, et al. A filamentous inclusion body within anterior horn neurones in motor neurone disease defined by immunocytochemical localisation of ubiquitin. *Neurosci Lett* 1988;94: 203–210.

22. Hirano A, Kurland L, Sayre G. Familial amyotrophic lateral sclerosis: a subgroup characterized by posterior and spinocerebellar tract involvement and hyalin inclusions in the anterior horn cells. *Arch Neurol* 1967; 16:232–243.

23. Nakano I, Hirano A, Kurland L, Mulder D, Holley P, Saccomanno G. Familial amyotrophic lateral sclerosis. Neuropathology of two brothers in American "C" family. *Neurol Med (Tokyo)* 1984;20:458–471.

24. Kato S, Hirano A. Involvement of the brain stem reticular formation in familial amyotrophic lateral sclerosis. *Clin Neuropathol* 1992;11:41–44.

25. Mizusawa H. Ubiquitinated inclusions in motor neuron diseases. *Adv Neurol Sci* 1996;40:5–15.

26. Mizusawa H, Hirano A, Yen S-H. Anterior horn cell inclusions in familial amyotrophic lateral sclerosis contain ubiquitin and phosphorylated neurofilament epitopes. *Neuropathology* 1991;11:11–20.

27. Murayama S, Ookawa Y, Mori H, et al. Immunocytochemical and ultrastructural study of Lewy body-like hyalin inclusions in familial amyotrophic lateral sclerosis. *Acta Neuropathol* 1989;78:143–152.

28. Shibata N, Hirano A, Kobayashi M, et al. Intense superoxide dismutase-1 immunoreactivity in intracytoplasmic hyaline inclusions of familial amyotrophic-lateral-sclerosis with posterior column involvement. *J Neuropathol Exp Neurol* 1996;55:481–490.

29. Takahashi K, Nakamura H, Okada E. Hereditary amyotrophic lateral sclerosis. Histochemical and electron microscopic study of hyaline inclusions in motor neuron. *Arch Neurol* 1987;27:292–299.

30. Tada J, Namikawa T, Wakayama I, Kihira T, Mizusawa H. An autopsy case of sporadic ALS with rapid clinical course and Lewy body-like intracytoplasmic inclusions in Onuf's nucleus. *Neurol Med (Tokyo)* 1994;44:377–384.

31. Kato T, Katagiri T, Hirano A, Sasaki H, Arai S. Sporadic lower motor neuron disease with Lewy body-like hyaline inclusions: a new subgroup? *Acta Neuropathol* 1988;76:208–211.

32. Kato T, Katagiri T, Hirano A, Kawanami T, Sasaki H. Lewy body-like hyaline inclusions in sporadic motor neuron disease are ubiquitinated. *Acta Neuropathol* 1989;77:391–396.

33. Murayama S, Mori H, Ihara Y, Bouldin T, Suzuki K, Tomonaga M. Immunocytochemical and ultrastructural studies of lower motor neurons in amyotrophic lateral sclerosis. *Ann Neurol* 1990;27:137–148.

34. Leigh P, Whitwell H, Garofalo O, et al. Ubiquitin-immunoreactive intraneuronal inclusions in amyotrophic-lateral-sclerosis—morphology, distribution, and specificity. *Brain* 1991;114:775–788.

35. Okamoto K, Hirai S, Shoji M, Harigaya Y, Fukuda T. Widely distributed Bunina bodies and spheroids in a case of atypical sporadic amyotrophic-lateral-sclerosis. *Acta Neuropathol* 1991;81:349–353.

36. Shibata N, Hirano A, Kobayashi M, et al. Cu/Zn superoxide dismutase-like immunoreactivity in Lewy body-like inclusions of sporadic amyotrophic lateral sclerosis. *Neurosci Lett* 1994;179:149–152.

37. Matsumoto S, Kusaka H, Ito H, Shibata N, Asayama T, Imai T. Sporadic amyotrophic lateral sclerosis with dementia and Cu/Zn superoxide dismutase-positive Lewy body-like inclusions. *Clin Neuropathol* 1996; 15:41–46.

38. Kusaka H, Matsumoto S, Imai T. Granulofilamentous profiles in lower motor neurons: a sporadic case of amyotrophic lateral sclerosis with many Lewy body-like inclusions. *Clin Neuropathol* 1992; 11:20–24.

39. Sasaki S, Sakuma H, Maruyama S, Yamane K. Sporadic motor neuron disease with Lewy body-like hyaline inclusions. *Acta Neuropathol* 1989;78:555–560.

40. Lowe J, Doherty F, Aldridge F, et al. Inclusion-bodies in motor cortex and brain-stem of patients with motor neuron disease are detected by immunocytochemical localization of ubiquitin. *Neurosci Lett* 1989;105:7–13.

41. Kihira T, Mizusawa H, Tada J, Namikawa T, Yoshida S, Yase Y. Lewy body-like inclusions in Onuf's nucleus from two cases of sporadic amyotrophic lateral sclerosis. *J Neurol Sci* 1993;115:51–57.

42. Mizusawa H, Nakamura H, Wakayama I, Yen S-H, Hirano A. Skein-like inclusions in the anterior horn cells in motor neuron disease. *J Neurol Sci* 1991;105:14–21.

43. Matsumoto S, Hirano A, Goto S. Ubiquitin-immunoreactive filamentous inclusions in anterior horn cells of Guamanian and non-Gua-manian amyotrophic lateral sclerosis. *Acta Neuropathol* 1990;80: 233–238.

44. Matsumoto S, Kusaka H, Ito H, Yamasaki M, Imai T. A comparative immunohistochemical study of ubiquitin-positive skein-like inclusions in anterior horn neurons in subgroups of adult-onset motor neuron diseases. *Clin Neurol (Tokyo)* 1993;33:1125–1130.

45. Suenaga T, Matsushima H, Nakamura S, Akiguchi I, Kimura J. Ubiquitin-immunoreactive inclusions in anterior horn cells and hypoglossal neurons in a case with Joseph's disease. *Acta Neuropathol* 1993;85: 341–344.

46. Bunina T. On intracellular inclusions in familial amyotrophic lateral sclerosis. *Korsakov J Neuropathol Psychiatry* 1962;62:1293–1299.

47. Hirano A. Pathology of amyotrophic lateral sclerosis. In: Gajdusek D, Gibbs CJ, Alpers M, eds. *Slow, latent and temperate virus infection.* Washington DC: National Institutes of Health, 1965:23–37.

48. Kusaka H, Imai T. Pathology of motor neurons in amyotrophic lateral sclerosis with dementia. *Clin Neuropathol* 1993;12:164–168.

49. Migheli A, Attanasio A, Schiffer D. Ubiquitin and neurofilament expression in anterior horn cells in amyotrophic lateral sclerosis: possible clues to the pathogenesis. *Neuropathol Appl Neurobiol* 1994;20:282–289.

50. Okamoto K, Hirai S, Amari M, Watanabe M, Sakurai A. Bunina bodies in amyotrophic lateral sclerosis immunostained with rabbit anti-cystatin C serum. *Neurosci Lett* 1993;162:125–128.

51. Hart M, Cancilla P, Frommes S, Hirano A. Anterior horn cell degeneration and Bunina-type inclusions associated with dementia. *Acta Neuropathol* 1977;38:225–228.

52. Tomonaga M, Saito M, Yoshimura H, Shimada H, Tohgi H. Ultrastructure of the Bunina bodies in anterior horn cells of amyotrophic lateral sclerosis. *Acta Neuropathol* 1978;42:81–86.

53. Mitsuyama Y. Presenile dementia with motor neuron disease in Japan: clinicopathological review of 26 cases. *J Neurol Neurosurg Psychiatry* 1984;47:953–959.

54. Kusaka H, Matsumoto S, Imai T. An adult-onset case of sporadic motor neuron disease with basophilic inclusions. *Acta Neuropathol* 1990;80: 660–665.

55. Kusaka H, Matsumoto S, Imai T. Adult-onset motor neuron disease with basophilic intraneuronal inclusion bodies. *Clin Neuropathol* 1993; 12:215–218.

56. Okamoto K, Hirai S, Amari M, et al. Oculomotor nuclear pathology in amyotrophic lateral sclerosis. *Acta Neuropathol* 1993;85:458–462.

57. Takahashi H, Oyanagi K, Ohama E, Ikuta F. Clarke's column in sporadic amyotrophic lateral sclerosis. *Acta Neuropathol* 1992;84:465–470.

58. Nakano I, Iwatsubo T, Hashizume Y, Mizutani T. Bunina bodies in neurons of the medullary reticular formation in amyotrophic lateral sclerosis. *Acta Neuropathol* 1993;85:471–474.

59. Takahashi H, Ohama E, Ikuta F, Tokiguchi S. An autopsy case of atypical motor neuron disease with Bunina bodies in the lower motor and subthalamic neurons. *Acta Pathol Jpn* 1991;41:45–51.

60. Takahashi H, Ohama E, Ikuta F. Are Bunina bodies of endoplasmic reticulum origin? An ultrastructural study of subthalamic eosinophilic inclusions in a case of atypical motor neuron disease. *Acta Pathol Jpn* 1991;41:889–894.

61. Knox C, Yates M, Chen I. Brain aging in normotensive and hypertensive strains of rats. *Acta Neuropathol* 1980;52:7–15.

62. Okamoto K, Shoji M, Harigaya Y, Yamazaki T, Hirai S. Fine structure of Bunina-like inclusion observed in neuron of olfactory bulb in the aged. *Neurol Med (Tokyo)* 1990;33:287–289.

63. Takahashi H, Egawa S, Ikuta F. Bunina body-like eosinophilic intracytoplasmic inclusions in a gangliocytomatous brain lesion. *Neuropathology* 1996;16:190–193.

64. Kawanami T, Ikemoto A, Llena J, Hirano A. Synaptophysin immunoreactivity pattern in the anterior horn cells in amyotrophic lateral sclerosis. *Can J Neuro Sci* 1993;20:75(abst).

65. Ikemoto A, Kawanami T, Llena J, Hirano A. Immunocytochemical studies on synaptophysin in the anterior horn of lower motor-neuron disease. *J Neuropathol Exp Neurol* 1994;53:196–201.

66. Sasaki S, Maruyama S. Decreased synaptophysin immunoreactivity of the anterior horns in motor neuron disease. *Acta Neuropathol* 1994;87: 125–128.

67. Kato T, Hirano A, Donnenfeld H. A Golgi study of the large anterior horn cells of the lumbar cords in normal spinal cords and in amyotrophic lateral sclerosis. *Acta Neuropathol* 1987;75:34–40.

68. Matsumoto S, Goto S, Kusaka H, Ito H, Imai T. Synaptic pathology of spinal anterior horn cells in amyotrophic lateral sclerosis: an immunohistochemical study. *J Neurol Sci* 1994;125:180–185.

69. Gonatas NK, Stieber A, Mourelatos Z, et al. Fragmentation of the Golgi apparatus of motor neurons in amyotrophic lateral sclerosis. *Am J Pathol* 1992;140:731–737.

70. Mourelatos Z, Hirano A, Rosenquist AC, Gonatas NK. Fragmentation of the Golgi apparatus of motor neurons in amyotrophic lateral sclerosis (ALS). Clinical studies in ALS of Guam and experimental studies in deafferented neurons and in beta,beta′-iminodipropionitrile axonopathy. *Am J Pathol* 1994;144:1288–1300.

71. Mourelatos Z, Gonatas N, Stieber A, Gurney M, Dal Canto M. The Golgi apparatus of spinal cord motor neurons in transgenic mice expressing mutant Cu, Zn superoxide dismutase becomes fragmented in early preclinical stages of the disease. *Proc Nat Acad Sci USA* 1996; 93:5472–5477.

72. Tascos N, Mourelatos Z, Gonatas NK. On the significance and reproducibility of the fragmentation of the Golgi apparatus of motor neurons in human spinal cords. *J Neuropathol Exp Neurol* 1995;54: 331–338.

73. Rosen DR, Siddique T, Patterson D, et al. Mutations in Cu/Zn superoxide dismutase gene are associated with familial amyotrophic lateral sclerosis. *Nature* 1993;362:59–62.

74. Bruijn L, Cleveland D. Mechanisms of selective motor neuron death in ALS: insights from transgenic mouse models of motor neuron disease. *Neuropathol Appl Neurobiol* 1996;22:373–387.

75. Dal Canto M, Gurney M. Development of central nervous system pathology in a murine transgenic model of human amyotrophic lateral sclerosis. *Am J Pathol* 1994;145:1271–1279.

76. Gurney ME, Pu H, Chiu AY, et al. Motor neuron degeneration in mice that express a human Cu,Zn superoxide dismutase mutation. *Science* 1994;264:1772–1775.

77. Kunst C, Mezey E, Brownstein M, Patterson D. Mutations in SOD1 associated with amyotrophic lateral sclerosis cause novel protein interactions. *Nat Genet* 1997;15:91–94.

78. Dal Canto M, Gurney M. Neuropathological changes in two lines of mice carrying a transgene for mutant human Cu,Zn SOD, and in mice overexpressing wild-type human SOD—a model of familial amyotrophic-lateral-sclerosis (FALS). *Brain Res* 1995;676:25–40.

79. Hirano A. Neuropathology of ALS: an overview. *Neurology* 1996;47: 63–66.

80. Bruijn L, Becher M, Lee M, et al. ALS-linked SOD1 mutant G85R mediates damage to astrocytes and promotes rapidly progressive disease with SOD1-containing inclusions. *Neuron* 1997;18:327–338.

81. Takahashi H, Makifuchi T, Nakano R, et al. Familial amyotrophic lateral sclerosis with a mutation in the Cu/Zn superoxide dismutase gene. *Acta Neuropathol* 1994;88:185–188.

82. Ince P, Shaw PJ, Slade JY, Jones C, Hudgson P. Familial amyotrophic lateral sclerosis with a mutation in exon 4 of Cu/Zn superoxide dismutase gene: pathological and immunocytochemical changes. *Acta Neuropathol* 1996;92:395–403.

83. Kato S, Shimoda M, Watanabe Y, Nakashima K, Takahashi K, Ohama E. Familial amyotrophic lateral sclerosis with a two base pair deletion in superoxide dismutase 1 gene: multisystem degeneration with intracytoplasmic hyaline inclusions in astrocytes. *J Neuropathol Exp Neurol* 1996;55:1089–1101.

84. Kato S, Kawata A, Oda M, Arai N, Komori T, Tanabe H. Absence of SOD1 gene abnormalities in familial amyotrophic lateral sclerosis with posterior column involvement without Lewy-body-like hyaline inclusions. *Acta Neuropathol* 1996;92:528–533.

85. Takahashi H, Oyanagi K, Ikuta F, Tanaka M, Yuasa T, Miyatake T. Widespread multiple system degeneration in a patient with familial amyotrophic lateral sclerosis. *J Neurol Sci* 1993;120:15–21.

86. Wohlfart G, Swank R. Pathology of amyotrophic lateral sclerosis: fiber analysis of the ventral roots and pyramidal tracts of the spinal cord. *Arch Neurol Psychiatry* 1941;46:783–799.

87. Matsumoto S, Kusaka H, Murakami N, Hashizume Y, Okazaki H, Hirano A. Basophilic inclusions in sporadic juvenile amyotrophic lateral sclerosis: an immunocytochemical and ultrastructural study. *Acta Neuropathol* 1992;83:579–583.

88. Hirano A, Iwata M. Pathology of motor neurons with special references to amyotrophic lateral sclerosis and related diseases. In: Tsubaki T, Toyokura Y, eds. *Amyotrophic lateral sclerosis.* Tokyo: University of Tokyo Press, 1979:107–133.

89. Mizutani T, Sakamaki S, Tsuchiya N, et al. Amyotrophic lateral sclerosis with ophthalmoplegia and multisystem degeneration in patients on long-term use of respirators. *Acta Neuropathol* 1992;84:372–377.

90. Ito H, Kusaka H, Matsumoto S, Imai T. Topographic involvement of the striatal efferents in basal ganglia of patients with adult-onset motor neuron disease with basophilic inclusions. *Acta Neuropathol* 1995;89: 513–518.

Motor Disorders,
edited by David S. Younger.
Lippincott Williams & Wilkins, Philadelphia © 1999.

CHAPTER 8

The Hypotonic Infant

Thornton B. Alex Mason II and Darryl C. De Vivo

The term *floppy infant syndrome* has been applied to infants with severe hypotonia. Hypotonia in an infant is identified first by inspection when supine, with the arms lying flail and the hips extended laterally, in the "frog-leg" posture. With gentle arm traction and elevation of the infant from the supine position, usually a prominent head lag is demonstrated with retroflexion of the neck (Fig. 1A). When supported in a sitting position, the infant veers forward because of poor axial tone (Fig. 1B). Upon vertical suspension, with the infant held upright under the arms, an infant with normal tone remains stable, but hypotonic infants begin to slip through the examiner's hands. When a hypotonic infant is suspended in the prone position with support of the trunk, the infant slumps over the examiner's hand in an inverted "U" posture with the head and limbs all hanging limply, "like a rag doll" (Fig. 1C). When movement at individual joints is examined by passive flexion and extension, resistance is decreased compared with normal infants. The infant's head should be kept in midline during this evaluation of limb tone, because head turning may produce a tonic neck reflex response and promote lateral tone asymmetries.

Muscle tone is controlled in part at the spinal cord level by gamma motor neurons, which are located in the ventral horn. Together with afferent muscle spindles and effector alpha motor neurons, they form a feedback loop to allow adjustment in muscle tone. If the alpha or gamma motor neurons are compromised, then hypotonia and weakness can occur. Muscle tone is also regulated by certain areas of the brain. The role of the upper motor neuron and corticospinal tract in the hypotonic infant is less

well understood, but experimental evidence supports the presence of cortical inhibition areas. One in particular is the supraorbital frontal lobe, which when stimulated produces diffuse nonreciprocal inhibition of mono- and polysynaptic reflexes and muscle tone (1). Clinically, the patient's state of alertness is important when assessing tone; for example, drowsiness is associated with decreased tone. The state of the maturation of the nervous system, in particular the corticospinal tracts, is important for the development of normal passive muscle tone and postures at rest (2). A premature neonate has less tone than a full-term newborn because these tracts are not completely myelinated until age 2 years. The status of the spinal cord motor neurons is also important because the motor unit is not compromised in central insults, wherein little or no true weakness ever occurs.

Symptomatic hypotonia or floppy infant syndrome is caused by a myriad of disorders. The differential diagnoses are shown in Table 1 (3). Certain studies listed in Table 2 should be considered in affected patients based on the specific clinical presentation.

In general, it is helpful to separate those conditions in the newborn period (first month of life) from those that more commonly affect infants later in the first year. Infantile spinal muscular atrophy has its onset in utero, but symptoms are usually delayed for 2 to 3 months, the time it takes for the limited compensation of initial motor neuron loss to beome clinically evident. Severe hypotonia and weakness are accompanied by difficulty with feedings, tongue fasciculation, and respiratory insufficiency. Muscle biopsy reveals hypertrophied fibers grouped among atrophic dying fibers. Mutation analysis of the *SMN* gene confirms the diagnosis. Death is usually caused by respiratory failure. Infants with congenital myotonic dystrophy, on the other hand, are severely affected at birth, usually requiring prolonged ventilatory support over several weeks and gavage feedings. Affected infants have prominent facial diplegia, including tenting

T.B.A. Mason II: Department of Neurology, Columbia University and New York Presbyterian Hospital, New York, New York 10032.

D.C. De Vivo: Department of Neurology and Pediatrics, Columbia University College of Physicians and Surgeons, and Neurological Institute and Babies Hospital, New York Presbyterian Hospital, New York, New York 10032.

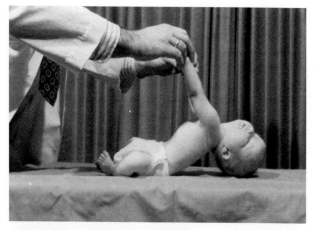

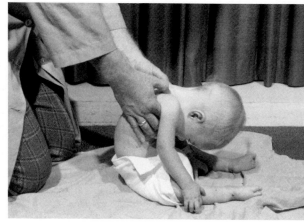

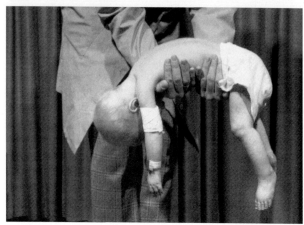

FIG. 1. Examination of the hypotonic infant. **A:** Gentle arm traction demonstrates a prominent head lag. **B:** In an upright seated position, there is decreased axial tone. **C:** Supported and elevated in a prone position, the floppy infant fails to right his head or to extend his extremities against gravity.

of the upper lip and a hatchet face when older. Genetic testing shows expansion of the CTG trinucleotide repeat of the myotonin-protein kinase gene (19q13). After a prolonged stay in the nursery, affected infants may be well enough to go home but generally remain symptomatic. Neonatal myasthenia gravis also affects newborn infants because of the transfer of anti-acetylcholine receptor antibodies from an affected mother. Clinical improvement of strength and muscle tone parallels clearance of the maternally derived antibodies over several weeks. Radioimmunoassay of anti-acetylcholine receptor antibodies from placental and newborn blood confirms the disorder. Small repeated doses of neostigmine, an acetylcholinesterase inhibitor, improves feeding.

One should also distinguish between hypotonic conditions without true limb weakness usually due to a central disorder and those infants with true limb weakness due to a neuromuscular cause. Floppy infants without true limb weakness may show signs of asphyxia, chromosomal abnormalities, metabolic disorders, or connective tissue disorders. Seizures are a clue to an underlying central nervous system disorder. In the absence of clinical seizures, an abnormal electroencephalogram provides support for cerebral dysfunction that usually correlates with the hypotonia. In central disorders, tendon reflexes are normal or

brisk, whereas they are generally absent in infants with true limb weakness. The presence of ankle clonus or Babinski sign points to an upper motor neuron lesion.

The history of asphyxia at birth as an explanation for hypotonia is suggested by low Apgar scores and the need for immediate resuscitation and respiratory support after birth. There may be signs of central nervous system impairment with decreased alertness and seizures. Over weeks to months, affected infants show signs of spastic quadriparesis, and those still hypotonic after 1 or 2 years can manifest a cerebellar syndrome with ataxia and incoordination (4). Severe asphyxia may also affect spinal cord lower motor neurons. Autopsy studies of fatally asphyxiated neonates with flaccid tone and areflexia demonstrate prominent ischemic necrosis of anterior spinal cord gray matter in a radially oriented watershed distribution consistent with hypoperfusion between the anterior spinal artery and the paired dorsal spinal arteries (5,6).

Dysmorphic features should lead to the investigation of chromosomal disorders. Profound hypotonia at birth and in infancy are seen in isochromosome 12p mosaicism or the Pallister mosaic aneuploidy syndrome. Clinical findings include coarse facies, prominent forehead, hypertelorism, sparse scalp hair, epicanthal folds, flat nasal bridge, and high-arched palate. Visualization under a

TABLE 1. *Etiologies of infantile hypotonia*

Disorders	Neuromuscular disorders (weakness prominent)	Central disorders; peripheral sparing motor unit (little or no weakness)
Neonatal	Infantile spinal muscular atrophy	Perinatal brain injury (ischemia, hemorrhage)
	Congenital myotonic dystrophy	Chromosomal disorders
	Neonatal myasthenia gravis	Congenital hypothyroidism
	Congenital myopathies	Genetic syndromes
	Multicore disease	Prader-Willi syndrome
	Central core disease	Lowe syndrome
	Nemaline myopathy	Smith-Lemli-Opitz syndrome
	Myotubular myopathy	Zellweger syndrome
	Congenital fiber type disproportion	Riley-Day syndrome
	Congenital muscular dystrophy	*In utero* toxin exposure and infection
	Fukuyama type	Failure to thrive syndromes
	"Occidental" type	Spinal cord injury or malformation
	Merosin deficient	Spinal dysraphism
	Metabolic myopathies	Sacral agenesis
	Pompe disease	Caudal regression syndrome
	MtDNA depletion syndrome	
	Cytochrome *c* oxidase deficiency	
	Glycogenosis type IV and V	
Age 1–6 mo (or later)	Infantile spinal muscular atrophy	Biotinidase deficiency
	Poliomyelitis	Metabolic cerebral degenerations
	Infantile botulism	Intoxication
	Acute peripheral neuropathies	Cervical spine trauma
	Infantile Guillain-Barré	
	Diphtheria	
	Tick-bite paralysis	
	Connective tissue disorders	
	Ehlers-Danlos syndrome	
	Marfan's syndrome	
	Subacute to chronic neuropathies	
Mucopolysaccharidoses	Metachromatic leukodystrophy	Metabolic and endocrine diseases
	Globoid cell leukodystrophy	Organic acidemia
	Neonatal adrenoleukodystrophy	Calcium abnormalities
	Infantile neuroaxonal dystrophy	Renal tubular acidosis
	Congenital myasthenic syndromes	Hypothyroidism

Adapted from Ref. 3, with permission.

Wood's lamp shows generalized pigmentary dysplasia (7). Terminal deletion of chromosome 2q is associated with infantile hypotonia, developmental delay, and craniofacial abnormalities, including frontal bossing and micrognathia (8). The inverted duplication 8p syndrome has hypotonia, feeding problems, and severe developmental delay. Dysmorphic features include low-set posteriorly rotated ears, high-arched palate, prominent forehead, and large mouth with thin upper lip (9). The diagnosis of Gillespie syndrome is suggested by the finding of partial aniridia and fixed dilated pupils in a hypotonic infant; severe cerebellar ataxia and mental retardation are also seen (10). Trisomy 21 is associated with a large variety of phenotypes that vary in prevalence and expression, including cardiac anomalies, Brushfield spots, and duodenal stenosis. Neonatal hypotonia and mental retardation are expected and present in close to 100% of individuals with Down syndrome (11). The Down syndrome chromosome region 1 (DCR1) on subband q22.2 of chromosome 21 contains genes that result in specific trisomy 21 phenotypes,

including hypotonia. Two recently discovered genes in DCR1 belong to a family of inward rectifier potassium channels (Kir), a class of channels that help to maintain resting membrane potential, modify excitability, and regulate muscle tone (12). Further study may elucidate what role these genes play in Down syndrome.

Hypothyroidism is a contributing cause of hypotonia, especially in Down syndrome. Congenital hypothyroidism presents with icterus, retardation of skeletal maturation and growth in length, abdominal distention, large tongue, skin mottling, hypotonia, and increased head size (13). Infants with Down syndrome have a 35-fold greater risk for primary hypothyroidism than other infants in the general population. The American Academy of Pediatrics Committee on Genetics recommends thyroid screening tests at 4 to 6 months, 12 months, and annually in patients with Down syndrome because of the increased risk for acquired hypothyroidism (14).

Prader-Willi syndrome is characterized by marked neonatal hypotonia and feeding problems. After the first

TABLE 2. *Important studies in diagnosis of hypotonia*

Nerve conduction studies
    Peripheral neuropathies
    Brachial plexus injuries
Tetanic nerve stimulation
    Botulism
    Neonatal myasthenia gravis
    Congenital myasthenic syndromes
Electromyography
    Congenital myopathies
    Myotonic dystrophy
    Spinal muscular atrophy
    Metabolic myopathies
Muscle biopsy
    Congenital myopathies
    Congenital muscular dystrophy
    Metabolic myopathies
Cultures
    Viral (polio, other enteroviruses; encephalitis)
    Bacterial (botulism, diphtheria, meningitis, sepsis)
Antibody titers
    Intrauterine infection (*Toxoplasmosis, Rubella,*
      cytomegalovirus, herpes)
    Neonatal myasthenia gravis (acetylcholine receptor
      antibodies)
Chromosomal studies
    Down syndrome
    Prader-Willi
    Other dysmorphic syndromes
Serum studies
    Endocrinopathies (hyper- and hypocalcemia,
      hypothyroidism)
    Congenital myopathies, muscular dystrophy (serum
      creatine kinase)
    Metabolic disorders (organic and amino acids, lactate,
      pyruvate, arterial blood gas)
    Neonatal adrenoleukodystrophy (very-long-chain fatty
      acids)
    Smith-Lemli-Opitz syndrome (hypocholesterolemia)
Cranial neuroimaging
    Asphyxia
    Hemorrhage
    Dysgenetic syndromes (especially with midline facial
      defects)
    Congenital muscular dystrophy (Fukuyama and merosin-
      negative)
    Leukodystrophies

year but before age 6, hyperphagia and obesity are present. Characteristic facial features include almond-shaped eyes, narrow bifrontal diameter, small mouth with thin upper lip, and down-turned corners of the mouth. In boys, there is often associated hypogenitalism, with micropenis, hypoplastic scrotum, and/or cryptorchidism (15,16). Prader-Willi syndrome results from a paternally derived deletion of 15q11-13 in approximately 70% of patients; the remainder have maternal uniparental disomy, that is, two maternal copies of 15q and no paternal copy, or an imprinting mutation. A DNA methylation-based test at the PW71 locus detects any of these three conditions (17). Conventional chromosome analysis, fluorescence in situ hybridization, and DNA polymorphism studies may distinguish the specific mutation in a given affected patient. High-resolution chromosome analysis is not recommended for diagnosis of Prader-Willi syndrome because of the high rates of false-positive and false-negative results (17). Other syndromes commonly associated with hypotonia are Lowe's syndrome, Smith-Lemli-Opitz syndrome, Zellweger's syndrome, and Riley-Day (familial dysautonomia) syndrome.

Biotinidase deficiency is a readily treatable metabolic disorder that should be considered in all infants with severe hypotonia, intractable seizures, and lactic acidosis (18,19). It first presents between 6 and 12 months of age but, in some, presents several weeks after birth. Affected patients display profound hypotonia, ataxia, visual and auditory impairment, developmental delay, alopecia, eczematous skin rash, and metabolic coma. Associated ketolactic acidosis and organic acidemia is caused by decreased activity of one of three biotin-dependent enzymes: pyruvate carboxylase, proprionyl CoA carboxylase, or β-methylcrotonyl CoA carboxylase. Biotinidase activity in serum can be assayed by quantitative calorimetric testing of blood-soaked filter paper samples as part of a newborn nursery screen. Untreated, it can be fatal; however, 10 to 20 mg/day of biotin dramatically stops anticonvulsant-unresponsive seizures in a few days. Other features also resolve quickly, especially if biotin therapy is instituted promptly. Because it is a treatable condition, biotinidase deficiency should be considered in all infants with severe hypotonia, intractable seizures, and lactic acidosis (18,19).

Ehlers-Danlos syndrome is a heritable connective tissue disorder and an important cause of infant hypotonia. It is characterized by excessively stretchable, fragile and easily bruised skin, and hyperextensible joints. The disease is transmitted in an autosomal dominant fashion. The clinical phenotype of Marfan's syndrome, another autosomal dominant disorder, includes long thin extremities, ectopia lentis, and aortic aneurysm. The mucopolysaccharidoses are rare lysosomal storage disorders of cartilage and bone, due to accumulation of one of several mucopolysaccharides such as dermatan sulfate, heparan sulfate, and keratan sulfate. Affected children have variable skeletal system, eye, liver, spleen, and central nervous system disease. Mucopolysaccharidoses should be suspected when coarse facial features, corneal opacities, developmental delay, kyphosis, growth failure, and stiff joints occur. Urinalysis screening and skin fibroblast or lymphocyte testing are useful methods of laboratory diagnosis (20).

The pregnancy, birth history, and family history can provide extremely important clues to the cause of infant hypotonia. Parental consanguinity increases the likelihood of autosomal recessive inherited disorders, including Pompe disease and congenital muscular dystrophy (CMD). An affected mother may be minimally symptomatic, and the diagnosis may emerge only after the birth of a severely affected child. The mother should be questioned about the quality and timing of fetal movements during pregnancy. Compared with infantile spinal muscular atrophy in which brisk movements decrease during pregnancy due to the progressive loss of motor neuron function, in CMD there are a paucity of movements throughout pregnancy that can also be a cause of arthrogryposis. In utero, toxin exposure may be revealed in the pregnancy history and can also produce dysmorphism and hypotonia. Common examples include fetal exposure to alcohol, heroin, phenytoin, and trimethadione. Drugs administered to the mother during labor and delivery can also affect the newborn, most dramatically upon birth, with gradual improvement afterward. Recovery may be hastened by the administration of the opioid antagonist, naloxone, or the benzodiazepine antagonist, flumazenil. Besides asphyxia, low Apgar scores and the need for delivery room resuscitation suggest prior sepsis or cerebral hemorrhage as the cause of central hypotonia. Appropriate cultures, acute and convalescent TORCH (toxoplasmosis, rubella, cytomegalovirus, herpes) titers, cranial ultrasound imaging, and toxicology screens may point to specific etiologies.

The pattern of clinical involvement is also important. Asymmetrically decreased leg tone and weakness, along with fever, meningeal signs, cerebrospinal fluid pleocytosis, and an elevated protein, suggests poliomyelitis or another enteroviral infection. Viral cultures and polymerase chain reaction may be helpful in identifying the responsible organism. Focal neonatal hypotonia is due to developmental anomaly or trauma. Flaccidity of one arm in infancy can result from brachial plexus injury, often encountered in association with dystocia and fetal macrosomia. Erb-Duchenne paralysis is an upper brachial plexopathy possibly associated with fracture of the clavicle or ipsilateral diaphragm paralysis. Lower brachial plexopathy of infancy, or Klumpke paralysis, may be accompanied by ipsilateral Horner's syndrome. The legs may be selectively involved as well because of spinal dysraphism, caudal regression syndrome, or sacral agenesis.

Guillain-Barré syndrome is a rare but important cause of acute ascending symmetric weakness, hypotonia, and areflexia in young infants (21). It leads to progressive proximal motor weakness of the legs, later followed by involvement of the arms, trunk, and face. Areflexia is common, although trace reflexes of the biceps and knee jerk may be present. Elevation of cerebrospinal fluid protein with few or no cells, so-called albuminocytologic dissociation, can be documented over several weeks (22). Electrophysiologic studies reveal reduced compound muscle action potential amplitudes often to 50% of normal, with prolongation of F-wave latencies even before the decrease in motor conduction velocities, which are maximal by the third week of illness. Denervation potentials on needle electromyogram occur late in the course and are associated with a poor outcome (23). Treatment

involves supportive care and careful monitoring of cardiac and respiratory status; plasmapheresis or intravenous immunoglobulin therapy is often beneficial. Diphtheria is caused by *Corynebacterium diphtheriae*. It produces a generalized demyelinating polyneuropathy clinically similar to Guillain-Barré syndrome. A protein exotoxin is secreted by the organism that inhibits myelin synthesis and may activate cytotoxic mechanisms in addition (24). Treatment of diphtheria consists of antitoxin administration and antimicrobial therapy. Tick paralysis is an acute illness like Guillain-Barré syndrome that presents in spring and summer months, and produces hypotonia. The paralysis is caused by a tick that is continuously attached and secreting toxin-laden saliva, and removal of the tick is rapidly curative (25).

The causes of acute descending weakness may be due to infantile botulism. The symptoms of botulism develop in a previously healthy infant, often age 2 to 6 months, although cases have been described in the first 2 weeks of life (26,27). The weakness is caused by ingestion of *Clostridium botulinum* spores, which are able to germinate in the infant gut and elaborate low levels of exotoxin usually below detectable levels on serum assay. The toxin impairs presynaptic axonal release of acetylcholine and produces weakness. Electrophysiologic studies show decreased miniature end-plate potentials due to a decrease in quantal release with nerve terminal depolarization (28). Clinical weakness typically begins with multiple cranial nerve palsies, leading to bilateral ptosis and dilated pupils with diminished light response. Poor feeding is due to a decreased suck ability and pooling of secretions in the pharynx. The weakness descends to the trunk and limbs; bowel sounds are hypoactive, and constipation is common. Deterioration can be rapid and lead to progressive respiratory compromise requiring ventilatory support (29). The most specific single electrophysiologic test for botulism is an incremental response on repetitive stimulation of 20 to 50 Hz. Concentric needle electromyography shows short-duration low-amplitude motor unit potentials (28). Fecal material should be sent for culture of *C. botulinum* and for exotoxin identification. Environmental cultures, including soil and dirt samples from the home, honey, or other products that may have been fed to the infant, are sometimes positive, suggesting the specific source of infection. Most infant botulism in America is caused by group I organisms that elaborate toxin types A and B (26). Treatment of infantile botulism is supportive. Attention should be paid to avoiding any medications that might exacerbate the neuromuscular transmission deficit, in particular aminoglycoside antibiotics, which are sometimes initiated empirically at presentation for possible sepsis (27). Full recovery is expected but may require several weeks to months.

Primary disorders of nerve and muscle can produce true limb weakness and hypotonia. Congenital myopathies are defined clinically and morphologically by the findings in a muscle biopsy specimen. They include multicore and central core disease, nemaline myopathy, myotubular or centronuclear myopathy, and congenital fiber type disproportion (small type I, large type II) (3,30). They commonly present with variable muscle weakness, feeding difficulty, decreased tendon reflexes, and respiratory failure often associated with mental retardation, dysmorphic physical features, scoliosis, and congenital hip dislocation.

By comparison, CMD shows primary myopathic changes in a skeletal muscle biopsy without distinctive histochemical or ultrastructural features. Infants with CMD are symptomatic from birth or the first few months of life. They manifest hypotonia, delayed motor milestones, early and severe contractures, and joint deformity. Serum creatine kinase (CK) is up to 30 times normal in early disease stages and then decreases rapidly. One type of CMD, frequent in Japan, is the Fukuyama type (linked to 9q31-33), characterized by severe mental retardation in all cases and seizures in about half. Magnetic resonance imaging reveals cerebral and cerebellar polymicrogyria, reflecting a neuronal migration defect. Although affected children never walk, they may live into adulthood (31). The occidental type of CMD occurs in infants from Western countries where only skeletal muscle appears to be involved clinically. A subset of both types has a specific absence of merosin (α_2 chain of laminin-2) by immunocytochemistry and immunoblot (32,33).

Metabolic myopathies cause myotonia and weakness. Pompe disease is an AR metabolic myopathy due to deficiency of the enzyme acid maltase. Affected infants are normal at birth but soon develop generalized hypotonia, weakness, macroglossia, and hepatomegaly. Electrocardiogram abnormalities include giant QRS complexes, short PR interval, and ventricular hypertrophy. Echocardiography reveals concentric hypertrophic cardiomyopathy. Electromyogram shows generalized myopathy with occasional positive sharp wave activity, fibrillation potentials, bizarre repetitive discharges, and myotonic discharges in the absence of clinically detectable myotonia (34,35). Muscle biopsy shows vacuolar myopathy that stains positively with the periodic acid-Schiff technique. Diastase digestion of fresh frozen tissue sections removes most vacuolar material, consistent with the presence of glycogen. Electron microscopy reveals glycogen sequestered into membrane-bound autophagic vacuoles (34,35). Other metabolic myopathies that present with infantile hypotonia include the mitochondrial DNA depletion syndrome, cytochrome c oxidase deficiency, glycogenosis type IV or debrancher enzyme deficiency, and glycogenosis type V or myophosphorylase deficiency. Lactic acidosis is a frequent associated finding in mitochondrial DNA depletion syndrome and cytochrome c oxidase deficiency.

Subacute and chronic diffuse neuropathies that cause hypotonia include metachromatic leukodystrophy, globoid cell leukodystrophy or Krabbe disease, neonatal adreno-leukodystrophy, and infantile neuroaxonal dystrophy. Clues to their diagnosis may include a known family history, upper motor neuron signs, cerebrospinal fluid protein elevation, and slow nerve conduction velocities. Metachromatic leukodystrophy, globoid cell leukodystrophy, and adrenoleukodystrophy all demonstrate white matter abnormalities on cranial magnetic resonance imaging. In neonatal adrenoleukodystrophy, moderate to severe hypotonia hepatomegaly and retinitis pigmentosa are noted at birth or shortly thereafter. Increased plasma levels of very-long-chain fatty acids are found, often with raised phytanic acid and bile fluid trihydrocoprostanic acid levels, consistent with a deficiency of multiple peroxisomal enzymes (36). Infantile neuroaxonal dystrophy is an AR disease, with marked generalized hypotonia in late infancy. There is an overall regression of motor and language milestones, which may be accompanied by bilateral pyramidal signs, esotropia, and pendular nystagmus. Electroencephalogram demonstrates an admixture of high-amplitude 18- to 20-Hz beta activity. Cranial imaging, electrophysiology studies, and serum amino acid screens are generally all normal (37). The diagnosis can be ascertained on skin and conjunctival biopsy, where axonal spheroids are found in unmyelinated nerve fibers near termination sites on skin appendages or dermal blood vessels. Electron microscopy reveals tuberomembranous and tuberocisternal profiles (37,38). The accumulation of this material in the axon terminal suggests impaired axonal transport in infantile neuroaxonal dystrophy (38).

The congenital myasthenic syndromes are a heterogeneous group of rare conditions caused by a variety of genetic defects affecting neuromuscular transmission. Unlike neonatal and juvenile myasthenia gravis, they are not antibody mediated. Affected children manifest weakness and abnormal fatigability on exertion in the first 2 years of life and sometimes at birth. Neither plasma exchange nor immune suppression offer a demonstrable benefit (39).

The possibility of an exogenous toxin should be considered in cases of acute and recurrent hypotonia. Although routine urine toxicology screens commonly detect drugs, one should remain alert to the continued possibility of a toxic substance when the initial screen is reported to be negative. In a report of Munchausen syndrome, chronic ipecac or emetine poisoning in infancy resulted in hypotonia, poor suck, and respiratory insufficiency (40). Carbamate and organophosphate poisoning results in pupillary changes, usually miosis; flaccid muscle tone; fasciculation; dyspnea; and stupor. Atropine sulfate in doses of 0.05 mg/kg repeated at regular intervals dramatically improves cholinergic crisis symptoms, including a depressed level of consciousness (41). Ingestion of ethylene glycol produces vomiting, irritability, acidosis, and hypotonia suggestive of a metabolic disorder. Organic acid analysis reveals glycolic acid and a positive anion gap, and urinalysis shows hematuria and calcium oxalate crystals (42).

Cervical spine trauma and spinal cord injury can lead to sudden unexplained hypotonia and quadriparesis. Cranial nerve function remains intact. Electromyography at the time of presentation may be normal and only later demonstrates denervation changes at affected spinal root segments. Immediate cervical spine immobilization with a hard collar is mandatory before imaging studies in clinically suspected cases. Skeletal survey may demonstrate other acute or healing fractures (43).

After excluding all other etiologies, a benign condition may be the cause of infant hypotonia. Essential hypotonia is applied to otherwise healthy infants with unexplained hypotonia, normal strength and tendon reflexes, and normal physical characteristics. The presence of an older sibling with infantile hypotonia as an isolated finding and normal tone later in childhood is supportive.

ACKNOWLEDGMENT

Supported by The Colleen Giblin Foundation.

REFERENCES

1. Sauerland EK, Knauss T, Nakamura Y, Clemente CD. Inhibition of monosynaptic and polysynaptic reflexes and muscle tone by electrical stimulation of the cerebral cortex. *Exp Neurol* 1967;17:159–171.
2. Sarnat HB. Do the corticospinal and corticobulbar tracts mediate functions in the human newborn? *Can J Neurol Sci* 1989;16:157–160.
3. De Vivo DC. The floppy infant syndrome. In: Rowland LP, ed. *Merritt's textbook of neurology*, 9th ed. Baltimore: Williams & Wilkins, 1995: 503–506.
4. Lesny IA. Follow-up study of hypotonic forms of cerebral palsy. *Brain Dev* 1979;1:87–90.
5. Clancy RR, Sladky JY, Rorke LB. Hypoxic-ischemic spinal cord injury following perinatal asphyxia. *Ann Neurol* 1989;25:185–189.
6. Rousseau S, Metral S, Lacroix C, Cahusac C, Nocton F, Landrieu P. Anterior spinal artery syndrome mimicking infantile spinal muscular atrophy. *Am J Perinatol* 1993;10:316–318.
7. Reynolds JF, Daniel A, Kelly TE. Isochromosome 12p mosaicism (Pallister mosaic aneuploidy or Pallister-Killian syndrome): report of 11 cases. *Am J Med Genet* 1987;27:257–274.
8. Gorski JL, Cox BA, Kyine M, Uhlmann W, Glover TW. Terminal deletion of the long arm of chromosome 2 in a mildly dysmorphic hypotonic infant with karyotype 46,XY,del(2)(q37). *Am J Med Genet* 1989; 32:350–352.
9. Feldman GL, Weiss L, Phelan MC, Schroer RJ, Van Dyke DL. Inverted duplication of 8p: ten new patients and review of the literature. *Am J Med Genet* 1993;47:482–486.
10. Nelson J, Flaherty M, Grattan-Smith P. Gillespie syndrome: a report of two further cases. *Am J Med Genet* 1997;71:134–138.
11. Kronenberg JR, Chen XN, Schipper R, et al. Down syndrome phenotypes: the consequences of chromosomal imbalance. *Proc Natl Acad Sci USA* 1994;91:4997–5001.
12. Gosset P, Ghezala GA, Korn P, et al. A new inward rectifier potassium channel gene (KCNJ15) localized on chromosome 21 in the Down syndrome chromosome region 1 (DCR1). *Genomics* 1997;44:237–241.
13. Virtanen M. Manifestations of congenital hypothyroidism during the 1st week of life. *Eur J Pediatr* 1988;147:270–274.
14. Roberts HE, Moore CA, Fernhoff PM, Brown AL, Khoury MJ. Population study of congenital hypothyroidism and associated birth defects, Atlanta, 1979–1992. *Am J Med Genet* 1997;71:29–32.
15. Greenberg F, Elder FF, Ledbetter DH. Neonatal diagnosis of Prader-Willi syndrome and its implications. *Am J Med Genet* 1987;28: 845–856.
16. Holm VA, Cassidy SB, Butler MG, et al. Prader-Willi syndrome: consensus diagnostic criteria. *Pediatrics* 1993;91:398–402.
17. Gillessen-Kaesbach G, Gross S, Kaya-Westerloh S, Passarge E, Horsthemke B. DNA methylation based testing of 450 patients suspected of having Prader-Willi syndrome. *J Med Genet* 1995;32:88–92.
18. Wolf B, Heard GS, Weissbecker KA, McVoy JR, Grier RE, Leshner RT. Biotinidase deficiency: initial clinical features and rapid diagnosis. *Ann Neurol* 1985;18:614–617.
19. Collins JE, Nicholson NS, Dalton N, Leonard JV. Biotinidase deficiency: early neurological presentation. *Dev Med Child Neurol* 1994; 36:268–270.
20. Dubowitz V. *The floppy infant*, 2nd ed. London: Spastics International Medical Publications, 1980.
21. al-Qudah AA, Shahar E, Logan WJ, Murphy EG. Neonatal Guillain-Barré syndrome. *Pediatr Neurol* 1988;4:255–256.
22. NINCDS ad hoc Guillain-Barré syndrome committee. Criteria for diagnosis of Guillain-Barré syndrome. *Ann Neurol* 1978;3:565–566.
23. Cornblath DR. Electrophysiology in Guillain-Barré syndrome. *Ann Neurol* 1990;27[Suppl]:S17–20.
24. Schaumburg HH, Kaplan JG. Toxic peripheral neuropathies. In: Asbury AK, Thomas PK, eds. *Peripheral nerve disorders 2*. Oxford: Butterworth-Heinemann, 1995:243–244.
25. Zanga JR. Tick paralysis: another lethal tick-borne disease. *Va Med* 1979;106:443–444.
26. Gay CT, Marks WA, Riley HD Jr, et al. Infantile botulism. *South Med J* 1988;81:457–460.
27. Hurst DL, Marsh WW. Early severe infantile botulism. *J Pediatr* 1993; 122:909–911.
28. Cornblath DR, Sladky JT, Sumner AJ. Clinical electrophysiology of infantile botulism. *Muscle Nerve* 1983;6:448–452.
29. Smith GE, Hinde F, Westmoreland D, Berry PR, Gilbert RJ. Infantile botulism. *Arch Dis Child* 1989;64:871–872.
30. Goebel HH. Congenital myopathies. *Acta Paediatr Jpn* 1991;33: 247–255.
31. Toda T, Segawa M, Nomura Y, et al. Localization of a gene for Fukuyama type congenital muscular dystrophy to chromosome 9q31-33. *Nat Genet* 1993;5:283–286.
32. Tome FMS, Evangelista T, Leclerc A, et al. Congenital muscular dystrophy with merosin deficiency. *CR Acad Sci III* 1994;317:351–357.
33. Helbling-Leclerc A, Zhang X, Topaloglu H, et al. Mutations in the laminin α_2-chain gene (LAMA2) cause merosin-deficient congenital muscular dystrophy. *Nat Genet* 1995;11:216–218.
34. Tsao CY, Boesel CP, Wright FS. A hypotonic infant with complete deficiencies of acid maltase and debrancher enzyme. *J Child Neurol* 1994; 9:90–91.
35. Engel AG, Gomez MR, Seybold ME, Lambert EH. The spectrum and diagnosis of acid maltase deficiency. *Neurology* 1973;23:95–106.
36. Aubourg P, Scotto J, Rocchiccioli F, Feldmann-Pautrat D, Robain O. Neonatal adrenoleukodystrophy. *J Neurol Neurosurg Psychiatry* 1986; 49:77–86.
37. Ozmen M, Caliskan M, Goebel HH, Apak S. Infantile neuroaxonal dystrophy: diagnosis by skin biopsy. *Brain Dev* 1991;13:256–259.
38. Kimura S. Terminal axon pathology in infantile neuroaxonal dystrophy. *Pediatr Neurol* 1991;7:116–120.
39. Shillito P, Angela V, Newsome-Davis J. Congenital myasthenic syndromes. *Neuromusc Disord* 1993;3:183–190.
40. Berkner P, Kastner T, Skolnick L. Chronic ipecac poisoning in infancy: a case report. *Pediatrics* 1988;82:384–386.
41. Sofer S, Tal A, Shahak E. Carbamate and organophosphate poisoning in early childhood. *Pediatr Emerg Care* 1989;5:222–225.
42. Woolf AD, Wynshaw-Boris A, Rinaldo P, Levy HL. Intentional infantile ethylene glycol poisoning presenting as an inherited metabolic disorder. *J Pediatr* 1992;120:421–424.
43. Thomas NH, Robinson L, Evans A, Bullock P. The floppy infant: a new manifestation of nonaccidental injury. *Pediatr Neurosurg* 1995; 23:188–191.

PART II

Nerve and Muscle Diseases

Motor Disorders,
edited by David S. Younger.
Published by Lippincott Williams & Wilkins, Philadelphia 1999.

CHAPTER 9

Clinical Features, Pathogenesis, Diagnosis, and Treatment of the Inflammatory Myopathies

Marinos C. Dalakas

The inflammatory myopathies comprise three major and distinct subsets: polymyositis (PM), dermatomyositis (DM), and inclusion body myositis (IBM) (1–8). Although the presence of moderate to severe muscle weakness and endomysial inflammation are common features in all these conditions, unique clinical, immunopathologic, and histologic criteria along with different prognosis and response to therapies characterize each subset.

The cause of PM, DM, and IBM is unknown, but an autoimmune pathogenesis is strongly implicated based on their association with other putative or definite autoimmune diseases or viral infections, evidence of T-cell–mediated myocytotoxicity and complement-mediated microangiopathy, and their varying response to immunotherapies (1–8). In IBM, autoimmune features coexist with degenerative signs consisting of vacuolization, amyloid deposition, and mitochondrial abnormalities. This chapter reviews the main clinical and histologic features of these diseases, their association with autoimmune conditions or viruses, and the underlying immunopathology. It also provides a practical approach to immunotherapeutic interventions.

CLINICAL FEATURES

Dermatomyositis

DM occurs in both children and adults. It is a distinct clinical entity identified by a characteristic rash accompanying or, more often, preceding the muscle weakness. The skin manifestations include blue-purple discoloration on the upper eyelids or heliotrope rash with edema, a flat red rash on the face and upper trunk, and erythema of the knuckles with a raised violaceous scaly eruption or *Got-*

tron rash that later results in scaling of the skin. An erythematous rash also occurs on other body surfaces, including the knees, elbows, malleoli, neck and anterior chest, often in a "V" sign, or on the back and shoulders, the so-called shawl sign; the latter can be exacerbated after exposure to the sun. In some patients the rash is pruritic, especially in the scalp, chest, and back. Dilated capillary loops at the base of the fingernails are characteristic of DM. The cuticles may be irregular, thickened, and distorted, and the lateral and palmar areas of the fingers may become rough and cracked, with irregular dirty horizontal lines, resembling mechanic's hands. The degree of weakness can be mild, moderate, or severe, leading to quadraparesis. At times, the muscle strength appears normal, hence the term "dermatomyositis sine myositis." When muscle biopsy is performed in such cases, however, significant perivascular and perimysial inflammation is seen (9) (Fig. 1). In children, DM resembles the adult disease, except for more frequent extramuscular manifestations. A common early abnormality in children is "misery," defined as an irritable child that feels uncomfortable, has a red flush on the face, is fatigued, does not feel well to socialize, and has a varying degree of proximal muscle weakness. A tiptoe gait due to flexion contracture of the ankles is also common. DM usually occurs alone or with systemic sclerosis and mixed connective tissue disease (1,2). Fasciitis and skin changes similar to those found in DM occurred in patients with the eosinophilia-myalgia syndrome associated with the ingestion of contaminated L-tryptophan (1,2).

Polymyositis

The actual onset of PM cannot be easily determined. Unlike in DM, in which the rash secures early recognition, patients with PM do not have unique heralding clinical features. In retrospect, affected patients present with subacute proximal muscle weakness and myalgia that

M. C. Dalakas: Neuromuscular Diseases Section, National Institute of Neurological Disorders and Stroke, National Institutes of Health, Bethesda, Maryland 20892.

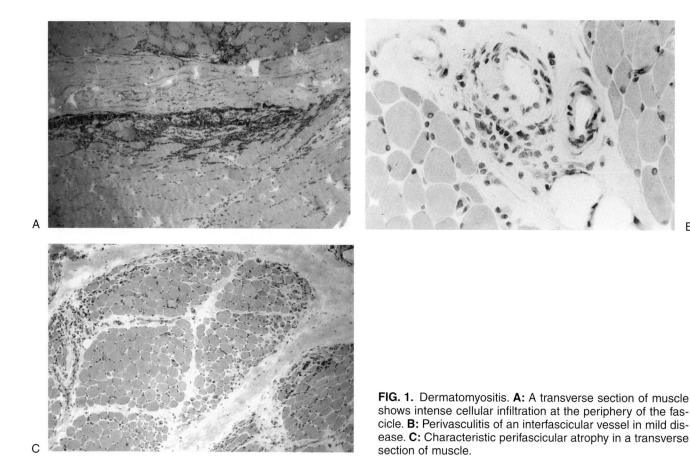

FIG. 1. Dermatomyositis. **A:** A transverse section of muscle shows intense cellular infiltration at the periphery of the fascicle. **B:** Perivasculitis of an interfascicular vessel in mild disease. **C:** Characteristic perifascicular atrophy in a transverse section of muscle.

exists for several months before they seek medical advice. In our judgement, the diagnosis of PM is one of exclusion. It is best diagnosed and defined as an inflammatory myopathy that develops subacutely, usually over weeks to months, and progresses steadily. PM occurs in adults without evidence of a rash, involvement of the extraocular and facial muscles, family history of a neuro-

muscular disease, history of exposure to myotoxic drugs or toxins, endocrinopathy, neurogenic disease, dystrophy, biochemical muscle disorder, or IBM as determined by muscle enzyme histochemistry and biochemistry (Fig. 2). PM can be viewed as a syndrome of diverse causes that occurs separately or in association with systemic autoimmune or connective tissue diseases and certain known

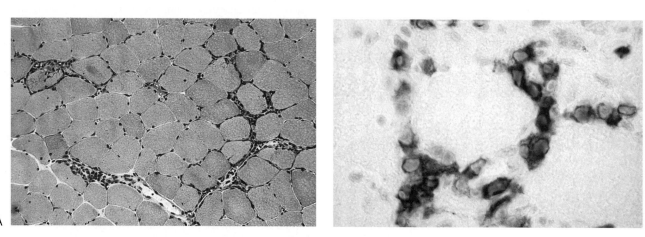

FIG. 2. Polymyositis. **A:** A longitudinal section of muscle shows intense cellular infiltration within the fascicle. **B:** Immunocytochemical staining reveals that the infiltrating cells invading the muscle fiber are mostly CD8+ T cells.

viral or bacterial infections. Other than D-penicillamine and zidovudine, in which the myopathy has endomysial inflammation, myotoxic drugs, such as emetine, chloroquine, steroids, cimetidine, ipecac, and lovostatin, are not a cause of PM. Instead, they can elicit a toxic noninflammatory myopathy that differs histologically from PM and does not require immunosuppressive therapy (1,2).

The animal parasites *Toxoplasma, Trypanosoma,* cysticerci, and trichinae may produce a focal or diffuse inflammatory myopathy known as parasitic PM. A suppurative myositis, known as tropical PM or pyomyositis, is caused by *Staphylococcus aureus, Yersinia, Streptococcus,* and other anaerobes. Pyomyositis is seen in rare patients with AIDS. Certain bacteria, such as *Borrelia burgdorferi* of Lyme disease and *Legionella pneumophila* of legionnaire's disease, are an infrequent cause of PM.

Inclusion Body Myositis

IBM affects men more often than women and is the most frequently acquired myopathy in men over age 50 years. It is commonly suspected in patients with presumed PM that do not respond to corticosteroid therapy. The involvement of distal muscles, especially foot extensors and deep finger flexors, which occurs in almost all patients, is a valuable clue to the early clinical diagnosis of IBM (1–7,10). Some patients present with falls and buckling of the knees due to proximal leg weakness. Others present with weakness in the small muscles of the hands, especially finger flexors, and complain of inability to hold certain objects such as golf clubs, play the guitar, turn keys, or tie knots. The weakness and accompanying wasting is often asymmetric with selective involvement of the quadriceps, iliopsoas, triceps, biceps, and finger flexor muscles of the forearm. Dysphagia occurs in up to 60% of patients, especially late in the dis-

ease. A lower motor neuron neurogenic disorder may be suspected, especially when the serum creatine kinase (CK) is not elevated. Sensory examination may be normal or show age-related vibratory sensory loss at the ankles. Contrary to early suggestions, distal weakness is not on a neurogenic basis but is a feature of the distal myopathy as shown by macroelectromyography (11). In contrast to PM and DM in which facial muscles are typically spared, mild facial muscle weakness occurs in 60% of patients with IBM (10). The diagnosis is always confirmed when the muscle biopsy shows the characteristic histopathologic changes (Fig. 3).

IBM can be associated with systemic autoimmune or connective tissue diseases in at least 20% of the cases. Inherited cases are often recessively transmitted and less frequently dominantly inherited, sometimes in association with leukoencephalopathy and others with quadriceps sparing. Hereditary IBM includes a variety of still ill-defined vacuolar distally greater than proximal myopathies with a clinical profile that differs from the sporadic IBM cases described above (12). Hereditary IBM with sparing of the quadriceps occurs not only in Iranian Jews but in other ethnic groups (13). Detailed description and genetic data on hereditary IBM are not provided in this review because these diseases lack inflammation in their muscles and do not represent a true inflammatory myopathy. There is, however, a subset of patients with familial IBM that have the typical phenotype of sporadic IBM with histologic and immunopathologic features identical to the sporadic form (14).

The progression of IBM is slow and steady, with a degree of disability that is generally related to the duration of the disease, although this has not been systematically studied. A review of 14 randomly chosen patients with symptoms for more than 5 years revealed that 10 required a cane or support for ambulation by the fifth year after onset of dis-

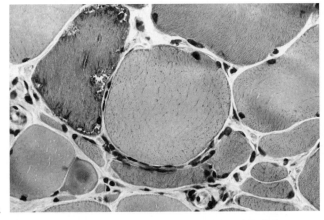

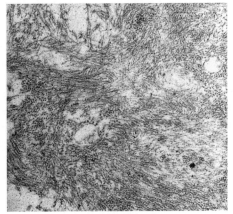

A   B

FIG. 3. Inclusion body myositis. **A:** A transverse section of muscle shows rimmed vacuoles and small atrophic fibers among big-size fibers. **B:** Characteristic filamentous inclusion seen by electron microscopy in the cytoplasm within one vacuole of myonuclei.

ease, whereas 3 of the remaining 5 with symptoms for 10 years or more required use of a wheelchair. Using quantitative muscle strength testing, we found a 10% drop in muscle strength over a 2-year period. In other studies from our institution, 86 consecutively studied patients showed progression that was faster with late disease onset. The patients whose disease begins in the sixth decade may require assistive devices at a statistically significant later time than those with disease onset in the eighth decade.

EXTRAMUSCULAR MANIFESTATIONS

In addition to the primary disturbance of skeletal muscles, there may be prominent extramuscular manifestations in patients with inflammatory myopathy: dysphagia, most prominent in IBM and DM, due to involvement of striated muscles of the oropharynx and distal esophagus; cardiac abnormalities consisting of atrioventricular conduction defects, tachyarrhythmias, low ejection fraction, and dilated cardiomyopathy alone or associated with hypertension or long-term steroid use; and respiratory involvement, resulting from weakness of chest-cage muscles, drug-induced pneumonitis as for example from methotrexate or interstitial lung disease. Interstitial lung disease can precede the myopathy or occur as an associated feature, overall in up to 10% of patients with PM or DM, most of whom have anti-Jo-1 antibodies. The latter may be at times associated with increased fatality resulting from adult respiratory distress syndrome in those with PM (15), emphasizing the diagnostic importance of these antibodies. Pulmonary capillaritis with varying degree of diffuse alveolar hemorrhage has also been described (16). Subcutaneous calcification, sometimes extruding on the skin and causing ulceration and infection, are found in children and some adults with DM (17). Gastrointestinal ulceration, seen more often in children with DM, is due to vasculitis and infection. Joint contractures are seen, especially in children with DM. General systemic disturbances are seen, such as fever, malaise, weight loss, arthralgia, and Raynaud's phenomenon, when the inflammatory myopathy is associated with a connective tissue disorder. Malignancy is also manifested with increased frequency in those with DM but not PM or IBM. Because tumors are usually uncovered not by a radiologic blind search but by abnormal findings on their medical history and physical examination, it is our practice to recommend only a complete annual physical examination, with breast, pelvic, and rectal examinations; urinalysis; complete blood cell count; blood chemistry tests; and a chest x-ray film.

DIAGNOSIS

The diagnosis of clinically suspected PM, DM, or IBM is confirmed by examination of serum muscle enzymes and compatible findings on electromyography and muscle biopsy.

Serum Muscle Enzymes

The most sensitive serum enzyme is CK, which in the presence of active disease can be elevated sometimes 50-fold or more. Although the CK usually parallels the disease activity, it can be normal in active DM and rarely even in active PM. In IBM, serum CK is usually elevated not more than tenfold, and in some cases may be normal even from the outset of the illness. The CK may also be normal in patients with untreated, even active, childhood DM and in some with PM or DM associated with a connective tissue disease, reflecting the concentration of the pathologic process in the intramuscular vessels and the perimysium. Along with CK, serum aspartate and alanine aminotranferases, lactate dehydrogenase, and aldolase levels may be elevated.

Electromyography

Electromyographic studies are generally useful for excluding neurogenic disorders and confirming either active or inactive myopathy. Needle electromyography shows myopathic potentials characterized by short-duration low-amplitude polyphasic units on voluntary activation and increased spontaneous activity with fibrillations, complex repetitive discharges, and positive sharp waves. This pattern also occurs in various acute and active toxic myopathic processes and should not be considered diagnostic for inflammatory myopathy. Polyphasic units of short and long duration suggestive of mixed myopathic and neurogenic disease are more often seen in IBM, but they can be seen in both PM and DM as a consequence of muscle fiber regeneration and the chronicity of the disease. With macroelectromyography, neurogenic involvement alone is not found in IBM (11).

Muscle Biopsy

Muscle biopsy is a potentially definitive test not only to establish the histologic diagnosis of DM, PM, and IBM, but also to exclude other morphologically distinct processes (Figs. 1–3). Although the presence of inflammation is the histologic hallmark for these diseases, there are additional unique histologic features characteristic for each group.

In DM, the endomysial inflammation is predominantly perivascular or in the interfascicular septae, around rather than within the muscle fascicles. Intramuscular blood vessels show endothelial hyperplasia with tuboloreticular profiles, fibrin thrombi especially in children, and obliteration of capillaries (1–6). There is muscle fiber necrosis, degeneration, and phagocytosis, often in groups, involving a portion of a muscle fasciculus in a wedgelike shape or at the periphery of the fascicle due to microinfarction. The latter results in perifascicular atrophy, characterized by two to ten layers of atrophic fibers at the periphery of the fascicles (Fig. 1).

The presence of perifascicular atrophy is diagnostic of DM, even in the absence of inflammation.

In PM there is no perifascicular atrophy and the blood vessels are normal. The endomysial infiltrates are mostly within the fascicles surrounding individual healthy myofibers, resulting in phagocytosis and necrosis. With chronic disease there is increased connective tissue formation and reaction with alkaline phosphatase stains.

The histologic hallmarks of IBM include basophilic granular inclusions distributed around the edge of slitlike vacuoles, so-called rimmed vacuoles (Fig. 3); angulated or round fibers, scattered or in small groups; eosinophilic cytoplasmic inclusions; primary endomysial inflammation with T cells invading muscle fibers in a pattern identical to, but often more severe than, those seen in PM; and tiny deposits of Congo red or crystal violet-positive amyloid in or adjacent to vacuoles. The amyloid, seen in approximately 80% of our patients, immunoreacts with β-amyloid protein, the type sequenced from the amyloid fibrils of blood vessels of patients with Alzheimer's disease (18–20). Characteristic filamentous inclusions seen by electron microscopy in the cytoplasm or in myonuclei and prominence in the vicinity of the rimmed vacuoles are also a hallmark. Although the demonstration of filaments by electron microscopy was at one time essential to the diagnosis of IBM, it is no longer necessary when all of the characteristic light microscopic features, including the amyloid deposits, are present. Furthermore, the filamentous inclusions are not specific for IBM but can be seen in other vacuolar myopathies. The cytoplasmic tubulofilaments within the vacuolated muscle fibers immunoreact strongly with tau, ubiquitin, chymothrypsin, and prion (18). Finally, abnormal mitochondria are seen as ragged red fibers that are often negative with cytochrome oxidase and contain mitochondrial DNA deletions (21).

IMMUNE-MEDIATED MECHANISMS

Presence of Autoantibodies

Various autoantibodies against nuclear and cytoplasmic antigens are found in up to 20% of patients with inflammatory myopathy (1–3,8,22). Antibodies to cytoplasmic antigens are directed against cytoplasmic ribonucleoproteins that are involved in RNA translation and protein synthesis. They include antibodies against various synthetases, translation factors, and proteins of the signal-recognition particles. The antibody directed against the histidyl-transfer RNA synthetase, called anti-Jo-1, accounts for 75% of all the anti-synthetases, and it is diagnostically useful because up to 80% of patients with anti-Jo-1 antibodies have interstitial lung disease. In general, they may not be specific because they are directed against ubiquitous targets and may represent epiphenomena without pathogenic significance; they occur in PM, DM, and IBM despite their clinical and immunopathologic differences; and they are almost always associated with interstitial lung disease even in patients who do not have active myositis.

Immunopathology of Dermatomyositis

It has been repeatedly shown that the primary antigenic targets in DM are components of the vascular endothelium of the endomysial blood vessels and the capillaries (23,24). The earliest pathologic alterations are changes in the endothelial cells consisting of pale and swollen cytoplasm with microvacuoles and undulating tubules in the smooth endoplasmic reticulum, followed by obliteration, microvessel necrosis, and thrombosis (24). The microvascular alterations occur early in the disease and are mediated by C5b-9 membranolytic attack complex (MAC), deposited along capillaries before the onset of inflammatory or structural changes in the muscle fibers (25). Using an in vitro assay system that measures C3 consumption by sensitized erythrocytes on the basis of radiolabeled anti-C3 antibodies (26), it is also known that patients with active, but not chronic, DM have a very high uptake of C3 in the serum. MAC and the active fragments of the early complement components C3b and C4b are also increased in the sera of patients using a radioimmunoassay (26).

Sequentially, the disease begins when putative antibodies are directed against endothelial cells of the endomysium (27) that activate the C3 component of the complement that forms C3b and C4b fragments and leads to formation and deposition of MAC on endomysial microvessels. The deposition of MAC leads to osmotic lysis of endothelial cells with capillary necrosis, perivascular inflammation, ischemia, and muscle fiber destruction resembling microinfarction. Perifascicular atrophy, seen more often in chronic stages, is a reflection of distal endofascicular hypoperfusion. Finally, there is marked reduction in the number of capillaries per each muscle fiber with dilatation of the remaining capillaries in an effort to compensate for the impaired perfusion.

Putative anti-endothelial cell antibodies that fix complement can be detected by an ELISA using human umbilical vein endothelial cells as antigen (28); however, characterization of the pathogenicity of these antibodies has not yet been performed. The presence of systemic features, with involvement of myocardium, pericardium, lungs, and the gut, suggests that the MAC-mediated microvascular injury may be more widespread and that the target antigen may be a ubiquitous component of the blood vessel endothelium. The activation of complement by putative anti-endothelial cell antibodies is believed to be responsible for the induction of cytokines (29) that in turn upregulate the expression of vascular and intercellular adhesion molecules (ICAM) type 1 on endothelial cells (30) and facilitate the exit of activated lymphoid cells to the perimysial and endomysial spaces.

Immunophenotypic analysis of the lymphocytic infiltrates in the muscle biopsies of patients with DM demonstrates a predominance of B cells and CD4+ cells in perimysial and perivascular regions, supporting a humoral-immune mediated process, as described above (4,31,32). In the perifascicular areas, however, the infiltrates contain mainly CD8+ cells and macrophages and invade major histocompatibility complex class I (MHC-I)–antigen-expressing muscle fibers, a sign of coexisting T-cell–mediated and MHC-I–restricted cytotoxic processes.

Immunopathology of Polymyositis and Inclusion Body Myositis

Cytotoxic T Cells

In PM and IBM, there is evidence of primarily antigen-directed cytotoxicity mediated by cytotoxic T cells (4,31,32). This is supported by the presence of CD8+ cells, which along with macrophages, initially surround healthy MHC-I class expressing nonnecrotic muscle fibers that eventually invade and destroy. The T cells are activated, as evidenced by their expression of ICAM-1 and MHC-I and -II antigens on their surface, and exert a cytotoxic effect against muscle fibers as supported by the following:

1. Cell lines established from muscle biopsies of PM patients exerted cytotoxicity to autologous myotubes in vitro (33).
2. With immunoelectron microscopy, CD8+ cells and macrophages send spikelike processes into nonnecrotic muscle fibers, which traverse the basal lamina and focally displace or compress the muscle fibers (31).
3. Cytotoxic autoinvasive CD8+ T cells contain perforin and granzyme granules (34) directed against the surface of myofibers and, upon release, they induce cell destruction.
4. On the basis of T-cell receptor analysis, there is clonal expansion of T cells with a restricted usage of the T-cell receptor variable region of certain T-cell receptor gene families, notably Va1, Vb15, and Vb6. This suggests that the T-cell response is driven by a muscle-specific antigen (35,36).
5. The cytotoxicity mediated by the CD8+ cells appears to be antigen-specific because, in addition to clonal expansion of certain T-cell receptor gene families described above, the T cells invade muscle fibers expressing MHC-I class antigen, a prerequisite for antigen recognition by the CD8+ cells. MHC-I class antigen is not present on normal muscle fibers but is ubiquitous to the sarcolemma of the muscle fibers in patients with PM and IBM (37). MHC-I expression is probably upregulated by cytokines secreted by activated T cells, macrophages, and viruses in a set-

ting of a viral infection. The nature of these antigenic peptides bound by the MHC-I for presentation to the CD8+ cells still remains unknown. It is believed that such antigens are probably endogenous sarcolemmal or cytoplasmic self proteins synthesized within the myofibers. The possibility of endogenous viral peptides appears unlikely because several laboratories have failed to amplify viruses within the muscle fibers not only in PM patients with a putative viral infection (38,39), but also in patients with classic PM associated with human immunodeficiency virus (HIV) type 1 or human T-cell lymphotropic virus type I (HTLV-I) infection (40,41).

6. In three rare cases, gamma/delta T cells or natural killer cells were the main participating cells in the myocytotoxicity of PM and IBM (42,43).

Cytokines and Adhesion Molecules

The T-cell–derived cytokines and interleukins (IL): IL-2, IL-4, IL-5; interferon-β; the macrophage-derived cytokines IL-1, IL-6, and tumor necrosis factor-α; and cytokines that are either T-cell– or macrophage-derived such as granulocyte-macrophage colony-stimulating factor and transforming growth factor-β can be amplified with the reverse transcriptase polymerase chain reaction (PCR) method in the muscles of patients with PM, DM, and IBM (44–46). The adhesion molecules and their receptors, ICAM-1, vascular cellular adhesion molecule type 1, and their respective ligands, integrins 1 and 2, are also upregulated on the endothelial cells or the infiltrating T cells in patients with PM, DM, and IBM and may facilitate the adhesion, penetration, and exit of activated T cells through the endothelial cell wall (32,44–46).

Association with Viral Infections

Coxsackie, influenza, paramyxoviruses, cytomegalovirus, Epstein Barr virus, and other viruses have been indirectly associated with chronic and acute myositis (47,48). The phenomenon of molecular mimicry has been proposed with the coxsakievirus because of structural homology between the Jo-1 and the genomic RNA of an animal picornavirus, the encephalomyocarditis virus. Sensitive PCR studies, however, have repeatedly failed to confirm the presence of such viruses in the muscle biopsies of patients we studied, suggesting that it is unlikely, although not impossible, for them to be replicated in the muscles of patients with PM, DM, and IBM (38,39).

The best evidence of a viral connection in PM and IBM is with retroviruses that were associated with PM in monkeys infected with the simian immunodeficiency virus (49,50) and in humans infected with HIV and HTLV-I (51,52). In HIV-positive patients, an inflammatory myopathy, HIV-PM, occurs as the first clinical indication of HIV infection or concurrent with other manifestations of AIDS (51,53,54). HIV seroconversion may coincide with myoglobulinuria and acute myalgia, suggesting that myotropism for HIV may be symptomatic early in the infection. In addition, HTLV-I does not only cause a myeloneuropathy, referred to as tropical spastic paraparesis, but also PM, which may coexist with tropical spastic paraparesis or may be the only clinical manifestation of HTLV-I infection (52–54). IBM also occurs with HIV or HTLV-I infection (55). Using either in situ hybridization, PCR, immunocytochemistry, or electron microscopy, we did not detect viral antigens within the myofibers of these patients' muscle but only in occasional endomysial macrophages (40,41,54,55). We interpreted these observations to suggest that in HIV-1 and HTLV-I PM and IBM, there is no evidence of persistent infection of the muscle fiber by the virus or viral replication within the muscle. The predominant endomysial cell in HIV-1 and HTLV-I PM and IBM are CD8+, non–viral-specific, cytotoxic T cells that along with macrophages invade or surround MHC-I–antigen-expressing nonnecrotic muscle fibers. We proposed that a T-cell–mediated and MHC-I–restricted cytotoxic process was a common pathogenetic mechanism in both retroviral negative and retroviral-positive PM and IBM, but in the latter, viral-induced cytokines might have triggered the process by breaking tolerance.

Role of Nonimmune Factors in Sporadic Inclusion Body Myositis

In IBM, the presence of amyloid-positive deposits within some of the vacuolated muscle fibers and the finding of abnormal mitochondria have generated reasonable concerns that, in addition to the autoimmune components mentioned earlier, there is also a degenerative process.

The amyloid deposits in IBM are accompanied by all of the other proteins seen in the β-amyloid of Alzheimer disease, including β-amyloid precursor protein, chymothrypsin, apolipoprotein E, and phosphorylated tau. Whether these deposits are secondarily related to the chronicity of the disease or are generated de novo and contribute to disease pathogenesis is unclear. The same can be said for mitochondrial abnormalities and mitochondrial DNA deletions that were observed in up to 70% of IBM muscles. Although such mitochondrial changes are more frequently seen in IBM than in normal aging, it is unclear if they are primary or secondary or if they are enhanced by the upregulated cytokines.

TREATMENT

Because the specific target antigens in DM, PM, and IBM are unknown, currently proposed forms of immunosuppressive therapy such as prednisone do not selectively target autoreactive T cells or the complement-mediated process on the intramuscular blood vessels. Instead, they induce nonselective immunosuppression or immunomodulation. Further, many of these therapies are empirical and mostly uncontrolled.

The goal of therapy in inflammatory myopathy is to improve muscle strength and thereby improve overall function in activities of daily living. When strength improves, the serum CK also tends to fall, but the reverse is not always true because most immunosuppressive therapies can result in decrease of serum muscle enzymes without necessarily improving muscle strength. Unfortunately, this has been misinterpreted as chemical improvement and has formed the basis for the common habit of chasing or treating the CK level instead of the muscle weakness, a practice that has led to a prolonged use of unnecessary immunosuppressive drugs and erroneous assessment of their efficacy. It is prudent to discontinue these nonspecific immunosuppressive drugs if after an adequate trial there has been only a reduction in the serum CK and not an objective improvement in muscle strength (1–3,56–59). Agents used in the treatment of PM and DM follow.

Corticosteroids, including prednisone, are the first-line agents. Its actions are unclear, but it may exert a beneficial effect by inhibiting recruitment and migration of lymphocytes to the areas of muscle inflammation and interfering with the production of lymphokines. Its effect on lymphokine IL-1 may be important because IL-1 is myotoxic (60) and is secreted by the activated macrophages that invade the muscle fibers. Steroid-induced suppression of ICAM-1 may also be relevant because downregulation of ICAM-1 can prevent the trafficking of lymphocytes across the endothelial cell wall toward the muscle fibers.

Because the effectiveness and relative safety of prednisone therapy will determine the future need for stronger immunosuppressive drugs, our preference has been to start with high dosages, such as 80 to 100 mg/day. After an initial period of 3 to 4 weeks, it is tapered over a 10-week period by reducing the alternate off-day dose by 10 mg/wk, or faster if necessary because of side effects, though the latter carries a greater risk of breakthrough of disease. If improvement occurs and there are no serious side effects, the dose can be gradually reduced by 5 to 10 mg every 3 to 4 weeks until the lowest possible dose that controls the disease is reached. If by the time the dose has been tapered to 80 to 100 mg alternating with 0 mg, approximately 14 weeks after initiating therapy (and there is no increase in muscle strength), the patient may then be considered unresponsive to prednisone, and tapering is accelerated while the next in line immunosuppressive drug is started (56–59).

Although almost all patients with bona fide PM or DM respond to steroids to some extent and for some period of time, a number of them fail to respond or become steroid resistant. The decision to start a nonsteroidal immunosuppressive drug in PM or DM is based on the need for its steroid-sparing effect, when despite steroid responsiveness the patient has developed significant complications; attempts to lower a high-steroid dosage have repeatedly resulted in a new relapse; an adequate dose of prednisone for 2 to 3 months was ineffective; and development of rapidly progressive disease with severe weakness and respiratory failure. The preference for selecting the immunosuppressive next in line is, however, empirical. The choice is usually based on individual experience and an assessment of the relative efficacy and safety ratio. The following immunosuppressive agents can be considered.

Azathioprine is an oral derivative of 6-mercaptopurine. Although daily dosages of 1.5 to 2 mg/kg are commonly given, we prefer 3 mg/kg. The drug is well tolerated, has few side effects, and empirically appears to be a useful long-term therapy for inflammatory myopathy.

Methotrexate is an antagonist of folate metabolism. Although a superiority to azathioprine has not been established, it has a faster mode of action. It can be given intravenously over 20 to 60 minutes at weekly doses of 0.4 mg/kg up to 0.8 mg/kg with sufficient fluids or orally. The starting dosage is 7.5 mg/wk for 3 weeks, given 2.5 mg three times daily, gradually increasing it by 2.5 mg/wk up to a total of 25 mg. Pneumonitis is a side effect that can be difficult to distinguish from the interstitial lung disease of primary myopathy, often associated with Jo-1 antibodies.

Cyclophosphamide is an alkylating agent that can be given intravenously or orally at dosages of 2 to 2.5 mg/kg in 50-mg tablets three times daily. It has not been effective in our experience (61) despite occasional promising results reported by others (62).

Chlorambucil is an antimetabolite that has been tried in some patients with variable results (63).

Cyclosporine is of uncertain value in PM and DM. Toxicity can be monitored by measuring trough serum levels that can vary between 100 and 250 ng/mL. A report that low dose cyclosporine was of benefit in childhood DM is still unconfirmed (64). An advantage of cyclosporine is that it acts faster than azathioprine and methotrexate and the results, whether positive or negative, are apparent early (65).

Plasmapheresis was not helpful in a double-blind placebo-controlled study (66).

Total lymphoid irradiation was helpful in selected patients and may have long-lasting benefit. The long-term side effects of this treatment, however, should be seriously considered before deciding on this experimental and rather extreme approach. Total lymphoid irradiation has been ineffective in IBM (67).

Intravenous immunoglobulin (IVIg) is a promising, but expensive, therapy. In uncontrolled studies of PM and DM, it was of reported benefit (68–70). We demonstrated the effectiveness of IVIg in a double-blind study of patients with refractory DM. Strength not only improves but the underlying immunopathology may resolve (71),

and this begins after the first infusion and is clearly evident by the second monthly dose. However, the benefit is short lived, usually for not more than 8 weeks and requiring repeated infusions at 6 to 8 weekly intervals to maintain improvement. The mechanism of action of IVIg in DM appears to be inhibition of the deposition and activation of complement components, especially MAC on the capillaries (26); suppression of cytokines, especially ICAM-1; saturation of Fc receptors; and interference with the action of macrophages (71,72).

A controlled double-blind study for PM is still underway, although uncontrolled studies showed effectiveness in up to 80% of the patients so treated. IVIg also exerted some benefit, although not statistically significant, in up to 30% of patients with IBM in a controlled double-blind study (73,74). Although the improvement was not dramatic, it made a difference in the lifestyles of some patients. A second study showed no further benefit when IVIg was combined with prednisone (75).

Until further control drug trials are completed, the following step-by-step empirical approach for the treatment of PM and DM is suggested:

Step 1—Start with high-dose prednisone.
Step 2—If there is a need for "steroid sparing," add azathioprine or methotrexate.
Step 3—*If step 2 fails, try high-dose IVIg therapy.*
Step 4—If step 3 fails, consider a trial, with guarded optimism, of cyclosporine, chlorambucil, or cyclophosphamide guided by the patient's age, degree of disability, tolerance, experience with the drug, and the patient's general health.

REFERENCES

1. Dalakas MC. Polymyositis, dermatomyositis, and inclusion-body myositis. *N Engl J Med* 1991;325:1487–1498.
2. Dalakas MC. Inflammatory myopathies: pathogenesis and treatment. *Neuropharmacology* 1992;5:327–351.
3. Dalakas MC, ed. *Polymyositis and dermatomyositis.* Boston: Butterworth, 1988.
4. Engel AG, Hohlfeld R, Banker BQ. The polymyositis and dermatomyositis syndrome. In: Engel AG, Franzini-Armstrong C, eds. *Myology.* New York: McGraw-Hill, 1994:1335–1383.
5. Hohlfeld R, Goebels N, Engel AG. Cellular mechanisms in inflammatory myopathies. In: Mastaglia FL, ed. *Bailliere's clinical neurology.* London: W.B. Saunders, 1993:617–636.
6. Karpati G, Carpenter S. Pathology of the inflammatory myopathies. In: Mastaglia FL, ed. *Bailliere's clinical neurology.* London: W.B. Saunders, 1993:527–556.
7. Dalakas MC. Inflammatory myopathies. *Curr Opin Neurol Neurosurg* 1990;3:689–696.
8. Plotz PH, Dalakas M, Leff RL, Love LA, Miller FW, Cronin ME. Current concepts in the idiopathic inflammatory myopathies: polymyositis, dermatomyositis and related disorders. *Ann Intern Med* 1989;111:143–157.
9. Otero C, Illa I, Dalakas MC. Is there dermatomyositis (DM) without myositis? *Neurology* 1992;42[Suppl]:388.
10. Sekul EA, Dalakas MC. Inclusion body myositis: new concepts. *Semin Neurol* 1993;13:256–263.
11. Luciano CA, Dalakas MC. A macro-EMG study in inclusion-body myositis: no evidence for a neurogenic component. *Neurology* 1997;48:29–33.

12. Sivakumar K, Dalakas MC. Inclusion body myositis and myopathies. *Curr Opin Neurol* 1997;10:413–420.
13. Sivakumar K, Dalakas MC. The spectrum of familial inclusion body myopathies in 13 families and description of a quadriceps sparing phenotype in non-Iranian Jews. *Neurology* 1996;47:977–984.
14. Sivakumar K, Semino-Mora C, Dalakas MC. An inflammatory, familial, inclusion body myositis with autoimmune features and a phenotype identical to sporadic inclusion body myositis: studies in 3 families. *Brain* 1997;120:653–661.
15. Clawson K, Oddis CV. Adult respiratory distress syndrome in polymyositis patients with the anti-Jo-I antibody. *Arthritis Rheum* 1995;38:1519–1523.
16. Schwarz MI, Sutarik JM, Nick JA, Leff JA, Emlen JW, Tuder RM. Pulmonary capillaritis and diffuse alveolar hemorrhage: a primary manifestation of polymyositis. *Am J Respir Crit Care Med* 1995;151:2037–2040.
17. Dalakas MC. Calcifications in dermatomyositis. *N Engl J Med* 1995;333:978.
18. Askanas V, Serdaroglu P, Engel WK, Alvarez RB. Immunocytochemical localization of ubiquitin in inclusion body myositis allows its light-microscopic distinction from polymyositis. *Neurology* 1992;42:460–461.
19. Mendell JR, Sahenk Z, Gales T, Paul L. Amyloid filaments in inclusion body myositis. *Arch Neurol* 1991;48:1229–1234.
20. Askanas V, Engel WK, Alvarez RB, Glenner GG. β-Amyloid protein immunoreactivity in muscle of patients with inclusion-body myositis. *Lancet* 1992;339:560–561.
21. Santorelli FM, Sciacco M, Tanji K, et al. Multiple mitochondrial DNA deletions in sporadic inclusion body myositis: a study of 56 patients. *Ann Neurol* 1996;39:789–795.
22. Targoff IN. Immune mechanisms of myositis. *Curr Opin Rheumatol* 1990;2:882–888.
23. Banker BQ. Dermatomyositis of childhood. Ultrastructural alterations of muscle and intramuscular blood vessels. *J Neuropathol Exp Neurol* 1975;35:46–75.
24. Carpenter S, Karpati G, Rothman S, Walters G. The childhood type of dermatomyositis. *Neurology* 1976;26:952–962.
25. Emslie-Smith AM, Engel AG: Microvascular changes in early and advanced dermatomyositis: a quantitative study. *Ann Neurol* 1990;27:343–356.
26. Basta M, Dalakas MC. High-dose intravenous immunoglobulin exerts its beneficial effect in patients with dermatomyositis by blocking endomysial deposition of activated complement fragments. *J Clin Invest* 1994;94:1729–1735.
27. Cervera R, Ramires G, Fernandez-Sola J, et al. Antibodies to endothelial cells in dermatomyositis: association with interstitial lung diseases. *Br Med J* 1991;302:880–882.
28. Stein DP, Jordan SC, Toyoda M, Gallera O, Dalakas MC. Anti-endothelial cell antibodies (AECA) in dermatomyositis (DM). *Neurology* 1993;43[Suppl]:356.
29. Lundberg I, Brengman JM, Engel AG. Analysis of cytokine expression in muscle in inflammatory myopathies, Duchennes dystrophy and non-weak controls. *J Neuroimmunol* 1995;63:9–16.
30. Stein DP, Dalakas MC. Intercellular adhesion molecule-I expression is upregulated in patients with dermatomyositis (DM). *Ann Neurol* 1993;34:268.
31. Arahata K, Engel AG. Monoclonal antibody analysis of mononuclear cells in myopathies. III. Immunoelectron microscopy aspects of cell-mediated muscle fiber injury. *Ann Neurol* 1986;19:112–125.
32. Dalakas MC. Immunopathogenesis of inflammatory myopathies. *Ann Neurol* 1995;37[Suppl]:74–86.
33. Hohlfeld R, Engel AG. Coculture with autologous myotubes of cytotoxic T cells isolated from muscle in inflammatory myopathies. *Ann Neurol* 1991;29:498–507.
34. Goebel N, Michaelis D, Engelhardt M, et al. Differential expression of perforin in muscle-infiltrating T cell in polymyositis and dermatomyositis. *J Clin Invest* 1996;12:2905–2910.
35. Bender A, Ernst N, Iglesias A, Dornmair K, Wekerle H, Hohlfeld R. T cell receptor repertoire in polymyositis: clonal expansion of autoaggressive CD8+ T cells. *J Exp Med* 1995;181:1863–1868.
36. O'Hanlon TP, Dalakas MC, Plotz PH, Miller FW. The alphabeta T-cell receptor repertoire in inclusion body myositis: diverse patterns of gene expression by muscle infiltrating lymphocytes. *J Autoimmun* 1994;7:321–333.
37. Karpati G, Pouliot Y, Carpenter S. Expression of immunoreactive major histocapability complex products in human skeletal muscles. *Ann Neurol* 1988;23:64–72.
38. Leff RL, Love LA, Miller FW, et al. Viruses in the idiopathic inflammatory myopathies: absence of candidate viral genomes in muscle. *Lancet* 1992;339:1192–1195.
39. Leon-Monzon M, Dalakas MC. Absence of persistent infection with enteroviruses in muscles of patients with inflammatory myopathies. *Ann Neurol* 1992;32:219–222.
40. Illa I, Nath A, Dalakas MC. Immunocytochemical and virological characterisics of HIV-associated inflammatory myopathies: similarities with seronegative polymyositis. *Ann Neurol* 1991;29:474–481.
41. Leon-Monzon M, Illa I, Dalakas MC. Polymyositis in patients infected with HTLV-I: the role of the virus in the cause of the disease. *Ann Neurol* 1994;36:643–649.
42. Hohlfeld R, Engel AG, Kunio Li, Harper MC. Polymyositis mediated by T lymphocytes that express the gamma and delta receptor. *N Engl J Med* 1991;324:877–881.
43. Dalakas MC, Illa I. Common variable immunodeficiency and inclusion body myositis: a distinct myopathy mediated by natural killer cells. *Ann Neurol* 1995;37:806–810.
44. Tews DS, Goebel HH. Cytokine expression profiles in idiopathic inflammatory myopathies. *J Neuropathol Exp Neurol* 1996;55:342–347.
45. Tews DS, Goebel HH. Expression of cell adhesion molecules in inflammatory myopathies. *J Neuroimmunol* 1995;59:185–194.
46. De Bleecker JL, Engel AG. Expression of cell adhesion molecules in inflammatory myopathies and Duchenne dystrophy. *J Neuropathol Exp Neurol* 1994;53:369–376.
47. Dalakas MC. Infection of human muscle, nerve and motor neurons with polioviruses and other enteroviruses. In: Rotbard HA, ed. *Human enteroviral infections*. Washington, DC: American Society for Microbiology (ASM) Press, 1995:387–398.
48. Hays AP, Gamboa ET. Acute viral myositis. In: Engel AG, Franzini-Armstrong C, eds. *Myology*. New York: McGraw-Hill, 1994:1399–1418.
49. Dalakas MC, London WT, Gravell M, Sever JL. Polymyositis in an immunodeficiency disease in monkeys induced by a type D retrovirus. *Neurology* 1986;36:569–572.
50. Dalakas MC, Gravell M, London WT, Cunningham G, Sever JL. Morphological changes of an inflammatory myopathy in rhesus monkeys with simian acquired immunodeficiency syndrome (SAIDS). *Proc Soc Exp Biol Med* 1987;185:368–376.
51. Dalakas MC, Pezeshkpour GH, Gravell M, Sever JL. Polymyositis in patients with AIDS. *JAMA* 1986;256:2381–2383.
52. Morgan O StC, Rodgers-Johnson P, Mora C, Char G. HTLV-I and polymyositis in Jamaica. *Lancet* 1989;2:1184–1187.
53. Dalakas MC, Pezeshkpour GH. Neuromuscular diseases associated with human immunodeficiency virus infection. *Ann Neurol* 1988;23[Suppl]:38–48.
54. Dalakas MC. Retroviral myopathies. In: Engel AG, Franzini-Armstrong C, eds. *Myology*. Vol. II. New York: McGraw-Hill, 1994:1419–1437.
55. Cupler EJ, Leon-Monzon M, Miller J, Semino-Mora C, Anderson TL, Dalakas MC. Inclusion body myositis in HIV-I and HTLV-I infected patients. *Brain* 1996;6:1887–1893.
56. Dalakas MC. Treatment of polymyositis and dermatomyositis. *Curr Opin Rheumatol* 1989;1:443–449.
57. Dalakas MC. How to diagnose and treat the inflammatory myopathies. *Semin Neurol* 1994;14:137–145.
58. Dalakas MC. Current treatment of the inflammatory myopathies. *Curr Opin Rheumatol* 1994;6:595–601.
59. Dalakas MC. Inflammatory myopathies: In: Rowland LP, and DiMauro S, eds. *Handbook of Clinical Neurology. Vol. 18. Myopathies*. Amsterdam: Elsevier Science Publishers, 1992:369–390.
60. Leon-Monzon M, Dalakas MC. Interleukin-1 (IL-1) is toxic to human muscle. *Neurology* 1994;44[Suppl]:132.
61. Cronin ME, Miller FW, Hicks JE, Dalakas M, Plotz PH. The failure of intravenous cyclophosphamide therapy in refractory idiopathic inflammatory myopathy. *J Rheumatol* 1989;16:1225–1228.
62. Bombardieri S, Hughes GRV, Neri R, Del Bravo P, Del Bono L. Cyclophosphamide in severe polymyositis. *Lancet* 1989;1:1138–1139.
63. Sinoway TA, Callen JP. Chlorambucil: an effective corticosteroid-sparing agent for patients with recalcitrant dermatomyositis. *Arthritis Rheum* 1993;36:319–324.
64. Heckmatt J, Hasson N, Saunders C, et al. Cyclosporin in juvenile dermatomyositis. *Lancet* 1989;1:1063–1066.

65. Grau JM, Herrero C, Casademont J, et al. Cyclosporine A as first choice for dermatomyositis. *J Rheumatol* 1994;21:381–382.

66. Miller FW, Leitman SF, Cronin ME, et al. A randomized double-blind controlled trial of plasma exchange and leukapheresis in patients with polymyositis and dermatomyositis. *N Engl J Med* 1992;326:1380–1384.

67. Kelly JJ Jr, Madoc-Jones H, Adelman LS, Andres PL, Munsat TL. Total body irradiation not effective in inclusion body myositis. *Neurology* 1986;36:1264–1266.

68. Cherin P, Herson S, Wechsler B, et al. Efficacy of intravenous immunoglobulin therapy in chronic refractory polymyositis and dermatomyositis. An open study with 20 adult patients. *Am J Med* 1991; 91:162–168.

69. Lang B, Laxer RM, Murphy G et al. Treatment of dermatomyositis with intravenous immunoglobulin. *Am J Med* 1991;91:169–172.

70. Jan S, Beretta S, Moggio M, Alobbati L, Pellegrini G. High-dose intravenous human immunoglobulin in polymyositis resistant to treat-ment. *J Neurol Neurosurg Psychiatry* 1992;55:60–64.

71. Dalakas MC, Illa I, Dambrosia JM, et al. A controlled trial of high-dose intravenous immunoglobulin infusions as treatment for dermatomyositis. *N Engl J Med* 1993;329:1993–2000.

72. Dalakas MC. Intravenous immunoglobulin therapy for neurological diseases. *Ann Intern Med* 1997;126:721–730.

73. Soueidan SA, Dalakas MC. Treatment of inclusion-body myositis with high-dose intravenous immunoglobulin. *Neurology* 1993;43:876–879.

74. Dalakas MC, Sekul EA, Cupler EJ, Sivakumar K. The efficacy of high dose intravenous immunoglobulin (IVIg) in patients with inclusion-body myositis (IBM). *Neurology* 1997;48:712–716.

75. Dalakas MC, Sonies B, Koffman B, Spector S, Sivakumar K, Cupler E, Lopez-Devine J. High-dose intravenous immunoglobulin (IVIg) combined with prednisone in the treatment of patients with inclusion-body myositis (IBM): a double blind, randomized controlled trial. *Neurology* 1997;48:332.

Motor Disorders,
edited by David S. Younger.
Lippincott Williams & Wilkins, Philadelphia © 1999.

CHAPTER 10

Metabolic Myopathies

Michio Hirano and Salvatore DiMauro

Metabolism is a Greek term that means "conversion" which has been used to denote all biochemical changes occurring in living organisms. Alternatively, it can be defined as the cellular functions related to energy production. Skeletal muscle is highly energy-dependent and therefore vulnerable to disorders of energy metabolism. The term metabolic myopathies refers to clinical disorders in which muscle weakness or dysfunction result from cellular defects in biochemical pathways of ATP production. This chapter reviews the main clinical and biochemical features of the major metabolic myopathies. Readers are referred to more comprehensive reviews for further details (1–6).

Skeletal muscle uses three major sources of ATP: high-energy phosphate compounds, for example, phosphocreatine; glycogen, and fatty acids (7). The type and duration of muscle activity dictates the relative proportions of energy derived from these three energy sources. At rest, fatty acid oxidation accounts for the bulk of ATP production, whereas during the first several minutes of moderate exercise, high-energy phosphate compounds regenerate ATP from ADP. After 5 to 10 minutes of exercise, glycogen becomes the major energy source, and after longer periods of exercise, fatty acids are the predominant sources of ATP. Both pyruvate, the end product of glycolysis, and fatty acids are transported into the mitochondrial matrix where they are processed to acetyl-CoA via the pyruvate dehydrogenase complex reaction and the sequential "turns" of beta-oxidation. Acetyl-CoA is metabolized through the Krebs cycle and oxidative phosphorylation to produce ATP. In the metabolic myopathies,

the specifically affected energy-producing pathway determines the type of exercise that will provoke symptoms. For example, defects of glycolysis, such as myophosphorylase deficiency (McArdle's disease), are evident after relatively short intervals of moderate to intense exercise, such as walking uphill or running at a rapid pace (8). By contrast, fatty acid metabolism disorders, such as carnitine palmitoyltransferase (CPT) II deficiency, are more likely to produce symptoms after exercising for extended periods of time (9).

The clinical manifestations of the metabolic myopathies are protean. Three general patterns can be discerned: progressive weakness; recurrent, acute, and reversible muscle dysfunction with exercise intolerance often accompanied by episodic elevated serum creatine kinase (CK) and myoglobinuria from muscle breakdown; and both patterns.

DEFECTS OF GLYCOGEN METABOLISM

During moderate- to high-intensity exercise, glycogen is the major source of stored energy for ATP production. The serum lactate rises in association with increased anaerobic glycogen catabolism. The associated muscular symptoms resulting from defects of glycogen metabolism include exercise intolerance, muscle cramps, and myoglobinuria. Of the 12 different glycogenoses that have been identified, 10 have associated neuromuscular syndromes (Table 1). Type I, due to glucose-6-phosphatase deficiency, causes liver and kidney dysfunction, whereas type VI due to hepatic phosphorylase deficiency affects the liver and erythrocytes. In this section, we describe the glycogenoses causing myopathy.

Type II: Acid Maltase Deficiency

Acid maltase deficiency (AMD) is distinct from other forms of glycogenoses because the enzyme is located in lysosomes. Three clinical disorders have been defined that differ in age at onset: infantile, childhood, and adult

M. Hirano: Department of Neurology, Columbia University School of Medicine and New York Presbyterian Hospital, New York, New York 10032.

S. DiMauro: H. Houston Merritt Clinical Research Center for Muscular Dystrophy and Related Diseases and Columbia University College of Physicians and Surgeons, New York, New York 10032.

TABLE 1. *Classification of glycogen storage diseases*

Type	Affected tissues	Clinical presentation	Enzyme defect	Inheritance pattern
II				
Infancy	Generalized	Cardiomegaly, weakness, hypotonia, death < age 1 yr	Acid maltase	AR
Childhood	Skeletal muscle	Myopathy simulating Duchenne dystrophy	Acid maltase	AR
Adult	Skeletal muscle	Myopathy simulating limb girdle dystrophy or polymyositis, respiratory insufficiency	Acid maltase	AR
III	Generalized	Hepatomegaly, fasting hypoglycemia, progressive weakness	Brancher	AR
IV	Generalized	Hepatosplenomegaly, liver cirrhosis, hepatic failure	Debrancher	AR
V	Skeletal muscle	Intolerance to intense exercise, cramps, myoglobinuria	Muscle phosphorylase	AR
VII	Skeletal muscle	Intolerance to intense exercise, cramps, myoglobinuria	Muscle phosphofructokinase	AR
VIII	Liver and skeletal muscle	Hepatomegaly, growth retardation, hypotonia	Phosphorylase kinase	AR
	Skeletal muscle	Exercise intolerance, myoglobinuria	Phosphorylase kinase	AR, XR
	Heart	Fatal infantile cardiomyopathy	Phosphorylase kinase	AR
IX	Generalized	Hemolytic anemia, seizures, mental retardation, intolerance to intense exercise, myoglobinuria	Phosphoglycerate kinase	AR
X	Skeletal muscle	Intolerance to intense exercise, myoglobinuria	Muscle phosphoglycerate mutase	XR
XI	Skeletal muscle	Intolerance to intense exercise, myoglobinuria	Muscle lactate dehydrogenase	AR

AR, autosomal recessive; XR, X-linked recessive.

AMD forms (1). Infantile AMD, or Pompe disease, presents in the first weeks or months of life with diffuse hypotonia and weakness including respiratory muscles; however, muscle bulk can be increased and macroglossia is common. There is marked cardiomegaly and mild hepatomegaly. The disease is usually fatal within the first year, and death occurs invariably before age 2 years due to pulmonary and cardiac failure. Childhood AMD typically presents with a delay in the onset of walking. The weakness of limb and axial muscles is slowly progressive, and in boys, the clinical picture with calf pseudohypertrophy can resemble Duchenne muscular dystrophy. Respiratory muscle weakness typically causes death in the second or third decade. Adult AMD is a slowly progressive myopathy beginning in the third or fourth decade without visceral organ involvement. Respiratory muscle weakness is out of proportion to the limb weakness and can be a clinical clue to the diagnosis. Serum CK is elevated in all forms of AMD. Electromyography (EMG) reveals small short-duration motor units with fibrillation, positive sharp waves, bizarre high-frequency discharges, and myotonic discharges. Muscle histology shows a vacuolar myopathy most prominent in the infantile form. The vacuoles are enlarged lysosomes engorged with periodic acid-Schiff (PAS)–positive diastase-digestible material and stains intensely for acid phosphatase. Electron microscopy confirms the presence of excess glycogen both within lysosomes and free in the cytoplasm.

Acid maltase activity is decreased in all tissues. Molecular genetic studies have revealed mutations in the lysosomal acid alpha-glucosidase gene. A T-to-G transition in the first intron is the most common pathogenic mutation and causes aberrant mRNA splicing; at least 20 other mutations have been identified in other pedigrees (10,11).

Type III: Debrancher Deficiency

Debrancher deficiency is clinically characterized by childhood-onset liver dysfunction with hepatomegaly, growth failure, fasting hypoglycemia, and occasionally hypoglycemic seizures. Symptoms resolve spontaneously at puberty, leading to more normal adult lives (12), although cirrhosis and hepatic failure may develop later (13). Myopathy presents in the third to fourth decade in 70% of patients and primarily affects distal leg and intrinsic hand muscles. The myopathy is slowly progressive and rarely incapacitating. Myoglobinuria occurred in one patient (14), and peripheral neuropathy and symptomatic cardiomyopathy were seen in others; however, laboratory evidence of myocardial ventricular hypertrophy is common. The serum CK is elevated in all patients with myopathy, and electrophysiological studies reveal myogenic changes but may also show decreased nerve conduction velocities.

Skeletal muscle biopsy shows severe vacuolar myopathy with PAS-positive vacuoles beneath the sarcolemma and between myofibrils. Ultrastructurally, they are mainly collections of free glycogen, although some glycogen-filled lysosomes are seen but are not as numerous as in AMD. The debrancher enzyme is a 160-kDa polypeptide with transferase and α-glucosidase catalytic functions. After muscle phosphorylase has shortened the peripheral chains of glycogen to about four glucosyl units, a partially digested polysaccharide is produced, called phosphorylase-limit-dextrin. The debrancher enzyme removes the residual oligosaccharide "twigs" through a two-step process catalyzed by 1,4-1,4-glucantransferase and amylo-1,6-glucosidase activities. At least seven different mutations in the gene for debrancher enzyme have been identified (15,16).

Type IV: Brancher Deficiency

Branching enzyme deficiency, or Andersen disease, is a severe rapidly progressive disease of infancy clinically dominated by liver dysfunction with hepatosplenomegaly, cirrhosis, and death by age 4 years due to hepatic failure or gastrointestinal bleeding. Muscle wasting, hypotonia, and contractures are common. Some children present primarily with cardiomyopathy. In two Israeli patients with adult polyglucosan body disease, brancher enzyme deficiency was identified in leukocytes (17). Bruno et al. (18) found the same abnormality in two Ashkenazi Jewish patients but not in a French Canadian patient with the same syndrome. Adult polyglucosan body disease is characterized by onset in the fifth to sixth decade of progressive upper and lower motor neuron dysfunction, sensory neuropathy, bladder and bowel incontinence, and, in some patients, dementia (19). In patients with liver involvement, the serum CK may be slightly elevated. Electrophysiologic testing of adult polyglucosan body disease patients demonstrates axonal sensorimotor neuropathy. Cytometric studies reveal a neurogenic bladder. Basophilic intensely PAS-positive polysaccharide bodies partially resistant to diastase digestion are found in skin, liver, muscle, heart, nerve, and central nervous system tissues. Ultrastructurally, the polysaccharide appears filamentous and finely granular. Branching enzyme catalyzes the final step of glycogen synthesis by adding short glucosyl chains of about seven glucosyl units with α-1,6-glucosidic bonds to linear peripheral chains of glycogen. The short glucosyl twigs are elongated by glycogen synthetase. Three pathogenic point mutations in branching enzyme were identified in two patients with the typical phenotype, whereas two other point mutations were found in a patient with nonprogressive hepatopathy (20).

Type V: Muscle Phosphorylase Deficiency

Myophosphorylase deficiency, or McArdle disease, is characterized by exercise intolerance with premature fatigue, myalgia, and cramps relieved by rest (2,21).

Symptoms generally occur during intense isometric exercise, such as lifting heavy weights, or during less-intense sustained dynamic exercise, such as walking up stairs. Most patients experience a "second wind" phenomenon; if they slow down or rest briefly at the onset of symptoms, exercising can resume at the original pace. About half of patients experience acute muscle necrosis and myoglobinuria after exercise; of these, another half develop renal failure (4). About a third develop fixed weakness, especially older patients. Atypical clinical presentations include "tiredness" or poor stamina, progressive limb weakness in the sixth to seventh decade, severe generalized neonatal weakness with respiratory insufficiency and death in infancy, and delayed psychomotor development and mild proximal weakness. The disease is transmitted in an autosomal recessive (AR) pattern, with men affected more often than women. Serum CK levels are elevated in more than 90% of patients. Nerve conduction studies are generally normal. EMG may be normal or show a myopathy. During spontaneous or exercise-induced contractures, the shortened muscles are electrically silent. ^{31}Phosphorous nuclear magnetic resonance spectroscopy reveals lack of cytoplasmic acidification during exercise with an excessive drop in the phosphocreatine:inorganic phosphate ratio.

Phosphorylase (α-1,4-glucan orthophosphate glycosyl transferase) initiates glycogen breakdown by removing 1,4-glucosyl residues phosphorylytically from the outer branches of glycogen and liberating glucose-1-phosphate (Fig. 1). Muscle phosphorylase activity is decreased to less than 10% of normal due to a specific defect in the muscle isoform; liver and brain isoforms also have been identified. Muscle glycogen levels may be normal or elevated. Molecular genetic studies have identified at least 11 point mutations in the muscle phosphorylase gene (6). The most common mutation in the United States and United Kingdom is a CGA(Arg) to TGA(Stop) at codon 49; this mutation is less common in northern Italian patients and not encountered in Japanese patients.

Therapies to bypass the metabolic defect by oral administration of glucose and fructose have shown inconsistent results. Slonim and Goans (22) tried a high-protein diet and demonstrated improvement in muscle endurance and strength. Phosphorylase requires a vitamin B_6 derivative as a cofactor, and myophosphorylase deficiency is associated with a secondary deficiency of that vitamin. In a study of four affected patients, pyridoxine administration led to improvement in muscle force generation (23).

Type VII: Phosphofructokinase Deficiency

Muscle phosphofructokinase (PFK) deficiency, or Tarui disease, is clinically indistinguishable from myophosphorylase deficiency (24). Vigorous exercise

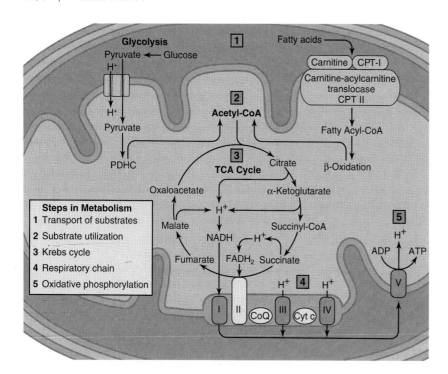

FIG. 1. Schematic representation of mitochondrial metabolism. Respiratory chain complexes or components encoded exclusively by the nuclear genome are light orange. Complexes containing some subunits encoded by the nuclear genome and others encoded by mitochondrial DNA are dark orange. CPT, carnitine palmitoyltransferase; PDHC, pyruvate dehydrogenase complex; CoA, coenzyme A; TCA, tricarboxylic acid; CoQ, coenzyme Q; Cyt c, cytochrome *c*. (Modified from Ref. 12, with permission of McGraw-Hill, New York.)

provokes cramps that are relieved by rest. PFK deficiency can also cause compensated hemolytic anemia, jaundice, and gouty arthritis, which may be helpful in making the diagnosis. Other clinical presentations include hemolytic anemia without myopathy, fixed weakness, and severe and often fatal infantile myopathy sometimes associated with encephalopathy. Laboratory studies generally reveal elevated serum CK, bilirubin, uric acid levels, and reticulocytosis. EMG shows myopathy with irritative features. Inheritance is AR, with men predominantly affected. In the United States, most patients have been of Ashkenazi Jewish origin. Muscle biopsy reveals accumulation of normal-appearing subsarcolemmal and intermyofibrillar glycogen and "pockets" of an abnormal polysaccharide that stains intensely with PAS but is resistant to diastase digestion. Ultrastructurally, this abnormal glycogen has a granular and filamentous appearance, similar to that in branching enzyme deficiency.

PFK (ATP:D-fructose 1-phosphotransferase) is a tetrameric enzyme. The three subunit forms are M (muscle), L (liver), and P (platelet). Muscle exclusively contains the M isoform, whereas erythrocytes contain both the L and M subunits. PFK deficiency causes a block distal to glucose and fructose metabolism that is not improved by administration of those substances. PFK-deficient patients depend on free fatty acids and ketones for ATP generation; therefore, exercise intolerance is worsened by high-carbohydrate meals that lower the blood levels of free fatty acid and ketones (25). The negative effect of glucose has been aptly described as an "out-of-wind" phenomenon (25). At least 12 distinct mutations in the muscle phosphorylase subunit have been identified (6). Treatment is problematic

as in myophosphorylase deficiency because glucose and fructose are not usable substrates.

Type VIII: Phosphorylase β Kinase Deficiency

Phosphorylase β kinase (PBK) deficiency is associated with four distinct phenotypes based on the mode of inheritance and tissue involvement: liver disease, typically a benign condition of infancy or childhood with hepatomegaly, growth retardation, delayed motor development, fasting hypoglycemia, and usually inherited as X-linked trait; liver and muscle disease with a static myopathy inherited as an AR trait; myopathy alone, inherited in an AR or X-linked recessive pattern; and fatal infantile cardiomyopathy. In patients with myopathy, serum CK is variably increased (9,26). EMG reveals myogenic abnormalities. Muscle biopsy reveals subsarcolemmal glycogen predominantly in type IIb fibers. Ultrastructurally, the glycogen is free in the cytoplasm and appears normal.

PBK is composed of the subunits α, β, γ, and δ and acts on two enzymes, glycogen synthetase and phosphorylase. Specifically, it converts phosphorylase from the less active β form to the more active α form while converting glycogen synthetase from the more active dephosphorylated form to a less active phosphorylated form. The genes encoding the PBK subunits have been cloned, and the molecular defects are under investigation. One 48-year-old man with distal limb weakness and low muscle enzyme had a point mutation in the muscle-specific α-subunit gene that converted a codon for glutamic acid to a stop codon (27). No specific therapy has been effective in this disorder; however, a high-protein diet may be helpful for reasons similar to myophosphorylase deficiency (22).

Type IX: Phosphoglycerate Kinase Deficiency

Phosphoglycerate kinase deficiency can be clinically asymptomatic or present with myopathy in association with hemolytic anemia, mental retardation, and seizures (28). Isolated myopathy with intolerance to vigorous exercise, cramps, and myoglobinuria, was reported in three patients (6). Laboratory findings include a variably increased resting serum CK level and a normal EMG. Muscle biopsy generally shows nonspecific morphologic changes and a normal glycogen content. Muscle phosphoglycerate kinase activity levels are decreased in patients. Phosphoglycerate kinase deficiency is an X-linked recessive disorder. Two different point mutations in this single polypeptide enzyme have been identified in patients with myopathy: a missense mutation and a splice junction mutation (6).

Type X: Phosphoglycerate Mutase Deficiency

Phosphoglycerate mutase (PGAM) deficiency has been identified in only 11 patients; all but 3 were African American (6). Symptoms generally include intolerance to strenuous exercise, cramps, and recurrent myoglobinuria. Muscle biopsies can be normal or show diffuse or patchy increased glycogen accumulation. PGAM activity in muscle tissue ranged from 2% to 6% of normal. The enzyme is a dimer composed of muscle-specific (M), brain-specific (B), or both isoforms. In patients with myopathy, mutations affect the M isoform. Cardiac muscle expresses both isoforms; hence, the BB isozyme protects the heart from symptoms in PGAM-M deficiency. The disease is transmitted in an AR pattern. Three point mutations have been identified in the PGAM-M gene (29,30). Interestingly, six of seven African American patients were found to be homozygous for a nonsense mutation in codon 79, whereas the seventh patient was a compound heterozygote for that mutation and a missense mutation. By contrast, two Italian patients were homozygous for a third missense mutation.

Type XI: Lactate Dehydrogenase Deficiency

Muscle lactate dehydrogenase (LDH-A) deficiency has been associated with exercise intolerance and myalgia after intense exercise, often followed by myoglobinuria. The first reported patient had serum LDH levels that did not rise proportionally with CK levels during a bout of myoglobinuria (31). Three affected women developed stiffness of the uterine muscle at the onset of delivery necessitating cesarean section, whereas a few patients had a dermatologic disorder characterized by follicular papules and erythematous patches (32). LDH is a tetrameric enzyme comprised of LDH-A and LDH-B subunits. The M4 tetramer predominates in skeletal muscle. In LDH-deficient patients with myopathy, the low residual LDH activity in muscle, about 5% of normal, is due to the small amount of retained LDH-B tetramers. Point mutations, splice junction and microdeletions in LDH-A have been identified in patients (32).

Type XII: Aldolase A Deficiency

In 1996, aldolase A deficiency was identified in a 4-year-old boy with exercise intolerance, mild weakness, developmental delay, hemolysis, and repeated bouts of rhabdomyolysis during febrile illnesses (33). The muscle biopsy did not reveal excess glycogen by histochemistry; however, it did show an aldolase activity level of 3.8% of normal by biochemical analysis and a homozygous point mutation was identified.

Forearm Ischemic Exercise Test

The forearm ischemic exercise test is useful in corroborating the diagnosis of defects in the glycogenolytic or the glycolytic pathways that impair lactate production during ischemic exercise. The protocol, as described by DiMauro and Bresolin (21), is shown in Table 2. An indwelling sterile needle is placed in a superficial antecubital vein and a baseline sample of blood is drawn for serum lactate, ammonia, and CK levels. A sphygmomanometer cuff is placed above the elbow and inflated to about 20 mm Hg above the systolic blood pressure. The patient vigorously squeezes a rolled-up sphygmomanome-

---

TABLE 2. *Forearm ischemic exercise test*

1. Explain the procedure to the patient.
2. Insert an indwelling sterile needle into the patient's antecubital vein. We prefer to use 23-gauge Butterfly needles. Collect blood for measurements of lactate, creatine kinase, and ammonia.
3. Place a sphygmomanometer cuff above the patient's elbow and inflate to about 20 mm Hg above the systolic blood pressure. In children, inflate to, but not above, the mean arterial pressure.
4. With constant encouragement, have the patient intermittently open and clench his or her fist for 1 min. We prefer to have the patient squeeze a rolled-up sphygmomanometer cuff. The patient should be encouraged to push the mercury column up as high as possible with each squeeze.
5. After 1 min of exercise, the blood pressure cuff is deflated and the patient rests.
6. If the patient develops a cramp, tell the patient to stop exercising immediately and deflate the sphygmomanometer cuff to avoid excess muscle necrosis.
7. Blood samples, drawn at 1, 3, 6, and 10 min after exercise and placed on ice, are sent for lactate, ammonia, and creatine kinase measurements.

ter cuff, pushing the mercury column to the top of the scale. After a minute of exercise, which can cause discomfort even in normal individuals and requires constant encouragement by the observer, the blood pressure cuff is deflated. Blood samples are each obtained at 1, 3, 6, and 10 minutes after cessation of exercise. In normal subjects, there is a three- to fivefold increase in blood lactate in the first two samples with a gradual decline to baseline level in later ones that does not generally occur in those with defects of the glycolytic pathway. Serum ammonia should normally rise three- to fivefold after exercise in both normal subjects and in patients with a glycogen metabolism defect. Patients with myophosphorylase deficiency generally show less than 1.5-fold increase in venous lactate levels (21). Many patients also develop muscle cramping during exercise and should immediately stop while the examiner deflates the sphygmomanometer cuff to reduce the risk of muscle necrosis. False-positive results arise because of suboptimal effort that may be suggested by the lack of rise in ammonia after ischemic exercise. If the patient's lactate rises after exercise but the ammonia fails to rise significantly, then the diagnosis of myoadenylate deaminase deficiency can be considered. The forearm ischemic exercise test can be difficult in children. For that reason, Bruno et al. (34) use a modified forearm semiischemic protocol inflating the sphygmomanometer cuff to the mean arterial pressure, which was reliable in patients ranging from ages 7 to 16 years.

DEFECTS OF LIPID METABOLISM

Lipids are the most important and efficient fuel source in the body. Fatty acids are vital during periods of fasting, particularly when liver glycogen stores are depleted a few hours after a meal. They serve three main functions: their partial oxidation in the liver produces ketones that are an important auxiliary fuel for almost all tissues and especially the brain; they provide a major energy source in cardiac and skeletal muscle, particularly during rest and during prolonged exercise; and ATP produced from fatty acid oxidation provides energy for gluconeogenesis and ureagenesis. The normal fatty acid oxidation pathway is outlined in Fig. 2. Adipocytes liberate free fatty acids that are bound to serum albumin or incorporated into triglyceride-rich lipoproteins and transported to other tissues. Short 4-carbon- and medium 8-carbon-chain fatty acids freely cross the outer and inner mitochondrial membranes into the mitochondrial matrix where they are metabolized to CoA esters before beta-oxidation. By contrast, the mitochondrial membranes are impermeable to long-chain fatty acids (LCFA); therefore, at the outer mitochondrial and endoplasmic reticulum membranes, LCFA must first be converted to CoA-thioesters by long-chain acyl-CoA synthetase. To cross the inner mitochondrial membrane, the very-long-chain acyl-CoA (VLCA-CoA) and long-chain acyl-CoA (LCA-CoA) molecules are converted into

acylcarnitine with release of free CoA by CPT I located on the inner side of the outer mitochondrial membrane. Carnitine:acylcarnitine translocase transports very long and long acylcarnitine across the inner mitochondrial membrane. Within the mitochondrial matrix, CPT II bound to the inner surface of the inner mitochondrial membrane exchanges CoA for carnitine to reform VLCA-CoA and LCA-CoA and liberate carnitine, which is shuttled back into the cytoplasm by the translocase.

VLCA-CoA, 14 to 24 carbon atoms in length, is processed by VLCA-CoA dehydrogenase bound to the inner mitochondrial membrane that creates 2-trans-enoyl-CoA molecules. The VLCA-CoA molecules are processed by a trifunctional enzyme, which is also bound to the inner mitochondrial membrane and possesses three beta-oxidation enzymatic activities: long-chain enoyl-CoA hydratase, long-chain-L-3-hydroxyacyl-CoA dehydrogenase, and long-chain thiolase enzymes. The process shortens the acyl-CoA by two carbon molecules.

Acyl-CoAs of 4 to 18 carbons in length are oxidized by the beta-oxidation pathway in the mitochondrial matrix. Each cycle the beta-oxidation system shortens the acyl-CoA by two carbon fragments through four catalytic steps: acyl-CoA dehydrogenase, 2-enoyl-CoA hydratase, L-3-hydroxyacyl-CoA dehydrogenase, and 3-ketoacyl-CoA thiolase. The acetyl-CoA moeity produced at each turn of the beta-oxidation spiral enters the Krebs cycle. There are three different mitochondrial matrix dehydrogenase enzymes, namely, short-chain acyl-CoA dehydrogenase, which acts on fatty acid of 4 to 6 carbon atoms; medium-chain acyl-CoA dehydrogenase (MCAD) for substrates of 4 to 14 carbon atoms, and long-chain acyl-CoA dehydrogenase for substrates of 10 to 18 carbon atoms. Defects of fatty acid oxidation can occur at various points along the pathway from the transport of fatty acid into mitochondria to the beta-oxidation cycle as described below.

Carnitine Deficiency

L-Carnitine or 3-hydroxy-4-N-trimethylammoniobutanoate is a vital molecule for the transport of LCFA into mitochondria. Other physiologic functions of L-carnitine include buffering of acyl-CoA:CoASH ratio, scavaging of potentially toxic acyl groups, and oxidation of branched-chain amino acids (35). About 75% of L-carnitine is derived from dietary sources, whereas the rest is synthesized in the liver and kidney; 95% of the total body carnitine is stored in muscle.

Primary deficiency of L-carnitine is manifested in three phenotypic forms: dilated cardiomyopathy, myopathy, and hypoketotic hypoglycemia with recurrent encephalopathy. Patients frequently show overlapping phenotypes. The age at onset of symptoms ranges from 1 month to 7 years with a mean of 2 years (4). The cardiomyopathy is progressive and rapidly fatal unless treated with L-carnitine supple-

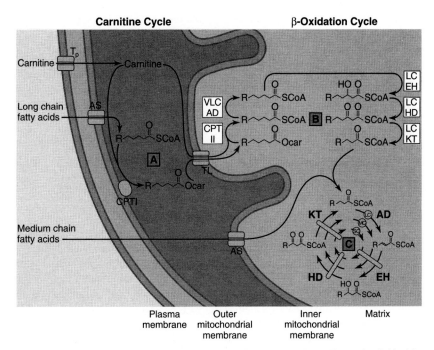

Carnitine Cycle

β-Oxidation Cycle

Plasma membrane | Outer mitochondrial membrane | Inner mitochondrial membrane | Matrix

FIG. 2. Schematic representation of fatty acid oxidation. This metabolic pathway is divided into the carnitine cycle (A), the inner mitochondrial membrane system (B), and the mitochondrial matrix system (C). The carnitine cycle includes the plasma membrane transporter, carnitine palmitoyltransferase I (CPT I). The reactions shown in B occur in the inner mitochondrial membrane. The carnitine-acylcarnitine translocase system and carnitine palmitoyltransferase II (CPT II). The inner mitochondrial membrane system includes the very-long-chain acyl-CoA dehydrogenase (VLCAD) and the trifunctional protein with three catalytically active sites. Long-chain acylcarnitines enter the mitochondrial matrix by the action of CPT II to yield long-chain acyl-CoAs. These thioesters undergo one or more cycles of chain shortening catalyzed by the membrane-bound system. Chain-shortened acyl-CoAs are degraded further by the matrix beta-oxidation system. Medium-chain fatty acids enter the mitochondrial matrix directly and are activated to the medium-chain acyl-CoAs before degradation by the matrix beta-oxidation system. T_p, carnitine transporter; TL, carnitine-acylcarnitine translocase; LC, long chain; EH, 2-enoyl-CoA hydratase; CoA, coenzyme A; VLC, very long chain; AD, acyl-CoA dehydrogenase; AS, arginosuccinate; HD, 3-hydroxyacyl-CoA dehydrogenase; CPT, carnitine palmitoyltransferase; KT, 3-ketoacyl-CoA thiolase; MC, medium chain; SC, short chain. (From Ref. 6, with permission.)

mentation. The myopathic form of L-carnitine deficiency is the least common phenotype and is usually associated with cardiomyopathy, encephalopathy, or both. It presents with motor delay, hypotonia, and slowly progressive proximal limb weakness. Acute metabolic encephalopathy is associated with hypoketotic hypoglycemia in younger infants. The episodes are typically triggered by intercurrent illnesses and stress, which are often complicated by recurrent vomiting and decreased oral dietary intake. Persistent central nervous system signs develop due to severe hypoglycemic encephalopathy and cardiac or respiratory arrest.

Laboratory studies reveal low total and free serum carnitine concentrations, usually less than 10% of normal. The diagnosis can be confirmed by documenting decreased carnitine uptake in cultured skin fibroblasts. Mutations in the sodium-ion dependent carnitine transporter gene have been identified as causes of primary carnitine deficiency (35a,35b). Primary carnitine deficiency responds dramatically to oral L-carnitine therapy at daily divided doses of 100 to 200 mg/kg of body weight. Primary carnitine deficiency is important to identify because it is potentially treatable, whereas secondary deficiencies are more common and due to a variety of underlying metabolic defects. Causes of secondary carnitine deficiency include defects of beta-oxidation; malnutrition; excessive carnitine loss, for example, in renal Fanconi syndrome; and valproic acid therapy that results in excessive carnitine excretion.

Carnitine Palmitoyltransferase Deficiency

Mitochondria contain two CPT enzymes, CPT I and II, that are vital in the transport of LCFA into mitochondria. CPT I is located in the inner aspect of the outer mitochondrial membrane, whereas CPT II is bound to the inner aspects of the inner mitochondrial membrane (Fig. 2). CPT I deficiency presents in infancy as attacks of potentially fatal, fasting-induced, hypoketotic hypoglycemia. The hypoglycemic episodes manifest as lethargy, coma, and seizures. They can lead to psychomotor developmental delay, hemiplegia, and generalized epilepsy. Myopathy is not a typical manifestation, and serum CK has been elevated in only two siblings (36); another patient had a lipid-storage myopathy (37). The diagnosis is confirmed by demonstrating decreased CPT I activity in cultured fibroblasts, leukocytes, or hepatocytes. CPT I activity is normal in skeletal muscle, accounting for the absence of clinical myopathy is probably due to tissue-specific isoforms. The first mutations in the CPT I gene have been identified in a patient with the hepatic form (37a).

In contrast, CPT II deficiency has variable clinical manifestations. Three forms of CPT II deficiency have been described: an infantile, late-infantile, and adult form. The early infantile phenotype is rare and presents at birth with severe hypoketotic hypoglycemia and generalized steatosis and can cause death in a few days. Multiple organ malformations are often present, including renal cystic dysplasia, nephromegaly, microgyria, neuronal heterotopia in the brain, and facial dysmorphism. The late-infantile hepatomuscular form is clinically similar to CPT I deficiency, with acute episodic fasting hypoglycemia and hypoketosis, lethargy, coma, and death. Seizures, hepatomegaly, cardiomegaly, arrhythmias, and pancreatitis have also been described (5). In both infantile forms, CPT II activity is less than 10% of normal.

The adult form of CPT II deficiency was first described in 1973 and is a common cause of exercise-induced myoglobinuria (9,38). It typically presents in young adulthood with complaints of muscle pain and pigmenturia after prolonged exercise. Severe bouts of rhabdomyolysis with myoglobinuria can cause acute renal failure. Some infants have presented with acute muscle breakdown induced by fever. Adult patients may also have rhabdomyolysis precipitated by fever or other stress. CPT activity is less than 30% of normal. CPT II is a homotetrameric enzyme and the gene (*CPT1*) encoding the subunit has been characterized. Missense, frameshift, and deletion mutations *CPT1* segregate with the clinical phenotypes. In the adult muscular form, the most common mutation is a C-to-T transversion at nucleotide (nt) 439, which changes a highly conserved serine to leucine (S113L) (39).

Carnitine-Acylcarnitine Translocase Deficiency

Rare patients with carnitine-acylcarnitine translocase deficiency (5) were first described clinically by Stanley et al. (41) in a young boy with stunted growth, recurrent vomiting, and coma from birth. At age 2.5 years, he had muscle weakness, cardiomyopathy, and fasting hypoglycemia. Hypoketosis, increased serum long-chain acylcarnitines, and normal CPT activity were later found. Carnitine-acylcarnitine translocase activity was less than 5% of normal control subjects.

BETA-OXIDATION DEFECTS

The breakdown of fatty acid in mitochondria requires two related systems: the inner mitochondrial membrane portion that metabolizes long-chain acyl-CoA and the mitochondrial matrix beta-oxidation spiral that acts on medium- and short-chain acyl-CoA (Fig. 2).

Beta-Oxidation Defects of the Inner Mitochondrial Membrane System

Very-long-chain acyl-CoA dehydrogenase (VLCAD) deficiency presents in infancy with hypoketotic hypoglycemia, hepatic steatosis, cardiomyopathy, and elevated plasma levels of long-chain acylcarnitines (42). Metabolic acidosis, dicarboxylic aciduria, and increased serum CK with myoglobinuria have also been noted. Patients with recurrent myoglobinuria have the same clinical phenotype as those with CPT II deficiency. Immunoblot analyses for VLCAD have shown absence of the protein in fibroblasts from patients (5). The cDNA for the human VLCAD has been cloned, and a 105-base pair (bp) deletion in the gene has been identified in two unrelated infants (5).

Patients with defects of trifunctional protein have isolated long-chain-L-3-hydroxyacyl-coA dehydrogenase (LCHAD) deficiency, whereas a small number of individuals have a combined defect of its three enzyme components. The clinical feature of LCHAD deficiency include onset in infancy, Reyes-like episodes, hypoketotic hypoglycemia with hepatic dysfunction, progressive myopathy, recurrent myoglobinuria, cardiomyopathy, and sudden infant death syndrome (4,5). Jackson et al. (43) first reported the combined defect of the three trifunctional enzyme activities in an infant with recurrent limb weakness, hypotonia, and anorexia precipitated by intercurrent illnesses, who died at age 4.5 years during a severe metabolic crisis with an elevated serum CK, hyperammonemia, and lactic acidosis.

The treatment of patients with inner mitochondrial membrane defects of fatty acid metabolism is mainly dietary. Affected patients should avoid prolonged fasts and long-chain fatty acid ingestion. Intravenous glucose should be given during acute intercurrent illnesses (4).

Beta-Oxidation Defects of the Mitochondrial Matrix System

The mitochondrial beta-oxidation matrix system shortens the fatty acid backbone of acyl-CoA by two carbon fragments during each turn though the beta-oxidation spiral. In this process, acetyl-CoA is produced and is oxidized in the Krebs cycle. In addition, electron transfer flavoprotein (ETF) is reduced; the reduced ETF provides reducing equivalents to the oxidative-phosphorylation pathway though the action of ETF CoQ oxidoreductase. Human diseases are caused by defects in several steps of this matrix system (Fig. 2).

Defects of long-chain, medium-chain, and short-chain acyl-CoA dehydrogenases generally occur in infancy. Medium-chain acyl-CoA dehydrogenase (MCAD) is, along with CPT II deficiency, the most frequent defect of beta-oxidation, with more than 200 identified patients and a disproportionately high incidence in Anglo-Saxon whites (44). MCAD typically begins in the first 2 years of life with fasting intolerance, nausea, vomiting, hypoketotic hypoglycemia, lethargy, and coma; however, clinical expression is variable and some patients are asymptomatic. MCAD activity in most tissues, including fibroblasts, lymphocytes, and liver, is low, generally 2% to 20% of normal. Early diagnosis and treatment can lead to a favorable outcome. Dietary therapy is aimed at avoidance of fasting and provision of adequate caloric intake. Most MCAD-deficient patients have an A-to-G transition mutation at nt 985 of the cDNA, causing a lysine-to-glutamate substitution at amino acid 304 of the mature protein, which leads to impaired homotetrameric assembly and instability of the protein (45,46). Long-chain acyl-CoA dehydrogenase deficiency is less common, and many reported patients instead have VLCAD deficiency. Short-chain acyl-CoA dehydrogenase deficiency has been documented in only a few patients with varying phenotypes, including one adult with progressive myopathy and massive lipid storage in type I muscle fibers and in several infants with failure-to-thrive and nonketotic hypoglycemia who died in early childhood (47,48).

Short-chain 3-hydroxyacyl-CoA dehydrogenase deficiency was identified in a 9-month-old child with episodes of hypoglycemia and Reyes-like encephalopathy (49). At age 16 years, she had an attack of hypoketotic hypoglycemia, acute myoglobinuria, and encephalopathy. She developed arrhythmia and died of a dilated cardiomyopathy. Deficiency of 2,4-dienoyl-CoA reductase was identified in muscle and liver of a dysmorphic infant with hypotonia who died at 4 months of age (50).

Multiple acyl-CoA dehydrogenase deficiency (MAD) or glutaric aciduria type II is a clinical syndrome characterized by metabolic acidosis, hypoketotic hypoglycemia, strong sweaty-feet odor, and early death. Three distinct clinical presentations of MAD deficiency exist: a severe neonatal form with congenital abnormalities, a severe neonatal form without congenital abnormalities, and a mild later-onset form (4,5). Pathology reveals fatty degeneration of kidney, liver, heart, and skeletal muscle. The biochemical abnormality is characterized by decreased activities of various acyl-CoA dehydrogenases with urinary excretion of large amounts of numerous organic acids. Three defects lead to MAD deficiency, namely, ETF deficiency, ETF CoQ oxidoreductase deficiency, and riboflavin (B$_2$)-responsive MAD.

DEFECTS OF MYOADENYLATE DEAMINASE

In 1978, myoadenylate deaminase (mAMPD) deficiency was first described in association with exercise-related myalgia and cramps (51). At present, it is also detected in 1% to 3% of skeletal muscle biopsies in asymptomatic patients so studied (52). Fishbein (53) proposed two forms of mAMPD deficiency: primary or hereditary mAMPD deficiency characterized by myopathy, exercise intolerance, myalgias, and cramps with negligible or less than 1% of normal residual activity and lack of cross-reactive material in muscle, and secondary or acquired mAMPD deficiency, associated with other well-defined neuromuscular disorders, higher residual enzyme activity, and detectable cross-reactive material. In the forearm ischemic exercise test, affected patients show a normal elevation of venous lactate, without a rise in ammonia and inosine monophosphate, the products of the mAMPD reaction.

DEFECTS OF OXIDATIVE-PHOSPHORYLATION

Since the initial discovery of mitochondrial DNA mutations in 1988, our understanding of the mitochondrial encephalomyopathies has advanced at an astoundingly rapid pace. This topic is reviewed extensively elsewhere. In this section, we illustrate some fundamental clinical and scientific themes.

Mitochondrial respiratory chain disorders often do not conform to single enzyme defects. The measured enzyme activities may be normal or multiple enzymes can be affected; therefore, a biochemical classification system can have limitations. Molecular genetics provides an alternative perspective of mitochondrial diseases. One can gain a better understanding of mitochondrial disorders by considering the several unusual genetic characteristics of mitochondria. They are unique organelles because they possess their own genetic material, mitochondrial DNA (mtDNA), which is a small circular molecule of 16.5 kilobases (kb) (58). Each mtDNA encodes 22 transfer RNAs, 13 polypeptides, and two ribosomal RNAs. The mtDNA-encoded polypeptides are functionally important because they are subunits of the respiratory chain. Most mitochondrial proteins are encoded in the nuclear DNA (nDNA); thus, mitochondria are the products of two genomes. Defects in either genome can cause mitochondrial dysfunction. To date, most respiratory chain defects characterized at the molecular genetic level are due to mtDNA mutations (59).

Four important characteristics of mtDNA contribute to the expression of a given mt gene defect. The first is heteroplasmy. Each mitochondrion contains 2 to 10 copies of mtDNA, and in turn, each cell contains multiple mitochondria. Therefore, there are numerous copies of mtDNA in each cell. Mutations of mtDNA may be present in some mtDNA molecules (heteroplasmy) or in all molecules (homoplasmy). As a consequence of heteroplasmy, the proportion of a deleterious mtDNA mutation can vary widely. An individual that harbors a large proportion of mutant mtDNA will be more severely affected than one with a low percentage of the same mutation. Therefore, there is a spectrum of clinical severity among patients with a given mitochondrial mutation.

A second factor that can influence the expression of an mtDNA mutation in a person is the tissue distribution of that mutation. In turn, variable tissue distribution broadens the clinical spectrum of pathogenic mtDNA mutations. The best example of tissue distribution variation is large-scale mtDNA deletions. Infants with a high proportion of deleted mtDNA in blood can develop Pearson anemia often accompanied by exocrine pancreatic dysfunction (60). Presumably, these infants have a high proportion of deleted mtDNA in the bone marrow stem cells. Some children survive the anemia with blood transfusions and subsequently recover because the stem cells, with a high proportion of deleted mtDNA, are under a negative selection bias. Later in life, however, those children can develop the multisystem mitochondrial disorder Kearns-Sayre syndrome (KSS) characterized by ophthalmoplegia, pigmentary retinopathy, and cardiac conduction block (61).

A third factor that determines clinical manifestations of a mtDNA mutation is the tissue threshold effect. Cells with high metabolic activities are severely and adversely affected by mtDNA mutations; therefore, these disorders tend to affect disproportionately brain and muscle (encephalomyopathies).

A fourth unusual characteristic of mtDNA is *maternal inheritance*. During the formation of the zygote, the mtDNA is derived exclusively from the oocyte. Thus, mtDNA is transmitted vertically in a non-Mendelian fashion from the mother to both male and female progeny. This inheritance pattern is important to recognize in determining whether a family is likely to harbor an mtDNA mutation. A caveat to this principle is the fact that maternal relatives who have a lower percentage of an mtDNA mutation may have fewer symptoms than the proband; thus, they may be oligosymptomatic or even asymptomatic. Therefore, in taking the family history, it is important to inquire about subtle symptoms and signs among maternally related family members that might be oligosymptomatic.

These peculiar features of "mitochondrial genetics" contribute to the clinical complexity of human mitochondrial disorders. Variable heteroplasmy of mtDNA mutations produces an extensive range of disease severity, whereas tissue distribution and tissue threshold of mtDNA mutations explain the frequent but variable involvement of multiple organ systems. In addition to mtDNA mutations, nDNA defects can also cause mitochondrial dysfunction. In fact, nDNA encodes most electron transport chain components, and recently the nDNA mutations associated with a defect in oxidative-phosphorylation have been identified (62). Finally, a third group of genetic mitochondrial disorders includes defects of intergenomic communication, presumably due to mutations of nDNA genes controlling replication and expression of the mitochondrial genome.

The evaluation, diagnosis, and treatment of the three major mitochondrial encephalomyopathy syndromes, namely, KSS; mitochondrial encephalomyopathy, lactic acidosis, with strokelike episodes (MELAS); and myoclonus epilepsy with ragged red fibers (MERRF) (61,63,64), have all been extensively characterized. On the whole, they comprise a heterogeneous group of multisystem disorders, but their proper classification has been the subject of vigorous debate. Accordingly, in the 1980s there were lively discussions between "splitters," who tried to define discrete clinical syndromes, and "lumpers," who thought that the clinical features of patients were too variable and often overlapping to allow easy clinical separation (65,66). The discovery of distinct mtDNA mutations demonstrated that, in general, clinical phenotypes had specific genotypes; however, some patients did not fit into any clinical syndrome or had an atypical presentation for a particular mtDNA mutation. Thus, both lumpers and splitters have been vindicated. Because clinicians are confronted with individual patients, clinical classification of the mitochondrial disorders still has pragmatic significance in guiding the diagnostic evaluation and in directing the therapy.

Kearns-Sayre Syndrome

Rowland and colleagues (65) defined KSS by the obligate triad of ophthalmoplegia, pigmentary retinopathy, and onset before age 20, with at least one of the following: cardiac conduction block, ataxia, and cerebrospinal fluid protein greater than 100 mg/dL. The existence of KSS as a distinct disorder is supported by the fact that more than 150 patients with these characteristics have been reported (67). Dementia is common, but seizures, seen in only 5 of 156 patients, are quite rare (67). Neuropathologic changes include basal ganglia calcifications and spongy changes of the brain white matter. About 90% of KSS patients have single large-scale rearrangements of the mtDNA; deletions, duplications, or both (68,69). Typically, KSS patients are sporadic, because the mtDNA rearrangements seem to originate in oogenesis or early zygote formation.

Syndrome of Myoclonus Epilepsy and Ragged Red Fibers

In contrast to KSS, MERRF includes epilepsy as a defining clinical feature, and therefore all patients with this diagnosis have seizures in addition to myoclonus, ataxia, and ragged red fibers in the muscle biopsy (63). Other common clinical manifestations associated with MERRF are hearing loss, dementia, peripheral neuropathy, short stature, exercise intolerance, lipomas, and lactic acidosis (70). Most MERRF patients have a history of affected maternally related family members, although not all have the full-blown syndrome.

In 1990, Shoffner et al. (71) identified an mtDNA A-to-G transition mutation at nt 8344 of the *tRNA^Lys* gene. That mutation was found in about 90% of MERRF patients tested (70). It was the first molecular genetic defect to be associated with a hereditary epilepsy syndrome. A second mutation in that gene at nt 8356 was identified in a pedigree with typical MERRF (72) and in another family with overlapping features of MERRF and MELAS (73). In families with a MERRF proband, oligosymptomatic and asymptomatic members harbor the same mtDNA mutation, but the phenotype is presumably attenuated by heteroplasmy and tissue distribution of the mtDNA mutation (70).

Syndrome of Mitochondrial Encephalomyopathy, Lactic Acidosis, and Strokelike Episodes

MELAS is another maternally inherited disorder whose defining clinical features include strokelike episodes typically before age 40, encephalopathy manifested as seizures or dementia, and mitochondrial dysfunction with lactic acidosis or ragged red fibers (64,74). In addition, at least two of the following clinical features should be present to secure the diagnosis: normal early development, recurrent headaches, or recurrent vomiting (74). Other commonly encountered manifestations include myopathic weakness, exercise intolerance, myoclonus, ataxia, short stature, and hearing loss (74). It is uncommon for more than one family member to have the full-blown MELAS syndrome. In most pedigrees, there is only one MELAS patient with oligosymptomatic or asymptomatic relatives in the maternal lineage.

In addition to these three phenotypes, many other clinical syndromes are associated with oxidative-phosphorylation defects (5,54). Despite the complexity and the heterogeneity of mitochondrial disorders, there are several clinical themes common to all. First, they tend to affect children and young adults. Second, they are often multisystemic. Third, maternal inheritance is pathognomonic of mtDNA point mutations, whereas patients with single large-scale rearrangements tend to be sporadic. Fourth, there is great variability of phenotypic expression in families with mtDNA point mutations.

Diagnostic Investigation

The diagnostic evaluation of a suspected mitochondrial encephalomyopathy begins with a detailed history relating to the possibility of abnormal infancy or early development, rapid exercise-induced fatigue, migrainous headaches, diabetes mellitus, short stature, hearing loss, or multiple lipomas; the latter is often seen in MERRF syndrome and while hypoparathyroidism is occasionally noted in KSS. Clues to an informative family history may be subtle, especially when dealing with an mtDNA point mutation. For example, in families with MELAS syndrome, relatives in the mater-

nal lineage may have migrainelike headaches or diabetes mellitus as the only manifestation of the genetic defect.

A careful general and neurologic examination will reveal clues to the correct diagnosis. Affected patients are often short and thin. Multiple lipomatosis can be disfiguring in patients with MERRF or their maternal relatives (75). Dementia can be a prominent finding in KSS, MELAS, and MERRF (67). Cranial nerve functions may be impaired and affect particularly extraocular muscles, with ptosis and progressive external ophthalmoplegia (PEO), which are necessary to diagnose KSS but are sometimes seen in MELAS patients. Fundoscopy may reveal pigmentary retinopathy in KSS and, less commonly, in MELAS and MERRF. Optic atrophy is sometimes detected in MERRF patients. Peripheral neuropathy is more frequent in MERRF than in the other two syndromes. Sensorineural hearing loss is common in many mitochondrial encephalomyopathies.

The laboratory evaluation should include a complete blood count, serum electrolytes, and calcium, phosphorous, liver function tests, blood urea nitrogen, creatinine, CK, and venous and arterial lactate and pyruvate levels. The latter are commonly elevated at rest in patients with mitochondrial encephalomyopathies and can increase dramatically after moderate exercise. An electrocardiogram may reveal preexcitation in MELAS or MERRF and heart block in KSS or MELAS. Lumbar puncture may show elevation of the cerebrospinal fluid protein, especially in KSS patients. Cerebrospinal fluid may also reveal elevated lactate and pyruvate levels. Electromyography and nerve conduction studies are typically consistent with a myogenic process, although neurogenic changes may be detected in MERRF or MELAS. Brain computed tomography or magnetic resonance imaging may reveal basal ganglia calcifications and atrophy in any of the three major syndromes. In patients with MELAS, there may be lesions compatible with stroke or infarction, typically in the posterior cerebrum, but they generally do not conform to the distribution of major named vessels (74). Clinical research has contributed greatly to our understanding of mitochondrial disorders and to our diagnostic capabilities. Specialized evaluation for oxidative-phosphorylation defects has evolved from laboratory research and includes histologic studies performed directly on skeletal muscle, including measurement of oxidative-phosphorylation enzyme activities, and molecular genetic analyses.

In the past, histologic research focused on morphologic abnormalities of skeletal muscle, but many characteristic microscopic changes have since been noted in other tissues. Accordingly, in the mid-1960s, Shy et al. (76) described the typical ultrastructural alterations seen in mitochondrial myopathies, including an overabundance of ultrastructurally normal mitochondria or "pleoconial myopathy," enlarged mitochondria with disoriented cristae or "megaconial myopathy," and inclusions within mitochondria or so-called "paracrystalline" and "osmiophilic" inclusions. Engel and Cunningham (77) developed the modified Gomori trichrome stain that is still commonly used to identify fibers with subsarcolemmal accumulations of mitochondrial, referred to as "ragged red fibers." Histochemical stains for mitochondrial enzymes are also used to identify excessive mitochondrial proliferation and to demonstrate specific enzyme defects. These stains include succinate dehydrogenase (SDH), nicotinamide dehydrogenase-tetrazolium reductase, and cytochrome *c* oxidase (COX). Immunohistochemical techniques are used to identify defects in specific mitochondrial polypeptides.

In KSS, MELAS, and MERRF, ragged-red fibers with ultrastructurally abnormal mitochondria are almost always identified in skeletal muscle by the Gomori trichrome stain. SDH histochemistry reveals mitochondrial proliferation as darker than normal staining in subsarcolemmal regions of muscle fibers. In MELAS patients, there is often excessive SDH staining within blood vessel walls, so-called strongly SDH-reactive vessels (78,79). Another characteristic of skeletal muscle in MELAS is the relative preservation of COX staining in ragged-red fibers, in contrast to the appearance from KSS and MERRF, which generally shows an abundance of COX-negative ragged-red fibers on serial or double-stained (SDH and COX) sections. However, the histologic abnormalities are neither specific nor sensitive enough to define all mitochondrial diseases. Morphologically abnormal muscle mitochondria have been detected in many conditions that are not primary oxidative-phosphorylation defects, for example, inflammatory myopathies (80) and myotonic dystrophy (81). Conversely, some conditions with defects of mitochondrial enzymes, mtDNA, or both do not have morphologically abnormal mitochondria, including CPT II deficiency. Even in the group of mtDNA-related diseases, not all are characterized by ragged-red fibers in muscle biopsies. As a rule, mutations in structural genes are not associated with ragged-red fibers, for example, Leber hereditary optic neuropathy (LHON) and neuropathy, ataxia, retinitis pigmentosa (NARP).

One can consider assaying the suspected abnormal respiratory chain enzyme in vitro by using crude extracts or isolated mitochondria. In KSS, MELAS, and MERRF, we can detect various combinations of respiratory chain enzyme deficiencies; however, the pattern is not consistent, and normal enzyme activities have been reported. A more reliable and specific next step is molecular genetic analysis.

Since the initial discoveries of the first mtDNA point mutation and large-scale deletions in 1988 (82–84), there has been an outburst of information relating molecular genetic defects to human disorders. Numerous mtDNA mutations have been identified, including duplications, depletions, multiple deletions, and more than 40 pathogenic point mutations (59,69,85,86). Holt et al. (82) first identified large-scale mtDNA deletions in mitochondrial myopathy patients and soon thereafter, Zeviani et al. (84)

pointed out the specific association with KSS. Approximately 90% of KSS patients have large-scale mtDNA deletions, duplications, or both (68,69). The mtDNA deletions generally range from about 2.0 to 10.4 kb in length (68,82) and are mainly confined to an 11-kb region that does not include the origins of mtDNA replication or mtDNA promoter regions. About a third of mtDNA deletions involve an identical 4977-bp segment that is often referred to as the "common deletion" (68). Most mtDNA deletions are flanked by direct DNA sequence repeats, which suggests that they may be created by homologous recombination events (87,88). The large-scale mtDNA deletions are often undetectable in leukocytes, so that molecular diagnosis requires muscle biopsy. MERRF was the first multisystemic disorder to be associated with an mtDNA point mutation, specifically, an adenine-to-guanine transition at nt 8344 (A8344G) in the transfer RNA lysine ($tRNA^{Lys}$) gene (71). A second $tRNA^{Lys}$ mutation at nt 8356 was associated with both MERRF and MERRF-MELAS phenotypes (72,73). These two point mutations can be easily identified in blood leukocytes from patients. Briefly, the leukocyte DNA is extracted, the $tRNA^{Lys}$ gene region is amplified by polymerase chain reaction, and the specific mutation is detected by a restriction enzyme fragment polymorphism length analysis (71,72). MELAS was also associated with a specific mtDNA point mutation, an adenine-to-guanine transition in the $tRNA^{Leu(UUR)}$ gene at nt 3243 (A3243G). About 80% of MELAS patients have been found to harbor this mutation. Five other point mutations have been identified in patients with MELAS. As in MERRF, blood leukocytes can be screened for MELAS-associated mtDNA point mutations.

Although the identification of mtDNA mutations has simplified diagnosis in most cases of mitochondrial encephalomyopathies, it has created new dilemmas. Genetic counseling of patients and their maternal relatives is difficult because heteroplasmy and variability of mutation tissue distribution make clinical outcome predictions tenuous. Similarly, prenatal diagnosis is also perilous. The molecular genetic information should be handled carefully because it can adversely affect medical insurability, employment opportunities, and the emotional status of patients.

Treatment

The medical management of mitochondrial myopathy has lagged behind research and diagnostic knowledge. Treatment can be divided into two types: symptomatic management and metabolic therapy. Seizures in MERRF and MELAS typically respond to conventional antiepilepsy drugs (89); however, they may be difficult to control in the setting of metabolic disarray. The electrolyte disturbances related to hypoparathyroidism and diabetes mellitus should be corrected. Thyroid hormone replacement will alleviate the hypothyroidism. Cardiac pacemaker placement can prolong life in KSS patients with cardiac conduction defects.

Treatments aimed at the primary biochemical defects in mitochondrial encephalomyopathies have been tried; however, the evidence of efficacy has been anecdotal. We generally recommend coenzyme Q10, 50 to 100 mg three times a day, and L-carnitine, 1,000 mg three times a day. Coenzyme Q10 is a quinone compound that normally shuttles electrons from complexes I and II to complex III and may stabilize the oxidative-phosphorylation enzyme complexes within the inner mitochondrial membrane (90). Dichloroacetate inhibits pyruvate dehydrogenase specific kinase, thus activating pyruvate dehydrogenase complex and reducing lactate (91,92). Vitamins that may donate electrons directly to COX include phylloquinone (vitamin K1), menadione (vitamin K3), and ascorbic acid (vitamin C) (54). Vitamin C has also been used as an antioxidant because the impaired oxidative-phosphorylation pathway may generate increased amounts of free radicals. Nicotinamide and riboflavin have been used to improve respiratory chain functions (93). No genetic therapy is presently available.

ACKNOWLEDGMENTS

Supported in part by grants from the National Institutes of Health (HD32062, NS28828, NS11766, NS01617, HL59657), the Muscular Dystrophy Association, and the Columbia-Presbyterian Medical Center Irving Scholar Program.

REFERENCES

1. DiMauro S, Tonin P, Servidei S. Metabolic myopathies. In: Rowland LP, DiMauro S, eds. *Myopathies*. Amsterdam: Elsevier Science Publishers B.V., 1992:479–526.
2. DiMauro S, Hirano M, Bonilla E, De Vivo DC. The mitochondrial disorders. In: Berg B, ed. *Pediatric neurology*. New York: McGraw-Hill, 1996:1201–1232.
3. Tein I. Metabolic myopathies. *Semin Pediatr Neurol* 1996;3:59–98.
4. De Vivo DC, Hirano M, DiMauro S. Mitochondrial disorders. In: Moser HW, ed. *Neurodystrophies and neurolipidoses*. Amsterdam: Elsevier Science B.V., 1997:389–446.
5. Di Donato S. Diseases associated with defects of beta-oxidation. In: Rosenberg RN, Prusiner SB, DiMauro S, Barchi RL, eds. *The molecular and genetic basis of neurological disease*. Boston: Butterworth-Heinemann, 1997:939–956.
6. DiMauro S, Servidei S, Tsujino S. Disorders of carbohydrate metabolism: glycogen storage diseases. In: Rosenberg RN, Prusiner SB, DiMauro S, Barchi RL, eds. *The molecular and genetic basis of neurological disease*. Boston: Butterworth-Heinemann, 1997:1067–1097.
7. Felig P, Wahren J. Fuel homeostasis in exercise. *N Engl J Med* 1975;293:1078–1084.
8. McArdle B. Myopathy due to a defect in muscle glycogen breakdown. *Clin Sci* 1951;10:13–33.
9. DiMauro S, DiMauro-Melis PM. Muscle carnitine palmitoyltransferase deficiency and myoglobinuria. *Science* 1973;182:929–931.
10. Raben N, Nichols RC, Boerkoel C, Plotz P. Genetic defects in patients with glycogenosis type II (acid maltase deficiency). *Muscle Nerve* 1995;S70–S74.
11. Nicolino M, Puech JP, Letourneur F, Fardeau M, Kahn A, Poenaru L. Glycogen-storage disease type II (acid maltase deficiency): identification of a novel small deletion (delCC482-483) in French patients. *Biochem Biophys Res Commun* 1997;235:138–141.
12. Smit GPA, Fernandes J, Leonard JV, et al. The long-term outcome of patients with glycogen storage diseases. *J Inherit Metab Dis* 1990;13:411–418.
13. Fellows IW, Lowe JS, Ogilvie AL, Stevens A, Toghill PJ, Atkinson M. Type III glycogenosis presenting as liver disease in adults with atypical histological features. *J Clin Pathol* 1983;36:431–434.
14. Brown BI. Debranching and branching enzyme deficiencies. In: Engel AG, Banker BQ, eds. *Myology*. New York: McGraw-Hill, 1986:1653–1661.
15. Okubo M, Aoyama Y, Murase T. A novel donor splice site mutation in the glycogen debranching enzyme gene is associated with glycogen storage disease type III. *Biochem Biophys Res Commun* 1996;224:493–499.
16. Shen J, Bao Y, Liu H-M, Lee P, Leonard JV, Chen Y-T. Mutations in exon 3 of the glycogen debranching enzyme gene are associated with glycogen storage disease type III that is differentially expressed in liver and muscle. *J Clin Invest* 1996;98:352–357.
17. Lossos A, Barash V, Soffer D, et al. Hereditary branching enzyme dysfunction in adult polyglucosan body disease: a possible metabolic cause in two patients. *Ann Neurol* 1991;30:655–662.
18. Bruno C, Servidei S, Shanske S, et al. Glycogen branching enzyme deficiency in adult polyglucosan body disease. *Ann Neurol* 1993;33:88–93.
19. Cafferty MS, Lovelace RE, Hays AP, Servidei S, DiMauro S, Rowland LP. Polyglucosan body disease. *Muscle Nerve* 1991;14:102–107.
20. Bao Y, Kishnani P, Wu J-Y, Chen Y-T. Hepatic and neuromuscular forms of glycogen storage disease type IV caused by mutations in the same glycogen-branching enzyme gene. *J Clin Invest* 1996;97:941–948.
21. DiMauro S, Bresolin N. Phosphorylase deficiency. In: Engel AG, Banker BQ, eds. *Myology*. New York: McGraw-Hill, 1986:1585–1601.
22. Slonim AE, Goans PJ. McArdle's syndrome: improvement with a high-protein diet. *N Engl J Med* 1985;312:355–359.
23. Beynon RJ, Bartram C, Hopkins P, et al. McArdle's disease: molecular genetics and metabolic consequences of the phenotype. *Muscle Nerve* 1995;3:S18–22.
24. Tarui S, Okuno G, Ikua Y, Tanaka T, Suda M, Nishikawa M. Phosphofructokinase deficiency in skeletal muscle. A new type of glycogenosis. *Biochem Biophys Res Commun* 1965;19:517–523.
25. Haller RG, Lewis SF. Glucose-induced exertional fatigue in muscle phosphofructokinase deficiency. *N Engl J Med* 1991;324:364–369.
26. Van der Berg LET, Berger R. Phosphorylase b kinase deficiency in man: a review. *J Inherit Metab Dis* 1990;13:442–451.
27. Wehner M, Clemens PR, Engel AG, Kilimann MW. Human muscle glycogenosis due to phosphorylase kinase deficiency associated with a nonsense mutation in the muscle isoform of the alpha subunit. *Hum Mol Genet* 1994;3:1983–1987.
28. Tsujino S, Shanske S, DiMauro S. Molecular genetic heterogeneity of phosphoglycerate kinase (PGK) deficiency. *Muscle Nerve* 1995;3:S45–S49.
29. Tsujino S, Shanske S, Sakoda S, Fenichel G, DiMauro S. The molecular genetic basis of muscle phosphoglycerate mutase (PGAM) deficiency. *Am J Hum Genet* 1993;52:472–477.
30. Tsujino S, Shanske S, Sakota S, DiMauro S. Molecular genetic studies in phosphoglycerate mutase (PGAM-M) deficiency. *Muscle Nerve* 1995;3:S50–S53.
31. Kanno T, Sudo K, Takeuchi I, et al. Hereditary deficiency of lactate dehydrogenase M-subunit. *Clin Chim Acta* 1980;108:267–276.
32. Kanno T, Maekawa M. Lactate dehydrogenase M-subunit deficiencies: clinical features, metabolic background, and genetic heterogeneities. *Muscle Nerve* 1995;3:S54–S57.
33. Kreuder J, Borkhardt A, Repp R, et al. Inherited metabolic myopathy and hemolysis due to a mutation in aldolase A. *N Engl J Med* 1996;334:1100–1104.
34. Bruno C, Bado M, Minetti C, Cordone G. Forearm semi-ischemic exercise test in pediatric patients. *J Child Neurol* 1998;6:288–290.
35. Hoppel C. The physiological role of carnitine. In: Ferrari R, DiMauro S, Sherwood G, eds. *L-Carnitine and its role in medicine: from function to therapy*. London: Academic Press, 1992:5–19.
35a. Lamhonwah A-M, Tein I. Carnitine uptake defect: frameshift mutations in the human plasmalemmal carnitine transporter gene. *Biochem Biophys Res Comm* 1998;252:396–401.
35b. Nezu J-I, Tamai I, Oku A, et al. Primary systemic carnitine deficiency is caused by mutations in a gene encoding sodium ion-dependent carnitine transporter. *Nature Genet* 1999;21:91–94.
36. Haworth JC, DeMagre F, Booth FA, et al. Atypical features of the hepatic form of carnitine palmitoyltransferase deficiency in a Huterite family. *J Pediatr* 1992;121:553–557.

37. Bonnefont JP, Haas R, Wolff J, et al. Deficiency of carnitine palmitoyltransferase I. *J Child Neurol* 1989;4:198–203.

37a. IJlst L, Mandel H, Oostheim W, Ruiter JPN, Gutman A, Wanders RJA. Molecular basis of human carnitine palmitoyltransferase I deficiency. *J Clin Invest* 1998;102:527–531.

38. Tonin P, Lewis LP, Servidei S, DiMauro S. Metabolic causes of myoglobinuria. *Ann Neurol* 1990;27:181–185.

39. Taroni F, Verderio E, Dworzak F, Willems PJ, Cavadini P, DiDonato S. Identification of a common mutation in the carnitine palmitoyltransferase II gene in familial recurrent myoglobinuria patients. *Nature Genet* 1993;4:314–320.

40. Kaufmann P, El-Schahawi M, DiMauro S. Carnitine palmitoyltransferase II deficiency: diagnosis by molecular analysis of blood. *Mol Cell Biochem* 1997;174:237–239.

41. Stanley CA, Hale DE, Barry GT, Deleeuw S, Boxer J, Bonnefont JP. A deficiency of carnitine-acylcarnitine translocase in the inner mitochondrial membrane. *N Engl J Med* 1992;327:19–22.

42. Bertrand C, Largiliere C, Zabot MT, Mathieu M, Vianey-Saban C. Very long-chain acyl-CoA dehydrogenase deficiency: identification of a new inborn error of mitochondrial fatty acid oxidation in fibroblasts. *Biochim Biophys Acta* 1992;1180:327–329.

43. Jackson S, Bartlett K, Land J, et al. Long-chain 3-hydroxyacyl-CoA dehydrogenase deficiency. *Pediatr Res* 1991;29:406–411.

44. Roe CR, Coates PM. Acyl-CoA dehydrogenase deficiency. In: Scriver CR, Beaudet AL, Sly WS, Valle D, eds. *The metabolic basis of inherited disease*. New York: McGraw-Hill, 1989:889–914.

45. Matsubara Y, Narisawa K, Miyabayashi S, et al. Identification of a common mutation in patients with medium-chain acyl-CoA dehydrogenase deficiency. *Biochem Biophys Res Commun* 1990;171:498–505.

46. Yokota I, Saijo T, Tanaka K. Impaired tetramer assembly of variant medium-chain acyl-CoA dehydrogenase with a glutamate or aspartate substitution for lysine 304 causing instability of the protein. *J Biol Chem* 1992;267:26004–26010.

47. Turnbull DM, Bartlett K, Stevens DL. Short-chain acyl-CoA dehydrogenase deficiency associated with a lipid storage myopathy and secondary carnitine deficiency. *N Engl J Med* 1984;311:1232–1236.

48. Amendt BA, Greene C, Sweetman L, et al. Short-chain acyl-coenzyme A dehydrogenase deficiency. Clinical and biochemical studies in two patients. *J Clin Invest* 1987;79:1303–1309.

49. Tein I, De Vivo DC, Hale DE, et al. Short-chain L-3-hydroxyacyl-CoA dehydrogenase deficiency in muscle: a new cause for recurrent myoglobinuria and encephalopathy. *Ann Neurol* 1991;30:415–419.

50. Roe CR, Millington DS, Norwood DL, et al. 2-4-Dienoyl-coenzyme A reductase deficiency: a possible new disorder of fatty acid oxidation. *J Clin Invest* 1990;85:1703–1707.

51. Fishbein WN, Armbrustmacher VW, Griffin JL. Myoadenylate deaminase deficiency: a new disease of muscle. *Science* 1978;200:545–548.

52. Sabina RL. Myoadenylate deaminase deficiency. In: Rosenberg RN, ed. *The molecular and genetic basis of neurological disease*. Stonham, CT: Butterworth-Heinemann, 1993:170–179.

53. Fishbein WN. Myoadenylate deaminase deficiency: inherited and acquired forms. *Biochem Med* 1985;33:158–169.

54. Shoffner JM, Wallace DC. Oxidative phosphorylation diseases. In: Schriver C, Beaudet A, Sly W, Valle D, eds. *The Metabolic and Molecular Bases of Inherited Diseases*. New York: McGraw-Hill, 1995:1535–1609.

55. Sato T, DiMauro S. *Mitochondrial encephalomyopathies*. New York: Raven Press, 1991.

56. DiMauro S, Wallace DC. *Mitochondrial DNA in Human Pathology*. New York: Raven Press, 1993.

57. Schapira AHV, DiMauro S. *Mitochondrial disorders in neurology*. Oxford: Butterworth-Heinemann Ltd., 1994.

58. Anderson S, Bankier AT, Barrel BG, et al. Sequence and organization of the human mitochondrial genome. *Nature* 1981;290:457–465.

59. Schon EA, Bonilla E, DiMauro S. Mitochondrial DNA mutations and pathogenesis. *J Bioenerg Biomembr* 1997;29:131–149.

60. Rötig A, Colonna M, Bonnefont JP, et al. Mitochondrial DNA deletion in Pearson's marrow/pancreas syndrome. *Genomics* 1989;10:502–504.

61. Kearns TP, Sayre GP. Retinitis pigmentosa, external ophthalmoplegia, and complete heart block. *Arch Ophthalmol* 1958;60:280–289.

62. Bourgeron T, Rustin P, Chretien D, et al. Mutation of a nuclear succinate dehydrogenase gene results in mitochondrial respiratory chain deficiency. *Nat Genet* 1995;11:144–149.

63. Fukuhara N, Tokigushi S, Shirakawa K, Tsubaki T. Myoclonus epilepsy associated with ragged-red fibers (mitochondrial abnormali-

ties): disease entity or syndrome? Light and electron microscopic studies of two cases and review of the literature. *J Neurol Sci* 1980;47:117–133.

64. Pavlakis SG, Phillips PC, DiMauro S, De Vivo DC, Rowland LP. Mitochondrial myopathy, encephalopathy, lactic acidosis, and strokelike episodes: a distinctive clinical syndrome. *Ann Neurol* 1984;16:481–488.

65. Rowland LP, Hays AP, DiMauro S, DeVivo DC, Behrens M. Diverse clinical disorders associated with morphological abnormalities of mitochondria. In: Cerri C, Scarlato G, eds. *Mitochondrial pathology in muscle diseases*. Padua: Piccin Editore, 1983:141–158.

66. Petty RKH, Harding AE, Morgan-Hughes JA. The clinical features of mytochondrial myopathy. *Brain* 1986;109:915–938.

67. Hirano M, DiMauro S. Clinical features of mitochondrial myopathies and encephalomyopathies. In: Lane R, ed. *Handbook of muscle disease*. New York: Marcel Dekker, 1996:479–504.

68. Moraes CT, DiMauro S, Zeviani M, et al. Mitochondrial DNA deletions in progressive external ophthalmoplegia and Kearns-Sayre syndrome. *N Engl J Med* 1989;320:1293–1299.

69. Poulton J, Deadman ME, Gardiner RM. Duplications of mitochondrial DNA in mitochondrial myopathy. *Lancet* 1989;1:236–240.

70. Silvestri G, Ciafaloni E, Santorelli F, et al. Clinical features associated with the A>G transition at nucleotide 8344 of mtDNA ("MERRF" mutation). *Neurology* 1993;43:1200–1206.

71. Shoffner JM, Lott MT, Lezza A, Seibel P, Ballinger SW, Wallace DC. Myoclonic epilepsy and ragged-red fiber disease (MERRF) is associated with a mitochondrial DNA tRNALys mutation. *Cell* 1990;61:931–937.

72. Silvestri G, Moraes CT, Shanske S, Oh SJ, DiMauro S. A new mtDNA mutation in the tRNALys gene associated with myoclonic epilepsy and ragged-red fibers (MERRF). *Am J Hum Genet* 1992;51:1213–1217.

73. Zeviani M, Muntoni F, Savarese N, et al. A MERRF/MELAS overlap syndrome with a new point mutation in the mitochondrial DNA tRNALys gene. *Eur J Hum Genet* 1993;1:80–87.

74. Hirano M, Pavlakis SG. Mitochondrial myopathy, encephalopathy, lactic acidosis, and strokelike episodes (MELAS): current concepts. *J Child Neurol* 1994;9:4–13.

75. Berkovic SF, Carpenter S, Evans A, et al. Myoclonus epilepsy and ragged-red fibres (MERRF): a clinical, pathological, biochemical, magnetic resonance spectrographic and positron emission tomographic study. *Brain* 1989;112:1231–1260.

76. Shy GM, Gonatas NK, Perez M. Childhood myopathies with abnormal mitochondria. I. Megaconial myopathy-pleoconial myopathy. *Brain* 1966;89:133–158.

77. Engel WK, Cunningham CG. Rapid examination of muscle tissue: an improved trichrome stain method for fresh-frozen biopsy sections. *Neurology* 1963;13:919–923.

78. Hasegawa H, Matsuoka T, Goto I, Nonaka I. Strongly succinate dehydrogenase-reactive blood vessels in muscles from patients with mitochondrial myopathy, encephalopathy, lactic acidosis, and stroke-like episodes. *Ann Neurol* 1991;29:601–605.

79. Sakuta R, Nonaka I. Vascular involvement in mitochondrial myopathy. *Ann Neurol* 1989;25:594–601.

80. Carpenter S, Karpati G, Eisen AA. *A morphologic study of muscle in polymyositis: clues to pathogenesis of different types*. Amsterdam: Excerpta Medica, 1975:374–379.

81. Fardeau M. *Ultrastructural lesions in progressive muscular dystrophies: a critical study of their specificity*. Amsterdam: Excerpta Medica, 1970:98–108.

82. Holt IJ, Harding AE, Morgan Hughes JA. Deletions of muscle mitochondrial DNA in patients with mitochondrial myopathies. *Nature* 1988;331:717-719.

83. Wallace DC, Singh G, Lott MT, et al. Mitochondrial DNA mutation associated with Leber's hereditary optic neuropathy. *Science* 1988;242:1427–1430.

84. Zeviani M, Moraes CT, DiMauro S. Deletions of mitochondrial DNA in Kearns-Sayre syndrome. *Neurology* 1988;38:1339–1346.

85. Moraes CT, Shanske S, Tritschler HJ, et al. MtDNA depletion with variable tissue expression: a novel genetic abnormality in mitochondrial diseases. *Am J Hum Genet* 1991;48:492–501.

86. Zeviani M, Servidei S, Gellera C, Bertini E, DiMauro S, DiDonato S. An autosomal dominant disorder with multiple deletions of mitochondrial DNA starting at the D-loop region. *Nature* 1989;339:309–311.

87. Schon EA, Rizzuto R, Moraes CT, Nakase H, Zeviani M, DiMauro S. A direct repeat is a hotspot for large-scale deletions of human mitochondrial DNA. *Science* 1989;244:346–349.

88. Mita S, Rizzuto R, Moraes CT, et al. Recombination via flanking

direct repeats is a major cause of large-scale deletions of human mitochondrial DNA. *Nucleic Acids Res* 1990;18:561–567.

89. So N, Berkovic S, Andermann F, Kuziencky R, Gendron D, Quesney L. Myoclonus epilepsy and ragged-red fibres (MERRF). *Brain* 1989;112: 1261–1276.

90. Lenaz G, De Santis A, Bertoli E. A survey of the function and specificity of ubiquinone in the the mitochondrial respiratory chain. In: Lenaz G, ed. *Coenzyme Q*. New York: Wiley, 1985:165–199.

91. De Vivo DC, Jackson A, Wade C, Altmann K, Stacpoole PW, DiMauro S. Dichloroacetate treatment of MELAS-associated lactic acidosis. *Ann Neurol* 1990;28:437.

92. Saito T, Naito E, Ito M, Takeda E, Hashimoto T, Kuroda Y. Therapeutic effects of sodium dichloroacetate on visual and auditory hallucinations in a patient with MELAS. *Neuropediatrics* 1991;22:166–167.

93. Penn AMW, Lee JWK, Thuillier P, et al. MELAS syndrome with mitochondrial tRNALeu(UUR) mutation: correlation of clinical state, nerve conduction, and muscle 31P magnetic resonance spectroscopy during treatment with nicotinamide and riboflavin. *Neurology* 1992;42:2147–2152.

94. DiMauro S. Disorders of carbohydrate metabolism. In: Rowland LP, ed. *Merritt's textbook of neurology*. Baltimore: Williams & Wilkins, 1995:572–575.

Motor Disorders,
edited by David S. Younger.
Lippincott Williams & Wilkins, Philadelphia © 1999.

CHAPTER 11

Childhood Muscular Dystrophies Sharing a Common Pathogenesis of Membrane Instability

Chang-Yong Tsao and Jerry R. Mendell

In the premolecular era, there were very few clues that different clinical and genetic forms of muscular dystrophy shared a common pathogenesis of membrane instability. Since the cloning of the gene for Duchenne muscular dystrophy (DMD) in late 1987 (1), our concepts have dramatically changed. Dystrophin is the product of the DMD locus, and we know that it is part of a complex of membrane-associated proteins, the dystrophin-glycoprotein complex (DGC), that span the muscle sarcolemma, providing linkage between the intracellular cytoskeleton and the extracellular matrix (2–4). In relation to human muscular dystrophies, it is useful to consider the constituents of the DGC: dystrophin, dystroglycans, and sarcoglycans. Laminin-2, a trilaminar molecular complex in the basal lamina, serves as the extracellular anchor for the DGC (5–7). The syntrophins represent another group of proteins bound to the DGC. They are composed of three isoforms, $\alpha 1$, $\beta 1$, and $\beta 2$, each the product of individual genes (8). Syntrophins are thought to function as modular adapters for recruitment of signaling proteins to the membrane. Their role in the pathogenesis of muscular dystrophy remains to be defined (9,10). This chapter reviews essential aspects of childhood muscular dystrophies that share a common pathogenesis of membrane instability.

DYSTROPHIN-GLYCOPROTEIN COMPLEX

Dystrophin is a large protein molecule of molecular weight 427 kDa, localized to the cytoplasmic face of the skeletal muscle membrane in a subsarcolemmal loca-

tion. The dystrophin domains include the amino terminus, the rod domain composed of 24-helical repeats, and a carboxy terminus (1). At the amino terminus, dystrophin is bound to the cytoskeletal protein, f-actin. The carboxy terminus includes a binding-site for the syntrophins, but more importantly its cysteine-rich region serves as a ligand to the dystroglycans. α/β-Dystroglycan is encoded by a single gene on chromosome 3p21 (1–4). Two proteins are proteolytically cleaved and undergo posttranslational modification. β-Dystroglycan serves as the ligand for the cysteine-rich region of dystrophin. α-Dystroglycan serves as the ligand for laminin-2 in the basal lamina. Thus, the dystroglycans establish a bridge across the membrane from the cytoskeleton and dystrophin to laminin-2 in the extracellular matrix.

The sarcoglycan subcomplex is an integral part of the DGC, composed of at least four transmembrane constituents: α-sarcoglycan (50 kDa, formerly called adhalin), β-sarcoglycan, λ-sarcoglycan, and δ-sarcoglycan (1–4). The precise relationship between the sarcoglycans and dystroglycans is not well established, but transgenic mice deleted for certain domains of dystrophin demonstrate that the sarcoglycan complex binds dystrophin via dystroglycan (8).

Laminins are ubiquitous integral constituents of the basal lamina of all tissues; laminins in skeletal muscle are designated laminin-2 (5–7). Laminin-2, as already noted, bears an integral relationship to the DGC but is considered to be a separate component (2–4,8). Its heterotrimeric molecular structure is arranged in the shape of a cross with one heavy α chain and two light chains, β and λ. Originally called merosin, the laminin heavy chain of skeletal muscle and Schwann cells is designated laminin $\alpha 2$. The gene for laminin $\alpha 2$ chain maps to chromosome 6q22-23 (11).

C.-Y. Tsao: Departments of Neurology and Pediatrics, Ohio State University and Children's Hospital, Columbus, Ohio 43205.

J.R. Mendell: Department of Neurology, Ohio State University, Columbus, Ohio 43210.

UNIFYING HYPOTHESIS OF MEMBRANE INSTABILITY

There is general agreement that the DGC confers stability to the muscle membrane (12). In DMD and the other muscular dystrophies, the serum CK elevation is usually seen at the time of birth and persists throughout life. Studies in DMD indicate that dystrophin deficiency disrupts the membrane localization for the dystroglycans and sarcoglycans. The same is true when the sarcoglycans are deficient, particularly α-sarcoglycan, where deficiency disrupts the integrity of localization for many components of the DGC. A strong argument favoring an integrated function of these proteins is the clinical picture of overlapping phenotypes as seen in the dystrophinopathy DMD and Becker muscular dystrophy (BMD), the sarcoglycanopathy limb girdle muscular dystrophy (LGMD), and the lamininopathy congenital muscular dystrophy, as presented. These findings support a unifying pathogenic concept for these muscular dystrophies as follows: Membrane tears from weakening of the sarcolemma cause excess calcium leak into the muscle fiber, initiating a cascade of events leading to muscle fiber necrosis. A combination of observations justifies the hypothesis that the disorders affecting structural proteins of the DGC and related proteins all have associated membrane instability leading to muscle fiber breakdown. The muscular dystrophy phenotype is the final outcome.

DYSTROPHINOPATHIES

Clinical Features

The features of DMD and BMD have been well described (13,14). Clinical symptoms of DMD are unusual in the neonatal period. Occasional patients, especially those with mental retardation, may exhibit delayed motor milestones. In most cases the disease becomes clinically apparent between ages 2 and 3 years. The condition shows relentless progression, with weakness and wasting more profoundly affecting the proximal lower extremity muscles. As the disease progresses, contractures develop that limit function, especially at the ankles and hips. Scoliosis is common after wheelchair confinement, which typically occurs about age 12. Most patients die of complications of respiratory insufficiency at about age 20 or slightly thereafter.

Cardiac involvement is a consistent part of DMD (15). The heart demonstrates fibrosis in the posterobasal portion of the left ventricular wall. The right ventricular septum and the right ventricular and atrial myocardium have much less involvement. Degenerative changes affecting the conduction system are infrequent. Despite known cardiac disease, most Duchenne patients remain surprisingly free of cardiovascular symptoms. Congestive heart failure and cardiac arrhythmias usually occur only in the late stages and especially during times of stress from intercurrent infections. Rarely, however, DMD patients have overt signs of congestive heart failure and, in fact, may die of cardiac failure with relative sparing of respiratory muscle function.

Clinical and pathologic involvement of smooth muscle of the gastrointestinal tract, although frequently overlooked, can be an important manifestation (16). A syndrome of acute gastric dilatation, also referred to as intestinal pseudo-obstruction, leads to sudden vomiting, abdominal pain and distention, and possibly death if untreated (16). Patients dying of this syndrome show degeneration of the outer longitudinal smooth muscle layer of the stomach; other regions of the gastrointestinal tract can be affected, causing symptoms such as severe constipation.

The average intelligence quotient falls approximately 1 standard deviation below the mean (17). The impairment of intellectual function appears to be nonprogressive and affects the verbal ability more than performance. The neuropathologic correlate for mental retardation in DMD has not been established.

In BMD, the pattern of muscle wasting closely resembles that seen in DMD. The natural history of the illness permits distinction between the two disorders. Most Becker patients experience difficulties between ages 5 and 15 years, although onset in the third to fourth decade or even later can occur. By definition, Becker patients ambulate beyond age 15, allowing clinical distinction from Duchenne dystrophy. Becker patients have a reduced life expectancy, but most patients survive at least into the fourth or fifth decade.

The preceding discussion implies a clear distinction between Duchenne and Becker patients, but a great heterogeneity of clinical presentation and course of illness can be recognized, emphasizing a continuous spectrum ranging from very severe to very mild (14). A well-recognized subgroup of patients with an intermediate course are referred to as outliers or the intermediate-form of dystrophinopathy. These patients can be recognized usually by age 3 years because of relative preservation of antigravity neck flexor muscle strength, whereas Duchenne patients lack this ability throughout their entire life. Patients with an intermediate phenotype retain the ability to climb stairs and walk after age 12 years but not beyond age 15 (18).

Other phenotypes of dystrophin deficiency have been recognized, adding to the clinical heterogeneity of the dystrophinopathies. A disorder of myalgia and myoglobinuria without persistent weakness has been described (19), and even a cardiomyopathy with few or absent skeletal muscle signs can occur (20). Perhaps the future will hold observations, indicating a selective deficiency of the brain dystrophin isoforms accounting for certain types of mental retardation.

Genetics

DMD is the most common X-linked recessive lethal disease with an incidence of approximately 1 in 3,500 newborns. It has been estimated that one third of the cases are the result of new mutations (18). The dystrophin gene spans more than 2,000 kilobases (kb) of genomic DNA and is composed of 79 exons that encode a 14-kb transcript (1); its enormity probably accounts for the high frequency of spontaneous mutations (21–29). Approximately 65% of DMD and BMD cases demonstrate large-scale deletions of several kilobases to greater than one million base pairs in the dystrophin gene. Duplications are found in approximately 5% of cases (23). The large gene size, particularly the introns, which average 35 kb, partly accounts for the high deletion rate. The deletions are nonrandomly distributed, occur primarily in the center, and less frequently near the 5' end of the gene; larger deletions usually begin at the 5' end of the gene. Deletions disrupting the open reading frame result in the more severe Duchenne phenotype in most cases. In the milder Becker dystrophy, the deletion maintains the translational reading frame, and a semifunctional truncated protein is produced. The reading frame rule explains the phenotypic differences observed in about 92% of the Duchenne/Becker cases. A major exception to the reading frame rule has been the identification of Becker patients with out-of-frame deletions of exons 3 to 7. It has been proposed that an alternate splicing mechanism or new cryptic translational start sites account for the milder phenotype observed with exons 3–7 deletions and the production of dystrophin (29).

There are several reports of point mutations, small deletions, and duplications in the dystrophin gene in DMD patients (24,26,27). Most of these point mutations have resulted in dystrophin truncation, consistent with the reading frame hypothesis. However, unlike the deletion hot spots, these small mutations are private and randomly distributed throughout the gene.

With the ability to perform direct DNA diagnostics on the deletion/duplication cases, the accuracy of carrier detection has significantly improved. Nevertheless, the carrier state of the mother of an isolated case should be interpreted cautiously from DNA testing. For example, when the mother has no detectable mutation of the dystrophin gene, the risk of carrier status still cannot be excluded because of the possibility of germline mosaicism (30). Mothers not harboring mutations of the dystrophin gene in peripheral blood leukocytes can still manifest mutations in a percentage of the oocytes. Such examples of germline mosaicism have important counseling implications. The sisters of Duchenne patients should be investigated independently of the outcome of DNA testing of the mother. Furthermore, a negative mutation result in the mother does not rule out a recurrence risk for future pregnancies, but the exact risk is unknown because there is no method to estimate the size of the mutant clone. The recurrence risk for the mother of a sporadic DMD case has been estimated to be as high as 14% (30).

Molecular Pathogenesis of the Dystrophinopathies

In DMD, the absence of dystrophin leads to a drastic reduction in all components of the DGC that are normally synthesized but not properly assembled or integrated into the sarcolemma (2–4,12). Based on these observations, it is proposed that disruption of the DGC plays a key role in the cascade of events, leading to muscle cell necrosis. The absence of dystrophin causes a disruption of the linkage between the subsarcolemmal cytoskeleton and the extracellular matrix, leading to sarcolemmal instability, membrane tears, and muscle cell necrosis.

Support for the delicate relationship within the components of the DGC is provided by experimental and clinical studies. For example, in transgenic *mdx* mice (the genetic mouse model with dystrophin deficiency), systematic studies replacing certain domains of dystrophin demonstrate the critical role of the cysteine-rich region (49–51). A dystrophin gene construct devoid of exons 64 to 70, responsible for transduction of the cysteine-rich domain, prevents localization of all components of the DGC. In clinical situations, even missense mutations can result in conformational changes of the molecular structure of dystrophin, preventing proper assembly of the DGC (27). These results support a model whereby dystrophin deficiency, or in some cases even small changes that alter the structural conformation of dystrophin, can disrupt the DGC, leading to membrane instability and predisposing the muscle to repeated insults, leading to muscle breakdown and a muscular dystrophy phenotype.

Treatment

Appropriate stretching of the heelcords, iliotibial bands, and hip flexors should be done to prevent contractures. Night splints may delay heelcord tightness. Scoliosis often occurs when patients lose ambulation. The segmental spinal stabilization described by Luque (31) is the procedure of choice to correct scoliosis. Patients with progressive curvatures measuring 35 to 45 degrees should be considered surgical candidates. A forced vital capacity of greater than 35% of predicted normal mean is recommended to prevent postoperative pneumonia. Anesthesia for patients with DMD should not include halogenated inhalational anesthetics or neuromuscular depolarizing agents such as succinylcholine because adverse reactions may occur that are similar, but not identical, to malignant hyperthermia (32).

Prednisone and deflazacort have been shown to benefit Duchenne dystrophy patients. In randomized, double-blind, controlled trials, both significantly increase muscle strength, pulmonary function, and functional ability (33,34). Improvement occurs as early as 10 days, with prednisone treatment reaching maximal improvement by 3 months. The recommended prednisone dosage is 0.75 mg/kg/day. Long-term studies indicate that a dose of 0.65 mg/kg/day can maintain improvement, but similar results cannot be achieved with alternate-day treatment (35,36). The major long-term benefits of prednisone are prolonged independent and braced ambulation. Both ambulatory and wheelchair-dependent patients maintain improved vital capacity measures for longer periods of time compared with control subjects. Significant side effects include growth retardation, weight gain, cushingoid facial appearance, excessive body hair, cataracts, and behavioral changes (33–36). Unacceptable weight gain is the most common reason for reducing or discontinuing prednisone (37).

Prednisone increases strength by increasing muscle mass (33,34) and decreasing muscle degradation (38). The decrease in muscle degradation may be due to an anti-inflammatory effect related to a reduction in total T cells and cytotoxic-suppressor T cells (39). Prednisone has no effect on dystrophin levels in muscle (40). Deflazacort, an oxazoline derivative of prednisone, has fewer side effects than prednisone, especially in bone osteoporosis and weight gain (41–44). In a randomized trial comparing deflazacort and prednisone, both drugs had equal efficacy after 1-year follow-up, but deflazacort-treated patients gained significantly less weight (45). Gene replacement therapy is on the horizon for dystrophin-deficient patients, but the results of clinical trials have not been reported. Alternative methods of dystrophin replacement by myoblast transfer have not been efficacious in controlled trials in DMD patients (46–48), as well as in mdx mice (49–51).

LIMB GIRDLE MUSCULAR DYSTROPHY

The term "limb girdle muscular dystrophy" initially referred to a heterogeneous group of disorders with both autosomal dominant (AD) and recessive (AR) inheritance patterns (52); that concept has been incorporated into current nosology (53,54). There are now at least eight diseases that have been classified as LGMDs (Table 1). This number is constantly expanding and will continue to grow. Fortunately, the new classification schema will accommodate change as explained in the discussion to follow.

LGMD1 refers to the dominantly inherited variants, whereas LGMD2 consists of disorders with AR transmission. Presently, linkage has been established for two dominantly inherited disorders, LGMD1A and LGMD1B (55–58). The recessively inherited forms of LGMD now number six. In five, the specific deficiency has been identified: LGMD2A [calpain 3 (CAPN3)] (59–62), 2B (unknown protein) (63), 2C (λ-sarcoglycan) (64–66), 2D (α-sarcoglycan) (67–72), 2E (β-sarcoglycan) (73,74), and 2F (δ-sarcoglycan) (75). One case of β-dystroglycan deficiency has been found but will probably not be officially assigned a number until the mutation is identified (76).

Clinical Features

There are features common to all LGMD disorders. Weakness is predominant in a limb girdle distribution with sparing of facial, extraocular, and pharyngeal muscles (53,54). It would be difficult to make a gene-specific diagnosis purely on clinical evaluation. In any of these conditions, the degree of weakness varies from an early onset, severe, Duchenne-like disorder to a mild Becker-like disorder. The heterogeneity of the Becker-like cases is every bit as diverse as that seen in the dystrophinopathies. Calf hypertrophy is common in the recessively inherited LGMDs but is not an invariable feature. The CAPN3-deficient patients are reported to have rather consistent calf muscle contractures resulting in "tiptoe" walking that often serves as the stimulus for the initial consultation (59–61).

Onset of weakness in distal muscles was considered to be tantamount to another diagnosis when criteria for LGMD were established (53,54). However, even this adage is weakening because evidence now indicates that

TABLE 1. *Limb girdle muscular dystrophy (LGMD)*

Disease	Protein	Size	Chromosomal localization
Autosomal dominant			
LGMD1A	Unknown	Unknown	5q31-33
LGMD1B	Unknown	Unknown	1q11-21
Autosomal recessive			
LGMD2A	Calpain 3	95 kDa	15q15.1-15.3
LGMD2B	Unknown	Unknown	2p13.3
LGMD2C	τ-Sarcoglycan	35kDa	13q12
LGMD2D	α-Sarcoglycan	50kDa	17q12-21.33
LGMD2E	β-Sarcoglycan	43kDa	4q12
LGMD2F	δ-Sarcoglycan	35kDa	5q33-34

the distal myopathy of Miyoshi appears to map to chromosome 2p in the same region as LGMD2B (77–79). Further, in some families, affected members can have either an LGMD-phenotype or a distal myopathy/phenotype. In contrast to dystrophinopathies, mentation is spared in the LGMDs. There appear to be few exceptions to this so far (68–70).

Several points should be made regarding patients with LGMD and cardiomyopathy. In AR LGMD, including deficiency of sarcoglycans, CAPN3, and β-dystroglycan, cardiomyopathy is unusual. At best, nonspecific T-wave changes may be seen. One exception has been reported in a patient with a Becker-like phenotype and a severe cardiomyopathy who underwent successful orthotopic heart transplant (71,72). Dystrophin was normal but both α- and β-sarcoglycans were deficient in the skeletal and cardiac muscle. Specific mutations were not reported in any skeletal muscle proteins so the primary defect remains unknown. Since this report, δ-sarcoglycan has been identified as the primary missing component of the DGC in the cardiomyopathic hamster, so suggesting that this patient and others may harbor a mutation in the δ-sarcoglycan gene similar to the hamster (80).

In the AD LGMD, only LGMD1B maps to chromosome 1q11-21 and is associated with a cardiomyopathy (57,58). In 62.5% of affected patients, cardiac conduction system disturbances occur at about age 50 years. Because of atrioventricular conduction system disturbances, patients present with bradycardia and syncopal attacks necessitating pacemaker implantation. Sudden death may occur. The neuromuscular symptoms precede cardiac involvement in nearly every instance.

Laboratory Features

The serum CK is elevated 2- to 350-fold above normal in patients with recessive inheritance and from normal to 6-fold increases in dominantly inherited LGMD. Myopathic electromyograms and muscle biopsy features with nonspecific myopathic or dystrophic changes are characteristic.

A specific diagnosis can be established for α- and β-sarcoglycan deficiency using commercially available antibodies on muscle biopsy sections. Western blot analysis can also be done and represents a better method to quantitate the amount of deficient protein. Antibodies to other sarcoglycan proteins (β and δ) are not available on a widespread basis. Antibody to CAPN3 is also not generally available except by contacting the authors of previous publications (60–62).

Genetics

The LGMDs are inherited as AD (LGMD1A and 1B) or AR (LGMD2A–F) disorders. The chromosomal linkage

and specific gene defect, if known, are listed in Table 1. β-Dystroglycan deficiency awaits further confirmation before being assigned a specific number (76).

It was predicted from the initial discovery of the DGC that defects in other membrane proteins would account for some forms of muscular dystrophy. This prophecy has been more than fulfilled, as exemplified by LGMDs with defects in the sarcoglycans (α, β, λ, δ) (67–75). α-Sarcoglycan deficiency is the most common of these disorders. A wide range of gene mutations has been found for each of these proteins: more than 40 mutations of the α-sarcoglycan gene have been found; β-sarcoglycan deficiency, 6 mutations; λ-sarcoglycan deficiency, 8 mutations; δ-sarcoglycan deficiency, 8 mutations. These numbers can be expected to change as new mutations are found.

The molecular defect in LGMD2A reveals a defect independent of the membrane-associated proteins (59–62). CAPN3 is a muscle-specific calcium-activated neutral protease. The disorder was first recognized in patients residing in a community living on Reunion Island in the Indian Ocean and in families in Brazil and in Amish patients of northern Indiana (59). Additional families were found in the French metropolitan area of Bern, Switzerland (60–62). CAPN3 deficiency is unique thus far among these dystrophic conditions because the disease is caused by mutations of a gene encoding for an enzyme rather than a structural protein. Over 40 mutations of the CAPN3 gene have been described (61).

Molecular Pathogenesis of the Sarcoglycanopathies and Calpainopathies

Absent, deficient, or altered sarcoglycans can severely effect the membrane localization of the other sarcoglycans and the constituents of the DGC. α-Sarcoglycan deficiency appears to have the most profound effect on other components of the sarcoglycan complex (81). The net result of deficiency is membrane instability. Repeated tears in the sarcolemma cause leakage of CK into the serum. More importantly, calcium enters through the membrane tears, resulting in a cascade of events leading to muscle fiber necrosis. Over time, the regenerative capacity of the muscle cannot keep up with the loss of muscle fibers, leading to replacement by fat and connective tissue. This is the essence of the dystrophic process, simulating the pathogenic events in DMDs and BMDs.

The disease pathogenesis resulting from loss of CAPN3 is poorly understood. How the loss of enzyme function causes muscle fiber breakdown remains baffling. There is no evidence for accumulation of toxic products as might be anticipated in an enzyme-deficient state. One hypothesis suggests that CAPN3 may be important in signal transduction (62).

Treatment

Only supportive treatment is available for LGMD patients. Children can benefit from long leg braces. Use of a wheelchair for shopping or recreational activities will help preserve vital energy. In patients with life-threatening cardiomyopathy, pacemaker implantation (58) or heart transplantation (82) are life-saving.

CONGENITAL MUSCULAR DYSTROPHIES

Laminin α2 Chain Deficiency

The congenital muscular dystrophies represent a heterogeneous and confusing group of diseases (Table 2). Laminin α2, formerly merosin, is the heavy chain component of the heterotrimeric laminin-2 complex (5–7). Laminin α2 chain deficiency is a very unique variant of infantile congenital muscular dystrophy (83–86).

Clinical Features

The disease usually comes to attention at birth or in the first few months of life because of hypotonia, delayed motor milestones, and joint contractures affecting elbows, hips, knees, and ankles. Severe contractures at birth are referred to as arthrogryposis multiplex congenita. Congenital hip dislocation may be seen in occasional patients. The loss of strength involves proximal more than distal muscles, and facial muscle weakness may be present; other cranial nerve musculature is spared. Some patients have a mild peripheral neuropathy manifesting as mild sensory loss or decreased reflexes (87). The severity of the disease varies greatly. Approximately one half remain severely disabled, never achieving the ability to stand independently. Rarely, patients die of respiratory insufficiency during the first few years of life. In contrast, some patients do not exhibit severe contractures and will learn to walk, although difficulty in running and stair climbing persist. It may be difficult to distinguish some of these patients from either the dystrophinopathies or sarcoglycanopathies.

One distinguishing feature of congenital muscular dystrophy with laminin α2 chain deficiency is the cerebral white matter hypomyelination recognized by computed tomography or magnetic resonance imaging (83–86). The low-density areas may be diffuse and symmetric or focal; the hypodensity may diminish or disappear with time, suggesting a delay in myelination. Cortical dysplasia and polymicrogyria, in addition to white matter changes, are seen in some patients (85,86). Most patients have no intellectual impairment. Occasional patients exhibit epilepsy or rarely mental retardation (85,86).

Laboratory Features

The serum CK is variably elevated in this disorder. It tends to rise early in the course, especially in the postnatal period where values are six- to sevenfold above normal. Late in the course, the CK may range from normal to fourfold.

Muscle biopsy shows the nonspecific features of a dystrophic process with fiber size variability, scattered hypercontracted fibers, and occasional necrotic muscle fibers. Endomysial connective tissue proliferation and fat replacement for lost muscle fibers would be typical. A specific diagnosis of laminin α2 chain deficiency can be made by immunohistochemical studies demonstrating absence of staining surrounding each muscle fiber (83). Presently, only a commercial antibody to the carboxy terminal of laminin α2 chain is available, making it very difficult to diagnose partial deficiency states that require an additional antibody that recognizes defects in the mid or amino terminal regions of the protein (88).

Skin biopsy represents an important alternative to muscle biopsy for diagnosis of laminin α2 chain deficiency. This basal lamina protein is also found in the skin, and therefore a less invasive procedure can be offered for diagnosis. A punch biopsy of the skin can show absence of laminin α2 deficiency and suffice for diagnosis (89).

The computed tomography or magnetic resonance imaging can be a valuable adjunctive laboratory study because the finding of hypomyelination in the setting of muscular dystrophy with no signs or at best subtle signs of central nervous system disease is highly indicative of laminin α2 chain deficiency.

TABLE 2. *Congenital muscular dystrophies*

	La α2D	FCMD	WWS	MEB
Inheritance	AR	AR	AR	AR
Chromosomal localization	6q22-23	9q31-33	Unknown	Unknown
CWM hypomyelination	Yes	Yes	Yes	Sometimes
Cortical dysplasia	Rare	Yes	Yes	Yes
Mental retardation	Rare	Yes	Yes	Yes
Eye abnormalities	No	Mild	Severe	Severe
400 kDa laminin-α2 reduction	Mild–severe	Mild	No	Mild

AR, autosomal recessive; CWM, cerebral white matter; La α2D, laminin α2 chain deficiency; FCMD, Fukuyama congenital muscular dystrophy; WWS, Walker-Warburg syndrome; MEB, muscle-eye-brain disease.

Genetics

Laminin α2 chain deficiency is inherited as an AR trait. The laminin α2 chain gene localizes to chromosome 6q22-23 (90), and specific mutations or point mutations, small deletions, and splice site of the gene have been identified in some patients (91–95).

Molecular Pathogenesis

The finding of laminin α2 chain deficiency is specific for congenital muscular dystrophy with hypomyelination. Laminin α2 chain serves as the ligand for α-dystroglycan of the DGC, and deficiency of this protein disrupts the extracellular anchor for the DGC. It provides another example of a childhood muscular dystrophy caused by disrupting the link between the subsarcolemmal cytoskeleton and the extracellular matrix. Additional studies are required to elucidate the relationship of the central hypomyelination to laminin α2 chain deficiency.

Other Forms of Congenital Muscular Dystrophies

Three variants of congenital muscular dystrophy present with a combination of central nervous system, ocular, and muscle abnormalities (96–104). The best characterized of these entities is Fukuyama congenital muscular dystrophy (FCMD), a condition predominantly found in Japan with a frequency of 7 to 12 per 100,000 (96,97). Functional disability is usually severe. The maximum level of acquired motor function achieved is crawling, and most affected patients never learn to walk. They become bedridden before age 10, and most die by age 20. Severe mental retardation is observed in all cases. IQ scores in most FCMD patients lie between 30 and 50. Seizures are common. The most characteristic neuropathologic change is polymicrogyria of the cerebrum and cerebellum due to defects in neuronal migration. Hydrocephalus, focal interhemispheric fusion, and hypoplasia of the corticospinal tracts are also observed. The eye findings in FCMD are relatively mild, including moderate to high myopia, mottling of retinal pigment epithelium, and variable optic nerve atrophy.

FCMD is inherited as an AR trait. Recent linkage studies demonstrate localization of the gene for FCMD to chromosome 9q31-33 (105). The specific gene causing FCMD has not been found, but chromosomal markers have been identified that are useful for presymptomatic, prenatal, and carrier diagnoses of family members. The chromosome 9 linkage excludes the laminin α2 chain as causative in this disease.

A partial deficiency of the laminin α2 chain has also been demonstrated by immunohistochemistry; abnormalities, however, are not exclusive to the laminin α2 chain and involve other laminin subunits including laminin β

and λ (106). The molecular pathogenesis of FCMD is not understood.

In addition to FCMD, two other conditions, Walker-Warburg syndrome (WWS) (99,103) and muscle-eye-brain (MEB) disease (98,101,104), enter into the differential diagnosis of central nervous system abnormalities, ocular defects, and muscular dystrophy. Whether WWS and MEB disease represent one entity best lumped under the designation cerebrooocular dysplasia with congenital muscular dystrophy (102) or separate nosologic entities will only be determined by identification of the gene or genes. Those who insist they are separate highlight several distinctions. In WWS or lissencephaly type II, the smooth cerebral surface is usually associated with cephalocele, hemispheric fusion, agenesis of the corpus callosum, and arrhinencephalia along with extensive ocular abnormalities, including microphthalmia, colobomas, corneal opacities, congenital cataracts, immature anterior chamber angle, retinal dysplasia, and nonattachment (107). Patients with WWS are severely affected at birth and usually die in the first few months of life. In MEB, the brain lesions are much less severe and show pachygyria and polymicrogyria and a cobblestone appearance with limited areas of lissencephaly confined to the occipital region (104). The eye manifestations are less pronounced, similar to those of FCMD (107).

In both WWS and MEB disease, the inheritance pattern appears to be AR. Chromosomal linkage has not been established for either disease (108). Immunohistochemical studies suggest that components of the DGC and laminins may be involved in the pathogenesis, but the primary defects have not been identified (109,110).

Treatment

The treatment for all forms of congenital muscular dystrophies is supportive. Anticonvulsant therapy is mandatory for those with seizures. Passive stretching to correct contractures, night splints, and serial plaster casts may be useful. Tenotomies may be necessary for some patients to facilitate standing and ambulation.

SUMMARY

New discoveries have dramatically changed the way we approach and think about patients with childhood muscular dystrophies. We have learned that not all young boys with proximal muscle weakness, large calves, and elevated serum CK levels have DMD. A host of muscle membrane protein abnormalities have now become candidate disorders. Other conditions such as CAPN3 deficiency must also be considered. Knowledge of how to approach these disorders is incumbent on the clinician caring for these patients. Diagnostic conclusions have important implications for prognosis, family planning, and possible future therapeutic intervention.

REFERENCES

1. Koenig M, Hoffman EP, Bertelson EP, et al. Complete cloning of the Duchenne muscular dystrophy cDNA and preliminary genomic organization of the DMD gene in normal and affected individuals. *Cell* 1987;50:509–517.
2. Campbell KP. Three muscular dystrophies: loss of cytoskeleton-extracellular matrix linkage. *Cell* 1995;80:675–679.
3. Worton R. Muscular dystrophies: diseases of the dystrophin-glycoprotein complex. *Science* 1995;270:755–756.
4. Bonnemann CG, McNally EM, Kunkel LM. Beyond dystrophin: current progress in the muscular dystrophies. *Curr Opin Pediatr* 1996;8: 569–582.
5. Engvall E. Laminin variants: why, where and when? *Kidney Int* 1993; 43:2–6.
6. Ehrig K, Leivo I, Argraves WS, et al. Merosin, a tissue-specific basement membrane protein is a laminin-like protein. *Proc Natl Acad Sci USA* 1990;87:3264–3268.
7. Burgeson RE, Chiquet M, Deutzman R. A new nomenclature for the laminins. *Matrix Biol* 1994;14:209–211.
8. Chamberlain JS, Corrado K, Rafael JA, et al. Interactions between dystrophin and the sarcolemmal membrane. *Soc Gen Physiol Ser* 1997;52:19–29.
9. Peters MF, Adams ME, Froehner SC. Differential association of syntrophin pairs with the dystrophin complex. *J Cell Biol* 1997;138: 81–93.
10. Ahn AH, Freener CA, Gussoni E, et al. The three human syntrophin genes are expressed in diverse tissues, have distinct chromosomal locations, and each bind to dystrophin and its relatives. *J Biol Chem* 1996;271:2724–2730.
11. Hillaire D, Leclerc A, Faure S, et al. Localization of merosin-negative congenital muscular dystrophy to chromosome 6q2 by homozygosity mapping. *Hum Mol Genet* 1994;3:1657–1661.
12. Mendell JR, Sahenk Z, Prior TW. The childhood muscular dystrophies: diseases sharing a common pathogenesis of membrane instability. *J Child Neurol* 1995;10:150–159.
13. Brooke MH, Fenichel GM, Griggs RC, et al. Clinical investigation in Duchenne dystrophy. 2. Determination of the "power" of therapeutic trials based on the natural history. *Muscle Nerve* 1983;6:91–103.
14. Brooke MH, Fenichel GM, Griggs RC, et al. Duchenne muscular dystrophy: patterns of clinical progression and effects of supportive therapy. *Neurology* 1989;39:475–481.
15. Griggs RC, Reeves W, Moxley RT. The heart in Duchenne dystrophy. In: Rowland LP, ed. *Pathogenesis of human muscular dystrophy.* Amsterdam: Excerpta Medica, 1977.
16. Barohn RJ, Levine EJ, Olson JO, Mendell JR. Gastric hypomotility in Duchenne muscular dystrophy. *N Engl J Med* 1988;319:15–18.
17. Leibowitz D, Dubowitz V. Intellect and behaviour in Duchenne muscular dystrophy. *Dev Med Child Neurol* 1981;23:577–590.
18. Hyser CL, Mendell JR. Recent advances in Duchenne and Becker muscular dystrophy. *Neurol Clin* 1988;6:429–454.
19. Samaha FJ, Quinlan JG. Myalgia and cramps: dystrophinopathy with wide-ranging laboratory findings. *J Child Neurol* 1996;11:21–24.
20. Muntoni F, Cau M, Ganau A, et al. Brief report: deletion of the dystrophin muscle-promoter region associated with X-linked dilated cardiomyopathy. *N Engl J Med* 1993;329:921–925.
21. Gillard EF, Chamberlain JS, Murphy EG, et al. Molecular and phenotypic analysis of patients with deletions within the deletion-rich region of the Duchenne muscular dystrophy (DMD) gene. *Am J Hum Genet* 1989;45:507–520.
22. Forrest SM, Cross GS, Speer A, et al. Preferential deletion of exons in Duchenne and Becker muscular dystrophies. *Nature* 1987;329: 638–640.
23. Hu X, Ray P, Murphy EG, et al. Duplication mutation at the Duchenne muscular dystrophin locus: Its frequency, distribution, origin, and phenotype/genotype correlation. *Am J Hum Genet* 1990;46: 682–695.
24. Prior TW. Perspectives and molecular diagnosis of Duchenne and Becker muscular dystrophies. *Clin Lab Med* 1995;15:927–941.
25. Gangopadhyay SB, Sheratt TG, Heckmartt JZ, et al. Dystrophin in frameshift deletion patients with Becker muscular dystrophy. *Am J Hum Genet* 1992;51:562–570.
26. Roberts RG, Gardner RJ, Bobrow M. Searching for the 1 in 2,400,000: a review of dystrophin gene point mutations. *Hum Mutat* 1994;4:1–11.
27. Prior TW, Bartolo C, Pearl DK, et al. Spectrum of small mutations in the dystrophin coding region. *Am J Hum Genet* 1995;57:22–33.
28. Beggs AH, Koenig M, Boyce FM, Kunkel LM. Detection of 98% of DMD/BMD gene deletions by PCR. *Hum Genet* 1990;86:45–48.
29. Winnard AV, Mendell JR, Prior TW, et al. Frameshift deletions of exons 3–7 and revertant fibers in Duchenne muscular dystrophy: mechanisms of dystrophin production. *Am J Hum Genet* 1995;56: 158–166.
30. Prior TW, Papp AC, Snyder PJ, Mendell JR. Germline mosaicism in carriers of Duchenne muscular dystrophy. *Muscle Nerve* 1992;15: 960–963.
31. Luque ER. Segmental correction of scoliosis with rigid internal fixation: preliminary report in orthopaedic transections. *J Bone Joint Surg* 1977;2:136.
32. Karpati G, Watters GV. Adverse anaesthetic reactions in Duchenne dystrophy. In: Angelini C, Danielli GA, Fontanari D, eds. *Muscular dystrophy research: advances and new trends.* Amsterdam: Excerpta Medica, 1980.
33. Mendell JR, Moxley RT, Griggs RC, et al. Randomized, double-blind six-month trial of prednisone in Duchenne's muscular dystrophy. *N Engl J Med* 1989;320:1592–1597.
34. Griggs RC, Moxley RT, Mendell JR, et al. Prednisone in Duchenne dystrophy: a randomized, controlled trial defining the time course and dose response. *Arch Neurol* 1991;48:383–388.
35. Fenichel GM, Florence JM, Pestronk A, et al. Long term benefit from prednisone therapy in Duchenne muscular dystrophy. *Neurology* 1991;41:1874–1877.
36. Fenichel GM, Mendell JR, Moxley RT, et al. A comparison of daily and alternate-day prednisone therapy in the treatment of Duchenne muscular dystrophy. *Arch Neurol* 1991;48:575–579.
37. Pandya S, Moxley RT, Griggs RC, et al. Long-term prednisone treatment of Duchenne muscular dystrophy: Side effects and effectiveness. *Neurology* 1996;46:A308(abst).
38. Moxley RT, Lorenson M, Griggs RC, et al. Decreased breakdown of muscle protein after prednisone therapy in Duchenne dystrophy. *J Neurol Sci* 1990;98[Suppl]:419.
39. Kissel JT, Burrow KL, Rammohan KW, Mendell JR, CIDD Study Group. Mononuclear cell analysis of muscle biopsies in prednisone-treated and untreated Duchenne muscular dystrophy. *Neurology* 1991; 41:667–672.
40. Burrow KL, Coovert DD, Klein CJ, et al. Dystrophin expression and somatic reversion in prednisone-treated and untreated Duchenne dystrophy. *Neurology* 1991;41:661–666.
41. Dubrovsky AL, Mesa L, Marco P, et al. Deflazacort treatment in Duchenne muscular dystrophy. *Neurology* 1991;41[Suppl]:136.
42. Angelini C, Pegoraro E, Perini F. A trial with a new steroid in Duchenne muscular dystrophy. In: Angelini C, Danieli GA, Fontanari D, eds. *Dystrophy research.* New York: Elsevier, 1991:173–179.
43. Mesa LE, Dubrovsky AL, Corderi J, et al. Steroids in Duchenne muscular dystrophy—deflazacort trial. *Neuromusc Disord* 1991;4:261–266.
44. Loftus J, Allen R, Hesp R, et al. Randomized double blind trial of deflazacort versus prednisone in juvenile chronic (or rheumatoid) arthritis: a relative bone sparing effect of deflazacort. *Pediatrics* 1991; 88:428–436.
45. Brooke MH. A randomized trial of deflazacort and prednisone in Duchenne muscular dystrophy: effect and toxicity. *Neurology* 1996; 46:A476(abst).
46. Karpati G, Ajdukovic D, Arnold D, et al. Myoblast transfer in Duchenne muscular dystrophy. *Ann Neurol* 1993;34:8–17.
47. Tremblay JP, Malouin F, Roy R, et al. Results of a triple blind clinical study of myoblast transplantations without immunosuppresive treatment in young boys with Duchenne muscular dystrophy. *Cell Transplant* 1993;2:99–112.
48. Mendell JR, Kissel JT, Amato AA, et al. Myoblast transfer in the treatment of Duchenne muscular dystrophy. *N Engl J Med* 1995;333: 832–838.
49. Rafael JA, Yoshihide S, Cole NM, et al. Prevention of dystrophic pathology in mdx mice by a truncated dystrophin isoform. *Hum Mol Genet* 1994;3:1725–1733.
50. Rafael JA, Cox GA, Corrado K, et al. Forced expression of dystrophin deletion constructs reveals structure-function correlations. *J Cell Biol* 1996;134:93–102.
51. Wells DJ, Wells KE, Asante G, et al. Expression of human full-length and minidystrophin in transgenic mdx mice: implications for gene ther-

apy of Duchenne muscular dystrophy. *Hum Mol Genet* 1995;4: 1245–1250.

52. Walton JN, Nattrass FJ. On the classification, natural history and treatment of the myopathies. *Brain* 1954;77:169–231.

53. Bushby K, Beckmann JS. Report on the Thirtieth and Thirty-first ENMC International Workshops on the limb-girdle muscular dystrophies: proposal for a new nomenclature. *Neuromusc Disord* 1995;5: 337–343.

54. Bushby KMD. Diagnostic criteria for the limb-girdle muscular dystrophy: report of the ENMC consortium on limb-girdle dystrophies. *Neuromusc Disord* 1995;5:71–74.

55. Gilchrest JM, Pericak-Vance MA, Silverman L, Roses AD. Clinical and genetic investigations in autosomal dominant limb girdle dystrophy. *Neurology* 1988;37:5–9.

56. Speer MC, Yamaoka LH, Gilchrest JM, et al. Confirmation of genetic heterogeneity in limb-girdle muscular dystophy: linkage of an autosomal dominant form to chromosome 5q. *Am J Hum Genet* 1992;50: 1211–1217.

57. van der Kooi AJ, van Meegen M, Ledderhof TM, et al. Genetic localization of a newly recognized autosomal dominant limb-girdle muscular dystophy with cardiac involvement (LGMD1B) to chromosome 1q11-21. *Am J Hum Genet* 1997;60:891–895.

58. van der Kooi AJ, Ledderhof TM, de Voogt WG, et al. A newly recognized autosomal dominant limb girdle muscular dystrophy with cardiac involvement. *Ann Neurol* 1996;39:636–642.

59. Fardeau M, Hillaire D, Mignard C, et al. Juvenile limb-girdle muscular dystrophy. Clinical, histopathological and genetic data from a small community living in the Reunion Island. *Brain* 1996;119:295–308.

60. Richard I, Broux O, Allamand V, et al. A novel mechanism leading to muscular dystrophy: mutations in calpain 3 cause limb-girdle muscular dystrophy type 2A. *Cell* 1995;81:27–40.

61. Fardeau M, Eymard B, Mignard C, et al. Chromosome 15-linked limb-girdle muscular dystrophy: clinical phenotypes in Reunion Island and French metropolitan communities. *Neuromusc Disord* 1996;6:447–453.

62. Spencer MJ, Tidball JG, Anderson LVB, et al. Absence of calpain 3 in a form of limb-girdle muscular dystrophy (LGMD2A). *J Neurol Sci* 1997;146:173–178.

63. Bashir R, Keers S, Stachan T, et al. Genetic and physical mapping at the limb-girdle muscular dystrophy locus (LGMD2B) on chromosome 2p. *Genomics* 1996;33:46–52.

64. Noguchi S, McNally EM, Ben Othmane K, et al. Mutations in the dystrophin-associated protein λ-sarcoglycan in chromosome 13 muscular dystrophy. *Science* 1995;270:819–822.

65. McNally EM, Passos-Bueno MR, Bonnemann CG, et al. Mild and severe muscular dystrophy caused by a single gamma-sarcoglycan mutation. *Am J Hum Genet* 1996;59:1040–1047.

66. McNally EM, Duggan D, Gorospe R, et al. Mutations that disrupt the carboxyl-terminus of λ-sarcoglycan cause muscular dystrophy. *Hum Mol Genet* 1996;5:1841–1847.

67. Roberds S, Leturcq F, Allamand V, et al. Missense mutations in the adhalin gene linked to autosomal recessive muscular dystrophy. *Cell* 1994;78:625–633.

68. Piccolo F, Roberds SL, Jeanpierre M, et al. Primary adhalinopathy: a common cause of autosomal recessive muscular dystrophy of variable severity. *Nat Genet* 1995;10:243–245.

69. Eymard B, Romero NB, Leturcq F, et al. Primary adhalinopathy (α-sarcoglycanopathy): clinical, pathologic, and genetic correlation in 20 patients with autosomal recessive muscular dystrophy. *Neurology* 1997;48:1227–1234.

70. Carrié A, Piccolo F, Leturcq F, et al. Mutational diversity and hot spots in the α-sarcoglycan gene in autosomal recessive muscular dystrophy (LGMD2D). *J Med Genet* 1997;34:470–475.

71. Fadic R, Sunada Y, Waclawik AJ, et al. Deficiency of a dystrophin-associated glycoprotein (adhalin) in a patient with muscular dystrophy and cardiomyopathy. *N Engl J Med* 1996;334:362–366.

72. McNally EM, Bonnemann CG, Kunkel LM, Bhattacharya SK. Deficiency of adhalin in a patient with muscular dystrophy and cardiomyopathy [letter]. *N Engl J Med* 1996;334:1610–1611.

73. Bonnemann CG, Modi R, Noguchi S, et al. β-Sarcoglycan (A3b) mutations cause autosomal recessive muscular dystrophy with loss of the sarcoglycan complex. *Nat Genet* 1995;11:266–273.

74. Lim LE, Duclos F, Broux O, et al. β-Sarcoglycan: characterization and role in limb-girdle muscular dystrophy linked to 4q12. *Nat Genet* 1995;11:257–265.

75. Nigro V, de Sá Moreira E, Piluso G, et al. Autosomal recessive limb-girdle muscular dystrophy, LGMD2F, is caused by a mutation in the δ-sarcoglycan gene. *Nat Genet* 1996:195–198.

76. Salih MAM, Sunada Y, Al-Nassar M, et al. Muscular dystrophy associated with β-dystroglycan deficiency. *Ann Neurol* 1996;40:925–928.

77. Bejaoui K, Hirabayashi K, Hentati F, et al. Linkage of Miyoshi myopathy (distal autosomal recessive muscular dystrophy) locus to chromosome 2p12-14. *Neurology* 1995;45:768–772.

78. Weiler T, Greenberg CR, Nylen E, et al. Limb-girdle muscular dystrophy and Miyoshi myopathy in an aboriginal Canadian kindred map to LGMD2B and segregate with the same haplotype. *Am J Hum Genet* 1996;59:872–878.

79. Illarioshkin SN, Ivanova-Smolenskaya IA, Tanaka H, et al. Refined genetic location of the chromosome 2p-linked progressive muscular dystropy gene. *Genomics* 1997;42:345–348.

80. Nigro V, Okazaki Y, Belsito A, et al. Identification of the Syrian hamster cardiomyopathic gene. *Hum Mol Genet* 1997;6:601–607.

81. Vainzof M, Passos-Bueno MR, Canovas M, et al. The sarcoglycan complex in the six autosomal recessive limb-girdle dystrophies. *Hum Mol Genet* 1996;5:1963–1969.

82. Fadic R, Yoshihida S, Waclawik AJ, et al. Brief report: deficiency of a dystrophin-associated glycoprotein (adhalin) in a patient with muscular dystrophy and cardiomyopathy. *N Engl J Med* 1996;334:362–366.

83. Tome FMS, Evangelista T, Leclerc A, et al. Congenital muscular dystrophy with merosin deficiency. *CR Acad Sci Paris* 1994;317:351–357.

84. Vainzof M, Marie SKN, Reed UC, et al. Deficiency of merosin (laminin M or α2) in congenital muscular dystrophy associated with cerebral white matter alterations. *Neuropediatrics* 1995;26:293–297.

85. Sunada Y, Edgar TS, Lotz BP, et al. Merosin-negative congenital muscular dystrophy associated with extensive brain abnormalities. *Neurology* 1995;45:2084–2089.

86. Pini A, Merlini L, Tome FMS, et al. Merosin-negative congenital muscular dystrophy, occipital epilepsy with periodic spasms and focal cortical dysplasia. Report of three Italian cases in two families. *Brain Dev* 1996;18:316–322.

87. Shorer Z, Philpot J, Muntoni F, et al. Peripheral nerve involvement in congenital muscular dystrophy. *J Child Neurol* 1995;10;472–475.

88. Sewry CA, Naom I, Dálessandro M et al. Variable clinical phenotype in merosin-deficient congenital muscular dystrophy associated with differential Immunolabeling of two fragments of the laminin α2 chain. *Neuromusc Disord* 1997;7:169–175.

89. Sewry CA, Philpot J, Sorokin LM, et al. Diagnosis of merosin (laminin 2) deficient congenital muscular dystrophy by skin biopsy. *Lancet* 1996;347:582–584.

90. Hillaire D, Leclerc A, Faure S, et al. Localization of merosin-negative congenital muscular dystrophy to chromosome 6q2 by homozygosity mapping. *Hum Mol Genet* 1994;3:1657–1661.

91. Helbling-Leclerc A, Zhang X, Topaloglu H, et al. Mutations in the laminin α2-chain gene (LAMA) cause merosin-deficient congenital muscular dystrophy. *Nat Genet* 1995;11:216–218.

92. Nissenen M, Helbling-Leclerc A, Zhang X, et al. Substitution of a conserved cysteine 996 in a cysteine rich motif of the laminin alpha2-chain in congenital muscular dystrophy with partial deficiency of the protein. *Am J Hum Genet* 1996;58:1177–1184.

93. Guicheney P, Vignier N, Helbling-Leclerc A et al. Genetics of laminin α2 chain (or merosin) deficient congenital muscular dystrophy: from identification of mutations to prenatal diagnosis. *Neuromusc Disord* 1997;7:180–186.

94. Allamand V, Sunada Y, Salih MAM, et al. Mild congenital muscular dystrophy in two patients with an internally deleted laminin α2-chain. *Hum Mol Genet* 1997;6:747–752.

95. Mendell JT, Feng B, Sahenk Z, et al. Novel laminin α2 mutations in congenital muscular dystrophy. *Hum Mutat* (in press).

96. Fukuyama Y, Kawazura M, Haruna H. A peculiar form of congenital progressive muscular dystrophy. Report of 15 cases. *Paediatr Univ Tokyo* 1960;4:5–8.

97. Fukuyama U, Osawa M, Suzuki H. Congenital progressive muscular dystrophy of Fukuyama type—clinical, genetic, and pathologic considerations. *Brain Dev* 1981;13:1–29.

98. Santavuori P, Leisti J, Kruus S. Muscle, eye and brain disease. A new syndrome. *Neuropediatrics* 1977;8[Suppl 8]:553.

99. Warburg M. The heterogeneity of microphthalmia in the mentally retarded. *Birth Defects* 1971;7:136–154.

100. Dambska M, Wisniewski K, Sher J, Solish G. Cerebrooculomuscular

syndrome: a variant of Fukuyama congenital cerebromuscular dystrophy. *Clin Neuropathol* 1982;1:93–98.

101. Korinthenberg R, Pal D, Schlake W, Klein J. Congenital muscular dystrophy, brain malformations and ocular problems (muscle, eye, and brain disease) in two German families. *Eur J Pediatr* 1984;142:64–68.

102. Towfighi J, Sassani JW, Suzuki K, Ladda RI. Cerebrooculardysplasia-muscular dystrophy (COM-MD). *Acta Neuropathol* 1984;65:110–123.

103. Williams RS, Swisher CN, Jennings M, et al. Cerebro-ocular dysgenesis (Walker-Warburg syndrome): neuropathologic and etiologic analysis. *Neurology* 1984;34:1531–1541.

104. Haltia M, Leivo I, Somer H, et al. muscle-eye-brain disease: a neuropathological study. *Ann Neurol* 1997:41:173–180.

105. Toda T, Segawa M, Nomura Y, et al. Localization of a gene for Fukuyama type congenital muscular dystrophy to chromosome 9q31-33. *Nat Genet* 1993;5:283–286.

106. Hayashi Y, Engvall E, Arikawa-Hirasawa E, et al. Abnormal localization of laminin subunits in muscular dystrophies. *J Neurol Sci* 1993; 119:53–64.

107. Dobyns W, Pagon R, Armstrong D, et al. Diagnostic criteria for Walker-Warburg syndrome. *Am J Med Genet* 1989;32:195–210.

108. Ranta S, Pihko H, Santavuori P, et al. Muscle-eye-brain disease and Fukuyama type congenital muscular dystrophy are not allelic. *Neuromusc Disord* 1995;5:221–225.

109. Wever UM, Durkin ME, Shang X, et al. Laminin 2 chain and adhalin deficiency in the skeletal muscle of Walker-Warburg syndrome (cerebroocular dysplasia muscular dystrophy). *Neurology* 1995;45: 2099–2111.

110. Voit T, Sewry CA, Meyer K, et al. Preserved merosin M-chain (or laminin-α2) expression in skeletal muscle distinguishes Walker-Warburg syndrome from Fukuyama muscular dystrophy and merosin-deficient congenital muscular dystrophy. *Neuropediatrics* 1995;26: 148–155.

Motor Disorders,
edited by David S. Younger.
Lippincott Williams & Wilkins, Philadelphia © 1999.

CHAPTER 12

Distal Myopathies

Richard J. Barohn and Anthony A. Amato

Myopathic disorders generally produce proximal arm and leg weakness, a so-called limb girdle pattern. This is the most common presentation of inflammatory myopathies; muscular dystrophies; and congenital, endocrine, and toxic myopathies. Accordingly, patients with limb girdle weakness complain of difficulty in climbing stairs, rising from a chair or toilet, and other activities that require the arms to be raised. However, occasional patients will present with a pattern of distal arm and leg weakness due to myopathy, which is the subject of this chapter.

HISTORICAL PERSPECTIVE

Gowers (1) first described distal myopathy in two patients. One was an 18-year-old man with hand, foot, sternocleidomastoid, and facial weakness that some believe may have had myotonic dystrophy (2,3). The second patient was a 23-year-old woman with shoulder and distal leg weakness, most likely a scapuloperoneal syndrome. Gowers realized that it was remarkable that in both patients, leg weakness was confined to distal muscles.

In the few reports of the first half of the century of myopathic disorders with predominantly distal weakness, there was obvious difficulty in differentiating them from cases of Charcot-Marie-Tooth disease (4–9), but the absence of sensory symptoms involvement and lack of pathologic changes in the spinal cord and peripheral nerves at autopsy supported myopathy.

Wilson (2) raised the dilemma in this manner: "The question at issue is simply posed: does a distal *myogenic* type occur, analogous to the known *myelogenic* (neural) form termed **peroneal muscular atrophy**? At present, no definite answer can be returned, but no good reason for denying the possibility has been adduced. Of the genuineness of the type, 'I am myself convinced'."

Welander (10) clarified the existence of a true distal myopathy in her 1951 monograph describing a large Scandinavian cohort. This scholarly article has been so influential that many physicians describe any case of distal myopathy as "Welander myopathy." However, as discussed, in the years after Welander's publication, several other distinct forms of distal muscular dystrophy have since been described (Table 1).

WELANDER DISTAL MYOPATHY: LATE-ADULT ONSET TYPE 1

Welander (10) described 249 cases of distal myopathy in 72 families. The pattern of inheritance was autosomal dominant (AD). Affected patients developed symptoms in the fifth decade (mean, 47 years), with onset as late as 77 years, rarely before 30. Thus, Welander myopathy has been classified as a late-onset adult disorder differentiated from early adult-onset distal myopathies (11,12). Patients nearly always develop weakness first in the finger and wrist extensors and later in toe and ankle extensors. Only rarely does proximal limb involvement occur even with disease progression. Tendon reflexes remain present except for ankle jerks that are lost late in the disease. Sensation is normal, although recent studies have shown some deficits on quantitative temperature and vibration testing (13). The early studies did not report serum creatine kinase (CK) levels, because this test was not routinely used at that time (10,14,15). It has subsequently been shown that the CK is normal or slightly elevated in the disorder (16,17). Electrodiagnostic studies show normal motor and sensory nerve conduction results. Needle electromyography (EMG) shows myopathic motor units, although some authors have reported mixed myopathic and neuropathic patterns (16–19). Fibrillations are often, but not always, present.

R. J. Barohn: Department of Neurology, University of Texas Southwestern Medical Center at Dallas, Dallas, Texas 75235.

A. A. Amato: Department of Medicine/Neurology, University of Texas Health Science Center at San Antonio, San Antonio, Texas 78284.

TABLE 1. *Classification of distal myopathies*

Type	Inheritance	Gene localization	Initial weakness	CK	Biopsy
Welander—late adult type I	Autosomal dominant	2p13	Hands, fingers/wrist extensors	Normal or slightly increased	Myopathic; vacuoles in some cases
Markesbery—late adult type II	Autosomal dominant	2q31	Legs, anterior compartment	Normal or slightly increased	Vacuolar myopathy
Nonaka—early adult onset type I (familial IBM)[a]	Autosomal recessive or sporadic	9p1-q1	Legs, anterior compartment	Slightly to moderately increased, usually <5× normal	Vacuolar myopathy
Miyoshi—early adult onset type II (LGMD 2B)[b]	Autosomal recessive or sporadic	2p13	Legs, posterior compartment	Increased 10–150× normal	Myopathic, usually without vacuoles; gastrocnemius often "end stage"
Laing—early adult onset type III	Autosomal dominant	Chromosome 14	Legs, anterior compartment and neck flexors	Slightly increased, <3× normal	Moderate myopathic changes/no vacuoles
Myofibrillar (Desmin) myopathy—onset in childhood to fourth decade	Autosomal dominant or sporadic ? autosomal recessive / ? X linked	11q21–23 2q35 Chromosome 12	Hands or legs	Moderately increased, <5× normal	Myopathy, usually with vacuoles; subsarcolemmal granules or cytoplasmic bodies; desmin accumulations with antibody assay

[a]Autosomal recessive familial IBM, also known as quadriceps sparing myopathy, has been genetically linked with the Nonaka distal myopathy (50–52).
[b]LGMD type 2B has been genetically linked with Miyoshi distal myopathy (63).
CK; creatine kinase; IBM, inclusion body myopathy; LGMD, limb girdle muscular dystrophy.

Muscle biopsy shows dystrophic features, including variability in fiber size, increased connective tissue and fat, central nuclei, and split fibers (10). Vacuoles, a common feature in several of the distal dystrophies, were observed by some (10,16,17,20) but not all authors (14,15,19). When present, they are in some muscle fibers and are often not a conspicuous histologic feature. In the more recent Scandinavian reports in which rimmed vacuoles were also seen, 15- to 18-nm cytoplasmic and nuclear filaments were observed on electron microscopy (16,17). These filaments are commonly seen in inclusion body myositis (IBM) but not specific to it alone. According to Lindberg et al. (17), the main pathologic features that distinguish IBM from Welander myopathy are inflammatory cell infiltrates in IBM. Groups of small angular fibers occur, so suggesting a neurogenic component (20). The sural nerve can show a moderate reduction in myelinated fibers but not axonal degeneration or demyelination/remyelination (20). Mild neuropathic features, suggested clinically, electrophysiologically, and histopathologically, are a pattern seen often in some other forms of distal myopathy. Welander patients experience very slow progression of weakness. Many continue to work, and the duration of life is not reduced (10). Patients in Welander's group with a rapid aggressive course developed proximal weakness and were thought to be homozygous for the genetic defect (10,21). The genetic localization of Welander myopathy is unknown. Initially, the disorder was reported to not be linked to other distal myopathy gene loci on chromosome 2 and 14q (21a), however a preliminary communication recently found linkage at 2p13 (21b).

MARKESBERY DISTAL MYOPATHY: LATE ADULT ONSET, TYPE 2

Non-Scandinavian autosomal dominant (AD) late-onset distal myopathy has been described in English (22) and French-English (23) families. The large pedigrees and several sporadic cases recently reported from Finland described as "tibial muscular dystrophy" also fall into this category (24–26). Weakness begins in ankle dorsiflexor muscles of the anterior compartment of the distal leg in contrast to Welander myopathy in which weakness first affects the hands. Patients first develop weakness after age 40, and as the disease progresses, distal finger and wrist extensors of the upper extremities can become involved (Fig. 1), and much later, proximal weakness can occur. The patients described by Markesbery et al. (23) appeared to progress more quickly than those with Welander myopathy. One of Markesbery's patients had a cardiomyopathy with heart block and failure requiring a pacemaker. At autopsy, vacuoles were present in both cardiac and skeletal muscle (23). Whereas most Finnish patients progressed more slowly and rarely involved the upper extremity or proximal muscles (26), some from the pedigree in western Finland exhibited severe limb girdle syndrome (24,25). Udd et al. (25) suggested that those with typical limb girdle dystrophy might be a phenotype homozygous for the dominant gene. Serum CK is normal or slightly elevated. EMG

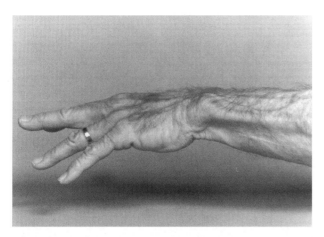

FIG. 1. Markesbery distal myopathy (late adult onset type 2). Note extensive forearm atrophy and weakness of finger extensors as patient attempts to raise fingers.

to Japan, although similar ones have since been reported from America (34–36), South America (37), and possibly from Italy (38), although the exact classification of the Italian family is unclear (39). Two cases reported by Walton and Nattras (40) probably fall into this category. Weakness begins late in the second or third decade with an average age at onset of 26 years. Initial weakness is in ankle dorsiflexor and toe extensor muscles, leading to foot drop and a steppage gait. Early in the disease, the finger and hand muscles can be weak but not as severe as the leg weakness. The degree of progression seems to be more aggressive in the non-Japanese cases. Weakness often remains distal in the Japanese cases, whereas non-Japanese cases eventually develop significant proximal weakness in the legs, arms, and neck muscles, and most lose the ability to walk (34). This degree of progression can also occur in Japanese patients (41). Complete heart block producing syncope and requiring a pacemaker has been reported (33).

Serum CK is slightly or moderately elevated but usually not more than five times normal. EMG studies reveal myopathic motor units and fibrillation potentials. The muscle biopsies from both Japanese and non-Japanese cases show vacuolar dystrophic myopathy (34–38,41) (Fig. 2A and B). The vacuoles are lined with granular material that is basophilic on staining with hematoxylin and eosin and purple-red with the modified Gomori trichrome stain, or so-called rimmed vacuoles. They exhibit acid phosphatase activity. On electron microscopy, in addition to autophagic vacuoles, some patients have nuclear or cytoplasmic 15- to 18-nm filamentous inclusions (42–44). Thus, these filaments, which were originally believed to be characteristic of IBM (see below), are seen in both Welander and Nonaka distal myopathies (45).

In this regard, it is interesting to discuss the cases that have been described as both "vacuolar myopathy sparing the quadriceps" (46) and some cases of "familial inclusion body myopathy" (47) (Table 1). The original cases

reveals small, brief, myopathic motor units with increased recruitment. Histologic findings reveal a dystrophic process. The striking feature in some patients was the presence of single or multiple vacuoles within many muscle fibers (23). In the Finnish patients, vacuoles were also occasionally present (24–26). The genetic defect in the Finnish families and in the Markesbery-Griggs kindred has recently been localized to 2q 31 (26a,26b).

NONAKA DISTAL MYOPATHY: EARLY ADULT ONSET, TYPE 1

Both forms of early adult-onset AR distal muscular dystrophy were first reported in the Japanese literature between 1963 and 1975 (27–30). They were not widely known in the West until Nonaka and colleagues published a series of papers on AR distal myopathy with rimmed vacuole formation (31–33). The cases have not been confined

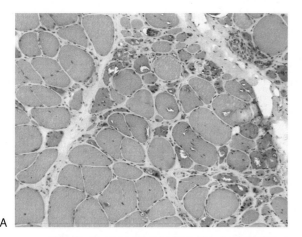
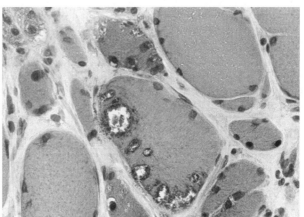

A   B

FIG. 2. Nonaka distal myopathy (early adult onset type 1). **A:** Muscle fiber size variability and rimmed vacuoles (hematoxylin & eosin; ×143). (From Ref. 11, with permission.) **B:** Multiple rimmed vacuoles at periphery of fiber (hematoxylin & eosin; ×575). (From Ref. 11, with permission.)

were described in Iranian Jews (46,48,49); however, the most recent ones are white American and Asian Indian (47). Clinically and histologically, they are indistinguishable from Nonaka distal myopathy. Like Nonaka myopathy, the inheritance pattern of hereditary IBM/quadriceps sparing myopathy is autosomal recessive (AR). Patients develop distal weakness in the anterior compartment of the legs as young adults, usually with a mean age at onset of 31 years (46). The weakness spreads to both proximal and distal muscles in the arms and legs, producing significant disability. A consistent clinical finding is the sparing of quadriceps muscle strength despite profound weakness of other proximal muscles at later stages. Mizusawa et al. (41) emphasized that the quadriceps were spared in their cases when proximal progression occurred. The pathology is identical in Nonaka myopathy and vacuolar myopathy sparing the quadriceps/familial IBM. In both disorders there is a vacuolar myopathy, no inflammation, and cytoplasmic and intranuclear 15- to 18-nm filaments. Given the striking clinical and pathologic similarity between Nonaka myopathy and vacuolar myopathy sparing the quadriceps/familial IBM, it is not surprising that both conditions have been localized to the 9p1-q1 gene locus by independent researchers (50–52). Thus, these disorders are the same and may be considered early adult-onset distal myopathy type 1.

It should be emphasized that the features that separate all these cases from sporadic IBM (see below) are early onset, initial symptoms in the ankle dorsiflexors, quadriceps sparing, AR inheritance, and lack of inflammation on muscle biopsy. Otherwise, routine light and electron microscopy findings are similar in all these disorders.

MIYOSHI DISTAL MYOPATHY: EARLY ADULT ONSET, TYPE 2

The early reports by Miyoshi et al. (29,30) of this disorder were largely unnoticed until their cases appeared in the Western literature (53). Since then, similar patients have been reported in the West (54–58a). As in Nonaka distal myopathy, symptoms develop between the ages of 15 and 25 and the disorder is transmitted in an AR pattern. However, in Miyoshi myopathy, the initial symptoms are in the gastrocnemius muscles, not the anterior compartment of the leg. Thus, patients notice that they cannot walk on their toes or climb stairs. Aching discomfort in the calves can occur. The gastrocnemius muscles become atrophic, and ankle muscle stretch reflexes are lost (Fig. 3). The muscles of the anterior compartment remain relatively spared early in the disease. The predilection for early involvement of the gastrocnemius muscles is the clinical hallmark of Miyoshi myopathy that distinguishes it from other distal dystrophies. Involvement of arms and hands is also unusual early in the disease. With progression, however, patients develop proximal arm and leg weakness of varying degrees. The hamstring muscle group (knee flexors) weaken more than

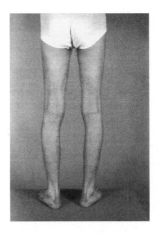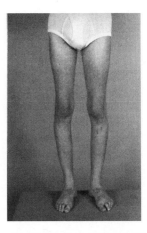

FIG. 3. Miyoshi distal myopathy (early adult onset type 2). Distal tapering with posterior compartment (gastrocnemius) atrophy. (From Ref. 57, with permission.)

the quadriceps muscles (knee extensors), and this may have implications for choice of biopsy site (57). Progression is variable with some patients remaining fairly stable with distal weakness, whereas others can have a more aggressive pattern involving both proximal and distal muscles (53).

The most characteristic laboratory finding in all Japanese and Western cases is a striking elevation of the serum CK from 20 to 150 times normal and usually between 5,000 and 20,000 IU/L. In some cases, an extremely high CK preceded clinical weakness or atrophy and was found during routine blood tests (56). Needle EMG reveals myopathic motor units and recruitment. However, in extremely weak and atrophic gastrocnemius muscles, motor units can be very sparse, and long-duration/polyphasic motor units with a decreased recruitment pattern can be seen. Muscle imaging has confirmed that the posterior compartment muscles of the distal lower extremity are generally more severely involved than those of the anterior compartment (58).

If a weak atrophic gastrocnemius muscle is biopsied, the usual finding is extensive fibrosis and fatty replacement with loss of most muscle fibers, a so-called end-stage muscle. On the other hand, if a relatively strong quadriceps muscle is biopsied, one can find minimal myopathic changes, including fiber size variability and central nuclei. Biopsy of an asymptomatic proximal arm muscle may also be relatively uninformative. We have found it useful to biopsy the biceps femoris in those cases with presumed intermediate histologic changes that includes striking fiber size variability and numerous necrotic and regenerating fibers (Fig. 4A–C). Both dystrophin and dystrophin-associated proteins are expressed normally on the muscle fibers (59). Although most cases of Miyoshi myopathy have not had vacuoles, we recently saw rimmed vacuoles in two cases (60). Thus, it appears that vacuole formation, although it may be more dramatic in some of

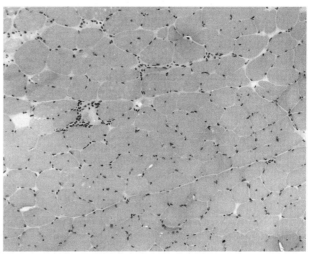

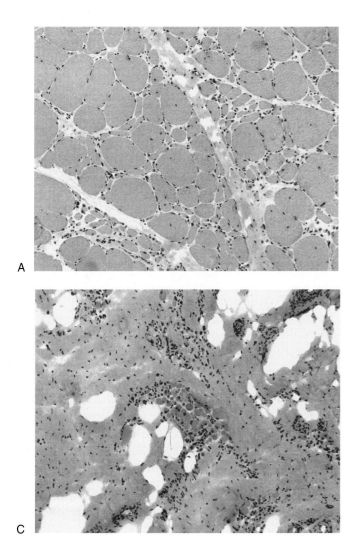

FIG. 4. Miyoshi distal myopathy (early adult onset type 2). **A:** Lateral gastrocnemius. Extensive fiber loss with replacement by connective and adipose tissue (hematoxylin & eosin; ×143). (From Ref. 11, with permission.) **B:** Vastus lateralis. Slight muscle size variability and a single necrotic fiber undergoing phagocytosis (hematoxylin & eosin). (From Ref. 11, with permission.) **C:** Biceps femoris. Changes intermediate to **A** and **B**, with variable muscle size, groups of small round fibers, and central nuclei (hematoxylin and eosin; ×143). (From Ref. 11, with permission.)

the distal myopathies, as for example, Nonaka myopathy, is ultimately a nonspecific histologic feature (45).

Miyoshi myopathy has recently been linked to chromosome 2p13; the gene has been cloned (61). The protein product of this gene has been called dysferlin (61a,61b); limb girdle muscular dystrophy (LGMD) type 2B has also been linked to this locus (62). Illarioshkin et al. (63) reported a large family in whom seven members had the typical LGMD clinical phenotype and three family members had distal myopathies. Both the LGMD and distal myopathy in this family were genetically linked to chromosome 2p13. The distal myopathy patients were different from the classic Miyoshi myopathy patients in that the anterior and posterior compartments of the legs were equally affected. Serum CK levels were elevated in both the LGMD and distal myopathy cases but more so in the patients with distal weakness, usually up to 56-fold normal. Muscle biopsy revealed nonspecific myopathic features, including autophagic vacuoles. Therefore, the clinical spectrum of chromosome 2p13 linked myopathies appears to be broad, and it is intriguing to speculate how different mutations in the chromosomal area and perhaps in the same gene give such disparate clinical phenotypes.

LAING DISTAL MYOPATHY: EARLY ONSET TYPE 3

Laing et al. (64) recently reported an Australian family of English/Welsh origin in which weakness begins in the anterior compartment of the legs and the neck flexors, followed by distal finger extensor involvement. Patients developed weakness between 4 and 25 years of age in an AD pattern. The serum CK was one to three times normal, and muscle biopsy showed moderate myopathic changes without vacuoles. The pedigree had nine affected members over four generations. The importance of this family is that genetic studies revealed linkage to chromosome 14. Although other cases with similar clinical features have not been described in the modern era, Laing et al. (64) believe their cases resemble the male patient Gowers described in 1902 (1). As previously mentioned, some authors believe the Gowers case may have had myotonic dystrophy (2,3,12). Whether or not the Gowers and Australian cases are the same disorder is primarily of historical interest and cannot be proven. However, these new cases are important because they provide us with another potential genetic region to explore in other distal myopathy patients. Hopefully, additional early adult-onset AD families will be reported to confirm the findings of Laing et al. (64). It is possible that the recent report of AD distal myopathy presenting in the first decade of life (65) and other early reports of childhood-onset distal myopathy may represent the same disorder (see below).

The genetic linkage of Miyoshi and Laing myopathies to 2p12-14 and 14, respectively, are important first steps toward a molecular understanding of these rare disorders. Until the genetic defects for the various distal muscular dystrophies have been discovered, we will need to continue to distinguish them based on their different clinical and laboratory features. The somewhat arbitrary nature of this type of classification is due to the overlapping clinical and histologic features. One can either lump all distal myopathies into one or two groups or split them into many categories. We have grouped them into six categories, the organization of which can expand or contract with subsequent understanding on a molecular level.

MYOFIBRILLAR MYOPATHY WITH ABNORMAL FOCI OF DESMIN

Another new category of distal myopathy has been proposed that is characterized by the pathologic finding of excessive desmin accumulation in muscle fibers (66–71). Desmin is not the only protein that accumulates in this disorder, and Nakano et al. (72) recommend the term "myofibrillar myopathy" because it may be a more accurate description of the spectrum of the pathogenic features. This was reported as desmin myopathy (73), desmin storage myopathy (74), spheroid body myopathy (75), cytoplasmic body myopathy (76), Mallory body myopathy and intermediate filament myopathy (77), familial cardiomyopathy with subsarcolemmal vermiform deposits (78), and myopathy with intrasarcoplamic accumulation of dense granulofilamentous material (79). In addition, some cases previously diagnosed with other forms of distal myopathy probably had myofibrillary myopathy. Of note is the family by Horowitz and Schmalbruch (69) with myofibrillary myopathy that was reported earlier by Milhorat and Wolff in 1943 (9) as distal myopathy. The latter was considered to have Markesbery myopathy (11) until the desmin stains were performed.

The clinical features are to an extent heterogeneous, and it is unclear if myofibrillar myopathy is a distinct entity. There is a wide clinical spectrum in the myopathies associated with focal desmin accumulation (66), the manifestations of which are extensively reviewed elsewhere (68). Most patients develop weakness between age 25 and 45, although there are reports of onset in infancy and later in life. In the Scandinavian cases of Edström et al. (67), weakness began at about age 40 in the distal upper arms (Fig. 5). In other cases, the distal legs exhibited weakness first, usually in the anterior compartment (68,69). A scapuloperoneal pattern was reported in a large pedigree (69a). Most patients have had an associated cardiomyopathy with heart block and arrhythmias, often requiring a pacemaker, and congestive heart failure. Progression to proximal muscles usually occurs, and some patients develop respiratory involvement requiring mechanical ventilation (69). Some patients develop cardiac symptoms before skeletal muscle weakness occurs. Children as young as 1 year can have diffuse primarily proximal or distal weakness. Several pediatric cases have been described with a giant axonal neuropathy associated with a desmin in cardiac and skeletal muscle; the family of Muntoni et al. (70) with cardiac and respiratory involvement and distal weakness also had mental retardation (70).

Most pedigrees have shown AD transmission, although X-linked inheritance was suspected in one family (70). There are also reports of sporadic and AR inheritance (68). Desmin is encoded by a single gene at 2q35 (66). Recently cases have been linked to desmin gene mutations (79a,79b). In a large AD scapuloperoneal pedigree, linkage was demonstrated to chromosome 12 (69a). Further, in an autosomal dominant family with myofibrillar myopathy a missense mutation on chromosome 11q21–23 in the α B-crystallin chaperone gene was identified (79c).

Serum CK levels are modestly elevated, usually less than five times normal. EMG shows a myopathic pattern with complex repetitive, myotonic, or pseudomyotonic discharges. Muscle biopsy demonstrates variability in fiber size, fiber splitting, increased central nuclei, and increased

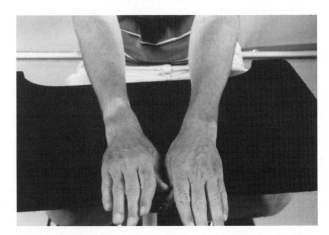

FIG. 5. Myofibrillary myopathy with abnormal foci of desmin. Note atrophy of the extensor forearm muscles.

connective tissue. Muscle fibers with rimmed vacuoles may also be evident. Subsarcolemmal cytoplasmic granular inclusions are seen, which are eosinophilic on hematoxylin and eosin stains and reddish or dark blue-green on the modified Gomori trichrome stain (Fig. 6A). In addition, dark-green smudges of amorphous material are also seen in Gomori trichrome stains (Fig. 6B). Immunohistochemistry reveals that these accumulations contain desmin (Fig. 6C). These deposits are amyloidogenic with Congo red staining (71). Excessive desmin accumulation has also been shown in cardiac muscles in patients with cardiomyopathy (70). Besides desmin, gelsolin, β-amyloid precursor protein, dystrophin, and neural cell adhesion molecule are also overexpressed (80).

Electron microscopy demonstrates two major types of lesions: foci of myofibrillar destruction and hyaline structures that appear as spheroidal bodies (72). The foci of myofibrillary destruction consist of disrupted myofilaments, Z-disk–derived bodies, dappled dense structures of Z-disk origin, and streaming of the Z-disk (78). The spheroidal bodies are composed of compacted and degraded remnants of thick and thin filaments (72). Although some authorities have demonstrated the accumulation of 8- to 10-nm filaments (81), others have not found these intermediate-sized filaments despite extensive searching (72).

Desmin is an intermediate filament protein of skeletal, cardiac, and some smooth muscles cells (66). This cytoskeletal protein links Z-bands with the plasmalemma and the nucleus. Although it seems clear that some distal myopathy patients do have abnormal desmin deposits, desmin accumulation is a nonspecific finding and can be seen in a variety of neuromuscular conditions, including X-linked myotubular myopathy, congenital myotonic dystrophy, spinal muscular atrophy, nemaline rod disease, fetal myotubes, and in regenerating muscle fibers of any etiology (66,82). Therefore, we can tentatively add myofibrillar myopathy, with abnormal foci of desmin, to the distal myopathy category scheme, keeping in mind the above caveats. Perhaps other previously reported cases of distal myopathy with cardiac abnormalities (23,36) should be restudied for desmin accumulation. Desmin antibody is commercially available, and immunohistochemical staining should probably be done on muscle biopsy specimens from all distal myopathy. Only in this manner can we determine if the presence of desmin accumulation actually is a marker for a unique myopathic condition.

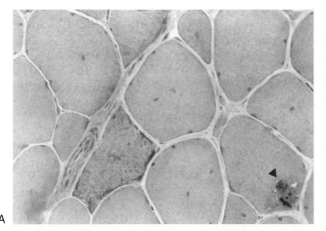

A

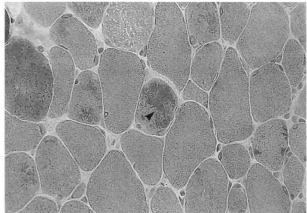

B

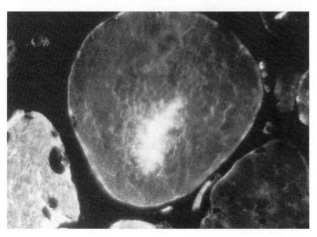

C

FIG. 6. Myofibrillary myopathy with abnormal foci of desmin. **A:** Focal granular cytoplasmic bodies and early vacuole formation (arrowhead) (modified trichrome, ×460). **B:** Dark green smudgy amorphous region (arrowhead) (modified trichrome, ×460). **C:** Focal nodular accumulations of desmin (immunofluorescence stain for desmin, ×800).

OTHER MYOPATHIES WITH DISTAL WEAKNESS

There are other myopathies that cause distal weakness; these are presented below and in Table 2.

Childhood-onset Distal Myopathy

There were early reports of infants that developed foot drop and finger/hand weakness before the age 2 years (83–85). This weakness was predominantly in ankle dorsiflexors, and wrist and finger extensor muscles, with AD transmission. Muscle biopsy and EMG supported a myopathic process but vacuoles were not seen. These cases remained either static after the teenage years or were very slowly progressive. All patients were ambulatory and quite active, and some were employed at work requiring extensive manual labor. The family recently described by Scoppetta et al. (65) can probably be placed in this clinical group.

One family with so-called juvenile-onset distal myopathy was also described (86). In this large Dutch pedigree, 19 members developed distal weakness in the hands and feet between ages 5 and 15 years. An AD inheritance was suspected. Both flexor and extensor distal muscle groups were affected. The disease progressed so slowly that the patients remained functional and active during adult life. Both myopathic and neuropathic features were seen on muscle biopsy and autopsy. These reports of childhood-onset distal myopathy preceded the availability of desmin staining, but there were no clues on light microscopy to suggest that excessive desmin may have been present. On the other hand, we mentioned earlier that the family

TABLE 2. *Other myopathies that can have distal weakness*

Childhood onset distal myopathy
Infantile onset (before age 2 yr)
Juvenile onset (before age 15 yr)
(? if these are Laing myopathy)
Myotonic dystrophy
Facioscapulohumeral dystrophy[a]
Scapuloperoneal myopathy[a]
Oculopharyngeal dystrophy
Emery-Dreifuss humeroperonal dystrophy[a]
Inflammatory myopathies
Inclusion body myositis
Polymyositis
Metabolic myopathy
Debrancher deficiency
Acid-maltase deficiency[a]
Congenital myopathy
Nemaline myopathy[a]
Central core myopathy[a]
Centronuclear myopathy
Nephropathic cystinosis
Myasthenia gravis

[a]Scapuloperoneal distribution of weakness can occur.

described by Scoppetta et al. (65) had many clinical similarities to Laing myopathy. It is possible that these early reports of childhood-onset distal myopathy could represent cases of Laing myopathy.

Other Muscular Dystrophies

Weakness of distal muscle groups may be prominent in some forms of muscular dystrophy. In myotonic dystrophy, wrist and finger extensors and ankle dorsiflexors are typically weaker than proximal limb muscles, especially early in the disease (87). Because the prevalence of myotonic dystrophy is 5 per 100,000 (88), it is probably the most commonly seen myopathic condition with prominent distal weakness, especially in the young and middle-aged groups. Rare patients with the phenotypic appearance of myotonic dystrophy and distal weakness but without clinical or electrical myotonia have been described (89). Patients with fascioscapulohumeral (FSH) dystrophy can develop weakness of ankle dorsiflexion and wrist and finger extension along with typical facial and scapular muscle involvement. Rarely, they can present with ankle weakness (90). Indeed, the presence of foot dorsiflexor weakness is included in the diagnostic criteria for FSH dystrophy (91). FSH dystrophy has been mapped to chromosome 4q35 (92). Patients with the so-called myopathic form of the scapuloperoneal syndrome have significant ankle weakness (93). Now that we know the genetic localization of FSH dystrophy, it can be shown that some, but not all, patients with scapuloperoneal myopathy may be variants of FSH (94,95). Recently, a large family with a scapuloperoneal myopathy was found to have genetic linkage to chromosome 12 (96). Patients with the X-linked Emery-Dreifuss disease, also known as humeroperoneal muscular dystrophy, present with ankle dorsiflexion, triceps and biceps weakness, along with contraction at the elbow and ankle (97). Some pedigrees of oculopharyngeal muscular dystrophy also have significant distal extremity weakness (98–101).

Inflammatory Myopathies

Rare cases of polymyositis have been described in which patients first develop weakness of the hands and ankles (102,103). Biopsy of proximal muscles revealed an inflammatory myopathy, and patients improved with steroid therapy. A more frequent situation in which an inflammatory myopathy presents with early distal weakness occurs with sporadic cases of IBM (104–107). Sporadic IBM accounts for approximately a third of all cases of inflammatory myopathy and is probably the most common cause of distal weakness due to a myopathy in elderly patients. IBM patients develop slowly progressive weakness, usually after the age of 50. The slow evolution of the disease is one of the primary reasons for the delay in diagnosis, which averages approximately 6 years from the onset of symptoms. The pattern of weakness in IBM is unique in that the clinical hallmark is early weakness and atrophy of wrist and finger flexors, quadriceps, and ankle dorsiflexors (Fig. 7A and B). Toe flexors are also frequently weak, sometimes producing a position of chronic great toe extension, or a pseudo-Babinski sign (Fig. 7C). Some degree of asymmetry in muscle weakness is the rule. Because of the dramatic knee extensor involvement, it is not exclusively a distal myopathy, although distal upper extremity flexor weakness is an invariable component of the disease. Both knee extensor and forearm and finger flexor weakness are included in the new clinical diagnostic criteria for IBM (105). Severe weakness in these muscle groups is so characteristic of

IBM that even if the classic histologic findings are not present on muscle biopsy, a presumptive diagnosis of "possible" IBM should be considered (106).

Classic light microscopy features are endomysial inflammation with invasion of nonnecrotic muscle fibers, eosinophilic cytoplasmic inclusions, and rimmed vacuoles within the muscle fibers that contain amyloid deposits (Fig. 8A) (105). On electron microscopy, there is an accumulation of cytoplasmic and intranuclear 15- to 21-nm filaments (Fig. 8B). Although inflammation is nearly always present, the other pathologic features may not be identified on the initial muscle biopsy, often requiring a second or third biopsy for confirmation (106). The histologic similarities between IBM and both Welander and Nonaka

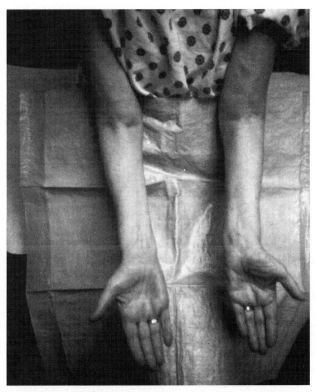

A

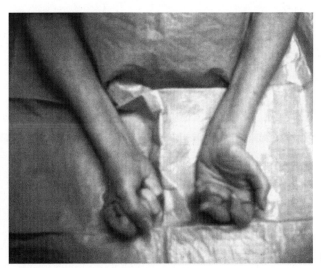

B

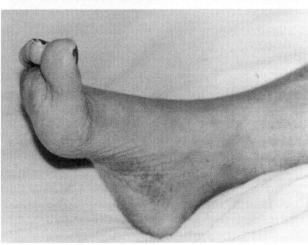

C

FIG. 7. Inclusion body myositis. **A:** Note bilateral atrophy of the flexor forearm muscles. **B:** Same patient as in A. Note inability to flex fingers completely in the left hand. **C:** Pseudo-Babinski sign with chronic toe extension due to weakness of toe flexors.

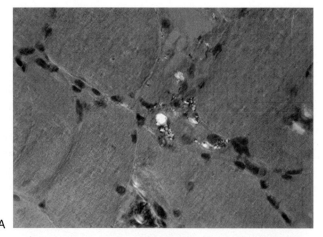

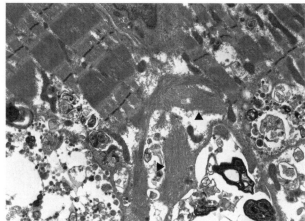

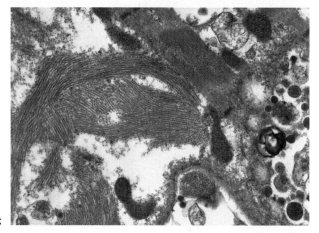

FIG. 8. Inclusion body myositis. **A:** Apple green birefringence indicating amyloid deposition (Congo red under polarized light, ×675). **B:** Electron microscopy showing the edge of a vacuole (with adjacent normal sarcomeres) containing cytoplasmic debris and 15- to 18-nm filaments (arrowheads) (×10,800). (Courtesy of Dennis Burns, MD.) **C:** Higher magnification of 15- to 18-nm filaments (×20,000) (Courtesy of Dennis Burns, MD.)

myopathy have already been described. Mendell et al. (108) found amyloidogenic green-birefringent deposits with Congo red stain in IBM biopsies. However, in that series, the single case of distal myopathy with rimmed vacuoles in the control group also showed these deposits. On histologic grounds, the presence of inflammation may be the only pathologic findings to differentiate IBM from distal muscular dystrophies.

On the other hand, despite the presence of inflammation in IBM, the disease is typically refractory to immunosuppressive therapy. The lack of response to immunosuppressive treatment distinguishes IBM from polymyositis and dermatomyositis. When patients with IBM are placed on prednisone therapy, strength continues to deteriorate, despite a decrease in serum CK and the suppression of inflammation on repeat muscle biopsy (109). In addition, although the inflammation decreases, the number of fibers with vacuoles and amyloid deposits increases over time (109). Finally, it has been shown that there is an accumulation of "Alzheimer-characteristic" proteins in vacuolated muscle fibers such as β-amyloid and paired helical filament-tau in IBM tissue (105). These observations suggest that IBM may be a degenerative rather than an autoimmune inflammatory myopathy and that the inflammation is a secondary response. Seen in this way, it may not be sur-

prising that there are many pathologic similarities between the distal muscular dystrophies and IBM.

AR familial inclusion body myopathy (47) was described in the section regarding Nonaka distal myopathy as recent linkage analyses support that they are the same myopathic disorder (51,52).

Table 3 lists the diseases that have been reported to have both vacuoles and 15- to 18-nm filaments. These filaments can be seen in both the cytoplasm or nucleus in all disorders except oculopharyngeal dystrophy and its distal variant, oculopharyngodistal dystrophy. In the oculopharyngeal dystrophies, the nuclear filaments are 8 to 10 nm and the cytoplasmic filaments are 15 to 18 nm.

Metabolic and Congenital Myopathies

Debrancher enzyme deficiency has been reported with severe distal leg weakness (110). We have recently observed a 30-year-old man with adult-onset acid-maltase deficiency who presented with a scapuloperoneal pattern of weakness (111).

Patients with nephropathic cystinosis develop a distal myopathy as a late complication of the disease. This is an AR lysosomal storage disorder in which cystine accumulates and leads to renal failure. Patients who survive child-

TABLE 3. *Myopathies with vacuoles and 15 to 18 nm filaments*

Inclusion body myositis
Welander myopathy
Nonaka myopathy/familial inclusion body myopathy/quadriceps sparing myopathy
Oculopharyngeal/adystrophy
Oculopharyngodistal dystrophy[a]

[a]Intranuclear nuclear filaments 8–10 nm also present.

hood due to renal transplantation develop weakness and wasting in the hand muscles. Electrodiagnostic studies are consistent with a myopathic process, and muscle biopsy of hand muscles shows a vacuolar myopathy (112).

Nonprogressive congenital muscle diseases such as nemaline rod (113–115), central core (116), and centronuclear myopathy (117) can have significant involvement of distal muscles. AD nemaline myopathy has been shown to be due to a mutation of the α-tropomyosin gene on chromosome 1 (114,115). In the Australian pedigree, patients first develop symptoms in late childhood, and ankle dorsiflexion weakness is the initial and most significant manifestation of the disease (114,115).

Myasthenia Gravis

Most patients with myasthenia gravis present with ocular, bulbar, and proximal limb muscle weakness (118). Rarely, their weakness can be distally prominent. We identified 7 of 234 (3%) patients with myasthenia gravis and primarily distal muscle weakness, mainly in finger extensors, followed by finger interossei. One patient had distal lower extremity weakness of the ankle dorsiflexors. In addition to the distal weakness, all had ocular and/or bulbar involvement and circulating antibodies to the acetylcholine receptor. The distal weakness in six patients improved with immunosuppressive therapy.

REFERENCES

1. Gowers WR. A lecture on myopathy and a distal form. *Br Med J* 1902;2:89–92.
2. Wilson SAK. *Neurology.* Vol. 2. London: Edward Arnold & Co., 1940:982–983.
3. Gardner-Medwin D, Walton J. The muscular dystrophies. In: Walton J, Karpati G, Hilton-Jones D, eds. *Disorders of voluntary muscle,* 6th ed. Edinburgh: Churchill Livingston, 1994:580.
4. Dejerine J, Thomas A. Un cas de myopathie a topographie type Aran-Duchenne suivi d'autopsie. *Rev Neurol* 1904;12:1187–1190.
5. Cambell CM. A case of muscular dystrophy affecting hand and feet. *Rev Neurol Psychiatry* 1906;4:192–202.
6. Spiller WG. Myopathy of a distal type and its relation to the neural form of muscular atrophy (Charcot-Marie-Tooth type). *J Nerv Mend Dis* 1907;34:14–30.
7. Batten FE. Distal type of myopathy. *Proc R Soc Med* 1910;3:92–93.
8. Batten FE. Distal type of myopathy in several members of a family. *Proc R Soc Med* 1910;3:93–95.
9. Milhorat AT, Wolff HG. Studies in diseases of muscle. XII. Progressive muscular dystrophy of atrophic distal type; report on a family; report of an autopsy. *Arch Neurol Psychiatry* 1943;49:655–664.
10. Welander L. Myopathia distalis tarda hereditaria. *Acta Med Scan* 1951;141[Suppl 265]:1–124.
11. Barohn RJ. Distal myopathies and dystrophies. *Sem Neurol* 1993;13:247–255.
12. Griggs RC, Markesbery WR. Distal myopathies. In: Engel A, Franzini-Armstrong C, eds. *Myology,* 2nd ed. New York: McGraw-Hill, 1994:1246–1257.
13. Borg K, Borg J, Lindblom U. Sensory involvement in distal myopathy (Welander). *J Neurol Sci* 1987;80:323–332.
14. Dahlgaard E. Myopathia distalis tarda hereditaria. *Acta Psychiatr Neurol Scand* 1960;35:440–447.
15. Barrows HS, Duemler LP. Late distal myopathy. Report of a case. *Neurology* 1962;12:547–550.
16. Borg K, Tome F, Edström L. Intranuclear and cytoplasmic filamentous inclusions in distal myopathy (Welander). *Acta Neuropathol* 1991;82:102–106.
17. Lindberg C, Borg K, Edström L, et al. Inclusion body myositis and Welander distal myopathy: a clinical, neurophysiological and morphological comparison. *J Neurol Sci* 1991;103:76–81.
18. Borg K, Åhlberg G, Borg J, Edström L. Welander's distal myopathy: clinical, neurophysiological and muscle biopsy observations in young and middle aged adults with early symptoms. *J Neurol Neurosurg Psychiatry* 1991;54:494–498.
19. Edström L. Histochemical and histopathological changes in skeletal muscle in late-onset hereditary distal myopathy (Welander). *J Neurol Sci* 1975;26:147–157.
20. Borg K, Solders G, Borg J, et al. Neurogenic involvement in distal myopathy (Welander). *J Neurol Sci* 1989;91:53–70.
21. Welander L. Homozygous appearance of distal myopathy. *Acta Genet* 1957;7:321–325.
21a. Åhlberg G, Borg K, Edstrom L, Anvret M, Welander distal myopathy is not linked to other defined distal myopathy gene loci. *Neuromusc Disord* 1997;7:256–260.
21b. Åhlberg G, Borg J, Ansved L, Edström L, Anvent M. Welander distal myopathy: genetic linkage and candidate gene on chromosome 2p. *Muscle Nerve* 1998;21:56.
22. Sumner D, Crawfurd Md'A, Harriman DGF. Distal muscular dystrophy in an English family. *Brain* 1971;94:51–60.
23. Markesbery WR, Griggs RC, Leach RP, et al. Late onset hereditary distal myopathy. *Neurology* 1974;23:127–134.
24. Udd, B, Kääriänen H, Somer H. Muscular dystrophy with separate clinical phenotypes in a large family. *Muscle Nerve* 1991;14:1050–1058.
25. Udd B, Partanen J, Halonen P, et al. Tibial muscular dystrophy: late adult-onset distal myopathy in 66 Finnish patients. *Arch Neurol* 1993;50:604–608.
26. Partanen J, Laulumaa V, Paljärve, et al. Late onset foot-drop muscular dystrophy with rimmed vacuoles. *J Neurol Sci* 1994;125:158–167.
26a. Haravuori H, Mäkelä-Bengs P, Figlewicz D, et al. Tibial muscular dystrophy and late-onset distal myopathy are linked to the same locus on chromosome 2q. *Neurology* 1998;50:A186.
26b. Havavuori H, Mäkelä-Bengs P, Udd B, et al. Assignment of the tibial muscular dystrophy locus to chromosome 2q31. *Am J Hum Genet* 1998;62:620–626.
27. Murone I, Sato T, Shirakawa K, et al. Distal myopathy—a case of non-hereditary distal myopathy. *Clin Neurol (Tokyo)* 1963;:378–386 (in Japanese with English abstract).
28. Sasaki K, Mori H, Takahashi K, et al. Distal myopathy—report of four cases. *Clin Neurol (Tokyo)* 1969;9:627–637 (in Japanese with English abstract).
29. Miyoshi K, Saijo K, Kuryu Y, et al. Four cases of distal myopathy in two families. *Jpn J Human Genet* 1967;12:113 (abstract in Japanese).
30. Miyoshi K, Tada Y, Iwasa M, et al. Autosomal recessive distal myopathy observed characteristically in Japan. *Jpn J Human Genet* 1975;20:62–63 (abstract in English).
31. Nonaka I, Sunohara N, Ishiura S, et al. Familial distal myopathy with rimmed vacuole and lamellar (myeloid) body formation. *J Neurol Sci* 1981;51:141–155.
32. Nonaka I, Sunohara N, Satoyoshi E, et al. Autosomal recessive distal muscular dystrophy: a comparative study with distal myopathy with rimmed vacuole formation. *Ann Neurol* 1985;17:51–59.
33. Sunohara N, Nonaka I, Kamei N, et al. Distal myopathy with rimmed vacuole formation: a follow-up study. *Brain* 1989;112:65–83.
34. Markesbery WR, Griggs RC, Herr B. Distal myopathy: electron microscopic and histochemical studies. *Neurology* 1977;27:727–735.

35. Miller RG, Blank NK, Layzer RB. Sporadic distal myopathy with early adult onset. *Ann Neurol* 1979;5:220–227.

36. Krendel D, Gilchrist J, Bossen E. Distal vacuolar myopathy with complete heart block. *Arch Neurol* 1988;45:698–699.

37. Isaacs H, Badenhorst M, Whistler T. Autosomal recessive distal myopathy. *J Clin Pathol* 1988;41:188–194.

38. Scoppetta C, Vaccario ML, Casali C, et al. Distal muscular dystrophy with autosomal recessive inheritance. *Muscle Nerve* 1988;7:478–481.

39. Somer H. Distal myopathies: 25th ENMC international workshop. *Neuromusc Disord* 1995;5:249–252.

40. Walton JN, Nattras FJ. On the classification, natural history and treatment of the myopathies. *Brain* 1954;77:169–231.

41. Mizusawa H, Kurisaki H, Takatsu M, et al. Rimmed vacuolar distal myopathy: a clinical, electrophysiological, histopathological and computed tomographic study of seven cases. *J Neurol* 1987;234:129–136.

42. Kumamota T, Fukuhara N, Naguishima M, et al. Distal myopathy: histochemical and ultrastructural studies. *Arch Neurol* 1982;51:141–155.

43. Matsubara S, Tannabe H. Hereditary distal myopathy with filamentous inclusions. *Acta Neurol Scand* 1982;65:363–368.

44. Mizusawa H, Kurisaki H, Takatsu M, et al. Rimmed vacuolar distal myopathy. An ultrastructural study. *J Neurol* 1987;234:137–145.

45. Jongen PJH, Laak HJT, Stadhouders AM. Rimed basophilic vacuoles and filamentous inclusions in neuromuscular disorders. *Neuromusc Disord* 1995; 5:31–38.

46. Sadeh M, Gadoth N, Hadar H, et al. Vacuolar myopathy sparing the quadriceps. *Brain* 1993;116:217–232.

47. Sivakumar K, Dalakas MC. The spectrum of familial inclusion body myopathies in 13 families and a description of a quadriceps-sparing phenotype in non-Iranian Jews. *Neurology* 1996;47:977–984.

48. Argov Z, Yarom R. "Rimmed vacuole myopathy" sparing the quadriceps: a unique disorder in Iranian Jews. *J Neurol Sci* 1984;64:33–43.

49. Massa R, Weller W, Karpati G, et al. Familial inclusion body myositis among Kurdish-Iranian Jews. *Arch Neurol* 1991;48:519–522.

50. Askanas V. New developments in hereditary inclusion body myopathies. *Ann Neurol* 1997;41:421–422.

51. Ikeuchi T, Asaka T, Saito M, et al. Gene locus for autosomal recessive distal myopathy with rimmed vacuoles maps to chromosome 9. *Ann Neurol* 1997;41:432–437.

52. Argov Z, Tiram E, Eisenberg I, et al. Hereditary inclusion body myopathy maps to chromosome 9p1-q1. *Ann Neurol* 1997;41:548–551.

53. Miyoshi K, Kawai H, Iwasa M, et al. Autosomal recessive distal muscular dystrophy. *Brain* 1986;109:31–54.

54. Kuhn E, Schroder M. A new type of distal myopathy in two brothers. *J Neurol* 1981;226:181–185.

55. Alderson MK, Ziter F. Distal muscular dystrophy [Letter]. *Muscle Nerve* 1985;8:7235.

56. Galassi G, Rowland LP, Hays A, et al. High serum levels of creatine kinase: asymptomatic prelude to distal myopathy. *Muscle Nerve* 1987;10:346–350.

57. Barohn RJ, Miller RG, Griggs RC. Autosomal recessive distal dystrophy. *Neurology* 1991;41:1365–1370.

58. Meola G, Sansone V, Rotondo G, et al. Computerized tomography and magnetic resonance muscle imaging in Miyoshi's myopathy. *Muscle Nerve* 1996;19:1476–1480.

58a. Linssen WHJP, Notermans NC, Van der Graaf Y, et al. Miyoshi-type distal muscular dystrophy. Clinical spectrum in 24 Dutch patients. *Brain* 1997;120:1989–1996.

59. Yamanouchi Y, Ozawa E, Nonaka I. Autosomal recessive distal muscular dystrophy: normal expression of dystrophin, utrophin and dystrophin-associated proteins in muscle fibers. *J Neurol Sci* 1994;126:70–76.

60. Shaibani A, Harati Y, Amato A, Ferrante M. Miyoshi myopathy with vacuoles. *Neurology* 1997;47[Suppl]:A195.

61. Bejaoui K, Hirabayashi K, Hentati F, et al. Linkage of Miyoshi myopathy (distal autosomal recessive muscular dystrophy) locus to chromosome 2p12-14. *Neurology* 1995;45:768–772.

61a. Liu J, Aoki M, Illa I, et al. Dysferlin, a novel skeletal muscle gene, is mutated in Miyoshi myopathy and limb girdle muscular dystrophy. *Nature Genetics* 1998:20:31–36.

61b. Bashir R, Britton S, Strachan T, et al. A gene related to caenorhabditis elegans spermatogenesis factor Fer-1 is mutated in limb-girdle muscular dystrophy type 2B. *Nature Genetics* 1998;20:37–42.

62. Bashir R, Strachan T, Keers S, et al. A gene for autosomal recessive limb-girdle muscular dystrophy maps to chromosome 2. *Hum Mol Genet* 1994;3:455–457.

63. Illarioshkin SN, Ivanova-Smoleskaya IA, Tanaka H, et al. Clinical and molecular analysis of a large family with 3 distinct phenotypes of progressive muscular dystrophy. *Brain* 1996;119:1895–1909.

64. Laing NG, Laing BA, Meredith C, et al. Autosomal dominant distal myopathy: Linkage to chromosome 14. *Am J Hum Genet* 1995;56:422–427.

65. Scoppetta C, Casali C, La Cesa I, et al. Infantile autosomal dominant distal myopathy. *Acta Neurol Scand* 1995;92:122–126.

66. Goebel HH. Desmin-related neuromuscular disorders. *Muscle Nerve* 1995;18:1306–1320.

67. Edström L, Thornell LE, Eriksson A. A new type of hereditary distal myopathy with characteristic sarcoplasmic bodies and intermediate (Skeletin) filaments. *J Neurol Sci* 1980;47:171–190.

68. Helliwell TR, Green ART, Green A, et al. Hereditary distal myopathy with granulo-filamentous cytoplasmic inclusions containing desmin, dystrophin and vimentin. *J Neurol Sci* 1994;124:174–187.

69. Horowitz S, Schmalbruch H. Autosomal dominant distal myopathy with desmin storage: a clinicopathologic and electrophysiologic study of a large kinship. *Muscle Nerve* 1994;17:151–160.

69a. Wilhelmsen KC, Blake DM, Lynch T, et al. Chromosome 12-linked autosomal dominant scapuloperoneal muscular dystrophy. *Ann Neurol* 1996;39:507–520.

70. Muntoni F, Catani G, Mateddu A, et al. Familial cardiomyopathy, mental retardation and myopathy associated with desmin-type intermediate filaments. *Neuromusc Disord* 1994;4:233–241.

71. Amato AA, Kagan-Hallet K, Jackson CE, Lampkins S, Wolfe GI, Ferrante M, Bigio E, Barohn RJ. The wide-spectrum of myofibrillar myopathy suggests a multifactorial etiology and pathogenesis. *Neurology* 1998;51:1646–1655.

72. Nakano S, Engel AG, Waclwik AJ, Emslie-Smith AM, Busis NA. Myofibrillary myopathy with abnormal foci of desmin positivity. I. Light and electron microscopy analysis of 10 cases. *J Neuropath Exp Pathol* 1996;55:549–562.

73. Cameron CHS, Mirakhur M, Allen IV. Desmin myopathy with cardiomyopathy. *Acta Neuropath* 1995;89:560–566.

74. Fardeau M, Tomé FMS. Congenital myopathies. In: Engel AG, Fanzini-Armstron C, eds. *Myology,* 2nd ed. New York: McGraw-Hill Inc., 1994: 522–526.

75. Goebel HH, Muller J, Gillen HW, Merrit AD. Autosomal dominant "spheroidal body myopathy." *Muscle Nerve* 1978;1:14–26.

76. Caron A, Viaer F, Lechevalier B, Chapon F. Cytoplasmic body myopathy: familial cases with accumulation of desmin and dystrophin. A immunohistochemical, immunoelectron microscopic and biochemical study. *Acta Neuropathol* 1995;90:150–157.

77. Fidzianska A, Goebel HH Osborn M, Lenard HG, Osse G, Langenbeck U. Mallory body-like inclusions in a hereditary congenital neuromuscular disease. *Muscle Nerve* 1983;6:195–200.

78. Carderon A, Becker LE, Murphy EG. Subsarcolemmal vermiform deposits in skeletal muscle associated with familial cardiomyopathy: report of two cases of a new entity. *Pediatr Neurosci* 1987;13:108–113.

79. Fardeau M, Godet-Guillain J, Tom F, et al. Une nouvelle affection musculaire familiale, e finie par l'accumulation intrasarcoplasmique d'un mat riel graunulofilmentaire dense en microscopie lectronique. *Rev Neurol* 1978;134:411–425.

79a. Muñoz-Mármol AM, Strasser G, Isamet M, et al. A dysfunctional desmin mutation in a patient with severe generalized myopathy. *Proc Nat Acad Sci USA* 1998;95:11312–11317.

79b. Goldfarb LG, Park K-Y, Cervenaková L, et al. Missense mutations in desmin associated with familial cardiac skeletal myopathy. *Nature Genetics* 1998;19:402–403.

79c. Vicart P, Caron A, Guicheney P, et al. A missense mutation in the αB-crystallin chaperone gene causes a desmin-related myopathy. *Nature Genetics* 1998;20:92–95.

80. DeBleecker JL, Engel AG, Ertl BB. Myofibrillary myopathy with abnormal foci of desmin positivity. II. Immunocytochemical analysis reveals accumulation of multiple other proteins. *J Neuropath Exp Pathol* 1996;55:563–577.

81. Porte A, Stoeckel ME, Sacrez A, Batzenschager A. Unusual cardiomyopathy characterized by aberrant accumulation of desmin-type intermediate filaments. *Virchows Arch* 1980;386:43–58; 1981;393:53.

82. Sarnat HB. Vimentin and desmin in maturing skeletal muscle and developmental myopathies. *Neurology* 1992;42:1616–1624.

83. Magee KE, DeJong RN. Hereditary distal myopathy with onset in infancy. *Arch Neurol* 1965;13:387–390.

84. Van der Does de Willebois AEM, Bethlem J, Meyer AEFH, et al. Distal myopathy with onset in early infancy. *Neurology* 1968;18:383–390.

85. Bautista J, Rafel E, Castilla J, et al. Hereditary distal myopathy with onset in early infancy. *J Neurol Sci* 1978;37:149–158.

86. Biemond A. Myopathia distalis juvenilis hereditaria. *Acta Psychiatr Neurol Scand* 1955;30:25–38.

87. Morgenlander JC, Massey JM. Myotonic dystrophy. *Semin Neurol* 1991;11:236–243.

88. Harper PS, Rüdel R. Myotonic dystrophy. In: Engel AG, Franzini-Armstrong C, eds. *Myology,* 2nd ed. New York: McGraw-Hill, 1994: 1192–1219.

89. Schotland D, Rowland L. Muscular dystrophy: features of ocular myopathy, distal myopathy, and myotonic dystrophy. *Arch Neurol* 1964;10:433–445.

90. Munsat TL. Fascioscapulohumeral dystrophy and the scapuloperoneal syndrome. In: Engel A, Franzini-Armstrong C, eds. *Myology,* 2nd ed. New York: McGraw-Hill, 1994:1220–1232.

91. Tawil R, McDermott MP, Mendell JR, et al. Fascioscapulohumeral muscular dystrophy (FSHMD): Design of natural history study and results of baseline testing. *Neurology* 1994;44:442–446.

92. Wijmenga C, Padberg GW, Moerer P, et al. Mapping of fascioscapulohumeral muscular dystrophy gene to chromosome 4q35-qter by multipoint linkage analysis and in situ hybridization. *Genomics* 1991;9: 570–575.

93. Thomas PK, Schott GD, Morgan-Hughes JA. Adult onset scapuloperoneal myopathy. *J Neurol Neurosurg Psychiatry* 1975;38:1008–1015.

94. Tawil R, Myers GJ, Weiffenbach B, Griggs RC. Scapuloperoneal syndromes: absence of linkage to the 4q35 FSHMD locus. *Arch Neurol* 1995;52:1069–1072.

95. Lunt PW, Jardine PE, Koch M. Phenotypic-genotypic correlation will assist genetic counseling in 4q35-fascioscapulohumeral muscular dystrophy. *Muscle Nerve* 1995;[Suppl 2]:S103–S109.

96. Wihelmsen KC, Blake DM, Lynch T. Chromosome 12-linked autosomal dominant scapuloperoneal muscular dystrophy. *Ann Neurol* 1996;39:507–520.

97. Rowland LP, Fetell M, Olarte M, et al. Emery-Dreifuss muscular dystrophy. *Ann Neurol* 1979;5:111–117.

98. Satoyoshi E, Kinoshita M. Oculopharyngodistal myopathy. *Arch Neurol* 1977;34:89–92.

99. Fukuhara N, Kumamoto T, Tadao T, et al. Oculopharyngeal muscular dystrophy and distal myopathy: intrafamilial difference in the onset and distribution of muscular involvement. *Acta Neurol Scand* 1982; 65:458–467.

100. Vita G, Dattola R, Santoro M, et al. Familial oculopharyngeal muscular dystrophy with distal spread. *J Neurol* 1983;230:57–64.

101. Amato AA, Jackson CE, Ridings L, Barohn RJ. Childhood-onset oculopharyngodistal myopathy with chronic intestinal pseudo-obstruction. *Muscle Nerve* 1995;18:842–847.

102. Hollinrake K. Polymyositis presenting as a distal muscle weakness—a case report. *J Neurol Sci* 1969;8:479–484.

103. Van Kasteren BJ. Polymyositis presenting with chronic progressive distal muscular weakness. *J Neurol Sci* 1979;41:307–310.

104. Lotz BP, Engel AG, Stevens JC, et al. Inclusion body myositis: observations in 40 patients. *Brain* 1989;112:727–747.

105. Griggs RC, Askanas V, DiMauro S, et al. Inclusion body myositis and myopathies. *Ann Neurol* 1995;38:705–713.

106. Amato AA, Gronseth GS, Jackson CE, Wolfe GI, Katz JS, Bryan WW, Barohn RJ. Inclusion body myositis: clinical pathologic boundaries. *Ann Neurol* 1996;40:581–586.

107. Amato AA, Barohn RJ. Idiopathic inflammatory myopathies. *Neurol Clin* 1997;3:615–648.

108. Mendell JR, Sahenk Z, Gales T. Amyloid filaments inclusion body myositis: novel findings provide insight into nature of filaments. *Arch Neurol* 1991;48:1229–1234.

109. Barohn RJ, Amato AA, Sahenk Z, Kissel JT, Mendell JR. Inclusion body myositis: explanation for poor response to immunosuppressive therapy. *Neurology* 1995;45:1302–1304.

110. DiMauro S, Hartwig G, Hays A, et al. Debrancher deficiency: neuromuscular disorder in 5 adults. *Ann Neurol* 1979;5:422–436.

111. Barohn RJ, McVey AL, DiMauro S. Adult acid maltase deficiency. *Muscle Nerve* 1993;16:672–676.

112. Charnas LR, Luciano CA, Dalakas M, et al. Distal vacuolar myopathy in nephropathic cystinosis. *Ann Neurol* 1994;35:181–188.

113. Hausmanowa-Petrusewicz I, Fidzianska A, Badurska B. Unusual course of nemaline myopathy. *Neuromusc Disord* 1992;2:413–418.

114. Laing NG, Majda BT, Akkari PA, et al. Assignment of a Gene (NEM1) for autosomal dominant nemaline myopathy to chromosome 1. *Am J Hum Genet* 1992;50:576–583.

115. Laing NG, Wilton SD, Akkari PA, et al. A mutation n the α-tropomyosin gene TPM3 associated with autosomal dominant nemaline myopathy. *Nat Genet* 1995;9:75–79.

116. Kratz R, Brooke MH. Distal myopathy. In: Vinken PJ, Bruyn GW, eds. *Handbook of clinical Neurology.* Vol. 40. Amsterdam: North-Holland, 1980:471–483.

117. Moxley RT, Griggs RC, Markesbery WR, et al. Metabolic implications of distal atrophy. Carbohydrate metabolism in centronuclear myopathy. *J Neurol Sci* 1978;39:247–259.

118. Nations SP, Wolfe GI, Amato AA, Jackson CE, Bryan WB, Barohn RJ. Clinical features of patients with distal myasthenia gravis. *Neurology* 1997;48[Suppl]:A64.

Motor Disorders,
edited by David S. Younger.
Lippincott Williams & Wilkins, Philadelphia © 1999.

CHAPTER 13

Myasthenia Gravis and Myasthenic Syndromes

Mark B. Bromberg

The neuromuscular junction (NMJ) has a complex anatomy and physiology but usually functions with extraordinary reliability. The uniqueness of the NMJ becomes apparent in the expression of clinical disease that results when junctional transmission fails.

This chapter reviews the normal and clinically relevant anatomy and physiology of the NMJ followed by essential features of the clinical and laboratory diagnosis, pathology, therapy, and prognosis of the NMJ disorders, especially myasthenia gravis (MG). The chapter then considers the major NMJ disorders. There are many excellent reviews of MG in the recent literature (1).

THE MOTOR UNIT

The motor unit consists of a motor neuron, its peripheral axon process, and the muscle fibers it innervates (Fig. 1). The motor axon ends in an arborization of terminal branches, which each make synaptic contact with a muscle fiber at the NMJ. The number of muscle fibers innervated by a single motor axon varies from 20 to 1,500 (2). With rare exception, each muscle fiber is innervated by a single motor axon terminal branch (3). However, a small percentage of extraocular muscle fibers are multiply innervated (4). The NMJ is located midway along the length of an individual fiber, in the region called the motor point (3).

In disorders of NMJ transmission, the associated weakness results from failure of muscle fiber activation. Symptoms can at times be highly regional among muscle groups, within a muscle, and within motor units. For example, NMJs from neighboring muscle fibers may show stable transmission, variable transmission, or complete block of transmission (5).

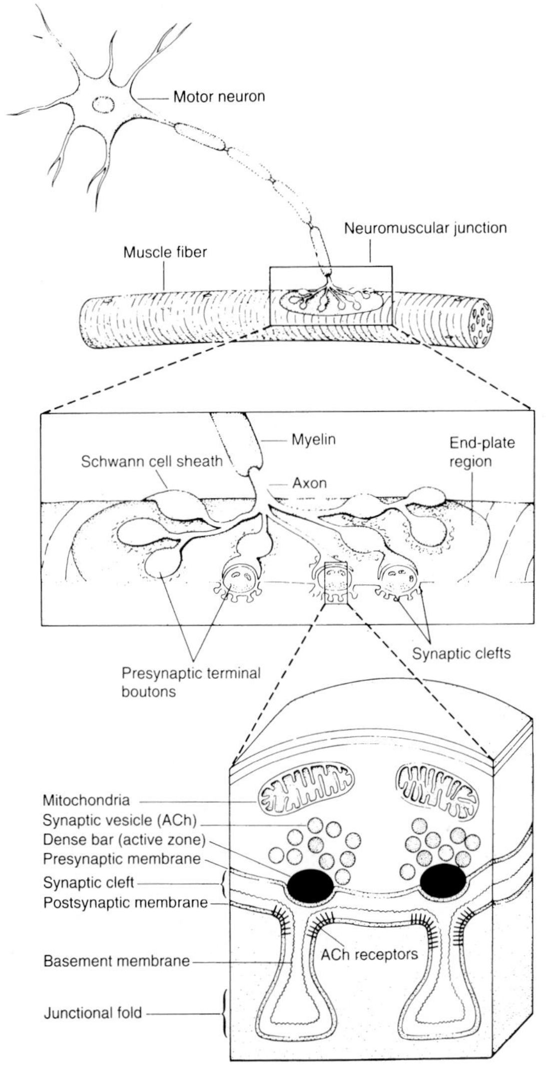

FIG. 1. Schematic diagram of the motor unit and neuromuscular junction. Only a single terminal branch of the motor unit is shown. (From Ref. 7, with permission.)

M. B. Bromberg: Department of Neurology, University of Utah School of Medicine, Salt Lake City, Utah 84132.

NEUROMUSCULAR JUNCTION ANATOMY

Presynaptic

Terminal branches of the motor axon end over a region of the muscle fiber called the end-plate (Fig. 1). The end-plate is a specialized segment of muscle fiber membrane with a high concentration of junctional acetylcholine (ACh) receptors. There are also extra-junction ACh receptors distributed along the membrane in low numbers that do not have a role in normal NMJ function. The terminal axon branches remain covered by Schwann cells until they lose their myelin covering. At the end-plate region, the axon expands into a complicated array with varicosities called synaptic boutons (Fig. 1). These are complex entities with many organelles, including mitochondria and enzymes for synthesis and release of ACh. The synaptic vesicles contain ACh and specialized areas of the presynaptic membrane called active zones that contain calcium channels, where vesicular release occurs.

ACh is synthesized from acetyl-CoA and choline by the enzyme choline acetyl transferase. Fifty percent of the choline in ACh is recycled by an active presynaptic reuptake mechanism (6). After synthesis, ACh is sequestered within membrane-bound vesicles. Each vesicle contains about 5,000 molecules of ACh. There are a tremendously large number of synaptic vesicles in each bouton. Boutons cluster in rows along specialized regions of the presynaptic membrane that facilitate the secretion of ACh, called active zones, where vesicles fuse and ACh is released by exocytosis (7). Exocytosis is a complex process that depends on the influx of calcium into the presynaptic terminal (Fig. 2). The active zone also includes rows of large particles thought to be the calcium channels. To prevent an increase in presynaptic membrane area by fusion of the membrane-bound vesicles, there is a recycling of excess membrane.

Postsynaptic

The presynaptic and postsynaptic membranes are separated by a gap of about 20 nm. The postsynaptic membrane is also highly specialized (8) and is thrown into deep folds that lie below presynaptic active zones (Fig. 1). The shoulders of the folds contain approximately 10,000 ACh receptors/μm^2, and voltage-sensitive sodium channels are situated beneath them. Clusters of molecules of acetylcholinesterase (AChE) are located in the depths of the folds. The primary mechanism of ACh inactivation is via the rapid hydrolysis of ACh into choline and acetate by AChE. Diffusion of ACh away from receptor sites is a lesser mechanism. The choline is actively taken up by the presynaptic membrane.

ACh receptors are pentomeric protein complexes consisting of α_2, β, γ, and δ subunits (Fig. 3). The receptor complex spans the postsynaptic membrane, and the subunits form a pore which is the ion channel of the action potential (AP) along the muscle fiber (9). There is a constriction in the pore that opens when ACh binds to the external portions of the α subunits, allowing sodium, potassium, or chloride to pass. The density of ACh receptors falls off away from the end-plate region. Between the end-plate and the muscle fiber membrane, there is a perijunctional region that contains a mixture of ACh receptors and sodium channels where the muscle fiber action potential (AP) is initiated. The muscle fiber membrane contains voltage-dependent sodium channels that participate in the propagation of the AP along the muscle fiber (7). ACh receptors are nonstatic protein structures that are degraded and renewed in about 12 days.

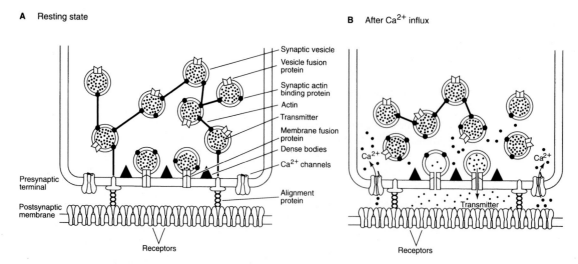

FIG. 2. Schematic diagram of the role of calcium on the release and mobilization of synaptic vesicles in the presynaptic terminal. **A:** Vesicles from the immediately available pool are docked at the active zone. Calcium channels are closed. **B:** The nerve action potential opens voltage-sensitive channels and the calcium influx facilitates vesicular release and mobilization of bound vesicles. (From Ref. 7, with permission.)

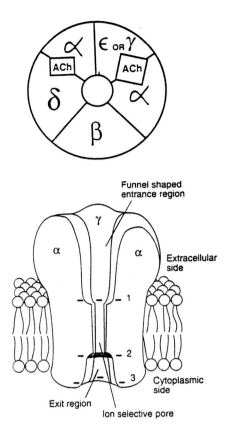

FIG. 3. Schematic diagram of the acetylcholine receptor complex. Top diagram shows the pentomeric structure of the receptor complex and binding sites for acetylcholine molecules to the α subunits. Bottom diagram shows the transmembrane position of the receptor and the ion pore or channel. (From Refs. 7 and 10, with permission.)

NEUROMUSCULAR JUNCTION PHYSIOLOGY

Presynaptic

Voltage-gated calcium channels along the presynaptic membrane in the vicinity of the active zone initiate the process of NMJ transmission that begins with a motor nerve fiber AP (Fig. 2). Graded degrees of terminal depolarization result in graded influxes of calcium into the presynaptic terminal. The release of ACh, in turn, is dependent on and proportional to the concentration of calcium in the terminal. The release of ACh is not smoothly graded but occurs in quantile units. These are the number of ACh molecules contained in a single vesicle. The postsynaptic response includes the number of vesicles released and the nature of the interaction of ACh with the receptors. The number of vesicles released with each motor fiber AP, in turn, is related to the probability of release. The role of calcium in the presynaptic terminal is to enhance the probability of ACh release, and the magnitude of release is exponential with the concentration of calcium (9). The spontaneous release of vesicles produces a very small postsynaptic potential called the miniature end-plate potential (MEPP), which can be recorded during routine needle electromyography (EMG)

studies as end-plate noise when the electrode tip is in the vicinity of NMJs at the motor point.

Calcium is required for the fusion of vesicles to the presynaptic membrane at the active zone and contributes to the dilation of the fusion pore between the vesicle and membrane, allowing release of ACh into the synaptic cleft (Fig. 2). Calcium is also involved in the mobilization of vesicles. The availability of vesicles for release of ACh can be considered to be distributed among several pools of ACh discussed later. In essence there is an immediately available pool, comprised of vesicles in the active zone; others are bound to the cytoskeleton. The influx of calcium frees the vesicles from a binding protein, making them available to move to the active zone for subsequent fusion and release of ACh (7). AChE is a molecule that floats above the end-plate membrane similar to a tethered balloon. There is competition between the ACh receptor and the AChase enzyme, and the initial high concentration of ACh favors the receptor. As molecules of ACh diffuse from the receptor, the enzyme hydrolyzes them into the precursors choline and acetic acid (6). Approximately 50% of the choline is taken up by the presynaptic membrane.

During a motor nerve AP, the concentration of calcium can rise a thousandfold within several hundred microseconds at the active zone where the calcium channels are most dense. The calcium buffering systems in presynaptic terminals are limited, and the repeated influx of calcium follows a train of high-frequency APs that saturates the system, leading to a residual calcium buildup. This increases the probability of vesicular release when the next nerve AP arrives. The buildup of calcium underlies the phenomena of posttetanic potentiation. The antagonism of calcium channels by high serum magnesium concentration blocks calcium-dependent release of ACh (7).

Postsynaptic

The α subunits are the sites where ACh attaches to open the receptor channel. One ACh molecule binds to each of the two subunits to bring about a conformational change in the receptor that increases the diameter of the pore or channel (Fig. 3). The concentration gradients of sodium, potassium, and chloride are such that sodium is the predominant ion flowing into the muscle fiber at the end-plate region. Normally, there is a rapid release of ACh from the presynaptic terminal that results in a near synchronous opening of approximately 20,000 receptor channels. The resultant end-plate current causes an EPP that depolarized the end-plate membrane (Fig. 4). The ACh concentration in the synaptic cleft falls rapidly due to hydrolysis by AChE and diffusion, and within a millisecond the channels close, causing a fall off of end-plate current flow. The EPP decays more slowly due to passive membrane properties of the muscle (7,9).

Under normal conditions the rising phase of the EPP reaches threshold, upon which voltage-dependent sodium

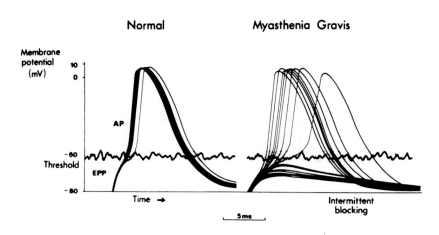

FIG. 4. Schematic diagram of an intracellular muscle fiber recording showing the generation of end-plate potentials (EPPs) and muscle fiber action potential (APs). On the left, normal neuromuscular junction function ensures that the rise time and amplitude of successive EPPs are sufficient to generate APs. Note the fluctuating threshold for generating an AP and resultant variability of the AP latency. This is normal jitter. On the right, in myasthenia gravis, there are insufficient acetylcholine receptors and the EPP rise times and amplitudes vary markedly. This results in increased jitter and at times failure to initiate an AP. This is called blocking. (From Ref. 5, with permission.)

channels open and a muscle fiber AP is initiated (Fig. 4). The AP is propagated along the muscle fiber membrane to the ends of the fiber, leading to muscle fiber shortening and the development of force via excitation–contraction coupling.

Muscle fiber APs are clinically and electrodiagnostically important for two reasons. First, they are prerequisites for the development of force and shortening in a muscle. Second, electrodiagnostic studies record the extracellular AP as the compound muscle action potential (CMAP) during nerve conduction studies or as the motor unit action potential during needle EMG. Routine electrodiagnostic testing detects abnormalities of the NMJ only if there is a failure to initiate the muscle fiber AP. Single-fiber EMG (SFEMG) detects less severe abnormalities of the NMJ. A number of factors govern endplate current flow and the shape of the EPP that are important in diseases of the NMJ. The rising phase of the EPP depends on the nearly simultaneous opening of a large number of channels in the AChR. In turn, the probability that a pore opens is largely determined by the concentration of ACh and the number of ACh receptors. Con-

sequently, the rise time and amplitude of the EPP depends on the probability of release of ACh and the total number of receptors available.

General Considerations

Normally, the NMJ functions with complete reliability, transforming each motor nerve AP into muscle fiber APs in all muscle fibers of the motor unit. There are various mechanisms within the complexity of the NMJ, collectively called the "safety factor," that ensure reliable NMJ transmission (10). These include an overabundance of ACh in the presynaptic terminals and more than adequate numbers of postsynaptic receptors. There is an immediately releasable pool of ACh in vesicles along the active zone (Fig. 2). There is another pool of vesicles bound to the cytoskeleton that are freed by calcium and that can be mobilized to the active zone for release. If the reuptake of choline is blocked experimentally by hemicholinium and the NMJ is activated to functional depletion of ACh, approximately 20% of the total ACh store still remains, presumably in a pool unavailable for release. The number

TABLE 1. *Descriptive model of the dynamics of normal NMJ transmission during low-frequency repetitive nerve stimulation*

Stimulus number	ACh pool	Available ACh quanta	ACh quanta released	Resultant EPP amplitude[a] (mV)	Action potential threshold reached
1	Immediate	1,000	200	60	Yes
2	Immediate	800	160	48	Yes
3	Immediate	640	128	38	Yes
4	Mobilizable	>640	>128	>38	Yes
5	Mobilizable	>640	>128	>38	Yes

Two ACh pools (immediately available and mobilizable) are under the influence of the influx of calcium into the presynaptic terminal. Mobilization of ACh ensures the release of an adequate number of ACh quanta. Because there are normal numbers of ACh receptors, each EPP exceeds the threshold for generating an action potential.

[a]In this model, the EPP amplitude must be greater than 30 mV to reach threshold for generation of a muscle fiber action potential.

NMJ, neuromuscular junction; ACh, acetylcholine; EPP, end plate potential.

Modified from Albers JW, AAEM Workshop on Repetitive Stimulation.

of vesicles and the amount of ACh released varies from transmission to transmission, but activation of the various pools ensures a sufficient amount to depolarize the postsynaptic membrane to threshold.

Calcium has a leading role in the release of ACh and in mobilization of ACh pools. Depolarization of the presynaptic terminal opens voltage-sensitive calcium channels. There is a linear relationship between terminal calcium concentration and the amount of presynaptic ACh released. Under normal circumstances, raising the terminal calcium concentration increases the amount of presynaptic ACh released but does not augment NMJ transmission (Table 1). This is because sufficient amount of ACh is normally released to ensure the generation of a muscle fiber AP. There are maneuvers that increase calcium availability that are important in the diagnosis and treatment of NMJ disorders. The postsynaptic ACh receptors interact with varying amounts of ACh. Under normal conditions there is always a sufficient amount of ACh to ensure depolarization of the end-plate to threshold with the generation of an AP (Fig. 4). The variability in the time to reach threshold in microseconds is of no clinical significance, but it can be measured by SFEMG.

MYASTHENIA GRAVIS

MG is an autoimmune disorder that affects the postsynaptic portion of NMJ transmission due to a reduction in the number or functioning ACh receptors.

Clinical Spectrum

MG is characterized by easy fatigability and weakness, primarily of ocular, bulbar, truncal, or proximal limb muscles (11), and can be fatal when respiratory muscles weaken enough to require mechanical, so-called myasthenic crisis. It is also characterized by fluctuations that occur over a day, weeks, months, and years, resulting in exacerbations and remissions. The distribution and severity varies among individuals. There are a large number of available treatments, the choice of which is guided by clinical factors. The onset may be sudden or insidious, with mild symptoms that wax and wane. Early symptoms may be so subtle as to escape detection for years such as double vision or mild ptosis. The areas of involvement increase over time. The first useful clinical classification system was developed by Osserman (12) (Table 2) and thereafter modified.

Ocular MG generally includes ptosis and diplopia. Bulbar symptoms of dysphagia and dysphonia may occur early in the course or follow generalized limb involvement. Respiratory involvement is a late manifestation and never occurs alone; however, some patients can have isolated vocal cord paralysis. Muscle weakness in MG is characterized by fatigability. Strength is near normal at the onset, but with effort, particularly against firm resis-

TABLE 2. *Osserman clinical classification of myasthenia gravis*

Stage	Symptoms
Neonatal	Transient symptoms from myasthenic mother
Juvenile	
Adult group I	Localized, usually ocular only
Adult group II	Generalized, both bulbar and generalized
Adult group III	Acute fulminating, bulbar and generalized with respiratory failure
Adult group IV	Late severe, evolving from groups I and II
Adult group V	With muscle atrophy, evolving from group II

Modified from Ref. 12.

tance testing, muscle weakness is detectible due to fatigue. Respiratory fatigue is more complex but can precipitously worsen after a period of compensation.

Natural History

Untreated, the natural history of MG is difficult to determine because many current therapies such as prednisone were available even early in the clinical description of the disease. In an early series at the turn of the century, it was found that a third of affected patients progressively worsened. Another one third had relapsing and remitting symptoms, and the remainder improved and led active lives for a period of time (13).

The contemporary natural history includes several important clinical points. Despite a large number of therapeutic regimens to enhance strength and promote remission, the most important improvement in clinical care has been the advent of positive pressure ventilation and respiratory critical care units to reduce mortality and morbidity from myasthenic crisis (14) and to permit safe performance of thymectomy. When the clinical course of a large number of patients are plotted, the maximal state of weakness during an exacerbation is usually experienced within the first 3 years, and the extent and severity will be evident during this time. Therefore, if ocular MG has not progressed to generalized involvement within 3 years, it is unlikely that it will do so (14).

Pathology

The pathologic alterations in MG are at the postsynaptic membrane and include simplification of the postsynaptic end-plate region with fewer and more shallow folds and a reduction in the number of ACh receptors. These changes result from antibody attachment to the receptors and activation of the complement cascade and receptor lysis by membrane attack complex (15,16). There are undoubtedly other mechanisms involved because some antibodies detected in the serum do not directly bind to the ACh receptor. In normal individuals, the half-life of the ACh receptor is approximately 12 days, but 3 days in MG.

The various types of ACh receptor antibodies in MG are operationally defined and based on laboratory testing procedures. *Binding* antibodies are detected by reaction of the patient serum with solubilized human skeletal muscle ACh receptor. *Modulating* antibodies are detected by reactivity with ACh receptor on living muscle and may be positive when the binding antibody is negative. *Blocking* antibodies are detected by binding of sera at or near the neurotransmitter binding site on solubilized human ACh receptors. There is a hierarchy of testing based on the frequency of occurrence (Table 3). Despite testing for three types of antibodies, only 80 to 86% of patients are seropositive. The false-positive rate is extremely low (17), and the specificity for MG is high.

Approximately 15% of patients with MG are seronegative based on the antibody panel described above. Seronegative patients are believed to have an autoimmune pathogenesis similar to the seropositive cases because defects in NMJ transmission can be passively transferred to experimental animals by serum or by the IgG fraction (18), but their diagnosis can be problematic because 50% have ocular symptoms alone and other diagnostic tests may be equivocal (19). Other organ-specific autoantibodies occur at a higher than expected frequency in patients with MG (20), including those to thyroid microsomes, thyroglobulin, and to gastric parietal cells. In seronegative patients with equivocal but suggestive symptoms of MG, these antibodies are supportive of the diagnosis of autoimmune MG (21).

Autoimmune Features

MG is a prototypic autoimmune autoantibody-mediated disease. Although the clinical focus is on the humoral arm of the immune system and autoantibodies to the ACh receptor, the disease starts with the cellular arm of the immune system, perhaps with a breakdown of T-cell tolerance. The normal process of T-cell tolerance is not fully understood, but it takes place in the thymus gland (22), as does the loss of tolerance in MG. While awaiting a full understanding of the physiologic and pathophysiologic processes of autoantibody diseases, several points are pertinent to the clinical diagnosis and management of MG. Because it is a specific autoantibody disease, there must

be exposure of T cells to the ACh receptor, either from myoid cells in the thymus or peripherally. The exposure and subsequent breakdown of self-tolerance is a complex process and probably involves genetic susceptibility. The result is activation of B cells and the production of specific autoantibodies. Once this process has begun, there are immune mechanism that regulate T-cell activity that affect the production of specific autoantibodies (22).

Pathophysiology

The pathophysiologic abnormality in MG results from a reduced number of ACh receptors. Fewer sodium channels open and the resultant EPPs have a slower rising phase and reduced amplitude. If the EPP amplitude does not depolarize the end-plate membrane to threshold, a muscle fiber AP will not be produced, NMJ transmission will fail, and the fiber will not contract or generate force (Table 4). A slower rise phase of the EPP, if it has sufficient amplitude to reach threshold, will have no clinical effect, although the slight delay in initiating the muscle fiber AP can be detected by SFEMG.

When NMJ transmission fails in MG, any method to increase the concentration of ACh at the receptor site increases the number of channel openings and improves amplitudes. There are two methods to increase the concentration of ACh. One is to increase the quantal release of ACh, which can be accomplished physiologically by increasing the concentration of calcium in the presynaptic terminal. A high-frequency train of presynaptic APs will overcome the calcium buffering capacity and result in greater quantal release. The second method is by reducing the rate of ACh hydrolysis by inhibiting the enzyme AChE. This can be accomplished by several drugs such as edrophonium and pyridostigmine. The effect of increasing the ACh concentration on a model of NMJ transmission can be seen in Table 4.

Diagnosis

The diagnosis of a defect in NMJ transmission may be clear when the history indicates and examination findings reveal fluctuating weakness and fatigue, especially of ocular, bulbar, and proximal limb muscles. The physical examination should include prolonged testing of strength

TABLE 3. *Muscle-specific autoantibodies associated with myasthenia gravis*

ACh receptor antibody type	Percentage positive	Clinical features	False-positive conditions
Binding	86	71% ocular MG	Thymoma, LEMS, small cell lung cancer, D-penicillamine
Modulating	86	71% ocular MG. Helpful when AChR binding antibodies are negative	May be caused by extraneous causes
Blocking	52	30% ocular MG	When curare-like agents are used

ACh, acetylcholine; MG, myasthenia gravis; LEMS, Lambert-Eaton myasthenic syndrome.
Modified from Ref. 17.

TABLE 4. *Descriptive model of the dynamics at an abnormal NMJ due to myasthenia gravis during low-frequency repetitive stimulation*

Stimulus number	ACh pool	Available ACh quanta	ACh quanta released	Resultant EPP amplitude[a] (mV)	Action potential threshold reached
1	Immediate	1,000	200	36	Yes
2	Immediate	800	160	28	No
3	Immediate	640	128	24	No
4	Mobilizable	>640	>128	>30	Yes
5	Mobilizable	>640	>128	>30	Yes

The effects of higher calcium concentration on the release of ACh are normal in MG. However, there are fewer functioning ACh receptors and the resultant EPP is lower than normal. The greater amount of ACh released with mobilization has some effect on the EPP amplitude, resulting in a greater likelihood of an EPP reaching threshold for an action potential. Numbers representing ACh quanta are approximate.

[a]In this model, the EPP amplitude must be greater than 30 mV to reach threshold for generation of a muscle fiber action potential.

NMJ, neuromuscular junction; ACh, acetylcholine; EPP, end plate potential.

if necessary to bring out fatigue, particularly when the patient is already medicated with prednisone. It is essential to determine whether an NMJ disorder is due to a postsynaptic or a presynaptic defect, such as Lambert-Eaton myasthenic syndrome (LEMS). Elevated titers of ACh receptor antibodies are highly correlated with MG but can also occur in LEMS (22a). It is important therefore to carry out electrodiagnostic testing to recognize a presynaptic defect by facilitation of the CMAP after exercise. Positive ACh receptor antibodies in patients with LEMS are thought to represent a nonpathologenic epiphenomenon and not the coexistence of both diseases.

Tensilon Test

Defects in NMJ transmission can be demonstrated by showing a brief improvement in transmission in the form of restoration of strength by giving a short acting AChase inhibitor. The rationale is based on demonstration of a clear difference comparing before, during, and after the intravenous administration of Edrophonium (Tensilon), which blocks AChase for two or three minutes. It is important that there be clearly weak muscle groups to follow because when symptoms and signs are mild and limited to ocular muscles, false positive diagnoses of MG may occur (22b). There are protocols for performing the Tensilon test in a double-blinded, placebo-controlled manner (39). It is emphasized that a positive Tensilon test does not distinguish between the various forms of presynaptic and post synaptic NMJ transmission failure.

Repetitive Stimulation

For there to be a demonstrable decrement to repetitive stimulation, a finite number of NMJs must have a failure of transmission. Abnormal NMJs fail during even low levels of repetitive stimulation, which forms the basis for this electrophysiologic test. A practical and effective testing paradigm is to measure the amplitude of the CMAPs

to five shocks at 2 to 4 Hz (23,24). The NMJ safety factor ensures sufficient ACh released to produce APs in all muscle fibers, and the CMAP amplitude will not change from shock to shock. However, when there is a reduction in the number of receptors due to a postsynaptic defect or a reduction in ACh release resulting from the presynaptic defect, there may be failure of transmission at some NMJs. This will be evident by a reduction in the CMAP amplitude by the third shock, as the immediate pool of ACh is depleted. This is termed the decremental response (Fig. 5). The extent of the CMAP amplitude decrement depends on the number of NMJs that fail and may not be

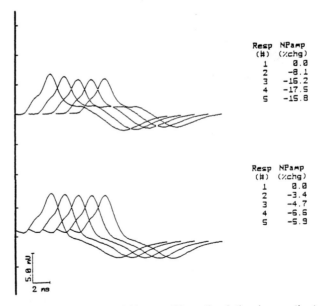

Resp (#)	NPamp (%chg)
1	0.0
2	-8.1
3	-16.2
4	-17.5
5	-15.8

Resp (#)	NPamp (%chg)
1	0.0
2	-3.4
3	-4.7
4	-6.6
5	-5.9

FIG. 5. Response to 3-Hz repetitive stimulation in a patient with myasthenia gravis. Top trace illustrates the decremental response with a maximal decrement of 17.5% with the fourth response. Bottom trace illustrates partial repair after 10 seconds of maximal muscle activation with a maximal decrement of 5.9%.

evident in very mild defects in NMJ transmission. The increase in ACh release by the activation of the mobilizable ACh pool after the third shock will, in turn, result in an increase in the number of NMJs successfully transmitting, and the CMAP amplitude to the fourth shock will show an increase. This results in a U-shaped decremental pattern to the five CMAPs (Fig. 5).

Increasing the presynaptic calcium concentration increases the amount of ACh released and restores NMJ transmission at some failed junctions. This can be accomplished by having the patient voluntarily maximally activate the muscle group being tested for 10 to 15 seconds. If repetitive nerve testing is repeated in 1 to 2 seconds after exercise, there will be partial repair of the initial decrement.

NMJ transmission is most prone to failure 2 to 4 minutes after 10 to 15 seconds of maximal exercise. If repetitive nerve stimulation is performed at this time, a greater degree of decrement will be observed or the subtle defect will be evident (Fig. 5) (24), so-called posttetanic exhaustion.

A number of procedural and technical issues increase the sensitivity of repetitive stimulation. Physiologically, the safety factor suggests that there should be no decrement to repetitive stimulation in a normal muscle (Table 1). However, many texts and reference manuals allow for some decrement in normal muscles and consider up to 8% normal. There are a number of possible reasons for the low percentage decrement in normal muscle. One is a change in stimulation current during the stimulation train due to movement of the limb. This can be reduced by using stimulus intensities of 150% of maximum and by immobilizing the limb (25). Most EMG machines calculate decrement from the negative peak CMAP amplitude. Many also use the isolectric line before the first CMAP as their baseline for amplitude measurement. If there is movement of the isolectric line for subsequent shocks, there may be calculation errors. Measurement of peak-to-peak CMAP amplitude is less susceptible to these types of errors (26).

Repetitive stimulation can be incorporated into routine nerve conduction studies that are usually performed on distal limb muscles. Decrement may not be observed in these muscles if the MG is mild or affects ocular muscles alone; however, testing of a proximal muscle such as trapezius muscle along the spinal accessory nerve may be informative (27). Stimulation of the facial nerve is associated with movement artifact and is therefore technically more difficult. There are issues yet unresolved of the mathematic expression of decrement (25) and the separation of true decrement and facilitation from pseudofacilitation (28).

Several practical guidelines can be offered to enhance the accuracy of repetitive stimulation and to reduce false-positive decremental responses to as low as 3%. First, a true decremental response must be properly pathologic with a U-shaped response, that is, less decrement by the fourth shock. Second, it should be reproducible with the same pathologic decrement seen with varying percentages on several separate trials. Third, it should show a physiologic response to an increase in presynaptic termi-

nal calcium after 10 seconds of exercise, an improvement in the decremental response.

Single-Fiber Electromyography

This is an electrophysiologic technique that analyzes the variability of NMJ transmission as a discharge-to-discharge variability in timing of single muscle fiber APs (5,29) (Fig. 6). This variability, called jitter, which is measured in microseconds, reflects slow EPP rise times and delayed generation of muscle fiber APs. When the EPP fails to reach threshold, jitter is infinite and the AP is blocked. It should be clear that SFEMG can detect abnormal jitter without blocking, whereas repetitive nerve stimulation only detects blocking (30,31). It requires a special concentric EMG needle with the exposed active electrode surface along the side of the needle and computer software to measure the variability. As most commonly measured, NMJ transmission is initiated by weak voluntary contraction, and the covariability of two NMJs is recorded. Alternatively, transmission can be initiated by electrical stimu-

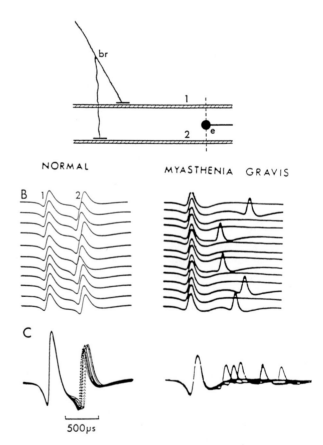

FIG. 6. Schematic diagram of single-fiber electromyography (SFEMG) recording technique and illustrative responses. Top diagram shows two muscle fibers (1 and 2) from the same motor unit. The SFEMG electrode, e, is positioned to record single fiber action potentials from each fiber. The higher amplitude of action potential 1 is used as the trigger potential. Lower traces show jitter from a normal and myasthenia gravis (MG) neuromuscular junction. Jitter is extreme in MG, with blocking of action potential 2. (Modified from Ref. 5, with permission.)

lation of motor nerve branches, and the variability of one NMJ is recorded. The normal range of jitter values has been determined empirically and differs among muscles and according to age (32). Abnormal jitter does not distinguish between presynaptic and postsynaptic defects of transmission. However, by stimulation of the motor nerve electrically, the discharge frequency at which maximal jitter occurs can help distinguish patterns suggestive of pre- or postsynaptic defects (33).

Comparison of Diagnostic Techniques

A suggestive clinical history and examination provides the impetus to proceed with confirmatory clinical, electrophysiologic, and serologic laboratory studies in MG. Diagnostic specificity for MG comes close to 100% when ACh receptor antibody titers are present, although their absence does not exclude the diagnosis. The edrophonium test, repetitive nerve stimulation, and SFEMG are specific for the defect in NMJ transmission. The sensitivity of the edrophonium test and repetitive nerve stimulation depends on the distribution and severity of symptoms. Ocular and mild generalized MG may present difficultly when the findings are subtle or mild. SFEMG is more sensitive in ocular MG and mild generalized involvement because it detects abnormalities that do not cause blocked transmission. A direct comparison of antibody testing, the Tensilon test, repetitive nerve stimulation, and SFEMG performed in the same patients has been made (Table 5) (34). SFEMG was the most sensitive for both ocular and generalized weakness when affected muscles were studied (99% to 89%). Antibody tests were more sensitive for generalized MG (80%) and less for ocular MG (55%). Repetitive nerve stimulation was almost as sensitive in the generalized form (76%), but least in the ocular form (48%).

Mediastinal Imaging

Approximately 10% of patients with MG will have evidence of a thymoma on computed tomography (CT) of the chest. Thymomas are clinically silent except for their association with weakness in MG; even so, only 40% of thymomas are associated with MG (35). Their presence cannot be predicted by the clinical features of MG, and therefore imaging is necessary. CT of the chest, not magnetic resonance imaging, is still the test of choice (36).

Treatment

Concepts

MG is a chronic disease with no cure at this time. The goal of treatment is sustained and complete remission, defined as the absence of symptoms and signs, with no medication. For many patients, complete remission may be elusive, and partial remission is a more practical goal (37). Therapy can be divided into three categories: drugs that improve NMJ transmission and the symptoms of weakness but do not affect the course of the disease, including the AChE inhibitors; procedures that affect the immune system over a limited time period but probably do not affect the natural history of the disease, such as plasmapheresis and intravenous immunoglobulin (IVIg); and drugs and procedures that modify the course of MG such as the immunosuppressants prednisone and azathioprine, and thymectomy.

Quantitative Testing

In certain patients, it may be difficult to determine if a particular therapeutic regimen is effective. For example, some may report worsening of symptoms, whereas strength appears unchanged or even improved. Under these circumstances, it is helpful to have quantitative data for objective comparisons. One quantitative scale that was developed as an end-point measure in a drug trial can be used clinically to determine overall function (38); however, it is important to try to carry out the measurements at the same time of the day or regularly at the time of the last dose of pyridostigmine. A frequently encountered problem is the differentiation of steroid myopathy from MG, especially when weakness advances on prednisone. Summing the values of decrement to repetitive nerve stimulation of several nerves or average neuromuscular jitter from SFEMG measurements can be helpful. Electrodiagnostic values are usually unchanged or improved in steroid myopathy and worse during an exacerbation of MG, so emphasizing the importance of establishing baseline electrodiagnostic values even in those whose diagnosis is made on the basis of elevated ACh receptor antibody titers.

TABLE 5. *Comparison of a series of diagnostic tests performed in 550 patients with myasthenia gravis*

	SFEMG in any muscle		SFEMG in ext dig com		Rep Stim in any muscle		Acetylcholine receptor antibody at any time	
	Gen MG	Ocular MG	Gen MG	Ocular MG	Gen MG	Ocular MG	Gen MG	Ocular MG
Percent abnormal	99	97	89	60	76	48	80	55

Gen MG, generalized weakness; Ext dig com, extensor digitorum communis muscle, commonly used studied with SFEMG; Ocular MG, weakness restricted to ocular muscles; SFEMG, single-fiber electromyogram; Rep Stim, repetitive stimulation.
Modified from Ref. 34.

Acetycholinesterase Inhibitors

Pyridostigmine (Mestinon) is the most commonly used AChE inhibitor. It reversibly binds to AChase and slows the hydrolysis of ACh, raising the concentration of ACh at the junctional folds and increasing the probability of ACh remaining attached to functional receptors. This leads to EPPs with a more rapid rise time and a higher amplitude and thus a greater likelihood of generating APs in previously blocked muscle fibers. It reaches peak serum concentrations in 90 to 120 minutes and has a similar half-life. Doses of 60 to 120 mg every 3 to 4 hours are most effective, but patients may modify their dose to match their level of activity and to reduce the common adverse side effects of cramping and diarrhea. It is rare for pyridostigmine alone to improve transmission to a satisfactory level, and therefore most patients require more definitive therapy (39).

Plasmapheresis and Intravenous Immunoglobulin

Plasmapheresis and IVIg rapidly influence the immune system but are of limited duration (40). A recent comparison of plasmapheresis and IVIg demonstrated equal effectiveness (41) and probably equivalent expense; however, they differ in their proposed mechanisms of action and thus may be complementary therapies in MG. Plasmapheresis removes antibodies, presumably those that act at the NMJ, but may also modulate the immune system. The response to plasmapheresis occurs over hours to days and is useful to treat or abort myasthenic crisis, but it requires special equipment to separate blood into components and trained personnel and is thus not widely available. A therapeutic trial usually consists of four to six exchanges on alternate days. The procedure is well tolerated but requires good venous access, and patients may require placement of a central venous catheter. Most complications are those associated with central catheters. IVIg consists of pooled exogenous antibodies from thousands of donors. Although the precise mechanisms of action are not well understood, exogenous antibodies interact at several different sites, including binding to the autoantibodies, to idiotypic antigenic sites, and to T cells to modulate the immune system (42,43). It does not require special equipment, and infusions can be performed easily with routine nursing care. The recommended total monthly dose is 2 g/kg in five daily doses, administered slowly enough to avert rate-related side effects. Repeat doses are usually 1 g/kg over 1 to 2 days. The most effective schedule has not yet been determined; however, the half-life of IVIg is about 4 weeks, and monthly doses are reasonable, with the goal of slowly tapering the frequency of treatments based on the clinical status. Clinical responses occur over 2 to 4 weeks.

Corticosteroids

Corticosteroids occupy a central role in the treatment of MG because of their effectiveness and reliability in initi-ating and maintaining a prolonged remission. Corticosteroids affect the immune system at several different levels (44), but the mechanism of influence on MG has not been established. Prednisone is the most widely used oral agent given initially at doses of 40 to 60 mg daily for 3 to 6 weeks and then slowly tapered after a beneficial response is seen. For unclear reasons, a high percentage of MG patients experience temporary worsening of their weakness that sometimes culminates in crisis after high initial doses; accordingly, patients receiving 100 g or more should probably be monitored initially in a hospital setting. Alternatively, the patient can be given a low dose and slowly increased over weeks (40). Although many prednisone taper protocols are followed, one goal is to convert relatively early in the taper schedule to alternative-day dosing to reduce the short-term side effects of weight gain and hyperglycemia, osteopenia, gastric and duodenal erosion, and cataracts (45). A short course of 2 g intravenous methylprednisolone followed by a second infusion 5 days later is sometimes effective in aborting myasthenic crisis, but this has never been formally studied (46).

Azathioprine

Azathioprine (Imuran) has been used in patients with poor responsiveness, intolerance, or frequent relapses with corticosteroids and as a steroid-sparing agent in conjunction with prednisone to reduce the long-term side effects (47); however, azathioprine is less effective than prednisone as monotherapy (48). Dosage varies, with some investigators raising the dose to achieve an elevation in the mean corpuscular volume or a drop in the white blood cell count, whereas others give a fixed dose based on weight, usually 3 to 5.0 mg/kg/day (49). There are several caveats of azathioprine therapy. First, there is a long delay in the onset of action, 24 months for the steroid-sparing effects to become evident (50). Second, side effects occur in about 10% of patients, including flu-like symptoms with nausea, fever, chills, arthralgias, or gastrointestinal complaints that usually resolve promptly with cessation of therapy (51). Third, bone marrow suppression occurs in all patients but is rarely a reason to stop therapy with careful monitoring. Fourth, there is the concern for an increased risk of cancers, primarily lymphomas after 10 to 20 years of therapy (52).

Thymectomy

The thymus has a central position in the pathogenesis of MG, and thymectomy has been an important treatment of MG. The earliest transsternal thymectomies for MG were performed for the removal of thymic tumors (53); however, the beneficial results in nonthymomatous patients were appreciated afterward. Nonetheless, it has been difficult to judge the efficacy of thymectomy for several reasons. First, there has not been a placebo-controlled trial. Second, it has been difficult to ascertain the absolute effectiveness of one type of operative procedure over another and the optimal extent of thymic resection necessary to obtain a maximal clinical response. The surgical approaches to the thymus gland include cervical, transsternal, combined cervical and transsternal, and thoracoscopic procedures (54). Third, there is a delay in the effectiveness that may be prolonged for years after surgery, yet long-term it carries the best likelihood for a sustained remission. Whether all thymic tissue needs to be removed to guarantee the best outcome is not truly known, although most authorities agree that the transsternal approach reduces the risk of leaving thymic tissue behind (54,55,56).

Thymectomy should be included in the initial and primary therapy of patients with generalized limb and bulbar involvement. In one study (56), two thirds of patients were asymptomatic after transsternal surgery, and of those, one sixth had ocular symptoms alone, whereas the remainder had mild generalized weakness. Younger patients, including those with juvenile MG, and older patients respond equally well. Plasmapheresis can improve the preoperative status and later immediate outcome of patients with bulbar weakness and a poor cough that may be a risk for prolonged postoperative intubation. One series (54), based on extensive surgical exploration of the anterior mediastinum and neck for thymic tissue, reported a progressive number of patients in full remission of up to 90% after 7 years of follow-up.

The role of the thymus and thymectomy is one of the more controversial therapeutic issues in MG. Nonetheless, the following guidelines appear to be reasonable. Radiographic evidence of an anterior mediastinal mass on chest CT warrants a thymectomy at any age because approximately 10% of patients with MG will have a thymoma. When there is no mediastinal mass, it seems appropriate to counsel the patient to undergo thymectomy to increase the probability of sustained remission. Plasmapheresis, corticosteroids, and IVIg can be used to optimize the clinical status in the meantime. Transsternal procedures that maximally visualize the anterior mediastinum are preferable to cervical and thoracoscopic procedures that remove less thymic tissue and can miss thymic tissue or a small thymoma.

Cyclosporine

Cyclosporine was found to be effective in a small trial as a steroid-sparing agent (38); however, the associated side effects include renal insufficiency, hypertension, headache, and hirsuitism.

It must be emphasized that MG is a highly variable disease and therefore treatment of the myasthenic patient is an art and must be individualized. There are very refractory patients who remain weak and require a variety of medications for unpredicted exacerbations. In these situations, finding the optimum combination of medications can be a challenge.

JUVENILE MYASTHENIA GRAVIS

Clinical Features

Juvenile MG is an immune-mediated disorder that has its onset before age 20 (57). Although similar to the disorder of adults, there are clinical differences. Juvenile MG is less likely to have an ocular presentation. Patients with an onset before puberty are more likely to be seronegative, with the percentage of seropositivity increasing with older age. This is probably due to the propensity of the mature immune system to produce circulating antibodies and the effect of sex hormones on immunoglobulin levels (58). The ACh receptor antibody titer may be a clue in distinguishing between congenital, genetic, or acquired forms of MG. The racial differences in juvenile MG are minor; African-American patients have a female-to-male affected sex predictor of 2:1, whereas in white patients the ratio is nearly equal. Disease severity and long-term prognosis is better when onset is before puberty. White patients have more frequent spontaneous remissions than African-American patients (59).

Treatment

The specific therapy is similar for juvenile and adult MG patients because seronegative and seropositive children and adult patients with acquired MG respond equally well to treatment (57). However, plasmapheresis may be more difficult to perform in young patients because of their small blood volumes. In children, there is an additional concern of the effect of prednisone on growth retardation. Azathioprine is a second-choice drug in this group because of the long-term risk of lymphoma. Thymectomy is effective in children; in fact, patients with juvenile MG may even have a more favorable prognosis than adults (56,58). There are racial differences that may affect the surgical outcome. The remission rate in African-American children is lower than in whites (59). Although concerns have been voiced for the long-term effects of thymectomy on the maturation of the immune system, such has never been seen in children with MG or among children that have had the thymus gland removed in the course of cardiac surgery for other reasons (56).

NEONATAL MYASTHENIA GRAVIS

Clinical Features

Neonatal MG is a transient form of NMJ transmission failure due to the passive transfer of maternal antibodies across the placenta. Symptoms include a poor suck, cry, facial weakness, dysphagia, and hypotonia (60). Clues to the diagnosis in utero may be the presence of reduced fetal movements. These infants appear to have more severe weakness, including respiratory failure at birth. Weakness in utero may also lead to joint contractures, and neonatal MG is included in the differential diagnosis of arthrogryposis. Although the overall probability of neonatal MG is low, it occurs in about 1 in 10 births to myasthenic mothers, and most infants born to myasthenic mothers are normal (61). Neonatal MG can occur in infants of myasthenic mothers who are in remission (62). The antibody type can be different between mother and affected infant, suggesting that affected infants can synthesize ACh receptor antibodies. Host factors are probably important in determining whether an infant becomes symptomatic, but the nature of these factors is unclear (61). There are no reliable predictive factors based on maternal severity of disease. However, mothers that have had an infant with neonatal MG have a higher likelihood of another affected child (60). Thus, every infant born to a myasthenic mother should be watched carefully in an intensive care unit for weakness and respiratory failure. Conversely, if there is no sign of neonatal MG after 5 to 10 days, the likelihood of an infant developing weakness because negligible. Once weakness begins, respiratory failure can occur precipitously; however, the course is usually a self-limited disorder with symptoms lasting weeks to months. Diagnosis is made by a test dose of edrophonium or diagnostic repetitive nerve stimulation (63,64).

Treatment

Treatment is based on severity of symptoms (65). Pyridostigmine alone is generally sufficient. Exchange transfusions have been performed with variable results, presumably because some infants with neonatal MG synthesize their own ACh receptor antibodies (61). Respiratory support may be necessary.

CONGENITAL OR GENETIC MYASTHENIA GRAVIS

Congenital MG represents a different spectrum of disorders, each due to a unique genetic defect in NMJ transmission (65). Most are genetic mutations with autosomal dominant and recessive modes of inheritance that alter NMJ structure or enzymatic function (66). Table 6 lists the known forms of congenital MG. Antibodies to the ACh receptor are never present. Before the acquired autoimmune nature of MG was realized, families of patients with congenital MG were known as familial infantile myasthenia.

Congenital MG is clinically characterized by early and relatively fixed degrees of weakness. The pattern of weakness is similar to immune-mediated MG and includes ptosis and extraocular, proximal limb, oropharyngeal, and even respiratory muscle weakness. There can be clinical exacerbations with marked increases that culminate in crisis. Weakness or hypotonia in early childhood may erroneously be ascribed to other genetic or

TABLE 6. *Classification of congenital myasthenic syndromes*

Presynaptic defects
ACh resynthesis or packaging
Paucity of vesicles
Synaptic defects
End-plate AChE deficiency
Postsynaptic defects
Slow-channel syndrome
AChR deficiency
Mutations of AChR subunit
Low-affinity fast-channel syndrome
High-conductance fast-channel syndrome
Severe AChR deficiency
Partially characterized defects
Congenital myasthenic syndrome resembling LEMS
AChR deficiency with paucity of secondary synaptic clefts
Familial limb girdle myasthenia

ACh, acetylcholine; AChE, acetylcholinesterase; AChR, acetylcholine receptor; LEMS, Lambert-Eaton myasthenic syndrome.
Modified from Refs. 65 and 66.

birth problems. Alternatively, early weakness may be so mild as to escape appreciation and not come to clinical attention again until childhood or even adulthood. Under these circumstances, a diagnosis of immune-mediated MG may be entertained.

Congenital MG responds poorly to pyridostigmine and usually not at all to immunomodulating therapy. A course of ephedrine given 15 mg orally three times daily may be effective in suspected cases.

The diagnosis of congenital MG should be entertained in any child with a diagnosis of MG that has been refractory to all modes of therapy. Further support for the diagnosis comes from inspection of early childhood pictures, looking for ptosis or hyperextension of the neck to achieve forward gaze. It should also be considered when other family members have had similar symptoms. Routine electrodiagnostic testing does not differentiate between immune-mediated and congenital cases; however, certain presynaptic forms of congenital MG may show facilitation after exercise, and two forms, one due to end-plate AChE deficiency and the other to a slow channel syndrome, may show a repetitive discharge after the CMAP following a single shock (Table 6). The meaningful investigation of these syndrome requires sophisticated morphologic and electrophysiologic studies of the NMJ usually available at only a few centers with a specific interest in these disorders.

LAMBERT-EATON MYASTHENIC SYNDROME

The association of small cell lung cancer (SCLC) and a myasthenic syndrome clinically and electrophysiologically was described by Lambert and coworkers in 1957 (67). The so-called LEMS is one of the best examples of an antibody-mediated paraneoplastic disease.

Clinical Features

Approximately 50 to 60% of patients with LEMS have an associated SCLC; other tumors have been described, including adenocarcinoma and breast cancer, and some may be unrelated to cancer (68). The disorder can thus be divided into two groups based on the presence of a cancer (68). Those without a tumor are generally of younger age, although most patients with LEMS are over age 40 at the onset of symptoms. Male sex is more common in the group with tumors.

The most common symptoms of LEMS are proximal leg and truncal weakness; ptosis and bulbar muscle weakness are less common. Respiratory failure is rare but can occur (68). Some patients have the warming up phenomena where by the first portion of a repetitive movement is more difficult than later ones. This may be apparent clinically with manual muscle testing that culminates in near-normal strength despite easily fatigability. Tendon reflexes may be absent with first testing and later normal after a brief agonist muscle contraction. Autonomic symptoms are common but may be overlooked and can include impotence in men, dry mouth, constipation, and urinary retention.

Natural History

The symptoms of LEMS can begin insidiously and can go undiagnosed for months to years. The most common initial diagnosis is MG (68). Among those with an associated tumor, the prognosis is largely determined by tumor progression and response to tumor treatment. In one series (68), three quarters of patients with a cancer died within a year compared with 80% of patients without a tumor who were alive 7 years after diagnosis. The cancer in LEMS may be inapparent for up to 4 years after onset of neurologic symptoms. Accordingly, it is important to differentiate between MG and LEMS and to perform an evaluation for occult SCLC if LEMS is diagnosed. This should include a history for cancer risk factors, a thorough medical evaluation, and CT of the chest with yearly repeat evaluations for the first 5 years after initial detection.

Pathophysiology

The disorder is due to autoantibodies directed against presynaptic voltage-gated calcium channels (VGCC) or related structures. This affects the regulation of channels in both those with and without an associated cancer (69,70). The antibodies are of the IgG class and are heterogeneous in their specificity against the several types of calcium channels (71). The etiology of antibodies in patients without an associated cancer is unclear, but there is likely antigenic similarity between presynaptic VGCC and those on tumors cells (72). In patients with an SCLC, antibody production is probably triggered by the tumor (73). These antibodies reduce the influx of calcium into the presynaptic terminal and reduce the amount of ACh released, in turn decreasing the size of EPPs and the likelihood of reaching threshold for a given muscle fiber AP (Table 7). The result is a low CMAP amplitude in most muscles that is also a measure of the severity of NMJ blockade (72). Similar calcium channels present on autonomic presynaptic nerve parasympathetic and sympathetic terminals account for the autonomic symptoms.

TABLE 7. *Descriptive model of the dynamics at an abnormal NMJ in LEMS after repetitive nerve stimulation*

Stimulus number	ACh pool	Available ACh quanta	ACh quanta released	Resultant EPP amplitude[a] (mV)	Action potential threshold reached
Before exercise					
1	Immediate	1,000	80	18	No
2	Immediate	800	72	12	No
3	Immediate	640	58	8	No
4	Mobilizable	>640	>58	>8	No
5	Mobilizable	>640	>58	>8	No
After exercise					
1	Immediate	1,000	200	36	Yes
2	Immediate	800	160	28	No
3	Immediate	640	128	24	No
4	Mobilizable	>640	>128	>30	Yes
5	Mobilizable	>640	>128	>30	Yes

Top of table shows the effects of reduced influx of calcium leading to a small number of ACh released. This results in lower amplitude EPPs that fail to elicit muscle fiber action potentials. Bottom of table shows how increased ACh released through enhanced calcium influx will facilitate transmission to normal. Numbers representing ACh quanta are approximate.

*In this model, the EPP amplitude must be greater than 30 mv to reach threshold for generation of a muscle fiber action potential.

NMJ, neuromuscular junction; LEMS, Lambert-Eaton myasthenic syndrome; ACh, acetylcholine; EPP, end plate potential.

Diagnosis

Electrodiagnostic testing is important in identifying LEMS and distinguishing it from MG. A low CMAP amplitude, often less than 10% of the lower limit of normal and in a diffuse distribution, is an important electrodiagnostic clue (Fig. 7). Repetitive motor nerve stimulation at rates of 2 to 4 Hz may show a decrement as in MG; however, the distinguishing feature of LEMS is a marked facilitation after 10 seconds of exercise or with high-frequency stimulation at 50 Hz. The degree of facilitation depends on the size of the first CMAP but will generally restore the CMAP amplitude to normal. The increment after high-frequency activation may reach 10,000-fold if the first CMAP is extremely small (68).

There is a serum assay for antibodies reactive to P/Q- and N-type VGCCs that are detected infrequently except in LEMS or in the context of other paraneoplastic neurologic disorders (70). There is an association between LEMS and both organ-specific and nonorgan-specific autoantibodies in patients with LEMS (20,68). The discovery of VGCC antibodies in a clinically affected patient should prompt a search for occult SCLC; generally, a chest CT or magnetic resonance image will suffice.

Treatment

Many of the same drugs and procedures used to treat MG are also effective in LEMS; however, there are drugs that specifically enhance presynaptic function that are unique to the treatment of LEMS. A laboratory measure that can be used to quantify therapeutic response and has predictive value is the amplitude of the CMAP at the start of therapy; a very low CMAP amplitudes generally suggests a poorer outcome with therapy (73).

Patients with LEMS may benefit from AChE drugs in doses used for MG, although the improvement in strength is likely to be mild. A trial of plasmapheresis may be effective, with rapid improvement in most patients (74,75), and the response may be sustained without an associated cancer. The IgG fraction collected from the plasma separation has been used to transfer symptoms of LEMS to experimental animals (75). IVIg in doses of 2 g/kg over 2 days was temporarily effective in a placebo-controlled crossover trial in LEMS patients without cancer (76). Prednisone was effective in small cohorts with or without cancer (77,78). Azathioprine was tried in patients with LEMS but usually in conjunction with other drugs; accordingly, its effectiveness was difficult to assess (75). There is concern that treatment of patients without an associated cancer could precipitate the development of a later cancer. In one study, several patients treated with azathioprine later showed evidence of SCLC, but several arguments suggest that azathioprine was not the cause. First, it is generally associated with the development of lymphoid tumors, not SCLC. Second, the time interval between initiation of azathioprine and development of cancer in the LEMS patients was 2 to 3 years, a

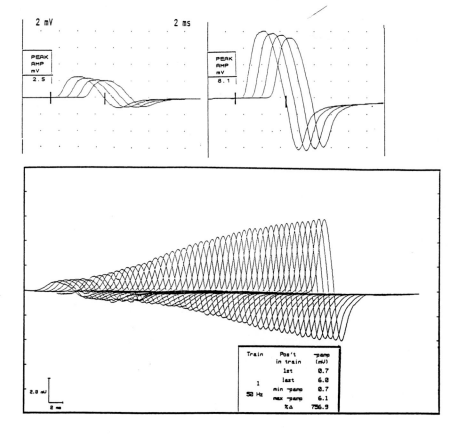

FIG. 7. Responses to repetitive stimulation in LEMS. Top: Left trace shows low amplitude response to 3-Hz repetitive stimulation; right trace shows 245% facilitation after 10 seconds of maximal muscle activation. Bottom: Facilitation of the response to 50-Hz repetitive stimulation with a 750% increase in amplitude.

period during which malignant cell changes could progress to a radiographically detectable lesion (68).

3,4-Diaminopyridine enhances synaptic transmission and increases ACh release by blocking potassium channels that prolongs nerve APs and in turn prolongs the activation of VGCC (79). In a double-blinded, placebo-controlled, crossover study, 3,4-Diaminopyridine doses of 25 mg orally four times daily significantly improved strength in patients with LEMS, with or without cancer (80). The drug remains effective after several years of follow-up. Mild side effects include perioral and acral paresthesias, epigastric distress, and rarely seizures. 3,4-Diaminopyridine is an orphan drug. It is not approved and is available in the United States at only a few institutions, such as the Mayo Clinic in Rochester, Minnesota, and Duke University in Durham, North Carolina. Availability outside of the United States is unknown.

Treatment of the underlying SCLC is an option with chemotherapy, radiation therapy, and rarely surgery. The response to primary treatment of the cancer has been variable but most show some initial improvement (73). Apparent cures of the cancer and LEMS after 7 years of follow-up have been reported. In some the cancer may respond but the symptoms of LEMS remained unchanged, whereas others have had initial improvement of their weakness but with later relapse.

CONCLUSION

The diagnosis and management of NMJ disorders is ever challenging. It requires understanding of the anatomy, physiology, pathology, immunology, and pharmacology of the motor unit. Diagnostic errors can be reduced by viewing disorders of the NMJ as a family of diseases, in which systematic electrophysiologic studies separate presynaptic from postsynaptic disorders. A battery of serologic, radiographic, and genetic studies provide support to the exact etiologic diagnosis. When thoughtful evaluation and management principles are followed, it will be apparent that each patient is unique, and some patients will continue to challenge the most experienced clinicians.

REFERENCES

1. Younger DS. Myasthenia gravis: historical perspective and overview. *Neurology* 1997;48[Suppl 5]:S1–7.
2. Feinstein B, Lindegrd B, Nyman E, Wohlfart G. Morphologic studies of motor units in normal human muscles. *Acta Anat* 1955;23:127–142.
3. Cors C, Woolf AL. *The innervation of muscle.* Springfield, IL: Charles C Thomas, 1959:12–14.
4. Porter JD, Baker RS. Muscles of a different color: the unusual properties of the extraocular muscles may predispose or protect them in neurogenic and myogenic disease. *Neurology* 1996;46:30–37.
5. Stålberg E, Trontelj JV. *Single fiber electromyography*, 2nd ed. New York: Raven Press, 1994.
6. Taylor P, Brown JH. Acetylcholine. In: Siegel GJ, Agranoff BW, Albers RW, Molinoff PB, eds. *Basic neurochemistry*, 5th ed. New York: Raven Press, 1994:231–260.
7. Kandel ER, Schwartz JH, Jessell TM. *Principles of neural science*, 3rd ed. Norwalk, CT: Appleton & Lange, 1991.

8. Engel AG, Sahashi K, Fumagalli G. The immunopathology of acquired myasthenia gravis. *Ann NY Acad Sci* 1981;377:158–174.
9. Katz B. *Nerve, muscle, and synapse.* New York: McGraw-Hill, 1966.
10. Kaminski HJ, Suarez JI, Ruff RL. Neuromuscular junction physiology in myasthenia gravis: isoforms of the acetylcholine receptor in extraocular muscles and the contribution of sodium channels to the safety factor. *Neurology* 1997;48[Suppl 5]:S8–S17.
11. Drachman DB. Myasthenia gravis. *N Engl J Med* 1994;330:1797–1810.
12. Osserman KE. *Myasthenia gravis.* New York: Grune & Stratton, 1958.
13. Campbell H, Bramwell E. Myasthenia gravis. *Brain* 1900;23:277–336.
14. Grob D, Brunner NG, Namba T. The natural course of myasthenia gravis and effect of therapeutic measures. *Ann NY Acad Sci* 1981;377:652–669.
15. Lennon VA, Lambert EH. Monoclonal autoantibodies to acetylcholine receptors: evidence for a dominant idiotype and requirement of complement for pathogenicity. *Ann NY Acad Sci* 1981;377:77–96.
16. Engel AG, Tsujihata M, Lindstrom IM, et al. The motor end plate in myasthenia gravis and in experimental autoimmune myasthenia gravis: a quantitative ultrastructural study. *Ann NY Acad Sci* 1976;274:60–79.
17. Howard FM, Lennon VA, Finley J, Matsumoto J, Elveback LR. Clinical correlations of antibodies that bind, block, or modulate human acetylcholine receptors in myasthenia gravis. *Ann NY Acad Sci* 1987;505:526–538.
18. Burges J, Vincent A, Molenaar PC, Newsom-Davis J, Peers C, Wray D. Passive transfer of seronegative myasthenia gravis to mice. *Muscle Nerve* 1994;17:1393–1400.
19. Soliven BC, Lange DJ, Penn AS, et al. Seronegative myasthenia gravis. *Neurology* 1988;38:514–517.
20. Lennon VA, Lambert EH, Whittingham S, Fairbanks V. Autoimmunity in the Lambert-Eaton myasthenic syndrome. *Muscle Nerve* 1982;5:S21–S25.
21. Lennon VA. Serological diagnosis of myasthenia gravis and the Lambert-Eaton myasthenic syndrome. In: Lisak RP, ed. *Handbook of myasthenia gravis and myasthenic syndromes.* New York: Marcel Dekker, 1994:149–164.
22. Sprent J. The thymus and T-cell tolerance. *Ann NY Acad Sci* 1993;68:1–15.
22a. Katz JS, Wolfe GI, Bryan WW, Tintner R, Barohn RJ. Acetylcholine receptor antibodies in the Lambert-Eaton myasthenic syndrome. *Neurology* 1998;50:470–475.
22b. Moorthy G, Behrens MM, Drachman DB, et al. Ocular pseudomyasthenia or ocular myasthenia "plus": a warning to clinicians. *Neurology* 1989;39:1150–1154.
23. Harvey AM, Masland RL. A method for the study of neuromuscular transmission in human subjects. *Bull J Hopkins Hosp* 1941;68:81–93.
24. Desmedt JE. The neuromuscular disorder in myasthenia gravis. I. Electrical and mechanical responses to nerve stimulation in hand muscles. In: Desmedt JE, ed. *New concepts of the motor unit, neuromuscular disorders, electromyographic kinesiology.* Basel: S Karger, 1973:241–304.
25. Oh SJ. *Electromyography. Neuromuscular transmission studies.* Baltimore: Williams & Wilkins, 1988.
26. Hansen SL, Singleton JR, Liow K, Chowdhury A, Bromberg MB. Minimizing trial-to-trial error in repetitive stimulation for neuromuscular junction disorders. *Muscle Nerve* 1997;20:1086(abst).
27. Schumm F, Stöhr M. Accessory nerve stimulation in the assessment of myasthenia gravis. *Muscle Nerve* 1984;7:147–151.
28. Tim RW, Sanders DB. Repetitive nerve stimulation studies in the Lambert-Eaton myasthenic syndrome. *Muscle Nerve* 1994;17:995–1001.
29. Sanders DB, Howard JF. AAEE minimonograph #25: Single-fiber electromyography in myasthenia gravis. *Muscle Nerve* 1986;9:809–819.
30. Schwartz MS, Stålberg E. Single fibre electromyographic studies in myasthenia gravis with repetitive nerve stimulation. *J Neurol Neurosurg Psychiatry* 1975;38:678–682.
31. Gilchrist MH, Massey JM, Sanders DB. Single fiber EMG and repetitive stimulation of the same muscle in myasthenia gravis. *Muscle Nerve* 1994;17:171–175.
32. Bromberg MB, Scott DM. Single fiber EMG reference values: reformatted in tabular form. AD HOC Committee of the AAEM Single Fiber Special Interest Group. *Muscle Nerve* 1994;17:820–821.
33. Trontelj JV, Stålberg E. Single motor end-plates in myasthenia gravis and LEMS at different firing rates. *Muscle Nerve* 1990;14:226–232.

34. Sanders DB. Electrophysiological and pharmacological tests in neuromuscular junction disorders. In: Lisak RP, ed. *Handbook of myasthenia gravis and myasthenic syndromes.* New York: Marcel Dekker, 1994:103–148.

35. Aarli JA. Myasthenia gravis and thymoma. In: Lisak RP, ed. *Handbook of myasthenia gravis and myasthenic syndromes.* New York: Marcel Dekker, 1994:207–224.

36. Batra P, Herrmann C, Mulder D. Mediastinal imaging in myasthenia gravis: correlation of chest radiography, CT, MR and surgical findings. *AJR Am J Roentgenol* 1987;148:515–519.

37. Rowland LP. Controversies about the treatment of myasthenia gravis. *J Neurol Neurosurg Psychiatry* 1980;43:644–659.

38. Tindall RSA, Rollins JA, Phillips TJ, Greenlee RG, Wells L, Belendiuk G. Preliminary results of a double-blind, randomized, placebo-controlled trial of cyclosporine in myasthenia gravis. *N Engl J Med* 1987;316:719–724.

39. Riggs JE. Pharmacologic enhancement of neuromuscular transmission in myasthenia gravis. *Clin Neuropharmacol* 1982;5:277–292.

40. Miller RG, Milner-Brown HS, Mirka A. Prednisone-induced worsening of neuromuscular function in myasthenia gravis. *Neurology* 1986;36:729–732.

41. Gajdos P, Chevret S, Clair B, Tranchant C, Chastang C. Clinical trial of plasma exchange and high-dose intravenous immunoglobulin in myasthenia gravis. *Ann Neurol* 1997;41:789–796.

42. Liblau R, Gajdos PH, Bustarret FH, El Habib R, Bach JF, Morel E. Intravenous γ-globulin in myasthenia gravis: interaction with anti-acetylcholine receptor autoantibodies. *J Clin Immunol* 1991;11:128–131.

43. Dwyer JM. Manipulating the immune system with immune globulin. *N Engl J Med* 1992;326:107–116.

44. Parrillo JE, Fauci AS. Mechanisms of glucocorticoid action of immune processes. *Annu Rev Pharmacol Toxicol* 1979;19:179–201.

45. Pascuzzi RM, Coslett BH, Johns TR. Long-term corticosteroid treatment of myasthenia gravis: report of 116 patients. *Ann Neurol* 1984;15:291–298.

46. Arsura E, Brunner NG, Namba T, Grob D. High-dose intravenous methylprednisolone in myasthenia gravis. *Arch Neurol* 1985;42:1149–1153.

47. Miano MA, Bosley TM, Heiman-Patterson TD, et al. Factors influencing outcome of prednisone dose reduction in myasthenia gravis. *Neurology* 1991;41:919–921.

48. Bromberg MB, Wald JJ, Forshew DA, Feldman EL, Albers JW. Randomized trial of azathioprine or prednisone for initial treatment of myasthenia gravis. *J Neurol Sci* 1997;150:59–62.

49. Matell G. Immunosuppressive drugs: azathioprine in the treatment of myasthenia gravis. *Ann NY Acad Sci* 1987;505:588–594.

50. Palace J, Newsom-Davis J, Lecky B, and the Myasthenia Study Group. A randomized double-blind trial of prednisolone or with azathioprine in myasthenia gravis. *Neurology* 1998;50:1778–1783.

51. Hohlfeld R, Michels M, Heininger K, Besinger U, Toyka KV. Azathioprine toxicity during long-term immunosuppression of generalized myasthenia gravis. *Neurology* 1988;38:258–261.

52. Krueger JG, Tallent MB, Richie RE, Johnson HK, MacDonnel RC, Turner B. Neoplasia in immunosuppressed renal transplant patients: a 20-year experience. *So Med J* 1985;78:501–505.

53. Blalock A, Mason MF, Morgan HJ, Riven SS. Myasthenia gravis and tumor of the thymus region. Report of a case in which the tumor was removed. *Ann Surg* 1939;110:544–559.

54. Jaretzki A. Thymectomy for myasthenia gravis: analysis of the controversies regarding technique and results. *Neurology* 1997;48[Suppl 5]:S52–S63.

55. Jaretzki A, Penn AS, Younger DS, et al. Maximal thymectomy for myasthenia gravis. *J Thorac Cardiovasc Surg* 1988;95:747–757.

56. Olanow CW, Wechsler AS, Sirotkin-Roses M, Stajich J, Roses AD. Thymectomy as primary therapy in myasthenia gravis. *Ann NY Acad Sci* 1987;505:595–606.

57. Snead OC, Benton JW, Dwyer D, et al. Juvenile myasthenia gravis. *Neurology* 1980;30:732–739.

58. Andrews PI, Massey JM, Sanders DB. Acetycholine receptor antibodies in juvenile myasthenia gravis. *Neurology* 1993:43:977–982.

59. Andrews PI, Massey JM, Howard JF, Sanders DB. Race, sex, and puberty influence onset, severity, and outcome in juvenile myasthenia gravis. *Neurology* 1994;44:1208–1214.

60. Morel E, Eymard B, Vernet-der Garabedian B, Pannier C, Dulac O, Bach JF. Neonatal myasthenia gravis: a new clinical and immunologic appraisal on 30 cases. *Neurology* 1988;38:128–142.

61. Lefvert AK, Osterman PO. Newborn infants to myasthenic mothers: a clinical study and an investigation of acetylcholine receptor antibodies in 17 children. *Neurology* 1983;33:223–238.

62. Elias SB, Butler I, Appel SH. Neonatal myasthenia gravis in the infant of a myasthenic mother in remission. *Ann Neurol* 1978;6:72–75.

63. Fenichel GM. Clinical syndromes of myasthenia in infancy and childhood. *Arch Neurol* 1978;35:97–103.

64. Cornblath DR. Disorders of neuromuscular transmission in infants and children. *Muscle Nerve* 1988;9:606–611.

65. Engel AG. Congenital myasthenic syndromes. In: Lisak RP, ed. *Handbook of myasthenia gravis and myasthenic syndromes.* New York: Marcel Dekker, 1994:33–62.

66. Engel AG, Ohno K, Milone M, Sine SM. Congenital myasthenic syndromes caused by mutations in acetylcholine receptor genes. *Neurology* 1997;48[Suppl 5]:S28–S35.

67. Eaton LM, Lambert EH. Electromyography and electric stimulation of nerves in diseases of motor unit. Observations on myasthenic syndrome associated with malignant tumors. *JAMA* 1957;163:1117–1124.

68. O'Neill JH, Murray NMF, Newsom-Davis J. The Lambert-Eaton myasthenic syndrome. *Brain* 1988;111:577–596.

69. Newsom-Davis J, Murray N, Wray D, et al. Lambert-Eaton myasthenic syndrome: electropysiological evidence for a humoral factor. *Muscle Nerve* 1982;5:S17–S20.

70. Lennon VA, Kryzer TJ, Griesmann GY, et al. Calcium-channel antibodies in the Lambert-Eaton syndrome and other paraneoplastic syndromes. *N Engl J Med* 1995;332:1467–1474.

71. Johnston I, Lang B, Leys K, Newsom-Davis J. Heterogeneity of calcium channel autoantibodies detected using a small-cell lung cancer line derived from a Lambert-Eaton myasthenic syndrome patient. *Neurology* 1994;44:334–338.

72. Lang B, Vincent A, Murray NMF, Newsom-Davis J. Lambert-Eaton myasthenic syndrome: immunoglobulin G inhibition of Ca^{2+} flux in tumor cells correlates with disease severity. *Ann Neurol* 1989;25:265–271.

73. Chalk CH, Murray NMF, Newsom-Davis J, O'Neill JH, Spiro SG. Response of the Lambert-Eaton myasthenic syndrome to treatment of associated small-cell lung carcinoma. *Neurology* 1990;40:1552–1556.

74. Dau PC, Denys EH. Plasmapheresis and immunosuppressive drug therapy in the Eaton-Lambert syndrome. *Ann Neurol* 1982;11:570–575.

75. Newsom-Davis J, Murray NMF. Plasma exchange and immunosuppressive drug treatment in the Lambert-Eaton myasthenic syndrome. *Neurology* 1984;34:480–485.

76. Bain PG, Motomura M, Newsom-Davis J, et al. Effects of intravenous immunoglobulin on muscle weakness and calcium-channel autoantibodies in the Lambert-Easton myasthenic syndrome. *Neurology* 1996;47:678–683.

77. Streib EW, Rothner AD. Eaton-Lambert myasthenic syndrome: long-term treatment of three patients with prednisone. *Ann Neurol* 1981;10:448–453.

78. Ingram DA, Davis GR, Schwartz MS, Traub M, Newland AC, Swash M. Cancer-associated myasthenic (Eaton-Lambert) syndrome. Distribution of abnormality and effect of treatment. *J Neurol Neurosurg Psychiatry* 1984;47:806–812.

79. Thomsen RH, Wilson DF. Effects of 4-aminopyridine and 3,4-diaminopyridine on transmitter release at the neuromuscular junction. *J Pharmacol Exp Ther* 1983;227:260–265.

80. McEvoy KM, Windebank AJ, Daube JR, Low PA. 3,4-Diaminopyridine in the treatment of Lambert-Eaton myasthenic syndrome. *N Engl J Med* 1989;321:1567–1571.

Motor Disorders,
edited by David S. Younger.
Lippincott Williams & Wilkins, Philadelphia © 1999.

CHAPTER 14

Membrane Motor Disorders (Channelopathies)

Michael Rose and Robert C. Griggs

There has been a virtual explosion in the recognition of disorders of membrane ion channels: the channelopathies. Ion channel function may be modulated by changes in voltage (voltage gated), chemical interaction (ligand gated), or by mechanical perturbation. Channelopathies can affect both the peripheral and central nervous system and may be inherited or acquired.

Disturbance of muscle ion channel function may result in muscle membrane hyperexcitability, leading to myotonia as the dominant feature, or alternatively it may result in muscle membrane inexcitability, leading to the weakness seen in periodic paralysis. The myotonias have traditionally been divided into dystrophic and nondystrophic disorders. The nondystrophic myotonias have myotonia as the prominent symptom and have been shown to be directly due to muscle membrane channelopathies. They may be divided into sodium or chloride channelopathies. Dystrophic myotonias usually have myotonia as one of several muscle symptoms, with muscle atrophy and weakness usually more prominent. These include myotonic dystrophy and proximal myopathy with myotonia. Their precise pathophysiology remains unclear; although there may not be a primary channel gene defect, it seems likely that there will be at least indirect disturbance of channel function to account for the myotonia. The Schwartz Jampel syndrome, or chondrodystrophic myotonia, has distinctive clinical features with prominent and severe continuous motor activity. The Schwartz Jampel syndrome may include two or more disorders. Neurophysiology shows heterogeneous features with a neurogenic origin for the continuous motor activity, at least in some cases, which are, therefore, not true myotonia. In other cases, physiologic and genetic studies suggest that a muscle sodium channel defect is present.

The periodic paralyses have been traditionally divided into those associated with a high or normal serum potassium or hyperkalemic periodic paralysis and those with a low serum potassium concentration or hypokalemic periodic paralysis. The serum potassium concentration is more a consequence than the cause of the periodic paralysis. This traditional separation has been vindicated by the demonstration that they are due to disorders of different ion channels with hyperkalemic periodic paralysis being a sodium channelopathy and hypokalemic periodic paralysis being a calcium channelopathy. Periodic paralysis may be secondary to changes in potassium concentration, and although these are not primary channelopathies, they merit inclusion in this chapter because they are important in differential diagnosis of the primary periodic paralyses. Andersen syndrome is a separate familial periodic paralysis with cardiac dysrhythmias and distinctive facial features. The genetic basis for Andersen syndrome remains unclear, but it is also a strong candidate for being a channelopathy.

The muscle channelopathies mentioned thus far are defects of voltage-gated channels. A defect of mechanically regulated channels may be responsible for rippling muscle syndrome. Defects in a ligand-gated channel, the nicotinic acetylcholine receptor, result in myasthenia gravis (MG), and these may be due to a gene defect as in congenital MG or due to autoimmune disease as in acquired autoimmune MG. Autoimmune antibodies may affect the voltage-gated presynaptic calcium channels causing Lambert-Eaton myasthenic syndrome (LEMS). The latter are discussed in Chapter 13. The ryanodine receptor is a ligand-gated calcium release channel that facilitates the release of calcium from the sarcoplasmic reticulum into the cytoplasm; defects in this channel result in malignant hyperthermia.

In the peripheral nerve, channelopathies can cause nerve hyperactivity, a feature of neuromyotonia or Isaacs syndrome, and myokymia. In Isaacs syndrome, where neuromyotonia is a major feature, most cases are sporadic

M. Rose: Department of Neurology, Guys, Kings and St. Thomas's Medical School and King's College Hospital, Denmark Hill, London SE5 8AZ, United Kingdom.

R.C. Griggs: Department of Neurology, University of Rochester, Rochester, New York 14642.

and usually on an autoimmune basis. Myokymia is a feature of episodic ataxia type 1, which is due to mutations of a potassium channel gene. The marine toxin ciguatoxin ingested from contaminated fish or shellfish is a potent sodium channel blocker that causes a rapid onset of numbness, intense paraesthesia, and dysesthesia, and muscle weakness (1).

SODIUM CHANNELOPATHIES

These are disorders of the α1 subunit of the muscle sodium channel. Allelic abnormalities of this channel result in a number of disorders, including paramyotonia congenita, hyperkalemic periodic paralysis, normokalemic periodic paralysis, and the sodium channel myotonias. The sodium channel myotonias phenotypically resemble myotonia congenita but have atypical features distinguished by worsening of the myotonia with potassium challenge, hence their alternative name of potassium aggravated myotonias. There are a number of variants, including myotonia permanans, myotonia fluctuans, and acetazolamide-sensitive myotonia.

Clinical Features

Paramyotonia Congenita

The predominant symptoms are those of paradoxical myotonia, usually present from birth and persisting throughout life, and cold-induced weakness. The myotonia is paradoxical because unlike classic myotonia, it increases with repetitive movements. The myotonia of paramyotonia congenita is also exacerbated by cold exposure and particularly affects the face, neck, and forearms. The legs are less affected. Typically on relief of the myotonia, either spontaneously or on warming, there is a variable degree of weakness that can persist for hours. In a warm environment, patients may have no symptoms at all. Pain and muscle hypertrophy are usually not seen. In some affected families there is a tendency for attacks of paralysis to be independent of the myotonia and of the cold, and these can be precipitated by potassium ingestion in much the same way as hyperkalemic periodic paralysis. Such symptoms of episodic nontemperature provoked weakness tend to occur in adolescence, if at all.

Hyperkalemic Periodic Paralysis and Normokalemic Periodic Paralysis

As with paramyotonia congenita, hyperkalemic periodic paralysis normally appears in infancy or early childhood with frequent episodes of paralysis that are generally brief and mild and last 15 minutes to 4 hours. Attacks are often precipitated by a period of rest after exercise or the administration of potassium. They also commonly start in the morning before breakfast. Stress tends to make the attacks more easily provoked. Attacks can be diminished or aborted by carbohydrate intake or exercise.

Weakness is mainly proximal, but distal muscles can be involved. There is usually no ocular or respiratory weakness. Examination during an attack reveals a flaccid tetraparesis with absent reflexes and normal sensation. Serum potassium concentrations may rise during the attack but not necessarily above the upper limit of normal range and rarely into levels that cause cardiac dysrhythmia. Thus, so-called normokalemic periodic paralysis may be a sodium channelopathy and merely part of the spectrum of hyperkalemic periodic paralysis. At least one family with normokalemic periodic paralysis has the same Thr704Met sodium channel mutation commonly seen in hyperkalemic periodic paralysis. Generally between attacks, patients maintain normal strength, but in a few cases there is persistent mild weakness. The frequency of attacks may decline as the patient gets older. In some families with hyperkalemic periodic paralysis, there is coexistent myotonia that may be subclinical and only detected on electromyography (EMG). If symptomatic it is usually mild. In these patients, cooling may provoke weakness but does not provoke myotonia.

Sodium Channel Myotonias or Potassium Aggravated Myotonia

This is a group of recently classified myotonias that have been shown to be due to sodium channel gene mutations but which do not have the features of paramyotonia congenita or episodes of periodic paralysis.

Myotonia Permanans

This is characterized by permanent very severe myotonia. One case was originally diagnosed as having Schwartz Jampel syndrome. Another had myotonia severe enough to impair breathing.

Myotonia Fluctuans

In this condition, myotonia fluctuates on a daily basis, being undetectable on some days. When present, myotonia mainly affects eye closure, chewing, swallowing, and hand grip and shows a warm-up phenomenon. The myotonia may worsen after exercise typically after a delay of 20 to 40 minutes and sometimes to the point of causing immobility. Such exacerbations may persist for 30 minutes to 2 hours. Exercise after cooling of the forearm may lead to worsening of the myotonia in some, but weakness is uncommon. It is not aggravated by cold. Potassium loading worsens the myotonia but does not cause episodes of weakness.

Acetazolamide-responsive Myotonia

This is associated with painful myotonia that responds well to acetazolamide, which are both atypical features for myotonia congenita. In some cases the myotonia is worsened by the cold but without associated weakness or a decrease in the compound muscle action potential (CMAP) as seen in paramyotonia congenita. Potassium loading worsens the painful myotonia but does not cause weakness as in hyperkalemic periodic paralysis. Fixed interictal weakness does not occur.

Pathophysiology

All of the above disorders result from allelic point mutations in the sodium channel gene *SCN4A* on 17q23-25 that codes for an adult isoform of the skeletal muscle sodium channel α1 subunit. To date, 19 different point mutations have been found that result in amino acid substitutions in conserved portions of the gene (Table 1). These mutations are all inherited in an autosomal dominant (AD) pattern. The effects of these mutations can be measured by electrical recording of sodium currents in dissociated fibers of muscle biopsies obtained from patients and in cultured myotubules and fibroblasts transfected with cDNA coding for mutant channels. All mutations so studied show abnormalities of voltage gating, causing slowing of fast inactivation of the sodium channel. This finding is consistent with the sites of these mutations that are either situated in the intracellular loop, which is believed to inactivate the

channel by occluding the inner mouth of the pore, or else line inner vestibule of the ion conducting pore to which the inactivation gate binds. In vitro disruption of fast inactivation of just 2% of sodium channels using a specific toxin has shown that the resulting small persistent sodium current is sufficient to cause delayed relaxation of muscle twitch. A prolonged current pulse elicits a train of repetitive action potentials that persists beyond the duration of the current pulse. These effects are analogous to that seen in myotonia. The self-sustained train of discharges occurring after the stimulus depends on an intact T-tubule system. This is thought to occur partly by excess potassium accumulation in T tubules.

It has not yet been possible to produce an animal model with the higher proportion of abnormal sodium channel fast inactivation that is seen in hyperkalemic periodic paralysis. However, computer modeling experiments have shown that increasing the proportion of abnormal fast inactivating channels only slightly above 2% is sufficient to cause prolonged depolarization of the membrane. This depolarization would inactivate both mutant and wild-type sodium channels which would render the muscle refractory to further stimulus and cause weakness. As depolarization of the membrane inactivates wild-type and

TABLE 1. *Muscle channel gene mutations with their clinical features*

Sodium channelopathy SCN4A 17q23–25		
Thr704Met		
Ser906Thr		
Ala1156Thr	With features of paramyotonia	Hyperkalemic periodic paralysis
Met1360Val	With features of paramyotonia	
Met1592Val	With features of paramyotonia	
Val1293Ile		
Thr1313Met		
Leu1433Arg		
Arg1448Cys		
Arg1448His		Paramyotonia congenita
Arg1448Pro		
Val1458Phe		
Phel1473Ser		
Ser804Phe	Myotonia fluctuans	
Ile1160Val	Acetazolamide sensitive myotonia	
Gly1306Ala	Myotonia fluctuans	Potassium aggravated myotonia
Gly1306Val	Exercise-induced myotonia	
Gly1306Glu	Myotonia permanans	
Val1589Met	Cold-sensitive myotonia	
Calcium channelopathy CACNL1A3 1q31–32		
Arg528His		
Arg1239His		Hypokalemic periodic paralysis
Arg1239Gly		
Chloride channelopathy CLCN1 7q35		
Gln552Arg	Myotonia levior	
Ile290Met	Thomsen's myotonia	
Gly230Glu	Thomsen's myotonia	Myotonia congenita
Pro480Leu	Thomsen's myotonia	
Plus 13 or more additional mutations	Becker's myotonia	

mutant sodium channels, this offers a pathophysiologic explanation for the dominant effect of these mutations. Recovery from this situation would be facilitated by slow reactivation of the sodium channels. A defect of slow reactivation is an additional feature of the Thr704Met and Met1592Val mutations that may accentuate the propensity to attacks of weakness. The computer models show that a raised extracellular potassium does accentuate the sodium channel-gating deficits, but it remains unclear as to why this should be a phenomenon seen with some sodium channel mutations and not others. The pathophysiologic basis for cold sensitivity, triggering of attacks by rest or fasting, the warm-up phenomenon, and paradoxical myotonia are incompletely understood.

Genotype Phenotype Correlations

The *SCN4A* gene is only expressed in significant levels in skeletal muscle, thus explaining the lack of cardiac or central nervous system involvement in these disorders (2). Each point mutation has been correlated with a predominant phenotype (Table 1). However, the various mutations are not distributed along the gene in an obvious way that correlates with the phenotype. Indeed, even adjacent mutations can cause different phenotypes; the Met1592Val mutation causes hyperkalemic periodic paralysis, whereas the almost adjacent Val1589Met mutation causes cold-induced potassium-aggravated myotonia (3). The Thr704Met and the Met1592Val mutations account for 60% and 30%, respectively, of the genotyped families with hyperkalemic periodic paralysis. In one family, a Met1360Val mutation was found to cause hyperkalemic periodic paralysis in one male only; females had EMG evidence of myotonia but no attacks of periodic paralysis (4). Those cases having the Thr704Met mutation are more likely to have fixed progressive weakness and myotonia. The Thr1313Met mutation occurs in 45% of cases of paramyotonia congenita, whereas the Arg1448Cys accounts for 35% of cases. There is some overlap of phenotype with the Met1360Val (4), Ser804Phe, Ala1156Thr, and Val1592Met mutations showing features of hyperkalemic periodic paralysis and paramyotonia in some families.

The phenotypic expression of a *SCN4A* mutation also depends on the nature of the amino acid switch, as well as the site of the mutation. The best example of this is the trio of mutations at the glycine 1306 site. Substitution of the glycine for glutamine resulted in severe permanent myotonia, requiring treatment to prevent respiratory embarrassment in one sporadic case of myotonia permanans. Substitution of glycine for valine resulted in exercise-induced myotonia without cold provocation and not requiring treatment in two members of one family. When alanine was the substituted amino acid, family members had myotonia fluctuans (5). An elegant explanation for the descending severity of the myotonia with these mutations is that it appears to relate to decreasing length of the side chain of the substituted amino acid; glutamine has a large side chain, valine has an intermediate length side chain, whereas alanine has a small one. The glycine at position 1306 is highly conserved and occupies the cytoplasmic loop between domains III and IV at the proposed site of the "hinge" for the "lid" occluding the ion channel pore. Glycine, having no side chains, confers a high degree of flexibility at the hinge that is compromised by its substitution by amino acids having side chains. The restriction of the hinge increases with the length of the side chains and causes increasing impairment of channel inactivation and thus worsening myotonia (5). One family with apparent hyperkalemic periodic paralysis was described in which there was no linkage to the *SCN4A* locus, suggesting genetic heterogeneity (6).

CHLORIDE CHANNELOPATHIES

There are two similar forms of myotonia congenita due to disorders of the chloride channel: Thomsen disease, an AD disorder, and Becker disease, which is autosomal recessive (AR).

Clinical Features

Thomsen's Myotonia

The main symptom is painless generalized myotonia, perceived as muscle stiffness, which usually appears in the first and second decade of life. It is provoked by exertion after rest and thus can be demonstrated by asking the patient to rise from a seated position after a period of rest. The myotonia improves with exercise. Patients have well-developed muscles with particular hypertrophy of the lower limbs, giving them an athletic appearance. Muscle strength can be normal, possibly even stronger than normal, giving them advantage in power sports where speed is not a requirement. They have normal reflexes. Eyelid, grip, and percussion myotonia can be demonstrated.

Becker's Myotonia

This disease has some features similar to Thomsen disease. The myotonia comes on later in life but can be more severe than in Thomsen disease. In addition to severe myotonic stiffness, patients can also have disabling transient weakness not seen in Thomsen disease. Their muscles are initially strong and then rapidly weaken, and it then takes a period of activity before full strength returns. The length of time for strength to recover can be 30 minutes or longer, resulting in severe and incapacitating weakness and a misdiagnosis of muscular dystrophy or periodic paralysis. Untreated patients can become wheelchair confined. As in Thomsen disease, there may be hypertrophy of leg and buttock muscles with hyperlordosis of the spine.

Myotonia Levior

This may be considered a mild form of Thomsen myotonia. Myotonia began at 5 years of age in two siblings. The myotonia was worse with exercise. The mother had a similar degree of myotonia. Examination showed no evidence of muscle hypertrophy and no permanent or transient weakness. Lid lag, percussion myotonia, and grip myotonia with warm up phenomenon were present. The myotonia was not aggravated by cooling nor by potassium loading (7).

Pathophysiology

In both forms of myotonia congenita, the characteristic feature is that of a reduced muscle membrane chloride conductance that results in muscle membrane hyperexcitability with after depolarization and repetitive firing leading to the myotonia. This abnormal physiology can be reproduced in normal muscle by chloride channel blockers or by the substitution of impermeable ions for chloride. Normal physiologic activity in muscle results in accumulation of potassium in the T tubules. Where chloride conductance is normal, the depolarizing effect of this accumulated potassium is limited and has no significant consequence. When chloride conductance is reduced below 30% of the total membrane conductance, the accumulated potassium results in a significant afterdepolarization and repetitive self-triggering electrical activity of the muscle.

Thomsen and Becker disease and myotonia levior are allelic disorders of a chloride channel gene (CLCNI) on chromosome 7q32. To date, six missense and one nonsense mutation have been identified as causing Thomsen's disease. At least 18, mostly missense, mutations have been described in association with Becker disease (8). Some previously described pathologic recessive mutations have been subsequently demonstrated to be nonpathogenic polymorphisms (8). Studies of the G230E dominant mutation in three families suggested a founder effect (10). Dominant mutations do not interfere with protein translation or turnover but when coexpressed 1:1 with wild-type chloride channels in the Xenopus oocyte expression system result in a reduction of the chloride current to 30 to 40% of normal (9). Using the same expression system, recessive mutations result in lesser degrees of impairment of chloride conductance. Some mutations exert only a mild dominant negative effect. This may result in a dominant pattern of inheritance but with reduced penetrance as seen with the G239E mutation (9), or the mutation may be inherited in either dominant or recessive fashion as seen with the R894X mutation (8,11). Recessive mutations are either homozygous or may exist as compound heterozygotes. In some cases of AR Becker disease, no second mutation has been found. In one such family the apparent recessive pattern

of inheritance was revised when careful repeat EMG study showed subclinical myotonia in one parent and in the sibling of an index case. Both these individuals had very mild symptoms of myotonia that had not been previously appreciated, and all three affected members of this family had the G239E mutation (8,9). Disease expression in true cases of single recessive mutations may be influenced by polymorphisms or the expression levels of other channels. The recessive or dominant expression of mutations exerting a mild dominant negative effect may also be dependent on similar influences of genetic background.

Genotype Phenotype Correlations

The F413X mutation is the most common Becker's disease mutation. In one survey, three mutations (R894X, F413C, and the 14bp deletion in exon 13) accounted for nearly a third of mutations seen in Becker disease (8). A family with myotonia levior had a Gln552Arg mutation (7). Because a CLCN1 mutation can be either recessive or dominantly inherited, it becomes difficult to predict the phenotype and inheritance from mutational data alone unless the functional effects of the mutation are known.

CALCIUM CHANNELOPATHY

Clinical Features; Hypokalemic Periodic Paralysis

Primary hypokalemic periodic paralysis is the most common of the familial periodic paralyses with an estimated prevalence of between 0.4 and 1.25 per 100,000 (12,13). It is an AD disorder but with variable penetrance in females and thus appears to be more common in males. Sporadic cases, amounting to up to a third of patient cases in most series, represent new mutations and can transmit the disease to succeeding generations. Attacks usually start in adolescence with 60% occurring before age 16 years (14). Onset is invariably before age 30 years. Attacks may occur spontaneously, often at night, so that patients awake with a variable degree of weakness. Attacks are most commonly precipitated by carbohydrate intake and rest after exercise but may also be provoked by cold exposure, alcohol, or emotional stress. The frequency of attacks is generally less than that seen in hyperkalemic periodic paralysis and can vary from daily or only one or two in a lifetime. The frequency of attacks may diminish with age. Normally, attacks last between 1 and 4 hours, but they can occasionally persist for up to 3 days. Patients are often unaware of the presence of attacks of moderately severe weakness. Prodromal symptoms of muscle stiffness, heavy limbs, or sweating may be followed by proximal lower limb weakness that evolves into tetraparesis. Although respiratory failure is rare, this and hypokalemia-induced cardiac dysrhythmias can cause fatality. Oliguria can result from the sequestration of intracellular water. In younger subjects, the only interictal abnormality may be eyelid myotonia, but older subjects, despite having fewer attacks, may have persistent and sometimes fluctuating weakness. Fixed interattack weakness occurs in most patients with frequent attacks. During attacks there is a flaccid areflexic weakness; ocular or bulbar involvement and respiratory failure rarely occur.

Pathophysiology

In hypokalemic periodic paralysis, the weakness results from an abnormality of muscle membrane excitability. There is an influx of potassium into the muscle fiber with an accompanying influx of extracellular water that accounts for the oliguria that may be part of the attacks. There is increased sensitivity to the effect of insulin on the movement of potassium into cells independent of its glucopenic action. This may account for the precipitation of hypokalemic periodic paralysis with large carbohydrate meals. In contrast to normal muscle fibers, the influx of potassium in hypokalemic periodic paralysis causes the muscle fibers to become depolarized and inexcitable.

Genotype Phenotype Correlations

Hypokalemic periodic paralysis was found to be linked to a skeletal muscle dihydropyridine receptor (CACNL1A3) with at least three mutations of this calcium channel gene located on chromosome 1q (Table 1) (15–18). These mutations are all located in transmembrane (S4) segments and are responsible for the voltage sensing properties of the channel. The dihydropyridine receptor has a primary role in electrocontraction coupling with opening of the calcium channels of the sarcoplasmic reticulum, allowing an influx of calcium into the muscle sarcoplasm and triggering muscle contraction. Although the mutations described in hypokalemic periodic paralysis lead to a loss of function of the dihydropyridine receptor, it is not clear how this results in the abnormal response of muscle fibers to insulin with the consequent hypokalemia and weakness (19,20). These mutations have been found in both white and Japanese families. There is no evidence for a founder effect, and de novo mutations can occur (15,17). It has been suggested that the condition is genetically heterogeneous because two families did not show linkage to the CACNL1A3 locus (21); the possibility that these kindreds have Andersen's syndrome was, however, not excluded. The Arg1239Gly mutation has only been described in one family (15). The Arg528His and Arg1239His mutations are seen in half of the families linked to chromosome 1 with the Arg1239His mutation being slightly more common (17,22). Patients with the Arg1239His mutation were younger and had lower

potassium levels during attacks compared with those having the Arg528His mutation (17). One kindred with the Arg528His mutation had coexisting cardiac dysrhythmia (17). Incomplete penetrance in females is a characteristic of the Arg528His mutation (17).

SECONDARY PERIODIC PARALYSES

Faced with a patient having their first attack of paralysis, the differential diagnosis should include other causes of a flaccid areflexic tetraparesis without sensory involvement. The metabolic causes of hypercalcemia, hypocalcemia, hypophosphatemia, hypomagnesemia, and rhabdomyolysis should be excluded. Guillain-Barré syndrome, LEMS, and acute poliomyelitis can also produce this picture. In many cases the history and associated features will point to the correct diagnosis. Secondary hypokalemic periodic paralysis usually results from intracellular potassium depletion from either renal, endocrine, or gastrointestinal potassium loss (Table 2). These underlying conditions are usually obvious, but sometimes this is not the case, and the recurrent episodes of transient weakness can then be difficult to distinguish from primary hypokalemic periodic paralysis. Late-onset, after age 25, hypokalemic periodic paralysis should raise a strong suspicion of secondary rather than primary periodic paralysis. Thyrotoxic periodic paralysis results from an alteration of muscle membrane permeability and is more common in Asians but also occurs in whites. The clinical presentation is often indistinguishable from hypokalemic periodic paralysis but with additional and sometimes subtle evidence of hyperthyroidism. Paralytic

TABLE 2. *Causes of secondary hypokalemic periodic paralysis*

Endocrine
    Primary hyperaldosteronism (Conn syndrome)
    Thyrotoxic periodic paralysis
Renal
    Juxta-glomerular apparatus hyperplasia (Bartter's syndrome)
    Renal tubular acidosis
    Fanconi's syndrome
    Recovery from acute tubular acidosis
Gastrointestinal
    Villous adenoma
    Gastrointestinal fistula
    Pancreatic noninsulin-secreting tumors with diarrhea
    Nontropical sprue
    Laxative abuse
Drug induced
    Amphotericin B
    Liquorice
    Corticosteroids
    p-Aminosalicylic acid
    Carbenoxalone
    Potassium-depleting diuretics

episodes may precede the occurrence of obvious hyperthyroidism. Thyroid hormone levels may not be elevated; a depression of the serum thyroid-stimulating hormone is the most sensitive diagnostic test.

ANDERSEN SYNDROME

Clinical Features

Andersen et al. (23) described two patients with the triad of periodic paralysis, primary cardiac dysrhythmia unrelated to potassium concentration, and dysmorphic features. Four patients in three kindreds were later described in 1994 and the features further delineated in 11 others among five kindreds (24). Inheritance was AD, but there were three seemingly sporadic cases. Not all affected patients had the full clinical triad. Cardiac dysrhythmia was the most constant feature with long QT syndrome, ranging from 0.43 to 0.60 msec. Other cardiac manifestations included supraventricular and ventricular tachycardia, bidirectional ventricular tachycardia, premature ventricular contractions, and torsade de pointes. Only 4 of 15 patients presented with cardiac symptoms of palpitations, syncope, or nonfatal cardiac arrest, all of which occurred in the first or second decade of life.

Attacks of periodic paralysis during the first two decades also occurred and varied in frequency from one attack ever to one every 5 weeks, usually lasting a few hours. A recognized precipitant was rest after exercise. Fixed proximal weakness was seen in some cases. Initially it had been thought that the periodic paralysis was "hyperkalemic" in nature because patients were either hyper- or normokalemic during attacks, and the attacks could all be induced by potassium challenge. However, additional cases have showed definite hypokalemia during attacks. Provocative potassium challenges, particularly hypokalemic ones, are not advisable in the presence of preexisting cardiac dysrhythmia. The periodic paralysis of Andersen syndrome is therefore best regarded as being outside the traditional divisions of hyper- or hypokalemic periodic paralysis. Dysmorphic features have included hypertelorism, low-set ears, broad nose, small mandible, clindodactyly, syndactyly high-arched palate, and scoliosis. The facial features are often subtle and better described as distinctive rather than dysmorphic.

Pathophysiology

Linkage to the *SCN4A* gene has been excluded in these cases. Mutational analysis has not revealed any of the common mutations in the *CACNL1A3* gene associated with hypokalemic periodic paralysis. There are four ion channel genes known to cause isolated long QT syndrome, all of which have been excluded as the cause of Andersen syndrome. Another single gene defect may yet be found to cause this syndrome. Alternatively, it may be a multiple gene defect.

DYSTROPHIC MYOTONIAS

Clinical Features

Myotonic Dystrophy

This is the most common adult-onset muscular dystrophy with a prevalence of 5 per 100,000 persons and an incidence of 13.5 per 100,000 live births. It shows AD inheritance with high penetrance and a great deal of phenotypic variation within families. It is multisystemic, as illustrated in Table 3, and because of this, patients can present to almost any speciality.

Muscle wasting particularly affects the temporalis and masseter muscles, causing a "hachet face," and this together with the sternomastoid muscle atrophy, frontal balding, and ptosis results in a characteristic appearance. Distal muscle weakness is prominent in finger flexor, extensor, and intrinsic hand muscles and foot drop. Later, more proximal muscle groups become involved, but the distal emphasis persists. There may be particular atrophy and weakness of the quadricep muscles at any time. Some patients have respiratory insufficiency due to

TABLE 3. *Multisystem involvement in myotonic dystrophy*

	Symptoms
Skeletal muscle	Weakness
	Myotonia
Cardiac	Conduction block
	Mitral valve prolapse
	Atrial and ventricular dysrhythmias
	Dilated cardiomyopathy
	Sudden death
Respiratory	Diaphragmatic and intercostal weakness
	Reduced respiratory drive
Gastrointestinal	Dysphagia
	Aspiration
	Megacolon
	Gallstones
Central nervous system	Apathy
	Paranoia
	Hypersomnolence
	Mental retardation
	Hydrocephalus
	White matter changes
Endocrine	Insulin resistance
	Hypogonadism
Ocular	Cataract
	Retinal pigmentary degeneration
	Meibomian cysts
	Ptosis
	Ophthalmoplegia
Bone	Frontal bossing
	Small sella turcica
	Hyperostosis
	High arched palate
	Large paranasal sinuses
Dermatological	Frontal balding
	Multiple pilomatrixomas

diaphragmatic and intercostal muscle weakness. Dysphagia and a nasal dysarthria signify palatal, pharyngeal, and tongue involvement.

The myotonia of myotonic dystrophy is rarely symptomatic but is an important diagnostic feature. Evidence for it may be found in the form of percussion myotonia of the thenar eminence, the forearm extensors, and tongue. Grip myotonia may be present. The myotonia diminishes with repeated contractions, the so-called warm-up phenomenon, and becomes less easy to detect as the muscle weakness progresses.

Cardiac involvement is usual in myotonic dystrophy. Ninety percent of patients show electrocardiogram (ECG) abnormalities with first-degree heart block or more extensive cardiac conduction defects. Atrial and paroxysmal ventricular tachycardias are also seen. Complete heart block may occur, making prophylactic pacemaker insertion essential in those with second-degree heart block or worse and advisable in those with progressive lengthening of the PR interval. Sudden death is more common in those with tachycardias and is harder to predict in this group, so pacemaker insertion in these patients is best guided by a history of syncope and an abnormal 24-hour ECG recording rather than on a routine 12-lead ECG. Cardiac failure is usually the result of cor pulmonale secondary to respiratory failure. Otherwise, cardiac failure is rare despite demonstrable abnormalities of cardiac muscle contractility.

Respiratory complications can be an early feature in myotonic dystrophy. In addition to respiratory muscle weakness, there may be reduced central respiratory drive and an undue sensitivity to sedative drugs, depolarizing blocking agents, and general anesthetics. Gastrointestinal symptoms are frequent and include dysphagia and constipation due to megacolon and reflex myotonic contraction of the anal sphincter. Diabetes mellitus is uncommon despite the evidence of peripheral insulin resistance and the increased insulinemia after glucose challenge. Testicular atrophy is common, and some patients have reduced androgen levels with consequently high gonadotropin levels. Infertility is common in both males and females. There is a high rate of fetal loss, and due to uterine smooth muscle involvement, delivery may be delayed, quite apart from any additional delay due to hypotonia in an affected fetus. Personality change is common with paranoia, apathy, and lack of drive, often accentuated by hypersomnolence. These factors make regular follow-up a challenge because patients often fail to attend or follow advice. Structural changes in the brain are infrequent, but brain scans may show cerebral atrophy, hydrocephalus, or white matter changes. Cataracts are almost universal, especially in older patients where they may be the only feature of the disease. They are characteristic, being iridescent multicolored crystalline flecks in the posterior subcapsular part of the lens. Slit-lamp examination may be required to visualize them. Meibomian cysts are common. Rarer ocular manifestations include retinopathy and ophthalmoparesis.

Congenital myotonic dystrophy is a distinct phenotype of myotonic dystrophy occurring in the offspring of some affected women. Sometimes the diagnosis of myotonic dystrophy has been missed in the mother and is not appreciated until after the infant is born. Intrauterine fetal hypotonia causes reduced fetal movements, polyhydramnios, and delayed delivery. The floppy baby may require ventilation for respiratory distress and may have foot and joint deformities caused by contractures. Jaw and facial weakness gives a "tented" look to the mouth and causes feeding and sucking difficulties. Myotonia is not evident at this age. Those that survive have mental retardation and delayed motor milestones.

Pathophysiology

The genetic basis of myotonic dystrophy is an expansion of the CTG trinucleotide repeat in the 3′ untranslated region of a serine threonine protein kinase (*DMPK*) gene on chromosome 19q13.3. The normal CTGn repeat number ranges from 5 to 37, whereas patients with myotonic dystrophy have between 50 to thousands of repeats. Age of onset and severity of the disease correlates roughly with the repeat expansion size. Expansion size tends to increase with successive generations with the largest expansions being maternally transmitted. This provides a molecular basis for the phenomenon of anticipation and the almost exclusively maternal transmission of congenital myotonic dystrophy. The myotonic dystrophy mutation persists despite the reduced fertility of affected individuals and the loss of alleles from the gene pool by those having congenital myotonic dystrophy. Replenishment of the gene pool is thought to be due to preferential expansion of the CTGn repeat by healthy individuals having alleles containing greater than 19 repeats. Most of the CTGn=5 allele undergoes a small number of initial expansions. Expansions of between 11 and 13 repeats do not produce pathologic expansion, whereas those greater than 19 repeats do. In heterozygous individuals, the allele with CTGn>19 is preferentially transmitted. Enlargement of the abnormal CTGn expansion with successive generations is correlated with the expansion size for both paternal and maternal transmission where the repeat size is less than 0.5 kilobases (kb). When the repeat size exceeds 0.5 kb, intergeneration enlargement of the expansion size is more likely for maternal transmission. Paternal transmission of alleles with expansion size greater than 1.5 kb results in contraction of the expansion size, and thus paternal transmission of congenital myotonic dystrophy is a very rare but not unheard of event (25). This suggests a selection barrier during spermatogenesis rather than alternative explanations such as mitochondrial inheritance, maternal imprinting, or placental factors. Perhaps sperm with long repeat expansions do not survive.

Because the mutation is in an untranslated region of the *DMPK* gene, it is unlikely to have a direct effect on the structure of the DMPK protein. There are a variety of ways in which the mutation could affect the level of translation of the *DMPK* gene, but there is conflicting information on how the levels of DMPK expression in myotonic dystrophy actually differ from normal. Most available data suggest a reduction in DMPK mRNA levels but without clear evidence that this leads to reduction in DMPK protein levels in the heterozygous state. DMPK knockout mice or mice overexpressing DMPK have relatively minor skeletal muscle changes and do not have the profound phenotype associated with myotonic dystrophy. There is evidence that the triplet repeat expansion alters chromatin structure 3′ to the *DMPK* gene, causing loss of a DNase I sensitive site (26). Thus, an alternative explanation for the pathogenicity of the CTGn repeat expansion is that it may affect the expression of flanking genes rather than the *DMPK* gene itself. One such candidate gene is a conserved region encoding for homeodomain containing proteins and designated the DM locus associated homeodomain protein (DMAHP). Homeodomain proteins are transcription proteins that regulate gene expression by binding to DNA and RNA. The DNase I sensitive site referred to above is in the promotor region of the *DMAHP* gene and DMAHP expression in myoblasts, muscle, and myocardium is reduced by the abnormal expanded CTGn repeat of myotonic dystrophy. The reduced expression occurs in the *cis* allele and is proportional to the length of the CTGn repeat (27,28).

Genotype Phenotype Correlations

There is a broad correlation between CTGn expansion size and the age at onset and the severity of the disease (Table 4). Variations in the expansion size are seen in different tissues with larger repeat sizes being seen in muscle compared with leukocytes (29,30). Better correlation between tissue involvement and expansion size might therefore be found if the expansion size was measured in the affected tissue. Within a given tissue there may be a variation in expansion size, suggesting mitotic instability for the expansion. The smallest size expansion appears to be the original inherited allele that is therefore increasing with age, explaining the progressive nature of myotonic dystrophy. The smallest repeat length in blood is the one that correlates best with age at onset.

Proximal Myotonic Myopathy

Proximal myotonic myopathy (PROMM) is an AD disorder that although having some features in common with myotonic dystrophy, lacks the abnormal expansion of the CTG repeat in the myotonic dystrophy gene. Although sharing the common features of cataract, muscle weakness, and myotonia, there are sufficient differences that make PROMM a clinically distinct syndrome. Because it is a recently described entity, our knowledge of the full clinical spectrum and natural history of PROMM will undoubtedly change.

Patients with PROMM commonly present between 20 and 60 years of age. There is as yet no clear evidence of a neonatal presentation. In contrast to myotonic dystrophy where the myotonia is mild and rarely a presenting feature, patients with PROMM often present with complaints of muscle stiffness that is variable from day to day and may be focal, affecting one limb only. The myotonia seems to be associated with a distinctive jerky relaxation phase, particularly of the thumb and index finger, and shows a warm-up phenomenon. Lid lag may be seen. Because of its initially mild and intermittent nature, the myotonia of PROMM may be hard to detect clinically. Muscle pain, unrelated to the myotonia, is another distinctive presenting feature and is described as an unpleasant intrusive sore aching pain present at rest and resistant to aspirin or nonsteroidal anti-inflammatory medication. The pains may vary in intensity, sometimes disappearing for days at a time, without obvious explanation. Patients may have undue sensitivity to local muscle trauma. Several patients had severe chest pains that resulted in a normal cardiac investigation.

Weakness is proximal rather than distal and particularly affects the legs. There may be sternocleidomastoid weakness. The weakness can display slow variability over hours or days. These episodes do not relate to exercise or to rest after exercise; indeed, there may be transient improvement of weakness for half an hour after exercise. Initial reports suggested that weak muscles show only mild, if any, atrophy in contrast to the more severe atrophy seen in myotonic dystrophy, but this may reflect the

TABLE 4. *Myotonic dystrophy: features correlating with expansion repeat size*

Phenotype	Clinical features	CTG repeat expansion length
Mild	Cataracts Muscle wasting and weakness	40–170
Classic	Myotonia Multisystem involvement	100–1000
Congenital	Hypotonia Mental retardation	500 to more than 3,000

age of the cases. In two families, older patients in their 60s and 70s developed disabling weakness and marked muscle atrophy (31,32). In one case, there was marked temporalis atrophy (31). In another, there was severe dysphagia (31). Calf hypertrophy has been described in some others. Fluctuations in the severity of myotonia, pain, and weakness may be related to temperature as two siblings were described in whom these symptoms worsened in warm temperatures. On EMG, sparse myotonic discharges at room temperature became more profuse when the muscle was warmed up (33).

Cataracts are common and in most patients occur before the age of 50 years. They may be indistinguishable from those seen in myotonic dystrophy. Hypogonadism has been described. Three patients had hypothyroidism, initially thought to be the cause of their proximal muscle weakness before the features of PROMM became apparent (34). There are suggestions that insulin resistance may occur in some cases of PROMM, but this needs further investigation. Cardiac dysrhythmias have been described, but it is not clear whether this is specific for PROMM or merely a coincidental finding. One family had deafness as a feature (32). To date, there have not been reports of respiratory failure. Initial reports stressed the lack of mental changes of the sort seen in myotonic dystrophy, but three patients had apathy and hypersomnia, and one of them had parkinsonian features with dystonia as well (31,33). Three cases had strokelike events, including one with a completed stroke and two with adult-onset epileptic seizures (31). Six cases had white matter abnormalities seen on brain magnetic resonance imaging, with five having central nervous system manifestations, although the relationship between the two was unclear (31). There can be phenotypic variation within families with some having asymptomatic cataracts or weakness, but there is insufficient evidence to say whether anticipation is a feature of PROMM.

Pathophysiology

Historically, PROMM was recognized because of its lack of association with the abnormal CTG repeat expansion of the myotonic dystrophy gene. There was also no linkage to the myotonic dystrophy gene nor to the sodium (*SCN4A*) or chloride (*CLCN1*) channel genes responsible for other myotonias. Muscle fibers from patients with PROMM show normal resting potential and normal chloride conductance. Spontaneous activity in isolated muscle fibers reduces with increased extracellular potassium concentration, the converse of that seen with most myotonias (35). Myotonic discharges were reduced on muscle cooling and increased with muscle warming, again the converse of what is seen in several other myotonic syndromes (33). Repetitive stimulation caused a decrement in the CMAP amplitude, particularly in proximal muscles, and this may relate to the development of weakness or its variability (33).

SCHWARTZ JAMPEL SYNDROME

Clinical Features

In this syndrome, typical onset is before age 3 with severe continuous motor activity and muscle stiffness, particularly in the face. Patients have an unusual masklike face with continuous motor activity of the chin and lips. Eye closure provokes blepharospasm, whereas excitement can cause worsening of muscle contraction and even laryngeal spasm. Hypertrophy of the shoulder muscles with shortening of the neck can occur, as can hypertrophy of thigh muscles. The voice may be high pitched. They may have a variety of skeletal malformations, including contractures and short stature that may be a consequence of the continuous motor activity. There may not necessarily be any chondrodysplastic features despite the alternative name of chondrodystrophic myotonia. Limited information suggests that any progression, if it occurs, is slow (36).

Pathophysiology

The continuous motor activity has differing EMG characteristics in different cases. In some, it resembles the activity seen in myotonic dystrophy with prolonged runs of falling or unchanging frequency or amplitude of motor units and "dive bomber discharges." In others, the activity resembles that seen in myotonia congenita, whereas still others have continuous spontaneous motor activity with fluctuation of the frequency or the amplitude of motor units. Activity can be continuous in some or interspersed by periods of electrical silence. In some, the activity is abolished by curare, suggesting that it is of neurogenic origin, whereas in others the discharges continue and would therefore be of muscle origin. It seems likely therefore that this is a heterogeneous condition with various etiologies and perhaps the clinical similarities relate more to the early onset and severity of the continuous motor activity. In one case where the discharges resembled that of myotonic dystrophy and were myogenic in origin, sodium channel activity was abnormal with synchronized late openings (37). Subsequently, this case was found to have a Gly1306Glu mutation of the sodium channel gene *SCN4A* and is now reclassed as myotonia permanans (37).

INVESTIGATION OF THE MYOTONIAS AND PERIODIC PARALYSES

Myotonias

The serum creatine kinase (CK) is usually normal, but there may be borderline elevations in Thomsen and Becker disease reflecting the degree of muscle hypertrophy. EMG shows spontaneous myotonic discharges, but in paramyotonia congenita and myotonic dystrophy, provocation by cooling of the examined limb may be required to demonstrate this. Myotonic discharges may not be apparent in children with myotonic dystrophy who are under the age of 5 years. There is also decrement in the CMAP with exercise or with high-frequency 30-Hz stimulation, particularly in cases of myotonia congenita. The decrement in the CMAP amplitude is particularly marked in Becker disease, and this may be the substrate for the transient weakness seen in that condition. Myopathic EMG features may be seen in myotonic dystrophy and in PROMM. Muscle biopsy may show little abnormality. Variation in fiber size with fiber hypertrophy and increased central nuclei may be found. In myotonic dystrophy there may be selective type 1 fiber atrophy, whereas in myotonia congenita there may be a lack of 2B fibers. Ring fibers and sarcoplasmic masses may be seen in myotonic dystrophy, but muscle fiber necrosis and increased connective tissue is uncommon. In paramyotonia congenita with hyperkalemic periodic paralysis, vacuolated fibers and necrotic fibers may be seen. Study of family members may be valuable because there may be clinical or EMG evidence of disease in apparently asymptomatic individuals, which clarifies the mode of inheritance. Slit-lamp examination may be valuable for carrier detection and diagnosis in myotonic dystrophy and PROMM. ECG is strongly advisable in cases of myotonic dystrophy.

Periodic Paralysis

During an episode, blood tests should be taken for potassium, calcium, magnesium, phosphate, and CK to exclude the other causes of weakness mentioned above. Because the potassium level may be normal during hyperkalemic periodic paralysis and occasionally so in hypokalemic periodic paralysis, potassium levels needs to be checked sequentially every 15 to 30 minutes to determine the direction of change at time when muscle strength is either worsening or improving. An ECG may show changes consistent with hypo- or hyperkalemia and may also forewarn of cardiac complications. EMG shows reduced CMAP amplitudes proportionate to the degree of weakness. Nerve conduction studies are otherwise normal. The neurophysiology also serves to exclude other causes of paralysis such as Guillain-Barré syndrome, MG, and LEMS.

Patients who are seen between attacks need investigation to exclude causes of secondary hypokalemia. EMG may be helpful in showing evidence of myotonia that favors hyperkalemic periodic paralysis. In patients with fixed weakness, the EMG may be myopathic. Even in those with an initially normal EMG there may be a characteristic decrement of the CMAP amplitudes with high-frequency (30-Hz) stimulation or after repetitive muscle contraction. Muscle biopsy is often abnormal between attacks of hypokalemic periodic paralysis with pathognomonic changes of large central vacuoles and occasional necrotic fibers. In hyperkalemic periodic paralysis,

smaller vacuoles may be present and tubular aggregates may be seen. Provocative testing may be required to confirm the diagnosis. This must be performed with careful supervision, including monitoring of the potassium and the ECG. Hypokalemic challenge can be performed by giving intravenous glucose with or without insulin. Hyperkalemic challenge can be performed by giving repeated small doses of oral potassium.

TREATMENT OF THE MYOTONIAS AND PERIODIC PARALYSES

There are four clinical symptoms that demand treatment in the myotonias and periodic paralyses: attacks of weakness, persistent fixed weakness, muscle stiffness, and muscle pain. Satisfactory treatment is now available for all symptoms, with the exception of attacks of weakness. There is inadequate controlled data to defend a specific treatment regimen.

Myotonias

Myotonia can be exacerbated by certain muscle relaxant drugs and by anticholinesterase drugs; in addition, anesthesia for these patients needs to be planned accordingly. Potassium administration can exacerbate myotonia, particularly sodium channel disorders, and thus potassium supplementation should only be given where necessary and with caution. Although it has been stated that there is an association between myotonias and malignant hyperthermia necessitating anesthetic precautions, the documentation of this statement is not sufficient to warrant pretreatment with dantrolene. The treatment of myotonia congenita relies on membrane stabilizing drugs such as procainamide and quinine, and these can be used intermittently on an as-needed basis. Phenytoin is more useful for chronic administration and is less likely to have cardiac side effects. Occasional cases of myotonia, particularly sodium channel myotonia, are responsive to acetazolamide. Mexilitine is useful for both the myotonia and the weakness associated with paramyotonia congenita and for Becker's myotonia.

Periodic Paralysis

Attacks of hypokalemic periodic paralysis may be partially prevented by low carbohydrate and low sodium diet. Acetazolamide was initially noted to be effective in preventing paralytic attacks and improving residual weakness between attacks. Recently, dichlorphenamide has been studied in a randomized controlled trial and found to be effective (38). When hypokalemic periodic paralysis is secondary to thyrotoxicosis, this also needs to have treatment. In the interim, the paralytic attacks and persistent weakness can be very effectively treated with α-adrenergic blocking agents. During acute attacks of hypokalemic periodic paralysis, emergency parenteral potassium treatment may be required, but the preference is very much in favor of oral potassium in these patients. Supportive therapy may be required for respiratory impairment, and the ECG should be carefully monitored for any cardiac dysrhythmia. In hyperkalemic periodic paralysis, attacks are usually mild but are still worth treating to prevent the onset of permanent weakness. Thiazide diuretics are usually effective treatment. During acute attacks, treatment is rarely needed, but carbohydrate-containing food and fluid may aggravate the weakness and potassium-containing foods should be avoided. Inhaled β-adrenergic agonists such as salbutamol are effective treatments but may be contraindicated if there is a coexisting cardiac dysrhythmia.

NEUROMYOTONIA

Clinical Features

Isaacs Disease

This is a syndrome in which neuromyotonia or hyperexcitability of peripheral nerves results in spontaneous and continuous muscle activity. Although some are inherited, most are acquired. The syndrome is rare, and assessment of its frequency and definitive clinical features is hampered by the variable names given to it in the past. Typical patients have muscle stiffness, cramps, myokymia, and pseudomyotonias. They may also have generalized weakness and sweating. Onset can be any time during life, and the condition tends to be chronic. Motor features are most prominent in the limbs and trunk. Respiratory muscle involvement can cause breathing difficulty and laryngeal involvement can cause stridor. Examination may reveal mild weakness with reduced or absent tendon reflexes and evidence of myokymia with occasional muscle hypertrophy as a result.

Episodic Ataxia Type 1

Episodes of cerebellar dysfunction begin in childhood or adolescence. Their frequency can be variable but can number up to 15 per day with a duration of 30 seconds to 15 minutes. Attacks can occur spontaneously but are more commonly provoked by the initiation of movement, postural change, or exercise, particularly where there is associated emotional excitement or anxiety. Attacks may include dysarthria, unsteady gait, shaking or jerking of the limbs, and in some cases abnormal posturing of the limbs. Nausea and headache have not been described, and there is no impairment of consciousness. Attacks can vary in both severity and range of features and can be so mild as to be concealed by the patient. Examination during attacks reveals gait ataxia, limb incoordination with dysdiadokinesis, slurred speech, but no nystagmus (39). There are usually no cerebellar findings between attacks. The most common, but not invariable, interictal finding is

that of continuous motor activity and myokymia, particularly evident in the face and as a mild tremor of the fingers when the hands are placed in a relaxed prone position. Occasionally, myokymia of limb muscles produces rippling of the skin. Although the myokymia may be prominent enough for the patient to notice it or gross enough to be palpated (40), it is generally subtle and may not be detected unless specifically sought. EMG may be required to demonstrate its presence (39).

Pathophysiology

The continuous discharges may originate anywhere along the length of the peripheral nerve. There is an association between Isaacs disease and autoimmune disease, and it is believed that the acquired varieties are in fact autoimmune, perhaps due to antibodies against potassium channel. Hereditary cases of Isaacs disease may be due to a genetic defect of the potassium channel. AD episodic ataxia type I results from mutations in the *KCNA1* gene at chromosome 12p13 (41,42).

Investigation

EMG confirms the presence of neuromyotonia in the form of doublets, triplets, or multiplet spontaneous motor unit discharges that may be present even in the absence of visible myokymia. Nerve and muscle biopsies show nonspecific features. In a few cases of Isaacs disease, oligoclonal IgG was found in the cerebrospinal fluid.

Management

For Isaacs disease, anticonvulsant medication such as phenytoin and carbamazapine have been the first line of treatment. Plasma exchange may be appropriate where an autoimmune etiology is thought likely. In some of these latter cases, immune suppression with steroids and azathioprine has been tried.

Attacks of episodic ataxia show a variable response to phenytoin (39,43,44) and no response to clomipramine, phenobarbitone, clonazepam, or cinnarizine (39). There was a reduction in both the frequency and severity of attacks in one case treated with flunarizine (44). Poor tolerance of carbonic anhydrase inhibitors such as acetazolamide (39,42,44) and diclophenamide (39) has limited their use, but sulthiame was better tolerated and appeared to produce a sustained benefit (39).

MALIGNANT HYPERTHERMIA

Clinical Features

Malignant hyperthermias are hereditary skeletal muscle disease, characterized by a hypercatabolic reaction of muscle to anesthetic agents or to physical or emotional stress. It has a worldwide distribution with an incidence of 1 in 12,000 anesthetic incidents in children and 1 in 50,000 anesthetic events in adults. However, it is possible that many mild cases go unrecognized and are mistaken for other anesthetic complications. Males are more affected than females, and there is a peak incidence at the age of 30 years after which the incidence declines such that cases are virtually unheard of beyond the age of 75 years. The most common precipitating event is that of halothane general anesthesia. The muscle relaxant succinylcholine is a milder trigger of attacks when used alone but a more potent one when combined with halothane. The likelihood of triggering an attack with these agents is increased if the patient has been exercising vigorously beforehand or is under stress at the time of anesthetic induction.

In between attacks of malignant hyperthermia, patients rarely have any muscle symptoms, although some muscle diseases are associated with attacks of malignant hyperthermia (see below). In 50% of cases, previous anesthesia had no complication. Attacks often start with jaw spasm followed by generalized muscle spasm and rigidity. This is associated with hyperventilation, tachycardia, and an unstable blood pressure. A mottled, flushed, and cyanotic skin rash may appear, and after an interval of 15 to 60 minutes, the body temperature may start to rise precipitously. Metabolic and respiratory acidosis, hypoxemia, generalized vasoconstriction, and an increased cardiac output then occur. The serum potassium and CK may rise, the latter up to 100-fold. Consequent complications of myoglobinuria and disseminated intravascular coagulation may occur, either of which can lead to renal failure. During recovery, patients may have a further relapse.

Pathophysiology

The central event appears to be an increase in the calcium concentration that results in continuous activation of the actin-myosin contraction apparatus and sustained muscle contraction. This increase in calcium level is due to an increased release of calcium from the sarcoplasmic reticulum of the muscle together with a reduction in calcium reuptake. The continuous muscle activity results in the muscle rigidity, muscle necrosis, hyperpyrexia, and hypermetabolism. Linkage has been found to chromosome 19q13.1. A ryanodine receptor gene in this region has been shown to have mutations in 2 to 5% of cases. The ryanodine receptor is a calcium-released channel involved in calcium homeostasis. Linkage has also been found to chromosome 17q1.2-24, which codes for the subunit of the sodium channel, and to chromosome 7q and 3q.

Investigation

During the acute illness, the main emphasis of the evaluation is monitoring possible hyperkalemic, cardiac, respiratory, or renal complications so that appropriate measures can be taken. Evaluation of well patients thought to be at risk of developing malignant hyperthermia can be difficult. Only a few have a raised serum CK. The genetic heterogeneity and the fact that even the recognized point mutations only cover a small percentage of the patients at risk limit the value of genetic testing. A variety of in vivo tests have been purported to highlight at-risk individuals, but these are not particularly reliable. The recognized screening test is the in vitro caffeine and halothane contracture test in which one looks for an exaggerated response to caffeine or halothane in freshly isolated muscle. This test is performed only in specialized centers, even so the overlap between normal and affected individuals is such that false-positive tests are invariable.

Management

Preventative measures include the avoidance of precipitating agents, namely halothane and succinylcholine. Patients should be advised to wear Medicalert bracelets to warn of their susceptibility to malignant hypothermia. Narcotics, barbiturates, benzodiazepines, nitrous oxide, and depolarizing muscle relaxants are safe to use. Acute management consists of the removal of the triggering agents and supportive measures as required. Rapid measures to produce body cooling may be required in response to the hyperpyrexia that if allowed to continue aggravates metabolic derangements. Dantrolene is the mainstay of treatment and given intravenously results in reversal of the abnormalities. The improved recognition of this complication and better supportive measures with the availability of dantrolene have resulted in a dramatic drop in mortality from 65% to 2%.

RIPPLING MUSCLE DISEASE

Clinical Features

Patients notice rippling of the muscles or complain of muscle spasms, but these are rarely troublesome. The rippling may be self-induced, especially after a period of rest or in the cold. Percussion of the muscle may cause painless contraction, swelling, or mounding of the muscle that may then roll across the limb over a 10-second period. There is no associated muscle wasting or weakness. There may be modest elevations of the CK. Needle EMG shows no abnormality, and the rippling itself is electrically silent. Muscle biopsy shows nonspecific features of variation in fiber size and scatter atrophic fibers. One case had selective type I fiber atrophy (45). Familial AD and sporadic cases have been described (45,46).

Pathophysiology

The cause of the rippling remains unclear. It has been speculated that it may be due to slow propagation of an internal sarcoplasmic action potential. The mechanical sensitivity could be due to activation of stretch-sensitive channels. One sporadic case of rippling muscles also developed MG and both remitted with immunotherapy, leading to speculation of an autoimmune basis for rippling muscles (46). Some cases have shown linkage to chromosome 1q41-42.

REFERENCES

1. DiNubile MJ, Hokama Y. The ciguatera poisoning syndrome from farm-raised salmon. *Ann Intern Med* 1995;122:113–114.
2. Trimmer JS, Cooperman SS, Tomiko SA, et al. Primary structure and functional expression of a mammalian skeletal muscle sodium channel. *Neuron* 1989;3:33–49.
3. Heine R, Pika U, Lehmann-Horn F. A novel SCN4A mutation causing myotonia aggravated by cold and potassium. *Hum Mol Genet* 1993;2: 1349–1353.
4. Lehmann-Horn F, Rudel R, Ricker K. Workshop report; non-dystrophic myotonias and periodic paralyses. *Neuromusc Dis* 1993;3:161–168.
5. Lerche H, Heine R, Pica U, et al. Human sodium channel myotonia: slowed channel inactivation due to substitutions for a glycine within the III-IV linker. *J Physiol* 1993;470:13–22.
6. Wang J, Zhou J, Todorovic SM, et al. Molecular genetic and genetic correlations in sodium channelopathies: lack of founder effect and evidence for a second gene. *Am J Hum Genet* 1993;52:1074–1084.
7. Lehmann-Horn F, Mailander V, Heine R, George AL. Myotonia levior is a chloride channel disorder. *Hum Mol Genet* 1995;4:1397–1402.
8. Meyer-Kleine C, Steinmeyer K, Ricker K, Jentsch TJ, Koch MC. Spectrum of mutations in the major human skeletal muscle chloride channel gene (CLCN1) leading to myotonia. *Am J Hum Genet* 1995;57: 1325–1334.
9. Steinmeyer K, Lorenz C, Pusch M, Koch MC, Jentsch TJ. Multimeric structure of ClC–1 chloride channel revealed by mutations in dominant myotonia congenita (Thomsen). *EMBO J* 1994;13:737–743.
10. Koty PP, Pegoraro E, Hobson G, et al. Myotonia and the muscle chloride channel: dominant mutations show variable penetrance and founder effect. *Neurology* 1996;47:963–968.
11. George AL Jr, Sloan-Brown K, Fenichel GM, Mitchell GA, Spiegel R. Nonsense and missense mutations of the muscle chloride channel gene in patients with myotonia congenita. *Hum Mol Genet* 1994;3: 2071–2072.
12. Kantola IM, Tarssanen LT. Familial hypokalaemic periodic paralysis in Finland. *J Neurol Neurosurg Psychiatry* 1992;55:322–324.
13. Johnsen T. Familial periodic paralysis with hypokalaemia. Experimental and clinical investigations. *Danish Med Bull* 1981;28:1–27.
14. Steinlein O. Familial nocturnal frontal lobe epilepsy. Clinical aspects and genetics. *Nervenarzt* 1996;67:870–874. In German.
15. Ptacek LJ, Tawil R, Griggs RC, et al. Dihydropyridine receptor mutations cause hypokalemic periodic paralysis. *Cell* 1994;77:863–868.
16. Jurkat-Rott K, Lehmann-Horn F, Elbaz A, et al. A calcium channel mutation causing hypokalemic periodic paralysis. *Hum Mol Genet* 1994;3:1415–1419.
17. Elbaz A, Vale-Santos J, Jurkat-Rott K, et al. Hypokalemic periodic paralysis and the dihydropyridine receptor (CACNL1A3): genotype/phenotype correlations for two predominant mutations and evidence for the absence of a founder effect in 16 Caucasian families. *Am J Hum Genet* 1995;56:374–380.
18. Boerman RH, Ophoff RA, Links TP, et al. Mutation in DHP receptor alpha 1 subunit (CACNL1A3) gene in a Dutch family with hypokalaemic periodic paralysis. *J Med Genet* 1995;32:44–47.
19. Sipos I, Jurkat-Rott K, Harasztosi C, Fontaine B, Kovacs L, Melzer WLH. Skeletal muscle DHP receptor mutations alter calcium currents in human hypokalaemic periodic paralysis myotubes. *J Physiol* 1995; 483:299–306.
20. Lehmann-Horn F, Sipos I, Jurkat-Rott K, et al. Altered calcium currents in human hypokalemic periodic paralysis myotubes expressing mutant L-type calcium channels. *Soc Gen Physiol Ser* 1995;50:101–113.
21. Plassart E, Elbaz A, Santos JV, et al. Genetic heterogeneity in hypokalemic periodic paralysis (hypoPP). *Hum Genet* 1994;94:551–556.
22. Fouad G, Dalakas M, Servidei S, et al. Genotype-phenotype correlations of DHP receptor alpha 1-subunit gene mutations causing hypokalemic periodic paralysis. *Neuromusc Dis* 1997;7:33–38.
23. Andersen ED, Krasilnikoff PA, Overvad H. Intermittent muscular weakness, extrasystoles, and multiple developmental anomalies. A new syndrome? *Acta Paediatr Scand* 1971;60:559–564.
24. Sansone V, Griggs RC, Meola G, et al. Andersen's syndrome: a distinct periodic paralysis. *Ann Neurol* 1997;42:305–312.
25. Nakagawa M, Yamada H, Higuchi I, Kaminishi Y, Miki T, Johnson K. A case of paternally inherited congenital myotonic dystrophy. *J Med Genet* 1994;31:397–400.
26. Otten AD, Tapscott SJ. Triplet repeat expansion in myotonic dystrophy alters the adjacent chromatin structure. *Proc Natl Acad Sci USA* 1995; 92:5465–5469.
27. Klesert TR, Otten AD, Bird TD, Tapscott SJ. Trinucleotide repeat expansion at the myotonic dystrophy locus reduces expression of DMAHP. *Nat Genet* 1997;16:402–406.
28. Thornton CA, Wymer JP, Simmons Z, McClain C, Moxley RT. Expansion of the myotonic dystrophy CTG repeat reduces expression of the flanking DMAHP gene. *Nat Genet* 1997;16:407–409.
29. Anvret M, Ahlberg G, Grandell U, Hedberg B, Johnson K, Edstrom L. Larger expansions of the CTG repeat in muscle compared to lymphocytes from patients with myotonic dystrophy. *Hum Mol Genet* 1993;2: 1397–1400.
30. Thornton CA, Johnson K, Moxley RT. Myotonic dystrophy patients have larger CTG expansions in skeletal muscle than in leukocytes. *Ann Neurol* 1994;35:104–107.
31. Hund E, Jansen O, Koch MC, et al. Proximal myotonic myopathy with MRI white matter abnormalities of the brain. *Neurology* 1997;48:33–37.
32. Udd B, Krahe R, Wallgren-Pettersson C, Falck B, Kalimo H. Proximal myotonic dystrophy—a family with autosomal dominant muscular dystrophy, cataracts, hearing loss and hypogonadism: heterogeneity of proximal myotonic syndromes? *Neuromusc Dis* 1997;7:217–228.
33. Sander HW, Tavoulareas GP, Chokroverty S. Heat-sensitive myotonia in proximal myotonic myopathy. *Neurology* 1996;47:956–962.
34. Griggs RC, Sansone V, Lifton A, Moxley RT. Hypothyroidism unmasking proximal myotonic myopathy. *Neurology* 1997;48:A267(abst).
35. Ricker K, Koch MC, Lehmann-Horn F, Pongratz D, Otto M, Heine R. Proximal myotonic myopathy: a new dominant disorder with myotonia, muscle weakness, and cataracts. *Neurology* 1994;44:1448–1452.
36. Spaans F, Theunissen P, Reekers AD, Smit L, Veldman H. Schwartz-Jampel syndrome. I. Clinical, electromyographic, and histologic studies. *Muscle Nerve* 1990;13:516–527.
37. Lehmann-Horn F, Iaizzo PA, Franke C, Hatt H, Spaans F. Schwartz-Jampel syndrome. II. Na+ channel defect causes myotonia. *Muscle Nerve* 1990;13:528–535.
38. Griggs RC, Tawil R, Brown RH, et al. Dichlorphenamide is effective in the treatment of hypokalemic periodic paralysis. *Ann Neurol* 1997; 42:428.
39. Brunt ER, van Weerden TW. Familial paroxysmal kinesigenic ataxia and continuous myokymia. *Brain* 1990;113:1361–1382.
40. van Dyke DH, Griggs RC, Murphy MJ, Goldstein MN. Hereditary myokymia and periodic ataxia. *J Neurol Sci* 1975;25:109–118.
41. Browne DL, Brunt ER, Griggs RC, et al. Identification of two new KCNA1 mutations in episodic ataxia/myokymia families. *Hum Mol Genet* 1995;4:1671–1672.
42. Lubbers WJ, Brunt ER, Scheffer H, et al. Hereditary myokymia and paroxysmal ataxia, linked to chromosome 12 is responsive to acetazolamide. *J Neurol Neurosurg Psychiatry* 1995;4:400–405.
43. Hanson PA, Martinez LB, Cassidy R. Contractures, continuous muscle discharges and titubation. *Ann Neurol* 1977;1:120–124.
44. Vaamonde J, Artieda J, Obeso JA. Hereditary paroxysmal ataxia with neuromyokymia. *Mov Dis* 1991;6:180–182.
45. Burns RJ, Bretag AH, Blumbergs PC, Harbord MG. Benign familial disease with muscle mounding and rippling. *J Neurol Neurosurg Psychiatry* 1994;57:344–347.
46. Ansevin CF, Agamanolis DP. Rippling muscles and myasthenia gravis with rippling muscles. *Arch Neurol* 1996;53:197–199.

Motor Disorders,
edited by David S. Younger.
Lippincott Williams & Wilkins, Philadelphia © 1999.

CHAPTER 15

Multifocal Motor Neuropathy

Gareth J. Parry

In 1985, Parry and Clarke (1) described a predominantly motor disorder with weakness, atrophy, cramps, fasciculations, and preserved tendon reflexes. Sensory symptoms were minimal without objective sensory loss. On the surface, these findings resembled motor neuron disease (MND), but the similarity was superficial; certainly the disorder should not have been mistaken for amyotrophic lateral sclerosis (ALS). The disorder differed from MND in the electrodiagnostic finding of multifocal motor conduction block (MCB). Multifocal motor neuropathy (MMN), as it is now known, is rare but has stimulated considerable discussion because it is treatable, whereas most cases of MND are not. It has also highlighted the difficulty in defining conduction block, particularly in chronic denervation, and has resulted in attempts to establish better criteria for the definition of conduction block. Parry and Clarke (1,2) first emphasized the striking motor predominance and pointed out the resemblance to MND, but Lewis et al. (3) had previously described a similar disorder with strikingly multifocal slowly evolving neuropathy that differed from MMN in the finding of significant sensory abnormalities. It is likely that these disorders are pathogenetically identical and may both be variants of chronic inflammatory demyelinating polyneuropathy (CIDP).

CLINICAL FEATURES OF MULTIFOCAL MOTOR NEUROPATHY

The essential clinical feature of MMN is slowly progressive weakness that is strikingly multifocal. It is localized to individual peripheral nerves, which is in contrast to the pattern in MND that is myotomal. It is nearly always accompanied by muscle wasting that may be severe with other muscles normal in bulk despite severe weakness,

another feature that distinguishes MMN from MND. Cramps, fasciculations, and myokymia also occur (4). MMN has a predilection for the arms whether it begins there or spreads there from the legs. Weakness of cranial muscles has been rarely reported: One patient had widespread bulbar weakness after almost 20 years of slowly progressive limb weakness (5) and the other presented with hemiatrophy of the tongue (6). Respiratory muscle involvement is equally rare. One patient had tachypnea after several months of severe quadriparesis without overt respiratory failure (7), whereas another died of respiratory failure (5). Although conduction block may be found at almost any site along the length of an affected nerve, the resulting weakness is usually most severe distally. There can be palpable enlargement or tumorlike swellings of the nerve corresponding to sites of conduction block (8–10), which appears on magnetic resonance imaging as areas of high T2 signal and gadolinium enhancement (10,11).

Subtle clinical sensory abnormalities are common. Patients with MMN (2,7,12–14) can have sensory abnormality, such as numbness or paresthesia, with or without objective sensory loss, especially late in their course. Hypo- or areflexia in severely weak atrophic muscles is common, but reflex loss in normal or minimally weak muscles also occurs, suggesting involvement of afferent fibers from muscle spindles. The sensory abnormalities suggest that MMN is a predominantly motor form of CIDP.

MMN typically begins in the third to fourth decade; however, childhood and elderly cases also occur. The progression is typically so slow that patients may not recall when the weakness first began. (One personal patient was unaware of bicep involvement despite profound weakness and wasting, and he unwittingly used trick movements to flex his elbow.) Patients usually remain ambulatory and functional even after years of progression. Another personal patient had weakness for 20 years at the time of diagnosis of MMN and remained functional 10 years later. Progression may be subacute (7), resulting in quadriplegia (4,7). Two fatal cases, including one reported in

G. J. Parry: Department of Neurology, Fairview-University Medical Center, University of Minnesota, Minneapolis, Minnesota 55455.

the literature (5) and one personal patient, died after more than two decades of progressive weakness.

The similarities of MMN and MND have been exaggerated with resulting uncertainty as to the number of ALS patients that prove to have MMN. Lange et al. (15) found MMN in 6% of patients with the clinical diagnosis of MND, but in my experience it is far less common. The differences between the two disorders outweigh their similarities. MMN should never be mistaken for ALS, even on purely clinical grounds for five reasons. First, bulbar involvement, which is common in ALS, is extremely rare in MMN. Second, Babinski and Hoffman signs, clonus, and frank spasticity are not encountered in MMN, although the finding of preserved tendon reflexes in limbs with weak, atrophic, and fasciculating muscles certainly raises the specter of upper motor neuron involvement. Third, severe weakness without wasting is a feature of MMN but never MND. Fourth, the weakness progresses slowly over years and decades in MMN and is rarely fatal, as compared with ALS in which death supervenes usually within 3 to 5 years of diagnosis. Fifth, weakness in MMN conforms to the distribution of individual peripheral nerves, whereas in ALS it is myotomal or upper motor neuron in type. Despite these substantive differences, weakness, atrophy, fasciculations, cramps, preserved reflexes, and a paucity of sensory abnormalities are common to both disorders. In addition, rare cases involve bulbar muscles and progress rapidly and individual deficits may become confluent, masking the conformity to a peripheral nerve distribution. Such cases require detailed electrodiagnostic studies to distinguish MND from MMN.

ELECTROPHYSIOLOGIC STUDIES

Electrodiagnosis in Multifocal Motor Neuropathy

Motor Nerve Conduction Studies

The diagnosis of MMN relies on the findings of motor nerve conduction studies (Fig. 1). The electrophysiologic sine qua non is focal or multifocal conduction block, confined to motor axons (2,13). Sensory conduction is normal, both distal to and through nerve segments with severe or complete MCB. The latter is most often found in forearm and distal nerve segments but can occur at any level (2,12–14,16). It can be seen at multiple sites along the length of a single nerve (7). Distal motor latency and F-wave latencies may be normal or prolonged (17). Conduction block is usually severe (11) and may be complete (14). Maximal conduction velocity through blocked segments is severely slowed when measured over short segments. However, conduction slowing over longer lengths of nerve when evaluated by conventional nerve conduction studies is less severe, and the velocity may even be normal (2,7), suggesting that the slowing is highly focal. Krarup et al. (14) confirmed this by stimulating at multiple closely spaced sites along the nerve, showing that

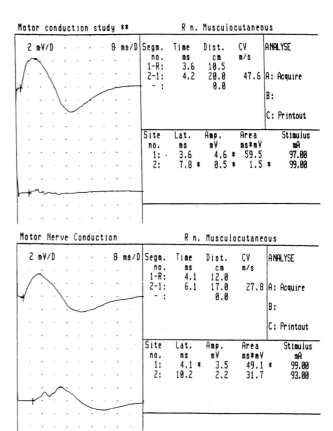

FIG. 1. The motor nerve conduction studies in the musculocutaneous nerve show severe conduction block between axilla and supraclavicular fossa (upper tracing). After treatment with several courses of high-dose intravenous immunoglobulin, there is partial resolution of the conduction block. (From Ref. 11, with permission.)

conduction slowing and block was confined to segments of 3 to 10 cm in length.

Sensory Nerve Conduction Studies

Sensory conduction is normal in MMN. Parry and Clarke (2) evaluated sensory conduction by means of ascending compound sensory nerve action potentials and somatosensory evoked potentials, which were normal despite more than 90% MCB; however, others found somatosensory evoked potential abnormalities in the face of normal distal sensory conduction (18). Krarup et al. (14) showed that the decline of the sensory nerve action potential amplitude across segments of severe motor block was no different from controls. In one case, sensory conduction proceeded normally despite complete motor block. Abnormalities of quantitative sensory testing have also been seen (19).

Electromyography

Needle electromyography shows denervation in weak and wasted muscles in MMN. Fibrillation activity is invariable and fasciculation is common. Weak nonwasted muscles can have a paucity of spontaneous activity, but voluntary motor unit potential (MUP) recruitment is reduced. Myokymia is occasionally seen and is an important clue to demyelination. In comparison with MND, denervation in MMN is confined to clinically weak muscles, whereas in MND and especially ALS, widespread denervation is invariably seen in clinically normal muscles.

Definition of Conduction Block

Conduction Block in Acute Demyelination

Normally only a small drop in the amplitude of the compound muscle action potential (CMAP) occurs along adjacent segments due to temporal dispersion. This amplitude drop should not exceed 15 to 20% along the wrist-to-elbow segment (20–22). In acute neuropathies, negative peak amplitude and duration criteria are sufficient to define conduction block. An amplitude drop of more than 20% is strongly suggestive of conduction block provided that temporal dispersion does not exceed 15%. When a demyelinating neuropathy progresses for more than a few days, the range of conduction velocities increases and abnormal temporal dispersion develops, resulting in decreased amplitudes and increased negative peak duration. Therefore, amplitude reduction alone is insufficient to define conduction block unless the negative peak duration increases by less than 15%.

The electrophysiologic features of acute conduction block due to pure demyelination can be examined by injecting antibodies to galactocerebroside, a component of myelin, into rat sciatic nerve (23,24). In the beginning, the distal response remains entirely normal. The proximal amplitude progressively falls to a nadir in 3 hours, but there is no temporal dispersion, and conduction remains normal using conventional techniques. Hence, a characteristic feature of acute demyelination is conduction block without slowing or temporal dispersion.

Conduction Block in Chronic Neuropathies

Changes in CMAP amplitude may be erroneously attributed to conduction block and can occur when the range of conduction velocities is increased or with chronic axon loss. As demyelinated axons remyelinate, there is an increased range of conduction velocities resulting in abnormal temporal dispersion and reduced CMAP amplitudes with proximal stimulation. The increased negative peak duration of the dispersed proximal response distinguishes this amplitude change from conduction block. However, amplitude reduction without an obvious increase in negative peak duration may occur due to interphase cancellation. The CMAP is comprised of summated MUP, and when there is a narrow range of conduction velocities and electrical impulses traverse a short distance, synchronous firing results in little opportunity for cancellation of the

negative phase by the positive phase of other motor units. With longer nerve segments, desynchronization leads to some phase interactions and cancellation is inevitable, resulting in loss of CMAP amplitude out of proportion to the increased negative peak duration. In normal motor nerves, this effect is negligible because the long duration of normal MUPs (5 to 15 msec) necessitates a large phase shift before significant phase interaction occurs (25). In hereditary demyelinating neuropathy, there is equal slowing in all fibers and the range of conduction velocities is minimally increased, so that amplitude loss due to interphase cancellation rarely occurs despite severe slowing (26). In acquired demyelinating neuropathies there is a marked increase in the range of conduction velocities with major phase shifts, and the CMAP amplitudes are often reduced out of proportion to the increased negative peak duration and thus mistaken for conduction block.

Amplitude changes due to phase cancellation also occur with chronic denervation. When motor units are lost, terminal collateral sprouting of remaining units causes polyphasia, increasing the likelihood of phase interaction and cancellation (27). With fewer motor units, phase cancellation has a larger effect on the CMAP amplitude. Therefore, patients with MND or chronic axonal neuropathies may have significant amplitude reductions that may be interpreted as conduction block. Apparent conduction block in ALS results from phase cancellation in partially denervated muscles. Computer simulation studies show that interphase cancellation can reduce the CMAP amplitude by 50% (28). However, the amplitude and waveform changes occur smoothly along the nerve as more distant sites are stimulated, whereas in focal demyelination they are confined to restricted nerve segments.

The difficulties wrought by dispersion and phase interaction leading to changes in amplitude alone should be interpreted with caution (29). Three steps should be undertaken to determine whether there is true conduction block. First, amplitude changes should occur over a short nerve segment rather than gradually along the length of the nerve. This can be demonstrated by incrementally stimulating short segments percutaneously or by a monopolar needle. Second, individual motor units may be present with distal stimulation, but not upon proximal stimulation or with volitional activation. Third, the waveform of the electrically evoked CMAP should resemble the summated individual surface recorded MUP, elicited by maximal volitional contraction. There is conduction block if the electrically elicited CMAP cannot be resynthesized from the surface recorded unitary volitional responses, especially if the patient is cooperative. Amplitude, and even area, changes should be interpreted with caution unless these criteria are met. From a diagnostic perspective, amplitude, waveform, and velocity changes have the same implication as conduction block provided they are focal or multifocal because both indicate acquired demyelination. Conduction block causes loss of function, whereas focal slowing and dispersion have negligible functional consequences.

Pathogenesis of Pure Motor Block

It is not known why conduction block in MMN is confined to motor axons. It may indicate a difference between the antigenic properties of the myelin of motor and sensory axons. The ceramide composition of gangliosides in human sensory and motor nerves is different, and that could impart antigenic differences to the myelin (30). There could be comparable demyelination in motor and sensory axons with a greater safety factor for impulse transmission in sensory axons, leading to conduction block in motor fiber alone (27). However, this is unlikely because the largest diameter axons have the most secure conduction and sensory axons are the largest. Demyelination could also be confined to motor fascicles within the nerve trunk, whereas the sensory fascicles are spared. Variation in the extent of the demyelination seen in different fascicles is common in CIDP, and the differences may occasionally be striking (31). On rare occasions, random demyelination may strike only motor fascicles, resulting in the clinical picture of MMN.

LABORATORY INVESTIGATION IN MULTIFOCAL MOTOR NEUROPATHY

The laboratory investigation of patients with MMN is seldom helpful. There is typically no associated systemic illness. Serum protein electrophoresis and immunoelectrophoresis are usually normal; however, some patients have antibodies to a variety of glycolipid determinants (see below). Cerebrospinal fluid protein is usually normal.

RELATIONSHIP OF MULTIFOCAL MOTOR NEUROPATHY TO ANTIGLYCOLIPID ANTIBODIES

Pestronk et al. (13) first described two patients with MMN that had IgG and IgM GM1 antibodies. Of 500 patients with various motor syndromes so studied (32), 74 had a progressive, asymmetric, pure lower motor neuron disorder, sparing bulbar muscles; 77% had antibodies to gangliosides, a much higher proportion than normal individuals or in those with neurologic or nonneurologic disorders. Three clinically distinct groups were identified as follows. Twenty-five patients had MMN with distal weakness and proximal conduction block, 21 of whom had elevated or very high anti-GM1 antibody titers. In 28 patients, the weakness was distal without conduction block, 64% of whom had elevated anti-GM1 antibodies. In a third group, the weakness was proximal without conduction block. Only 2 of 18 patients so studied had anti-GM1 antibodies, but some had antibodies to other gangliosides. On the basis of these observations, anti-GM1 antibodies were assigned

a critical pathogenetic role in MMN. However, others have been unable to confirm these results. Nobile-Orazio et al. (33) studied sera from 232 patients with MND; 23% had anti-GM1 antibodies, regardless of whether they had ALS, progressive bulbar palsy, or pure lower motor neuron disease. In addition, 19% of patients with other neuropathies had elevated antibodies. Others have also found antibodies to GM1 and other gangliosides in disorders of the lower motor neuron (34–36) and in ALS (37–39). Overall, about 70% of MMN patients have elevated GM1 antibody titers. The highest titers are found in MMN; however, a 10-fold elevation or more is characteristic of MMN. Lower titers are suggestive but nonspecific. Nonetheless, MMN should not be diagnosed on the basis of an elevated GM1 antibody titer nor excluded when normal or minimally elevated.

PATHOLOGY

Motor Nerve Pathology

Descriptions of the presumptive motor nerve pathology are derived from biopsies of mixed nerves in patients with MMN. One patient underwent biopsy of the right ulnar nerve in the axilla, along a site of documented MCB (40). More than half of the cross-sectional area of the nerve was normal, but there were patches of demyelination (Fig. 2). Many axons were thinly myelinated in relation to their diameter and some showed onion bulb formation, a feature of repeated demyelination and remyelination. Inflammatory cells were absent. A second patient had a biopsy of the medial pectoral nerve (10). At surgery, multifocal enlargements of the brachial plexus were seen and intraoperative nerve conduction studies across the site of enlargement in the medial cord documented severe MCB. The medial pectoral nerve, arising from the proximal medial cord at the site of focal enlargement, was removed. The low power light photomicrograph showed a patch

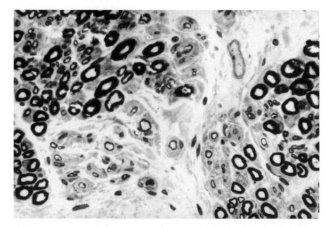

FIG. 2. Ulnar nerve biopsy from the axilla at a site of conduction block. There is an area of demyelination in the center, but adjacent fascicles are spared. (From Ref. 40, with permission.)

within the fascicle of severe demyelination. Electron microscopy showed large diameter axons with very thin myelin (Fig. 3A) and some axons that were completely devoid of myelin, being surrounded only by Schwann cell processes and redundant basal lamina (Fig. 3B). Some thinly myelinated axons were surrounded by supernumearry Schwann cells, forming rudimentary onion bulbs. There was an increase in the endoneurial interstitial space, concentrated in the subperineurial area, suggesting endoneurial edema, and the perineurium was thickened. Inflammatory cells were also absent. A third patient had a biopsy of a supraclavicular mass that was found to consist of nerve, and MMN was diagnosed several years later (41). The paraffin-embedded nerve showed exuberant onion bulb formation (Fig. 4A). The endoneurial interstitial space was markedly increased, and there was prominent mononuclear cell infiltration concentrated around endoneurial venules but also extending into the general endoneurial compartment (Fig. 4B). The infiltrate consisted mainly of lymphocytes with many macrophages.

The pathology in this case differed from those described by Kaji et al. (10) and Auer et al. (40) in the more severe onion bulb formation, the presence of prominent mononuclear cell inflammation, and the degree of interstitial edema but more closely resembled those described by Adams et al. (42) and Bradley et al. (43) in the lack of classic clinical and electrophysiologic features of MMN. The first report described two patients with steroid-responsive sensory and motor multifocal neuropathy with nerve hypertrophy, a clinical picture resembling the neuropathy described by Lewis et al. (3) ("Lewis-Sumner syndrome") that closely resembles MMN. Pathologically, the nerves showed marked interstitial hypertrophy and onion bulb formation with both focal and diffuse mononuclear inflammatory cell infiltration. The second report described a patient with a motor neuropathy that was asymmetric but not strikingly multifocal as is typical of MMN. Electrophysiologic studies showed multifocal MCB, but sensory nerve action potential amplitudes were reduced. Once again, the brachial plexus biopsy showed marked interstitial hypertrophy, onion bulb formation, and mononuclear cell inflammation.

The pathologic changes in mixed nerves support the concept that MMN is an autoimmune disorder. Mononuclear cell and macrophage infiltration with demyelination and onion bulb formation are features common to other autoimmune neuropathies, and identical abnormalities are seen in the sensory nerves of patients with CIDP. Impressed by the failure to reestablish normal conduction despite remyelination, Kaji et al. (10) postulated the pres-

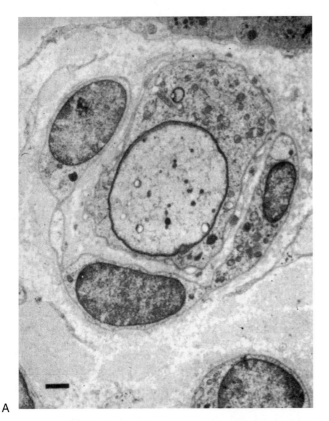
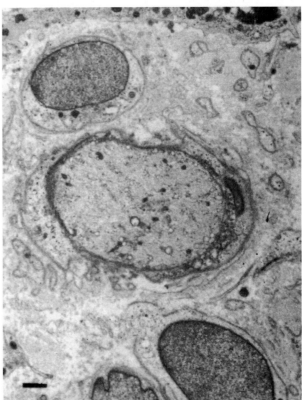

A

B

FIG. 3. Electron microscopy of a biopsy taken from the medial pectoral nerve adjacent to a site of conduction block in the medial cord of the brachial plexus. **A:** A thinly myelinated large-diameter axon surrounded by a small onion bulb. Bar, 1 m. **B:** A large-diameter axon entirely devoid of myelin. Bar, 1 m. (From Ref. 10, with permission.)

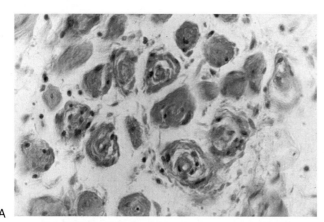 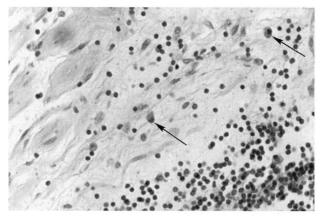

FIG. 4. Low power light microscopy of paraffin-embedded nerve taken from the brachial plexus of a woman with MMN. **A:** There is exuberant onion bulb formation and a marked increase in the endoneurial interstitial space. **B:** Prominent endoneurial mononuclear cell infiltration with occasional macrophages (arrows). (From GJ Parry. *Multifocal motor neuropathy: pathogenesis and treatment.* Amsterdam: Elsevier Science, 1997:73–83, with permission.)

ence of a factor that blocks sodium channels or prevents their redistribution. Further argument in favor of blocking antibodies comes from the often rapid response to treatment. Conduction block may result from minimal morphologic changes at the node of Ranvier, and conformational changes may remodel the paranodal apparatus sufficiently to reestablish conduction within days of starting treatment. Nonetheless, it is curious that fixed conduction block at one site may remain for years, suggesting the presence of a soluble factor that inhibits recovery, whether by blocking sodium channels or preventing remyelination. The remarkable similarity of the pathologic changes in patients with classic MMN or Lewis-Sumner syndrome and typical CIDP suggests that slight differences in similar primary antigens triggering the immune response may account for the clinical differences.

Sensory Nerve Pathology

Mild pathologic changes in sensory nerves also occur in MMN. Parry and Clarke (2) noted mild loss of myelinated axons in the sural nerve of the one patient, although quantitative morphometry was not done. Mild perivascular inflammatory cell infiltration (7,14), mild fiber loss (2,14), subtle demyelination (14,44), and regeneration (44) were described. There was only one systematic quantitative study of sensory nerves in MMN (45). The mean total fiber density in 10 patients so studied did not differ from normal control subjects, although one patient had a total fiber density of less than 50% of the normal mean. In six patients, there was a significant reduction in the number of large fibers measuring more than 7 m. The most common abnormality, seen in all 11 nerves, was mild demyelination consisting of an increased number of thinly myelinated fibers, miniature onion bulbs, rare demyelinated fibers, and active macrophage-mediated

demyelination, without endoneurial edema or endoneurial or epineurial inflammation. The abnormalities in sensory nerves underscore the extent of fiber type involvement and support the kinship of MMN to CIDP.

Treatment of Multifocal Motor Neuropathy

All effective treatments for MMN involve immune modulation or suppression. The rationale for immunotherapy in MMN derived from its similarity to CIDP. The discovery of high titers of GM1 antibodies often seen in MMN supported the concept of an immune basis, and the pathologic features, previously described, provided further support for this concept. Attempts to define the best treatment of MMN are still based on anecdotal reports and small controlled series. However, a consensus has emerged in favor of high-dose intravenous immunoglobulin (IVIg) therapy for most affected patients.

Intravenous Immunoglobulin

High-dose IVIg is the most widely used and effective treatment for MMN. The literature contains reports on such treatment in nearly 50 patients. Kaji et al. (46) reported improvement with IVIg in two patients that failed prednisone, plasmapheresis, and oral cyclophosphamide. In general, clinical improvement occurred in 2 to 4 weeks. One patient required monthly treatment, whereas the other was treated for 5 months with sustained benefit. Chaudhry et al. (47) treated nine patients and all improved, usually within hours to days, peaking at 2 weeks and lasting about 2 months, although one obtained sustained remission. The response to treatment was independent of the initial GM1 antibody titer, the change in GM1 antibody titer, or obvious change in conduction block. Nobile-Orazio et al. (48) noted dramatic and sustained improvement; one patient returned to normal within a few months of receiving a single course of IVIg and was in sustained remission at 12 month follow-up. Other patients treated, in addition, with oral cyclophosphamide increased the intertreatment interval of IVIg, but they generally had elevated GM1 antibody titers that were unaffected by immune suppression.

Several placebo-controlled observations soon followed. Yuki et al. (49) noted improvement with IVIg but not with placebo in a single-blinded protocol. Azulay et al. (50) treated five patients with MMN in a double-blind placebo-controlled trial and showed increased muscle strength. Van den Bergh et al. (51) treated six respondents in an open-label trial, who then received IVIg or placebo in a double-blind protocol. Five patients responded to IVIg but not placebo, whereas the sixth responded equally to both.

Our experience with IVIg has generally been similar. All seven of our patients responded to treatment (Table 1), but improvement was not sustained for more than 2 months after a single course, and long-term treatment was always needed. In three patients, there was improvement in MCB that paralleled treatment (Fig. 1) (11), whereas the others improved without demonstrable changes in MCB. The rapidity of the clinical improvement can only be explained by reversal of conduction block. The inability to document reversal of conduction block in some cases probably reflects conduction block at sites technically difficult to evaluate such as nerve roots and proximal nerve trunks. Segmental amplitude ratios may not improve with treatment because of the slowly conducting components, giving rise to dispersed responses that occur too late to contribute to the CMAP amplitude. There has not been a consistent relationship between treatment response and either the initial or later GM1 antibody titer. We found that response to treatment tended to be less over time but that no patient became unresponsive. Others also found that the effectiveness of IVIg diminished with longer treatment (44) and that some patients became refractory (52). In some of our patients, addition of azathioprine or prednisone enabled the intertreatment interval to be increased.

TABLE 1. *Quantitative muscle strength testing*

	June 1993	August 1993	November 1993
Shoulder flexion	10.4	18.6	22.0
Shoulder extension	25.0	40.0	44.0
Elbow flexion	7.3	12.9	14.6
Wrist extension	6.0	7.4	10.8

Improvement in strength in affected muscles after monthly treatment with high-dose intravenous immunoglobulin in a patient with multifocal motor neuropathy. Numbers refer to the weight in kilograms that the patient could lift. All values shown are from the right arm.

Cyclophosphamide

Pestronk et al. (13) reported responsiveness of MMN to cyclophosphamide. One patient was treated with a single course of 3 g/m^2 intravenous cyclophosphamide over 8 days, followed by oral therapy for 10 months. Strength improved to near normal even after discontinuation of treatment. A second patient received the same dose without additional oral therapy and relapsed after 8 months. He was later retreated with intravenous followed by oral therapy, and improvement was later maintained. The response to treatment was paralleled by a fall in GM1 antibody titers. These observations were extended to nine patients with similar results (53). However, cyclophosphamide dosages were high, incurring a significant risk of serious adverse effects. In recognition of this, Pestronk et al. (54) lowered the dose of intravenous cyclophosphamide preceded by 2 days of plasmapheresis and achieved similar benefits with a 50 to 70% reduction in drug dose. With either of these regimens there was 1 to 2 years of sustained improvement after cessation of treatment, although relapses were common and required retreatment. Tan et al. (55) administered intravenous cyclophosphamide, but the response in their patients was independent of a change in GM1 antibody titers.

Other treatments for MMN have generally been ineffective. A few patients respond to prednisone (55,56), but in most it was ineffective and occasionally caused rapid deterioration (57). In one atypical patient with rapidly evolving weakness there was improvement with prednisone and plasmapheresis (7). No other patient has responded to plasmapheresis.

RELATIONSHIP OF MULTIFOCAL MOTOR NEUROPATHY TO CHRONIC INFLAMMATORY DEMYELINATING POLYNEUROPATHY

There are clinical, electrophysiologic, morphologic, and immunologic similarities between MMN and CIDP. Classically, CIDP is a largely symmetric, sensory, and motor neuropathy (51); however, motor features predominate and can be strikingly asymmetric. The patients described by Lewis et al. (3) were similar to those with MMN in view of the motor predominance and predilection for the arms. Conversely, most patients with MMN have subtle sensory symptoms or signs and abnormalities of quantitative sensory testing, sensory nerve conduction, and frequent morphologic abnormalities in sensory nerves. Elevated GM1 antibody titers can be seen in both disorders, although they are always higher in MMN. Thus, in the autoimmune demyelinating neuropathies, there may be a continuum of features, including predominantly sensory, sensory-motor, and predominantly motor, which may be symmetric, asymmetric, or even strikingly multifocal.

SUMMARY

MMN is a strikingly asymmetric predominantly motor variant of CIDP. The resemblance of MMN to MND has been exaggerated, and the two can generally be readily distinguished on clinical and electrophysiologic grounds. Further studies are clearly needed to fully clarify the relationship between MMN and other motor syndromes associated with glycolipid antibodies.

REFERENCES

1. Parry GJ, Clarke S. Pure motor neuropathy with multifocal conduction block masquerading as motor neuron disease. *Muscle Nerve* 1985;8:167(abst).
2. Parry GJ, Clarke S. Multifocal acquired demyelinating neuropathy masquerading as motor neuron disease. *Muscle Nerve* 1988;11:103–107.
3. Lewis RA, Sumner AJ, Brown MJ, Asbury AK. Multifocal demyelinating neuropathy with persistent conduction block. *Neurology* 1982;32:958–964.
4. Roth G, Rohr J, Magistris MR, Ochsner F. Motor neuropathy with proximal multifocal persistent conduction block, fasciculations and myokymia. Evolution to tetraplegia. *Eur Neurol* 1986;25:416–423.
5. Magistris MR, Roth G. Motor neuropathy with multifocal persistent conduction blocks. *Muscle Nerve* 1992;15:1056–1057.
6. Kaji R, Shibasaki H, Kimura J. Multifocal demyelinating motor neuropathy: cranial nerve involvement and immunoglobulin therapy. *Neurology* 1992;42:506–509.
7. Van den Bergh P, Logigian EL, Kelly JJ Jr. Motor neuropathy with multifocal conduction blocks. *Muscle Nerve* 1989;11:26–31.
8. Bradley WG, Bennett RK, Good P, Little B. Proximal chronic inflammatory polyneuropathy with multifocal conduction block. *Arch Neurol* 1988;45:451–455.
9. Auer RN, Bell RB, Lee MA. Neuropathy with onion bulb formations and pure motor manifestations. *Can J Neurol Sci* 1989;16:194–197.
10. Kaji R, Oka N, Tsuji T, Mezaki T, Kimura J. Pathological findings at the sites of conduction block in multifocal motor neuropathy. *Ann Neurol* 1993;33:152–158.
11. Parry GJ. AAEM Case Report #30: Multifocal motor neuropathy. *Muscle Nerve* 1996;19:269–276.
12. Roth G, Magistris MR. Neuropathies with prolonged conduction block, single and grouped fasciculations, localized limb myokymia. *Electroencephalogr Clin Neurophysiol* 1987;67:428–438.
13. Pestronk A, Cornblath DR, Ilyas AA, et al. A treatable multifocal motor neuropathy with antibodies to GM1 ganglioside. *Ann Neurol* 1988;24:73–78.
14. Krarup C, Stewart MB, Sumner AJ, Pestronk A, Lipton SA. A syndrome of asymmetric limb weakness with motor conduction block. *Neurology* 1990;40:118–127.
15. Lange DJ, Trojaborg W, Latov N, et al. Multifocal motor neuropathy with conduction block: is it a distinct clinical entity? *Neurology* 1992;42:497–505.
16. Lange D, Blake DM, Hirano M, Burns SM, Latov N, Trojaborg W. Multifocal conduction block motor neuropathy: diagnostic value of stimulating cervical roots. *Neurology* 1990;40[Suppl 1]:182.
17. Chaudhry V, Corse AM, Cornblath DR, Kuncl RW, Freimer ML, Griffin JW. Multifocal motor neuropathy: electrodiagnostic features. *Muscle Nerve* 1994;17:198–205.
18. Valls-Sole' J, Cruz-Martinez A, Graus F, Saiz A, Arpa J, Grau JM. Abnormal sensory conduction in multifocal demyelinating neuropathy with persistent conduction block. *Neurology* 1995;45:2024–2028.
19. Pouget J, Azulay J-P, Bile-Turc F, et al. Sensory function study in 15 cases of multifocal motor neuropathy. *Muscle Nerve* 1994;17[Suppl]:S237(abst).
20. Kelly JJ Jr. The electrodiagnostic findings in the peripheral neuropathy associated with monoclonal gammopathy. *Muscle Nerve* 1983;6:504–509.
21. Albers JW, Donofrio PD, McGonagle TK. Sequential electrodiagnostic abnormalities in acute inflammatory demyelinating polyneuropathy. *Muscle Nerve* 1985;8:528–539.
22. Cornblath DR. Electrophysiology in Guillain-Barre syndrome. *Ann Neurol* 1990;27[Suppl]:S17–S20.
23. Saida K, Saida T, Brown MJ, Silberberg DH, Asbury AK. Antiserum-mediated demyelination in vivo. A sequential study using intraneural injection of experimental allergic neuritis serum. *Lab Invest* 1978;39:449–462.
24. Sumner AJ, Saida K, Saida T, Silberberg DH, Asbury AK. Acute conduction block associated with experimental antiserum-mediated demyelination of peripheral nerve. *Ann Neurol* 1982;11:469–477.
25. Kimura J, Machida M, Ishida T, et al. Relation between size of compound sensory or muscle action potentials, and length of nerve segment. *Neurology* 1986;36:647–652.
26. Lewis RA, Sumner AJ. The electrodiagnostic distinctions between chronic familial and acquired demyelinative neuropathies. *Neurology* 1982;32:592–596.
27. Sumner AJ. Separating motor neuron diseases from pure motor neuropathies. Multifocal motor neuropathy with persistent conduction block. *Adv Neurol* 1991;56:399–403.
28. Rhee RK, England JD, Sumner AJ. Computer simulation of conduction block: effects produced by actual block versus interphase cancellation. *Ann Neurol* 1990;28:146–156.
29. Cornblath DR, Sumner AJ, Daube J, et al. Conduction block in clinical practice. *Muscle Nerve* 1991;14:869–871.
30. Ogawa-Goto K, Funamoto N, Abe T, Nagashima K. Different ceramide compositions of gangliosides between human motor and sensory nerves. *J Neurochem* 1990;55:1486–1493.
31. Nukada H, Pollock M, Haas LF. Is ischemia implicated in chronic multifocal demyelinating neuropathy? *Neurology* 1989;39:106–110.
32. Pestronk A, Chaudhry V, Feldman EL, et al. Lower motor neuron syndromes defined by patterns of weakness, nerve conduction abnormalities, and high titers of antiglycolipid antibodies. *Ann Neurol* 1990;27:316–326.
33. Nobile-Orazio E, Carpo M, Legname G, Meucci N, Sonnino S, Scarlato G. Anti-GM1 IgM antibodies in motor neuron disease and neuropathy. *Neurology* 1990;40:1747–1750.
34. Nardelli E, Steck AJ, Barkas T, Schluep M, Jerusalem F. Motor neuron syndrome and monoclonal IgM with antibody activity against gangliosides GM1 and GD1b. *Ann Neurol* 1988;23:524–528.
35. Shy ME, Heimann-Patterson T, Parry GJ, Tahmoush A, Evans VA, Schick PK. Lower motor neuron disease in a patient with autoantibodies against Gal (b 1-3) GalNAc in gangliosides GM1 and GD1b: improvement following immunotherapy. *Neurology* 1990;40:842–844.
36. Pestronk A. Motor neuropathies, motoneuron disorders and antiglycolipid antibodies. *Muscle Nerve* 1991;14:927–936.
37. Pestronk A, Adams RN, Clawson L, et al. Serum antibodies to GM1 ganglioside in amyotrophic lateral sclerosis. *Neurology* 1988;38:1457–1461.
38. Pestronk A, Adams RN, Cornblath DR, Kuncl RW, Drachman DB, Clawson L. Patterns of serum IgM antibodies to GM1 and GD1a gangliosides in amyotrophic lateral sclerosis. *Ann Neurol* 1989;25:98–102.
39. Shy ME, Evans VA, Lublin FD, et al. Antibodies to GM1 and GD1b in patients with motor neuron disease without plasma cell dyscrasia. *Ann Neurol* 1989;25:511–513.
40. Auer RN, Bell RB, Lee MA. Neuropathy with onion bulb formations and pure motor manifestations. *Can J Neurol Sci* 1989;6:194–197.
41. Midani H, Parry GJ, Day JW: Electrophysiology and brachial plexus pathology in a woman misdiagnosed as HMSN-I. *Muscle Nerve* 1993;16:1103(abst).
42. Adams RD, Asbury AK, Michelsen JJ. Multifocal pseudohypertrophic neuropathy. *Trans Am Neurol Assoc* 1965;90:30–34.
43. Bradley WG, Bennet RK, Good P, Little B. Proximal chronic inflammatory polyneuropathy with multifocal conduction block. *Arch Neurol* 1988;45:451–455.
44. Bouche P, Moulonguet A, Younes-Chennoufi AB, et al. Multifocal motor neuropathy with conduction block: a study of 24 patients. *J Neurol Neurosurg Psychiatry* 1995;59:38–44.
45. Corse AM, Chaudhry V, Crawford TO, Cornblath DR, Kuncl RW, Griffin JW. Sensory nerve pathology in multifocal motor neuropathy. *Ann Neurol* 1996;39:319–325.
46. Kaji R, Shibasaki H, Kimura J. Multifocal demyelinating motor neuropathy: cranial nerve involvement and immunoglobulin therapy. *Neurology* 1992;42:506–509.

47. Chaudry V, Corse AM, Cornblath DR, et al. Multifocal motor neuropathy: response to human immune globulin. *Ann Neurol* 1993;33:237–242.
48. Nobile-Orazio E, Meucci N, Barbieri S, Carpo M, Scarlato G. High-dose intravenous immunoglobulin therapy in multifocal motor neuropathy. *Neurology* 1993;43:537–544.
49. Yuki N, Yamazaki M, Kondo H, Suzuki K, Tsuji S. Treatment of multifocal motor neuropathy with a high dosage of intravenous immunoglobulin. *Muscle Nerve* 1993;16:220–221.
50. Azulay J-P, Blin O, Pouget J, et al. Intravenous immunoglobulin treatment in patients with motor neuron syndromes associated with anti-GM1 antibodies: a double-blind, placebo-controlled study. *Neurology* 1994;44:429–432.
51. Van den Bergh LH, Kerkhoff H, Oey PL, et al. Treatment of multifocal motor neuropathy with high dose intravenous immunoglobulins: a double blind, placebo controlled study. *J Neurol Neurosurg Psychiatry* 1995;59:248–252.
52. Elliott JL, Pestronk A. Progression of multifocal motor neuropathy during apparently successful treatment with human immunoglobulin. *Neurology* 1994;44:967–968.
53. Feldman EL, Bromberg MB, Albers JW, Pestronk A. Immunosuppressive treatment in multifocal motor neuropathy. *Ann Neurol* 1991;30:397–401.
54. Pestronk A, Lopate G, Kornberg AJ, et al. Distal lower motor neuron syndrome with high-titer serum IgM anti-GM1 antibodies: improvement following immunotherapy with monthly plasma exchange and intravenous cyclophosphamide. *Neurology* 1994;44:2027–2031.
55. Tan E, Lynn J, Amato AA, et al. Immunosuppressive treatment of motor neuron disorders. Attempts to distinguish a treatable disorder. *Arch Neurol* 1994;51:194–200.
56. Olney RK, Pestronk A. Prednisone treatment of multifocal predominantly-motor neuropathy. *Neurology* 1992;42[Suppl 3]:178.
57. Donaghy M, Mills KR, Boniface SJ, et al. Pure motor demyelinating neuropathy: deterioration after steroid treatment and improvement with intravenous immunoglobulin. *J Neurol Neurosurg Psychiatry* 1994;57:778–783.

Motor Disorders,
edited by David S. Younger.
Lippincott Williams & Wilkins, Philadelphia © 1999.

CHAPTER 16

Charcot-Marie-Tooth Disorders and Other Hereditary Neuropathies

Robert E. Lovelace

Peripheral neuropathy is among the most common neurologic disorders after stroke and epilepsy. Up to 20% of all neuropathies have a confirmed or suggested inherited basis (1–3). The presenting symptoms of a genetic neuropathy are found distally in the limbs due to involvement of the longest nerve fibers, often with pes cavus and club foot and later claw hand deformities (4–6). The Charcot-Marie-Tooth (CMT) disorders comprise 80 to 90% of all genetic neuropathies (7,8) and have an incidence of more than 42 per 100,000, which represents more than 250,000 cases nationwide. The terms peroneal muscular atrophy (9), hereditary motor and sensory neuropathy (HMSN), and CMT are used interchangeably for the prototypic disorder that exhibits clinical and genetic heterogeneity (10,11).

BACKGROUND

The recent explosion in molecular genetics of the past 15 years has revolutionized our understanding and classification of the CMT disorders (Table 1), but on the whole it has not yet translated into useful therapy (12–15). The first major advance was the application of electrophysiologic studies to the nosology, with the designation of some conditions as axonal and others as demyelinating. Those with normal or slightly reduced compound muscle action potentials (CMAP) and sensory nerve action potentials (SNAP) and excessively slow nerve conduction velocity (NCV) were deemed demyelinating. Others with low-amplitude CMAP and SNAP and normal or mildly reduced NCV were deemed axonal (6,12–17). The classification of the CMT neuropathies begins with the main

division of demyelinating neuropathy, termed CMT1 or HSMN1, and the axonal type, termed CMT2, HSMN2, or "neuronal" form. Both have the same phenotypic presentation. The group of distal spinal muscular atrophies (SMA) (18,19) with a phenotype similar to peroneal muscular atrophy is known as the spinal type and lacks slowing of NCV or involvement of sensory fibers. Hereditary neuropathy with liability to pressure palsy (HNPP) (14,17,20,21) shares clinical features with CMT1A, and when all such cases are ascertained, HNPP probably has a similar incidence (Gareth Parry, personal communication, 1998).

Symmetric involvement of the hands and feet is important in the general presentation of an inherited neuropathy. It may be so insidious as to be overlooked or compensated by the patient for years. Progressive deformity of the legs is related to differential muscle imbalance and sensory deprivation. Even though a delay of several years may occur, hand involvement invariably manifests itself in a similar way with profound difficulty in handling small objects such as a button or pen. This is usually associated with atrophy of intrinsic hand muscles and the lower forearms. The absence of hand involvement should cast doubt on the diagnosis of a genetic neuropathy. Patients with HNPP present with multiple nerve lesions and prominent asymmetry reminiscent of chronic inflammatory demyelinating polyneuropathy (CIDP) (22–24).

The application of molecular genetics has more clearly defined the clinical and genetic diversity of CMT and its related disorders than ever before. Genetic investigations can be performed in utero to determine fetal involvement. Lebo et al. (25) pioneered methods of intrauterine diagnosis and described at least eight genetic abnormalities with abnormal membrane proteins. It is potentially useful in CMT syndromes, particularly CMT1A, wherein the effects of reduplications, particularly of a large segment

R. E. Lovelace: Columbia University College of Physicians and Surgeons and Neurological Institute, New York Presbyterian Hospital, New York, New York 10032.

TABLE 1. *Classification of CMT neuropathies*

Disorder	Chromosome/Locus	Gene
CMT type 1A	17p11.2-12	*PMP22*
CMT type 1B	1q22-23	*Po*
CMT type 1C	—	—
CMT type 2A	1q36	—
CMT type 2B	3q13-22	—
CMT type 2C	—	—
CMT type 3A	17p11.2-12	*PMP22*
CMT type 3B	1q22-23	*Po*
CMT type 4A	8q13-21.1	
CMT-X linked	Xq13.1	Connexin 32
HNPP type A	17p11.2-12	*PMP22*

CMT, Charcot-Marie-Tooth; HNPP, hereditary neuropathy with liability to pressure palsy.
Modified from Ref. 17.

of DNA, and increased gene dosage leads to increased clinical severity (25–28). Lupski (28) described use of genetic tests for each of the 10 different CMT syndromes, including the deletions in HNPP. If all of the individually mutated amino acid deletions in the gene for peripheral myelin protein (PMP) 22, myelin protein zero (MPZ) or P0, and connexin are counted, there are altogether more than 300 genetic defects in the CMT disorders. In a given family, the clinical manifestations of CMT can vary from asymmetric or pes cavus deformity to profound locomotor problems and limb deformity requiring Canadian crutches or a wheelchair (3,29). Slow NCV in hypertrophic nerves does not always define the dominant CMT1A phenotype because it also occurs in the recessive disorder Dejerine-Sottas disease or HMSN3, now termed CMT3 (30,31); in amyelinating neuropathy (32,33); and in CIDP (34), demyelinating neuropathy associated with antibodies to myelin-associated glycoprotein (MAG) (35), and HNPP. Unlike CMT, in both anti-MAG neuropathy and HNPP, distal motor latencies are disproportionately long for the degree of slowing (17,36). Genetic heterogeneity in CMT may also be manifested in a single family such as when CMT types 1 and 2 and the spinal form are simultaneously present (10).

NON-CHARCOT-MARIE-TOOTH GENETIC NEUROPATHIES

Other hereditary neuropathies that should be considered in a given patient include those associated with the recessively inherited disorders metachromatic leukodystrophy, abetalipoproteinemia or Bassen-Kornzweig disease, and polyglucosan body disease, all typified by chemical or storage products and specific neuropathologic changes. Acute intermittent porphyria (37) and familial amyloid polyneuropathy (FAP) (38) are dominantly inherited. Acute intermittent porphyria results from deficiency of uroporphyrin-1-synthetase and porphobilinogen deaminase due to 1 of 18 mutations in the

porphobilinogen gene (37); FAP is discussed in more detail below. Demyelinating neuropathy is occasionally associated with mitochondrial encephalomyopathy in which the mode of transmission is generally maternal; however, rare patients have demonstrated recessive and dominant Mendelian inheritance (39,40). The leukodystrophies generally present with symptoms and signs referable to the central nervous system (CNS) (2); however, abnormal nerve conduction studies with slowing of NCV indicates peripheral nervous system involvement as in childhood and adult-onset forms of metachromatic leukodystrophy (41,42).

Adrenoleukodystrophy and adrenomyeloneuropathy are X-linked disorders characterized by cerebellar ataxia, corticospinal tract degeneration, dementia, and slowing of NCV indicative of peripheral demyelinating neuropathy (43–45). Affected patients show increased levels of serum C24 and C26 saturated very-long-chain fatty acids due to a defect in fatty acid acyl-coenzyme A synthetase encoded at Xq28. Abetalipoproteinemia is a childhood cerebral demyelinating disorder resulting from vitamin E deficiency; however, the neuropathy is more axonal than demyelinating (46). There is more than one genetic type of Pelizaeus-Merzbacher disease, another rare X-linked leukodystrophy (47). In one family so studied, female carriers were identified by electrophysiologic studies (48), and the relationship was suggested for a PLP (proteolipid protein) gene dosage effect in the X chromosome, homologous to that of the *PMP22* gene in CMT1A for chromosome 17 (49). Krabbe's disease (50), Fabry's disease (51), giant axonal neuropathy (52,53), and Cockayne's syndrome (54,55) can have slow NCV indicating peripheral nerve involvement, as do patients with olivopontocerebellar degeneration, now termed spinocerebellar atrophy (SCA) (56), and others with myotonic muscular dystrophy (57), the latter of which maps to chromosome 19q13 (57). The several types of SCA are separable by clinical and genetic differences (14,58,59). A rare neuropathy described in association with Joseph-Machado degenerative disease involves anterior horn cells (60,61).

The five subtypes of FAP demonstrate extensive genetic and therefore phenotypic diversity. Affected patients generally show late-age onset, slow progression, autonomic involvement, fasciculation in wasted muscles, and, in some, carpal tunnel syndrome (62–64). The most common gene defect resides on chromosome 18 at q11.2 and q12.1, in the gene for prealbumin transthyretin in Portuguese-Cypriot patients (37,65). The gene defect in Iowa patients, FAP type IV, maps to chromosome 11 at q23-qter and is associated with apolipoprotein A1. Finnish, FAP type V, patients have a gene defect on chromosome 9 at q33 with abnormal production of gelsoline (38,66,67). Suspicion of FAP is an indication for nerve and muscle biopsy that should include immunofluorescence for amyloid apple-green birefringence (63,68).

CHARCOT-MARIE-TOOTH DISEASE AND RELATED DISORDERS

The incidence of 42 per 100,000 persons for the CMT disorders may be an underestimate if based on conventional clinical and electrophysiologic studies. When cases of HNPP and asymptomatic family members are included using sensitive nerve conduction studies and special sensory recording studies, the incidence doubles (2,4,5,14,69).

Our understanding of CMT has evolved over the past century. Charcot and Marie (70) favored an SMA basis, but Tooth (71) likened it to neuropathy. The acquired limb deformities include clubbed foot, talipes equina varus, pes cavus, flat feet, hammer toes, foot drop, and claw hand (Fig. 1). These lead to the characteristic gait disorder associated with foot slapping, unsteadiness, and frequent falls. The least manifestation, pes cavus, is found in patients with forme fruste who can also have NCV as slow as those with more severe clinical involvement (16,17,72–74). Stork-leg deformity describes the marked atrophic appearance of the lower leg beginning in the thigh, giving rise to the appearance of an inverted champagne bottle. Stork legs and clubbed feet are also found in patients with Friedrich's ataxia (FA) (75) or SCA1, which may resemble CMT in appearance. The gene for FA is located on chromosome 9 at q21 (76). Pes cavus and talipes equina varus by themselves do not indicate CMT because they are also a feature of anti-

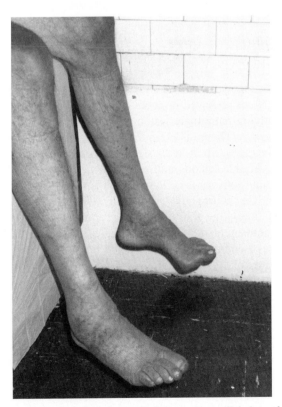

FIG. 1. Pes cavus foot deformity is seen in medial view of the left foot in a patient with CMT type 1A.

MAG, diabetic, amyloid neuropathy, myotonic muscular dystrophy, Welander's disease, scapuloperoneal syndrome, Duchenne muscular dystrophy, spastic paraplegia, and the nonneurologic disorder, idiopathic familial talipes equina varus (2,77). About one third of family propositi show additional features of CMT sufficient to warrant additional clinical subgroups (6). Patients with neuronal or CMT2C can have a hoarse voice due to vocal cord paresis (78). Others have proximal weakness of an SMA type with depressed or absent tendon reflexes and pes cavus. A recently examined patient with CMT2C in addition had bulbar palsy.

Patients with CMT are more sensitive to neurotoxic drugs and chemicals and can develop worsening of sensory function and walking ability. The CMT Association has published a list of these proscribed substances (79). Pregnancy and parturition can precipitate clinical worsening (2,80). Some affected patients may, for example, require a cane, crutches, or even a wheelchair postpartum due to interim worsening.

Primary complaints in the arms are infrequent (6,7), but atrophy and weakness of intrinsic hand muscles are an invariable finding on examination even when they are not apparent to the patient. Pain, paresthesia, numbness, dysesthesia, and burning sensations appear in late stages (3). Glove-and-stocking or distal vibratory loss occurs in most patients. In HNPP, the sensory loss is asymmetric, corresponding to individually affected nerves. Patients with CMT3 can have prominent sensory involvement leading to foot ulcers and osteomyelitis at sites of deformity. The fingers in such patients may be whittled away in a Motvan hand appearance or demonstrate the hypertrophic changes of the "main succulent." Proprioceptive defects also occur in FA (75) and in others with hereditary sensory and autonomic neuropathies (HSAN) (81), sometimes accompanied by autonomic vascular alterations. Myotonic Dystrophy may mimic the appearance of CMT in the legs (82).

Parents, siblings, and children should be included in the clinical evaluation of an index case. Hypertrophic supraclavicular, posterior and greater auricular, ulnar, superficial radial, and peroneal sensory nerves are frequently palpable or visible in CMT1 and -3 (30,31,83); the latter has a tapir face appearance (2,31). Scoliosis is sometimes found in CMT but more often in FA. Patients with CNS involvement can have normal or brisk reflexes and elicitable Babinski signs (2,82,84). Ocular involvement with optic atrophy and retinitis pigmentosa can occur in CMT (85) but is more common in FA (75,85), Refsum's disease, and abetalipoproteinemia (46). The association of optic atrophy and retinitis pigmentosa should lead to consideration of an underlying mitochondrial disorder (39). Cerebellar and extrapyramidal involvement should lead to consideration of SCA (56), Joseph's disease (60), and adrenomyeloneuropathy (44). Childhood axonal involvement should lead to careful consideration of CMT2C with vocal cord paralysis (78) but can also occur in Fabry's disease (51,87), giant axonal neuropathy (52,53), CMT3 (30,31,86,88), Krabbe disease's (50), and Cockayne's syndrome (54,55). One third of patients have an essential or familial tremor (89). Roussy and Levy (90) believed that the syndrome of CMT associated with tremor was a distinct entity, but most now consider it a variant of CMT1 (91,92). The differentiation of CMT1 from CMT2 is usually not clinically possible. In general, CMT1 has palpable hypertrophic nerves (2,84,93), and CMT2 has a later onset of disease typically in the second decade and is clinically less severe (17). Newborns with CMT3 may be hypotonic at birth and demonstrate severe generalized weakness, sensory loss, and hypertrophic nerves. A Tunisian autosomal recessive variant of CMT4 is even more severe (86) because of rapid advancement of muscular weakness in childhood, and severe gait disability often culminates in the need for a wheelchair (94). In addition, in CMT4 there is pes cavus, scoliosis, and slowing of NCV in the range found in CMT1 and CMT3.

In the fully developed state, HNPP is indistinguishable from CMT1 (95) and shares a common locus on chromosome 17 (96). Onset is usually in the second or third decade with episodes of multiple or recurrent mononeuropathies at sites prone to compression. Recovery from an episode may be complete, but subsequent ones have significant residua and coalescence of lesions leading to the appearance of generalized demyelinating neuropathy in the legs. The most common involved nerves are the ulnar at the elbow, peroneal at the fibular head, radial at the humeral spiral groove, median at the wrist, and involvement of the brachial and lumbar plexuses. Swollen demyelinated areas or tomaculi are composed of redundant myelin loops and reduplicated internodal myelin segments. The intermittent nature of HNPP can lead to an erroneous diagnosis of CIDP or conduction block neuropathy (23,24). Brachial plexus involvement in HNPP differs from neuralgic amyotrophy, brachial neuritis, and true familial brachial plexus neuropathy, respectively, by the absence of pain and dysmorphic features (97–99).

LABORATORY STUDIES

Electrodiagnostic studies are important in all patients with CMT (2,3,34,100,101) because it distinguishes the demyelinating and axonal forms and effectively screens index cases and minimally affected family members or those with forme fruste such as pes cavus deformity (2–4). The electrophysiologic features of CMT and other genetic neuropathies include uniform slowing of NCV along segments, proximal and distal (102); absence of motor conduction block or significant temporal dispersion (22,102); and with the exception of HNPP that resembles anti-MAG paraproteinemic neuropathy, pro-

portionate prolongation of distal latencies for the degree of slowing of NCV (35,36). CMAP and SNAP amplitudes correlate with the severity of clinical involvement, especially with slow progression over many years. Special stimulation and recording techniques using high voltage, near-nerve percutaneous electrodes, proximal stimulation, and various late responses such as the H reflex and F response are helpful to show the essential characteristics of CMT, especially the uniformity of slowing.

Nerve biopsy indicates the degree of neuropathy and reveals morphologically specific alterations, including demyelination, remyelination, and onion bulb formation (6,93). The latter are visible by light and electron microscopy as concentrically laminated Schwann cell processes in cotyledon layers (8,103). They are seen in CMT1, CMT3, and CMT4 and occasionally in CIDP (22), hypothyroid neuropathy (6,82), sensory neuropathy and multiple endocrine neoplasia (104), and in HNPP with tomaculi (95,105).

Serum for very-long-chain fatty acids, in addition, are useful in the diagnosis of adrenomyeloneuropathy and adrenoleukodystrophy. A blood smear can be inspected for acanthocytes in the evaluation of abetalipoproteinemia (46,106); ocular and CNS involvement may be estimated by the responses obtained in electroretinography and in somatosensory evoked potentials (46). Serum lysosomal enzymes can be used to exclude hexosaminidase A deficiency and the diagnosis of GM2 gangliosidosis (107,108), especially among cases of CMT resembling SMA.

HEREDITARY SENSORY AND AUTONOMIC NEUROPATHY

The clinical features and inheritance patterns of the HSAN are reviewed in detail elsewhere (6,7,81,88). The underlying pathologic lesion and gene products are still unknown. There is frequent association with CNS involvement, often with deformed and atrophic lower legs. Trophic lesions and ulcers of the feet result from profound sensory loss. Patients with HSAN1 are characterized by neurogenic arthropathy with recurring fractures, mutilating foot ulcers, onset in the second decade, and autosomal dominant inheritance. Affected patients typically complain of severe distal burning, aching, lancinating, and stabbing leg pains (109). Three types are congenital or recessive, including HSAN2 or Morvan syndrome with congenital insensitivity to pain (110), HSAN3 or Riley-Day syndrome with familial dysautonomia (109), HSAN4 with anhydrosis (111), and other solitary cases with insensitivity to pain. One was classified as HSAN5 because of type C fiber abnormality defined histologically by a nerve biopsy. Other cases similar to type 2 have had retinitis pigmentosa and sensory difficulty related to oral food handling (112). There is an X-linked form associated with hereditary ataxia. There are also cases defined by problems in DNA repair (113). The electrophysiologic diagnosis of HSAN has been facilitated by the four generations of computer-assisted sensory examination because it enables careful evaluation of automated sensory and autonomic parameters (114).

APPLICATION OF MOLECULAR GENETICS

Each year a new CMT-related chromosome deletion is discovered or redefined, and every month a new gene deletion or DNA protein mutation is reported. In 1991, Vance et al. (115) identified the gene locus of the most common form of hypertrophic demyelinating CMT along the short arm of chromosome 17 at p11.2 and designated 1A. Later studies showed a tandem duplication of 1.5 million base pairs or 6 cM in distance and subject to crossovers during meiosis (26,116,117). Changes in the proximal and distal breaking points during meiosis were related to misaligned chromosomes (118). A relation of the number of duplications to the severity of disease presentation was later apparent (24,26,119). An extra copy of the gene, termed trisomic overexpression, was related to increased severity of CMT1A (27), and the discovery of the gene for PMP22 in an area of duplication was later shown (120,121). In the mutant Trembler-J mouse, the gene for PMP22 had mutations causing a leucine-to-proline substitution at various positions along the first transmembrane protein domain of the gene (122,123). An identical mutation was associated with a neuropathy resembling CMT1A. The mouse was also an excellent model for hypomyelinating neuropathy (124,125). Whereas genetic duplication caused CMT1A and PMP overexpression, HNPP was due to deletions, and point mutations in the transmembrane protein domain of the PMP22 protein causes HNPP (69,126,127). The gene encoding P0 associated with CMT1B, CMT3, and congenital hypomyelinating syndrome was discovered on the long arm of chromosome 1 adjacent to the Duffy blood group locus (128–132). Like PMP22, it is subject to changes by mutation and point deletions in its extracellular domain. One unusual family with tomaculous neuropathy also mapped to this area (133). CMT1C is phenotypically similar to CMT1A and B, but the associated gene or chromosomal defect has not been identified.

CMT2A and 2B have phenotypes similar to 1A and B and respectively map to the short arm of chromosome 1 at p36 (134) and to the long arm of chromosome 3 at q1-22 (135). Clinically they differ in the presence of hyporeflexia and not areflexia, less severe weakness and tremor, nonpalpable nerves, and axonopathic pathologic changes in the nerve biopsy. Positional cloning has elucidated candidate genes (136). CMT2C has not shown chromosomal linkage; however, a fourth subtype, CMT2D, probably resides on chromosome 7 (137).

CMT3, once believed by Dejerine and Sottas as a distinct entity, is now considered a mixture of several different genetic demyelinating neuropathies (31). CMT3A has point mutations in the *PMP22* gene (132), but duplications also lead to gene dosage effects and more severely affected phenotypes (17). For example, one set of parents each with three copies of chromosome 17p11.2-12 led to a total of four copies of the *PMP22* gene in an affected child (26). Clinical and genetic heterogeneity can even be found in a given encoded family, as for example in the occurrence of several sporadic dominant and recessive forms of CMT3 and others later deemed to be related to genetic mosaicism. CMT3B is related to a deletion in P0 or MPZ, a 28-kDa glycoprotein comprising about one half of the myelin protein (138,139). Some deletions in this area have severe phenotypes, such as those that encode the congenital hypomyelination syndrome (140). Patients with CMT3C cannot be ascribed to either the PMP22 or P0 locus.

CMTX is sex linked and either recessive or dominantly inherited. The dominant form is the most common and linked to the X chromosome at q13 (141–144). This gene is responsible for the connexin gap junction protein that transports ions and small molecules through laminar myelin to the innermost layers and is located at the nodes of Ranvier and at the Schmidt Lanterman clefts; over 32 different deletions have been reported. In some dominant families with only female transmission the women have a milder involvement than the men. Patients with families of both CMT1 and -2 lineage should be screened for CMTX mutations and CMT P0 and PMP22 deletions because they have a more severe phenotype than CMT1A (28). There are four projected transmembrane positions similar to PMP22 in the connexin 32 molecule. However, all reported disease-producing mutations suggest that involvement of all regions of the protein are important in function. Mutations in both the coding and noncoding regions of the gene have also been described (145,146) Patients with families of CMT1 phenotype who prove negative for the CMT1a duplication should then be tested for CMTX, the next most common demyelinating type.

Clinical Genetic Cutting Edge

Further investigations (14) have yielded a region known as the CMT1A-REP, or repeat, a sequence of 24,000 nucleotides of ancestral primate origin (148) that has important implications for the mapping of breakpoints in HNPP (147). It is a transposon-associated recombination hot spot along which crossover points tend to be clustered in a rather narrow 700 base pair region. In essence, it allows the chromosome to mispair during meiosis (147). Another ancestral gene appears to be important in the cytochrome *c* oxidase system of mitochondrial metabolism (149). It is possible that pairing of the defective *COX* gene with a point mutation on another chromosome could explain the occurrence of both Mendelian and non-Mendelian mechanisms of inheritance in some cases of HNPP. The gene for CMTX recessive is not known; however, two suggested loci, one at Xp26 and the other at Xq22, encode CMT-like syndromes with slowing of NCV, spastic paraparesis, and mental retardation (150). An X-linked recessive axonal form encoded at Xq24-26 as well combines deafness and mental retardation (151). A recent study reported CNS dysfunction ascertained by trimodal evoked responses in similarly affected CMT cases (152).

Relapsing neuropathy was not confirmed in abnormalities of HLA testing, and is classified in the CIDP group of disorders. Some of these cases together with chronic CIDP patients referred for molecular genetics may eventually be ascertained as HNPP; forecast in the final paper of the late Anita Harding (153): Similar patients with typical CMT1 (demyelinating type) with higher than normal cerebrospinal fluid protein and evidence of inflammation on biopsy, respond to immune modulation and suppressive therapy in the same way as CIDP (154). Some of these patients with a satisfactory response reach their baseline level of neuropathy on immune modulation treatments (22,23), and are now being tested for HNPP. CMT syndromes may be associated with multiple endocrine neoplastic disorders, with inherent connective tissue defects as noticed in Marfau syndrome and with a number of disorders with defective DNA repair that have specific metabolic defects (1). Examples of the last are neuropathy in ataxia telangiectasia and xeroderma pigmentosa as well as Chediak-Higashi disease, an extremely rare and autosomal recessive early childhood disorder with mental retardation (155,156). Neuropathy can also occur in chorea-acanthocytosis of adult onset (157).

Kremer described genetic susceptibility to the production of neuropathy with toxins such as thalidamide, izoniazide, and pyridoxine by mechanisms which are poorly understood (158).

TREATMENT

Genetically engineered therapies are still the domain of experimental models; accordingly, the mainstay of management is a multidisciplinary care program. Dietary therapy, for example, is indicated in patients with Refsum's disease due to the overabundance of phytanic acid. Barbiturates should be avoided in acute intermittent porphyria because they can precipitate an attack. The neurotoxicity of isoniazid is preventable with pyridoxine. Vitamin E therapy can prevent or reverse visual and peripheral nerve involvement in abetalipoproteinemia (46,159). Immunosuppression is potentially important in the occasional patients with demonstrable inflammation on a nerve biopsy specimen (22,23,154). Known neurotoxins should be avoided in all patients with CMT (160).

Most neuromuscular clinics and local chapters of the Muscular Dystrophy Association and Charcot-Marie-Tooth Association have access to multidisciplinary care comprised by a pediatric or adult neurologist, geneticist, social worker, physiatrist, podiatrist, orthopedist, physi-

cal and occupational therapists, psychotherapists or psychiatrists, and other necessary consultants. The clinical aspects of rehabilitation are important because it requires proper timing of podiatric and orthopedic measures, orthotics, and assistive devices. With the exception of foot deformities that impede walking and cannot be overcome with passive manipulation, a useful approach is to defer surgeries of the joints and tendon problems of childhood until later in adolescence. Reactive psychological problems should be discussed with an appropriately trained therapist. Because a patient with CMT may deteriorate during pregnancy, it is useful for the obstetrician to keep close touch with the treating neurologist. One potentially promising therapy is the use of neurotrophic factors that may improve myelination and axonal flow in damaged nerves; however, they are still only available in selected controlled therapeutic trials (160).

ACKNOWLEDGMENTS

I am grateful to Professor Edward H. Lambert for stimulating my interest in this subject and for emphasizing the value of careful and comparative electrophysiologic studies in defining the peripheral neuropathies. Modern pioneers in the description and classification of the CMT group of disorders include, from the clinical and pathophysiological standpoint, the following: Drs. Peter Dyck, P.K. Thomas, George Serratrice, James McLeod, Robert Ouvrier, Walter Bradley, Fritz Buchthal, Fritz Behse, Austin Sumner, Gareth Parry, and Carlos Garcia. Without the seminal work in molecular genetics of Garth Nicholson, Jeffrey Vance, Roger Lebo, Thomas Bird, James Lupski, Kenneth Fischbeck, and Philip Chance, the great advances of the past 15 years would not have been possible. A new generation of molecular geneticists and experimental pathologists are restimulating these advances into the 21st century in the great tradition of the application of molecular genetics to neurologic diseases as set by the late Anita Harding.

REFERENCES

1. Harding AE, Thomas PK. Genetically determined neuropathy. In: Asbury AK, Gilliatt RW, eds. *Peripheral nerve disorders*. London: Butterworth, 1984:205–242.
2. Lovelace RE. Hereditary induced peripheral neuropathies. *Clin Podiatr Med Surg* 1993;7:37–50.
3. Lovelace RE. Hereditary peripheral neuropathies: nosology, pathophysiology, genetics and therapy. *Lower Extrem* 1994;1:145–158.
4. Dyck PJ. History, heterogeneity, classification and treatment of inherited neuropathy. In: Lovelace RE, Shapiro HK, eds. *Charcot-Marie-Tooth disorders: pathophysiology, molecular genetics and therapy*. New York: Wiley-Liss, 1989:1–15.
5. Lovelace RE, Shapiro HK. *Charcot-Marie-Tooth disorders: pathophysiology, molecular genetics and therapy*. New York: Wiley-Liss, 1989.
6. Brust JCM, Lovelace RE, Devi S. Clinical and electrodiagnostic features of Charcot-Marie-Tooth syndrome. *Acta Neurol Scand* 1978; 58[Suppl]:1–142.
7. Dyck PJ. Inherited neuronal degeneration and atrophy affecting peripheral motor, sensory and autonomic neurons. In: Dyck PJ, Thomas PK, Lambert EH, Bunge R, eds. *Peripheral neuropathy*. Philadelphia: W.B. Saunders, 1984:1600–1655.

8. Dyck PJ. Neuronal atrophy and degeneration predominantly affecting peripheral and sensory neurons. In: Dyck PJ, Thomas PK, Griffin JW, Low PA, Podulso JF, eds. *Peripheral neuropathy*, 3rd ed. Philadelphia: W.B. Saunders, 1993:1065–1095.

9. Serratrice G, Roux H, eds. *Peroneal atrophies and related disorders*. New York: Masson, 1979.

10. Lovelace RE. Charcot-Marie-Tooth PLUS and heterogeneity: clinical and electrophysiological studies. In: Lovelace RE, Shapiro HK, eds. *Charcot-Marie-Tooth disorders: pathophysiology*, molecular genetics and therapy. New York: Wiley Liss, 1989:49–58.

11. Lovelace RE. Charcot-Marie-Tooth disorders: an example of clinical and genetic heterogeneity. *Neurol Neurochir Pol* 1995;T20(XLV)[Suppl 1]:35–39.

12. Lovelace RE, Rowland LP. Hereditary neuropathies. In: Rowland LP, ed. *Merritt's textbook of neurology*, 9th ed. Baltimore: Williams & Wilkins, 1995:651–657.

13. Chance PF, Pleasure D. Charcot-Marie-Tooth syndrome. *Arch Neurol* 1993;50:1180–1184.

14. Murakami T, Garcia CA, Reiter L, Lupski JR. Charcot-Marie-Tooth disease and related inherited neuropathies. *Rev Mol Med* 1996;75:1–18.

15. Harding AE, Thomas PK. Inherited neuropathies: the interface between molecular genetics and pathology. *Brain Pathol* 1993;3:129–133.

16. Harding AE, Thomas PK. The clinical features of hereditary motor and sensory neuropathy types I and II. *Brain* 1980;103:259–280.

17. Mendell JR. Charcot-Marie-Tooth neuropathies and related disorders. *Semin Neurol* 1998;18:41–47.

18. Marsden CD. Inherited neuronal atrophy and degeneration predominantly of lower motor neurons. In: Dyck PJ, Thomas PK, Lambert EH, eds. *Peripheral neuropathy*. Philadelphia: W.B. Saunders, 1975: 771–790.

19. Harding AE, Thomas PK. Distal spinal muscular atrophy: a report on 34 cases and a review of the literature. *J Neurol Sci* 1980;45:337–348.

20. Shaffer LG, Kennedy GM, Spikes AS, Lupski JR. Diagnosis of CMT 1A duplications and HNPP deletions by interphase FISH: implications for testing in the cytogenetics laboratory. *Am J Med Genet* 1997; 69:325–331.

21. Tyson J, Makcolm S, Thomas PK, Harding AE. Deletions of chromosome 17 p11.2 in multifocal neuropathies. *Ann Neurol* 1996;39: 180–186.

22. Small GA, Lovelace RE. Chronic inflammatory demyelinating polyneuropathy. *Semin Neurol* 1993;13:305–312.

23. Lovelace RE. Chronic inflammatory demyelinating polyneuropathy. *Pediatr Sicily* 1991;46:577–587.

24. LeForestier N, LeGuern E, Coullin P, et al. Recurrent polyneuropathy with 17p 11.2 deletion. *Muscle Nerve* 1997;20:1184–1186.

25. Lebo RV, Martelli L, Su Y, et al. Prenatal diagnosis of Charcot-Marie-Tooth disease type 1 A by multicolor in situ hybridization. *Am J Med Genet* 1993;47:441–450.

26. Lupski JR, Montes de Oca-Luna R, Slaugenhaupt S, et al. DNA duplication associated with Charcot-Marie-Tooth disease type 1A. *Cell* 1991;66:219–232.

27. Chance PF, Bird TD, Matsunami N, Lensch MW, Brothnan AR, Feldman GM. Trisomy 17p associated with Charcot-Marie-Tooth neuropathy type 1A phenotype: evidence for gene dosage as a mechanism in CMT 1A. *Neurology* 1992;42:2295–2299.

28. Lupski JR. DNA diagnostics for Charcot-Marie-Tooth disease and related neuropathies [editorial]. *Clin Chem* 1996;42:995–998.

29. Garcia CA. The clinical features of Charcot-Marie-Tooth disorders. In: Parry GJ, ed. *Charcot-Marie-Tooth disorder: a handbook for primary care physicians*. Upland, PA: Charcot-Marie-Tooth Association, 1995:1–30

30. Ouvrier RA, McLeod JG, Conchin TE. The hypertrophic form of hereditary motor and sensory neuropathy. *Brain* 1987;110:121–148.

31. Ouvrier RA, McLeod JG. Hereditary motor and sensory neuropathy: type III. In: Lovelace RE, Shapiro HK, eds. *Charcot-Marie-Tooth disorders: pathophysiology, molecular genetics and therapy*. New York: Wiley-Liss, 1989:27–48.

32. Dyck PJ, Lambert EH, Sanders K, O'Brien PC. Severe hypomyelination and marked abnormality of conduction in Dejerine-Sottas hypertrophic neuropathy: myelin thickness and compound action potential of sural nerve in vitro. *Mayo Clin Proc* 1971;46:432–436.

33. Harati Y, Butler IJ. Congenital hypomyelinating neuropathy. *J Neurol Neurosurg Psychiatry* 1985;48:1264–1270.

34. Lovelace RE, Myers SJ. Nerve conduction and neuromuscular transmission. In: Downey JA, Myers SJ, Gonzalez EG, Lieberman JS, eds.

The physiological basis of rehabilitation medicine, 2nd ed. Stoneham, MA: Butterworth-Heinemann, 1994:215–242.

35. Trojaborg W, Hays AP, Van den Berg L, Latov N. Motor conduction parameters in neuropathies associated with anti-MAG antibodies and other types of demyelinating and axonal neuropathies. *Muscle Nerve* 1995;18:730–735.

36. Amato AA, Gronesth GS, Collarane KS, et al. Tomaculous neuropathy: a clinical and electrophysiological study in patients with and without 1.5-Mb deletion in chromosome 17p 11.2. *Muscle Nerve* 1996;19:16–22.

37. Sparkes RS, Sasaki H, Mohandes T, et al. Assignment of the prealbumin (PALB) gene (familial amyloidotic polyneuropathy) to human chromosome region 18q11.2 to q12.1. *Hum Genet* 1987;75: 151–154.

38. Gux F, DeRooij F, deBoor E, et al. Two novel mutations of the porphobilinogen deaminase gene in acute intermittent porphyria. *Hum Mol Genet* 1993;2:1735–1736.

39. Schroder JM. Neuropathy associated with mitochondrial disorders. *Brain Pathol* 1993;3:177–190.

40. DiMauro S, Moraes CT. Mitochondrial encephalopathies. *Arch Neurol* 1993;11:1197–1208.

41. Fullerton PM. Peripheral nerve conduction in metachromatic leucodystrophy (sulfatide lipidosis). *J Neurol Neurosurg Psychiatry* 1964; 27:100–105.

42. Baumann N, Masson M, Carreau V, et al. Adult forms of metachromatic leucodystrophy: clinical and biochemical approach. *Dev Neurosci* 1991;13:211–215.

43. Moser HW, Moser AB, Powers JM. The prenatal diagnosis of adrenoleucodystrophy demonstration of increased hexosanic acid levels in cultured aminocytes and fetal adrenal gland. *Pediatr Res* 1982; 26:172–175.

44. Schaumburg HH, Powers JM, Raine CS, et al. Adrenomyeloneuropathy: a probable variant of adrenoleukodystrophy. II. General pathology, neuropathology, and biochemical aspects. *Neurology* 1977;27: 1114–1119.

45. Gene locations. *Neuromusc Disord* 1993;3:83–87.

46. Brin MF, Pedley TA, Lovelace RE, et al. Electrophysiologic features of abetalipoproteinemia. Functional consequences of vitamin E deficiency. *Neurology* 1986;36:669–673.

47. Bornohofen JH, Sun CN, Araoz CH. Segmental peripheral nerve demyelination in classical Pelizaeus-Merzbacher disease type 1: an ultrastructural study. *Neurology* 1976;26:3884.

48. Lovelace RE, Johnson WT, Martin J. Peripheral nerve involvement and carrier detection in Pelizaeus-Merzbacher disease. *Nat Genet* 1994; *Proc AAEM* 1976:(Abstr.48).

49. Ellis D, Malcolm S. Proteolipid protein gene dosage in Pelizaeus-Merzbacher disease. *Nat Genet* 1994;6:333–334.

50. Dunn HG, Lake BD, Dolmen CL, et al. The neuropathy of Krabbe's infantile cerebral sclerosis (globoid cell dystrophy). *Brain* 1969;92: 329–344.

51. Sheth KJ, Swick HM. Peripheral nerve conduction in Fabry's disease. *Ann Neurol* 1980;71:319–323.

52. Asbury AK, Gale MK, Cox SC, et al. Giant axonal neuropathy. A unique case with segmental neurofilamentous masses. *Acta Neuropathol Scand* 1972;20:237–247.

53. Carpenter S, Karpati G, Auburn F, et al. Giant axonal neuropathy. A clinical and morphological distinct neurological disease. *Arch Neurol* 1974;31:312–316.

54. Moosa A, Dubowitz V. Peripheral neuropathy in Cockayne's syndrome. *Arch Dis Child* 1970;45:674–677.

55. Grunnet ML, Zimmerman AW, Lewis RA. Ultrastructure and electrodiagnosis of peripheral neuropathy in Cockayne's syndrome. *Neurology* 1983;33:1606–1609.

56. Roohi F, List T, Lovelace RE. Slow motor conduction in myotonic dystrophy. *Electromyogr Clin Neurophysiol* 1981;21:91–106.

57. Klesant TR, Otten AD, Bird TD, Tapscott SJ. Trinucleotide expansion of the myotonic dystrophy locus feducos espression of DMAHP. *Nat Gen* 1997;16:402–406.

58. Zoghili H, Jodice C, Sendkuiji L, et al. The gene for autosomal dominant spinocerebellar ataxia (SC1) maps telomeric to the HLA complex and is closely linked to D6S89 locus in three large kindreds. *Am J Hum Genet* 1991;49:23–30.

59. Gispert S, Twells R, Orozeo G, et al. Chromosome assignment of the second (Cuban) locus for autosomal dominant cerebellar ataxia (SCA2) to human chromosome 12q.23-24. *Nat Genet* 1992;4:257–259.

60. Nakano KK, Dawson DM, Sperce A. Machado disease: a hereditary ataxia in Portuguese immigrants to Massachusetts. *Neurology* 1972; 22:49–55.

61. Takiyama Y, Nishizawa M, Tonaka H, et al. The gene from Machado-Joseph disease maps to chromosome 14q. *Nat Genet* 1993;4:300–304.

62. Andrade C. A peculiar form of peripheral neuropathy: familial atypical generalized amyloidosis with special involvement of the peripheral nerves. *Brain* 1952;75:408–427.

63. Reilly MM, King RHM. Familial amyloid polyneuropathy. *Brain Pathol* 1993;3:165–176.

64. Rukavina JG, Block WD, Jackson CE, et al. Primary systemic amyloidosis: a review and experimental genetic and clinical study of cases with particular emphasis on the familial form. *Medicine* 1956;35:229–234.

65. Araki S, Mita S, Ide M, et al. Molecular genetics of familial amyloidotic polyneuropathy type 1. In: Lovelace RE, Shapiro HK, eds. *Charcot-Marie-Tooth disorders: pathophysiology, molecular genetics, and therapy.* New York: Wiley-Liss, 1989:263–268.

66. Nicholas W, Gregg R, Breuer J, et al. Characterization of the gene for familial amyloidotic polyneuropathy (FAP III/Iowa) and genotyping by allele-specific PCR. *Am J Hum Genet* 1989;45:A210.

67. Maury C, Alli K, Baumann M. Finnish hereditary amyloidosis: amino-acid sequence homology between the amyloid fibril protein and human plasma gelsolin. *FEBS Lett* 1990;280:85–87.

68. Araki S, Mawatari S, Ohta M, et al. Polyneuritic amyloidosis in a Japanese family. *Arch Neurol* 1968;18:593–602.

69. Chance PF, Abbas N, Lensch MW, et al. Two autosomal dominant neuropathies result from reciprocal DNA duplication/deletion of a region on chromosome 17. *Hum Mol Genet* 1994;3:223–228.

70. Charcot J-M, Marie P. Sur une forme particuliere d'atrophie musculaire progressive souvent familiale debutant par les pieds et les jambes et atteignant plus tards les maines. *Rev Med* 1886;6:97–138.

71. Tooth H. *The peroneal type of progressive muscular atrophy* [thesis]. London: Lewis HK Publishers, 1886.

72. Lovelace RE, Brust JCM, Devi S. The clinical and electrodiagnostic features of typical Charcot-Marie-Tooth disease. In: Serratrice G, Roux H, eds. *Peroneal atrophies and related disorders.* Paris: Masson, 1979:23–28.

73. Gabreels-Festen A, Gabreels F. Hereditary demyelinating motor and sensory neuropathy. *Brain Pathol* 1993;3:135–146.

74. Hahn AF. Hereditary motor and sensory neuropathy. HMSN II (neuronal type) and X-linked HMSN. *Brain Pathol* 1993;3:147–155.

75. Harding AE. Friedrich's ataxia: a clinical and genetic study of 90 families with an analysis of early diagnosis criteria and intrafamilial clustering of clinical features. *Brain* 1981;104:589–620.

76. Chamberlain S, Shaw J, Rowland A, et al. Mapping of mutation causing Friedrich's ataxia to human chromosome 9. *Nature* 1988;334:248–250.

77. Rebbeck TR, Ditz FR, Murray JC. A single gene explanation for the probability of having idiopathic talipes equina varus. *Am J Hum Genet* 1993;53:1051–1063.

78. Dyck PJ, Litchy WJ, Minnerath S, et al. Hereditary motor and sensory neuropathy with diaphragm and vocal cord paralysis. *Ann Neurol* 1994;35:608–615.

79. Parry GJ, ed. *Charcot-Marie-Tooth disorders: a handbook for primary care physicians.* Upland, PA: Charcot-Marie-Tooth Association, 1994.

80. Rudnik-Schoeneborn S, Rohrig D, Nicholson G, et al. Pregnancy and delivery in Charcot-Marie-Tooth disease type 1. *Neurology* 1993;43: 2011–2016.

81. Thomas PK. Hereditary sensory neuropathies. *Brain Pathol* 1993;3: 157–163.

82. Brust JCM, Lovelace RE, Devi S. Clinical and electrophysiologic features of Charcot-Marie-Tooth disease plus additional neurological features. In: Serratrice G, Roux H, eds. *Peroneal atrophies and related disorders.* New York: Masson, 1979:39–47.

83. Dejerine J, Sottas J. Sur le nevrite: interstitielle hypertrophique et progressive de l enfance. *CR Soc Biol* 1893;45:63–96.

84. Brust JCM, Lovelace RE, Devi S. Clinical and electrodiagnostic features of the Charcot-Marie-Tooth syndrome. *Acta Neurol Scand* 1978; 58[Suppl 68]:1–142.

85. Wapner F, Lovelace RE, Odell JG, et al. Charcot-Marie-Tooth disorder with optic atrophy. More genetic heterogeneity. *Ann Neurol* 1991; 30:264(abst).

86. Ouvrier RA, McLeod JG, Morgan GJ, et al. Hereditary motor and sensory neuropathy of neuronal type with onset in early childhood. *J Neurol Sci* 1981;51:181–197.

87. Desnick RJ, Sweeley CC. Fabry's disease (alpha-galactosidase A defi-

ciency). In: Stanbury JB, Wyngaarden JB, Fredrickson DS, Goldstein GL, Brown MS, eds. *The metabolic basis of inherited disease,* 5th ed. New York: McGraw-Hill, 1983:857–880.

88. Dyck PJ. Inherited neuronal degeneration and atrophy affecting peripheral motor, sensory, and autonomic neurons. In: Dyck PJ, Thomas PK, Lambert EH, eds. *Peripheral neuropathy.* Philadelphia: W.B. Saunders, 1975:825–867.

89. Yudell A, Dyck PJ, Lambert EH. A kinship with the Roussey-Levy syndrome. *Arch Neurol* 1965;13:432–440.

90. Roussy G, Levy G. Sept cas d une maladie familiale particuliere: troubles de la marche, pieds bots et areflexie tendineuse generalisee avec accessoirement, legere maladresse des mains. *Rev Neurol* 1926;1: 427–450.

91. LaPresle J. Contribution a l etude de la dystasie areflexique hereditaire. Etat actuel de quarte des sept cas princeps de Roussy et Mlle Levy, trente annees apres la premier publication de ces auteurs. *Sem Hop Paris* 1956;32:2473–2482.

92. Lupski JR, Garcia CA, Parry GJ, Patel PI. Charcot-Marie-Tooth polyneuropathy syndrome: clinical, electrophysiological, and genetic aspects. *Curr Neurol* 1991:1–25.

93. Dyck PJ, Lambert EH. Lower motor and primary sensory neuron diseases with peroneal muscular atrophy. 1. Neurologic, genetic, and electrophysiologic findings in hereditary polyneuropathies. *Arch Neurol* 1968;18:603–618.

94. Ben Othmane K, Hentati F, Lennon F, Ben Hmaida M. Linkage of a locus (CMT 4A) for autosomal recessive Charcot-Marie-Tooth disease to chromosome 8q21. *Hum Mol Genet* 1993;10:1625–1628.

95. Behse F, Buchthal F, Carlsen F, et al. Hereditary neuropathy with liability to pressure palsies. Electrophysiologic and histopathologic aspects. *Brain* 1972;95:777–797.

96. Vance JM, Nicholsen GA, Yamaoka LH, Stajich J, Steward CS, Spear MC. Linkage of Charcot-Marie-Tooth neuropathy type 1A to chromosome 17. *Exp Neurol* 1989;104:186–189.

97. Tsairis P, Dyck PJ, Mulder DW. Natural history of brachial plexus neuropathy. Report on 99 patients. *Arch Neurol* 1972;27:109–117.

98. Bosch EP, Chiu HC, Martin MA. Brachial plexus involvement in familial pressure sensitive neuropathy: electrophysiologic and morphological findings. *Ann Neurol* 1980;8:620–624.

99. Wiederholt WC. Hereditary brachial neuropathy. Report of two families. *Arch Neurol* 1974;30:252–254.

100. Myers SJ, Lovelace RE. The motor unit and muscle action potentials. In: Downey JA, Myers SJ, Gonzalez EG, Lieberman JS, eds. *The physiological basis of rehabilitation medicine,* 2nd ed. Massachusetts: Butterworth, 1994:243–282.

101. Lange DJ, Trojaborg W. Electromyography and nerve conduction studies. In: Rowland LP, ed. *Merritt's textbook of neurology,* 9th ed. Baltimore: Williams & Wilkins, 1995:77–82.

102. Lewis RA, Sumner AJ. The electrodiagnostic distinctions between chronic familial and acquired demyelinative neuropathies. *Neurology* 1982;32:592–596.

103. Ohnishi A, Murai Y, Ikeda M, Fujita T, Furuya H, Kuroiwa Y. Autosomal recessive motor and sensory neuropathy with excessive myelin-outfolding in sural nerve: subtype of HMSN type III. In: Lovelace RE, Shapiro HK, eds. *Charcot-Marie-Tooth disorders: pathophysiology, molecular genetics, and therapy.* New York: Wiley-Liss, 1989:217–224.

104. Dyck PJ, Low PH, Stevens JC. Burning feet as the only manifestation of dominantly inherited sensory neuropathy. *Mayo Clin Proc* 1983;58: 426–429.

105. Madrid R, Bradley WG. The pathology of neuropathies with focal thickening of the myelin sheath (tomaculous neuropathy). Studies on the formation of the abnormal myelin sheath. *J Neurol Sci* 1975;25:415–448.

106. Pollock M, Nukada H, Frith RW, et al. Peripheral neuropathy in Tangier disease. *Brain* 1983;106:911–928.

107. Johnson WG. The clinical spectrum of hexosaminidase deficiency disease. *Neurology* 1981;31:1453–1456.

108. Willner JP, Grabowski GA, Gordon RE, et al. Chronic GM2 gangliosidosis masquerading as a typical Friedrich's ataxia. Clinical, morphological and biochemical study of 9 cases. *Neurology* 1981;31:787–798.

109. Dyck PJ, Stevens JC, O'Brien PC, et al. Neurogenic arthropathy in recurring fractures with subclinical inherited neuropathy. *Neurology* 1983;33:357–367.

110. Nukada H, Pollock H, Haas LF. The clinical spectrum and morphology of type II hereditary sensory neuropathy. *Brain* 1982;105:647–665.

111. Swanson AG. Congenital insensitivity to pain with anhidrosis. *Arch Neurol* 1963;8:299–304.

112. Dyck PJ, Mellinger JF, Reagan TJ, et al. No indifference to pain but varieties of hereditary sensory and autonomic neuropathy. *Brain* 1983; 106:373–390.

113. Lockman JA, Kennedy WR, White JR. The Chediak-Higashi syndrome. Electrophysiology and electron microscopic observations on the peripheral neuropathy. *J Pediatr* 1967;70:942–951.

114. Dyck PJ, Zimmerman IR, O'Brien PC, et al. Introduction of automated systems to evaluate touch pressure, vibration, and thermal cutaneous sensation in man. *Ann Neurol* 1978;4:502–510.

115. Vance JM, Barker D, Yamaoka LH, et al. Localization of Charcot-Marie-Tooth disease type 1A (CMT1A) to chromosome 17p11.2. *Genomics* 1991;9:623–628.

116. Raeymaekers P, Timmerman V, et al. Duplication in chromosome 17p11.2 in Charcot-Marie-Tooth neuropathy type 1A (CMT1A). *Neuromusc Disord* 1991;1:93–97.

117. Rayemaekers P, Timmerman V, Nelis E, et al. Estimation of the size of the chromosome 17p11.2 duplication in Charcot-Marie-Tooth neuropathy type 1A (CMT1A). *J Med Genet* 1992;29:5–11.

118. Pentao L, Wise CA, Chinault AC, Patel DI, Lupski JR. Charcot-Marie-Tooth type 1A duplication appears to arise from recombination at repeat sequences flanking the 1.5Mb monomer unit. *Nat Genet* 1992; 2:292–300.

119. Lupski JR, Wise CA, Kuwane A, et al. Gene dosage is a mechanism for Charcot-Marie-Tooth disease type 1A. *Nat Genet* 1992;1:29–33.

120. Roa BB, Garcia CA, Pentao L, et al. Evidence for recessive PMP22 point mutation in Charcot-Marie-Tooth disease 1A. *Nat Genet* 1993; 5:189–196.

121. Roa BB, Garcia CA, Suter U, et al. Charcot-Marie-Tooth disease type 1A. Association with point mutation in the PMP22 gene. *N Engl J Med* 1993;329:96–101.

122. Suter U, Moskow JJ, Welcher AA, et al. A leucine-to-proline mutation in the putative first transmembrane domain of the 22-Kda peripheral myelin protein in the Trembler-J mouse. *Proc Nat Acad Sci USA* 1992; 89:4382–4386.

123. Suter U, Welcher AA, Ozcelik T, et al. Trember mouse carrier a point mutation in a myelin gene. *Nature* 1992;356:241–244.

124. Aguayo JA, Attiwell M, Trecarten J, Perkins S, Bray GM. Abnormal myelination in transplanted Trember mouse Schwann cells. *Nature* 1977;265:73–75.

125. Valentijn LJ, Bass F, Volterman RA, et al. Identical point mutations of PMP-22 in Trembler-J mouse and Charcot-Marie-Tooth disease type 1A. *Nat Genet* 1992;2:288–291.

126. Chance PF, Albersen MJ, Leppig KA, et al. DNA deletion associated with hereditary neuropathy with liability to pressure palsies. *Cell* 1993;72:143–151.

127. Lorenzetti D, Pareyson D, Sghirlanzoni A, et al. A 1.5 Mb in 17p11.2-p12 is frequently observed in Italian families with hereditary neuropathy with liability to pressure palsies. *Am J Hum Genet* 1995;56:91–98.

128. Lebo RV, Chance PF, Dyck PJ, et al. Chromosome 1 Charcot-Marie-Tooth disease (CMT1B) locus on the Fc receptor gene region. *Hum Genet* 1991;88:1–12.

129. Bird TD, Ott J, Giblett ER. Evidence for linkage of Charcot-Marie-Tooth neuropathy to the Duffy locus on chromosome 1. *Am J Hum Genet* 1982;34:388–394.

130. Lemke G, Lamar E, Patterson J. Isolation and analysis of the gene encoding peripheral myelin protein zero. *Neuron* 1988;1:73–78.

131. Hayasaka K, Himoro M, Sato W, et al. Charcot-Marie-Tooth neuropathy type 1B is associated with mutations of the Po gene. *Nat Genet* 1993;5:31–34.

132. Hayasaka K, Himoro M, Sawaishi Y, et al. De novo mutation of the myelin Po gene in Dejerine-Sottas disease (hereditary motor and sensory neuropathy type III). *Nat Genet* 1993;5:266–268.

133. Thomas FP, Lebo RV, Rosoklija G, et al. Tomaculous neuropathy in chromosome 1 Charcot-Marie-Tooth syndrome. *Acta Neuropathol Scand* 1994;87:91–97.

134. Ben Othmane K, Middleton LT, Loprest LJ, et al. Localization of a gene (CMT2A) for autosomal dominant Charcot-Marie-Tooth disease type 2 to chromosome 1p and evidence of genetic heterogeneity. *Genomics* 1993;17:370–375.

135. Kwon JM, Elliot JL, Yee W, et al. Assignment of a second Charcot-Marie-Tooth type II locus to chromosome 3q. *Am J Hum Genet* 1995; 57:853–858.

136. Timmerman V, DeJonghe P, Spoelders P, et al. Linkage and mutation analysis of Charcot Marie Tooth neuropathy type 2 families with chromosomes 1p35–p36 and Xq13. *Neurol* 1996;46:1311–1318.

137. Ionasescu V, Searby C, Sheffield VC, Rokina T, Nashimura D, Ionasescu R. 7p (CMT2D). *Hum Mol Genet* 1996;9:1373–1375.

138. Roa BB, Dyck PJ, Marks HG, Chance PF, Lupski JR. Dejerine-Sottas syndrome associated with point mutation in the PMP-22 gene. *Nat Genet* 1993;5:269–273.

139. Roa BB, Werner LE, Garcia CA, et al. Myelin protein zero (MPZ) gene mutations in a non-duplication type 1 Charcot-Marie-Tooth disease. *Hum Mutat* 1996;7:36–45.

140. Warner LE, Hilz MJ, Appel SH, et al. Clinical phenotype of different MPZ (Po) mutations may include Charcot-Marie-Tooth type 1B, Dejerine-Sottas and congenital hypomyelination. *Neuron* 1996;17:1–20.

141. Beckett J, Holden NE, Simpson BN, White BN, MacLeod PM. Localization of X-linked dominant Charcot-Marie-Tooth disease to Xq13.1. *J Neurogenet* 1986;3:225–231.

142. Ionasescu V, Burns TL, Serby CL, Ionasescu R. X-linked dominant Charcot-Marie-Tooth neuropathy with 15 cases in a family: genetic linkage study. *Muscle Nerve* 1988;11:1154–1156.

143. Bergoffem J, Scherer SS, Wang S, et al. Connexin mutation in X-linked Charcot-Marie-Tooth disease. *Science* 1993;262:2039–2042.

144. Ionasescu V, Searby CL, Ionasescu R. Point mutation of the connexin 32 (GJB1) gene in X-linked dominant Charcot-Marie-Tooth neuropathy. *Hum Mol Genet* 1994;3:355–358.

145. Ionasescu V, Ionasescu R, Searby C. Correlation between connexin 32 gene mutation and clinical phenotypes in X-linked dominant Charcot-Marie-Tooth neuropathy. *Am J Med Genet* 1996;63:486–491.

146. Ionasescu V, Searby C, Ionasescu R, Neuhaus IM, Werner R. Mutation of the non-coding region of the connexin 32 gene in X-linked dominant Charcot-Marie-Tooth neuropathy. *Neurology* 1996;47: 541–544.

147. Kiyosawa H, Lensch MV, Chance PF. Analysis of the CMT1A-REP repeat: mapping crossover breakpoints in CMT1A and HNPP. *Hum Mol Genet* 1995;4:2327–2334.

148. Kiyosawa H, Chance P. Primate origin of the CMT1A-REP repeat and analysis of a putative transposom-associated hotspot. *Hum Mol Genet* 1996;5:745–753.

149. Reiter LT, Murakami T, Koeuth T, Gibbs RA, Lupski JR. The human COX10 gene is disrupted during homologous recombination between the 24 kb proximal and distal CMT1A-REPs. *Hum Mol Genet* 1997; 6:1595–1603.

150. Ionasescu V, TrofatterJ, Haines JL, Summers AM, Ionasescu R, Searby C. Heterogeneity in X-linked recessive Charcot-Marie-Tooth neuropathy. *Am J Hum Genet* 1991;1:1075–1083.

151. Priest JM, Fischbeck KH, Nouri N, Keats BKB. A locus for axonal motor sensory neuropathy with deafness and mental retardation maps to Xq24-q26. *Genomics* 1995;29:409–412.

152. Ionasescu V. Charcot-Marie-Tooth neuropathies. From clinical description to molecular genetics. *Muscle Nerve* 19;18:267–275.

153. Harding AE. From the syndrome of Charcot-Marie and Tooth to disorders of peripheral myelin proteins. *Brain* 1995;118:809–818.

154. Dyck PJ, Swanson CJ, Low PA, Bartelson JD, Lambert EH. Prednisone responsive hereditary motor and sensory neuropathy. *Mayo Clin Proc* 1982;52:239–246.

155. Misra VP, King RH, Harding AE, Muddle JR, Thomas PK. Peripheral neuropathy in the Chediak-Higashi syndrome. *Acta Neuropathol (Berl)* 1991;81:354–358.

156. Pezeshkpour G, Kurent JS, Krarup C, et al. Peripheral neuropathy in the Chediak-Highashi syndrome. *J Neuropathol Exp Neurol* 1986;45: 353–359.

157. Ohnishi A, Sato Y, Nagara H, et al. Neurogenic muscular atrophy and low density of large myelinated fibers of sural nerve of chorea acanthocytosis. *J Neurol Neurosurg Psychiatry* 1981;44:645–648.

158. Kremer M. Clinical aspects of toxic neuropathy. In: Cummings JA, Kremer M, eds. *Biochemical aspects of neurological disorders*. Oxford: Blackwell, 1965:85–100.

159. Verhegen WIN, Gabreels-Festen AWM, Van Wensen PJM, et al. Hereditary neuropathy with liability to pressure palsy: a clinical electroneurophysiological and morphological study. *J Neurol Sci* 1993; 116:176–184.

160. Ben Hamida M, Belal S, Sirugo G. Friedrich's ataxia phenotype not linked to chromosome 9, and associated with selective autosomal recessive vitamin E deficiency in two inbred Tunisian families. *Neurology* 1993;43:2179–2183.

161. Williams LL, O'Dougherty MM, Wright FS, Bibulski RJ, Horrocks LA. Dietary essential fatty acids, vitamin E and Charcot-Marie-Tooth disease. *Neurology* 1986;36:1200–1205.

Motor Disorders,
edited by David S. Younger.
Lippincott Williams & Wilkins, Philadelphia © 1999.

CHAPTER 17

Acute and Chronic Inflammatory Demyelinating Polyneuropathy

Richard J. Barohn and David S. Saperstein

Immune-mediated acute and chronic inflammatory demyelinating polyneuropathies (AIDP, CIDP) represent an important group of neuropathic disorders. AIDP is characterized by rapidly evolving weakness, sensory loss, and areflexia (1–3) over days or several weeks. CIDP is not as common as AIDP and evolves over months (4,5). Most clinical neurologists will be involved in the management of these patients, and there are now a variety of reasonable therapies available for acquired demyelinating neuropathies. In this chapter, the clinical presentations, laboratory studies, diagnostic criteria, treatment, and prognosis for both disorders are reviewed.

ACUTE INFLAMMATORY DEMYELINATING POLYNEUROPATHY OR GUILLAIN-BARRÉ SYNDROME

Historical

The clinical features of a 43-year-old man with ascending paralysis and sensory loss that worsened over days and resulted in death from respiratory failure was first described by Landry in 1859 (6). The author stated that he had observed four similar cases and that spontaneous resolution occurred. Nineteen years later, Guillain et al. (7) reported two similar cases and described the characteristic cerebrospinal fluid (CSF) abnormalities. They demonstrated the loss of tendon reflexes both on the neurologic examination and with an electrophysiologic myogram and speculated the disorder was a "radiculoneuropathic syndrome." Although sometimes referred to as the Landry-

Guillain-Barré-Strohl syndrome, AIDP is most commonly called the Guillain-Barré-Strohl syndrome or, more often, the Guillain-Barré syndrome (GBS).

Immunopathology

In GBS, there is inflammation and demyelination with a predilection for roots and proximal nerve segments. Autopsy studies and nerve biopsies demonstrate lymphocyte and macrophage infiltration of nerves with segmental demyelination (8). Much of the evidence that GBS is immunologically mediated is derived from comparisons with the animal model experimental allergic neuritis (EAN) (9,10). Animals immunized with peripheral nerve tissue develop ataxia and paralysis approximately 2 weeks after injection. As in GBS, pathologically there is a marked cellular infiltration of the peripheral nerves by lymphocytes and macrophages with segmental demyelination; CSF shows an albuminocytologic dissociation. EAN can also be induced by a basic protein of peripheral nerve myelin, P2 protein (11). Most evidence indicates that EAN is a cell-mediated disease, because it can be passively transferred to naive rats by lymphocytes from sensitized animals. The role of circulating antibodies in EAN is not as clear, although some investigators have passively transferred the disease from serum (12). One group has been able to demonstrate complement-fixing antibodies to peripheral nerve myelin in the serum of GBS patients (13). The titer of peripheral nerve myelin antibodies reportedly declined with clinical improvement and correlated with the appearance of terminal complement complexes in the serum, CSF, and nerve (14).

Epidemiology and Antecedent Events

The incidence of GBS is 1 to 2 per 100,000 people (2,15), making it the most common cause of acute generalized weakness. The mean age at the onset of GBS is 40

R. J. Barohn: Department of Neurology, University of Texas Southwestern Medical Center at Dallas, Dallas, Texas 75235-8897.

D. S. Saperstein: Neuromuscular Disease Service, Department of Neurology, Wilford Hall Medical Center, San Antonio, Texas 78236.

years, but it can occur at any age. Known viral precipitants are Epstein-Barr virus (mononucleosis or hepatitis), cytomegalovirus, and human immunodeficiency virus (HIV) (Table 1). In HIV, GBS occurs at the time of seroconversion or early in the disease (16). However, specific viral etiologies are usually not identified. Bacterial infections rarely associated with a GBS-like illness include *Mycoplasma pneumoniae* and Lyme disease.

Campylobacter jejuni enteritis precedes GBS in approximately 25 to 38% of patients (17–19) and may be the most common antecedent infection. GBS in these cases develops about 9 days after the initial gastroenteritis, when stool cultures for *C. jejuni* are often negative. However, serologic antibody evidence of recent infection is present at this time. The prevalence of *C. jejuni* among healthy individuals in the United States is low, probably less than 1% (20). Approximately two million *Campylobacter* infections occur each year in the United States, although most of these patients do not develop GBS. Among Japanese patients, Yuki et al. (21) found that two rare serotypes of *C. jejuni* (PEN 19 and LIO 7) were isolated greater than 10 times more frequently from GBS patients compared with sporadic *C. jejuni* enteritis patients. This infection with a particular serotype may be an explanation for why so few patients who are infected with *C. jejuni* go on to develop GBS.

Other antecedent events associated with GBS include immunizations (22), surgery (23), epidural anesthesia (24), and concurrent illnesses such as Hodgkin's disease (25,26).

Clinical Features

Initial symptoms are usually numbness and tingling of the extremities. Aching or severe neuritic pain in the extremities and back is common, occurring in at least half of patients at some point in the disease (1,2). After the initial sensory symptoms, weakness involving proximal and distal muscles ensues over days. Usually the lower extremity muscles are affected first—the so-called

TABLE 1. *Guillain Barré syndrome: antecedent events*

Viral infections
  Unspecified
  Epstein-Barr virus—mononucleosis
  HIV—infection
  Others; measles, mumps, varicella-zoster
Bacterial infections
  Campylobacter jejuni
  Lyme disease
  Mycoplasma pneumoniae
Other events
  Immunizations
  Surgery
  Epidural anesthesia
  Hodgkin's disease

ascending pattern. However, descending presentations, with onset in the face or arms, also occurs. In the Boston series, 56% of patients had the onset of weakness in the legs, 12% in the arms, and 32% simultaneously in the arms and legs (1,2). Facial weakness involving orbicularis oculi and lower facial muscles is usually present. A small number of patients (approximately 5%) with otherwise typical GBS develop ophthalmoplegia and/or ptosis. GBS is a pure motor disorder in about a third of cases, and they are more likely to be associated with *C. jejuni*. Patients become hypo- or areflexic within the first several days, although in exceptional cases normal reflexes are retained through the first week of the illness.

Over 50% of patients reach their nadir by 2 weeks, 80% by 3 weeks, and 90% by 4 weeks (1,27,28). It is extremely unusual for symptoms to continue to worsen after 1 month. The tempo of progression is variable, and patients can become flaccid and ventilator dependent in a few days. Respiratory failure occurs in 30% of patients. Autonomic dysfunction has been estimated to occur in two thirds of patients (1). Manifestations of autonomic dysfunction include hyper- and hypotension, cardiac arrhythmias, neurogenic pulmonary edema, and bladder and gastrointestinal dysfunction.

Asbury and Cornblath (29) proposed diagnostic criteria for GBS, summarized in Table 2.

Guillain-Barré Syndrome Variants

In addition to the classic presentation of GBS, clinical variants have been described (Table 3). The syndrome described by Fisher (30) consisting of ophthalmoplegia, ataxia, and areflexia was the first recognized GBS variant. These patients do not have weakness, but the CSF protein is elevated. Patients with otherwise typical GBS who also have ophthalmoplegia do not have the Miller Fisher syndrome. A syndrome mimicking an acute spinal cord lesion occurs with back pain, bilateral lower extremity numbness, weakness, and areflexia, sparing the arms (31). Other regional variants include pharyngeal-cervical-brachial weakness with ptosis (mimicking botulism), ptosis without ophthalmoplegia, and facial diplegia or sixth nerve palsies with paresthesias (31,32). Pure sensory and autonomic variants have also been reported (1,33).

Both pure motor and severe axonal variants have been described, and there appears to be extensive overlap between these two presentations. Thus, pure axonal patients may also be pure motor clinically and vice versa, although this is not invariable. The axonal variant patients develop rapidly progressive weakness with prolonged paralysis and respiratory failure over a few days (34). The axonal variant is more often associated with antecedent *C. jejuni* enteritis and has a poor prognosis (19). The largest number of cases of pure motor axonal GBS come from northern China, although there have been descriptions from other countries as well (35–37). This variant has been

TABLE 2. *Diagnostic criteria for Guillain-Barré syndrome*

Required	Supportive	Features casting doubt	Exclusionary
Progressive weakness of >1 limb	Progression <4 weeks Symmetric weakness	Marked asymmetry	Other causes (toxins, botulism, porphyria, diphtheria)
Areflexia or hyporeflexia	Sensory symptoms or signs	Onset with or persistence of bladder/bowel dysfunction	
	Cranial nerve involvement, especially 7	>50 lymphocytes/mm^3 in CSF	
	Autonomic dysfunction	Polys in CSF	
	CSF protein elevation CSF cell count <20/mm^3	Sensory level	
	Electrophysiologic features of demyelination		
	Recovery		

CSF, cerebrospinal fluid.
Adapted from Ref. 29.

labeled acute motor axonal neuropathy (AMAN) (38). Recently, four cases of an acute motor-sensory axonal neuropathy (AMSAN) were reported, also from China (39). These cases were also associated with *C. jejuni* infection. However, evidence of *C. jejuni* infection can occur in cases of otherwise typical demyelinating motor-sensory GBS. It appears that prior infection with *C. jejuni* initiates an immune attack against peripheral nerves, probably by "molecular mimicry," producing GBS, and that these patients are more likely to develop a pure axonal or pure motor presentation with a poor prognosis.

Laboratory Features

CSF is remarkable for elevated protein with minimal, if any, lymphocytic pleocytosis, the so-called albuminocytologic disassociation. This is usually seen after the first week. In the Boston series (1,2), 34% of patients

TABLE 3. *Guillain-Barré syndrome variants*

Miller-Fisher syndrome
    Ophthalmoplegia, ataxia, areflexia
Areflexic parapareses with back pain (resembles cord lesion)
Pharyngeal–cervical–brachial weakness (resembles botulism)
Ptosis without ophthalmoplegia
Facial diplegia with paresthesias
Sixth nerve palsies with paresthesias
Pure axonal
    Rapidly progressive weakness
    Prolonged paralysis and respiratory failure
    Associated with *Campylobacter jejuni*
    Often pure motor (AMAN) but not always (AMSAN)
Pure motor
Pure sensory
Pure autonomic

AMAN, acute motor axonal neuropathy; AMSAN, acute motor-sensory axonal neuropathy.

had normal CSF protein in the first week, whereas only 18% had normal CSF after 2 weeks. In the proposed laboratory criteria, less than 10 lymphocytes/mm^3 are most supportive of the diagnosis and more than 50 cells/mm^3 should cast doubt on the diagnosis (29). If a there are more than 50 cells/mm^3, one should consider an underlying HIV infection in addition to GBS (16). An HIV antibody assay should be obtained in these cases and also in any GBS patients with risk factors for HIV infection.

The electrophysiologic hallmarks of demyelination are a prolonged distal latency, slowed conduction velocity, temporal dispersion, partial or complete conduction block, and prolonged F-wave latency (40–42). In the first week of GBS, nerve conduction studies may show only minimal changes. The earliest abnormal features include a low amplitude or prolonged latency of the compound muscle action potential (CMAP) and prolonged or absent F waves, indicating a disorder of terminal nerve fibers or the roots. Later, slowing of the conduction velocity, conduction block, and temporal dispersion can be demonstrated. The maximal degree of abnormalities in motor conduction studies occurs between the third and eighth week, and demyelinating criteria can be met in 87% of patients during the first 5 weeks (40). The changes in sensory conduction studies lag behind the motor abnormalities. A helpful clue is the preservation of a normal sural nerve sensory study even in the setting of severe leg weakness, abnormal motor studies, or when sensory symptoms are present (40). The initial needle electromyography changes include fast firing motor units with effort or a neurogenic recruitment pattern. After 2 to 4 weeks, fibrillation potentials can develop in weak muscles, indicating some degree of secondary axonal damage, even in cases that show primarily demyelinating motor nerve conduction features. In the axonal variant, CMAP amplitudes drop precipitously in the first several days of the illness and then become unevocable. Demyelinating conduction findings do not occur, and patients develop diffuse fibrillation potentials (34).

Electrophysiologic guidelines for establishing demyelination in GBS are essentially the same as those developed for CIDP (41,43). However, these criteria are not as useful in GBS as they are in CIDP, especially early in the course of the illness, during which electrophysiologic changes are unusual. These criteria are somewhat cumbersome to use because they were primarily developed for research protocols, and therefore clinicians should not expect each GBS patient to meet the strict criteria for demyelination.

Few other diagnostic laboratory studies need to be performed in typical GBS cases. Patients with risk factors for HIV should be so tested (43). If a preceding viral infection and lymphadenopathy is present, a monospot test can be obtained, but this will not alter management. Viral antibody panels, heavy metal measurements, and porphyria studies need not be routinely checked except when there is a suspicion of a particular disorder. In addition, it is unclear how stool cultures or antibody measurements for *C. jejuni* change the therapeutic plan except when positive, and then they may be a poor prognostic marker. Antibiotic treatment for *C. jejuni* is not routinely given, even if a prior infection can be documented. GBS is presumably an immune sequelae of the bacterial infection, and the clinical manifestations of the preceding infection usually resolve by the time symptoms of GBS arise (29). Most cases of *C. jejuni* enteritis are self-limited, resolving after several days, and require no treatment (20). Antimicrobial therapy can hasten the clearance of *C. jejuni* from the stool (44), but there is no evidence to suggest that such treatment has an effect on the course of GBS after the onset of neuropathic symptoms.

Antibodies to the various gangliosides GM1, GM1b, GD1b, and others have been documented in several series of GBS patients (9,45–47). Recent studies have shown that many, but not all, of the patients so studied had evidence of *C. jejuni* infection (48,49). In the British study (49), 25% of all GBS patients had GM1 antibodies, as did 52% of the patients with GBS and *C. jejuni* infection. *C. jejuni* has GM1-like oligosaccharides that can lead to cross-reacting antibodies, explaining why an antibody directed against the bacteria may also produce a neuropathy (48).

The diagnosis of GBS rests on the clinical presentation and CSF findings and is supported by the electrodiagnostic studies. Although most patients with GBS alone do not have antibodies to gangliosides, most patients with the Miller Fisher syndrome have increased titers of serum GQ1b antibodies (50,51). High levels of GQ1b were noted in cranial nerves 3, 4, and 6. They are specific for the Miller Fisher syndrome and have not been reported in GBS. Therefore, this assay, which is now commercially available, is extremely useful in supporting the clinical diagnosis of Miller Fisher syndrome.

Gadolinium-enhanced magnetic resonance imaging of the lumbosacral region can show root enhancement in GBS and CIDP (52–55). Although there is no need to obtain this study in routine cases, it can be useful in areflexic paraparetic/back pain GBS variants to establish the site of the lesion.

There is also little role for nerve biopsy in GBS; however, it is interesting to note that the pathology of AMAN in Chinese patients differs from typical GBS. In AMAN there is axonal degeneration of ventral roots and motor nerves without inflammation (56). In addition, macrophages are present in the periaxonal spaces of large motor fibers, between the axolemma and Schwann cell, a finding not typically seen in GBS. Acute motor-sensory axonal neuropathy cases have been shown to have similar pathology but with involvement of dorsal and ventral roots (39).

Treatment

General Supportive Care

The most important treatment of GBS is supportive care. Patients need to be monitored closely for respiratory and autonomic instability. Forced vital capacity should be followed, and values below 15 to 20 mL/kg should lead to consideration of endotracheal intubation. Progressive flexor and extensor neck weakness correlates closely with respiratory compromise and can be used to monitor impending respiratory failure. Leg stockings and miniheparin injections twice daily are indicated for prevention of deep venous thrombosis and pulmonary emboli. Aggressive physical therapy can help prevent muscle contractures in severely weak patients. A means for communication should be established in patients who are on mechanical ventilation.

Plasma Exchange

Plasmapheresis directly removes circulating antibodies, immune complexes, complement, and other nonspecific inflammatory mediators. In two large series (57,58), plasma exchange (PE) was shown to be an effective treatment in GBS (Table 4) as gauged by reducing the time to walk, both unaided and aided; time on the ventilator; time in the hospital; and time to improve one grade. Even though that study did not contain a sham-treated group and the investigators were not blinded, PE is still generally considered the gold standard for the treatment of GBS.

The "dose" or amount of PE is 200 to 250 mL/kg total exchange. Thus, a 70-kg patient should undergo a total exchange of 15,000 mL. This is usually done in four to six exchanges of 2 to 4 L each over 5 to 14 days, daily or every other day. The replacement fluid should be albumin or

TABLE 4. *Guillain-Barré syndrome: North American and French plasmapheresis trials*

	PE	Control
North American (1985)[a]		
Number of patients	122	123
Time to improve 1 grade (days)	19	40
Time to walk unaided—all patients (days)	53	85
Time to walk unaided—respirator (day)	97	169
Time on ventilator (days)	9	23
% improved 1 grade at 1 month	59	39
% improved at 6 months	97	87
French (1987)[b]		
Number of patients	109	111
Time to weaning (days)	18	31
Time to walk unaided (days)	70	111
Time in hospital (days)	28	45
% patients to ventilator after entry	21	42

PE, plasmapheresis.
All differences in both columns are statistically significant.
[a]From Ref. 57.
[b]From Ref. 58.

purified protein fraction. There is no need for further PE treatments after 200 to 250 mL/kg has been exchanged, even if the patient is still quite weak and ventilator dependent, and there is no evidence that further PE beyond this amount increases the likelihood of a beneficial effect (59).

Although the PE-treated groups in the North American and French studies did better than control subjects, the time spent on a ventilator was still fairly long, even in PE-treated patients. Therefore, physicians, patients, and family members need to have realistic expectations about the extent of the effect of both PE and intravenous immunoglobulin (IVIg). Dramatic improvement within days of beginning treatment is not the rule; however, if improvement does occur, it is probably likely to have happened in that patient without treatment.

One of the limitations of plasmapheresis is the need for a large double-lumen intravenous catheter to be placed in the subclavian or femoral vein, introducing the potential risks of pneumothorax, hemorrhage, and sepsis. The complications of PE include hypotension, pulmonary embolism, anemia, low platelets, and prolongation of clotting parameters.

Intravenous Immunoglobulin

IVIg is being used increasingly for the treatment of neurologic and nonneurologic immune-mediated diseases. Its mechanism of action is unknown. The first large study to show the effectiveness of IVIg in GBS was the Dutch trial (60) comparing the efficacy of IVIg to PE in 150 patients. That study had no control group and showed that IVIg was as effective as, and possibly better than, PE. Table 5 shows the results of the Dutch IVIg study in comparison with the North American Plasmapheresis Study. A criticism of the Dutch study was that the PE group did not do any better than the control group in the North American study; a subsequent larger study further showed no difference between the outcomes with IVIg or PE (61).

The total dose of IVIg is 2 g/kg. Therefore, for a 70 kg-patient this is 140 g. The dose can be given over 5 days (0.4 g/kg/day) or 2 days (1 g/kg/day). Because most GBS patients are in the hospital for longer than 2 days, there is probably no advantage to giving it in less than 5 days for this disorder. Although the side effects are usually mild, the infusions are generally better tolerated if given over 5 days (Table 6). The side effects of IVIg include flulike symptoms, with chills, fever, myalgia, diaphoresis, hypotension, fluid overload, nausea, vomiting, rash, headache, aseptic meningitis, and neutropenia. Renal insufficiency and stroke secondary to hyperviscosity may also occur, particularly in older patients with concomitant medical problems. Patients with IgA deficiency may experience anaphylaxis when given IVIg. Although it is generally good practice to obtain quantitative IgA levels before infusing the drug, in acute GBS this is often not practical. Hepatitis C outbreaks in patients who received IVIg occurred in Europe and the United States (62,63). Manufacturers now take steps to eliminate the possibility of hepatitis virus

TABLE 5. *Guillain-Barré syndrome: Dutch IVIg vs. plasmapheresis studies compared with the North American plasmapheresis study*

	DUTCH[a]		North American[b]	
	IVIg	PE	PE	Control
Total patients	74	73	108	120
Improved 1 grade (4 weeks) (%)	53	34	59	39
Days to improve 1 grade (median)	27	41	19	40
Days to grade 2	55	69	53	85
Number of multiple complications	5	16		
Ventilator dependent by week 2 (%)	27	42		

[a]From Ref. 60.
[b]From Ref. 57.
IVIg, intravenous immunoglobulin; PE, plasmapheresis.

TABLE 6. *IVIg side effects*

Chills/fever/myalgias ("flu-like")
Diaphoreses/flushing
Hypotension
Fluid overload
Nausea/vomiting
Headache/aseptic meningitis
Renal insufficiency
Allergic reaction
   Hives
   Macular rash
   Anaphylaxis (IgA deficient pts)
Stroke (hyperviscosity)
Hepatitis C
Neutropenia

IVIg, intravenous immunoglobulin.

TABLE 7. *Guillain-Barré syndrome: plasma exchange, IVIg, or both*

	PE	IVIg	Both
Number of patients	121	130	128
Days to walk unaided	49	51	40
% Unable to walk unaided after 48 weeks	16.7	16.5	13.7
Median days to hospital discharge	63	53	51
Median days to stop artificial ventilation	29	26	18
Deaths	4.1%	4.6%	6.3%

PE, plasma exchange; IVIg, intravenous immunoglobulin. From Ref. 61.

transmission by heat pasteurization or solvent/detergent inactivation, so this is no longer a concern. There has never been a reported case of HIV infection transmitted by IVIg.

Two reports raised the issue of relapses after treatment with IVIg (64,65), causing confusion among doctors trying to make a rational treatment decision for a GBS patient (66). Relapses were also reported with PE (57,67). The French study had a relapse rate of 5.5% compared with 1% for the control group with PE. Physicians have to accept that some GBS patients may have minor relapses. Although the relapse rate may be slightly higher with either IVIg and PE compared with no treatment, the weight of all available clinical evidence indicates it is better to treat GBS patients than not to.

Should Both Plasma Exchange and Intravenous Immunoglobulin Be Used in Guillain-Barré Syndrome Patients?

A question left unaddressed until recently was whether combined treatment with PE and IVIg was superior to treatment with either agent alone. Although there does not appear to be much sense in giving a patient IVIg and then removing it with PE, the converse could potentially be true. The Plasma Exchange Sandoglobulin Guillain-Barré (PSGBS) study group conducted a multicenter trial comparing monotherapy with PE or IVIg and PE followed by IVIg. Combined treatment produced no significant difference in outcome compared with either modality alone (Table 7) (61); accordingly, PE and IVIg therapy appear to be equally effective. A similar smaller study supported this view (68). The PSGBS study found no significant difference in the incidence of side effects from PE compared with IVIg.

Both PE and IVIg have strengths and weaknesses as therapies (Table 8). In older hemodynamically unstable patients, IVIg may be a better choice, as well as in hospitals where PE is not available. Both therapies are expen-

sive; a 5-day course of each costs about $10,000 to $20,000. In some institutions, IVIg is significantly more expensive than PE because of pharmacy charges.

Corticosteroids

Corticosteroids are probably not of benefit in the treatment of GBS; in fact, in an early study, steroid-treated patients did worse than control subjects (69). Intravenous methylprednisolone was evaluated in GBS by a large randomized British study in which 124 patients received 500 mg daily for 5 days within 15 days of onset compared with an equal number of placebo-treated control subjects (70). PE was given to some patients depending on the practice of the center, and about half of the patients in addition received PE. There was no difference between the two groups in the degree of improvement at 4 weeks or in secondary outcome measures. They concluded that "a short course of high-dose methylprednisolone given early in GBS is ineffective" (70). A smaller Dutch open-label pilot study of 25 patients receiving intravenous methylprednisolone and IVIg did better than 74 patients from the earlier Dutch study who received IVIg alone (71). A similar study is underway in Europe. Although the issue of intravenous corticosteroids in early GBS requires further investigation, at the present time this is not a recommended therapy.

Treatment of GBS Variants

Although there have been no controlled series addressing treatment of the GBS variant syndromes, in general, if such patients have significant clinical impairments, they should be treated as discussed above for GBS.

Prognosis

According to Ropper and colleagues (1,2), about 15% of patients have complete recovery without residual symptoms or signs; about 5% die of secondary complications, including aspiration pneumonia, adult respiratory

TABLE 8. *Plasma exchange vs. IVIg treatment*

Pro-PE	Con-PE	Pro-IVIg	Con-IVIg
It makes sense	Central line	It works	Makes less sense
It works	Morbidity	Easy to give	Not as long a track record
Longer track record	Need sophisticated equipment and PE team	Faster to give full course	Anaphylaxis
	Expense	No sophisticated equipment	Expense
	? Rebound	Fewer side effects	? Rebound

PE, plasma exchange; IVIg, intravenous immunoglobulin.

distress syndrome, sepsis, pulmonary embolism, and dysautonomia. Major residual neurologic deficits occur in 10% of patients. Most of the remaining 70% of patients have minor residual problems, such as distal numbness or weakness, that do not interfere with activities of daily living.

The North American GBS study (72) identified four factors that indicated a poor prognosis (regardless of whether or not patients received plasmapheresis), including age older than 50 to 60 years, a rapid onset before presentation, the need for mechanical ventilation, and severely reduced CMAP amplitudes. A preceding diarrheal illness with *C. jejuni* may probably be added to this list. A single report suggests that preceding cytomegalovirus infection can delay recovery (73) (Table 9).

Although most patients with the severe axonal motor variant of GBS (AMAN) would be expected to have a more prolonged recovery, this is not always the case. Two recent articles describing the Chinese experience found that some patients with AMAN can recover rapidly (74,75). Hypothetical mechanisms accounting for this include an immune attack on the nodes of Ranvier or autoantibody-mediated blockade of axonal sodium channels (74,75). A monophasic course occurs in 95% of patients. Minor "relapses" in which patients show signs of slight deterioration during the recovery phase are uncommon. Relapses occurred in about 1% of the control groups in controlled trials (57,58). What many physicians or patients may interpret as a "relapse" is more likely a long plateau phase showing little signs of improvement on a day-to-day basis. True relapsing GBS, in which a patient recovers and then deteriorates months or years later, occurs in about 5% of cases (76).

TABLE 9. *Guillain Barré syndrome: poor prognostic factors*

1. Older age (>50–60)
2. Rapid onset before presentation (<7 days)
3. Mechanical ventilation
4. Severely reduced distal motor amplitudes (CMAPs)
5. Preceding diarrheal illness with *C. jejuni*
6. ? Preceding infection with cytomegalovirus

CMAP, compound muscle action potential.

CHRONIC INFLAMMATORY DEMYELINATING POLYNEUROPATHY

Historical

In 1958, Austin (77) described the entity of recurrent steroid-responsive polyneuropathy. Dyck et al. (4) compiled the first large series of these patients and referred to the condition as chronic inflammatory demyelinating polyneuropathy. It is important to recognize because it statistically represents a significant number of all initially undiagnosed acquired neuropathies, with estimates varying from 10 to 20% (78), and it is treatable. In our series, CIDP comprised 10% of 402 consecutive neuropathy patients referred to our neuromuscular clinic.

Immunopathology

There is less laboratory evidence for an immune-mediated pathogenesis for CIDP compared with its acute counterpart, GBS. Inflammatory cell infiltration and demyelination with remyelination is generally not seen in sural biopsies in most patients (5); however, immuno-staining for T cells in nerve biopsies has been shown to yield a much higher incidence of inflammatory cell infiltration (79,80).

Clinical Features

Patients typically present with progressive, stepwise, or relapsing weakness (4,5). Diagnostic criteria for CIDP requires progressive weakness for *2 or more months*, so distinguishing it from GBS (5,43,81). Weakness can vary in severity but is generally symmetric, involving proximal and distal limb muscles; however, facial and neck flexor weakness can occur. The extraocular muscles are rarely involved. Sensory complaints usually consist of numbness and tingling, but painful paresthesias are not uncommon. Many patients describe loss of balance. Deep tendon reflexes are usually absent or depressed. Autonomic and respiratory insufficiency occurs infrequently compared with GBS.

Preceding infections are less common in CIDP as compared with GBS. Some suggest a role for preceding respiratory (82,83) and *C. jejuni* infection (47); however, the relationship of infection to CIDP is not as well substantiated as it is for GBS.

Laboratory Features

The most important laboratory studies for support of the diagnosis of CIDP are the CSF examination, electrophysiologic studies, and nerve biopsy. Of the three, lumbar puncture is generally the most useful because 94% of patients have an elevated CSF protein (71), and like GBS, the diagnosis of CIDP is supported by CSF with typical albuminocytologic disassociation.

Nerve conduction studies in CIDP are suggestive of demyelination, with slowed conduction velocities, prolonged or absent F waves, conduction block, and temporal dispersion (Figs. 1 and 2); however, only about 70% of patients meet strict criteria for demyelinaton (5,84). The electrophysiologic criteria established by an ad hoc subcommittee of the American Academy of Neurology (AAN) are most frequently used (Table 10) (43,84); however, they are somewhat cumbersome in daily practice.

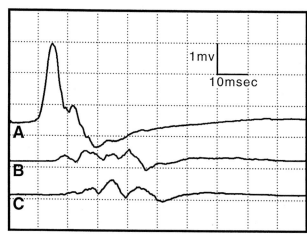

FIG. 2. Ulnar nerve conduction study from a patient with CIDP. (*A*) Stimulation at the wrist. (*B*) Stimulation below the elbow. (*C*) Stimulation above the elbow. There is prolonged distal latency (7.5 msec), slower conduction velocity in the below-elbow segment (33.3 m/sec) compared with the across-elbow segment (42.0 m/sec), and temporal dispersion. Although there is an 84% amplitude drop between the wrist and below-elbow segment, the area does not decrease and the duration increases by 79%. (From Barohn RJ, Saperstein DS. Guillain-Barré Syndrome and chronic inflammatory demyelinating polyneuropathy. *Semin Neurol* 1998;18:49–61, with permission, Thieme Publishing.)

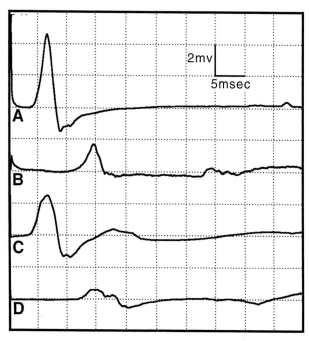

FIG. 1. Median (*A* and *B*) and ulnar (*C* and *D*) motor nerve conduction studies from a CIDP patient. Median nerve: (*A*) Stimulation at the wrist. (*B*) Stimulation at the elbow. There is a prolonged distal latency (7.8 msec), slow conduction velocity (20.0 m/sec), and conduction block (61% amplitude drop without significant temporal dispersion). Ulnar nerve: (*C*) Stimulation at the wrist. (*D*) Stimulation at the elbow. There is a prolonged distal latency (6.8 msec), slow conduction velocity (13 m/sec), and conduction block (76% amplitude drop). All values in both nerves meet demyelinating criteria. (From Barohn RJ, Saperstein DS. Guillain-Barré Syndrome and chronic inflammatory demyelinating polyneuropathy. *Semin Neurol* 1998;18:49–61, with permission, Thieme Publishing.)

TABLE 10. *Electrophysiologic guidelines for acquired demyelinating neuropathy*

Three of four are needed to meet demyelinating criteria:
1. Nerve conduction velocity
   Reduction of nerve conduction velocity in two or more motor nerves. [Reduced < 80% of the lower limit of normal (LLN) if the compound motor action potential (CMAP) amplitude exceeds 80% of LLN or reduced <70% of LLN if CMAP amplitude is <80% of LLN.]
2. Conduction block and temporal dispersion
   Partial conduction block (PCB) or temporal dispersion (TD) in one or more motor nerves. [PCB is present if there is a >20% drop in the negative peak (NP) area or peak-to-peak (PTP) amplitude between proximal and distal stimulation sites, provided there is a <15% change in NP duration. TD is present if there is a >20% drop in NP area or PTP amplitude but the change in NP duration exceeds 15%.]
3. Distal latency
   Prolonged distal latencies in two or more nerves. [Prolonged > 125% of the upper limit of normal (ULN) if CMAP amplitude exceeds 80% of LLN or prolonged >150% of ULN if CMAP amplitude is <80% of LLN.]
4. F-wave latency
   Absent or prolonged F-wave latencies in at least two nerves. [Prolonged > 125% of ULN if CMAP amplitude > 80% of LLN or prolonged > 150% of ULN if CMAP amplitude is <80% LLN.]

Adapted from Ref. 43.

Many neurologists may not readily know how slow a conduction velocity needs to be to reach 70% or 80% of the lower limit of normal or what constitutes a distal latency and F-wave prolongation of 125% and 150% above the upper limit of normal. A CMAP amplitude loss of less than or greater than 80% lower limit of normal is also critical in their use. Table 11 provides examples of the various nerve conduction study parameters that meet demyelinating criteria. We modified recommendations of the ad hoc subcommittee of the AAN criteria with respect to the definition of conduction block and temporal dispersion (85). For conduction block, we require a 50% drop in CMAP amplitude and area between proximal and distal stimulation sites with a change in CMAP duration of less than 30% compared with 20% and 15%, respectively (Table 10). Similarly, we describe abnormal temporal dispersion as an increase in CMAP duration of 30% or more with less than a 50% decrease in CMAP amplitude and area across a nerve segment. These more restrictive criteria are appropriate because a study of normal control subjects found CMAP area reductions of 25 to 30% and increases in CMAP duration of up to 30% between proximal and distal stimulation sites (86).

Sural nerve biopsy is helpful in excluding other etiologies such as amyloidosis, vasculitis, and various hereditary or toxic neuropathies. In classic CIDP, the nerve shows demyelination, remyelination, and occasionally inflammation (Fig. 3). However, of the three laboratory studies mentioned, sural nerve biopsy is probably the least useful in the diagnosis of CIDP, except if the CSF or electrophysiology are not supportive of the diagnosis in a patient who clinically resembles CIDP, in which case a sural nerve biopsy should be performed. In a series of 60 patients, 48% had evidence of demyelination or remyelination, 21% had axonopathy, 13% had mixed myelinopathy/axonopathy, and 18% were normal (5). Only 11% had histologic evidence for inflammation, although immunostaining for lymphocytes was not performed (79,80).

Few blood tests are required in patients with typical CIDP. All patients with suspected CIDP should be checked for a serum paraprotein. If a paraprotein is present, a search for lymphoma or osteosclerotic myeloma should be undertaken (87). We generally order anti-myelin-associated glycoprotein (anti-MAG) assays on patients with an IgM paraprotein, although they can rarely be seen in the absence of a serum paraprotein (88). When present, it suggests a more refractory course with therapy; however, our treatment approach is not altered. It can be argued that from a practical standpoint there is no need to obtain an anti-MAG antibody assay in CIDP patients other than to document its presence. There is also no need to obtain ganglioside antibody measurements in CIDP because, even if positive, they will not alter therapy.

Diagnostic Criteria

Barohn et al. (5) proposed inclusionary and exclusionary criteria for the diagnosis of CIDP in 1989. Cases categorized as "definite," "probable," and "possible" were based on laboratory features (Table 12) (82). Definite CIDP patients satisfy all three laboratory features: CSF, electrophysiology, and a nerve biopsy. In probable cases, two of three criteria are satisfied and one of three are met in possible CIDP (81). This classification differs slightly from that published by the ad hoc subcommittee of the AAN (43), and it is easier to use. Although the criteria are valuable for research purposes, they can also be used in routine patient management. It is important for clinicians to know that they can make a presumptive diagnosis of CIDP even if the electrophysiologic studies, nerve biopsy, or even the CSF do not have features fulfilling acquired demyelinaton. Patients with probable or possible CIDP should certainly be treated. Conversely, one should not withhold potentially beneficial therapy in a patient even if the nerve conduction studies do not fall in the demyelinating range or if the nerve biopsy instead shows noninflammatory axonopathy.

Clinical Variants

CIDP also occurs in the setting of a variety of other disorders (Table 13), which have been termed "CIDP with concurrent illness" (5,89–91), including those with clinical or laboratory evidence of central nervous system demyelination and overlap cases (92,93).

TABLE 11. *Nerve conduction study values needed to be considered "demyelinating"*

	NCV (m/sec)			DL (msec)			F waves (msec)		
	LLN	<80%[a]	<70%[b]	ULN	>125%[a]	>150%[b]	ULN	>120%[a]	>150%[b]
Median	48	38.4	33.6	4.5	5.6	6.7	31.0	37.2	46.5
Ulnar	48	38.4	33.6	3.6	4.5	5.4	32.0	38.4	48.0
Peroneal	42.0	33.6	29.4	6.6	8.2	9.9	56.0	67.2	84.0
Tibial	42.0	33.6	29.4	6.6	8.2	9.9	58.0	69.6	87.0

[a] = If Amp > 80% LLN.
[b] = If Amp < 80% LLN.
If median CMAP LLN 3.0 mV, then 80% LLN = 2.4 mV; ulnar CMAP LLN 5.0 mV, then 80% LLN = 4 mV; peroneal CMAP LLN 2.0 mV, then 80% LLN = 1.6 mV; tibial CMAP LLN 4.0 mV, then 80% LLN = 3.2 mV.
NCV, nerve conduction velocity; DL, distal latency; LLN, lower limit of normal; ULN, upper limit of normal.

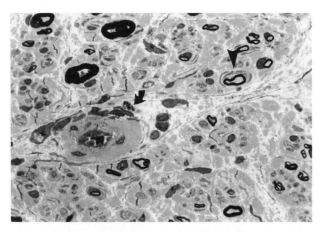

FIG. 3. Sural nerve biopsy from a patient with CIDP. A few mononuclear inflammatory cells surround the endoneurial blood vessel (curved arrow). There is a decrease in the number of large myelinated fibers. Some thinly myelinated fibers have excessive Schwann cell process proliferation ("onion bulbs") (arrowhead) (toluidine blue stain). (From Brey RL, Barohn RJ, et al. *Neurologist* 1996;2:25–52, with permission, Williams & Wilkins.)

TABLE 12. *Diagnostic criteria for CIDP*

Mandatory clinical features
    Progression of muscle weakness in proximal and distal muscles of upper and lower extremities for 2 months
    Areflexia or hyporeflexia
Major laboratory features
    Evidence of demyelination on nerve conduction studies (see Table 10)
    Cerebrospinal fluid (CSF) studies
        CSF protein > 45 mg/dL
        Cell count < 10/mm^3
    Nerve biopsy features
        Nerve biopsy with predominant features of demyelination that include segmental demyelination, remyelination, onion-bulb formation, and inflammation.
Mandatory exclusion criteria (patients must be devoid of these features)
    Clinical features of a hereditary neuropathy or history of exposure to drugs or toxins known to cause peripheral neuropathy.
    Laboratory evidence from blood, urine, or CSF examination of a potential etiology for the neuropathy other than CIDP.
    Evidence on nerve biopsy for a potential etiology for neuropathy other than CIDP.
    Electrodiagnostic features of neuromuscular transmission defect, myopathy, or anterior horn cell disease.
Diagnostic categories (must meet all mandatory exclusion criteria)
    Definite CIDP
        Mandatory clinical features
        All major laboratory features
    Probable CIDP
        Mandatory clinical features
        2 of 3 major laboratory features
    Possible CIDP
        Mandatory clinical features
        1 of 3 major laboratory features

Adapted from Refs. 5, 43, and 81.

TABLE 13. *CIDP with concurrent illness*

HIV infection
Monoclonal gammopathy
Chronic active hepatitis
Inflammatory bowel disease
Connective tissue disease
Bone marrow and organ transplants
Lymphoma
Hereditary neuropathy
Diabetes mellitus
Thyrotoxicosis
Nephrotic syndrome
CNS demyelination

CNS, central nervous system.

CIDP with a benign monoclonal gammopathy generally does not reveal an underlying lymphoma, osteosclerotic myeloma, or another malignancy to account for the paraprotein. The treatment of these patients should be similar to those without paraproteins.

Pure sensory and axonal variants of CIDP have been reported and both apparently respond to immunosuppressive therapy (33,94–96). These patients do not meet the diagnostic criteria for CIDP, and the existence of these variants is somewhat controversial.

Patients with subacute weakness of 4 to 8 weeks, so-called subacute demyelinating polyneuropathy (97), have also been reported. Treatment can be the same as that used for CIDP, although it is interesting that three of the cases reported by Hughes et al. (97) had spontaneous recoveries, suggesting a similarity to GBS.

Treatment

Randomized controlled trials confirmed the benefit of corticosteroids (98), PE (99,100), and IVIg (101) in CIDP. First line is prednisone, which was more effective than placebo in a controlled study (Table 14) (98). Therapy is initiated with 100 mg orally once daily. When improvement begins, usually within 2 to 4 weeks, it is switched to alternate days. When strength has returned to normal or improvement has plateaued, usually within 3 to

TABLE 14. *Therapeutic options in CIDP*

First line
    Prednisone
    ? IVIg
Second line
    Plasmapheresis
    IVIg
    Azathioprine
Third line:
    Cyclosporine
    Cyclophosphamide
Experimental:
    Interferon

IVIg, intravenous immunoglobulin.

6 months, the prednisone dose can be slowly tapered by 5 mg every 2 to 3 weeks. Some patients can be tapered off completely, but relapses often occur. It is important for both the patient and physician to realize that CIDP is a chronic disorder and may require one or more years of immunosuppressive therapy.

PE was more effective than "sham" pheresis for CIDP in two important studies (99,100). PE is typically used if patients are severely weak or if they relapse on prednisone. Five to 10 treatments are usually performed over 1 to 4 weeks at the initiation of therapy. Unlike the situation in GBS, however, there is no benchmark goal of how much total fluid to remove. We generally do not routinely repeat PE at fixed intervals but instead use repeat courses of five or six PE treatments as needed if the patient deteriorates again. When we initiate PE in a patient who has worsened while on prednisone, we usually increase the steroid dose or add a second oral immunosuppressive agent; otherwise, the patient may relapse when the effect of PE has worn off, usually in 4 to 8 weeks.

IVIg was recently introduced for the treatment of CIDP. Although early studies showed variable results (102–104), two important recent studies convincingly showed that IVIg had an important role in the treatment of CIDP. Dyck et al. (105) compared PE with IVIg in 20 patients with CIDP and found that both therapies were equally effective. In the report by Hahn et al. (101), 30 patients received IVIg at doses of 2 g/kg over 5 days or an intravenous placebo in a randomized, double-blind, crossover study. Nineteen of 30 patients improved on IVIg, including 9 chronic progressive and 10 patients with relapsing CIDP, whereas all worsened on placebo alone. Similar improvement was seen both on neurologic disability scale scores and nerve conduction studies. Eight of nine patients with chronic progressive CIDP improved to normal function and maintained this level with the single 5-day course of IVIg; five were maintained on small doses of oral prednisone.

The patients studied by Dyck et al. (105) and Hahn et al. (101) were generally not new in onset, and many had already been tried on prednisone therapy. A randomized placebo-controlled study of IVIg in CIDP patients who never received prior immunosuppressive therapy was just completed in North America, and the data are currently being analyzed. This study was designed to determine if IVIg should be a first-line therapy in CIDP. It is currently difficult to convince third-party payers to cover IVIg in CIDP. Hopefully, this will be less of a problem as further evidence accumulates regarding the effectiveness of IVIg therapy in CIDP. After 6 months of IVIg therapy, we generally try to stop the IVIg or extend the treatments by 1 to 2 months. The optimal duration of treatment with IVIg in this disorder is not known. Some chronic progressive patients in the study by Hahn et al. (101) required only the induction therapy; however, most were also on prednisone (101).

In the single controlled study of azathioprine in CIDP, the drug was no more effective than placebo (106). However, it is still occasionally used as a second-line therapy in patients who relapse on prednisone therapy, especially if IVIg cannot be used. Cyclosporine (107,108) and, less often, cyclophosphamide are third-line oral therapies that can be tried. Several small reports described benefit of interferon-α (109,110) or interferon-β (111). A recent open-label study of interferon-α treatment in 16 patients followed for 6 weeks found improvement in 56% (112). Although encouraging, further studies involving placebo control, larger patient members, and larger follow-up are needed.

Prognosis

In our retrospective series, greater than 90% of patients with CIDP initially improved with immunosuppressive treatment; however, the relapse rate was high, approaching 50% (5). Only 30% of patients in this series achieved a complete remission off medication (5). Two patients (3.3%) died. It appears the longer patients are followed, the more likely they will relapse (5). In the series of Dyck et al. (4), 64% of patients were improved or in remission and able to return to work, 8% were ambulatory but unable to work, 11% were bedridden or wheelchair bound, and 11% died of the disease. Gorson et al. (113) found that, overall, 66% of their patients responded to prednisone, PE, or IVIg. These three retrospective series found no factors predictive of a poor response. Two recent prospective studies may provide more reliable numbers regarding how often patients respond to treatment. In the controlled trial of IVIg in CIDP patients performed by Hahn et al. (101), 63% (19/32) responded favorably. Patients with an acute relapse or with a disease duration of 1 year or less were more likely to respond. In a separate study by this group (100), 80% (12/15) of patients who received PE also responded.

Most patients with monoclonal proteins and CIDP have the same response to therapy as CIDP patients without paraproteins. Patients with IgM paraproteins, particularly those that are anti-MAG, may be more resistant to therapy (114–117). However, much of this data is based on studies of patients with monoclonal protein-associated polyneuropathies, not patients meeting the diagnostic criteria for CIDP. A retrospective review comparing CIDP patients with a paraprotein with those without found no difference between patients with IgM, IgG, or IgA gammopathies (118,119). Some authors advocate treating neuropathy patients with IgM paraproteins with chemotherapeutic agents such as chlorambucil or cyclophosphamide (120–122). IVIg appeared beneficial in two small open studies of neuropathy patients with IgM gammopathy (123,124), whereas a small controlled trial (117) found a much more modest response. A recent controlled study comparing IVIg and interferon-α treatment in IgM gammopathy patients found little benefit from IVIg, whereas there was improvement in 80% of the interferon-treated group (125). There have been no prospective studies addressing treatment of CIDP with a monoclonal gammopathy of uncertain significance (MGUS); we currently treat them no differently from other CIDP patients.

REFERENCES

1. Ropper AH, Wijdicks EFM, Truax BT. *Guillain-Barré syndrome.* Philadelphia: F.A. Davis, 1991.
2. Ropper AH. The Guillain-Barré syndrome. *N Engl J Med* 1992;326: 1130–1136.
3. Parry GJ. *Guillain-Barré syndrome.* New York: Thieme Medical Publishers, Inc., 1993.
4. Dyck PJ, Lais AC, Ohta M, Bastron JA, Okazaki H, Groover RV. Chronic inflammatory demyelinating polyradiculoneuropathy. *Mayo Clin Proc* 1975;50:621–637.
5. Barohn RJ, Kissel JT, Warmolts JR, Mendell JR. Chronic inflammatory demyelinating polyradiculoneuropathy: clinical characteristics, course, and recommendations for diagnostic criteria. *Arch Neurol* 1989;46: 878–884.
6. Landry O. Note sur la paralysie ascendante aigue. *Gaz Hebd Med Paris* 1859;6:472–474.
7. Guillain G, Barré JA, Strohl A. Sur un syndrome de radiculonévrite avec hyperalbuminose du liquide céphalo-rachidien sans réaction cellulaire. Remarques sur les caractéres cliniques et graphiques de réflexes tendineux. *Bull Soc Med Hop Paris* 1916;40:1462–1470.
8. Asbury AK, Arnason BG, Adams RD. The inflammatory lesion in idiopathic polyneuritis. Its role in pathogenesis. *Medicine* 1969;48:173–215.
9. Hartung HP, Pollard JD, Harvey GK, Toyka KV. Immunopathogenesis and treatment of the Guillain-Barré syndrome. Part 1 and Part 2. *Muscle Nerve* 1995;18:137–164.
10. Waksman BH, Adams RD. Allergic neuritis: experimental disease rabbits induced by the injection of peripheral nervous tissue and adjuvants. *J Exp Med* 1955;102:213–236.
11. Kadlubowski M, Hucher RAC. Identification of the neuritogen for experimental allergic neuritis. *Nature* 1979;277:140–141.
12. Hahn AF, Gilbert JJ, Feasby RE. Passive transfer of demyelination by experimental allergic neuritis serum. *Acta Neuropathol (Berl)* 1980; 49:169–176.
13. Koski CL, Gratz E, Sutherland J, Mayer RF. Clinical correlation with anti-peripheral-nerve myelin antibodies in Guillain-Barré syndrome. *Ann Neurol* 1986;19:575–577.
14. Koski CL. Characterization of complement-fixing antibodies to peripheral nerve myelin in Guillain-Barré syndrome. *Ann Neurol* 1990;27[Suppl]:S44–S47.
15. Alter M. The epidemiology of Guillain-Barré syndrome. *Ann Neurol* 1990;27[Suppl]:S7–12.
16. Cornblath DR, McArthur JC, Kennedy PG, Witte AS, Griffin JW. Inflammatory demyelinating peripheral neuropathies associated with human T-cell lymphotrophic virus type III infection. *Ann Neurol* 1987; 21:32–40.
17. Rees JH, Soudain SE, Gregson NA, Hughes RA. *Campylobacter jejuni* infection and Guillain-Barré syndrome. *N Engl J Med* 1995; 333:1415–1417.
18. Bolton CF. The changing concepts of Guillain-Barré syndrome. *N Engl J Med* 1995;333:1415–1417.
19. Griffin JW, Ho TW. The Guillain-Barré syndrome at 75: the *Campylobacter* connection. *Ann Neurol* 1993;34:125–127.
20. Blaser MJ. *Campylobacter* species. In: Mandell GL, Douglas RG, Bennett JE, eds. *Principles and practice of infectious diseases,* 4th ed. New York: Churchill Livingstone, 1995:1649–1658.
21. Yuki N, Takahashi M, Tagawa Y, et al. Association of *Campylobacter jejuni* serotype with antiganglioside antibody in Guillain-Barré syndrome and Fisher's syndrome. *Ann Neurol* 1997;42:28–33.
22. Schonberger LB, Hurwitz ES, Katona P, et al. Guillain-Barré syndrome: its epidemiology and associations with influenza vaccination. *Ann Neurol* 1981;9[Suppl]:31.
23. Arnason BG, Asbury AK. Idiopathic polyneuritis after surgery. *Arch Neurol* 1968;18:500–507.
24. Steiner I, Argov Z, Cahan C, et al. Guillain-Barré syndrome after epidural anesthesia: direct nerve root damage may trigger disease. *Neurology* 1985;35:1473–1475.
25. Cameron DG, Howell DA, Hutchinson JL. Acute peripheral neuropathy in Hodgkin's disease. Report of a fatal case with histologic features of allergic neuritis. *Neurology* 1958;8:575.
26. Lisak RP, Mitchell M, Zweiman B, et al. Guillain-Barré syndrome and Hodgkin's disease: three cases with immunological studies. *Ann Neurol* 1977;1:72–78.
27. Loffel NB, Rossi LN, Mumenthaler M. Lutschg J, Ludin HP. The Landry-Guillain-Barré syndrome. Complications, prognosis, and natural history in 123 cases. *J Neurol Sci* 1977;33:71–79.
28. Gibbles E, Giebisch U. Natural course of acute and chronic monophasic inflammatory demyelinating polyneuropathies (IDP). *Acta Neurol Scand* 1991;85:282–291.
29. Asbury AK, Cornblath DR. Assessment of current diagnostic criteria for Guillain-Barré syndrome. *Ann Neurol* 1990;27[Suppl]:S21–24.
30. Fisher CM. An unusual variant of acute idiopathic polyneuritis (syndrome of ophthalmoplegia, ataxia, and areflexia). *N Engl J Med* 1956; 255:57–65.
31. Ropper AH. Unusual clinical variants and signs in Guillain-Barré syndrome. *Arch Neurol* 1986;43:1150–1152.
32. Ropper AH. Further regional variants of acute immune polyneuropathy. *Arch Neurol* 1994;51:671–675.
33. Simmons Z, Tivakaran S. Acquired demyelinating polyneuropathy presenting as a pure clinical sensory syndrome. *Muscle Nerve* 1996; 19:1174–1176.
34. Feasby TE, Gilbert JJ, Brown WF, et al. An acute axonal form of Guillain-Barré polyneuropathy. *Brain* 1986;109:1115–1126.
35. Ramos-Alvarez M, Bessudo L, Sabin A. Paralytic syndromes associated with non-inflammatory cytoplasmic or nuclear neuronopathy: acute paralytic disease in Mexican children, neuropathologically distinguishable from Landry-Guillain-Barré syndrome. *JAMA* 1969;207: 1481–1492.
36. Valencio L, Najera E, Perez Gallardo F, et al. Outbreak of paralytic illness of unknown etiology in Albacete, Spain. *Am J Epidemiol* 1971; 94:450–456.
37. Jackson CE, Barohn RJ, Mendell JR. Acute paralytic syndrome in three American men: comparison with Chinese cases. *Arch Neurol* 1993;50:732–735.
38. McKhann GM, Cornblath DR, Griffin JW, et al. Acute motor axonal neuropathy: a frequent cause of acute flaccid paralysis in China. *Ann Neurol* 1993;33:333–342.
39. Griffin JW, Li CY, Ho TW, et al. Pathology of the motor-sensory axonal Guillain-Barré syndrome. *Ann Neurol* 1996;39:17–28.
40. Albers JW, Donofrio PD, McGonable TK. Sequential electrodiagnostic abnormalities in acute inflammatory demyelinating polyradiculoneuropathy. *Muscle Nerve* 1985;8:528–539.
41. Cornblath D. Electrophysiology in Guillain-Barré syndrome. *Ann Neurol* 1990;27[Suppl]:S17–20.
42. Cornblath DR, Mellits Ed, Griffin JW, et al. Motor conduction studies in Guillain-Barré syndrome: description and prognostic value. *Ann Neurol* 1988;23:354–359.
43. Ad Hoc Subcommittee of the American Academy of Neurology AIDS Task Force. Research criteria for diagnosis of chronic inflammatory demyelinating polyneuropathy (CIDP). *Neurology* 1991;41:617–618.
44. Anders BJ, Lauer BA, Paisley JW, Reller LB. Double-blind placebo controlled trial of erythromycin for treatment of *Campylobacter* enteritis. *Lancet* 1982;1:131–134.
45. Vriesendorp FJ, Mishu B, Blaser MJ, Koski CL. Serum antibodies to GM1, GD1b, peripheral nerve myelin, and *Campylobacter jejuni* in patients with Guillain-Barré syndrome and controls: correlation and prognosis. *Ann Neurol* 1993;34:130–135.
46. Ilyas AA, Willison HG, Quarles RH, et al. Serum antibodies to gangliosides in Guillain-Barré syndrome. *Ann Neurol* 1988;23:440–447.
47. van der Meché FGA, van Doorn PA. Guillain-Barré syndrome and chronic inflammatory demyelinating polyneuropathy: immune mechanisms and update on current therapies. *Ann Neurol* 1995;37[Suppl 1]: S14–31.
48. Oomes PG, Jacobs BC, Hazenberg MP, Banffer JR, van der Meche FG. Anti-GM$_1$ IgG antibodies and *Campylobacter* bacteria in Guillain-Barré syndrome: evidence of molecular mimicry. *Ann Neurol* 1995;38:170–175.
49. Rees JH, Gregson NA, Hughes RA. Anti-ganglioside GM1 antibodies

in Guillain-Barré syndrome and their relationship to *Campylobacter jejuni* infection. *Ann Neurol* 1995;38:809–816.

50. Willison HJ, Veitch J, Paterson G, Kennedy PG. Miller Fisher syndrome is associated with serum antibodies to GQ1b ganglioside. *J Neurol Neurosurg Psychiatry* 1993;56:204–206.

51. Yuki N, Sato S, Tsuji S, Ohsawa T, Miyatake T. Frequent presence of anti-GQ1b antibody in Fisher's syndrome. *Neurology* 1993;43:414–417.

52. Morgan GW, Barohn RJ, Bazan C, King RB, Klucznik RP. Nerve root enhancement with MRI in inflammatory demyelinating polyradiculoneuropathy. *Neurology* 1993;43:618–620.

53. Perry JR, Fung A, Poon P, Bayer N. Magnetic resonance imaging of nerve root inflammation in the Guillain-Barré syndrome. *Neuroradiology* 1994;36:139–140.

54. Crino PB, Zimmerman R, Laskowitz D, Raps EC, et al. Magnetic resonance imaging of the cauda equina in Guillain-Barré syndrome. *Neurology* 1994;44:1334–1336.

55. Gorson KC, Ropper AH, Muriello A, Blair R. Prospective evaluation of MRI lumbosacral nerve root enhancement in acute Guillain-Barré syndrome. *Neurology* 1996;47:813–817.

56. Griffin JW, Li CY, Ho TW, et al. Guillain-Barré syndrome in northern China: The spectrum of neuropathologic changes in clinically defined cases. *Brain* 1995;118:577–595.

57. Guillain-Barré Syndrome Study Group. Plasmapheresis and acute Guillain-Barré syndrome. *Neurology* 1985;35:1096–1104.

58. French Cooperative Group on Plasma Exchange in Guillain-Barré Syndrome. Role of replacement fluids. *Ann Neurol* 1987;22:753–761.

59. The French Cooperative Group on Plasma Exchange in Guillain-Barré Syndrome. Appropriate number of plasma exchanges in Guillain-Barré syndrome. *Ann Neurol* 1997;41:298–306.

60. van der Meché FGA, Schmitz PIM, the Dutch Guillain-Barre Study Group. A randomized trial comparing intravenous immune globulin and plasma exchange in Guillain-Barre Syndrome. *N Engl J Med* 1992;326:1123–1129.

61. Plasma Exchange/Sandoglobulin Guillain Barré Syndrome Trial Group. Randomized trial of plasma exchange, intravenous immunoglobulin, and combined treatments in Guillain Barré syndrome. *Lancet* 1997;349:225–230.

62. Bjoro K, Froland SS, Yun Z, Samdal HH, Haaland T. Hepatitis C infection in patients with primary hypogammaglobulinemia after treatment with contaminated immune-globulin. *N Engl J Med* 1994;331:1607–1611.

63. Schiff RI. Transmission of viral infections through intravenous immune globulin [editorial]. *N Engl J Med* 1994;331:1649–1650.

64. Irani DN, Cornblath DR, Chaudhry V, Borel C, Hanley DF. Relapse in Guillain-Barré syndrome after treatment with human immune globulin. *Neurology* 1993;43:872–875.

65. Castro LHM, Ropper AH. Human immune globulin infusion in Guillain-Barré syndrome: worsening during and after treatment. *Neurology* 1993;43:1034–1036.

66. Bleck TP. IVIG for GBS: Potential problems in the alphabet soup. *Neurology* 1993;43:857–858.

67. Ropper AH, Albers JW, Addison R. Limited relapse in Guillain-Barré syndrome after plasma exchange. *Arch Neurol* 1988;45:314–315.

68. Bril V, Ilse WK, Pearce R, Dhanani A, Sutton D, Kong K. Pilot trial of immunoglobulin versus plasma exchange in patients with Guillain-Barré syndrome. *Neurology* 1996;46:100–103.

69. Hughes RAC, Newsom-Davis J, Perkin GD, Pierce JM. Controlled trial of prednisolone in acute polyneuropathy. *Lancet* 1978;2:750–753.

70. Guillain-Barré Syndrome Steroid Trial Group. Double-blind trial of intravenous methylprednisolone in Guillain-Barré syndrome. *Lancet* 1993;341:586–590.

71. The Dutch Guillain-Barré Study Group. Treatment of Guillain-Barré syndrome with high-dose immune globulins combined with methylprednisolone: a pilot study. *Ann Neurol* 1994;35:749–752.

72. McKhann GM, Griffin JW, Cornblath DR, et al. Plasmapheresis and Guillain-Barré syndrome: analysis of prognostic factors and the effect of plasmapheresis. *Ann Neurol* 1988;23:347–353.

73. Visser LH, van der Meché FGA, Meulstee J, et al. Cytomegalovirus infection and Guillain-Barré syndrome: the clinical, electrophysiologic, and prognostic features. *Neurology* 1996;47:668–673.

74. Ho TW, Hsieh ST, Nachamkin I, et al. Motor nerve terminal degeneration provides a potential mechanism for rapid recovery in acute motor axonal neuropathy after *Campylobacter* infection. *Neurology* 1997;48:717–724.

75. Ho TW, Li CY, Cornblath DR, et al. Patterns of recovery in the Guillain-Barré syndromes. *Neurology* 1997;48:695–700.

76. Wijdicks EFM, Ropper AH. Acute relapsing Guillain-Barré syndrome after long asymptomatic intervals. *Arch Neurol* 1990;47:82–84.

77. Austin JH. Recurrent polyneuropathies and their corticosteroid treatment. *Brain* 1958;81:157–194.

78. Dyck PC, Oviatt KF, Lambert EH. Intensive evaluation of referred unclassified neuropathies yields improved diagnosis. *Ann Neurol* 1981;10:222–226.

79. Cornblath DR, Griffin DE, Welch D, Griffin JW, McArthur JC. Quantitative analysis of endoneurial T-cells in human sural nerve biopsies. *J Neuroimmunol* 1990;26:113–118.

80. Matsummuro K, Izumo S, Umehara F, Osame M. Chronic inflammatory demyelinating polyneuropathy: histological and immunopathological studies in biopsied sural nerves. *J Neurol Sci* 1994;127:170–178.

81. Mendell JR. Chronic inflammatory demyelinating polyradiculoneuropathy. *Annu Rev Med* 1993;44:211–219.

82. Prineas JW, McLeod JG. Chronic relapsing polyneuritis. *J Neurol Sci* 1976;27:427–458.

83. Steck AJ. Inflammatory neuropathy: pathogenesis and clinical features. *Curr Opin Neurol Neurosurg* 1992;5:633–637.

84. Bromberg MB. Comparison of electrodiagnostic criteria for primary demyelination in chronic polyneuropathy. *Muscle Nerve* 1991;14:968–976.

85. Katz JS, Wolfe GI, Bryan WW, et al. Electrophysiologic findings in multifocal motor neuropathy. *Neurology* 1997;48:700–707.

86. Oh SJ, Kim DE, Koruoglu AR. What is the best diagnostic index of conduction block and temporal dispersion. *Muscle Nerve* 1994;17:489–493.

87. Kissel JT, Mendell JR. Neuropathies associated with monoclonal gammopathies. *Neuromusc Disord* 1995;6:3–18.

88. Nobile-Orazio E, Latov N, Hays AP, Takatsu M, et al. Neuropathy and anti-MAG antibodies without detectable serum M-protein. *Neurology* 1984;34:218–221.

89. Romanick-Schmiedl S, Kiprov D, Chalmers AC, Miller RG. Extraneural manifestations of chronic inflammatory demyelinating polyradiculoneuropathy. *Am J Med* 1990;89:531–534.

90. Stewart JD, McKelvey R, Durcan L, Carpenter S, Karpati G. Chronic inflammatory demyelinating polyneuropathy (CIDP) in diabetics. *J Neurol Sci* 1996;142:59–64.

91. Amato AA, Barohn RJ, Sahenk Z, Tutschka PJ, Mendell JR. Polyneuropathy complicating bone marrow and solid organ transplantation. *Neurology* 1993;43:1513–1518.

92. Mendell JR, Kolkin S, Kissel JT, Weiss KL, Chakeres DW, Rammohan KW. Evidence for central nervous system demyelination in chronic inflammatory demyelinating polyradiculoneuropathy. *Neurology* 1987;37:1291–1294.

93. Thomas PK, Walker RWH, Rudge P, et al. Chronic demyelinating peripheral neuropathy associated with multifocal central nervous system demyelination. *Brain* 1987;110:53–76.

94. Oh SJ, Joy JL, Sunwoo IN, Kuruoght R. A case of chronic sensory demyelinating neuropathy responding to immunotherapies. *Muscle Nerve* 1992;15:255–256.

95. Chroni E, Hall SM, Hughes RAC. Chronic relapsing axonal neuropathy: a first case report. *Ann Neurol* 1995;37:112–115.

96. Uncini A, Sabatelli M, Mignogna T, Lugaresi A, Liguori R, Montagna P. Chronic progressive steroid responsive axonal polyneuropathy: a CIDP variant or a primary axonal disorder? *Muscle Nerve* 1996;19:365–371.

97. Hughes R, Sanders E, Hall S, Atkinson P, Colchester A, Payan P. Subacute idiopathic demyelinating polyradiculoneuropathy. *Arch Neurol* 1992;49:612–616.

98. Dyck PJ, O'Brien PC, Oviatt KF, et al. Prednisone improves chronic inflammatory demyelinating polyradiculoneuropathy more than no treatment. *Ann Neurol* 1982;11:136–141.

99. Dyck PJ, Daube J, O'Brien P, et al. Plasma exchange in chronic inflammatory demyelinating polyradiculoneuropathy. *N Engl J Med* 1986;314:461–465.

100. Hahn AF, Bolton CF, Pillay N, et al. Plasma-exchange therapy in chronic inflammatory demyelinating polyneuropathy: A double-blind, sham-controlled, cross-over study. *Brain* 1996;119:1055–1066.

101. Hahn AF, Bolton CF, Zochodne D, Feasby TE. Intravenous immunoglobulin treatment in chronic inflammatory demyelinating

polyneuropathy: a double-blind, placebo-controlled, cross-over study. *Brain* 1996;119:1067–1077.

102. van Doorn PA, Brand A, Strengers PFW, Meulstee J, Vermeulen M. High-dose intravenous immunoglobulin treatment in chronic inflammatory demyelinating polyneuropathy: a double-blind, placebo-controlled crossover study. *Neurology* 1990;40:209–212.

103. van Doorn PA, Vermeulen M, Brand A, Mulder PGH, Busch HFM. Intravenous immunoglobulin treatment in patients with chronic inflammatory demyelinating polyneuropathy. Clinical and laboratory characteristics associated with improvement. *Arch Neurol* 1991;48:217–220.

104. Vermeulen M, van Doorn PA, Brand A, Strengers PFW, Jennekens FG, Busch HFM. Intravenous immunoglobulin treatment in patients with chronic inflammatory demyelinating polyneuropathy: a double-blind, placebo-controlled study. *J Neurol Neurosurg Psychiatry* 1993;56:36–39.

105. Dyck PJ, Litchy WJ, Kratz KM, et al. A plasma exchange versus immune globulin infusion trial in chronic inflammatory demyelinating polyradiculoneuropathy. *Ann Neurol* 1994;36:838–845.

106. Dyck PJ, O'Brien P, Swanson C, Low P, Daube J. Combined azathioprine and prednisone in chronic inflammatory demyelinating polyneuropathy. *Neurology* 1985;35:1173–1176.

107. Kolkin S, Nahman, NS, Mendell JR. Chronic nephrotoxicity complicating cyclosporine treatment of chronic inflammatory demyelinating polyradiculoneuropathy. *Neurology* 1987;37:147–149.

108. Mahattanakul WO, Crawford T, Griffin JW, Goldstein JM, Cornblath DR. Treatment of chronic inflammatory demyelinating polyneuropathy with cyclosporin-A. *J Neurol Neurosurg Psychiatry* 1996;60:186–187.

109. Sabatelli M, Mignona T, Lippi G, Milone M, et al. Interferon-alpha may benefit steroid unresponsive chronic inflammatory demyelinating polyneuropathy. *J Neurol Neurosurg Psychiatry* 1995;58:638–639.

110. Gorson KC, Allam G, Simovic D, Ropper AH. Improvement following interferon-alpha 2A in chronic inflammatory demyelinating polyneuropathy. *Neurology* 1997;48:777–780.

111. Choudhary PP, Thompson N, Hughes RAC. Improvement following interferon-beta in chronic inflammatory demyelinating polyneuropathy. *J Neurol* 1995;242:252–253.

112. Gorson KC, Ropper AH, Clark BD, et al. Treatment of chronic inflammatory demyelinating polyneuropathy with interferon-α 2a. *Neurology* 1998;50:84–87.

113. Gorson KC, Allam G, Ropper AH. Chronic Inflammatory demyelinating polyneuropathy: clinical features and response to treatment in 67 consecutive patients with and without a monoclonal gammopathy. *Neurology* 1997;48:321–328.

114. Dyck PJ, Low PA, Windebank AJ, et al. Plasma exchange in polyneuropathy associated with monoclonal gammopathy of undetermined significance. *N Engl J Med* 1991;325:1482–1486.

115. Yeung KB, Thomas PK, King RHM, et al. The clinical spectrum of peripheral neuropathies associated with benign monoclonal IgM, IgG and IgA paraproteinaemia. *J Neurol* 1991;238:383–391.

116. Notermans NC, Wokke JHJ, van den Berg LH, et al. Chronic idiopathic axonal polyneuropathy comparison of patients with and without monoclonal gammopathy. *Brain* 1996;119:421–427.

117. Dalakas MC, Quarles RH, Farrer RG, et al. A controlled study of intravenous immunoglobulin in demyelinating neuropathy with IgM gammopathy. *Ann Neurol* 1996;40:792–795.

118. Simmons Z, Albers JW, Bromberg MB, Feldman EL. Presentation and initial clinical course in patients with chronic inflammatory demyelinating polyradiculoneuropathy: comparison of patients without and with monoclonal gammopathy. *Neurology* 1993;43:2202–2209.

119. Simmons Z, Albers JW, Bromberg MB, Feldman EL. Long-term followup of patients with chronic inflammatory demyelinating polyradiculoneuropathy, without and with monoclonal gammopathy. *Brain* 1995;118:359–368.

120. Latov N, Sherman WH, Hays AP. Peripheral neuropathy and anti-MAG antibodies. *CRC Crit Rev Neurobiol* 1988;3:301–332.

121. Nobile-Orazio E, Baldini L, Barbieri S, et al. Treatment of patients with neuropathy and anti-MAG M-proteins. *Ann Neurol* 1988;24:93–97.

122. Blume G, Pestronk A, Goodnough LT. Anti-MAG antibody-associated polyneuropathies: improvement following immunotherapy with monthly plasma exchange and IV cyclophosphamide. *Neurology* 1995;45:1577–1580.

123. Cook D, Dalakas M, Galdi A, et al. High-dose intravenous immunoglobulin in the treatment of demyelinating neuropathy associated with monoclonal gammopathy. *Neurology* 1990;40:212–214.

124. Leger JM, Younes-Chennoufi AB, Chassandro B, et al. Human immunoglobulin treatment of multifocal motor neuropathy and polyneuropathy associated with monoclonal gammopathy. *J Neurol Neurosurg Psychiatry* 1994;57[Suppl]:46–49.

125. Mariette X, Chastang C, Clavelou P, et al. A randomised clinical trial comparing interferon-α and intravenous immunoglobulin in polyneuropathy associated with monoclonal IgM. *J Neurol Neurosurg Psychiatry* 1997;63:28–34.

Motor Disorders,
edited by David S. Younger.
Lippincott Williams & Wilkins, Philadelphia © 1999.

CHAPTER 18

Lyme Neuroborreliosis

John J. Halperin

Infectious causes of nervous system disease are surprisingly common. Worldwide, leprosy is one of the most frequent causes of peripheral neuropathy. Human immunodeficiency virus infection obviously is a widespread disorder with frequent and prominent nervous system involvement. In the past two decades, a relatively novel but far less common infection, Lyme disease, has gained tremendous notoriety as a potential cause of nervous system dysfunction. Although now the most common vectorborne disease in the United States, this tickborne spirochetosis only affects about 16,000 patents in the United States, the most recent year for which final data are available (1). The nervous system is thought to be involved in about 15% of untreated infected individuals (2), resulting in an annual incidence of nervous system Lyme disease, or neuroborreliosis, of about 0.6 per 100,000, slightly less than that of amyotrophic lateral sclerosis. In most patients, the involvement consists of a self-limited and readily treatable lymphocytic meningitis.

One might well ask then why this disease has been the subject of so much concern and debate. To some extent, these numbers are misleading in that this disease is very focally prevalent, that is, in regions of high prevalence, as many as 0.1% of the population may be infected annually. In these areas, this obviously is a legitimate source of concern. In other areas, however, the likelihood of acquiring the disease is extremely improbable, although it is always worth inquiring if affected patients have traveled to endemic areas.

EPIDEMIOLOGY

Because the epidemiology is such an important component of diagnosis, it is worthwhile to start by reviewing the unusual zoonosis that puts patients at risk for infection. The responsible spirochete, *Borrelia burgdorferi*, is transmitted essentially exclusively by the bite of infected hard-shelled *Ixodes* ticks. These ticks occur only in specific locales in which appropriate hosts are available. Larval ticks hatch uninfected, insomuch as transovarial transmission of *B. burgdorferi* rarely if ever occurs. The larva then typically feeds on a small mammal such as a field mouse and matures into a nymph. If this initial host is infected, the tick will generally become infected as well. When the nymphal tick partakes of its blood meal, it can transmit infection or it can become infected if it was not previously and its second host was. Infecting this second host requires a complex process and prolonged attachment. Ingestion of blood triggers spirochete proliferation in the tick gut and subsequent dissemination to its salivary glands. From there the tick can inject spirochetes into the new host, typically a deer or bear but sometimes inadvertently humans. Because this proliferation and dissemination of spirochetes within the tick takes some time, the tick must typically be attached for at least 48 to 72 hours before the host is at significant risk of becoming infected.

Endemic cycles have become established in discrete areas of North America, Europe, and Asia. Along the eastern coast of the United States, from Maryland to Massachusetts, infected *Ixodes scapularis* ticks, known colloquially as "deer ticks" for the preferred host of the adult forms, are widely prevalent. The same ticks are also found in Minnesota and Wisconsin, where they are known as "bear ticks." Related ticks, *I. ricinus*, known as the "sheep tick," are found in Europe, whereas *I. persulcatus* predominates in Asia. In general, the tick lives where its animal hosts are widespread, usually in relatively undeveloped areas. People are at greatest risk of infection when their habitat infringes on these regions, for example, in rural and exurban environments.

Although the spirochete and the specifics of its life cycle have only been characterized within the last two decades (3), many of the clinical disorders it causes have

J. J. Halperin: Department of Neurology, New York University School of Medicine, New York, New York and North Shore University Hospital, Manhasset, New York 11030.

been well known for many years. After infection, most patients develop the characteristic erythema migrans or erythema chronica migrans rash (4). This slowly enlarging erythroderm, which may reach many inches in diameter, is often asymptomatic. It typically develops over days to weeks at the site of the tick bite; in some patients the spirochetes disseminate early and cause multifocal erythema migrans. Either at this stage or subsequently, patients may develop fever, arthralgias, and malaise and a flulike syndrome, but not flulike in the sense of having upper respiratory or gastrointestinal symptoms. Because the tick bite and rash are often both asymptomatic and because both may occur on parts of the body that are not easily seen, many patients are unaware of either. However, prospective studies in children suggest that the rash occurs in as many as 90% of infected individuals (5).

The rash was first described early in this century (4). Shortly thereafter, the neurologic consequences were well described (6). The first clearly identifiable patient with neuroborreliosis in the literature developed a painful polyradiculopathy with prominent segmental weakness and a lymphocytic meningitis. The authors postulated that the illness was caused by a tickborne spirochete, treated the patient with arsenicals, and he recovered. By the 1950s, European physicians were quite familiar with this disorder and routinely treated it with penicillin. In the United States, the disease was first recognized as a form of childhood arthritis, occurring in near-epidemic proportions in the towns surrounding Lyme, Connecticut (7). Detailed epidemiologic studies demonstrated that this disorder occurred in children with histories of *Ixodes* tick bites and erythema migrans. Additional studies demonstrated that these same individuals frequently developed a constellation of neurologic disorders (8) quite similar to those described in Europe years before, that is, lymphocytic meningitis, painful radiculitis, and cranial neuritis. These studies ultimately led to the isolation and identification of a novel spirochete, named *B. burgdorferi*, as the causative organism (9,10). The following year, an apparently identical organism was isolated in Europe (11).

Clinical manifestations of this infection appear to differ in different parts of the world. In Europe, most studies have emphasized neurologic and cutaneous abnormalities, including several rather unusual dermatologic abnormalities, known as acrodermatitis chronica atrophicans and lymphocytoma cutis, which have rarely been recognized in the United States. Cardiac and rheumatologic abnormalities were not emphasized in early European patients, but a clue to this may be found in a sentinel paper describing the neurologic manifestations, which referred to rheumatism in the title (12). In fact, they appear to be far less prominent in European patients, in contrast to the United States where rheumatologic involvement has received a great deal of emphasis, whereas neurologic complications were, at least initially, believed to be less important (7).

Several factors have contributed to these apparent differences. In part, it undoubtedly represents a bias of ascertainment, because rheumatologists have been in the forefront of dealing with this disease in the United States, whereas in Europe this disease has historically been treated primarily by neurologists. At least equally important, though, it is now known that there are important differences in the prevalent strains of infecting organisms in different parts of the world; the broad group of organisms is now known as *B. burgdorferi sensu lato*. In Europe two strains are most prevalent; *B. garinii* is responsible for most neurologic disease and *B. afzelii* causes the unusual dermatologic manifestations. In North America one strain predominates, known as *B. burgdorferi sensu stricto*. Presumably different strains have tropisms for different organ systems, leading to the observed clinical differences.

DIAGNOSIS

The spectrum of neurologic and behavioral disorders ascribed to Lyme neuroborreliosis has been the subject of much debate. For some, clear epidemiologic associations have been established, whereas the causal nature in others has been the subject of anecdotal case reports or small series. Determining a true cause and effect relationship in a given disorder has been difficult because of the limitations of currently available diagnostic techniques. They have led to attribution of all manner of symptoms to this infection, often despite a lack of definitive data.

In general, the laboratory diagnosis of Lyme disease has relied on the demonstration of peripheral blood immunoreactivity against the causative organism. Microbiologic culture has not been useful for several reasons. The spirochete, *B. burgdorferi*, is fastidious, requiring specific media, known as BSK II, which is not commonly stocked by most microbiology laboratories. The bacterial load is probably rather small except in skin lesions, for which microbiologic diagnosis is usually superfluous, giving rise to problems of sampling and limiting sensitivity (13). The organism grows slowly in vitro, requiring that cultures be maintained for several weeks before being considered clearly positive or negative. This approach is impractical in all but research laboratories devoted to this effort.

Other organism-based techniques have similarly proven to be disappointing. Polymerase chain reaction, which detects genetic material from one or a small number of organisms, has typically been positive in 50 to 75% of patients (14–18), depending on the primer set chosen, the laboratory performing the assay, and the sample size. Antigen-based assays have been quite variable, and none to date has stood the test of time. As a result, most laboratory-based support for the diagnosis has been based on serologic testing, using primarily an enzyme-linked immunosorbent assay (ELISA) and Western blots.

Serologic testing has several inherent limitations. First, after the immune system is exposed to a new antigen, it takes time for a specific detectable immune response to develop—typically 3 to 6 weeks. During this time, even a very specific and sensitive antibody-based assay will generally be negative. Second, because antibody responses in general persist for an extended period of time, a single positive serologic test can at best be taken as evidence of prior exposure and not necessarily of active infection. Although in other infections it is commonplace to look at evolving titers, using an acute change in titer as evidence of active infection has not generally been done in Lyme disease. Perhaps this has been accepted by analogy to diagnosis in syphilis, the other well-known spirochetosis, in which a single positive Venereal Disease Research Laboratory (VDRL) or fluorescent treponemal antibody test is taken as evidence of infection in need of treatment.

Although the combination of a positive reagin-based test such as a VDRL or rapid plasma reagin and a positive fluorescent treponemal antibody-absorbed is quite specific for syphilis, the same cannot be said for a positive Lyme ELISA. For example, there is cross-reactivity with other organisms. Some are due to antigenically similar organisms, such as other spirochetoses including syphilis, relapsing fever, and periodontal disease from *Treponema denticola*. Other cross-reactions are due to nonspecific polyclonal B-cell activation, such as occurs in subacute bacterial endocarditis, parvovirus infection, or infectious mononucleosis. The laboratory can have great difficulty differentiating true positives from false positives due to related organisms. Nonspecific false positives can often be addressed by using Western blots, which examine the specific antigens with which the host's antibodies react.

Consensus criteria have been developed for Western blots (Table 1), which have very high specificity, that is, in patients with what appears to be acute Lyme disease, a positive IgM Western blot provides very compelling confirmation that the disorder is indeed due to *B. burgdorferi* infection (19,20). Similarly, a positive IgG blot provides

strong evidence in support of a more long-standing infection. Notably, though, the sensitivity of neither is very high. In the original study giving rise to these criteria (19), only 32% of patients with acute disease met IgM criteria, whereas 83% of those with chronic disease met IgG criteria. It is important to emphasize that this technique should be used primarily to improve the *specificity* of serologic testing, not the *sensitivity*; for example, a positive Western blot in a patient with a negative ELISA is unlikely to be meaningful.

Other general limitations of serologic testing relate to the concept of positive and negative predictive values. In most assays, the normal range is defined by assuming that most values cluster within a range extending either 2 or 3 standard deviations from the mean. Approximately 95% of all values will fall within 2 standard deviations, 99% within 2.5 standard deviations, and 99.7% within 3 standard deviations. This becomes important if serologic testing is performed indiscriminately. Nationwide the incidence of Lyme disease is approximately 5 per 100,000 (1). Using a 3 standard deviation cutoff, 3 individuals per 1,000 will fall outside the normal range, purely due to statistical variation; half of these values will exceed the upper limit of normal. As a result, in 100,000 samples, 150 will be false positives, whereas 5 will be true positives, even with this very restrictive statistical definition. Even in an endemic area, where the annual incidence is typically about 1 per 1,000, 100 of every 100,000 samples will be true positives compared with 150 false positives. In such areas, interpretation is made more difficult by the fact that seroprevalence rates are about 10% (21,22). In other words, of the 100,000 samples, 10,000 will be true positives but 9,000 of these will presumably reflect past exposure and not necessarily active infection. All of this makes interpretation of a positive result difficult in an endemic area and virtually impossible in a nonendemic area.

Finally, there are limitations peculiar to serologic testing for Lyme disease. Different laboratories have used highly divergent technical approaches to this procedure, ranging from testing against a single highly purified antigen from the flagellae of the organism (23), to the use of whole spirochete sonicates, to other combinations in between. Most laboratories use conventional ELISA kits, and some use a capture ELISA. There is no agreement on how to define positive or negative results, and because each of these approaches has some validity, there is as yet limited agreement on how best to perform and interpret these assays, resulting in significant divergence of results among different labs (24,25).

Serologic diagnosis of central nervous system (CNS) infection is actually easier and potentially more informative because little or no antibody is normally produced and the local production of specific antibody within the CNS can be measured (26–28). Although cross-reactivity does occur with other infections, only syphilis causes

TABLE 1. *Consensus criteria for Western Blot confirmation*

IgM (2 of 3 required)	IgG (5 of 10 required)
23 kDa	18 kDa
39 kDa	23 kDa
41 kDa	28 kDa
	30 kDa
	39 kDa
	41 kDa
	45 kDa
	58 kDa
	66 kDa
	93 kDa

From Refs. 19 and 20.

both prominent cross-reactivity and a CNS infection; hence, if the CSF VDRL is negative, a positive result can be assumed to be indicative of CNS Lyme disease. The major limitation of this technique from a diagnostic point of view is that it can remain positive for years after cure of the CNS infection (29), making it difficult to use to follow treatment response. However, because most individuals with active infection have other CSF evidence of active inflammation, such as an elevated CSF protein or a pleocytosis, these less specific markers can be used to assess response.

Different laboratories have used different approaches in assessing CSF Lyme serologies. The one important consideration is that the proportion of specific antibody in CSF must be compared with that in blood. Some laboratories do not do this but rather compare CSF results to serum normals. Such an approach is valid in all but two circumstances. Patients with positive peripheral blood serologies will typically have positive CSF results by this approach, because some antibody diffuses into the CSF. Only by comparing the two values, demonstrating proportionately more specific antibody in the CSF, can CNS infection be inferred. The other source of confusion is patients with blood–brain barrier breakdown or other causes of increased CSF immunoglobulin, as for example, multiple sclerosis (MS). In such patients the standard techniques underdilute CSF, so that the proportion of specific antibody appears to be much greater than it is. This allows small amounts of nonspecific cross-reacting antibody to appear to cause significant positives; however, these are obviously meaningless. Consequently, proper interpretation of the results of CSF Lyme testing requires appropriate comparison with serum antibody results.

CLINICAL MANIFESTATIONS

Among the large range of neurologic disorders that has been attributed to Lyme disease, some occur with such frequency that they can be considered firmly linked. Others are uncommon but have compelling laboratory support for a linkage and therefore can be considered as real. Others are plausible, based on what is known of the pathophysiology. Others must be considered highly speculative.

The syndrome first described by Garin and Bujadoux (6) 75 years ago and named in their honor consists of a lymphocytic meningitis and painful polyradiculitis clearly due to the Lyme spirochete (2,8). In about 10% of such patients, the organism can be cultured from CSF (13), and intrathecal antibody production is demonstrable in over 90% (27). The lymphocytic meningitis—which can occur in isolation or in combination with cranial or peripheral nerve involvement—is indistinguishable clinically from viral meningitis. Patients develop varying degrees of headache, neck stiffness, and photophobia. CSF demonstrates a lymphocytic pleocytosis, typically up to a few hundred cells, mild elevation of protein, and typically normal glucose. Symptoms can be self-limited but probably resolve more quickly with antibiotics. Radicular involvement is similarly common. This can precisely mimic a mechanical monoradiculopathy or may be more widespread, resembling either a plexopathy, a mononeuritis multiplex, or even a disseminated polyneuropathy clinically similar to the Guillain-Barré syndrome. However, neurophysiologic testing does not usually demonstrate typical demyelinating changes, and a CSF pleocytosis is usually present (30). Cranial nerve involvement also occurs frequently. The facial nerve is probably the most commonly involved and may be affected bilaterally. The nerves to the extraocular muscles also are affected with some frequency, as are the trigeminal and the VIIIth. Lower cranial nerves seem to be the least likely to be involved. In most instances, cranial nerve involvement probably occurs as part of a basilar meningitis, with nerves affected as they pass through the inflamed subarachnoid space. However, Lyme disease also commonly causes a mononeuropathy multiplex; in many instances at least facial nerve involvement may occur as part of this peripheral nervous system (PNS) disorder, even in the absence of meningitis (30).

All these disorders tend to occur fairly early in disease. Common to all is a vigorous immune response, prominent symptoms of radicular-type pain, focal weakness, and acute to subacute onset, typically within a few months of the onset of the infection. Other patients may develop much more indolent syndromes. In contrast to the more acute syndromes, symptoms tend to be mild and develop slowly. Patients commonly describe mild positive and negative sensory symptoms with mild paresthesias, sensory loss, perhaps gait instability, and minimal weakness (31). This may occur in as many as a third of untreated patients with chronic infection. Why some patients develop acute dramatic syndromes whereas others develop a more protracted and subtle disorder is not clear. Presumably it reflects a combination of factors, including differences in host immunity, both in terms of human leukocyte antigen-dictated immune characteristics and prior immune experience, strain differences in spirochetes, and perhaps coinfection with other tickborne organisms such as ehrlichia, babesia, or tickborne encephalitis virus.

Interestingly, in patients with both acute and indolent PNS involvement, neurophysiologic studies are usually indicative of a mononeuropathy multiplex (30). Nerve biopsies in both populations typically show axon loss and perivascular inflammatory infiltrates (31,32). Patients generally do not develop frank necrotizing vasculitis with vessel wall necrosis. In the only good animal model of human neuroborreliosis, the tick-infected rhesus macaque monkey, all untreated monkeys studied to date developed mononeuropathy multiplex (33). As in humans, it has not been possible to demonstrate spirochetes, immune complexes, or other proof of a pathophysiologic mechanism.

CNS involvement is more varied. Conceptually, this can be divided into extra-axial disease such as meningitis, parenchymal disease such as encephalomyelitis, and CNS dysfunction without obvious structural CNS change. As with PNS involvement, when patients become symptomatic fairly early in infection, involvement tends to develop fairly rapidly with a prominent inflammatory response. Lymphocytic meningitis is the most common form of CNS involvement. Far more dramatic, but fortunately rare, is an encephalomyelitis. Patients develop focal inflammation of the brain or spinal cord parenchyma (34–36). This disorder occurs in perhaps 0.1% of patients with untreated *B. burgdorferi* infection, both in Europe and in North America. Involvement primarily involves the white matter; experimental evidence indicates that the spirochete preferentially adheres to oligodendroglia (37), perhaps accounting for this tropism. Typically, most patients present with a myelopathic picture with progressive gait spasticity and sphincter dysfunction. Others develop focal inflammation in the brain, with symptoms and findings appropriate to the site of inflammation. Seizures occur rarely if at all. Brain magnetic resonance imaging typically demonstrates areas of inflammation within white matter. Antibiotic therapy will generally arrest disease progression, and in many patients leads to some improvement. In some, in whom significant structural damage has occurred, residua will occur.

The mechanism underlying this disorder remains unclear. The few pathologic studies available demonstrate focal perivascular inflammation (38), similar to that seen in the peripheral nerve. There is some evidence to suggest that organisms are present in the region of inflammation (38), but this cannot yet be considered conclusive. The observation that patients can improve significantly after antibiotic treatment certainly supports the conclusion that viable bacteria play an essential role in this process. However, it has been extraordinarily difficult to culture spirochetes from such patients. To date, comparable lesions have not occurred in the monkey model. Although transient bacterial seeding of the neuraxis has been demonstrated in several animal models, in none has parenchymal brain or spinal cord damage been demonstrable (39).

Far more common is a mild confusional state, without focal neurologic signs. This phenomenon was originally reported in patients with systemic nonneurologic Lyme disease, typically patients with chronic arthritis (27,35). These individuals described difficulty with memory and cognitive functioning. Originally thought to be a peculiarly American phenomenon, similar observations have now been made in European patients (40). Mini-Mental Status testing and more formal neuropsychologic testing typically demonstrate significant, although not profound, cognitive deficits, all of which generally improve after antimicrobial therapy (41–43). Other evaluations in these patients are generally less informative. Magnetic resonance images in some demonstrate small regions of abnormality in the white matter. In most, scans are negative. CSF in some is negative; in others mild nonspecific abnormalities or occasionally even intrathecal antibody production is found. In some affected patients, this appears to be a mild version of the more dramatic encephalomyelitis. In others, there is little compelling evidence of CNS infection. In such individuals it has been postulated that this might be a toxic-metabolic encephalopathy secondary to infection outside the neuraxis. In one study, elevated concentrations of quinolinic acid were demonstrated in serum, with parallel elevations in the CSF (44). Quinolinic acid, a tryptophan metabolite, is produced in response to inflammation under the control of γ-interferon and tumor necrosis factor-α and is pharmacologically active at NMDA receptors where it can affect neuronal function. This model suggests a mechanism by which a soluble neuroimmunomodulator is produced in the periphery, diffuses into the CNS, and there has a pharmacologic action altering CNS function. Whether this or some other cytokine or other molecule actually plays such a role remains to be confirmed.

Finally, much has been said about how Lyme disease can masquerade as other neurologic diseases—an observation that stems in large part from the lack of specific, unique, gold standard diagnostic tests both for Lyme disease and for many other neurologic syndromes. The disorder that has most frequently been confused with neuroborreliosis has been MS. Because Lyme encephalomyelitis and MS both involve acute inflammation in the white matter, it is clear why some confusion could arise. Moreover, there is suggestive evidence that Lyme disease may be one of numerous nonspecific stimuli to inflammation within the CNS, which, perhaps by increasing local production of γ-interferon can trigger MS attacks. However, it is extremely unusual for Lyme encephalomyelitis to relapse after being definitively treated, and it is even more uncommon for patients with MS to have evidence of intrathecal production of antibodies against *B. burgdorferi*.

The confusional state has similarly led to concerns that Lyme disease could cause Alzheimer disease. Although, like many other infections, Lyme disease can lead to a transient worsening of cognitive functioning in affected patients, there is little to suggest that it causes a permanent progressive dementing illness resembling Alzheimer disease.

There has also been interest in the potential overlap of Lyme neuroborreliosis with motor neuron disease (45). The radiculoneuropathy of Lyme disease commonly has a more prominent motor than sensory component, leading to some potential for confusion. If, in addition, the patient has myelopathic involvement, the combination of upper and lower motor neuron signs may resemble amyotrophic lateral sclerosis. However, assessment of CSF and careful clinical analysis will usually differentiate between these disorders.

Finally, anecdotal reports have suggested associations with Parkinson's disease and a variety of psychiatric disorders. No systematic studies have substantiated these associations to date, so for now these associations must be considered conjectural.

TREATMENT

There continues to be considerable controversy concerning the optimal treatment of Lyme neuroborreliosis (Tables 2 and 3). Several randomized blinded studies demonstrated that oral treatment with either doxycycline or amoxicillin for 3 weeks is highly effective in early disease (46). In patients with Lyme arthritis, oral regimens can also be effective (47). In patients with more long-standing or more severe disease or involvement of the CNS, parenteral treatment is generally chosen, typically a third-generation cephalosporin such as ceftriaxone or cefotaxime. Most studies have shown the two agents to be equally effective. Studies comparing 2- and 4-week regimens also failed to prove that a longer course was more beneficial (48,49). However, anecdotally, many centers that treat large numbers of patients have observed CNS relapses in patients who have received just 2 weeks of therapy; it has consequently become commonplace to treat for 4 weeks when using parenteral therapy. Although some recommend substantially longer courses, there is no scientific evidence that this confers any additional benefit; however, because of this widespread feeling that such prolonged courses are needed, the National Institutes of Health has recently initiated a study to address this issue.

Two other regimens may be useful in the treatment of CNS disease. One European study demonstrated that oral doxycycline was highly effective in most patients with Lyme meningitis (50); however, long-term follow-up in this group was limited. Similarly, in patients with PNS disease, including some with facial nerve paralysis, oral regimens may be effective. However, this has not been studied extensively, and at this point treatment of these patients must be individualized. Finally, parenteral penicillin has been used for years, with considerable efficacy. The organism does tend to be more sensitive to ceftriaxone and cefotaxime, particularly at concentrations achieved by these drugs in the CNS. Ceftriaxone has generally become the preferred agent for parenteral therapy both because of some studies suggesting greater efficacy and also because of ease of dosing.

CONCLUSION

Lyme disease, a recently described spirochetosis, frequently affects the CNS and PNS. It does so in one of several distinct manners. PNS involvement is due to a mononeuropathy multiplex but may be manifest as a monoradiculopathy, mononeuritis, or more diffuse process. CNS involvement is most frequently manifest as a benign lymphocytic meningitis. Rare patients develop a focal or multifocal leukoencephalomyelitis. Some patients develop encephalopathy that may be due to either a mild encephalitis or the remote effects of a non-CNS infection. Accurate diagnosis of CNS infection requires assessment of CSF, with measurement not just of CSF anti-*Borrelia* antibody but of actual intrathecal antibody production. When the diagnosis is secure, antimicrobial therapy is usually successful.

TABLE 3. *Treatment suggestions*

Disorder	Suggested treatment
Meningitis	IV ceftriaxone *or* cefotaxime *or* penicillin *or?* po doxycycline
Encephalomyelitis	IV ceftriaxone *or* cefotaxime *or* penicillin
PNS (peripheral neuropathy, radiculoneuropathy, cranial neuropathy)	CSF−; oral regimens *may* be effective CSF+; as encephalomyelitis
Encephalopathy	CSF−; oral regimens *may* be effective CSF+; as encephalomyelitis

PNS, peripheral nervous system; CSF, cerebrospinal fluid.

TABLE 2. *Treatment regimens*

Agent	Dose	Duration (days)
Ceftriaxone[a]	2 g IV q24h	14–28
Cefotaxime	2 g IV q8h	14–28
Penicillin	3–4 MU IV q4h	14–28
Doxycycline[b]	100–200 mg po b.i.d.	21–30
Amoxicillin	500–1,000 mg po t.i.d.	10–30

[a]Ceftriaxone should probably not be used in the third trimester of pregnancy.
[b]Doxycycline should not be used in pregnant women or in children age 8 or under.
From Ref. 51.

REFERENCES

1. Summary of notifiable diseases, United States, 1996. *MMWR Morb Mortal Wkly Rep* 1997;45:3.
2. Pachner AR, Steere AC. The triad of neurologic manifestations of Lyme disease. *Neurology* 1985;35:47–53.
3. Burgdorfer W, Barbour AG, Hayes SF, Benach JL, Grunwaldt E, Davis JP. Lyme disease: a tick-borne spirochetosis? *Science* 1982;216:1317–1319.
4. Afzelius A. Erythema chronicum migrans. *Acta Derm Venereol (Stockh)* 1921;2:120–125.
5. Pediatric Lyme Disease Study Group, Gerber MA, Shapiro ED, Burke GS, Parcells VJ, Bell GL. Lyme disease in children in southeastern Connecticut. *N Engl J Med* 1996;335:1270–1274.
6. Garin C, Bujadoux A. Paralysie par les tiques. *J Med Lyon* 1922;71:765–767.
7. Steere AC, Malawista SE, Hardin JA, Ruddy S, Askenase W, Andiman WA. Erythema chronicum migrans and Lyme arthritis. The enlarging clinical spectrum. *Ann Intern Med* 1977;86:685–698.
8. Reik L, Steere AC, Bartenhagen NH, Shope RE, Malawista SE. Neurologic abnormalities of Lyme disease. *Medicine* 1979;58:281–294.
9. Benach JL, Bosler EM, Hanrahan JP, et al. Spirochetes isolated from the blood of two patients with Lyme Disease. *N Engl J Med* 1983;308:740–742.

10. Steere AC, Grodzicki RL, Kornblatt AN, et al. The spirochetal etiology of Lyme disease. *N Engl J Med* 1983;308:733–740.
11. Asbrink E, Hovmark A, Hederstedt B. Serologic studies of erythema chronicum migrans afzelius and acrodermatitis chronica atrophicans with indirect immunofluorescence and enzyme-linked immunosorbent assays. *Acta Derm Venereol (Stockh)* 1985;65:509–514.
12. Bannwarth A. Chronische lymphocytare meningitis, entzundliche polyneuritis und rheumatismus. *Arch Psychiatr Nervenkr* 1941;113:284–376.
13. Karlsson M, Hovind HK, Svenungsson B, Stiernstedt G. Cultivation and characterization of spirochetes from cerebrospinal fluid of patients with Lyme borreliosis. *J Clin Microbiol* 1990;28:473–479.
14. Rosa PA, Schwan TG. A specific and sensitive assay for the Lyme disease spirochete *Borrelia burgdorferi* using the polymerase chain reaction. *J Infect Dis* 1989;160:1018–1029.
15. Halperin JJ, Keller T, Whitman M. PCR-based detection of CSF *B. burgdorferi* in the assessment of treatment response in CNS Lyme borreliosis. *Neurology* 1993;43[Suppl 2]:A186–187.
16. Nocton JJ, Dressler F, Rutledge BJ, Rys PN, Persing DH, Steere AC. Detection of *Borrelia burgdorferi* DNA by polymerase chain reaction in synovial fluid from patients with Lyme arthritis. *N Engl J Med* 1994; 1994:229–234.
17. Lebech AM, Hansen K. Detection of *Borrelia burgdorferi* DNA in urine samples and cerebrospinal fluid samples from patients with early and late Lyme neuroborreliosis by polymerase chain reaction. *J Clin Microbiol* 1992;30:1646–1653.
18. Nocton JJ, Bloom BJ, Rutledge BJ, et al. Detection of *Borrelia burgdorferi* DNA by polymerase chain reaction in cerebrospinal fluid in Lyme neuroborreliosis. *J Infect Dis* 1996;174:623–627.
19. Dressler F, Whalen JA, Reinhardt BN, Steere AC. Western blotting in the serodiagnosis of Lyme disease. *J Infect Dis* 1993;167:392–400.
20. Recommendations for test performance and interpretation from the Second National Conference on Serologic Diagnosis of Lyme Disease. *MMWR Morb Mortal Wkly Rep* 1995;44:590–591.
21. Hanrahan JP, Benach JL, Coleman JL, et al. Incidence and cumulative frequency of endemic Lyme disease in a community. *J Infect Dis* 1984; 150:489–496.
22. Steere AC, Taylor E, Wilson ML, Levine JF, Spielman A. Longitudinal assessment of the clinical and epidemiologic features of Lyme disease in a defined population. *J Infect Dis* 1986;154:295–300.
23. Hansen K, Hindersson P, Pedersen NS. Measurement of antibodies to the *Borrelia burgdorferi* flagellum improves serodiagnosis in Lyme disease. *J Clin Microbiol* 1988;26:338–346.
24. Bakken LL, Case KL, Callister SM, Bourdeau NJ, Schell RF. Performance of 45 laboratories participating in a proficiency testing program for Lyme disease serology. *AMA* 1992;268:891–895.
25. Lane RS, Lennette ET, Madigan JE. Interlaboratory and intralaboratory comparisons of indirect immunofluorescence assays for serodiagnosis of Lyme disease. *J Clin Microbiol* 1990;28:1774–1779.
26. Stiernstedt GT, Granstrom M, Hederstedt B, Skoldenberg B. Diagnosis of spirochetal meningitis by enzyme linked immunosorbent assay and indirect immunofluorescence assay in serum and cerebrospinal fluid. *J Clin Microbiol* 1985;21:819–825.
27. Halperin JJ, Luft BJ, Anand AK, et al. Lyme neuroborreliosis: central nervous system manifestations. *Neurology* 1989;39:753–759.
28. Steere AC, Berardi VP, Weeks KE, Logigian EL, Ackermann R. Evaluation of the intrathecal antibody response to *Borrelia burgdorferi* as a diagnostic test for Lyme neuroborreliosis. *J Infect Dis* 1990;161: 1203–1209.
29. Hammers-Berggren S, Hansen K, Lebech AM, Karlsson M. *Borrelia burgdorferi*-specific intrathecal antibody production in neuroborreliosis: a follow-up study. *Neurology* 1993;43:169–175.
30. Halperin JJ, Luft BJ, Volkman DJ, Dattwyler RJ. Lyme neuroborreliosis—peripheral nervous system manifestations. *Brain* 1990;113: 1207–1221.
31. Halperin JJ, Little BW, Coyle PK, Dattwyler RJ. Lyme disease- a treatable cause of peripheral neuropathy. *Neurology* 1987;37:1700–1706.
32. Vallat JM, Hugon J, Lubeau M, Leboutet MJ, Dumas M, Desproges-Gotteron R. Tick bite meningoradiculoneuritis. *Neurology* 1987;37:749–753.
33. England JD, Bohm RP, Roberts ED, Philipp MT. Mononeuropathy multiplex in rhesus monkeys with chronic Lyme disease. *Ann Neurol* 1997; 41:375–385.
34. Ackermann R, Rehse KB, Gollmer E, Schmidt R. Chronic neurologic manifestations of erythema migrans borreliosis. *Ann NY Acad Sci* 1988;539:16–23.
35. Halperin JJ, Pass HL, Anand AK, Luft BJ, Volkman DJ, Dattwyler RJ. Nervous system abnormalities in Lyme disease. *Ann NY Acad Sci* 1988; 539:24–34.
36. Broderick JP, Sandok BA, Mertz LE. Focal encephalitis in a young woman 6 years after the onset of Lyme disease. *Mayo Clin Proc* 1987; 62:313–316.
37. Garcia Monco JC, Fernandez-Villar B, Benach JL. Adherence of the Lyme disease spirochete to glial cells and cells of glial origin. *J Infect Dis* 1989;160:497–506.
38. Oski J, Kalimo H, Marttila RJ, et al. Inflammatory brain changes in Lyme borreliosis. A report on three patients and review of literature. *Brain* 1996;119(Pt 6):2143–2154.
39. Pachner AR, Delaney E, O'Neill T, Major E. Inoculation of nonhuman primates with the N40 strain of *Borrelia burgdorferi* leads to a model of Lyme neuroborreliosis faithful to the human disease. *Neurology* 1995;45:165–172.
40. Benke T, Gasse T, Hittmair-Delazer M, Schmutzhard E. Lyme encephalopathy: long-term neuropsychological deficits years after acute neuroborreliosis. *Acta Neurol Scand* 1995;91:353–357.
41. Halperin JJ, Krupp LB, Golightly MG, Volkman DJ. Lyme borreliosis-associated encephalopathy. *Neurology* 1990;40:1340–1343.
42. Krupp LB, Masur D, Schwartz J, et al. Cognitive functioning in late Lyme borreliosis. *Arch Neurol* 1991;48:1125–1129.
43. Kaplan RF, Meadows ME, Vincent LC, Logigian EL, Steer AC. Memory impairment and depression in patients with Lyme encephalopathy: comparison with fibromyalgia and nonpsychotically depressed patients. *Neurology* 1992;42:1263–1267.
44. Halperin JJ, Heyes MP. Neuroactive kynurenines in Lyme borreliosis. *Neurology* 1992;42:43–50.
45. Halperin JJ, Kaplan GP, Brazinsky S, et al. Immunologic reactivity against *Borrelia burgdorferi* in patients with motor neuron disease. *Arch Neurol* 1990;47:586–594.
46. Dattwyler RF, Volkman DJ, Conaty SM, Platkin SP, Luft BJ. Amoxycillin plus probenecid versus doxycycline for treatment of erythema migrans borreliosis. *Lancet* 1990:336:1404–1406.
47. Steere AC, Levin RE, Molloy PJ, et al. Treatment of Lyme arthritis. *Arthritis Rheum* 1994;37:878–888.
48. Dattwyler RJ, Halperin JJ, Volkman DJ, Luft BJ. Treatment of late Lyme disease. *Lancet* 1988;1:1191–1193.
49. Dattwyler RJ, Luft BJ, Maladorno D, et al. Treatment of late Lyme disease—a comparison of 2 weeks vs 4 weeks of ceftriaxone. VII International Congress on Lyme Borreliosis. San Francisco, California, 1996, p. 186.
50. Karlsson M, Hammers-Berggren S, Lindquist L, Stiernstedt G, Svenungsson B. Comparison of intravenous penicillin G and oral doxycycline for treatment of Lyme neuroborreliosis. *Neurology* 1994;44: 1203–1207.
51. Wormser GP. Treatment and prevention of Lyme disease, with emphasis on antimicrobial therapy for neuroborreliosis and vaccination. *Semin Neurol* 1997;17:45–52.

Motor Disorders,
edited by David S. Younger.
Lippincott Williams & Wilkins, Philadelphia © 1999.

CHAPTER 19

Motor Neuropathy and Monoclonal Gammopathy

Thomas H. Brannagan III and Norman Latov

Motor neuropathy is manifested by weakness, wasting, fasciculation, and normal sensations; thus, it resembles motor neuron disease (MND) clinically (1–3). It can be generalized or involve one or more individual nerves, with acute, subacute, or slowly progressive onset. Motor nerve axons are primarily affected, not the perikaryon. Motor neuropathy is often immunologically mediated and, in contrast to MND, may respond to immunosuppressive therapy.

Laboratory investigations can aid in the diagnosis of motor neuropathy and provide clues as to its etiology. Electrophysiologic studies often reveal conduction abnormalities, including conduction block. Serologic studies may reveal high titers of anti-GM1 or GD1a ganglioside autoantibodies often in association with an IgM paraprotein. This chapter review aspects of motor neuropathy due to monoclonal gammopathy.

CLINICAL FEATURES

Motor neuropathy begins at almost any age from the second to eighth decade, with a predilection for men. The neuropathy can be generalized or involve only one or several nerves, and is frequently asymmetric. The arms are more frequently involved than the legs (4,5), and unlike MND, bulbar involvement and respiratory failure rarely if ever occur (6,7). It is usually slowly progressive, sometimes over 20 years or more (7,8). Deep tendon reflexes may be absent or hypoactive but are sometimes active in weak and wasted limbs (9–11); Babinski signs are never a feature of motor neuropathy, and myokymia rarely occurs (12,13).

T. H. Brannagan III: Department of Neurology, MCP-Hahnemann University, Philadelphia, Pennsylvania 19102-1192.

N. Latov: Department of Neurology, Columbia University and Peripheral Neuropathy Center, New York Presbyterian Hospital, New York, New York 10032.

ELECTRODIAGNOSTIC STUDIES

In both motor neuropathy and MND, electrophysiologic studies show reduced compound motor action potentials (CMAP) amplitudes, with fibrillation and fasciculation activity, and long duration neurogenic motor unit potentials on needle electromyography consistent with axonal degeneration and denervation. There may be associated demyelinating features that help distinguish it from MND, including slowing of motor nerve conduction velocities, prolongation of distal motor and F-wave latencies (into a demyelinating range), temporal dispersion, or motor conduction block. Some patients with motor neuropathy exhibit minimal electrical abnormalities in life and thus may be difficult to diagnose.

Multifocal demyelinating neuropathy with persistent conduction block was first described electrophysiologically in 1982 by Lewis et al. (14) among several patients with chronic sensorimotor demyelinating polyneuropathy characterized clinically by mononeuritis multiples and electrophysiologically by persistent multifocal conduction block. In 1985, Parry and Clark (15,16) described several patients with a syndrome resembling MND, but with multifocal motor conduction block and normal sensory conduction. Persistent motor conduction block is one feature that unequivocally identifies a patient as having a neuropathy, although its demonstration may be technically difficult. Paranodal and internodal demyelination increases the transverse capacitance and reduces the resistance at the internode. This increases outward leakage current, increasing the time the internal longitudinal current must flow to generate an impulse at the next node of Ranvier. If the transverse current leakage is excessive, not enough current may be available to depolarize the next node of Ranvier and the impulse blocks (17,18). The demonstration of a drop in the CMAP \amplitude from proximal to distal stimulation is insufficient by itself to conclude the presence of conduction block because similar findings can result from submaximal stimulation along sites where the nerve trunk is deep to the skin such as at Erb's point (19). Interphase shift and cancellation of the negative phase of the motor unit action potential with the positive phase of another motor unit potential also results in significant drops in amplitude, particularly with chronic partial denervation. There is no definitive consensus as to the required amplitude or area loss for the block in multifocal motor neuropathy (MMN), with published figures ranging from 20 to 50% (4,5,13,20–26). However, an amplitude loss of up to 41% and area loss of 29% can be seen in normal subjects (27). Computer modeling indicates that temporal dispersion can result in a drop in amplitude of greater than 50%, but a drop in the area of greater than 50% is due to conduction block (28). The analysis of short nerve segments is most helpful in demonstrating conduction block because a gradual change in amplitude is also likely to be caused by temporal dispersion (29).

Motor conduction block may be verified by comparing the partially blocked CMAP with the surface-recorded potential obtained during maximal volitional effort. This is accomplished by triggering on the largest peak of the recruitment pattern during maximal effort (30). If the volitional summated potential is larger than the proximal CMAP, than true conduction block has not occurred and the reduced proximal amplitude may be due to submaximal stimulation.

Patients with motor neuropathies, diagnosed by presence of conduction block or elevated titers of anti-GM1 antibodies, frequently exhibit other conduction abnormalities. In nine patients with motor conduction block, the only features of demyelination were seen in the same or other nerves: temporal dispersion in five, slowed motor conduction velocity in seven, and prolonged distal motor latencies in four; all had prolonged F waves in at lease one nerve (21). In a study of 16 patients with MMN including 9 with elevated anti-GM1 antibodies and 5 with motor conduction block, 15 patients had other features of demyelination: 5 had prolonged distal latencies, 7 had abnormal temporal dispersion, 8 had prolonged F waves not explained by distal slowing, and 13 had conduction velocity slowing. Eight patients had at lease one nerve with pure axonal features but had other nerves meeting demyelinating criteria. The one patient that did not meet formal criteria for demyelinating neuropathy instead had a prolonged F-wave latency and a 31% drop in the median CMAP area across the forearm. Two thirds each of patients treated with intravenous immunoglobulin (IVIg) with or without conduction block improved (31).

Sensory conductions across the site of motor conduction block should be normal (16,26), but that generally requires special techniques to ensure that pure motor conduction is present (32,33).

PATHOLOGIC STUDIES

Nerve biopsy can be helpful in supporting the diagnosis of motor neuropathy. Noninflammatory demyelination was seen at the site of conduction block in two patients with anti-GM1 antibodies (34). Similar findings were seen in the peripheral nerves of other patients, although not at the site of conduction block (22,35). IgM deposits at the nodes of Ranvier were seen in the neural nerve of a patient with MMN and anti-GM1 antibodies (23); however, other reported cases were normal (25,36) or showed minimal abnormalities (36,37). Obturator motor nerve biopsy shows increased regenerative clusters of small myelinated fibers in comparison with those with MND (35).

There is limited postmortem data of patients with motor neuropathy; however, four patients (24,38–40) with a lower motor neuron syndrome resembling spinal muscular atrophy (SMA) were studied at postmortem examination. One patient with motor neuropathy and an IgM monoclonal gammopathy without known conduction block or elevated GM1 titers was reported by Rowland et al. (38). There was central chromatolysis of anterior horn cells accompanied by severe loss of nerve fibers in the ventral roots. Another patient with motor neuropathy and an IgM polyclonal gammopathy, in addition, showed endoneurial perivascular lymphocytic infiltration (39). A third patient with elevated anti-GM1 antibodies revealed immunoglobulin deposits on myelin sheaths with predominant involvement of the anterior roots, explaining the lack of correlation between the presence of distal conduction block and the distribution or severity of weakness (24). A fourth patient with motor neuropathy without anti-GM1 antibodies or conduction block had perineurial perivascular mononuclear inflammation in peripheral motor nerves (40).

Nonetheless, the differentiation of motor neuropathy from MND may be difficult even after extensive evaluation. Clinical features that may distinguish motor neuropathy from MND include the multifocal or asymmetric involvement, and prolonged time course. Electrophysiological may show persistent multifocal conduction block (16) or other signs of demyelination on electrophysiologic studies (21,31). High titers of anti-GM1 and anti-GD1a antibodies often seen in motor neuropathy are rarely found in MND (11,41).

Motor neuropathy may also be difficult to distinguish from motor forms of CIDP and, as discussed in Chapter 15, both respond to immunosuppressive therapy (42). Unlike CIDP, however, motor nerve velocities in motor neuropathy are normal between regions of block as are sensory conduction studies, and the cerebrospinal fluid (CSF) protein is not commonly elevated. Corticosteroids are frequently helpful in CIDP but not in MMN (43–45).

MOTOR NEUROPATHY AND MONOCLONAL GAMMOPATHY

Monoclonal gammopathy results from the abnormal proliferation of monoclonal B cells that secrete excessive IgM, IgG, or IgA antibodies (46). The monoclonal antibodies are detected and characterized by serum protein immunoelectrophoresis or immunofixation electrophoresis and are called M-proteins or paraproteins. They may be autoreactive and cause autoimmune disease; however, 1% of normal adults have serum M-proteins, and the monoclonal gammopathy may be coincidental and unrelated to the motor neuropathy.

The incidence of peripheral neuropathy in patients with IgM monoclonal gammopathies is 5 to 50% (47–50). In most patients with peripheral neuropathy and IgM M-proteins, the monoclonal gammopathy is nonmalignant, and the M-proteins have autoantibody activity and react with oligosaccharide determinants of glycolipids or glycoproteins or glycoconjugates concentrated in peripheral nerve. Occasionally, it is sometimes associated with Waldenström's macroglobulinemia, B-cell lymphoma, or chronic lymphocytic leukemia.

Structure of Glycolipids

Glycosphingolipids are composed of the long-chain aliphatic amine sphingosine, an acylated ceramid attached to one or more sugars. Gangliosides are complex glycosphingolipids containing sialic acid. Sialic acid is a generic term for *N*-acylneuraminic acid. Gangliosides are designated G for ganglioside followed by M, D, T, or Q for mono, di, tri, or quad, respectively, referring to the number of sialic acids. Arabic numbers and lowercase letters follow and refer to the sequence of migration by thin-later chromatography (51,52).

IGM MONOCLONAL GAMMOPATHIES

In 1968, Peters and Clatanoff (53) described a patient with SMA and IgM monoclonal gammopathy who improved with chlorambucil treatment. However, that patient probably had a motor neuropathy rather than MND. The first documented case of a patient with motor neuropathy and an IgM monoclonal gammopathy was reported by Rowland et al. in 1982 (38). That patient presented with progressive weakness, wasting, and fasciculation and had an IgM-k monoclonal gammopathy. Motor conduction velocities were slow, with normal sensory conductions.

Motor Neuropathy and Anti-GM1 Antibodies

In 1986, Freddo et al. (54) described a patient with SMA clinically, anti-GM1 antibodies, and an IgM monoclonal gammopathy. A second similar patient improved with intravenous cyclophosphamide therapy (55). In 1988, Pestronk et al. (20) demonstrated that patients with MMN and conduction block had high titers of IgM anti-GM1 antibodies. In 1990, Yuki et al. (56) reported IgG anti-GM1 antibodies in patients with acute motor axonal neuropathy, a variant of the Guillain-Barré syndrome (GBS). Estimates of the frequency of increased IgM anti-GM1 antibody titers in patients with MMN range from 18 to 84% (11). In most patients, they are polyclonal, but some are monoclonal, and the total serum IgM concentration is often increased.

In a review of 14 patients chosen for the presence of highly elevated anti-GM1 antibody titers, 5 had a single site of conduction block, 4 had multiple conduction blocks, 1 had diffusely slowed motor conductions, and the remaining had normal motor conductions.

In most patients, the anti-GM1 antibodies recognize the Gal(B1-3)GalNAc determinant that is shared by asialo GM1 (AGM1) and the ganglioside GDLB. The same determinant is also present on some glycoproteins and is recognized by the lectin peanut agglutinin. Some of the antibodies, however, are highly specific for GM1 or recognize internal determinants shared by GM2 (57–60). Although GM1 and other Gal(B1-3)GalNAc bearing glycoconjugates are highly concentrated and widely distributed in the central and peripheral nervous systems, they are generally cryptic and unavailable to the antibodies. However, anti-GM1 antibodies bind to spinal cord gray matter and to GM1 on the surface of isolated bovine spinal motor neurons but not to dorsal root ganglia neurons (61). In peripheral nerve, GM1 ganglioside and Gal(B1-3)GalNAc–bearing glycoproteins are expressed at the nodes of Ranvier (62). Two glycoproteins have been identified as the oligodendroglial-myelin glycoprotein in paranodal myelin and a versican-like glycoprotein in the nodal gap (63). The antibodies also bind to the presynaptic terminals at the motor end-plate in skeletal muscle, where the antibodies might also exert an effect (55,64).

It is not known whether the anti-GM1 antibodies cause or contribute to the disease or whether they are only an associated abnormality. The binding to motor but not sensory neurons correlates with the clinical syndrome. GM1 is highly enriched in myelin sheaths of motor nerves and differs in its ceramides in comparison with sensory nerves (65,66). This might render the anterior roots more susceptible to the autoantibody effects. In one study, rabbits immunized with GM1 or Gal(1-3)GalNAc-BSA developed conduction abnormalities with immunoglobulin deposits at the nodes of Ranvier (67), and in another, serum from a patient with increased titers of anti-GM1 antibodies and IgM deposits at the nodes of Ranvier produced demyelination and conduction block when injected into rat sciatic nerve (68). The human anti-GM1 antibodies have also been shown to bind to, and kill, mammalian spinal motor neurons in culture (69) and at the motor end-plate (70). Serum from patients with MMN both with and without anti-GM1 antibodies block nerve conduction in the mouse phrenic nerve-diaphragm preparation (71). Anti-GM1 antibodies alter potassium current and, in the presence of complement, block sodium channels in rat myelinated nerve fibers (72). Based on the persistence of the motor conduction block and the pathologic findings of axons devoid of myelin and only minimal onion bulbs, Kaji et al. (73) suggested that anti-GM1 antibodies impair remyelination. The variable regions of anti-GM1 antibodies from normal individuals or patients with neuropathy exhibit multiple somatic mutations in their hypervariable regions, suggesting that they have been derived from a process of antigenic stimulation (74,75).

In contrast to the IgM anti-GM1 antibodies in patients with chronic motor neuropathies, increased titers of polyclonal IgG or IgA anti-GM1 antibodies are associated with acute motor axonal neuropathy. These have been reported to occur after infection with *Campylobacter jejuni* (56,76–79), which bears GM1-like oligosaccharides (80–82), or after parenteral injection of GM1-containing gangliosides (83–85a). Postmortem studies in some of the patients who died of GBS after *C. jejuni* infection showed noninflammatory degeneration of the anterior roots and chromatolytic changes in spinal motor neurons (78) similar to the chronic disease associated with IgM anti-GM1 antibodies.

IgM Anti-GD1a Autoantibodies

Several patients with motor neuropathy and anti-GD1a antibodies have been described. The first patient was a 73-year-old man with 3 years of lower limb weakness and an IgM-k monoclonal gammopathy. He had absent leg and reduced arm reflexes. CSF examination was normal, and nerve conduction velocity was slow. During 2 years of treatment with melphalan and corticosteroids, he did not progress (86). The other two patients had high titers of anti-GD1a IgM antibodies. One was a 66-year-old woman with 8 months of progressive weakness and wasting in distal muscles in the arms and legs. The second was a 63-year-old woman with 6 months of asymmetric weakness who was unable to walk or use her upper limbs. Sensation was normal in both, and reflexes were absent except for reduced ankle reflexes in the second patient. CSF revealed one to three white blood cells, and the protein content was between 60 and 78 mg/dL. CMAP amplitudes and motor conduction velocities were reduced, the latter into a demyelinating range. Some sensory responses were abnormal in the first patient, although they were normal in the other. The first patient did not respond to IVIg or oral cyclophosphamide. There was a slight but progressive improvement with prednisone leading to the ability to stand and walk with a cane. The other patient improved with IVIg and later rapidly deteriorated despite prednisone and plasma exchange, but reinstitution of IVIg and oral cyclophosphamide led to improvement. In two other

patients with IgG anti-GD1a antibodies and GBS, the clinical improvement was accompanied by a corresponding decline in anti-GD1a titers (87).

IgG AND IgA MONOCLONAL GAMMOPATHIES

Patients with motor neuropathies and nonmalignant IgA monoclonal gammopathies have also been reported (88,89) including several with IgA-δ monoclonal gammopathies (90–92). One patient had motor neuropathy with an IgG-k paraprotein and the Crow-Fukase syndrome of gynecomastia, hypertrichosis, leg edema, impotence, and a raised CSF protein (93). It is not known whether the monoclonal gammopathy in these patients were coincidental or related to the neuropathy.

TREATMENT OF MOTOR NEUROPATHY

The treatment of choice for motor neuropathy is IVIg, which has been shown effective in placebo-controlled trials (4,94). A favorable response of IVIg was reported in 67 to 100% of patients (95,96), including reduction of the degree of conduction block and an increase in the amplitude of the CMAP (21). However, its effect is transient, and prolonged therapy is often required. Frank remissions with (95) or without therapy (97) have also been reported, with benefit lasting up to 4 years (95). Patients can occasionally have a diminished response after prolonged treatment (95,98), but responsiveness to IVIg can sometimes be restored with plasmapheresis, similarly to that of CIDP (99). Of the patients with motor neuropathy and anti-GM1 antibodies, those with conduction block have the best response to IVIg (4), and of those with MMN, the presence of anti-GM1 antibodies is associated with a better therapeutic response (95). Patients without anti-GMI antibodies or conduction block also respond to IVIg (31,35).

The mode of action of IVIg in motor neuropathy is probably multifactorial. Although titers of anti-GM1 antibodies remain unchanged after IVIg treatment, it probably exerts anti-idiotypic activity (100,101) or blocks Fc-receptor-mediated recruitment of macrophages and inhibits complement activation and the action of various cytokines, as suggested in other autoimmune diseases (102–104).

Motor neuropathy is also responsive to the chemotherapeutic agents chlorambucil (55), cyclophosphamide (20, 32,43), and fludarabine (105), which lower autoantibody titers and serum IgM concentrations and lessen dependency on IVIg. Oral cyclophosphamide or plasmapheresis have generally been ineffective (6,34). Corticosteroids are rarely beneficial and have been associated with disease exacerbations (43–45).

Rare patients with motor neuropathy without nerve conduction abnormalities suggesting demyelination also respond to immunosuppressive medications, including chlorambucil (55); plasmapheresis followed by cyclophosphamide (106); IVIg (107); or plasmapheresis, dexamethasone, and cyclophosphamide (39).

REFERENCES

1. Rossi O. La neurite sistematizzata motrice. *Rassegna Clin Sci* 1928; VI:3–7.
2. Hyland HH, Russell WR. Chronic progressive polyneuritis, with report of a fatal case. *Brain* 1930;53:278–289.
3. Wilson SAK. Motor neuritis. In: Wilson SAK, eds. *Neurology*. Baltimore: Williams & Wilkins, 1940:305–307.
4. Azulay JP, Blin O, Pought J, et al. Intravenous immunoglobulin treatment in patients with motor neuron syndromes associated with anti-GM1 antibodies: a double-blind, placebo-controlled study. *Neurology* 1994;44:429–432.
5. Lange DJ, Trojaborg W, Latov N, et al. Multifocal motor neuropathy with conduction block: is it a distinct clinical entity? *Neurology* 1992;42:497–505.
6. Kaji R, Shibasaki H, Kimura J. Multifocal demyelinating motor neuropathy: cranial nerve involvement and immunoglobulin therapy. *Neurology* 1992;42:506–509.
7. Magistris M, Roth G. Motor neuropathy with multifocal persistent conduction blocks [letter]. *Muscle Nerve* 1992;9:1056–1057.
8. Parry GJG. Motor neuropathy with multifocal persistent conduction blocks [reply]. *Muscle Nerve* 1992;1057.
9. Evangelista T, Carvalho M, Conceicao I, Pinto A, de Lurdes M, Luis ML. Motor neuropathies mimicking amyotrophic lateral sclerosis/motor neuron disease. *J Neurol Sci* 1996;139:95–98.
10. Kaji R, Mezaki T, Hirota N, Kimura J, Shibasaki H. Multifocal motor neuropathy with exaggerated deep tendon reflexes. *Neurology* 1994; 44:A180(abst).
11. Kinsella LJ, Lange DJ, Trojaborg W, Sadiq SA, Younger DS, Latov N. Clinical and electrophysiologic correlates of elevated anti-GM1 antibody titers. *Neurology* 1994;44:1278–1282.
12. Roth G, Rohr J, Magistric MR, Ochsner F. Motor neuropathy with proximal multifocal persistent conduction block, fasciculations, and myokymia. Evolution to tetraplegia. *Eur Neurol* 1986;25:416–423.
13. Bouche P, Moulonguet A, Younes-Chennoufi AB, et al. Multifocal motor neuropathy with conduction block: a study of 24 patients. *J Neurol Neurosurg Psychiatry* 1995;59:38–44.
14. Lewis RA, Sumner AJ, Brown MJ, Asbury AK. Multifocal demyelinating neuropathy with persistent conduction block. *Neurology* 1982; 32:958–964.
15. Parry GJ, Clarke S. Pure motor neuropathy with multifocal conduction block masquerading as motor neuron disease. *Muscle Nerve* 1985;8: 617(abst).
16. Parry GJ, Clarke S. Multifocal acquired demyelinating neuropathy masquerading as motor neuron disease. *Muscle Nerve* 1988;11: 103–107.
17. Brown WF. Acute and chronic inflammatory demyelinating neuropathies. In: Brown WF, Bolton CF, eds. *Clinical electromyography*, 2nd ed. Boston: Butterworth Heinemann, 1993.
18. Koles ZJ, Rasminsky M. A computer simulation of conduction in demyelinated nerve fibers. *J Physiol* 1972;227:351–364.
19. Cornblath DR, Sumner AJ. Conduction block in neuropathies with necrotizing vasculitis. *Muscle Nerve* 1991;2:185–186.
20. Pestronk A, Cornblath DR, Ilyas AA, et al. A treatable multifocal motor neuropathy with antibodies to GM1 ganglioside. *Ann Neurol* 1988;24:73–73.
21. Chaudhry V, Corse AM, Cornblath DR, Kuncl RW, Freimer ML, Griffin JW. Multifocal motor neuropathy: electrodiagnostic features. *Muscle Nerve* 1994;17:198–205.
22. Auer RN, Bell RB, Lee MA. Neuropathy with onion bulk formations and pure motor manifestations. *Can J Neurol Sci* 1989;16:194–197.
23. Santoro M, Thomas FP, Fink ME, et al. IgM deposits at nodes of Ranvier in a patient with amyotrophic lateral sclerosis, anti-GM1 antibodies, and multifocal motor conduction block. *Ann Neurol* 1990;28: 273–377.
24. Adams D, Kuntzer T, Steck AJ, Lobrinus A, Janzer RC, Regli F. Motor conduction block and high titers of anti-GM1 ganglioside antibodies:

25. pathological evidence of a motor neuropathy in a patient with lower motor neuron syndrome. *J Neurol Neurosurg Psychiatry* 1993;56: 982–987.
25. Van Den Bergh P, Logigian EL, Kelly JJ. Motor neuropathy with multifocal conduction blocks. *Muscle Nerve* 1989;12:26–31.
26. Krarup C, Stewart JD, Sumner AJ, Pestronk A, Lipton SA. A syndrome of asymmetrical limb weakness and motor conduction block. *Neurology* 1990;40:118–127.
27. Oh SJ, Kim DE, Kuruoglu HR. What is the best diagnostic index of conduction block and temporal dispersion. *Muscle Nerve* 1994;17: 489–4983.
28. Rhee EK, England JD, Sumner AJ. A computer simulation of conduction block: effects produced by actual block versus interphase cancellation. *Ann Neurol* 1990;28:146–156.
29. Cornblath DR, Sumner AJ, Daube J, et al. Conduction block in clinical practice. *Muscle Nerve* 1991;14:869–871.
30. Lange DJ, Trojaborg W, McDonald TD, Blake DM. Persistent and transient conduction block in motor neuron diseases. *Muscle Nerve* 1993;16:896–903.
31. Katz JS, Wolfe GI, Bryan WW, Jackson CE, Amato AA, Barohn RJ. Electrophysiologic findings in multifocal motor neuropathy. *Neurology* 1997;48:700–707.
32. Krarup C, Sethi RK. Idiopathic brachial plexus lesion with conduction block of the ulnar nerve. *Electroencephalogr Clin Neurophysiol* 1989; 72:259–267.
33. Parry GJG. Motor Neuropathy with multifocal conduction block. In: Dyck PJ, Thomas PK, et al., eds. *Peripheral neuropathy*, 3rd ed. Philadelphia: W.B. Saunders, 1993:1343–1353.
34. Kaji R, Oka N, Tsuji T, et al. Pathological findings at the site of conduction block in multifocal motor neuropathy. *Ann Neurol* 1993; 33:152–158.
35. Corbo M, Abouzahr MK, Latov N, et al. Motor nerve biopsy studies in motor neuropathy and motor neuron disease. *Muscle Nerve* 1997; 20:15–21.
36. Hays AP. Separation of Motor Neuron diseases from pure motor neuropathies: pathology. In: Rowland LP, ed. *Amyotrophic lateral sclerosis and other motor neuron diseases*. New York: Raven Press, 1991: 385–398.
37. Corse AM, Chaudry V, Crawford TO, Cornblath DR, Kuncl RW. Sensory nerve pathology in multifocal motor neuropathy. *Ann Neurol* 1996;3:319–325.
38. Rowland LP, Defendini R, Sherman W, et al. Macroglobulinemia with peripheral neuropathy simulating motor neuron disease. *Ann Neurol* 1982;11:532–536.
39. Parry GJ, Holtz SJ, Ben-Zeev D, Drori JB. Gammopathy with proximal motor axonopathy simulating motor neuron disease. *Neurology* 1986;36:273–276.
40. Ropper AH, Gorson KC. Autopsy of chronic inflammatory axonal motor radiculoneuropathy resembling motor neuron disease. *Neurology* 1997;48:A226(abst).
41. Taylor BV, Gross L, Windebank AJ. The sensitivity and specificity of anti-GM1 antibody testing. *Neurology* 1996;47:951–955.
42. Krendal DA. Biopsy findings link multifocal motor neuropathy to chronic inflammatory demyelinating polyneuropathy. *Ann Neurol* 1996; 40:948–950(letter).
43. Feldman EL, Bromberg MB, Albers JW, Pestronk A. Immunosuppressive treatment in multifocal motor neuropathy. *Ann Neurol* 1991;30: 397–401.
44. Donaghy M, Mills KR, Boniface SJ, et al. Pure motor demyelinating neuropathy: deterioration after steroid treatment and improvement with intravenous immunoglobulin. *J Neurol Neurosurg Psychiatry* 1994;57:778–783.
45. Thomas PK, Claus DJ, Workman JM, et al. Focal upper limb demyelinating neuropathy. *Brain* 1996;119:765–774.
46. Latov N. Pathogenesis and therapy of neuropathies associated with monoclonal gammopathies. *Ann Neurol* 1995;37:S32–42.
47. Logothetis J, Silverstein P, Coe J. Neurological aspects of Waldenström's macroglobulinemia. *Arch Neurol* 1960;3:564–573.
48. Harbs H, Arfmann M, Frick E, et al. Reactivity of sera and isolated monoclonal IgM from patients with Waldenström's macroglobulinemia with peripheral nerve myelin. *J Neurol* 1985;232:43–48.
49. Kyle RA, Garton JP. The spectrum of IgM monoclonal gammopathy in 430 cases. *Mayo Clin Proc* 1987;62:719–731.
50. Nobile-Orazio E, Marmiroli P, Baldini L, et al. Peripheral neuropathy

in macroglobulinemia: incidence and antigen specificity of M-proteins. *Neurology* 1987;37:1506–1514.

51. Svennerholm L. Designation and schematic structure of gangliosides and allied glycosphingolipids. *Progr Brain Res* 1994;101:xi–xiv.

52. Willison HJ. Antiglycolipid antibodies in peripheral neuropathy: fact or fiction? *J Neurol Neurosurg Psychiatry* 1994;57:1303–1307.

53. Peters HA, Clatanoff DV. Spinal muscular atrophy secondary to macroglobulinemia: reversal of symptoms with chlorambucil therapy. *Neurology* 1968;18:101–108.

54. Freddo L, Yu RK, Latov N, et al. Gangliosides GM1 and Gd1b are antigens for IgM M-protein in a patient with motor neuron disease. *Neurology* 1986;36:454–458.

55. Latov N, Hays AP, Donofrio PD, et al. Monoclonal IgM with a unique specificity to gangliosides GM1 and GD1b and to lacto-*N*-tetraose associated with human motor neuron disease. *Neurology* 1988;33:763–768.

56. Yuki N, Yoshino H, Sato S, Miyatake T. Acute axonal polyneuropathy associated with anti-GM1 antibodies following *Campylobacter* enteritis. *Neurology* 1990;40:1900–1902.

57. Ilyas AA, Willison HJ, Dalakas M, Whitaker JN, Quarles RH. Identification and characterization of gangliosides reacting with IgM paraproteins in three patients with neuropathy and biclonal gammopathy. *J Neurochem* 1988;51:851–858.

58. Kusunoki S, Shimizu T, Matsumura K, Maemura K, Mannen T. Motor dominant neuropathy and IgM paraproteinemia: the IgM M-protein binds to specific gangliosides. *J Neuroimmunol* 1989;21:177–181.

59. Baba H, Daune GC, Ilyas AA, et al. Anti-GM1 ganglioside antibodies with differing specificities in patients with multifocal motor neuropathy. *J Neuroimmunol* 1989;25:143–150.

60. Sadiq SA, Thomas FP, Kilidireas K, et al. The spectrum of neurological disease associated with anti-GM1 antibodies. *Neurology* 1990;40:1067–1072.

61. Corbo M, Quattrini A, Lugaresi A, et al. Patterns of reactivity of human anti-GM1 antibodies with spinal cord and motor neurons. *Ann Neurol* 1992;32:487–493.

62. Corbo M, Quattrini A, Latov N, Hays AP. Localization of GM1 and Gal(B1-3)GalNAc antigenic determinants in peripheral nerve. *Neurology* 1993;43:809–816.

63. Apostolski S, Sadiq SA, Hays A, et al. Identification of Gal(B1-3)GalNAc bearing glycoproteins at the nodes of Ranvier in peripheral nerve. *J Neurosci Res* 1994;38:134–141.

64. Thomas FP, Adapon PH, Goldberg GP, Latov N, Hays AP. Localization of neural epitopes that bind to IgM monoclonal autoantibodies (M-proteins) from two patients with motor neuron disease. *J Neuroimmunol* 1989;21:31–39.

65. Ogawa-Goto K, Funamoto N, Abe T, Nagashima K. Different ceramide compositions of gangliosides between human motor and sensory nerves. *J Neurochem* 1990;55:1486–1492.

66. Ogawa-Goto K, Funamoto N, Ohta Y, Abe T, Nagashima K. Myelin gangliosides of human peripheral nervous system: an enrichment of GM1 in the motor nerve myelin isolated from cauda equina. *J Neurochem* 1992;59:1844–1848.

67. Thomas FP, Trojaborg W, Nagy C, et al. Experimental autoimmune neuropathy with anti-GM1 antibodies and immunoglobulin deposits at the nodes of Ranvier. *Acta Neuropathol* 1991;82:278–383.

68. Santoro M, Uncini A, Corbo M, et al. Experimental conduction block induced by serum from a patient with anti-GM1 antibodies. *Ann Neurol* 1992;31:385–390.

69. Heiman-Patterson T, Krupa T, Thompson P, Nobile-Orazo E, Tahmoush AJ, Shy ME. Anti-GM1/GDLB M-proteins damage human spinal cord neurons co-cultured with muscle. *J Neurol Sci* 1991;30:38–45.

70. Willison HJ, Roberts M, O'Hanlon G, Paterson G, Vincent A, Newsom Davis J. Human monoclonal anti-GM1 ganglioside antibodies interfere with neuromuscular transmission. *Ann Neurol* 1994;36:289.

71. Roberts M, Willison HJ, Vincent A, Newsom-Davis J. Multifocal motor neuropathy human sera block distal motor nerve conduction in mice. *Ann Neurol* 1995;38:111–118.

72. Takigawa T, Yasuda H, Kikkawa R, Shigeta Y, Saida T, Kitasato H. Antibodies against GM1 ganglioside affect K+ and Na+ currents in isolated rat myelinated nerve fibers. *Ann Neurol* 1995;37:436–442.

73. Kaji R, Hirota N, Oka N, et al. Anti-GM1 antibodies and impaired blood-nerve barrier may interfere with remyelination in multifocal motor neuropathy. *Muscle Nerve* 1994;17:108–110.

74. Weng NP, Yu-Lee LY, Sanz I, Patten BM, Marcus DM. Structure and specificities of anti-ganglioside autoantibodies associated with motor neuropathies. *J Immunol* 1992;149:2518–2529.

75. Marcus DM, Went N. The structure of human anti-ganglioside antibodies. *Progr Brain Res* 1994;101:289–293.

76. Walsh FS, Cronin M, Koblar S, et al. Association between glycoconjugate antibodies and *Campylobacter* infection in patients with Guillain-Barré syndrome. *J Neuroimmunol* 1991;34:43–51.

77. Van den Berg LH, Marrink J, de Jager AEJ, et al. Anti-GM1 antibodies in patients with Guillain-Barré syndrome. *J Neurol Neurosurg Psychiatry* 1992;55:6–11.

78. McKhann GM, Cornblath DR, Griffin JW, et al. Acute motor axonal neuropathy: a frequent cause of acute flaccid paralysis in China. *Ann Neurol* 1993;33:333–342.

79. Kornberg A, Pestronk A, Bieser K, et al. The clinical correlates of high-titer IgG anti-GM1 antibodies. *Ann Neurol* 1994;35:234–237.

80. Aspinall GO, McDonald AG, Raju TS, et al. Serological diversity and chemical structure of *Campylobacter jejuni* low-molecular weight lipopolysaccharides. *J Bacteriol* 1992;174:1324–1332.

81. Yuki N, Handa S, Taki T, et al. Cross-reactive antigen between nervous tissue and bacterium elicits Guillain-Barré syndrome: molecular mimicry between ganglioside GM1 and lipopolysaccharide from Penner's serotype 19 of *Campylobacter jejuni. Biomed Res* 1992;13:451–453.

82. Wirguin I, Suturkova-Milosevic LJ, Della-Latta P, Fisher T, Brown RH Jr, Latov N. Monoclonal IgM antibodies to GM1 and asialo-GM1 in chronic neuropathies cross-react with *Campylobacter jejuni* lipopolysaccharides. *Ann Neurol* 1994;35:698–703.

83. Latov N, Koski CL, Walicke PA. Guillain-Barré syndrome and parenteral gangliosides [letter]. *Lancet* 1991;338:757.

84. Nobile-Orazio E, Carpo M, Meucci N, et al. Guillain-Barré syndrome associated with high titers of anti-GM1 antibodies. *J Neurol Sci* 1992;109:200–206.

85. Landi G, D Alessandro R, Dossi BC, Ricci S, Simone IL, Cioccone A. Guillain-Barré syndrome after exogenous gangliosides in Italy. *BMJ* 1993;307:1463–1464.

85a. Illa I, Ortiz N, Gallard E, Juarez C, Grau J, Dalakas MC. Acute axonal Guillain-Barré syndrome with Ig antibodies against motor axons following parenteral gangliosides. *Ann Neurol* 1995;38:218–224.

86. Bollensen E, Schipper HI, Steck AJ, et al. Motor neuropathy with activity of monoclonal IgM antibody to GD1a ganglioside. *J Neurol* 1989;236:353–355.

87. Carpo M, Nobile-Orazio E, Neucci N, et al. Anti-GD1a ganglioside antibodies in peripheral motor syndromes. *Ann Neurol* 1996;39:539–543.

88. Yeung KB, Thomas PK, King RHM, et al. The clinical spectrum of peripheral neuropathies associated with benign monoclonal IgM, IgG, IgA paraproteinaemia. Comparative clinical, immunological and nerve biopsy findings. *J Neurol* 1991;238:383–391.

89. Chazot G, Berger B, Carrier H, et al. Manifestations neurologiques des gammopathies monoclonales. *Rev Neurol* 1976;132:195–212.

90. Bosch EP, Ansbacher LE, Goeken JA, Cancilla PA. Peripheral neuropathy associated with monoclonal gammopathy. Studies of intraneural injections of monoclonal immunoglobulin sera. *J Neuropathol Exp Neurol* 1982;41:446–459.

91. Nemni R, Mamoli A, Fazio R, et al. Polyneuropathy associated with IgA monoclonal gammopathy: a hypothesis of its pathogenesis. *Acta Neuropathol* 1991;81:371–376.

92. Hemachudha T, Phanuphak P, Phanthumchinda K, Kasempimolpron S. Proximal motor neuropathy, IgA paraproteinaemia and anti-myelin-associated glycoprotein reactivity. *Postgrad Med J* 1989;65:662–664.

93. Berkovic SF, Scarlett JD, Symington GR, Dennett X, Woodruff RK. Proximal motor neuropathy, dermato-endocrine syndrome, and IgGk paraproteinemia. *Arch Neurol* 1986;43:845–848.

94. Van den Berg LH, Kerkhoff H, Oey PL, et al. Treatment of multifocal motor neuropathy with high dose intravenous immunoglobulins: a double blind, placebo controlled study. *J Neurol Neurosurg Psychiatry* 1995;59:248–252.

95. Azulay J, Rihet P, Pouget J, et al. Long term follow up of multifocal motor neuropathy with conduction block under treatment. *J Neurol Neurosurg Psychiatry* 1997;62:391–394.

96. Chaudhry V, Corse AM, Cornblath DR, et al. Multifocal motor neuropathy: Response to human immune globulin. *Ann Neurol* 1993;33:237–242.

97. Chad DA, Hammer K, Sargent J. Slow resolution of multifocal weak-

ness and fasciculation: a reversible motor neuron syndrome. *Neurology* 1986;36:1260–1263.

98. Elliott JL, Pestronk A. Progression of multifocal motor neuropathy during apparently successful treatment with human immunoglobulin. *Neurology* 1994;44:967–968.

99. Berger AR, Herskovitz S, Scelsa S. The restoration of IVIg efficacy by plasma exchange in CIDP. *Neurology* 1995;45:1628–1629.

100. Yuki N, Miyagi F. Possible mechanism of intravenous immunoglobulin treatment on anti-GM1 antibody-mediated neuropathies. *J Neurol Sci* 1996;139:160–162.

101. Mali U, Oleksowicz L, Latov N, Cardo LJ. Intravenous g-globulin inhibits binding of anti-GM1 to its target antigen. *Ann Neurol* 1996; 39:136–139.

102. Kurlander RJ. Reversible and irreversible loss of Fc receptor function of human monocytes as a consequence of interaction with immunoglobulin G. *J Clin Invest* 1980;66:776–781.

103. Basta M, Dalakas MC. High-dose intravenous immunoglobulin exerts its beneficial effect in patients with dermatomyositis by blocking endomysial depostition of activated complement fragments. *J Clin Invest* 1994;94:1729–1735.

104. Abe Y, Horiuchi A, Miyake M, Kimura S. Anti-cytokine nature of natural human immunoglobulin;one possible mechanism of the clinical effect of intravenous immunoglobulin therapy. *Immunol Rev* 1994; 139:5–19.

105. Sherman WH, Latov N, Lange D, Hays AP, Younger D. Fludarabine for IgM antibody mediated neuropathies. *Ann Neurol* 1994;36:326.

106. Pestronk A, Lopate G, Kornberg AJ, et al. Distal lower motor neuron syndrome with high-titer serum IgM anti-GM1 antibodies: improvement following immunotherapy with monthly plasma exchange and intravenous cyclophosphamide. *Neurology* 1994;44:2027–2031.

107. Van den Berg LH, Franssen H, Van Doorn PA, Wokke JHJ. Intravenous immunoglobulin treatment in lower motor neuron disease associated with highly raised anti-GM1 antibodies. *J Neurol Neurosurg Psych* 1997;63:674–677.

Motor Disorders,
edited by David S. Younger.
Lippincott Williams & Wilkins, Philadelphia © 1999.

CHAPTER 20

Peripheral Nerve Vasculitis

John T. Kissel and Michael P. Collins

Disturbances of motor function are the most prominent manifestations of peripheral nerve vasculitis. Although occasional patients have predominantly, or exclusively, sensory symptoms and signs, most patients present with complaints related to the motor system (1–15). Weakness resulting from ischemic damage to the motor nerves is obviously the most common source of motor disturbance in these patients, but other factors are also important. Because peripheral nerve vasculitis frequently occurs in the setting of an underlying collagen vascular disease, superimposed involvement of the joints, as with vasculitis in rheumatoid arthritis, can also seriously impair motor function. In addition, the severe dysesthetic pain frequently seen in vasculitic neuropathy patients can itself limit normal motor function because of the patient's reluctance to move the affected painful limb.

All these facets of motor dysfunction generally respond to immunosuppressive therapy and supportive measures. Vasculitic neuropathy is one of the most treatable causes of neurologic morbidity. Neuropathy often represents the earliest, and at times the only, manifestation of vasculitis that when severe can be life threatening. Therefore, it is important to recognize patients with both disorders. This chapter reviews the classification, presentation, immunopathogenesis, diagnosis, treatment, and prognosis of peripheral nerve vasculitis.

DEFINITION AND CLASSIFICATION

Vasculitis refers to a heterogeneous group of diseases characterized by inflammation and necrosis of blood vessel walls. It leads to narrowing and thrombosis of vessel lumina and secondary ischemia of dependent tis-

J. T. Kissel and M. P. Collins: Department of Neurology, Ohio State University, Columbus, Ohio 43210.

TABLE 1. *Classification of vasculitides*

A. Vasculitides resulting from direct infection
  1. Bacterial (e.g., syphilis, tuberculous, ?Lyme)
  2. Fungal (e.g., cryptococcus, aspergillosis)
  3. Rickettsial (e.g., Rocky Mountain Spotted Fever)
  4. Viral (e.g., herpes zoster, cytomegalovirus, ?HIV)
B. Vasculitides resulting from immunologic mechanisms
  1. Systemic necrotizing vasculitis
    a. Classic polyarteritis nodosa (PAN)
    b. Antineutrophil cytoplasmic antibody-associated
      ii Wegener's granulomatosis
      ii. Churg-Strauss syndrome
      iii. Microscopic polyangiitis
    c. Vasculitis with connective tissue disease (CTD)
    d. PAN related to hepatitis B virus
    e. Polyangiitis overlap syndrome
  2. Hypersensitivity vasculitis
    a. Primary
      i. Henöch-Schonlein purpura
      ii. Cutaneous leukocytoclastic angiitis
    b. Secondary[a]
      i. Vasculitis associated with infections
      ii. Vasculitis associated with malignancy
      iii. Drug-induced vasculitis (e.g., amphetamines, cocaine)
      iv. Vasculitis with CTD
      v. Essential mixed cryoglobulinemia
  3. Giant-cell arteritis
    a. Temporal arteritis
    b. Takayasu's arteritis
  4. Localized vasculitis
    a. Isolated peripheral nerve vasculitis (nonsystemic vasculitic neuropathy)
    b. Isolated central nervous system vasculitis
    c. Localized vasculitis of other organs (e.g., gastrointestinal tract, testicles, uterus, retina, skin, kidney)

[a]Each of these entities can also produce a systemic necrotizing vasculitis less commonly.

TABLE 2. *Clinical and pathologic features of primary and secondary vasculitides associated with peripheral nerve involvement*

Disorder	Histopathology	Vessels affected	Other organs involved (%)	Laboratory studies (%)	PNS, CNS changes	Tissues to biopsy	References
Group 1							
Classic polyarteritis nodosa	Necrotizing vasculitis; mixed infiltrate	Small and medium arteries	Kidneys (not GN) ~70 Skin ~50 Muscles ~40 GI ~30 Testes 5–30 Heart ~15	↑ ESR ~90 RF 40–50 ↓ Comp ~25 Hep B ~30 Hep C 5–20 ANCA 10–20 Angio (+) 70%	PNS ~60 CNS 10–20	Nerve Muscle Skin Kidney Rectum Testis	16, 18–21, 23–28, 52
Microscopic polyangiitis	Necrotizing vasculitis; mixed infiltrate[a]	Arterioles, capillaries, venules	Glomerulonephritis ~100 Lungs 40–50 GI, skin ~50 Eye ~30 Spleen ~30 Muscles ~20	ANCA 75–90 (p > c) RF 40–50 ↓ Comp—rare Hep B (-) Angio ~ rare (+)	PNS ~20 CNS 10–15	Kidney Lungs Skin Nerve	16, 20, 21, 24, 29, 52
Churg-Strauss syndrome	Necrotizing vasculitis; eosinophils; granulomas[a]	Small and medium-sized vessels	Lungs 100 Skin ~60 GI ~50 Heart ~50 Kidneys (GN) ~40 ENT ~25	ANCA 60–75 (p > c) ↑ eos ~100 ↑IgE ~75 RF ~50	PNS ~65 CNS ~25	Nerve Skin Lungs Kidney ENT	16, 19–21, 24, 25, 27, 30, 52
Wegener's granulomatosis	Necrotizing vasculitis; granulomas[a]	Small and medium arteries, arterioles, capillaries, venules, veins	ENT > 90 Lungs ~85 Kidneys (GN) ~75 Eyes ~50 Skin 40–50	ANCA 60–90 RF ~60	PNS ~15 CNS 4–8	ENT Lungs (open) Kidney Orbit Skin Nerve	16, 19–21, 25, 26, 31–33,52
Rheumatoid vasculitis	Necrotizing vasculitis; small-vessel intimal hyperplasia[a]	All sizes, types	Skin ~75 Muscle ~50 Heart 30–40 Spleen ~25 GI ~10	RF > 95 ↓ Comp ~60 ANCA 15–75 ANA 20–60	PNS 40–50 CNS—rare	Nerve Muscle Skin Rectum Salivary gland	16, 20, 23, 25, 34–36, 52
Lupus vasculitis	Necrotizing vasculitis[a]	Small, and medium-sized vessels	Skin ~90 Other organs rare	ANA 99 dsDNA 50–70 Sm 20–30 Ro 25–60 La 10–35 RF ~30	PNS ~10 CNS 5–10	Skin Nerve Kidney	16, 20, 23, 25, 35, 37, 38, 52, 53
Sjögren's— associated vasculitis	Necrotizing Small-vessel endarteritis[a]	Small-medium arteries, arterioles, capillaries, venules	Skin ~75 GI ~50 Glomerulonephritis ~50 Muscle ~50 Lungs, spleen, ENT rare	ANA ~90 Ro 40–95 La 70–90 RF ~60 ↓ Comp > 50	PNS ~40 CNS—?	Nerve Kidney	16, 23, 25, 35, 39, 40, 53
Group 2							
Hypersensitivity vasculitis	LCV in skin	Arterioles, capillaries, venules	Skin 100 (GN) 7–40 GI 5–10 Heart 0–25	↑ ESR 40–70 RF ~15 ANA ~15 ↓ Comp—rare	PNS—rare CNS—rare	Skin Kidneys	16, 18, 25, 26, 43, 44, 46
Henoch-Schönlein purpura	LCV in skin; IgA vascular deposits	Arterioles, capillaries, venules	Skin 100 GI 40–70 Kidneys (GN) 20–60	↑ ESR ~20 ↑ IgA ~50 ↓ Comp—rare	PNS—rare CNS—rare	Skin Kidney	
Mixed[a] cryoglobulinemic vasculitis	Necrotizing vasculitis; occlusive microangiopathy; LCV in skin	Small arteries, arterioles, capillaries, venules	Skin ~75 GN ~20 Raynaud's 20–45 GI (pain) ~10	RF > 80 ↓ Comp > 50 Hep C ~80 Hep B ~5	PNS ~50 CNS—rare	Skin Nerve Kidney	16, 20, 21, 47–49
Group 3							
Temporal arteritis	Necrotizing vasculitis; granulomas and giant cells ~50%	Medium-large arteries	PMR ~50 ↑LFTs 30 Subclavian, brachial, vertebral, abdominal aorta ~10	↑ ESR > 85 ANCA—rare Angio— infrequent (+)	Optic nerve 20–35 PNS ~20(?) CNS ~4	Temporal artery Nerve	19, 21, 25, 26, 50-52
Group 4							
Isolated peripheral nerve vasculitis	Necrotizing vasculitis; epineurial > perineurial	Small arteries, arterioles	Muscle 80	↑ ESR ~60	PNS 100 CNS 0	Nerve Muscle	4, 7–15, 25, 56

[a]All may be associated with leukocytoclastic vasculitis in skin.

ANCA, antineutrophil cytoplasmic autoantibodies; angio-abdominal angiographically demonstrated microaneurysms; CNS, central nervous system; comp, circulating complement factors; ENT, upper respiratory tract involvement; GN, glomerulonephritis; LCV, leukocytoclastic vasculitis; PMR, polymyalgia rheumatica; PNS, peripheral nervous system; RA, rheumatoid arthritis; RF, rheumatoid factor; SLE, systemic lupus erythematosus.

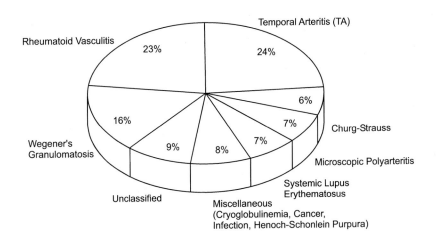

FIG. 1. Graph illustrating relative annual incidence of the various types of vasculitis. Numbers given are in percent of all cases. (From Refs. 54 and 55.)

sues (16). Since the initial description of "periarteritis nodosa" by Kussmaul and Maier in 1866 (17) in a patient with peripheral neuropathy, the clinical and pathologic features of numerous vasculitic syndromes have been described, and multiple classification schemes have been proposed to provide a conceptual framework for these diseases (16,18–20). Although all the proposed schemes are slightly different, most classify the syndromes predominately on the basis of the size and location of involved vessels. In addition, most systems distinguish between the primary and secondary vasculitides.

In 1994, the Chapel Hill Consensus Conference on the Nomenclature of Systemic Vasculitis (21) proposed a classification scheme with many advantages over prior schemes. However, our categorization, as outlined in Table 1, is more comprehensive, stresses etiologies, and groups the disorders along common management approaches. It generally follows the scheme of Jennette and Falk (22), wherein two major groups of disorders are recognized: those associated with direct infection of the vessels or primary immunologic phenomenon. The immune-mediated disorders are divided into four additional groups as follows: group 1, those typically associated with multiorgan failure and an ominous prognosis; group 2, hypersensitivity vasculitis with skin involvement and of a specific initiating factor or identifiable antigen; group 3, giant cell arteritides which are infrequently associated with neuropathy; and group 4, localized vasculitis, including nonsystemic vasculitic neuropathy. Peripheral neuropathy is a common feature in most systemic vasculitides occurring in up to 65% of patients with these syndromes (24). A summary of key distinguishing features for the primary and selected secondary disorders is outlined in Table 2 (16,18,20,21, 23–53).

Figure 1 illustrates the average annual incidence rates for the common vasculitides based on the new Chapel Hill Consensus Conference nomenclature and several recent epidemiologic studies (54,55). Temporal arteritis and rheumatoid vasculitis are the most common forms of systemic vasculitis. The relative frequency of vasculitic *neuropathy,* however, is quite different because of the differing prevalence of neuropathy in each disorder. Neuropathy is more common in systemic necrotizing vasculitis, excluding Wegener's granulomatosis, than in temporal arteritis. Moreover, nonsystemic vasculitic neuropathy cases are not accounted for in epidemiologic studies of systemic vasculitis. The combined incidence of each category of vasculitic neurpathy, abstracted from series dedicated to such patients, is compiled in Table 3 (2–12,15,56).

TABLE 3. *Relative prevalence of conditions reported in association with vasculitic neuropathy*

Type of vasculitis	Relative prevalence (%)
Classic polyarteritis nodosa or microscopic polyangiitis	31
Nonsystemic vasculitic neuropathy	28
Rheumatoid vasculitis	16
Connective tissue diseases not otherwise specified	7
Churg-Strauss syndrome	7
Lupus vasculitis	3
Primary Sjögren's syndrome	3
HIV infection	1
Mixed cryoglobulinemia	1
Wegener's granulomatosis	1
Miscellaneous (malignancy, scleroderma, temporal arteritis, hypereosinophilic syndrome, monoclonal gammopathy of undetermined significance)	2

Data based on review of 505 reported cases of vasculitic neuropathy (2–12,15,56).

CLINICAL FEATURES AND PRESENTATION

The clinical presentation of a patient with peripheral nerve vasculitis depends on three factors: distribution of the involved neural vessels, spectrum of extraneurologic organ involvement, and severity and rate of progression of the underlying vasculitic process. Patients with systemic necrotizing vasculitis (Table 1, group 1) will have other involved tissues besides the peripheral nerve, for example, skin, joints, kidneys, lungs, gastrointestinal tract, and central nervous system, although the dysfunction may be extremely mild or subclinical and detectable only after extensive laboratory evaluation (1–3,5,8,10, 12). Constitutional symptoms such as fever, weight loss, anorexia, myalgias, arthralgias, and nonspecific fatigue and "weakness" occur in about 80% of patients (2,4,5,9, 11). A careful general examination is mandatory to look for systemic abnormalities that may suggest a more generalized process. Although patients with nonsystemic vasculitic neuropathy (Table 1, group 4) lack systemic organ involvement, constitutional symptoms occur in about one half of patients (4,9,11,15).

The neuropathy associated with necrotizing arteritis has a characteristic clinical presentation whether it occurs alone or in association with systemic vasculitis. The onset is usually subacute, with symptoms present for weeks to months before presentation (6,14). Some patients may present with an onset so acute as to mimic Guillain-Barré syndrome, whereas others have an indolent course with mild symptoms present for years before presentation (4). Because ischemia does not have a predilection for motor and sensory fibers, both modalities are nearly always affected. Rare patients have exclusively sensory involvement, particularly in association with rheumatoid arthritis and human immunodeficiency virus infection (36,57). Focal weakness and numbness are the most common presenting symptoms, resulting from ischemic damage to mixed nerve trunks. The ischemia is painful, and most patients complain of deep aching discomfort in the affected limb that later evolves into burning dysesthetic pain (4,8,10,11).

There can be restricted symptomology such as unilateral foot drop or intrinsic hand muscle weakness due to single nerve involvement. However, because of the random and widespread nature of vasculitis, multifocal nerve involvement is more typical at the outset, with about one half of patients presenting with mononeuropathy multiplex (1,2,4, 5,7,10–14,56). Although in most cases of mononeuropathy multiplex the nerve deficits can be accurately localized to specific named nerves, in 25% there is extensive asymmetric or "overlapping" bilateral involvement. Untreated, mononeuropathy multiplex classically evolves in a step-wise fashion with progressive weakness and disability due to additional nerve lesions. Certain nerves appear to have a particular propensity for involvement, most likely because of their primary and collateral vascular supply (Table 4).

TABLE 4. *Most commonly involved nerves in vasculitic neuropathies*

Nerve	Frequency of involvement[a] (%)
Peroneal	90
Posterior tibial	38
Ulnar	35
Median	26
Radial	12
Femoral	6
Sciatic	3

[a]Numbers represent percent of reported cases with involvement of the particular nerve. Data are cumulative and based on review of five series involving 272 patients where the distribution of involvement was given (3,7,8,15,18).

Slowly progressive distal symmetric polyneuropathy occurs in about a third of all cases (1–15,56) and results from extensive ischemic involvement at many levels of multiple nerve trunks.

DIFFERENTIAL DIAGNOSIS

Conditions other than vasculitis can have a similar pattern of asymmetric or multifocal peripheral nerve involvement and should be considered as alternate diagnostic possibilities (Table 5). A careful history, examination, and diagnostic evaluation, including electrodiagnostic studies, serologies, and cerebrospinal fluid analysis supplemented by nerve and muscle biopsy, are all generally necessary to prove vasculitis and exclude other disorders. The more common disorders in this differential include multifocal sensorimotor chronic inflammatory demyelinating polyradiculoneuropathy, idiopathic plexopathy, sarcoidosis, Lyme disease in endemic areas, hereditary neuropathy with liability to pressure palsies, and diabetes mellitus. The latter can mimic vasculitis by producing cranial mononeuropathies, truncal neuropathies, entrapment neuropathies such as carpal tunnel syndrome and ulnar neuropathies, and rare nonentrapment limb mononeuropathies (58). Subacute, often asymmetric weakness and wasting of pelvifemoral muscles accompanied by thigh and hip pain may also occur in diabetic patients (58,59). This entity has been referred to as diabetic amyotrophy, proximal diabetic neuropathy, and the Bruns-Garland syndrome. The distal lower extremities and rarely the proximal upper extremities may also be affected. An ischemic pathogenesis related to changes in the endoneurial microvessels is the most likely proximate cause, but metabolic factors may also be important (59). Several recent reports of T-cell predominant perivascular inflammation, vascular complement deposition, and multifocal fiber loss with axonal degeneration in cutaneous nerve biopsies, along with anecdotal reports of responsiveness to immunotherapy, have prompted some investigators to propose a vasculitic basis for this particular diabetic condi-

TABLE 5. *Differential diagnosis of multifocal neuropathy*

A. Ischemic neuropathies
  1. Peripheral nerve vasculitis
  2. Diabetes mellitus
    a. Diabetic amyotrophy (proximal diabetic neuropathy)
    b. Mononeuropathy multiplex (cranial nerve, thoracic, limb)
  3. Bland microvasculopathy of scleroderma
B. Inflammatory/immune-mediated neuropathies[a]
  1. Sarcoidosis
  2. Multifocal demyelinating neuropathy with persistent conduction block
  3. Multifocal motor neuropathy
  4. Multifocal variants of Guillain-Barré syndrome
  5. Idiopathic brachial or lumbosacral plexopathy
  6. Eosinophilic syndromes
    a. Eosinophilia-myalgia syndrome
    b. Eosinophilic fasciitis (Shulman syndrome)
    c. Idiopathic hypereosinophilic syndrome
C. Infection-related neuropathies[a]
  1. Leprosy
  2. Lyme disease
  3. Retroviral (HIV, HTLV-1)
  4. Herpes virus (herpes-zoster, cytomegalovirus)
  5. Infective endocarditis
  6. Other (leptospirosis, hepatitis A, *M. pneumoniae*, ascaris, *Plasmodium falciparum*)
D. Drug-induced neuropathies[a]
  1. Antibiotics (penicillin, sulfonamides)
  2. Cromolyn
  3. Thiouracil
  4. Allopurinol
  5. Interferon-alpha
  6. Drugs of abuse (amphetamines, cocaine, heroin)
E. Hereditary neuropathies
  1. Hereditary neuropathy with liability to pressure palsies (HNPP)
  2. Hereditary neuralgic amyotrophy (HNA)
  3. HNA with relapsing multifocal sensory neuropathy
  4. Porphyria
  5. Tangier's disease
F. Traumatic neuropathies
  1. Multiple peripheral nerve injuries
  2. Burns
  3. Multifocal entrapments
    a. Diabetes mellitus
    b. HNPP
G. Neoplasia-related neuropathies
  1. Infiltrative processes
    a. Non-Hodgkin's lymphoma (B > T cell)
    b. Leukemia (T, B, NK cell)
    c. Angiocentric lymphoproliferative lesions
      (1) Lymphomatoid granulomatosis
      (2) Angiotropic lymphoma (B >> T cell)
    d. Hodgkin's lymphoma (rare)
    e. Multiple myeloma (rare)
    f. Carcinoma (with leptomeningeal metastases)
  2. Mass lesions
    a. Schwannomas (neurofibromatosis-1, -2)
    b. Extranodal lymphoma
    c. Chloroma (granulocytic sarcoma)
H. Other poorly validated or rare associations
  1. Wartenberg's migrant sensory neuritis
  2. Sensory perineuritis
  3. Cholesterol emboli syndrome
  4. Idiopathic thrombocytic purpura
  5. Gastrointestinal conditions (Crohn's, ulcerative colitis, celiac sprue)

[a]Some associated with vasculitis.
HTLV-I, human T-cell lymphotropic virus type I; NK, natural killer.

tion (60–62). However, frank necrotizing vasculitis is rare in these patients and multifocal fiber loss can also be observed in other types of diabetic neuropathy (60–63). Moreover, a beneficial response to treatment in patients with proximal diabetic neuropathy should be interpreted with caution because spontaneous recovery frequently occurs, even in those with inflammatory nerve lesions (64). Further studies are urgently needed to resolve these important issues.

EVALUATION AND DIAGNOSIS

Vasculitic neuropathy usually occurs in one of three clinical settings. The first is in the context of a previously diagnosed systemic vasculitis or another collagen vascular disease. Therein, the diagnosis is straightforward, and careful consideration of the clinical, electrophysiologic, and pathologic data will confirm the diagnosis of vasculitic neuropathy. The second scenario is the presentation of neuropathy as the predominant manifestation of an undiagnosed systemic condition affecting multiple organ systems. The clinician then attempts to define the extent and distribution of the involved organs and determines the most appropriate tissue to biopsy for diagnosis. In the third presentation, the most difficult to recognize, neuropathy is the only manifestation of vasculitis without other organ involvement. Although each of these clinical scenarios presents in a slightly different fashion, the evaluation of a patient with a suspected vasculitic neuropathy should always include blood work, electrodiagnostic studies, and, in most cases, cutaneous nerve and muscle biopsy. The suggested routine diagnostic tests for patients with an uncertain diagnosis are listed in Table 6, in addition to other tests that are useful in certain specific clinical situations. Approximately 25% of patients with vasculitic neuropathy will have cerebrospinal fluid protein elevation, but this finding is nonspecific and not usually helpful in making a definite diagnosis (5–7,9,10).

Nerve conduction studies and needle electromyography are mandatory in the evaluation of vasculitic neuropathy to document the extent and severity of individual nerve involvement. Patients with distal symmetric

TABLE 6. *Laboratory studies in patients with suspected vasculitic neuropathy*

Test	Associated conditions
Nonspecific measures of inflammation and organ involvement	
Complete blood count	Anemia: all systemic vasculitides ~40–50%
	Leukocytosis: all systemic vasculitides ~70%
	Thrombocytosis: all systemic vasculitides 40–65%
Erythrocyte sedimentation rate	Mild ↑ in ~60% of isolated PNS vasculitis; marked ↑ in ~85% of all systemic vasculitides
Chemistry panel	↑ BUN, creatinine: renal involvement
	↑ LFTs: liver involvement; hepatitis
	↑ Glucose: diabetes mellitus
Urinalysis	Proteinuria, hematuria, RBC casts: renal involvement or underlying connective tissue disease/malignancy
Chest films	Pulmonary involvement, sarcoidosis, malignancy, or lymphoproliferative lesions
Antinuclear antibody (ANA)	(+)>90% connective tissue diseases; ~30% systemic and ~20% nonsystemic vasculitis
Serum complements	↓ in >60% SLE, RV, EMC, Sjögren's; ~25% classic PAN
Rheumatoid factor	(+) >90% RV, EMC; 40–60% Wegener's, Sjögren's, PAN, MPA, CSS
More specific studies frequently useful	
Cryoglobulins	(+) in EMC/hepatitis C, plasma cell dyscrasias, lymphoproliferative disorders, PAN, connective tissue diseases, hepatitis B, other chronic infections
Eosinophil count	↑ in CSS (>>MPA, PAN), eosinophilia-myalgia syndrome, eosinophilic fasciitis, hypereosinophilic syndrome, some infections and drug reactions
Protein immunofixation, electrophoressis	Monoclonal protein: plasma cell dyscrasia, lymphoma, leukemia
Anti-dsDNA	(+) in SLE
Anti-Ro and -La	(+) in SLE and Sjögren's syndrome
Anti-Sm	(+) in SLE
Anti-Sc 70 and -centromere	(+) in scleroderma
Hepatitis B serologies	Surface antigen (+) in hepatitis B-associated PAN
Hepatitis C serology or RNA	(+) circulating antibodies and/or RNA in hepatitis C-associated EMC
Glycosylated hemoglobin	↑ in diabetes mellitus
More specific studies obtained selectively	
HIV serology	(+) in HIV infection, CMV multifocal neuropathy
HTLV-I serology	(+) in HTLV-I infection
Lyme serology	(+) in Lyme disease
cANCA (anti-proteinase 3)	(+) in Wegener's >> MPA, CSS (pANCA is too nonspecific to be useful)
Serum angiotensin-converting enzyme	↑ in sarcoidosis (leprosy, chronic hepatitis, lymphoma, diabetes, RV, scleroderma)

BUN, blood urea nitrogen; cANCA, classic antineutrophil cytoplasmic autoantibody; CSS, Churg-Strauss syndrome; EMC, essential mixed cryoglobulinemia; HNPP, hereditary neuropathy with liability to pressure palsies; LFTs, liver function tests; MPA, microscopic polyangiitis; PAN, polyarteritis nodosa; pANCA, perinuclear antineutrophil cytoplasmic autoantibody; PNS, peripheral nervous system; RV, rheumatoid vasculitis; SLE, systemic lupus erythematosus; HTLV-I, human T-cell lymphotropic virus type I; RBC, red blood cell.

polyneuropathy on clinical examination have significant asymmetry on electrodiagnostic studies suggesting overlapping multiple mononeuropathy (5,65). Electrical studies can also establish a baseline for the degree and pattern of axon loss to serve as a reference in monitoring the patient's response to therapy (2). This is particularly important in patients with severe disease because it may be difficult to assess their progression on clinical grounds alone. These studies also assist in the choice of the best nerve and muscle for biopsy (2). The specific findings on electrodiagnostic studies reflect the primary underlying pathology of vasculitic neuropathy, namely ischemic axonal damage that typically involves motor and sensory nerves (1–7,10,11,23,65). Compound sensory and motor action potentials are usually reduced in amplitude or unevokable, whereas conduction velocities are normal or mildly reduced and distal latencies are normal or mildly prolonged. Transient "conduction block" can be seen 6 to 10 days after ischemic injury but disappears as the axon degenerates (23,65). Persistent conduction block is uncommon in vasculitic neuropathy but can occur as a result of ischemia-induced metabolic failure or secondary paranodal and segmental demyelination (66–68). However, a predominance of demyelinating features is distinctly unusual and should prompt reconsideration of the diagnosis. The most commonly affected nerves in the legs are the peroneal and sural (2,4,10). The ulnar nerve followed by the median and radial nerves are the most frequently affected in the arms (23,65).

Electromyography reveals fibrillation potentials and positive sharp waves in about half of cases and decreased motor unit recruitment in clinically affected muscles (2,4,5). Proximal muscles can be affected to a similar degree as more distal ones, because vasculitis is not a length-dependent neuropathy (4). Chronic "neurogenic" potentials can be seen in patients with long-standing disease.

Although the clinical picture, laboratory testing, and electrophysiologic data may strongly suggest vasculitic neuropathy, definitive diagnosis requires pathologic confirmation in a sensory nerve. The sural and superficial peroneal nerves are most commonly chosen for biopsy; however, the latter is preferred because a peroneus brevis muscle biopsy can be obtained through the same incision (69). Combining nerve with a muscle biopsy increases the diagnostic yield, even in cases of "nonsystemic" vasculitic neuropathy (8). The sensitivity of diagnosing vasculitic neuropathy by combined biopsy is about 60 to 70% (13,70). The pathologic appearance of vasculitis in a peripheral nerve varies with the age of the lesion. Active lesions are characterized by inflammatory cells that invade the vessel wall associated with necrosis (Fig. 2). Chronic lesions show evidence of vascular repair, including intimal hyperplasia with variable lumenal narrowing, thrombosis, vascular recanalization, and perivascular macrophages filled with hemosiderin (Fig. 3) (16,25,56,71). Endothelial cell disruption and hemorrhage can occur but are not sufficient or required for diagnosis. Vasculitis of the nerve has a predilection for epineurial blood vessels with a diameter of 75 to 250 µm. For reasons that are unclear, endoneurial vessels are usually spared (4,7,10).

The pathologic changes in the nerve fascicles themselves, although not pathognomonic, are often distinctive

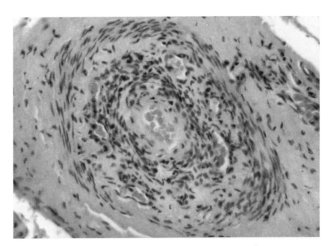

FIG. 3. Superficial peroneal nerve biopsy from patient with vasculitic neuropathy and more chronic vascular lesions. There are several small recanalization channels in the wall of the inflamed and damaged vessel (hematoxylin and eosin, ×500).

enough to strongly support the diagnosis of vasculitis in the appropriate clinical setting. There is nearly always a loss of myelinated nerve fibers that occurs asymmetrically between and within fascicles (Fig. 4) (4,7,56,71,72). Multiple fibers undergoing Wallerian degeneration are typically present (7,72). Large myelinated fibers are more susceptible to ischemia, but small myelinated fibers and unmyelinated fibers can also be affected in severe cases (72). In fulminant cases, Schwann cells, fibroblasts, and all other cellular elements may be lost, and the nerve can appear totally infarcted. Immunofluorescent staining is useful in confirming the diagnosis of vasculitis. Immune deposits of IgG, IgA, IgM, C3, and C5b-9 membrane

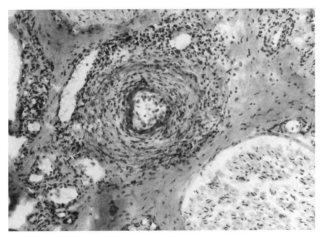

FIG. 2. Sural nerve biopsy from a patient with nonsystemic vasculitic neuropathy showing perivascular and transmural mononuclear cell infiltration in an epineurial vessel producing fibrinoid necrosis of the vessel wall (hematoxylin and eosin, ×350).

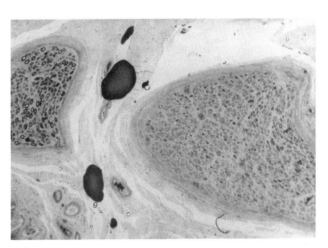

FIG. 4. Superficial peroneal nerve specimen from patient with rheumatoid vasculitis and vasculitic neuropathy showing marked asymmetry in the degree of myelinated fiber loss. The fascicle on the right demonstrates severe myelinated fiber loss, whereas that on the left is less affected (epoxy resin-embedded, toluidine blue stained, ×450).

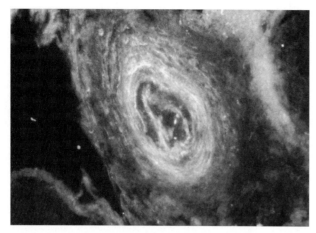

FIG. 5. Immunofluorescent staining of sural nerve in a case of systemic necrotizing vasculitis showing a single epineurial vessel with transmural deposition of IgM (fluorescein-conjugated anti-human IgM, ×375).

attack complex (MAC) are found in approximately 80% of patients (Fig. 5) (9,10,14,73) and appear to be specific for vasculitis (74). Perls' ferrocyanide test for perivascular iron may also be a sensitive and specific marker for vasculitic neuropathy (75).

PATHOGENESIS

Approximately 50% of vasculitic neuropathy cases occur in the setting of a systemic disease, most commonly polyarteritis nodosa or rheumatoid arthritis (Table 3). Another 10% are associated with infection, malignancy, or drug ingestion. An antigen-antibody complex related to the systemic illness presumably triggers the immunologic processes that result in vessel damage. In the remaining 40%, the neuropathy occurs without an associated condition or etiology. Although in all of these

settings, the pathogenesis is presumed to involve autoimmunity, the vasculitides must still be considered idiopathic in that very little is understood concerning their etiology or the antigens that trigger the immunological processes (except for some of the secondary syndromes such as polyarteritis nodosa related to hepatitis B) (22). The clinical, laboratory, and pathologic features of the various vasculitides are so protean that a single immunopathogenic mechanism cannot underlie all the syndromes and etiologies. It is likely that diverse mechanisms specific for the proximate disorder trigger and perpetuate equally diverse sequences of downstream immunologic events (76,77).

There has been remarkable progress in the past decade in the elucidation of effector mechanisms in systemic and peripheral nerve vasculitis (77,78). Table 7 summarizes the principal categories of immunologic phenomena that can cause vasculitis. Although these may seem mutually exclusive, in fact there are many similarities, and more than one may operate simultaneously in a given patient to produce vasculitis.

On a fundamental level, the postulated immunopathogenic mechanisms of vasculitis (Table 7) begin with antigen recognition by the host, initiating either a humoral or cellular immune response (or both), with the vascular endothelium assuming a pivotal role as the result of a disruption in the normal homeostasis between circulating leukocytes and endothelial cells (79). Selected leukocytes adhere to the endothelial surface, the cell type and specificity of which are determined by a complex network of cellular adhesion molecules and soluble mediators that affect their expression (80,81). An equally complex array of cytokines, chemotactic agents, and other inflammatory regulators are locally elaborated that mediate leukocyte and endothelial cell activation, adherence of additional effector cells, and transendothelial migration of leuko-

TABLE 7. *Proposed pathogenic mechanisms in vasculitides involving peripheral nerves*

Category	Antigen	Mechanisms	Effectors	Examples
Direct infection of blood vessels	Organism	Activation of inflammatory mediators, host's humoral and cellular response Cytopathic effect by virus	Neutrophils (bacteria) Lymphs, macrophages (most viruses; Lyme)	Cytomegalovirus Herpes zoster ?HIV, Lyme
Immune complexes	Viruses, drugs, IgG, tumor Unknown in most	Deposition of complexes in vessel walls, complement activation, effector cell recruitment	Neutrophils early Monocytes and macrophages late	Hypersensitivity Hep B-assoc PAN Rheumatoid vasculitis
ANCA-mediated	Proteinase 3 Myeloperoxidase	Activation of circulating neutrophils and monocytes; endothelial cell activation	Neutrophils early Eosinophils (CSS)	Wegener's MPA, CSS
T-cell–mediated	Unknown (? vessel wall)	Sensitization and activation of CD4+ T cells, release of pro-inflammatory cytokines	CD8+ cytotoxic T cells Monocytes and macrophages	? Temporal arteritis ? Wegener's, CSS, PAN ? Isolated PNS vasculitis

ANCA, antineutrophil cytoplasmic autoantibody; CSS, Churg-Strauss syndrome; MPA, microscopic polyangiitis; PAN, polyarteritis nodosa.

cytes (76,77,79–82). Effector cells damage the vessel wall by degradative enzyme release, respiratory burst-induced production of toxic oxygen free radicals, perforin- or MAC-mediated cytolysis, and enzyme-induced apoptosis (22,79). The cellular participants continue to express and release new cytokines that recruit new effector and regulatory immune cells to the site, promote procoagulant tendencies, and induce connective tissue reactions. Regulatory anti-inflammatory cytokines later assume a predominant role and downregulate the inflammatory process. Endothelial cell, fibroblast, and smooth muscle cell proliferation results in a thickened, scarred, and possibly thrombosed or occluded blood vessel (76, 81,83,84).

Irrespective of the exact immunopathogenesis, the expression and regulation of surface adhesion molecules on both endothelial cells and lymphocytes is crucial to the pathogenesis of all forms of vasculitis (76–82,85,86). Three large families of cellular adhesion molecules have been characterized, the selectins, integrins, and immunoglobulin superfamily, each of which includes multiple classes of adhesion molecules that are each expressed by differing groups of inflammatory and endothelial cells. Together they account for the bulk of inflammatory cell adhesion to and migration through endothelial cells. The role of cytokines and other inflammatory mediators in the activation of both the endothelium and the circulating and adherent effector cells is equally important (75–79,83,84). Given the extreme complexity of cytokine secretion and function, their specific role in the vasculitides is still difficult to elucidate. This has been reviewed extensively elsewhere (83,84).

The principal differences in the immunopathogenic mechanisms for the vasculitides lie in the cells and molecules that initially recognize the pathogenic antigens and those cells and molecules most important in effecting the final vessel damage (22,76,77). In immune complex-mediated vasculitides, circulating antibodies recognize an endogenous or exogenous antigen, forming complexes that deposit locally along blood vessel walls. The primary effector pathway results from complement activation, formation of MAC, and the recruitment of neutrophils to the site of blood vessel wall damage from which proteolytic enzymes are locally discharged, and activation of the coagulation system occurs. The immune complex mechanism appears to be of primary importance only in neuropathies that occur in the setting of hypersensitivity vasculitis or vasculitis with some connective tissue diseases and infections (22,77,78,87).

In other antibody-mediated vasculitides, autoantibodies are directed against antigens present in microvessels and other cells rather than circulating antigens. Anti-endothelial cell antibodies have been detected in some cases of systemic vasculitis, and antibodies to neutrophil cytoplasmic antigens have been demonstrated in most patients with Wegener's granulomatosis, classic and microscopic pol-

yarteritis, and Churg-Strauss syndrome (52,88). Anti-neutrophil cytoplasmic antibodies have a broad spectrum of activity and regulate a wide range of neutrophil functions that could result in endothelial cell damage, but their role in the pathogenesis of vasculitic neuropathy seems limited based on current evidence (22,52,89).

A primary cell-mediated process involving cytotoxic T cells now appears to be the predominant immunopathogenic mechanism for most cases of peripheral nerve vasculitis. Immunohistochemical analyses of peripheral nerve vasculitic lesions reveal that T cells and macrophages are the predominant cell types, whereas B cells and neutrophils, both important in the antibody-mediated mechanisms, are uncommon (9,73,90). Most T cells are CD8+ cytotoxic/suppressor cells, suggesting that direct cell-mediated mechanisms, possibly directed against the endothelium, are of primary pathogenic significance in this disorder (73). Similar findings have been reported in the pulmonary and temporal artery lesions of patients with Wegener's granulomatosis and temporal arteritis (91,92). The endothelial cells probably serve as antigen-presenting cells, with subsequent vascular damage mediated by degradative enzyme release, free radical production, perforin-mediated cytolysis, and induced apoptosis (81).

All vasculitic processes invariably result in narrowing or occlusion of affected vessels, with reduced blood flow and ischemic damage to the affected organs. Because of its rich anastomotic blood supply, the peripheral nerve is injured only after extensive involvement of the vasa nervorum and then frequently in the "watershed" zones of relatively poor perfusion (93). In the upper limb, the median and ulnar nerves frequently receive no nutrient arteries between the axilla and elbow, whereas in the lower limb, the sciatic nerve has few collateral feeding vessels between the inferior gluteal and popliteal arteries (71). The clinical relevance of these anatomic features has never been formally studied. However, large-vessel vasculitis might render these territories more susceptible to ischemic nerve damage.

TREATMENT

The remarkable achievements of the past 15 years in the immunopathogenic mechanisms of systemic and peripheral nerve vasculitis have not yet translated into an equally diverse array of therapeutic options. Current treatment of vasculitic neuropathy is far from satisfactory and reflects the intrinsic difficulties encountered in treating vasculitis in general. Most patients are treated with relatively non-specific immunosuppressive agents such as prednisone that result in global immunosuppression. Treatment decisions are still based largely on anecdotal evidence, because there are few prospective double-blind trials (94–96). Therapy has also been complicated by the difficulty involved in treating multiple organ systems in a given patient and the differing approaches by subspecialists.

The cornerstone of therapy for vasculitic neuropathy involves the removal of the inciting antigen, if it can be identified, and the prompt institution of aggressive immunosuppressive therapy for a duration sufficient to ensure that the inflammatory processes have been suppressed. Antigen removal is possible for relatively few of the vasculitides, particularly those related to drugs and infections. For example, there are several reports of a 70 to 80% response to antiviral therapy with vidarabine or interferon-α2, with or without concurrent plasma exchange, in patients with neuropathy and either hepatitis B associated-polyarteritis nodosa or hepatitis C-associated cryoglobulinemia (28,49,97,98).

In most patients with vasculitic neuropathy, however, the pathogenic antigen is not known; even in those patients where an inciting antigen can be identified, general immunosuppressive therapy is usually given (96). Many different regimens and agents have been used with varying success; however, the most consistently effective one for patients with systemic necrotizing vasculitis (group 1, Table 1) involves the combination of oral prednisone or intravenous methylprednisolone and cyclophosphamide (24,94,95). Patients with nonsystemic vasculitic neuropathy (group 4, Table 1) can be treated with prednisone alone if the clinical involvement is relatively mild. However, it has been our experience that more mistakes are made by undertreating vasculitic neuropathy than by overtreating it with combination therapy.

The standard regimen of prednisone 1.5 mg/kg/day and cyclophosphamide 1.5 to 2.5 mg/kg/day can each be taken in a single morning dose. In fulminant cases, there is a theoretical advantage in commencing with 1 g of intravenous methylprednisolone daily or on alternate days for five or six doses to control the inflammatory process more quickly (69,96,99). After 3 to 4 weeks of daily oral therapy, the prednisone can be switched to an alternate-day regimen at the same dose. The combination regimen is then maintained for 3 to 12 months or more, depending on the clinical response.

Several modifications of the above protocol have been described with varying degrees of success. Oral pulse therapy with doses of cyclophosphamide of up to 5 mg/kg/day for 2 to 5 days was used in patients with severe Wegener's granulomatosis (33), and intravenous pulsing has also been used in dose ranges of 350 to 1,000 mg/m^2 at 1- to 4-week intervals (94,99–101). These regimens appear to have fewer long-term side effects than daily oral therapy, including less hemorrhagic cystitis and bladder carcinoma, but their comparative efficacy is uncertain.

The primary goals of treatment are to stop progression of neurologic deficits, reduce pain related to ischemia, and restore an appropriate microenvironment to the nerve so that axonal regeneration can take place. Because this may be an extremely slow process, particularly if extensive and proximal axonal damage has occurred, actual clinical improvement in strength or sensation may not be evident for months after initiation of therapy. A common mistake in treatment is to assume that the immunosuppressive regimen is "not working" because the patient has noticed no clinical improvement and to switch to alternative agents. The first signs of improvement may only be reduced pain and a mild increase in proximal strength. Once the clinical status is stable and improvement maximized, the prednisone can be slowly tapered, as for example, by 5 mg every 2 to 3 weeks to avert disease exacerbation. If it does relapse, the patient can be pulsed with prednisone or methylprednisolone at doses equivalent to the initial therapy until control of the disease is again attained, and tapering is then resumed. Cyclophosphamide is continued for at least 1 year after disease stabilization and then tapered off over 4 to 8 weeks.

Patients who are not candidates for cyclophosphamide because of unacceptable or anticipated side effects or who progress while on it require alternative therapy (Table 8). In these instances, azathioprine or methotrexate are the suitable alternatives, but there is no clear evidence favoring one over the other (94,102,103). Cyclosporine has been used in resistant patients and should be considered in those refractory to all other agents or with tenuous bone marrow function (104).

Controlled trials of plasma exchange with standard immunosuppression in polyarteritis nodosa and Churg-Strauss syndrome showed no benefit (99), although it has been used with some success in combination with antiviral therapy for patients with hepatitis B-associated polyarteritis and cryoglobulinemia (96,98). Intravenous immunoglobulin has been tried in several different types of vasculitis. The initial results are encouraging, but controlled trials have not yet been reported, and no information exits regarding its effect on vasculitic neuropathy (105).

Comprehensive management of the patient with vasculitic neuropathy requires more than immunosuppressive treatment. A program of supportive measures is crucial in optimizing recovery. The most important of these include limiting the side effects of the immunosuppressive drugs by careful monitoring, pain management, controlling other conditions that may be contributing to ischemia, and providing optimal physical and occupational therapy.

Patients treated with prednisone must be carefully monitored for hypertension, weight gain, glucose intolerance, electrolyte imbalance, cataracts, glaucoma, osteoporosis, superimposed myopathy, and avascular necrosis of the hip (106). A tuberculin skin test should be placed before treatment, and antituberculosis prophylaxis should be given to positive responders. A low-sodium, low-simple-sugar, calorie-restricted diet limits weight gain in most patients. Calcium, vitamin D or calcitriol, biphosphonates, and estrogen supplements in postmenopausal women limit osteoporosis (107). Bone mineral density measurements should be obtained at baseline and repeated at 6- to 12-month intervals in appropriate

TABLE 8. *Alternative immunosuppressive agents in treatment of vasculitic neuropathies*

Drug	Mechanisms	Dose	Side effects	Laboratory monitoring
Azathioprine	Inhibits purine metabolism DNA/RNA synthesis Inhibits T, B, NK cell function	2–3 mg/kg/day	Marrow suppression, Hepatotoxicity, GI intolerance Systemic hypersensitivity Susceptibility to infection, Pancreatitis Malignancy (?)	CBC, LFTs, CXR
Methotrexate	Folate antagonist ↓ DNA/RNA synthesis	7.5–20 mg/wk (oral) 25–50 mg/wk (IM or IV)	Marrow suppression, GI intolerance Mucositis, hepatotoxicity, Alopecia Susceptibility to infection Pneumonitis, malignancy (?):	CBC, LFTs, CXR, creatinine Hep B and C
Cyclosporine	Suppression of T-cell activation and proliferation	3–5 mg/kg/day (oral)	Nephrotoxicity/hypertension HyperK, hypoMg, Gingival hyperplasia GI intolerance, hepatotoxicity Tremor, paresthesias, edema Encephalopathy/seizures·	CBC, LFTs, BUN, creatinine Electrolytes, Mg, urinalysis Blood pressure, drug levels
IVIg	Blocks F_c receptors on effector cells	0.4 mg/kg/day for 5 days	Fever, chills, myalgias, Headache, aseptic meningitis Nausea, rash, leukopenia	CBC, BUN, creatinine Quantitative immunoglobulins Urinalysis, hepatitis C transmission
	Inhibits complement deposition Idiotype/anti-idiotype interactions		Acute renal failure Anaphylaxis (IgA ↓)	Retinal necrosis

CBC, complete blood count; BUN, blood urea nitrogen; LFTs, liver function tests; CXR, chest x-ray; IVIg, intravenous immunoglobulin; NK, natural killer.

patients (107). The potential toxicity of cyclophosphamide, includes hemorrhagic cystitis in up to 40% of patients and bladder cancer in 5%, which can be minimized by aggressive oral hydration and frequent urination (108). The risk of *Pneumocystis carinii* pneumonia can be reduced with trimethoprim/sulfamethoxazole prophylaxis given three times weekly in patients taking *daily* glucocorticoids and a cytotoxic agent (108). The principal side effects of the other medications are given in Table 8.

Effective pain management is an important, and often neglected, aspect to the care of these patients. Aside from the obvious benefit to the patient's overall well-being, it permits more aggressive physical therapy to be performed and also allows the treating physician to more accurately assess changes in muscle strength by manual muscle testing. Agents such as the tricyclic antidepressants, carbamazepine, gabapentin, mexilitine, clonazepam, and topical lidocaine cream have all been used with varying degrees of success (109). Opioid therapy is often necessary to achieve adequate pain control.

Strenuous efforts should be made to limit the possible ischemia-enhancing effects of other conditions. Smoking should be discontinued, and diabetes should be controlled as tightly as possible. This is frequently a difficult task because prednisone therapy exacerbates glucose intolerance. Hyperlipidemia and hypertension should also be

treated. Antiplatelet agents should be considered in patients with signs of progressive neurologic injury despite aggressive immunosuppression (95).

Physical therapy is important for patients with significant motor impairments, not only to maintain range of motion and strength but also to improve functional status. There is convincing data that exercise that involves compressive force both reduces osteoporosis and minimizes the risk of steroid myopathy (110). Judicious bracing and the use of ambulatory aids in conjunction with physical therapy can be crucial in maintaining ambulation, although bracing can be extremely difficult in patients with joint deformities due to superimposed collagen-vascular disease. Occupational therapy can assist patients in their recovery of upper limb function and reacquisition of daily living skills.

PROGNOSIS

The value of combination immunosuppression therapy in patients with certain vasculitides is unquestionable. In Wegener's granulomatosis, a remission rate of 75% is now achievable, compared with a mean *survival* of only 5 months before the introduction of immunosuppressive agents (31). Similar results have been reported for polyarteritis nodosa and isolated central nervous system angiitis (95,102).

Although the prognosis is less well defined for patients with vasculitic neuropathy, three retrospective series have examined long-term outcome (7,10,14). These studies clearly demonstrate that patients with nonsystemic vasculitic neuropathy have a more benign prognosis than those with a systemic necrotizing vasculitis. Mortality, in particular, is much higher in the systemic group, with a 60% mortality within 5 years in one study (10). In contrast, patients with nonsystemic vasculitic neuropathy had an 85% survival after a mean follow-up of 11 years in one study and a 96% survival after 3 to 4 years in other series (7,14). The neurologic status of the patients with nonsystemic vasculitic neuropathy was also more likely to improve than the status of those with systemic disease.

Although there is strong support for the use of aggressive immunosuppression in vasculitic neuropathy patients, several long-term studies have identified disturbing aspects to the standard regimen that have a serious impact on prognosis (31,111). For example, about 50% of patients with Wegener's granulomatosis on chronic combination therapy suffer a disease relapse and 40% experience serious drug-induced side effects, with a 50% rate of significant infection. Even more ominously, there was a 2.4-fold increase in malignancy, a 30-fold increased risk of bladder cancer, and an 11-fold increase in lymphoma compared with a control population (31). These findings indicate that more effective and less toxic treatments are urgently needed for this group of diseases.

REFERENCES

1. Moore PN, Fauci AS. Neurologic manifestations of systemic vasculitis: a retrospective study of the clinicopathologic features and responses to therapy in 25 patients. *Am J Med* 1981;71:517–524.
2. Wees SJ, Sunwoo IN, Oh SJ. Sural nerve biopsy in systemic necrotizing vasculitis. *Am J Med* 1981;71:525–532.
3. Chang RN, Bell CC, Hallett M. Clinical characteristics and prognosis of vasculitic mononeuropathy multiplex. *Arch Neurol* 1984;41:618–621.
4. Kissel JT, Slivka AP, Warmolts JR, Mendell JR. The clinical spectrum of necrotizing angiopathy of the peripheral nervous system. *Ann Neurol* 1985;18:251–257.
5. Bouche P, Leger JM, Travers MA, Cathala HP, Castaigne P. Peripheral neuropathy in systemic vasculitis: clinical and electrophysiologic study of 22 patients. *Neurology* 1986;36:1598–1602.
6. Harati Y, Niakan E. The clinical spectrum of inflammatory-angiopathic neuropathy. *J Neurol Neurosurg Psychiatry* 1986;49:1313–1316.
7. Dyck PJ, Benstead TJ, Conn DL, Stevens JC, Windebank AJ, Low PA. Nonsystemic vasculitic neuropathy. *Brain* 1987;110:843–854.
8. Said G, Lacroix-Ciaudo C, Fujimura H, Blas C, Faux N. The peripheral neuropathy of necrotizing arteritis: a clinicopathological study. *Ann Neurol* 1988;23:461–465.
9. Panegyres PK, Blumbergs PC, Leong AS-Y, Bourne AJ. Vasculitis of peripheral nerve and skeletal muscle: clinicopathological correlation and immunopathogenic mechanisms. *J Neurol Sci* 1990;100:193–202.
10. Hawke SHB, Davies L, Pamphlett R, Guo Y-P, Pollard JD, McLeod JG. Vasculitic neuropathy: a clinical and pathological study. *Brain* 1991;114:2175–2190.
11. Nicolai A, Bonetti B, Lazzarino LG, Ferrari S, Monaco S, Rizzuto N. Peripheral nerve vasculitis: a clinico-pathological study. *Clin Neuropathol* 1995;14:137–141.
12. Singhal BS, Khadilkar SV, Gursahani RD, Surya N. Vasculitic neuropathy: profile of twenty patients. *J Assoc Physic India* 1995;43:459–461.
13. Chia L, Fernandez A, Lacroix C, Adams D, Plante V, Said G. Contribution of nerve biopsy findings to the diagnosis of disabling neuropathy in the elderly: a retrospective review of 100 consecutive patients. *Brain* 1996;119:1091–1098.
14. Davies L, Spies JM, Pollard JD, McLeod JG. Vasculitis confined to peripheral nerves. *Brain* 1996;119:1441–1448.
15. Said G. Peripheral neuropathy in polyarteritis nodosa. *Springer Semin Immunopathol* 1996;18:75–84.
16. Lie JT. Systemic and isolated vasculitis: a rational approach to classification and pathologic diagnosis. *Pathol Annu* 1989;24:25–114.
17. Kussmaul A, Maier R. Ueber eine bisher nicht bescriebene eigenthumliche Arterienerkrankung (Periarteritis nodosa), die mit Morbus Brightii und rapid fortschreitender allgemeiner Muskellahmung einhergeht. *Dtsch Arch Klin Med* 1866;1:484–517.
18. Fauci AS, Haynes BF, Katz P. The spectrum of vasculitis: clinical, pathological, immunologic, and therapeutic considerations. *Ann Intern Med* 1978;89:660–676.
19. Hunder GG, Arend WP, Bloch DA, et al. The American College of Rheumatology 1990 criteria for the classification of vasculitis: introduction. *Arthritis Rheum* 1990;33:1101–1107.
20. Valente RM, Hall S, O'Duffy JD, Conn DL. Vasculitis and related disorders. In: Kelley WN, Harris ED, Ruddy S, Sledge CB, eds. *Textbook of rheumatology,* 5th ed. Philadelphia: W.B. Saunders, 1997: 1079–1122.
21. Jennette JC, Falk AJ, Andrassy K, et al. Nomenclature of systemic vasculitides: proposal of an international concensus conference. *Arthritis Rheum* 1994;37:187–192.
22. Jennette JC, Falk RJ. Update on the pathobiology of vasculitis. In: Schoen FJ, Gimbrone MA, eds. *Cardiovascular pathology clinicopathologic correlations and pathogenetic mechanisms.* Baltimore: Williams & Wilkins, 1995:156–172.
23. Olney RK. AAEM minimonograph #38: neuropathies in connective tissue disease. *Muscle Nerve* 1992;15:531–542.
24. Lhote F, Guillevin L. Polyarteritis nodosa, microscopic polyangiitis, and Churg-Strauss syndrome: clinical aspects and treatment. *Rheum Dis Clin North Am* 1995;21:911–947.
25. Chalk CH, Dyck PJ, Conn DL. Vasculitic neuropathy. In: Dyck PJ, Thomas PK, Griffin JW, Low PA, Poduslo JF, eds. *Peripheral neuropathy,* 3rd ed. Philadelphia: W.B. Saunders, 1993:1424–1436.
26. Moore PM, Calabrese LH. Neurologic manifestations of systemic vasculitides. *Semin Neurol* 1994;14:300–306.
27. Guillevin L, Le Thi Huong D, Godeau P, Jais P, Wechsler B. Clinical findings and prognosis of polyarteritis nodosa and Churg-Strauss angiitis: a study in 165 patients. *Br J Rheumatol* 1988;27:258–264.
28. Guillevin L, Lhote F, Cohen P, et al. Polyarteritis nodosa related to hepatitis B virus: a prospective study with long-term observation of 41 patients. *Medicine* 1995;74:238–253.
29. Lhote F, Cohen P, Genereau T, Gayraud M, Guillevin L. Microscopic polyangiitis: clinical aspects and treatment. *Ann Med Intern* 1996;147: 165–177.
30. Sehgal M, Swanson JW, DeRemee RA, Colby TV. Neurologic manifestations of Churg-Strauss syndrome. *Mayo Clin Proc* 1995;70: 337–341.
31. Hoffman GS, Kerr GS, Leavitt RY, et al. Wegener granulomatosis: an analysis of 158 patients. *Ann Intern Med* 1992;116:488–498.
32. Nishino H, Rubino FA, DeRemee RA, Swanson JW, Parisi JE. Neurological involvement in Wegener's granulomatosis: an analysis of 324 consecutive patients at the Mayo Clinic. *Ann Neurol* 1993;33:4–9.
33. Duna GF, Galperin C, Hoffman GS. Wegener's granulomatosis. *Rheum Dis Clin North Am* 1995;21:949–986.
34. Vollertsen RS, Conn DL. Vasculitis associated with rheumatoid arthritis. *Rheum Dis Clin North Am* 1990;16:445–461.
35. Bacon PA, Carruthers DM. Vasculitis associated with connective tissue disorders. *Rheum Dis Clin North Am* 1995;21:1077–1096.
36. Puechal X, Said G, Hilliquin P, et al. Peripheral neuropathy with necrotizing vasculitis in rheumatoid arthritis: a clinicopathologic and prognostic study of thirty-two patients. *Arthritis Rheum* 1995;38: 1618–1629.
37. Omdal R, Mellgren SI, Husby G, Salvesen R, Henriksen OA, Torbergsen T. A controlled study of peripheral neuropathy in systemic lupus erythematosus. *Acta Neurol Scand* 1993;88:41–46.
38. Drenkard C, Villa AR, Reyes E, Abello M, Alarcon-Segovia D. Vasculitis in systemic lupus erythematosus. *Lupus* 1997;6:235–242.
39. Mellgren SI, Conn DL, Stevens JC, Dyck PJ. Peripheral neuropathy in primary Sjögren's syndrome. *Neurology* 1989;39:390–394.
40. Fox RI. Sjögren's syndrome. In: Kelley WN, Harris ED, Ruddy S,

Sledge CB, eds. *Textbook of rheumatology,* 5th ed. Philadelphia: W.B. Saunders, 1997:955–968.

41. Oddis CV, Eisenbeis CH, Reidbord HE, Steen VD, Medsger T. Vasculitis in systemic sclerosis: association with Sjögren's syndrome and the CREST syndrome variant. *J Rheumatol* 1987;14:942–948.

42. Seibold JR. Scleroderma. In: Kelly WN, Harris ED, Ruddy S, Sledge CB, eds. *Textbook of rheumatology,* 5th ed. Philadelphia: W.B. Saunders, 1997:1133–1162.

43. Calabrese LH, Michel BA, Bloch DA, et al. The American College of Rheumatology 1990 criteria for the classification of hypersensitivity vasculitis. *Arthritis Rheum* 1990;33:1108–1113.

44. Michel BE, Hunder GG, Bloch DA, Calabrese LH. Hypersensitivity vasculitis and Henoch-Schonlein purpura: a comparison between the 2 disorders. *J Rheumatol* 1992;19:721–728.

45. Robson WLM, Leung AKC. Henoch-Schonlein purpura. *Adv Pediatr* 1994;41:163–194.

46. Martinez-Taboada VM, Blanco R, Garcia-Fuentes M, Rodriguez-Valverde V. Clinical features and outcome of 95 patients with hypersensitivity vasculitis. *Am J Med* 1997;102:186–191.

47. Gemignani F, Pavesi G, Manganelli P, Ferraccioli G, Marbini A. Peripheral neuropathy in essential mixed cryoglobulinemia. *J Neurol Neurosurg Psychiatry* 1992;55:116–120.

48. Monti G, Galli M, Invernizzi F, et al. Cryoglobulinemias: a multi-centre study of the early clinical and laboratory manifestations of primary and secondary disease. *Q J Med* 1995;88:115–126.

49. David WS, Peine C, Schlesinger P, Smith SA. Nonsystemic vasculitic mononeuropathy multiplex, cryoglobulinemia, and hepatitis C. *Muscle Nerve* 1996;19:1596–1602.

50. Caselli RJ, Hunder GG. Neurologic complications of giant cell (temporal) arteritis. *Semin Neurol* 1994;14:349–353.

51. Hunder GG. Giant cell arteritis and polymyalgia rheumatica. *Med Clin North Am* 1997;81:195–219.

52. Kallenberg CGM, Brouwer E, Weening JJ, Cohen Tervaert JW. Antineutrophil cytoplasmic antibodies: current diagnostic and pathophysiological potential. *Kidney Int* 1994;46:1–15.

53. von Muhlen CA, Tan EM. Autoantibodies in the diagnosis of systemic rheumatic disease. *Semin Arthritis Rheum* 1995;24:323–358.

54. Watts RA, Scott DGI. Classification and epidemiology of the vasculitides. *Bailliere's Clin Rheumatol* 1997;11:191–217.

55. Watts RA, Carruthers DM, Scott DGI. Epidemiology of systemic vasculitis: changing incidence or definition? *Semin Arthritis Rheum* 1995;25:28–34.

56. Midroni G, Bilbao JM. *Biopsy diagnosis of peripheral neuropathy.* Boston: Butterworth-Heinemann, 1995:241–265.

57. Bradley WG, Verma A. Painful vasculitic neuropathy in HIV-1 infection: relief of pain with prednisone therapy. *Neurology* 1996;47:1446–1451.

58. Bruyn GW, Garland H. Neuropathies of endocrine origin. In: Vinken PJ, Bruyn GW, eds. *Handbook of clinical neurology.* Vol. 8. New York: North-Holland, 1970:29–71.

59. Barohn RJ, Sahenk Z, Warmolts JR, Mendell JR. The Bruns-Garland syndrome (diabetic amyotrophy) revisited 100 years later. *Arch Neurol* 1991;48:1130–1135.

60. Said G, Goulon-Goeau C, Lacroix C, Moulonguet A. Nerve biopsy findings in different patterns of proximal diabetic neuropathy. *Ann Neurol* 1994;35:559–569.

61. Dyck PJ, Giannini C. Pathologic alterations in the diabetic neuropathies of humans: a review. *J Neuropathol Exp Neurol* 1996;55:1181–1193.

62. Younger DS, Rosoklija G, Hays AP, Trojaborg W, Latov N. Diabetic peripheral neuropathy: a clinicopathologic and immunohistochemical analysis of sural nerve biopsies. *Muscle Nerve* 1996;19:722–727.

63. Dyck PJ, Lais A, Karnes JL, O'Brien P, Rizza R. Fiber loss is primary and multifocal in sural nerves in diabetic polyneuropathy. *Ann Neurol* 1986;19:425–439.

64. Said G, Elgrably F, LaCroix C, et al. Painful proximal diabetic neuropathy: inflammatory nerve lesions and spontaneous favorable outcome. *Ann Neurol* 1997;41:762–770.

65. Wilbourn AJ, Levin KH. Ischemic neuropathy. In: Brown WF, Bolton CF, eds. *Clinical electromyography,* 2nd ed. Boston: Butterworth-Heinemann, 1993:369–390.

66. Jamieson PW, Giuliani MJ, Martinez AJ. Necrotizing angiopathy presenting with multifocal conduction blocks. *Neurology* 1991;41:442–444.

67. Nukada H, Dyck PJ. Acute ischemia causes axonal stasis, swelling, attenuation and secondary demyelination. *Ann Neurol* 1987;22:311–318.

68. Parry GJ, Linn DJ. Conduction block without demyelination following acute nerve infarction. *J Neurol Sci* 1988;84:265–273.

69. Kissel JT, Mendell JR. Vasculitic neuropathy. *Neurol Clin* 1992;101:761–781.

70. Collins MP, Kissel JT, Sahenk Z, et al. Diagnostic value of combined superficial peroneal/peroneus brevis muscle biopsy in suspected vasculitis. *Ann Neurol* 1996;40:545–546(abst).

71. Dyck PJ, Conn DL, Ozaki H. Necrotizing angiopathic neuropathy: three-dimensional morphology of fiber degeneration related to sites of occluded vessels. *Mayo Clin Proc* 1972;47:461–475.

72. Fujimura H, LaCroix C, Said G. Vulnerability of nerve fibers to ischaemia: a quantitative light and electron microscopic study. *Brain* 1991;114:1929–1942.

73. Kissel JT, Riethman JL, Omerza J, Rammohan KW, Mendell JR. Peripheral nerve vasculitis: immune characterization of the vascular lesions. *Ann Neurol* 1989;25:291–297.

74. Schenone A, DeMartini I, Tabaton M, et al. Direct immunofluorescence in sural nerve biopsies. *Eur Neurol* 1988;28:262–269.

75. Adams CWM, Buk SJA, Hughes RAC, Leibowitz S, Sinclair E. Perls' ferrocyanide test for iron in the diagnosis of vasculitic neuropathy. *Neuropathol Appl Neurobiol* 1989;15:433–439.

76. Cid MC. New developments in the pathogenesis of systemic vasculitis. *Curr Opin Rheumatol* 1996;8:1–11.

77. Sneller MC, Fauci AS. Pathogenesis of vasculitic syndromes. *Med Clin North Am* 1997;81:221–242.

78. Haynes BF. Vasculitis: pathogenic mechanisms of vessel damage. In: Gallin JI, Goldstein IM, Snyderman R, eds. *Inflammation: basic principles and clinical correlates.* New York: Raven Press, 1992:921–941.

79. Ali H, Haribabu B, Richardson RM, Snyderman R. Mechanisms of inflammation and leukocyte activation. *Med Clin North Am* 1997;81:1–28.

80. Cohen Tervaert JW, Kallenberg CGM. Cell adhesion molecules in vasculitis. *Curr Opin Rheumatol* 1997;9:16–25.

81. Cotran RS, Briscoe DM. Endothelial cells in inflammation. In: Kelley WN, Harris ED, Ruddy S, Sledge CB, eds. *Textbook of rheumatology,* 5th ed. Philadelphia: W.B. Saunders, 1997:183–198.

82. Springer TA. Traffic signals for lymphocyte recirculation and leukocyte emigration: the multistep paradigm. *Cell* 1994;76:301–314.

83. Pober JS, Cotran RS. Cytokines and endothelial cell biology. *Physiol Rev* 1990;70:427–451.

84. Mosman T. Cytokines and immune regulation. In: Rich RR, Fleisher TA, Schwartz BD, Shearer WT, Strober W, eds. *Clinical immunology: principles and practice.* St. Louis: Mosby, 1996;217–230.

85. Imhof BA, Dunon D. Leukocyte migration and adhesion. *Adv Immunol* 1995;58:345–416.

86. Smith CW. Cellular adhesions and interactions. In: Rich RR, Fleisher TA, Schwartz BD, Shearer WT, Strober W, eds. *Clinical immunology: principles and practice.* St. Louis: Mosby, 1996;176–191.

87. Mannik M. Serum sickness and pathophysiology of immune complexes. In: Rich RR, Fleisher TA, Schwartz BD, Shearer WT, Strober W, eds. *Clinical immunology: principles and practice.* St. Louis: Mosby, 1996;217–230.

88. Del Papa N, Gambini D, Meroni PL. Anti-endothelial cell antibodies and autoimmune disease. *Clin Rev Allerg* 1994;12:275–286.

89. Locke IC, Cambridge G. Autoantibodies to neutrophil granule proteins: pathogenic potential in vasculitis? *Br J Biomed Sci* 1996;53:302–316.

90. Cid M-C, Grau JM, Casademont J, et al. Immune histochemical characterization of inflammatory cells and immunologic activation markers in muscle and nerve biopsy specimens from patients with systemic polyarteritis nodosa. *Arthritis Rheum* 1994;37:1055–1061.

91. Gephardt GN, Ahmad M, Tubbs RR. Pulmonary vasculitis (Wegener's granulomatosis): immunohistochemical study of T and B cell markers. *Am J Med* 1983;74:700–704.

92. Shiki H, Shimokama T, Watanabe T. Temporal arteritis: cell composition and the possible pathogenic role of cell-mediated immunity. *Hum Pathol* 1989;20:1057–1064.

93. McManis PG, Low PA, Lagerlund JD. Microenvironment of nerve: blood flow and ischemia. In: Dyck PJ, Thomas PK, Griffin JW, Low PA, Poduslo JF, eds. *Peripheral neuropathy,* 3rd ed. Philadelphia: W.B. Saunders, 1993:453–473.

94. Duna GF, Hoffman GS. Immunosuppression: new perspectives in the treatment of the systemic vasculitides. *Ann Intern Med* 1994;145:581–594.

95. Moore PM. Vasculitis: diagnosis and therapy. *Semin Neurol* 1994;14: 159–167.

96. Calabrese LH, Hoffman GS, Guillevin L. Therapy of resistant systemic necrotizing vasculitis: polyarteritis, Churg-Strauss syndrome, Wegener's granulomatosis, and hypersensitivity vasculitis group disorders. *Rheum Dis Clin North Am* 1995;21:41–57.

97. Ferri C, Marzo E, Longombardo G, et al. Interferon-alpha in mixed cryoglobulinemia patients: a randomized, crossover-controlled trial. *Blood* 1993;81:1132–1136.

98. Guillevin L, Lhote F, Gherardi R. The spectrum and treatment of virus-associated vasculitides. *Curr Opin Rheumatol* 1997;9:31–36.

99. Guillevin L, Lhote F, Cohen P, et al. Corticosteroids plus pulse cyclophosphamide and plasma exchanges versus corticosteroids plus pulse cyclophosphamide alone in the treatment of polyarteritis nodosa and Churg-Strauss syndrome patients with factors predicting poor prognosis. *Arthritis Rheum* 1995;38:1638–1645.

100. Hoffman GS, Leavitt RY, Fleisher TA, Minor JR, Fauci AS. Treatment of Wegener's granulomatosis with intermittent high-dose intravenous cyclophosphamide. *Am J Med* 1990;89:403–410.

101. Adu D, Pall A, Luqmani RA, et al. Controlled trial of pulse versus continuous prednisolone and cyclophosphamide in the treatment of vasculitis. *Q J Med* 1997;90:401–409.

102. Leib ES, Restivo C, Paulus HE. Immunosuppressive and corticosteroid therapy of polyarteritis nodosa. *Am J Med* 1979;67:941–947.

103. Sneller MC, Hoffman GS, Talar-Williams C, Kerr GS, Hallahan CW, Fauci AS. An analysis of forty-two Wegener's granulomatosis patients treated with methotrexate and prednisone. *Arthritis Rheum* 1995;38: 608–613.

104. Allen NB, Caldwell DS, Rice JR, McCallum RM. Cyclosporin A therapy for Wegener's granulomatosis. In: Gross WL, ed. *ANCA-associated vasculitides: immunological and clinical aspects.* New York: Plenum Press, 1993:473–476.

105. Lockwood CM. New treatment strategies for systemic vasculitis: the role of intravenous immune globulin therapy. *Clin Exp Immunol* 1996; 104[Suppl 1]:77–82.

106. Boumpas DT. Glucocorticoid therapy for immune diseases: basic and clinical correlates. *Ann Intern Med* 1993;119:1198–1208.

107. Hochberg MC, Prashker MJ, Greenwald M, et al. Recommendations for the prevention and treatment of glucocorticoid-induced osteoporosis (American College of Rheumatology Task Force on Osteoporosis Guidelines). *Arthritis Rheum* 1996;39:1791–1801.

108. Langford CA. Chronic immunosuppressive therapy for systemic vasculitis. *Curr Opin Rheum* 1997;9:41–47.

109. Galer BS. Neuropathic pain of peripheral origin: advances in pharmacologic treatment. *Neurology* 1995;45[Suppl 9]:S17–S25.

110. Dalakas M. Pharmacologic concerns of corticosteroids in the treatment of patients with immune-related neuromuscular diseases. *Neurol Clin* 1990;8:93–118.

111. Gordon M, Luqmani RA, Adu D, et al. Relapses in patients with a systemic vasculitis. *Q J Med* 1993;86:779–789.

Motor Disorders,
edited by David S. Younger.
Lippincott Williams & Wilkins, Philadelphia © 1999.

CHAPTER 21

Critical Illness Neuropathy and Myopathy

Charles F. Bolton

Weakness of limb and respiratory muscles is a serious and increasingly common problem in intensive care units (ICU). Its management demands neurologic consultation, creatine kinase (CK) measurements, electrophysiologic testing, magnetic resonance imaging (MRI) of the spinal cord, and sometimes biopsy of a muscle and nerve to diagnose this problem in the ICU of which there is a variety of causes. This chapter describes the general approach to the evaluation of neuromuscular disorders in the ICU.

NEUROMUSCULAR EVALUATION IN CRITICALLY ILL AND INJURED PATIENTS

Neuromuscular History

If the patient is alert and able to write, an adequate history can be obtained by having the patient respond by handwriting. If limb paralysis precludes this, the patient may respond by nodding or shaking the head for yes or no answers. If the patient is stuporous, confused, or comatose, the history of neuromuscular symptoms can generally be obtained from the referring physician, emergency room or ICU physician, hospital chart, relatives, friends, or an employer.

Spinal or radicular pain, bulbar or limb weakness, breathing difficulties, impaired sensation, bladder dysfunction, muscle cramping, fasciculation, and fatigability are important clues to an underlying neuromuscular disorder. The neuromuscular problem may follow a major surgical procedure, for example, surgery on the thoracic aorta that may accompany spinal cord ischemia and resulting paraplegia. Neuromuscular blocking agents, even short-acting ones such as vecuronium, can have an action of several hours in the setting of renal failure. It is

important to recognize the reasons for intubation and mechanical ventilation, whether for airway protection or weakness of the respiratory muscles, and the type of mechanical ventilation, frequency of intermittent mandatory ventilation, degree of pressure support, blood gas results, and the ability to breath while off the ventilator.

Neuromuscular Physical Examination

General inspection of the skin may reveal localized edema and redness at sites of compression that are likely to occur in patients with drug-induced coma lasting hours. Pressure at the site of an underlying peripheral nerve can cause mononeuropathy. Signs of sympathic insufficiency such as increased temperature, redness, and dry skin in a paretic lower limb compared with the opposite limb suggest a lesion of the lumbar plexus because sympathetic fibers bypass the caudal nerve roots.

Ptosis, asymmetric ocular palsies, and facial weakness require exclusion of a neuromuscular transmission defect. The response to a tracheal tug on the endotracheal tube assesses the ability to swallow and cough. Abnormalities of this type are seen in motor neuron disease, Guillain-Barré syndrome (GBS), and neuromuscular junction disorders.

Assessment of the respiratory system should be done in the presence of the intensivist and if necessary assisted by the respiratory technologist. The ability to breathe independently is assessed by discontinuing or altering mechanical ventilation by stopping intermittent mandatory ventilation while keeping the patient on pressure support or continuous positive airway pressure to overcome airway/ventilator resistance; a maximum of 15 minutes maintains reasonable oxygenation. Mechanical ventilation is warranted when there is respiratory distress, arterial oxygen saturation of < 90% based on an oximeter reading, or a significant rise in breath rate or blood pressure. Needle electromyogram (EMG) of the diaphragm can accurately assess the pattern of respiration by observ-

C.F. Bolton: Department of Clinical Neurological Sciences, University of Western Ontario and London Health Sciences Centre, London, Ontario N6A 4G5, Canada.

ing the bursts of motor unit potentials (MUPs) with each inspiration and may be of localizing value (Fig. 1). The overall strength and rate of respiratory effort should be ascertained. The signs of reduced movement of chest wall muscles on attempted inspiration with forced outward movement of the abdominal muscles as the diaphragm descends are important clinical clues of an underlying neuromuscular disorder.

Generalized or focal muscle wasting is difficult to determine in the presence of limb edema. An affected patient can have voluntary or semivoluntary movements in bulbar and limb muscles in a pattern that suggests hemiplegia, quadriplegia, or paraplegia. If there are no such movements, compression of the nail beds with a pencil may induce one of several involuntary motor responses. Simple flexion movement of the stimulated ipsilateral or contralateral limbs occurs on a reflex basis at the level of the spinal cord level and even in brain death. More complex movements of a voluntary nature require intact cerebral function. If the opposite hand accurately moves in a coordinated way to attempt to remove the painful stimulus, reasonable function of that limb must be present. In addition, the patterns of limb movement may offer further clues as to the presence or absence of coexisting neuromuscular disease. For example, painful stimulation that induces vigorous facial grimacing without limb movement often seen in severe forms of CIP implies normal afferent and efferent cranial conduction of the painful stimulus along peripheral and central nervous system (CNS) pathways. Similar findings are often seen in high cervical cord lesions, but because severe pain impulses are not transmitted through the spinal cord, facial grimacing is not present. Vigorous upward movement of the great toe

on plantar stimulation may be absent on the side of a peroneal nerve palsy. There may be absence of a knee jerk, suggesting lumbosacral plexopathy with particular involvement of the femoral nerve.

Laboratory Studies

The neurologic findings of lesions at various sites along the neuroaxis are shown in Fig. 2A through E. Acute spinal cord dysfunction, trauma, ischemia, infection, and spinal shock cause flaccid quadriplegia and areflexia simulating polyneuropathy unless careful testing with a pin reveals a clear sensory level. MRI is often necessary on a emergency basis to exclude a spinal cord lesion, followed by electrophysiologic studies over the next few days to exclude a polyneuropathy. Technical challenges to EMG can arise in the ICU due to electrical interference from adjacent machines, poorly grounded plug-ins, inadequate shielding of cables, and other electrical devices. The skin should be adequately prepared to reduce resistance. The 60-cycle notch filter on the EMG machine may have to be used. It may not be possible to electrically stimulate certain nerves due to the presence of intravascular lines, surgical wounds and dressings, casts, and splints. Cardiac arrhythmias may be induced if an electrical stimulus is applied along a limb with an intravascular line that resides distally in the heart, in which case it may be wise to test the opposite side. The ground electrode should be on the same side of the body that is being stimulated to avoid transmission of the electrical impulse through the heart. Virtually all EMG studies including those of the diaphragm are quite safe. In our experience, these various technical challenges can be eas-

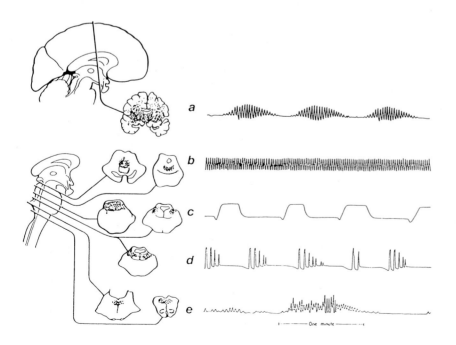

FIG 1. Abnormal respiratory patterns associated with pathologic lesions (shaded areas) at various locations in the brain. (*a*) Cheyne-Stokes respiration. (*b*) Central neurogenic hyperventilation. (*c*) Apneusis. (*d*) Cluster breathing. (*e*) Ataxic breathing. Here, respiratory movements were recorded with a chest-abdomen pneumograph, but we found such patterns can be detected from needle EMG recordings of the diaphragm. (From Ref. 70, with permission.)

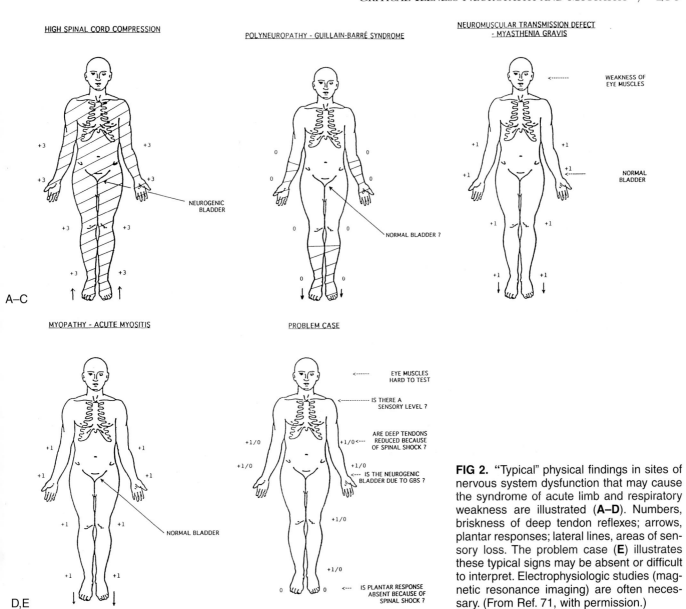

HIGH SPINAL CORD COMPRESSION

POLYNEUROPATHY - GUILLAIN-BARRÉ SYNDROME

NEUROMUSCULAR TRANSMISSION DEFECT - MYASTHENIA GRAVIS

NEUROGENIC BLADDER

NORMAL BLADDER ?

WEAKNESS OF EYE MUSCLES

NORMAL BLADDER

MYOPATHY - ACUTE MYOSITIS

PROBLEM CASE

NORMAL BLADDER

EYE MUSCLES HARD TO TEST

IS THERE A SENSORY LEVEL ?

ARE DEEP TENDONS REDUCED BECAUSE OF SPINAL SHOCK ?

IS THE NEUROGENIC BLADDER DUE TO GBS ?

IS PLANTAR RESPONSE ABSENT BECAUSE OF SPINAL SHOCK ?

A–C

D,E

FIG 2. "Typical" physical findings in sites of nervous system dysfunction that may cause the syndrome of acute limb and respiratory weakness are illustrated (**A–D**). Numbers, briskness of deep tendon reflexes; arrows, plantar responses; lateral lines, areas of sensory loss. The problem case (**E**) illustrates these typical signs may be absent or difficult to interpret. Electrophysiologic studies (magnetic resonance imaging) are often necessary. (From Ref. 71, with permission.)

ily overcome, and a complete electrophysiologic assessment can almost always be achieved.

ACUTE LIMB AND RESPIRATORY WEAKNESS DEVELOPING BEFORE ADMISSION TO THE CRITICAL CARE UNIT

This category includes patients who present with rapidly developing paralysis of limb and respiratory muscles requiring endotracheal intubation and mechanical ventilation. Their course may be so rapid that time is insufficient for an accurate diagnosis or screening diagnostic studies before admission to the ICU. In this acutely developing situation, clinical signs may be confusing. The differential diagnosis should be systematically approached (Table 1) and the relevant conditions eliminated (Fig. 3).

Spinal Cord Compression

In acute disorders of the high cervical spinal cord (Fig. 2), compression due to neoplasm, infection, or acute transverse myelitis, the traditional signs of localized spinal cord disease may be absent. Hyperreflexia is usually abolished by spinal shock, and the sensory level may be difficult to determine, particularly in high cervical lesions. Thus, MRI of the spinal cord on an emergency basis is generally necessary. Motor conduction studies show decreased compound muscle action potential (CMAP) amplitudes due to anterior horn cell injury if 5 days have already elapsed since the injury. If sensory nerve conduction studies (NCS) are normal and if clinical sensory loss is present, the lesion lies proximal to the dorsal root ganglion, usually indicating a myelopathy. Needle EMG abnormalities appear 10 to 20 days afterward in direct relation to the distance from the

TABLE 1. *Differential diagnosis in the intensive care unit (ICU) of the syndrome of rapidly developing weakness of limb and respiratory muscles*

Weakness before admission to the ICU	Weakness after admission to the ICU
Disorders of the spinal cord	
Traumatic myelopathy	
Acute epidural compression due to neoplasm, infection	
Acute transverse myelitis	
Acute ischemia	
Motor neuron disease	
Acute polyneuropathy	
Guillain-Barré syndrome (GBS)	Critical illness polyneuropathy
Axonal forms of GBS	Motor neuropathy (N-M blockers)
Acute motor and sensory neuropathy (AMSAN)	
Acute motor axonal neuropathy (AMAN)	
Miller-Fisher syndrome	
Chronic polyneuropathies	
Chronic inflammatory demyelinating polyneuropathy	Chronic polyneuropathies plus sepsis
Neuromuscular transmission defects	
Myasthenia gravis	N-M blockers
Lambert-Eaton myasthenic syndrome	
Hypocalcemia	
Hypermagnesemia	
Organophosphate poisoning	
Wound botulism	
Tick bite paralysis	
Myopathy	
Muscular dystrophy—Duchenne's, myotonic, etc.	Cachectic myopathy
Acute necrotizing myopathy-myoglobinuria	Necrotizing myopathy of intensive care
	Thick filament myopathy

From Ref. 71, with permission.

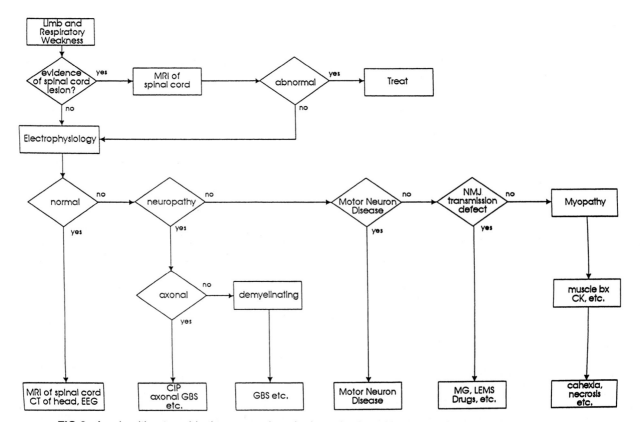

FIG 3. An algorithm to guide the approach to the investigation of intensive care unit patients who have weakness of limb and respiratory muscles. Note: Positive serology or stool culture for *C. jejuni* may be the earliest warning of the axonal form of GBS. MRI, magnetic resonance imaging; NMJ, neuromuscular junction; bx, biopsy; CK, creatine phosphokinase; CT, computed tomography; CIP, critical illness polyneuropathy; GBS, Guillain-Barré syndrome; MG, myasthenia gravis; LEMS, Lambert-Eaton myasthenic syndrome. (From Ref. 71, with permission.)

site of injury to the muscle examined. The pattern of needle EMG signs of denervation assists in localization of the segmental level, whether unilateral or bilateral, although it may not be precise due to considerable overlap of paraspinal muscle innervation. Scalp somatosensory evoked potential recordings generally reveal delayed or absent responses. Normal peripheral nerve and T12 responses localize the lesion to above the T12 level. Absent or delayed T12 responses suggest that the lesion is in the region of the cauda equina or lumbosacral plexus if peripheral nerve somatosensory evoked potentials are normal. Unless the spinal cord lesion clearly involves the somaesthetic pathways, somatosensory evoked potential results may be normal in the presence of a spinal cord lesion of considerable size.

Motor Neuron Disease

Motor neuron disease may present, for the first time and initially undiagnosed, as severe respiratory insufficiency (1). The combination of clinical upper and lower motor neuron signs, including hyperreflexia, weakness, wasting and fasciculation, makes the diagnosis inescapable; however, lingual signs my be overlooked in an intubated patient. Electrophysiologic studies confirm the diagnosis and exclude motor neuropathy with multifocal conduction block (2). Phrenic nerve conductions and needle EMG of the chest wall and diaphragm can be helpful in selected patients.

Acute Polyneuropathy

Polyneuropathy is generally suspected (Fig. 2) in the presence of weakness, hyporeflexia, and distal sensory loss.

Acute Inflammatory Demyelinating Polyneuropathy and Guillain-Barré Syndrome

The electrophysiologic features of GBS reflect peripheral nerve demyelination. In the initial stages, conduction velocities are mildly depressed or normal, F waves are prolonged or absent, and there may be evidence of conduction block and rapidly firing MUPs without spontaneous needle activity (3). NCS and EMG of the diaphragm are particularly valuable in establishing the type and severity of phrenic nerve and diaphragm involvement (4,5). Serial electrophysiologic studies are valuable in following the course of the disease and response to treatment, after plasmapheresis, intravenous immunoglobulin, or corticosteroids. In our experience, symptomatic improvement precedes electrophysiologic improvement. Except for the Miller Fisher syndrome comprising ophthalmoplegia, ataxia and areflexia, primarily axonal variants of GBS (Table 1), require management in the ICU. Serology or stool culture evidence of

Campylobacter jejuni may be a proximal precipitating factor in these axonal forms (6).

Acute Motor and Sensory Axonal Neuropathy

This form (7) of rapidly developing paralysis reaches completion over hours and requires prompt admission to the ICU for ventilatory assistance. With varying severity, virtually all muscles of the body, including cranial musculature, may be totally paralyzed. At the worst extreme, it clinically simulates brain death; however, the electroencephalogram is normal. The peripheral cranial nerves may be unresponsive to high-voltage and long-duration electrical stimulation. Sensory nerve action potential (SNAP) and CMAP are reduced or absent.

Acute Motor Axonal Neuropathy

This is an acute paralytic syndrome of children and young adults (8). It ascends symmetrically over days with normal sensation and often preserved deep tendon reflexes. The cerebrospinal fluid protein is increased without pleocytosis. Electrophysiologic studies reveal motor axonopathy. CMAP amplitudes are reduced with normal distal latencies and SNAP responses. There are varying degrees of denervation on needle EMG. There may be significant respiratory paralysis. Good recovery eventually occurs. This variant of GBS may be related to *C. jejuni* enteritis arising through cross-reacting anti-GM antibodies (9). Acute porphyria, Lyme disease, and human immunodeficiency virus infection may present with a similar syndrome.

Chronic Polyneuropathies

Chronic polyneuropathies occasionally evolve rapidly with respiratory insufficiency. Although rare, it may occur in chronic inflammatory demyelinating polyneuropathy and diabetic polyneuropathy. In addition to the more typical clinical and electrophysiologic signs of these polyneuropathies, phrenic NCS and needle EMG of the diaphragm confirm the neuropathic basis of the respiratory insufficiency.

Neuromuscular Transmission Defects

Defects in neuromuscular transmission (Fig. 2) are rare but present particular challenges in diagnosis. Respiratory insufficiency may be the presenting feature of myasthenia gravis or Lambert-Eaton myasthenic syndrome (10,11) accompanied by weakness in swallowing and breathing muscles. There is an experimental model of a rare variant of myasthenic crisis (12). The unequivocal diagnosis of myasthenia gravis rests on the presence of fluctuation of weakness in eye, facial, and limb muscles; a positive edrophonium test; and decremented response of sequential CMAP with 3 per second supramaximal stimulation; and elevated titers of acetylcholine receptor antibodies. Phrenic NCS and needle EMG studies of the diaphragm may reveal partial denervation. Immunomodulating therapy improves all aspects of myasthenia gravis, including respiratory muscles, that precedes successful weaning from the ventilator.

The Lambert-Eaton myasthenic syndrome, hypocalcemia, hypermagnesemia, organophosphate poisoning, and wound botulism may affect presynaptic neuromuscular transmission and may be identifiable on electrophysiologic studies.

Myopathies

Patients with chronic myopathy (Fig. 2) may require intubation and admission to the ICU because of respiratory muscle weakness, although the diagnosis is usually evident as in the case of muscular dystrophy. In more acute myopathies, such as necrotizing myopathy with myoglobinuria, the diagnosis is later evident because of high serum levels of CK, myoglobinuria, and necrosis on a muscle biopsy.

ACUTE LIMB AND RESPIRATORY WEAKNESS DEVELOPING AFTER ADMISSION TO THE INTENSIVE CARE UNIT

At least 50% of patients in large medical and surgical ICUs have significant involvement of the nervous system. Neuromuscular problems are much more frequent than is generally recognized. Sepsis and multiple organ failure now occur in 20 to 50% of patients in a medical ICU (13), and 70% of such patients have CIP (14). Neuromuscular blocking agents and steroids may cause further distinctive neuromuscular syndromes (15,16). The difficulty in clinically evaluating patients with neuromuscular problems, often with difficulty in weaning from the ventilator, has led to increased reliance on electrophysiologic studies (17) and occasionally muscle and nerve biopsy. This subject has been recently reviewed (15,16,18,19).

Myelopathy

Myelopathies seen in the ICU are usually due to trauma, compression by neoplasm, hemorrhage, or infection in the epidural space or infarction of the spinal cord infarction secondary to surgical procedures on the aorta. In most instances the myelopathy occurs before admission to the ICU.

Acute Polyneuropathy

Critical Illness Polyneuropathy

Since its initial description 13 years ago (20), CIP has been recognized as a common polyneuropathy, occurring in 50 to 70% of critically ill or injured patients (14,21, 22). Such patients are now included in the syndrome termed systemic inflammatory response syndrome (SIRS) (23). It occurs in response to both infection and several forms of trauma, including major surgery and burns. Because SIRS occurs in half of all patients in a general medical or surgical ICU, it should be regarded as a common polyneuropathy (Table 2). Indeed, we encounter it almost as frequently as GBS. CIP has been reviewed by Leijten and de Weerd (18), Hund (19), Bolton (23), and Leijten (24). The latter investigator described 150 cases reported in the literature up to 1993 and added 50 cases of his own. Hund et al. (25) recently identified a low-molecular-weight humoral neurotoxic factor in the sera of patients with CIP.

The earliest nervous system manifestation of SIRS is septic encephalopathy, characterized by inattention and disorientation (26). The patient gradually slips into coma, usually without focal signs, seizures, myoclonus, or asterixis. The electroencephalogram is a sensitive indicator of the presence and severity of septic encephalopathy. Computed tomography (CT) and MRI of the brain and serial neurologic examinations are usually unremarkable (27).

If SIRS can be treated specifically with antibiotics, surgical drainage of an infected focus, inotropic drugs, or fluid replacement, the encephalopathy improves rapidly, but difficulty in weaning from the ventilator often persists. In our unit, CIP is the most common neuromuscular cause of ventilator dependency after cardiac and pulmonary etiologies have been excluded (10,28,29). Clinical signs of polyneuropathy are present in about half of patients. Electrophysiologic studies are therefore necessary to firmly establish the diagnosis of CIP.

Central respiratory drive may be assessed by decreasing ventilatory support to 5 to 8 cm H_2O of pressure support or continuous positive airway pressure to overcome airway and ventilator resistance, for a maximum of 15 minutes. Mechanical ventilation is restored if there is evidence of respiratory distress, arterial oxygen saturation less than 90% based on a pulse oximeter reading, or a significant rise in heart rate or blood pressure. This is done at the time of needle EMG of the diaphragm.

The earliest electrophysiologic sign, usually within 1 week, is a reduction of CMAP amplitudes, with little or no change in distal latencies, typical of axonal damage. Fibrillation potentials and positive sharp waves do not generally appear for 3 weeks. MUPs, if they can be voluntarily activated by the patient, often appear normal or somewhat low in amplitude with increased polyphasia, suggestive of primary involvement of muscle by sepsis. These electrophysiologic changes are also consistent with primary myopathy; hence, it is important to demonstrate depression of SNAP amplitudes before a firm diagnosis of CIP is made. Repetitive nerve stimulation studies may be abnormal by coincidence if neuro-

TABLE 2. *Neuromuscular conditions in the critical care unit associated with the systemic inflammatory response syndrome*

Condition	Incidence	Clinical feature	Electromyography	Creatine phosphokinase
Polyneuropathy Critical illness polyneuropathy	Common	Flaccid limbs and respiratory weakness	Axonal degeneration of motor and sensory fibers	Near normal
Motor neuropathy	Common with neuromuscular blocking agents	Flaccid limbs and respiratory weakness	Axonal degeneration of motor fibers	Near normal
Neuromuscular transmission defect Transient neuromuscular blockade	Common with neuromuscular blocking agents	Flaccid limbs and respiratory weakness	Abnormal repetitive nerve stimulation studies	Normal
Myopathy Thick filament myopathy	Common with steroids, neuromuscular blocking agents, and asthma	Flaccid limbs and respiratory weakness	Abnormal spontaneous activity	Elevated
Disuse (cachectic myopathy)	Common (?)	Muscle wasting	Normal	Normal
Necrotizing myopathy of intensive care	Rare	Flaccid weakness, myoglobinuria	Abnormal spontaneous activity in muscle	Markedly elevated

CK, creatine kinase. Reproduced from Ref. 23, with permission.

muscular blocking agents have been given, and their effects may persist beyond several hours to a number of days if the patient is in renal or liver failure (30). Phrenic NCS and needle EMG of the chest wall and diaphragm are useful in showing that CIP is the probable proximate cause of difficulty in weaning from the ventilator (31).

Knowledge of the presence of CIP aids management on the ventilator and, in particular, indicates that the patient has a neuromuscular problem, which may prolong care in the ICU. If it is mild, recovery occurs within a matter of weeks, but if severe, recovery may be prolonged by several months and incomplete (32). Physiotherapy and rehabilitation should be tailored to the severity of the polyneuropathy. In a prospective study by Leijten et al. (32), CIP was associated with increased mortality and rehabilitation problems. Other than management of the septic syndrome, there is no specific treatment of CIP. Wijdicks and Fulgham (33) failed to observe improvement after treatment with high-dose intravenous immunoglobulin. Even though sepsis and multiple organ failure are less common in pediatric patients, a few instances of pediatric CIP have been reported (34–36).

The morphologic aspects of CIP have been examined in peripheral nerve and muscle biopsies and in postmortem studies of the CNS and peripheral nervous system (28). They reveal evidence of a noninflammatory motor and sensory axonopathy. Muscle tissue shows acute and chronic denervation, with scattered grouped atrophic myofibers and occasional necrotic myofibers, suggesting associated primary myopathy as well. The only CNS manifestation is central chromatolysis of anterior horn cells and loss of dorsal root ganglion neurons, secondary to the axonopathy.

Acute Motor Neuropathy Associated with Competitive Neuromuscular Blocking Agents

Patients with forms of this polyneuropathy (37–43) have generally been in an ICU for days to weeks and have received competitive neuromuscular blocking agents, such as pancuronium bromide or the shorter acting agent vecuronium, for 48 hours or more and occasionally for days or weeks to ease mechanical ventilation. When the agents are discontinued, difficulty weaning from the ventilator and limb paralysis ensue. The serum CK level is mild or moderately elevated. There is electrophysiologic evidence of severe primary motor axonopathy with or without a defect in neuromuscular transmission on slow rates of stimulation. Muscle biopsy shows varying degrees of denervation atrophy and muscle necrosis.

The mechanism of the neuropathy is unknown, but sepsis appears to be an underlying factor in most if not all cases (16), because when the various contributing systemic complications are successfully treated, the neuromuscular condition itself improves and rapid recovery sometimes occurs. We (14) and others (21,22,44) have failed to implicate neuromuscular blocking agents as a cause of CIP.

Neuromuscular Transmission Disorders and Myopathies

Transient neuromuscular blockade, thick filament myopathy, cachetic myopathy, and acute necrotizing myopathy, in the order of their severity, may be the cause of difficulty in weaning from the ventilator in critical illness and injury.

Competitive neuromuscular blocking agents, often used to ease mechanical ventilation, are metabolized or cleared by the liver and kidney. In the presence of multiorgan failure, neuromuscular blockage may be prolonged for days after discontinuation (30). Repetitive stimulation studies will correctly identify the defect in neuromuscular transmission; however, by the time of testing, many patients will already have developed underlying CIP. Recovery may occur over a short period of time but may be prolonged for weeks or even months in severe cases.

Thick filament myopathy (41,45–49) occurs in children and adults during exacerbations of severe asthma or after organ transplantation (50). Endotracheal intubation and placement on a ventilator is usually necessary, accompanied by high-dose corticosteroids to treat the asthma and neuromuscular blocking agents to ease mechanical ventilation, often for days. On attempted weaning from the ventilator, the patient is found to have severe neuromuscular respiratory insufficiency and limb weakness. Ophthalmoplegia may be present (51). CK levels are often considerably increased. Repetitive nerve stimulation and sensory NCS are usually normal; however, motor NCS reveal low CMAP amplitudes. On needle EMG, MUPs tend to be low in amplitude, with short duration and excessive polyphasia, indicative of primary myopathy. Direct electrical stimulation of the muscle membrane may reveal inexcitability (52). Muscle biopsy shows central pallor of muscle fibers, which ultrastructurally is due to destruction of thick myosin filaments (46). It is possible that the administration of corticosteroids activates an ATP–ubiquitin-dependent proteolytic system that leads to myosin degradation, as postulated in two patients (49). Another possible mechanism of proteolysis postulated in five patients reported by Showalter and Engel (53) was increased expression of calpain, which itself alters calcium homeostasis. All patients were critically ill and suffered from SIRS, including one that had not received steroids or neuromuscular blocking agents. Thus, SIRS again appears to be the common etiologic factor. Recovery typically occurs rapidly. The clinical and electrophysiologic features are usually so distinctive in this syndrome that muscle biopsy is often not necessary. Although controversial, neuromuscular blocking agents at low doses and for short intervals can still be useful to ease mechanical ventilation in asthmatics.

Cachectic myopathy, disuse atrophy, and catabolic myopathy are terms used interchangeably (54) to describe this syndrome of muscle weakness and wasting (15,16). Motor and sensory NCS, needle EMG, and CK levels are all generally normal. Muscle biopsy may be normal or show nonspecific type 2 muscle fiber atrophy. An exception is the recent report by Gutmann et al. (55) of two critically ill patients, both of whom received prolonged neuromuscular blockage, but only in the one that received corticosteroids did severe muscle weakness and unusually severe atrophy of type 2 muscle fibers ensue, with regenerative changes on muscle biopsy.

Acute necrotizing myopathy of intensive care is a rare disorder (56,57). It is precipitated by a wide variety of infective, chemical, and other insults and enters in the differential diagnosis of acute myoglobinuria (15,16). Ramsay et al. (57) and Zochodne et al. (56) reported 11 such cases with severe weakness, high CK levels, and myoglobinuria. Electrophysiologic studies were consistent with severe myopathy, and muscle biopsy showed widespread fiber necrosis. Rapid and spontaneous recovery occurs in mild cases, but in more severe ones, notably the ones reported by Ramsay et al. (57), the prognosis was generally poor.

My colleagues and I have observed mild increases in CK levels, scattered necrosis of muscle fibers, and denervation atrophy on muscle biopsy in some critically ill patients, suggesting primary involvement of muscle and mild CIP. This may be due to a reduction in bioenergetic reserves, as measured by ^{31}P nuclear MR spectroscopy. Two of our patients had very low ratios of phosphocreatine/inorganic phosphate, more than would be expected from denervation of muscle alone (15,16). These abnormalities returned toward normal as the patients recovered from the critical illness and from the polyneuropathy. Nonetheless, muscle biopsies performed in 11 patients were notable for denervation atrophy, presumably secondary to a CIP (58).

Difficulty Weaning from the Ventilator and Electrophysiologic Studies of The Respiratory System

Techniques of phrenic NCS and needle EMG of the diaphragm (31) have proved to be of great value in establishing a neuromuscular basis for respiratory insufficiency and failure to wean from the ventilator. In patients with GBS, NCS complemented vital capacity in determining the need for respiratory assistance (5). Documenting the degree of axonal degeneration or demyelination of phrenic nerves also aids in long-term prognostication. In a recent study of 40 patients with difficulty in weaning from the ventilator when a neuromuscular cause was suspected, 95% had diaphragmatic abnormalities (10). In an earlier study, Spitzer et al. (59) found a high incidence of both polyneuropathy and myopathy as causes of prolonged difficulty in weaning. Most had CIP, but there were varying combinations of unilateral phrenic nerve damage, neuromuscular transmission defects, and primary myopathies. Combined electrophysiologic studies of the limbs and respiratory system were of great assistance in identifying these conditions and rendering a prognosis.

Mononeuropathies

Lumbosacral or brachial plexopathies may be secondary to direct trauma, usually from motor vehicle accidents or surgery. Insertion of catheters into the iliac arteries or aorta may dislodge thrombi, and the resulting embolization impairs vascular supply to nerves and, in this manner, induces focal ischemic plexopathy (60). Direct surgical trauma to vessels may also induce vascular insufficiency. Motorcycle accidents commonly traumatize the brachial plexus. Proximal lesions are suggested by Horner's syndrome, winging of the scapular, and diaphragm paralysis. Electrophysiologic studies ideally performed after 3 weeks will further help localize the lesion. Myelography, CT myelography, or MRI may provide more positive evidence of root avulsion, which would preclude attempts at operative nerve repair. Fractures of the pelvis may cause varying patterns of damage to the lumbosacral plexus. Observations of focal weakness on reflex or voluntarily induced movement, plus abnormalities of the deep tendon reflexes, may provide an initial clue to the presence of such damage. Thus, weakness of hip adduction and flexion, knee extension, and an absent ankle jerk suggest damage to L2-4 roots of the lumbosacral plexus. Electrophysiologic studies should successfully demonstrate abnormalities on motor and sensory NCS and needle EMG that localize the lesion to the brachial or lumbosacral plexus.

There are several types of mononeuropathies. If the primary reason for admission to the ICU was the postoperative state, the initial surgery may have induced a mononeuropathy when operating room equipment or perhaps the surgery itself directly damaged a peripheral nerve. For example, weakness of dorsiflexion of the wrist and digits and an absent brachioradialis reflex suggests radial nerve damage in the spinal groove of the humerus by fracture or direct compression. Phrenic nerves, either bilaterally or unilaterally, may be damaged at the time of surgery by direct trauma or by the application of cold, as occurs in the hypothermia associated with cardiac surgery (61). Distal nerves may be damaged as a result of impairment of nutrient blood supply and distal embolization, as for example in the occurrence of femoral or sciatic neuropathy after cardiac or vascular surgery. Electrophysiologic studies show a relatively pure axonopathy affecting motor and sensory fibers.

Patients who are being anticoagulated run the risk of hemorrhage because a sudden rise in tissue pressure produces a compartment syndrome and severe compression results in nerve ischemia. The compartments most commonly involved are the iliopsoas and gluteal, producing acute femoral or sciatic neuropathies (62). Fractures and soft tissue trauma may also induce compartment syndromes. An immediate CT should be ordered, which will show the location of the hemorrhage. Then, surgical decompression may successfully decompress the nerve. The situation is so acute and emergent that electrophysiologic studies are of little value.

PATHOPHYSIOLOGY OF CRITICAL ILLNESS NEUROPATHY AND MYOPATHY

The microcirculation is disturbed in sepsis (Fig. 3). Blood vessels supplying the peripheral nerves lack autoregulation (63), rendering these vessels susceptible to such disturbances. Moreover, cytokines that are secreted in sepsis have histamine-like properties that may increase microvascular permeability (28). The resulting endoneurial edema induces hypoxia by an increase in intercapillary distance and other mechanisms. Severe energy deficits can induce a primarily distal axonal degeneration if highly energy-dependant systems involve axonal transport of structural proteins. The predominantly distal involvement may explain why recovery in some patients can be surprisingly short, conforming to the short length of nerve through which axonal regeneration takes place. It is possible that cytokines themselves may have a direct toxic effect on peripheral nerves. Tumor necrosis factor decreases the resting transmembrane potential of skeletal muscle fibers in vitro (64) and induces muscle proteolysis in animals (65). Hund et al. (25) used a bioassay method to extract a low-molecular-weight fraction of the serum of patients with CIP that proved to be toxic to rat spinal motor neurons.

Disturbances of the microcirculation to nerve and muscle may also explain the effects of neuromuscular blocking agents and corticosteroids. Through increased capillary permeability induced by sepsis, neuromuscular blocking agents, notably vecuronium or its metabolite, 3 desacetyl-vecuronium (30), could have a direct toxic effect on peripheral nerve axons. These neuromuscular blocking agents may also cause functional denervation through their prolonged neuromuscular blocking action (66). The result would be denervation atrophy of muscle and a relatively pure motor neuropathy.

We have always been concerned that antibiotics, particularly aminoglycosides, with their known neural toxicity, might cause CIP. These drugs might gain access to the peripheral nerve as a result of increased capillary permeability. However, there has been no statistical proof that antibiotics cause peripheral nerve dysfunction in sepsis (14). Nonetheless, this possibility should be explored by basic science experiments.

The schema shown in Fig. 4 explains the acute quadriplegic myopathy that develops when critically ill patients are treated with neuromuscular blocking agents and corticosteroids. Animal experiments by Karpati et al. (67) showed that if muscle was first denervated by nerve transection and then corticosteroids given, a thick filament myopathy similar to that myopathy seen in humans could

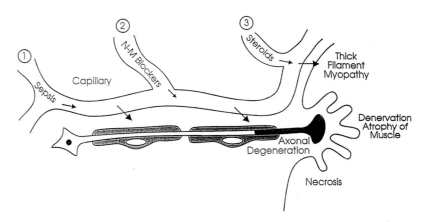

FIG 4. Theoretical mechanisms of neuromuscular complications of the systemic inflammatory response syndrome (SIRS). (*1*) Sepsis induces a release of cytokines that cause increased capillary permeability. This effect, and other microvascular mechanisms, induce a critical illness polyneuropathy, with distal axonal degeneration of nerve and denervation atrophy of muscle. (*2*) Neuromuscular (N-M) blocking agents in the presence of SIRS traverse the hyperpermeable capillary membrane and have a direct toxic effect on nerve or cause "functional denervation" to increase denervation of muscle. (*3*) Steroids gain access to muscle by this mechanism and, in the presence of denervation due to *1* and *2*, induce a thick filament myopathy and varying degrees of necrosis. Combinations of *1, 2,* and *3* may occur in the same patient. (From Ref. 69, with permission.)

be induced. In humans, CIP and neuromuscular blocking agents combine to denervate muscle, and steroids in turn induce myopathic changes. The rapidly evolving myopathy reported recently by Al-Lozi et al. (68) is characterized by destruction of thick filaments throughout the muscle fibers and acute necrotizing myopathy (56,57) and may simply represent a further stage of this process. Two postulated mechanisms of protein degradation in critically ill patients prompted by corticosteroids include the activation of ubiquitin (49) and alterations of calpain with abnormal calcium homeostasis (53).

REFERENCES

1. Chen R, Grand'Maison F, Strong MJ, Ransay DA, Bolton CF. Motor neuron disease presenting as acute respiratory failure: a clinical and pathological study. *J Neurol Neurosurg and Psychiatry* 1996;60:455–458.
2. Preston DC, Kelly JJ. Atypical motor neuron disease. In: Brown WF, Bolton CF, eds. *Clinical electromyography*, 2nd ed. Boston: Butterworth-Heinemann, 1993:451–476.
3. Kimura J. Proximal versus distal slowing of motor nerve conduction velocity in the Guillain-Barré syndrome. *Ann Neurol* 1978;3:344–350.
4. Markand ON, Kincaid JC, Pourmand RA, et al. Electrophysiologic evaluation of diaphragm by transcutaneous phrenic nerve stimulation. *Neurology* 1984;34:604–614.
5. Zifko U, Chen R, Remtulla H, Hahn AF, Koopman W, Bolton CF. Respiratory electrophysiologic studies in Guillain-Barré syndrome. *J Neurol Neurosurg Psychiatry* 1996;60:191–194.
6. Bolton CF. Editorial: The changing concepts of Guillain-Barré syndrome. *N Engl J Med* 1995;333:1415–1417.
7. Feasby TE, Gilbert JJ, Brown WF, et al. Acute axonal form of Guillain-Barré polyneuropathy. *Brain* 1986;109:1115–1126.
8. McKhann GM, Cornblath DR, Ho T, et al. Clinical and electrophysiological aspects of acute paralytic disease of children and young adults in northern China. *Lancet* 1991;338:593–597.
9. Hartung HP, Pollard JD, Harvey GK, Toyka KV. Immunopathogenesis and treatment of the Guillain-Barré syndrome. Part II. *Muscle Nerve* 1995;18:154–164.
10. Maher J, Rutledge F, Remtulla H, Parkes A, Bernardi L, Bolton C. Neu-

romuscular disorders associated with failure to wean from the ventilator. *Intensive Care Med* 1995;21:737–743.
11. Nicolle MW, Stewart DJ, Remtulla H, Chen R, Bolton CF. Lambert-Eaton myasthenic syndrome presenting with severe respiratory failure. *Muscle Nerve* 1996;10:1328–1333..
12. Burges J, Vicent A, Moienaar PC, Newsom-Davis J, Peers C, Wray D. Passive transfer of seronegative myasthenia gravis to mice. *Muscle Nerve* 1994;17:1393–1400.
13. Tran DD, Groeneveld ABJ, van der Meuien J, et al. Age, chronic disease, sepsis, organ system failure, and mortality in a medical intensive care unit. *Crit Care Med* 1990;18:474–479.
14. Witt NJ, Zochodne DW, Bolton CF, Wells G, Young GB, Sibbald WJ. Peripheral nerve function in sepsis and multiple organ failure. *Chest* 1991;99:176–184.
15. Bolton CF, Young GB, Zochodne DW. Neurological changes during severe sepsis. In: Dobb GJ, ed. *Current topics in intensive care*. Philadelphia: W.B. Saunders, 1994:180–217.
16. Bolton CF. Muscle weakness and difficulty in weaning from the ventilator in the critical care unit. *Chest* 1994;106:1–2.
17. Bolton CF. Electrophysiological studies in critically ill patients. *Muscle Nerve* 1987;10:129–135.
18. Leijten FSS, de Weerd AW. Critical illness polyneuropathy: a review of the literature, definition and pathophysiology. *Clin Neurol Neurosurg* 1994;96:10–19.
19. Hund EF. Neuromuscular complications in the ICU: the spectrum of critical illness-related conditions causing muscular weakness and weaning failure. *Neurosciences* 1996;136:10–16.
20. Bolton CF, Gilbert JJ, Hahn AF, Sibbald WJ. Polyneuropathy in critically ill patients. *J Neurol Neurosurg Psychiatry* 1984;47:1223–1231.
21. Leijten FS, De Weerd AW, Poortvliet DC, De Riddler VA, Ulrich C, Harink-De Weerd JE. Critical illness polyneuropathy in multiple organ dysfunction syndrome and weaning from the ventilator. *Intensive Care Med* 1996;22:856–861.
22. Berek K, Margreiter J, Willeit J, Berek A, Schmotzhard E, Mutz NJ. Polyneuropathies in critically ill patients: a prospective evaluation. *Intensive Care Med* 1996;22:849–855.
23. Bolton CF. Sepsis and systemic inflammatory response syndrome (SIRS): neuromuscular manifestations. *Crit Care Med* 1996;8:1408–1416.
24. Leijten FSS. Critical illness polyneuropathy—a longitudinal study. Doctoral thesis. Rijksuniversiteit te Leiden, The Netherlands, 1996.
25. Hund E, Herbert M, Becker CM, Hacke W. A humoral neurotoxic factor in sera of patients with critical illness polyneuropathy. *Ann Neurol* 1996;40:539.

26. Young GB, Bolton CF, Austin TW, et al. The encephalopathy associated with septic illness. *Clin Invest Med* 1990;13:297–304.

27. Young GB, Bolton CF, Austin TW, et al. The electroencephalogram in sepsis associated with encephalopathy. *J Clin Neurophysiol* 1991;9:145–152.

28. Zochodne DW, Bolton CF, Wells GA, et al. Critical illness polyneuropathy: a complication of sepsis and multiple organ failure. *Brain* 1987;110:819–842.

29. Maher J, Rutledge F, Remtulla H, Parkes A, et al. Neurophysiological assessment of failure to wean from a ventilator. *Can J Neurol Sci* 1993;20:S28.

30. Segredo V, Caldwell JE, Matthay MA, et al. Persistent paralysis in critically ill patients after long-term administration of vecuronium. *N Engl J Med* 1992;327:524–528.

31. Bolton CF. Clinical neurophysiology of the respiratory system. AAEM Minimonograph #40. *Muscle Nerve* 1993;16:809–818.

32. Leijten FSS, Harinck-de Weerd JE, Poortvliet DCJ, de Weerd AW. The role of polyneuropathy in motor convalescence after prolonged mechanical ventilation. *JAMA* 1995;274:1221–1225.

33. Wijdicks EF, Fulgham JR. Failure of high dose intravenous immunoglobulins to alter the clinical course of critical illness polyneuropathy. *Muscle Nerve* 1994;17:1494–1495.

34. Sheth RD, Pryse-Philips WEM: Post-ventilatory quadriplegia: critical illness polyneuropathy in childhood. *Neurology* 1994;44:A169.

35. Dimachkie M, Austin SG, Slopis JM, Vriesendorp FJ. Critical illness polyneuropathy in childhood. *J Child Neurol* 1994;9:207.

36. Bolton CF. EMG in the paediatric critical care unit. In: Jones HR, Bolton CF, Harper M, eds. *Paediatric electromyography*. New York: Raven Press, 1996:445–466.

37. Subramony SH, Carpenter DE, Raju S, et al. Myopathy and prolonged neuromuscular blockade after lung transplant. *Crit Care Med* 1991;19:1580–1582.

38. Rossiter A, Souney PF, McGowan S, et al. Pancuronium-induced prolonged neuromuscular blockade. *Crit Care Med* 1991;12:1583–1587.

39. Gooch JL, Suchyta MR, Balbierz JM. Prolonged paralysis after treatment with neuromuscular junction blocking agents. *Crit Care Med* 1991;9:1125–1131.

40. Kupfer Y, Namba T, Kaldawi E, et al. Prolonged weakness after long-term infusion of vecuronium-bromide. *Ann Intern Med* 1991;117:484–486.

41. Barohn RJ, Jackson CE, Rogers SJ, Ridings LW, McVey AL. Prolonged paralysis due to nondepolarizing neuromuscular blocking agents and corticosteroids. *Muscle Nerve* 1994;17:647–654.

42. Giostra E, Magistris MR, Pizzolato G, Cox J, Chevrolet J-C. Neuromuscular disorder in intensive care unit patients treated with pancuronium bromide. *Chest* 1994;106:1:210–220.

43. Op de Coul AAW, Werheul GAM, Leyten ACM, et al. Critical illness polyneuromyopathy after artificial respiration. *Clin Neurol Neurosurg* 1991;93:27–33.

44. Latronico N, Fenzi F, Recupero D, et al. Critical illness myopathy and neuropathy. *Lancet* 1996;347:1579–1582.

45. Lacomis D, Smith TW, Chad DA. Acute myopathy and neuropathy in status asthmaticus: case report and literature review. *Muscle Nerve* 1993;16:84–90.

46. Danon MJ, Carpenter S. Myopathy and thick filament (myosin) loss following prolonged paralysis with vecuronium during steroid treatment. *Muscle Nerve* 1991;14:1131–1139.

47. Douglass JA, Tuxen DV, Horne M, et al. Myopathy in severe asthma. *Am Rev Respir Dis* 1991;146:517–519.

48. Hirano M, Ott BR, Raps EC. Acute quadriplegic myopathy: complication of treatment with steroids, nondepolarizing blocking agents, or both. *Neurology* 1992;42:2082–2087.

49. Minetti C, Hirano M, Morreale G, et al. Ubiquitin expression in acute steroid myopathy with loss of myosin thick elements. *Muscle Nerve* 1996;19:94–96.

50. Lacomis D, Giuliani MJ, Van Cott A, Dramer DJ. Acute myopathy of intensive care: clinical, electromyographic, and pathological aspects. *Ann Neurol* 1996;40:645–654.

51. Sitwell LD, Weinshenker BG, Monpetit V, et al: Complete ophthalmoplegia as a complication of acute corticosteroid- and pancuronium-associated myopathy. *Neurology* 1991;41:921–922.

52. Rich MM, Teener JW, Raps EC, Schotland DL, Bird SJ. Muscle is electrically inexcitable in acute quadriplegic myopathy. *Neurology* 1996;46:731–736.

53. Showalter CJ, Engel AG. Acute quadriplegic myopathy: Analysis of myosin isoforms and evidence for calpain-mediated proteolysis. *Muscle Nerve* 1997;20:316–322.

54. Clowes GHA, George BC, Villee CA. Muscle proteolysis induced by a circulating peptide in patients with sepsis or trauma. *N Engl J Med* 1983;308:545–552.

55. Gutmann L, Blumenthal D, Gutmann L, Schochet S. Acute type II myofiber atrophy in critical illness. *Neurology* 1996;46:819–821.

56. Zochodne DW, Ramsay DA, Saly V, et al. Acute necrotizing myopathy of intensive care: electrophysiological studies. *Muscle Nerve* 1994;17:285–292.

57. Ramsay DA, Zochodne DW, Robertson DM, et al. A syndrome of acute severe muscle necrosis in intensive care unit patients. *J Neuropathol Exp Neurol* 1993;52:387–398.

58. Pringle CE, Bolton CF, Ramsay DA, et al. Muscle biopsy in critical illness: electrophysiological and morphological correlations. *Can J Neurol Sci* 1992;2:297(abst).

59. Spitzer AR, Giancarlo T, Maher L, et al. Neuromuscular causes of prolonged ventilator dependency. *Muscle Nerve* 1992;15:682–686.

60. Wilbourne AJ, Furlan AAJ, Helley N, Ruschaupt W. Ischemic monomelic neuropathy. *Neurology* 1983;33:447–451.

61. Abd AG, Braun NMT, Baskin MI, O'Sullivan MM, Alkaitis DA. Diaphragmatic dysfunction after open heart surgery: treatment with a rocking bed. *Ann Intern Med* 1989;111:881–886.

62. Matsen FA. *Compartmental syndromes*. New York: Grune & Stratton, 1980.

63. Low PA, Tuck RR, Takeuchi M. Nerve microenvironment in diabetic neuropathy. In: Dyck PJ, Thomas PK, Asbury AK, et al., eds. *Diabetic neuropathy*. Philadelphia: W.B. Saunders, 1987:268–277.

64. Tracey KJ, Lowry SF, Beutler B, et al. Cachectin/tumor necrosis factor mediates human muscle denervation: topical 31-P spectroscopy studies. *Magn Reson Med* 1988;7:373–383.

65. Fong Y. Cachectin/TNF or Il-1a induces cachexia with redistribution of body proteins. *Am J Physiol* 1989;256:659–665.

66. Wernig A, Pecot-Dechavassine M, Stover H. Sprouting and regression of the nerve at the frog neuromuscular junction in normal conditions and after prolonged paralysis with curare. *J Neurocytol* 1980;9:277–303.

67. Karpati G, Carpenter S, Eisen AA. Experimental core-like lesions and nemaline rods: a correlative morphological and physiological study. *Arch Neurol* 1972;27:247–266.

68. Al-Lozi MT, Pestronk A, Yee WC, et al. Rapidly evolving myopathy with myosin-deficient muscle fibers. *Ann Neurol* 1994;35:273–279.

69. Bolton CF. Neuromuscular complications of sepsis. *Intensive Care Med* 1993;19:S58–S63.

70. Plum F, Posner JB. *The diagnosis of stupor and coma*, 3rd ed. Philadelphia: F.A. Davis, 1980:53–54.

71. Bolton CF, Young GB. The neurological consultation and neurological syndromes in the intensive care unit. *Baillieres Clin Neurol* 1996;5:447–475.

Motor Disorders,
edited by David S. Younger.
Lippincott Williams & Wilkins, Philadelphia © 1999.

CHAPTER 22

Hereditary Spastic Paraplegia

Hugo W. Moser

PREVALENCE AND CLASSIFICATION OF HEREDITARY SPASTIC PARAPLEGIA

In a series of 672 patients with spastic paraparesis admitted to Columbia-Presbyterian Medical Center in New York between 1960 and 1976, spinal cord trauma was the most common cause (27%), followed by tumors, multiple sclerosis, and congenital anomalies (1); 2.3% were familial and in 6.5% no etiology could be identified. The causes to be discussed in this chapter clearly encompass the familial cases plus an unknown proportion of the cases in which no etiology was established. Hereditary spastic paraplegia (HSP) constituted 11.7% of 60 "pure spastic paraplegia" seen at the Mayo Clinic (2). HSP thus may account for approximately 10% of cases of spastic paraparesis. The prevalence of pure HSP, which is discussed in more detail below, has been estimated to be 9.6 per 100,000 (1).

The HSP syndromes are heterogeneous in respect to patterns of neurologic change, severity, mode of inheritance, gene localization, and gene defects. HSP has been subdivided into a more common "pure" form (pHSP) in which progressive spasticity of the legs is the main abnormality and rarer "complicated" forms in which it is combined with additional neurologic or nonneurologic features (3,4). This subdivision is still used (5) and is applied in this chapter, even though both forms are heterogeneous and there may be dispute as to the range of other neurologic abnormalities seen in patients with pHSP (3). Although recent advances in genetics and biochemistry have permitted exact delineation of some causes of HSP, much still remains to be learned about the causes and classification of most cases.

H. W. Moser: Departments of Neurology and Pediatrics, Johns Hopkins University and Neurogenetics Research, Kennedy Krieger Institute, Baltimore, Maryland 21205.

PURE HEREDITARY SPASTIC PARAPLEGIA

Clinical Features and Pathology

The prevalence of pHSP is estimated to be 9.6 per 100,000 (6). Seventy to 80% of cases show an autosomal dominant (AD) mode of inheritance, with autosomal recessive (AR) inheritance responsible for most of the remainder (5). X-linked recessive forms are rare, but, as discussed below, the gene defects in three forms have now been defined (7–9). The AD forms of pHSP have been the subject of detailed clinical and pathologic analyses, which have led to relatively consistent findings (3,10), even though, as discussed below, genetic linkage analyses suggest that even this group is heterogeneous. Harding (3,4) subdivided the AD forms of pHSP into two types on the basis of age at onset, which in type 1 was below age 35 and type 2 above that age. Spasticity was the predominant handicap in type 1, whereas in type 2, muscle weakness, urinary symptoms, and impaired vibration and joint position sense were frequently present. Progression of the illness was slow in both groups, and very few had to give up work because of their disability, even though 13 of 21 patients examined by Behan and Maia (11) eventually required a cane or were chairbound. In the series of Bell and Carmichael (12), the mean age at death was 57 ± 3.02 years and the mean duration was 57.5 ± 13.69 years. The main pathologic changes were in the spinal cord, including degeneration of corticospinal tracts from the medullary pyramids downward and increasing caudally; posterior column degeneration, particularly the fasciculus gracilis, increasing rostrally; and to a lesser extent the lateral spinocerebellar tracts (10,11). This process has been described as a "dying back" of nerve fiber endings. Magnetic resonance imaging (MRI) generally shows atrophy of the spinal cord, particularly in the cervical region (13). The degree of sensory tract involvement on postmortem examination does not always correlate with clinical findings. One patient in whom the sensory tracts were involved pathologically did not have clinically evident sensory changes. In other patients the pathologic changes were confined to the corticospinal tracts (14). pHSP patients do not show abnormalities of brain or peripheral nerves and there is no primary demyelination. Motor and sensory conduction studies in peripheral nerves are normal (15).

Genetics of Pure Hereditary Spastic Paraplegia

The fact that pHSP can be associated with AD, AR, and X-linked recessive modes of inheritance indicates the genetic heterogeneity of this syndrome.

Autosomal Dominant Pure Hereditary Spastic Paraplegia

Linkage studies have been published in complete form in 34 families (5,16–24). Of those families showing evidence of linkage, most are linked to chromosome 2 (2p21-p24). Three families showed linkage to chromosome 14 (19,22) and one to chromosome 15 (20). Linkage to all three loci has been excluded in a number of families, suggesting the existence of at least one further locus (5). Analysis of ages at onset provided evidence of anticipation in 11 families where the gene mapped to chromosome 2 (17,18,21) and 14 (19), suggesting the possibility that the underlying abnormality might involve a trinucleotide repeat expansion. Chromosome 2-linked families have shown both early- and late-onset pHSP, whereas the family linked to chromosome 14 had early-onset disease (17). Candidate genes have not yet been identified.

Autosomal Recessive Forms of Pure Hereditary Spastic Paraplegia

Only a few pHSP families with an AR pattern of inheritance have been reported. Bruins and Simons (25) reported a family with 179 members among four generations in which 15 members had pHSP and several consanguineous marriages had occurred. Four other families with an AR form of inheritance were summarized in a previous review (10). In Harding's survey of 22 families with pHSP, AR mode of inheritance appeared to be present (3). The clinical findings in these three families did not differ from those with AD forms.

It has been recently demonstrated that the juvenile and adult forms of globoid or Krabbe leukodystrophy, in which there is a deficiency of the lysosomal enzyme galactocerebrosidase, can present initially as pHSP (26,27). Cognitive function is often intact. At later stages, other features that distinguish it from pHSP, such as optic atrophy, dementia, and paralysis of bulbar muscles, supervene.

X-linked Pure Hereditary Spastic Paraplegia

Thirteen families with X-linked pHSP were cited by Ulku et al. (28). Cambi et al. (29) reported an additional

family. MRI in those cases demonstrated discrete white matter lesions in the periatrial regions that were more prominent posteriorly.

Our understanding of X-linked pHSP increased greatly when it was demonstrated that X-linked HSP and Pelizaeus-Merzbacher disease were in fact allelic (8). Pelizaeus-Merzbacher disease is an X-linked dysmyelinating disorder, which in its classic form presents in early childhood with nystagmoid eye movements; slowly progressive psychomotor retardation; and progressive pyramidal, dystonic, and cerebellar signs (30). The gene defect, which causes defective synthesis of proteolipid protein (31,32), the major structural protein of central nervous system myelin, has been mapped to Xq21.3-22. The demonstration that defects in proteolipid synthesis could also be associated with a milder adult phenotype, such as pHSP (8), came as a surprise and has led to a reevaluation of previously reported families with X-linked pHSP. Kobayashi et al. (33) demonstrated a mutation of the proteolipid gene in one of the X-linked pHSP kindreds previously reported in 1961 (34). The gene defect in the family reported by Keppen et al. (35) mapped to Xq21-22 and likely involved the same gene. Mutations in the proteolipid gene can also cause spastic paraparesis in heterozygous females (36) and may also cause the complicated form of HSP (37). The types of mutations of the proteolipid gene associated with either Pelizaeus-Merzbacher disease or pHSP can vary widely (38). The proportion of X-linked pHSP due to mutations in the proteolipid protein gene is not known, because suitable genetic studies have not been performed in all reported families.

Adrenomyeloneuropathy (AMN) can also cause X-linked pHSP (39). In this disorder it is common for heterozygous females also to show signs of spastic paraparesis. It represents one of the phenotypes of the adrenoleukodystrophy–AMN complex (40). The gene codes for a peroxisomal membrane protein that has been mapped to Xq28. The disease can be diagnosed by the demonstration of abnormally high levels of plasma very-long-chain fatty acids (41). The clinical presentation of AMN varies widely, and the diagnosis may be missed. Up to 50% of patients have normal adrenal function (42). It is recommended that the assay for plasma very-long-chain fatty acids be performed in all patients with familial spastic paraparesis, except those kindreds in which male to male transmission has been demonstrated, because this excludes an X-linked disorder such as AMN.

COMPLICATED FORMS OF HEREDITARY SPASTIC PARAPARESIS

In the complicated forms of HSP, the spastic paraparesis is associated with a variety of other neurologic or somatic abnormalities. These are listed in Table 1. Recent advances have been made in the study of the MASA syn-

TABLE 1. *Classification of complicated spastic paraplegias*

Type	Clinical features	Inheritance pattern
With amyotrophy		
Resembling peroneal muscular atrophy	Mild paraparesis accompanied by features resembling Charcot-Marie-Tooth disease.	AD
Of small hand muscles	Mild paraparesis with moderate/severe amyotrophy of small hand muscles.	AD
Troyer syndrome	Early onset with motor and speech delay; severe spasticity and distal amyotrophy of all four limbs. Pseudobulbar palsy, dysarthria, and emotional lability. Described in Amish.	AR
Charlevoix-Saguenay syndrome	Early onset. Dysarthria, nystagmus, cerebellar ataxia. Amyotrophy in all four limbs. Spasticity prominent in legs. Defective vertical pursuit eye movements. Occurs in an isolated area of Quebec.	AR
Resembling amyotrophic lateral sclerosis		AR/AD
Sjögren-Larsson syndrome	Congenital ichthyosis, severe mental retardation, and usually nonprogressive spastic paraplegia.	AR, caused by mutations in fatty aldehyde dehydrogenase gene
MASA syndrome	Mental retardation, aphasia, spasticity, and adducted thumbs. Allelic with X-linked hydrocephalus.	XLR, caused by mutations in L1-gene
With cerebellar signs	Cerebellar dysarthria, mild upper limb ataxia, and spastic paraplegia. Distal wasting may occur.	AR/AD
Kjellin syndrome	Mental retardation, progressive spastic paraplegia from 20s, distal neurogenic atrophy of limbs, dysarthria, central retinal degeneration	AR
With optic atrophy	Rare. Associated with a variety of additional features in different family reports.	AR/AD
With choreoathetosis dystonia	Additional features may occur in some families. Consider dopa responsive dystonia as an alternative diagnosis.	AR/AD
Mast syndrome	Dementia, dysarthria, athetosis, and spastic paraplegia. Described in Amish population.	
With sensory neuropathy	Sensory neuropathy often affects all modalities and may lead to trophic ulceration and mutilation. Trophic ulcers may have early onset.	AR/AD
With disordered skin pigmentation	Two separate conditions reported. First with generalized depigmentation at birth, becoming patchily pigmented. Second with hypopigmented skin below knee.	AR/AD
With hyperekplexia	A single family described in which hyperekplexia and spastic paraplegia cosegregate.	AD, caused by mutations in gene for the *u*1 subunit of glycine receptor

AR, autosomal recessive; AD, autosomal dominant; XLR, X-linked recessive.
Modified from Ref. 5, with permission.

drome (mental retardation, aphasia, shuffling gait, and adducted thumbs) (43), HSAS (X-linked hydrocephalus due to aqueductal stenosis) (44), and the Sjögren-Larsson syndrome (45).

The MASA syndrome is an X-linked disorder in which mental retardation and adducted thumbs are the most striking features. Spastic paraparesis is evidenced by shuffling gait and hyperreflexia in the legs. It is one of 33 syndromes in which X-linked mental retardation is associated with spastic paraplegia (46). Schrander-Strumpel et al. (46) performed a detailed analysis of six families with MASA, HSAS, and other mixed phenotypes. They found clinical overlap of MASA and HSAS (Table 2) and proposed that they be referred to as the HSAS/MASA spectrum. HSAS and MASA co-occur in the same family. Both conditions were mapped to Xq28 and have been shown to be associated with the gene that codes for cell adhesion molecule L1 (9). Fourteen independent mutations have been reported and shown to be disease causing. The same mutation may be associated with either MASA or HSAS or with intermediate phenotypes.

TABLE 2. Clinical manifestations in families from the literature, reported as having MASA syndrome or HSAS (patients surviving beyond age 1 year)

Finding	MASA syndrome (n = 98)	HSAS (n = 70)
Male:female ratio	93:5	70:0
Head circumference in centiles	n = 25	n = 41
<P3	—	1
P3–P50	12	5
P50	7	6 (2 × shunted)
P50–P98	6	9
>P98	—	20
Mental retardation IQ	98/98 (100%)	69/70 (98%)
	n = 30	n = 36
<20 (profound)		7
20–35 (severe)	2	17
35–50 (moderate)	10	7
50–70 (mild)	9	2
70–85 (borderline)	9	1 (IQ 85)
Spastic paraplegia	58/63 (92%)	35/41 (85%)
Speech delay	45/50 (90%)	?[a]
Adducted thumbs	63/68 (93%)	27/31 (87%)
Brain abnormality		
Hydrocephaly	9/17 (53%)	30/70
Corpus callosum agenesis	4/13 (31%)	Common

[a]Not reported in general.
From Ref. 46, with permission.

DIFFERENTIAL DIAGNOSIS AND DIAGNOSTIC WORKSHOP

The familial spastic paraplegias are highly heterogeneous and should be distinguished from a large number of nongenetic disorders. Precise diagnosis is of key importance for genetic counseling and in some instances can lead to specific therapies. Although recent advances in genetics, biochemistry, and neuroimaging have increased the capacity to achieve precise diagnosis, in a large number of cases, such as the AD pHSP, this is not yet possible, and further efforts to define the gene defects are to be encouraged. Emphasis will be placed on the disorders for which there is, or may be, specific therapy, such as Refsum disease (47), dopamine responsive dystonia (48), AMN (40), and globoid leukodystrophy (26).

The *AD forms of pHSP* must be distinguished from other disease entities and, because they are heterogeneous, also from each other. They can be distinguished from the spinocerebellar degenerations (49) and disorders such as the Machado-Joseph disease by the prominence of cerebellar dysfunction in these syndromes. The molecular abnormalities in the cerebellar ataxias have been recently defined (50). Dopamine-sensitive dystonia is another entity that should be considered. Nygaard et al. (48) reported 16 of 66 patients with this syndrome that had been diagnosed initially as spastic paraplegia or spastic diplegia.

It is an AD trait, in which dystonia and diurnal variation of the severity of symptoms are common features, and often shows a striking response to levodopa therapy.

AD pHSP disorders are heterogeneous and, as already noted, have been linked to at least three distinct loci. Genetic linkage analysis cannot as yet be used for diagnosis or counseling, but it is likely that the gene defects and mutations in some of these families will be defined in the next few years, and this will provide powerful new tools for counseling.

Patients with *AR forms of pHSP* should be tested for inborn errors of metabolism. It has already been noted that adult globoid leukodystrophy may present as a spastic paraparesis (26) and can be identified by an assay for galactocerebrosidase activity in peripheral blood leukocytes. Points of distinction from pHSP are the clinical evidence of cerebral involvement and white matter lesions on brain MRI. Adult forms of metachromatic leukodystrophy, Tay-Sachs, or Sandhoff disease may also be associated with spastic paraparesis, but there is usually evidence of cerebral involvement and, in the case of metachromatic leukodystrophy, peripheral nerve abnormalities. Both conditions can be diagnosed by assays of appropriate enzymes in peripheral blood leukocytes. Adult Refsum's disease can be distinguished by the associated pigmentary degeneration of the retina, peripheral nerve involvement, and elevated levels of plasma phytanic acid (47). Sjögren-Larsson syndrome is associated with ichthyosis and psychomotor degeneration in addition to spastic quadriparesis and can be diagnosed by the assay of fatty aldehyde dehydrogenase in cultures of skin fibroblasts (Table 3) (51).

Friedreich ataxia can usually be distinguished by the absence of deep tendon reflexes and ataxia. However, a recent survey of cases confirmed by genetic analysis

TABLE 3. Clinical features of Sjögren-Larsson syndrome

Major Features
Congenital ichthyosis[a]
Mental retardation[a]
Spastic diplegia or tetraplegia[a]
Glistening white dots on the retina
Short stature
Seizure disorder
Speech defects
Minor associated features
Kyphoscoliosis
Macular degeneration
Hypertelorism
Wide-spaced teeth
Enamel hypoplasia
Metaphyseal dysplasia

[a]These feature are present in virtually all Sjögren-Larsson syndrome patients.
From Ref. 51, with permission.

indicated that the range of phenotypes was wider than had been previously recognized. Deep tendon reflexes may be retained or even increased (52). Diagnosis is based on the demonstration of expansion of GAA repeats in chromosome 9.

Specific diagnostic approaches to *X-linked HSP* have been recently developed. These include the demonstration of deletions, mutations, or duplications of the gene on Xq21-22 that encodes proteolipid protein (38). As already noted, X-linked HSP syndromes are allelic with Pelizaeus-Merzbacher disease. The MASA–HSAS complex is associated frequently with a mutation of the cell adhesion molecule 1 in Xq28 (9). Finally, AMN can present as familial spastic paraparesis (40) and is diagnosed easily by demonstration of abnormally high levels of plasma very-long-chain fatty acids (41). It is likely that, considered together, these three entities account for a significant proportion of X-linked familial spastic paraparesis.

The differential diagnosis of *sporadic spastic paraparesis* is extensive. Sporadic cases may be the only known example of one of the familial entities described above or due to nongenetic causes described in chapters of this book (see chapters 18,23,24,27 and 28), such as multiple sclerosis, tumors, infections, or deficiencies of vitamins B_{12} and E.

Therapy and Counseling

The most important aspects of therapy are the general supportive and rehabilitative measures presented in the other chapters of this book (see chapters 41–45). Specific therapies are available for a few of the disorders, such as dietary therapy for Refsum's disease (47), levodopa for dopamine responsive dystonia (48), and bone marrow transplantation for the adult form of globoid leukodystrophy (26).

Genetic counseling is of great importance and can be specific and accurate for AMN, Sjögren-Larsson syndrome, globoid and metachromatic leukodystrophy, and the disorders cited above in which the gene defects and mutations have been identified. Counseling for those HSPs in which the gene or metabolic defects have not yet been defined continues to represent a challenge. In respect to the AD pHSP syndromes, it should be noted that most of these disorders are compatible with personally and professionally satisfactory quality of life (3) and can be helped by rehabilitative measures.

REFERENCES

1. Ungar-Sargon JY, Lovelace RE, Brust JCM. Spastic paraplegia-paraparesis. *J Neurol Sci* 1980;46:1–12.
2. Stark FM, Moersch FP. Primary lateral sclerosis: a distinct clinical entity. *J Nerv Ment Dis* 1945;102:332–337.
3. Harding AE. Hereditary "pure" spastic paraplegia: a clinical and genetic study of 22 families. *J Neurol Neurosurg Psychiatry* 1981;44:871–883.
4. Harding AE. Classification of the hereditary ataxias and paraplegias. *Lancet* 1983;1:1151–1155.
5. Reid E. Pure hereditary spastic paraparesis. *J Med Genet* 1997;34:499–503.
6. Polo JM, Calleja J, Combartos O, et al. Hereditary ataxias and paraplegias in Cantabria, Spain. An epidemiological and clinical study. *Brain* 1991;114:855–866.
7. Mosser J, Lutz Y, Stoeckel ME, et al. The gene responsible for adrenoleukodystrophy encodes a peroxisomal membrane protein. *Hum Mol Genet* 1994;3:265–271.
8. Saugier-Veber P, Munnich A, Bonneau D, et al. X-linked spastic paraplegia and Pelizaeus-Merzbacher disease are allelic disorders at the proteolipid protein locus. *Nat Genet* 1994;6:257–262.
9. Jouet M, Moncla A, Paterson J, et al. New domains of neural cell-adhesion molecule L1 implicated in X-linked hydrocephalus and MASA syndrome. *Am J Hum Genet* 1995;56:1304–1314.
10. Bruyn RPM, Scheltens P. Hereditary spastic paraparesis (Strumpell-Lorrain). In: Vinken PJ, Bruyn GW, Klawans HL, deJong JMBV, eds. *Handbook of clinical neurology*. Vol. 59. Amsterdam: Elsevier, 1991:301–318.
11. Behan WMH, Maia M. Strumpell's familial spastic paraplegia: genetics and neuropathology. *J Neurol Neurosurg Psychiatry* 1974;37:8–20.
12. Bell J, Carmichael EA. On hereditary ataxia and spastic paraplegia. *Treasury Hum Inherit* 1939;IV(Pt III):141–156.
13. Harding AE. Hereditary spastic paraplegias. *Semin Neurol* 1993;13:333–336.
14. Younger DS, Chou S, Hays AP, et al. Primary lateral sclerosis: a clinical diagnosis reemerges. *Arch Neurol* 1988;45:1304–1307.
15. McLeod JG, Morgan A, Reye C. Electrophysiological studies in familial spastic paraplegia. *J Neurol Neurosurg Psychiatry* 1977;40:611–615.
16. Hentati A, Pericac-Vance MA, Lennon F, et al. Linkage of a locus for autosomal dominant familial spastic paraplegia to chromosome 2p markers. *Hum Mol Genet* 1994;3:1867–1871.
17. Raskind WH, Pericac-Vance MA, Lennon F, Wolff J, Lipe HP, Bird TD. Familial spastic paraparesis: evaluation of locus heterogeneity, anticipation, and haplotype mapping of the SPG4 locus on the short arm of chromosome 2. *Am J Med Genet* 1997;74:26–36.
18. Burger J, Metzke H, Paternotte C, Schilling F, Hazan J, Reis A. Autosomal dominant spastic paraplegia with anticipation maps to 4-cM interval on chromosome 2p21-p24 in a large German family. *Hum Genet* 1996;98:371–375.
19. Gispert S, Santos N, Damen R, et al. Autosomal dominant familial spastic paraplegia: reduction of the FSP 1 candidate region on chromosome 14q to 7cM and locus heterogeneity. *Am J Hum Genet* 1995;56:183–187.
20. Fink JK, Brocade-Wu CT, Jones SM, et al. Autosomal dominant familial spastic paraplegia: tight linkage to chromosome 15q. *Am J Hum Genet* 1995;56:188–192.
21. Hazan J, Fontaine B, Bruyn RPM, et al. Linkage of a new locus for autosomal dominant familial spastic paraplegia to chromosome 2p. *Hum Mol Genet* 1994;3:1569–1673.
22. Hazan J, Lamy C, Meki J, Munnich A, deRecondo J, Weissenbach J. Autosomal dominant familial spastic paraplegia is genetically heterogeneous and one locus maps to chromosome 14q. *Nat Genet* 1993;5:163–167.
23. DeJonge P, Krols L, Michalik A, et al. Pure familial spastic paraplegia: clinical and genetic analysis of nine Belgian pedigrees. *Eur J Hum Genet* 1996;4:260–266.
24. Kobayashi H, Garcia CA, Alfonso G, et al. Molecular genetics of familial spastic paraplegia: A multitude of responsible genes. *J Neurol Sci* 1995;137:131–138.
25. Bruins JW, Simons X. Paraplegia spastica hereditaria. *Ned Tijdschr Geneesk* 1958;45:2210–2218.
26. Kolodny E. Globoid leukodystrophy. In: Moser HW, Vinken PJ, Bruyn GW, eds. *Neurodystrophies and neurolipidoses, handbook of clinical neurology*. Amsterdam: Elsevier, 1996:187–210.
27. Koyabashi T, Furuya X, Fukuyama H, Saito Y, Fushi N, Yamashita Y. Adult-type Krabbe's disease: clinical, radiological and molecular analyses of four patients. *Ann Neurol* 1995;38:349.
28. Ulku A, Karasoy H, Karatepe A, Gokcay F. X-linked spastic paraplegia. *Acta Neurol Scand* 1991;83:403–406.
29. Cambi F, Tartaglino L, Lublin F, McCarren X. X-linked pure familial spastic paraparesis. *Arch Neurol* 1995;53:665–669.
30. Boulloche J, Aicardi J. Pelizaeus-Merzbacher disease: clinical and nosological study. *J Child Neurol* 1986;1:233–239.
31. Koeppen AH, Ronca NA, Greenfield EA, Hans MB. Defective biosyn-

thesis of proteolipid protein in Pelizaeus-Merzbacher disease. *Ann Neurol* 1987;21:159–170.

32. Hudson LD, Puckett C, Berndt J, Chan J, Gencic S. Mutation of the proteolipid protein gene PLP in a human X chromosome-linked myelin disorder. *Proc Natl Acad Sci USA* 1989;86:8128–8131.

33. Kobayashi H, Hoffman EP, Marks HG. The rumpshaker mutation in spastic paraplegia. *Nat Genet* 1994;7:351–352.

34. Johnston AW, McKusick VA. A sex-linked recessive form of spastic paraplegia. *Am J Hum Genet* 1961;14:83–93.

35. Keppen LD, Leppert MF, O'Connel O, et al. Etiological heterogeneity in X-linked spastic paraplegia. *Am J Hum Genet* 1987;41:933–943.

36. Nance MA, Boyadjiev S, Pratt VM, Taylor S, Hodes ME, Dlouhy SP. Adult-onset neurodegenerative disorder due to proteolipid protein gene mutation in the mother of a man with Pelizaeus-Merzbacher disease. *Neurology* 1996;47:1333–1335.

37. Bonneau D, Rozet JM, Bulteau C, et al. X-linked spastic paraplegia (SPG2): clinical heterogeneity at a single locus. *J Med Genet* 1993;30:381–384.

38. Hodes ME, Dlouhy SR. The proteolipid protein gene: double, double, . . . and trouble. *Am J Hum Genet* 1996;59:12–15.

39. Maris T, Androulidakis EJ, Tzagournissakis M, Papavassiliou S, Moser H, Plaitakis A. X-linked adrenoleukodystrophy presenting as neurologically pure familial spastic paraparesis. *Neurology* 1995;45:1101–1104.

40. Moser HW. Adrenoleukodystrophy: genetics, pathogenesis and therapy. *Brain* 1997;120:1485–1508.

41. Moser HW, Moser AB, Frayer KK, et al. Adrenoleukodystrophy: increased plasma content of saturated very long chain fatty acids. *Neurology* 1981;31:1241–1249.

42. Brennemann W, Kohler W, Zierz S, Klingmuller D. Occurrence of adrenocortical insufficiency in adrenomyeloneuropathy. *Neurology* 1996;47:605.

43. Blanchine JW, Lewis RC. The MASA syndrome: a new heritable mental retardation syndrome. *Clin Genet* 1974;5:298–306.

44. Bickers DS, Adams RD. Hereditary stenosis of the aqueduct of Sylvius as a cause of congenital hydrocephalus. *Brain* 1949;72:246–262.

45. Sjögren Y, Larsson T. Oligophrenia in combination with congenital ichthyosis and spastic disorders: a clinical and genetic study. *Acta Psychiatr Neurol Scand* 1957;32[Suppl 113]:1–112.

46. Schrander-Stumpel C, Howeler C, Jones M, et al. Spectrum of X-linked hydrocephalus HSAS syndrome, and complicated spastic paraplegia (SPG1): clinical review with six additional families. *Am J Med Genet* 1995;57:107–116.

47. Steinberg D. Refsum disease. In: Scriver CR, Beaudet AL, Sly WS, Valle DE, eds. *The metabolic and molecular basis of inherited disease*, 7th ed. New York: McGraw-Hill, 1994:2351–2369.

48. Nygaard TG, Marsden CD, Fahn S. Dopa-responsive dystonia: long-term treatment response and prognosis. *Neurology* 1991;41:174–181.

49. DeJong VJMB, Bolhuis PA, Barth PG. Differential diagnosis of the patient with hereditary and spinocerebellar disorders in hereditary neuropathies and spinocerebellar atrophies. In: DeJong VJMB, ed. *Handbook of clinical neurology*. Amsterdam: Elsevier, 1991:643–699.

50. Zoghbi H. The expanding world of ataxins. *Nat Genet* 1996;14:237–238.

51. Rizzo W. Sjögren-Larsson syndrome. In: Moser HW, Vinken PJ, Bruyn GW, eds. *Neurodystrophies and neurolipidoses: handbook of clinical neurology*. Vol. 22. Amsterdam: Elsevier, 1996:615–621.

52. Durr A, Cossee M, Agid Y, et al. Clinical and genetic abnormalities in patients with Friedreich's ataxia. *N Engl J Med* 1996;335:1169–1174.

Motor Disorders,
edited by David S. Younger.
Lippincott Williams & Wilkins, Philadelphia © 1999.

CHAPTER 23

Tropical Myeloneuropathies

Gustavo C. Román

The pattern of neurologic disease occurrence in the tropics appears to be determined primarily by socioeconomic factors rather than by geography or climate (1–3). In fact, tropical diseases such as malaria and cysticercosis were common in Europe and North America a century ago. Deficiencies in environmental sanitation, lack of potable water, overcrowding, malnutrition, and exposure to neurotoxins are some of the determinants of spinal cord and peripheral nerve diseases in the tropics (4).

MYELOPATHIES

Acute Myeloneuropathies

Bilharziasis (schistosomiasis) is the most common cause of acute adult myelopathy in the tropics due to spinal cord involvement by *Schistosoma haematobium*, particularly in Africa and the Middle East, and by *S. mansoni* in the Caribbean, Venezuela, and Brazil. Bilharziasis is a major health problem in the tropics, with 600 million people estimated to be at risk (1,2,5). It occurs when the cercariae, released from a freshwater intermediate snail host, pierce and penetrate human skin or mucosal surfaces with invasion of the bloodstream, usually while the human host swims in a pond or a river. Magnetic resonance imaging shows hyperintense lesions due to parasitic involvement in the region of the conus medullaris. An enzyme-linked immunosorbent assay is available to confirm the etiology. Praziquantel is the drug of choice in uncomplicated cases, but corticosteroids and decompressive laminectomy may be necessary in those with severe compression or cerebrospinal fluid (CSF) block on myelogram.

Transverse Myelitis

Acute transverse myelitis is the most common cause of back pain in children presenting with a spinal cord syndrome that evolves over hours or days after a viral infection or vaccination. The diagnosis remains one of exclusion. Treatment with corticosteroids is recommended. Human rabies may present as a postviral transverse myelitis after a bat bite. African children that survive on a diet of cassava are at risk for konzo, a form of acute spastic paraplegia due to excessive cyanide consumption and poor dietary intake of sulphur-containing amino acids (6,7).

Multiple sclerosis is rare in the tropics; however, a number of well-documented cases have been reported from Africa and Latin America. Devic's disease, or neuromyelitis optica, includes bilateral optic neuritis and transverse myelitis and is the form of multiple sclerosis most commonly observed in India, Japan, and the Caribbean. Subacute myelo-optic neuropathy was due to consumption of clioquinol; related halogenated quinolines present in plants of the Annonaceae family and in herbal teas of the Caribbean may cause a similar disease (8).

Chronic Myelopathies

Tropical Spastic Paraparesis

Infection with the human T-lymphotropic virus type I (HTLV-I) causes tropical spastic paraparesis, the most common late-onset spastic paraplegia in the tropics (9). Also, HTLV-I is also the cause of adult T-cell leukemia-lymphoma. Cases occur endemically in South America, the Caribbean, the Seychelles Islands in the Indian Ocean, Africa, and nontropical areas of Japan. It presents clinically with leg stiffness and cramps, accompanied by incapacitating gait difficulty due to proximal weakness of the legs, with urinary frequency, constipation, and impotence in men. Serum and CSF shows typical segmented leukocytes or "flower cells," and high titers of anti-HTLV-I antibodies. Rare cases of tropical spastic paraparesis have also been reported with HTLV-II infection. There may be a striking resemblance to amyotrophic lateral sclerosis because of muscle weakness, wasting, and fasciculation in distal hand, shoulder, and tongue muscles.

G. C. Román: Department of Neurology, University of Texas Health Sciences Center, San Antonio, Texas 78284-7883.

PERIPHERAL NEUROPATHIES

Peripheral neuropathies are relatively common in the tropics (4). In addition to leprosy, other common forms include diabetes, genetic diseases, alcoholism, and a number of inflammatory, postinfectious, neurotoxic, and nutritional neuropathies due to deficiencies of micronutrients as listed in Table 1.

Leprosy is the most common cause of neuropathy worldwide due to infection with *Mycobacterium leprae*. Its prevalence in the 1980s was estimated by the World Health Organization to be 10 to 12 million cases; in the 1990s it fell to 2.4 million cases due to widespread use of combined antimicrobial therapy (2). It occurs throughout the tropics and subtropics of southeast Asia, Africa, Central and South America, the western Pacific, the eastern Mediterranean, Japan, Korea, China, Hawaii, Florida, and Louisiana. The tuberculoid, lepromatous, and borderline forms are all characterized by palpable nerve thickening, usually accompanied by skin areas of anesthesia. Multidrug treatment includes dapsone, rifampicin, and clofazimine. Corticosteroids and thalidomide are often required for the treatment of erythema nodosum leprosum and other reactions to the treatment. Prevention of eye complications, joint erosion, and deformities is mandatory.

With the decline of poliomyelitis as a cause of acute flaccid paralysis, Guillain-Barré syndrome (GBS) is now the most frequent cause of acute paralysis in children in the tropics, with an incidence greater than in industrialized countries. In Central America, poisoning with *Karwinskia calderoni* and *K. humboldtiana* resembles GBS. Clusters of GBS cases have occurred in association with swine flu vaccination, poliomyelitis vaccination, and after exposure to rabies vaccination in Latin America, India, and Thailand. Infectious agents believed to play a role in cases of GBS in the tropics include cytomegalovirus, Epstein-Barr virus, the human immunodeficiency virus, dengue, varicella-zoster, measles, and *Mycoplasma pneumoniae*. Also, rabies may present as an ascending or descending paralysis identical to GBS, and the typical hydrophobia and aerophobia may be mistaken for bulbar and respiratory paralysis.

A seasonal syndrome resembling GBS has been observed in China. Clinically, it is a pure motor axonopathy, probably associated with *Campylobacter* infection. Neuropathologic changes similar to those observed in China have also been noted in fatal cases of GBS in patients from Mexico, Colombia, and Cuba. Other conditions presenting with acute flaccid paralysis in the tropics include botulism, elapid snake envenoming, and epidemic paralysis from dietary consumption of gossypol, a phenolic compound present in cottonseed oil leading to renal loss of potassium, and licorice (*Glycyrrhiza glabra*).

Nutritional deficiency can be a proximate cause of a variety of axonal neuropathies such as beriberi, due to thiamine B deficiency, and subacute combined degenera-

TABLE 1. *Peripheral neuropathies in the tropics*

Inflammatory and postinfective neuropathies
Leprosy
Guillain-Barré syndrome
    Acute demyelinating neuropathy
    Acute motor axonal neuropathy (Chinese paralytic syndrome)
    Postrabies vaccine paralysis
Other postinfectious neuropathies
Neuropathies of infectious diseases
    Campylobacter jejuni
    Rabies
    Diphtheria
    Mycoplasma
    Lyme borreliosis (Bannwarth's syndrome)
    HIV (AIDS)
    HTLV-I/II
Toxic neuropathies
Heavy metals
    Arsenic
    Lead
    Thalium
Insecticides
    Organophosphorous esters
Plant poisons
    Manihot (cassava)
    Karwinskia humboldtiana
    Gloriosa superba
    Podophyllum pelatum
Animal poisons
    Ciguatoxin
    Paralytic shellfish poisoning (saxitoxin)
    Tick-bite paralysis
Systemic diseases
Diabetes mellitus
Amyloidosis
Uremia
Sarcoidosis
Myxedema
Connective tissue diseases
Acute intermittent porphyria
Critical illness neuropathy
Nutritional neuropathy
Beriberi and other B-group vitamin deficiencies
Strachan's syndrome
Tropical malabsorption-malnutrition
Alcoholic neuropathy
Other etiologies
Trauma, neoplasia, genetic neuropathies
Disorders of neuromuscular transmission
Myasthenia gravis
Botulism
Animal poisons
    Neurotoxic snake bite
    Marine neurotoxins
    Dart-poison frogs (South America)
    Tick-bite paralysis
Plant Poisons
    Curare
Insecticide intoxication (intermediate syndrome)

Modified from Román GC. Tropical neuropathies. *Baillière's Clin Neurol* 1995;4:469–487.

tion due to cyanocobalamin or B_{12} deficiency. There are a number of less well-defined predominantly sensory neuropathies, usually accompanied by optic, auditory, and spinal cord involvement, that have been clinically classified under the broad term of Strachan's syndrome. Although the B-group vitamins and vitamin E have been experimentally shown to cause predominantly axonal neuropathies, they rarely occur in isolation in tropical conditions because most instances of human malnutrition are usually due to overall dietary deficiency. Tropical malabsorption also plays a significant role by decreasing the availability of vitamins.

Nutritional neuropathies are endemic in subpopulations of Africa, Asia, and Latin America due to chronically deficient diets and widespread malnutrition; however, the number of cases seeking medical attention is relatively low. When a population precariously at risk is exposed to an added factor that precipitates the expression of marginally asymptomatic cases, epidemic outbreaks may occur. There may be an interaction of toxic and nutritional factors, such as in superimposed alcoholic neuropathy, tobacco–alcohol amblyopia, and cases associated with the consumption of cyanide-producing tropical foodstuffs such as cassava. Precipitating factors include pregnancy and lactation, infectious diarrhea, malaria, and the increased metabolic requirements for thiamine due to increased carbohydrate intake and intense physical activity under hot and humid weather conditions. Neurologic signs in nutritional disorders occur relatively late because of a combination of factors. There may be a severe deficiency of essential or protective nutrients such as sulfur-containing amino acids and the antioxidant carotenoid, lycopene. Dorsal root ganglia, neurons, large myelinated distal axons, bipolar retinal neurons, and cochlear neurons are the most sensitive elements of the peripheral nervous system and the first to suffer damage and manifest symptoms.

Strachan's Syndrome

First recognized by Strachan in Jamaica (1888, 1897), the syndrome named in his honor is characterized by orogenital dermatitis, painful sensory neuropathy, amblyopia, and deafness (10). With regional variations, Strachan's syndrome has been reported in malnourished populations in Africa, India, and the Caribbean and most recently in Cuba, where it affected over 50,000 persons (11–13). It was observed during World War II in prisoners of war in tropical camps under conditions of dietary restriction and forced labor (14). In Africa, affected patients were relatively young with a mean age of 35 years and generally from low socioeconomic environments in sub-Saharan Africa. Sensory neuropathy, decreased vision, and hearing loss along with sensory ataxia and spastic paraparesis were the predominant presenting features. In a fourth of the cases, malnutrition was

evident, with skin and mucosal pellagroid changes. Most were women; pregnancy was a precipitating factor in a third. Gastrointestinal problems were frequent, including chronic diarrhea, gastric achlorhydria or hypochlorhydria, and abnormal liver biopsy. CSF was usually normal. Slow peroneal motor nerve conduction velocities were found in all patients, and sural nerve biopsies showed changes consistent with axonal neuropathy. With parenteral vitamin B-complex treatment, 65% of patients improved.

In India, patients had a predominantly sensory neuropathy associated with chronic malnutrition, alcohol abuse, and pellagra, in addition to low blood levels of thiamine, riboflavin, nicotinic acid, pantothenic acid, pyridoxine, and folic acid. Absorption and levels of vitamin B_{12} were normal. Withdrawal of alcohol, balanced diet, and vitamin B-group treatment led to neurologic improvement. Traditionally, pernicious anemia and neuropathy and myelopathy caused by vitamin B_{12} deficiency have been rare in the tropics, even among strict vegetarians or vegans. These conditions are probably underdiagnosed because most vegan Indian patients with megaloblastic anemia studied in England had dietary B_{12} deficiency and some had pernicious anemia.

In the Caribbean, a cluster of nutritional neuropathies was recently observed in Cuba (11). This epidemic neuropathy affected 50,862 patients between 1992 and 1993 with an incidence of 462 per 100,000. Most cases occurred in patients age 25 to 64 years, whereas children, adolescents, pregnant women, and the elderly were rarely affected. The highest rates were found in the tobacco-growing province of Pinar del Río (11–13). Clinical manifestations included retrobulbar optic neuropathy, sensorineural deafness, sensory and autonomic neuropathy, and dorsolateral myelopathy. Less often, dysphonia, dysphagia, and spastic paraparesis were present and frequent in mixed forms. Neurologic symptoms were preceded by weight loss, anorexia, chronic fatigue, lack of energy, irritability, sleep disturbances, and difficulties with concentration and memory. Optic neuropathy consisted of blurred vision, photophobia, central and cecocentral scotomata, deficit of color vision for red and green, and loss of axons in the maculopapillary bundle with temporal disc pallor in advanced cases (11,15,16). Approximately a third of patients had skin and mucous membrane lesions, peripheral nerve and spinal cord involvement, and 20% had hearing loss. Neuropathic symptoms (11) included painful and burning dysesthesias in soles and palms, numbness, cramps, paresthesiae, and hyperhidrosis. The nerves were sensitive to pressure. Motor involvement was minimal. Objective sensory signs were mild and included stocking and glove vibratory, light touch, and pinprick sensory loss. Achilles tendon reflexes were decreased or absent. Motor nerve conduction velocities were normal, and sensory nerve potential amplitudes were decreased only in severe cases. Sural nerve biopsies showed an axonal neuropathy with predominant loss of large myelinated fibers (17).

Patients with dorsolateral myelopathy (11) presented with sensory gait ataxia due to proprioceptive loss, imbalance, and proximal leg weakness, brisk knee reflexes, and crossed adductor responses despite decreased or absent ankle reflexes, Babinski signs, and frank spasticity. Sensorineural deafness was usually symmetric, with high-pitch tinnitus and deafness (11). Pure tone audiometry demonstrated 4- to 8-kHz hearing loss. There were no associated vestibular symptoms. Affected patients were generally farmers of lower income and had less education compared with healthy control subjects. The use of tobacco, in particular at least four cigars per day, was the factor most associated with the highest risk of optic neuropathy (12,13). Other factors included lack of food for several days, eating lunch less than 5 days per week, and eating breakfast less than once per week. Protective factors included having relatives overseas to buy supplementary food and raising chickens at home for the ingestion of B-group vitamins and sulfur-containing amino acids. High levels of lycopene, a nonvitamin A carotenoid antioxidant found in tomatoes, guavas, watermelons, and other red fruits, conferred the strongest protection (13); consumption of riboflavin, an antioxidant, was also protective (13). Marked improvement of vision was obtained with parenteral B-group vitamins and folic acid. Therefore, despite the absence of overt malnutrition in Cuba, a deficit of B-group vitamins, mainly cobalamin and thiamine, compounded by lack of essential sulfur-amino acids in the diet, was the cause of the outbreak. The relative absence of cases in children, pregnant women, and the elderly, those so often affected by nutritional neuromyelopathies in the tropics, was explained by the availability of nutritional supplements for them.

Beriberi

Until early in this century, beriberi was a major public health problem in China, Japan, Indonesia, the Philippines, and Africa and among populations dependent on polished rice for their staple diet. Food supplementation with thiamine practically eliminated beriberi around the world. Most cases are currently observed in alcoholic patients and in the elderly on poor diets; however, beriberi continues to occur in the tropics when conditions of low thiamine intake, high carbohydrate diet, and high energy expenditure are met (4). Wet beriberi presents clinically with dysesthesias and foot drop. The more prominent systemic illness is cardiac failure, suggested by pedal edema, that accounts for the high fatality rate. Typical lesions in the heart include myocardial edema, central necrosis of fibers, and mitochondrial lesions. Sural nerve biopsies show axonopathy. The diagnosis is confirmed by low serum levels of thiamine and thiamine pyrophosphate activity. The dietary history usually reveals low intake of thiamine in the diet or consumption of thiaminase present, for example, in raw fish. There is no effective body storage of thiamine, and dietary deficiency leads to symptoms in a month or two. Thiamine plays a central role in energy production, and thiamine requirements depend on the metabolic rate of the body. High energy expenditures in the hot and humid conditions of the tropics and a diet based on complex carbohydrates contribute to outbreaks of beriberi. It responds rapidly to parenteral thiamine.

Toxic Neuropathies

A large number of industrial or environmental products selectively affect the nerves. In the tropics, widespread and indiscriminate use of toxic pesticides, compounded by a lack of education on their proper handling and storage, increases the problem of toxic exposure. This is amplified by inherent malnutrition, infection, and genetic susceptibility (18,19).

The most common heavy metal compounds that cause peripheral neuropathy are arsenic, lead, and thallium (20). Pharmacologic products (21), such as isoniazid, ethambutol, sulfonamides, nitrofurantoin, metronidazole, chloroquine, clioquinol, chloramphenicol, dapsone, and aromatic diamines, used in the treatment of leishmaniasis and trypanosomiasis, can cause peripheral nerve disease in the tropics. Neurotoxic industrial agents include n-hexane, methyl-n-butyl ketone, carbon disulfide, acrylamide, and trichloroethylene (20).

Tri-ortho-cresyl phosphate intoxication was the cause of Jamaica ginger paralysis. Epidemics also occurred in Morocco, Durban, Bombay, and Sri Lanka due to contamination or adulteration of food or cooking oils with tri-ortho-cresyl phosphate. The clinical disorder includes symmetric weakness and wasting of distal muscles of the arms with claw-hand deformity wrist drop, minimal sensory abnormalities, and late pyramidal signs. Organophosphorous pesticides produce a delayed distal axonopathy. A postsynaptic neuromuscular junction disorder occurs 2 to 3 days after toxic exposure. Ocular toxicity, or Saku's disease, occurs with fenthion, dichlorovos, fenitrothion, malathion, parathion, and methyl-parathion exposure.

Neurologic Problems Associated with Dietary Cyanide Intoxication

A number of staple foods in the tropics contain large amounts of cyanogenic glycosides. They include cassava, yams, sweet potatoes, corn, millet, bamboo shoots, and beans, particularly small black lima beans, which grow wild in Puerto Rico and Central America. Inhaled tobacco smoke contains 150 to 300μg of cyanide per cigarette. The hydrolysis of plant glycosides also releases cyanide in the form of hydrocyanic acid. Intoxication occurs by rapid cyanide absorption through the gastrointestinal tract or the lungs. Detoxification is mainly due to thiocyanate in a reaction mediated by a sulfur-transferase or rhodanase, which converts thiosulfate into thiocyanate and sulfite. Thiocyanate is a goitrogenic agent that may be responsible for endemic cretinism in some tropical areas. The sulfur-containing essential amino acids cystine, cysteine, and methionine provide the sulfur for these detoxification reactions.

Cassava is a root crop consumed in large quantities throughout the tropics and constitutes the major source of calories for some 300 million people. It contains linamarin, a cyanogenic glycoside. Cassava is the staple diet in western Nigeria, Zaire, Tanzania, Senegal, Uganda, and Mozambique. In these countries, a number of neurologic disorders have been associated with high dietary intake of cassava in association with depletion of sulfur-containing amino acids. However, it should be noted that these problems are not common in Latin America, even though cassava consumption in countries such as Brazil is among the highest in the world.

The clinical syndromes associated with chronic cyanide intoxication are tropical ataxic neuropathy, a form of spastic paraparesis known as konzo, tropical amblyopia, and nerve deafness. Tropical ataxic neuropathy was first observed in Nigeria, in areas where the diet depended almost exclusively on cassava (22). It reached an estimated prevalence of 18 to 26 per 1,000, with equal sex distribution. Onset was usually in the third and fourth decades. It consists of chronic and slowly progressive predominantly sensory polyneuropathy, associated with posterior column involvement, optic atrophy, and sensorineural deafness. Symptoms include distal painful burning paresthesiae, numbness, and cramps. On examination there is impaired vibratory perception in the feet, with loss of knee and ankle reflexes. Two thirds of affected patients have incoordination and a broad-based ataxic gait. Weakness and atrophy of distal leg muscles, especially of the peroneal group, also occurs. Other symptoms include blurring of vision due to bilateral optic atrophy (81%) and tinnitus followed by bilateral nerve deafness (36%). Few patients demonstrate corticospinal tract pyramidal signs. About 40% of patients present with skin and mucosal lesions suggestive of vitamin deficiency. In other African countries such as Senegal, similar syndromes have been observed in malnourished populations, although not necessarily in association with high cassava intake. The frequency of visual loss (19%), deafness (13%), and mucocutaneous lesions (15%) is much lower in these patients than in those from Nigeria.

Konzo is the traditional name given in Kwango, Zaire to a form of epidemic spastic paraparesis described during times of drought and famine in cassava-staple areas (6,7). Epidemics have occurred in rural areas of Mozambique, Tanzania, Zaire, and the Central African Republic. The disease occurs in up to two thirds of children and lactating women with a prevalence of 29 to 34 per 1,000.

Women and children eat raw and sun-dried uncooked bitter cassava, whereas men normally eat well-cooked cassava. Traditional methods of cassava preparation in Africa include soaking, fermentation, and sun drying, which leaves substantial amounts of cyanogenic glycosides in the cassava meal. Signs of acute cyanide intoxication are followed by sudden nonprogressive spastic paraparesis with later flexion contractures of hamstrings and Achilles tendons. Scissoring gait and toe walking are frequently present, and patients require one or two sticks to walk. Increased tone in the lower limbs, hyperreflexia, ankle clonus, and Babinski signs are usually present. There is no light touch or pinprick sensory loss. Impairment of rapid movements and hyperreflexia in the upper limbs are also present. Nystagmus and dysarthria may occur. There is minimal recovery with a nutritious diet and vitamin therapy.

Tropical amblyopia has been described in association with chronic cassava intake (23). The condition, initially described in Cuba in 1898 by Mádan, is variously known as tobacco amblyopia, tobacco-alcohol amblyopia, West Indian amblyopia, and Jamaican optic neuropathy. Cases similar to those observed in Cuba were recently reported in Tanzania in association with peripheral neuropathy (24). All are probably clinically identical to the retrobulbar neuropathy of pernicious anemia due to vitamin B_{12} deficiency and to the nutritional amblyopia described above. The common element is an underlying deficiency of micronutrients, in particular B-group vitamins, folic acid, and sulfur amino acids. For these reasons, the term nutritional or deficiency amblyopia is preferred. The differential diagnosis should include methyl alcohol intoxication, a common cause of epidemic blindness in the tropics resulting from consumption of adulterated alcohol.

As with tropical amblyopia, sensorineural deafness was commonly found in patients from Nigeria in association with cassava intake and micronutrient deficiencies (22). Also, this lesion is probably primarily nutritional in origin.

REFERENCES

1. Román GC. Tropical neurology. In: Bradley WG, Daroff RB, Fenichel GM, Marsden CD, eds. *Neurology in clinical practice*, 2nd ed. Boston: Butterworth-Heinemann, 1996:2103–2128.
2. Román GC. Neurology in public health. In: Detels R, Holland WW, McEwen J, Omenn GS, eds. *Oxford textbook of public health*, 3rd ed. Oxford: Oxford University Press, 1997:1195–1223.
3. Toro G, Román GC, Navarro de Román LI. *Neurologia tropical*. Bogota: Printer, 1983.
4. Román GC. Tropical neuropathies. *Baillière's Clin Neurol* 1995;4: 469–487.
5. Shakir RA, Newman PK, Poser CM, eds. *Tropical neurology*. London: W.B. Saunders, 1996.
6. Rosling H. Cassava, cyanide, and epidemic spastic paraparesis. *Acta Univ Upsaliensis* 1986;19:1–52.
7. Tylleskär T. The causation of konzo. Studies on a paralytic disease in Africa. *Acta Univ Upsaliensis* 1994;43:1–67.
8. Caparros-Lefebre D, Charpentier D, Joseph H, Strobel M, Bequet D,

Berchel C. High prevalence of SMON after use of tropical herbal medicine. *Neurology* 1997;48[Suppl 2]:A95.

9. Román GC, Vernant JC, Osame M. *HTLV-I and the nervous system.* New York: Liss, 1989.

10. Román GC. Epidemic neuropathies of Jamaica. *Trans Stud Coll Phys Philadelphia Med Hist* 1985;7:261–274.

11. Román GC. An epidemic in Cuba of optic neuropathy, sensorineural deafness, peripheral sensory neuropathy and dorsolateral myeloneuropathy. *J Neurol Sci* 1994;127:11–28.

12. Centers for Disease Control and Prevention. Epidemic neuropathy—Cuba, 1991–1994. *MMWR Mortal Morb Wkly Rep* 1994;43:183–192.

13. Cuba Neuropathy Field Investigation Team. Epidemic optic neuropathy in Cuba—clinical characterization and risk factors. *N Engl J Med* 1995;333:1176–1182.

14. Román GC, Spencer PS, Schoenberg BS. Tropical myeloneuropathies: the hidden endemias. *Neurology* 1985;35:1158–1170.

15. Newman NJ, Torroni A, Brown D, et al. Epidemic neuropathy in Cuba not associated with mitochondrial DNA mutations found in Leber's hereditary optic neuropathy patients. *Am J Ophthalmol* 1994;118:158–168.

16. Sadun AA, Martone JF, Muci-Mendoza R, et al. Epidemic optic neuropathy in Cuba: eye findings. *Arch Ophthalmol* 1994;112:691–699.

17. Borrajero I, Pérez JL, Domínguez C, et al. Epidemic neuropathy in Cuba: morphological characterization of peripheral nerve lesions in sural nerve biopsies. *J Neurol Sci* 1994;127:68–76.

18. Senanayake N, Román GC. Disorders of neuromuscular transmission due to natural environmental toxins. *J Neurol Sci* 1992;107:1–13.

19. Senanayake N, Román GC. Toxic neuropathies in the tropics. *J Trop Geograph Neurol* 1991;1:3–15.

20. Ludolph AC, Spencer PS. Toxic neuropathies and their treatment. *Baillière's Clin Neurol* 1995;4:505–527.

21. Windebank AJ. Drug-induced neuropathies. *Baillière's Clin Neurol* 1995;4:529–573.

22. Osuntokun BO. An ataxic neuropathy in Nigeria: a clinical, biochemical and electrophysiological study. *Brain* 1968;91:215–248.

23. Osuntokun BO, Osuntokun O. Tropical amblyopia in Nigerians. *Am J Ophthalmol* 1971;71:708–716.

24. Plant GT, Mtanda AT, Arden GB, Johnson GJ. An epidemic of optic neuropathy in Tanzania: characterization of the visual disorder and associated peripheral neuropathy. *J Neurol Sci* 1996;145:127–140.

PART III

Spinal Cord Diseases

Motor Disorders,
edited by David S. Younger.
Lippincott Williams & Wilkins, Philadelphia © 1999.

CHAPTER 24

Motor Dysfunction in Multiple Sclerosis

Steven R. Schwid, Peter A. Calabresi, and Andrew D. Goodman

Multiple sclerosis (MS) is a chronic, immune-mediated, demyelinating disease of the central nervous system (CNS). MS is characterized pathologically by plaques of inflammation, demyelination, and gliosis disseminated in space, that is, in different locations in the CNS, and in time, namely, separate attacks. The signs and symptoms depend on the location of the lesions within the brain and spinal cord. Motor dysfunction in MS can include of spasticity, weakness, tremor, and ataxia and is one of the most common and disabling symptoms. In this chapter, we review the epidemiology, pathology, pathophysiology, diagnosis, clinical manifestations, and treatment of MS with an emphasis on motor system manifestations.

EPIDEMIOLOGY

The prevalence of MS is difficult to estimate because of several constraints: ascertainment bias, the lack of definitive tests to diagnose MS, and the tendency of patients and physicians to overlook milder forms. The best estimates come from population-based samples in which referral bias is minimized. They find prevalence rates of 2 per 100,000 in Japan to 100 or more persons per 100,000 in northern Europe and North America (1,2). The disease is twice as common in temperate regions than in the tropics. Migration studies suggest that a critical environmental exposure occurs before age 15 (3,4), although the exact nature of this environmental exposure has yet to be defined.

S. R. Schwid: Department of Neurology, University of Rochester Medical Center, Rochester, New York 14642.

P. A. Calabresi: Department of Clinical Neurosciences, Brown University and Multiple Sclerosis Program, Rhode Island Hospital, Providence, Rhode Island 02903.

A. D. Goodman: Department of Neurology, University of Rochester and Multiple Sclerosis Center, Strong Memorial Hospital, Rochester, New York 14642.

Women are affected twice as often as males, and whites have a much higher incidence rate than other races. The incidence of MS peaks in the fourth decade of life, but the disease commonly presents between ages 15 and 60. Childhood onset occurs but is uncommon. Overall, MS is the third most common cause of disability in the United States in the 15- to 50-year-old group after trauma and musculoskeletal disease (5).

GENETICS

Although the prevalence of MS is roughly 1 per 1,000 in the general population, siblings of affected patients have a 2 to 5% lifetime risk, whereas parents and children of MS patients have a 1% risk. Monozygotic twins have a 30% risk, whereas dizygotic twins have a risk similar to that of another sibling (6,7). Linkage studies implicate the major histocompatibility complex (MHC) and other immunoregulatory genes as important determinants of this hereditary risk (8,9). Genetic factors may also relate to different forms of the disease. Asians are more likely to develop disease restricted to the optic nerves and spinal cord, whereas whites tend to develop disseminated disease. Affected whites have an increased frequency of the HLA-DR2 haplotype but not Asians (10).

PATHOLOGY AND PATHOPHYSIOLOGY

MS plaques occur throughout the CNS, but they are particularly common in the optic nerves, cerebral periventricular white matter, brainstem, and spinal cord tracts. Acute lesions have marked perivascular inflammatory cell infiltrates, comprised predominantly of mononuclear cells, T lymphocytes, and macrophages, with occasional B cells and plasma cells. As the lesion progresses, demyelination ensues, with macrophages and microglial cells that phagocytose myelin debris. Initially, oligodendrocytes, the myelin-producing cells, proliferate, but they are destroyed as infiltration and astrocytic gliosis extend. When this process is more severe and long-standing, axonal loss may also be evident (11).

Although the ultimate etiology of MS remains poorly understood, pathologic and experimental evidence suggests that damage is mediated by the immune system. Current theories support an undefined activating process that triggers the immune response against one or more myelin antigens, including myelin basic protein, proteolipid protein, myelin/oligodendrocyte glycoprotein, myelin-associated glycoprotein, and other gangliosides. Cytokines released from activated T cells may amplify the immune response within the CNS by promoting the expression of adhesion molecules on adjacent blood vessels and by the propagation of further T-cell activation through upregulation of class II MHC molecules. A variety of inflammatory mediators, including tumor necrosis factor and other cytokines; oxygen radicals; and nitric oxide play a role in demyelination. Systemic immune dysregulation has been demonstrated in vitro and in vivo, but their significance is unclear (12,13). Demyelination causes symptoms through slowed axonal conduction, conduction block, and ectopic signal transmission (14). Cytokines may also modulate axonal conduction and synaptic transmission in addition to causing structural myelin damage (15).

Motor dysfunction from MS is manifested as spasticity, weakness, tremor, and ataxia. Spasticity is defined as a velocity-dependent increase in muscular tone. It is caused by the loss of inhibitory inputs from corticospinal and other descending motor pathways to gamma motoneurons and interneuron networks that participate in spinal cord reflex arcs. Hyperreflexia, muscle spasms, and other upper motor neuron (UMN) signs are related to similar mechanisms (16). Weakness and impairment of fine motor control are caused more directly by interruption of input to alpha motoneurons. Rarely, muscle atrophy and other lower motor neuron signs may be present. Tremor and ataxia are related to lesions of the cerebellum and cerebellar pathways through the brainstem, red nucleus, thalamus, and basal ganglia. Classically, lesions have been attributed to Mollaret's triangle, comprised of the dentate nucleus of the cerebellum, inferior olive, and red nucleus. In some cases, proprioceptive loss may be the primary cause for impairment (17). The neural circuitry involved in the pathogenesis of tremor is complex and variable, as evidenced by the mixed results of ablative procedures such as thalamotomy (18).

Motor fatigue, defined as a loss of force-generating capacity during sustained motor activity, can also contribute to motor dysfunction and disability, even in patients without other signs of motor dysfunction. If fatigability was related to demyelination in central motor pathways, this would likely be caused by frequency-dependent conduction block with successive action potential transmissions. Laboratory evidence supporting this hypothesis stems from observations of the refractory period between transmissions that increases from 1 msec

in myelinated axons to 4 msec or more after demyelination (19). A similar refractory period was not demonstrated in patients with MS nor was there a change in central motor conduction velocity or amplitude during fatiguing exercise (20). These studies suggest that motor fatigue may be caused by impaired drive to the primary motor cortex from premotor areas rather than an impairment in UMN or lower motor neuron transmission.

DIAGNOSIS

The diagnosis of MS is made by the history, serial examinations, and appropriate laboratory studies. Two or more white matter lesions on brain imaging studies due to multiple clinical attacks disseminated in time and space that cannot be explained by another disease process is definite evidence of MS. Criteria have been published to define the certainty of diagnosis for the purposes of epidemiologic studies and clinical trials (21).

In patients whose history and examination suggest less than two CNS lesions, ancillary tests can be used to establish the presence of disseminated disease. Magnetic resonance imaging (MRI) of the brain is the most useful test in this regard for two reasons: it excludes compressive or mass lesions and it detects symptomatic lesions in the brain and spinal cord (22). Over 95% of patients with clinically definite MS have abnormalities on brain MRI. The typical pattern of lesions includes multiple irregular lesions within the white matter, particularly adjacent to the lateral ventricles, in the corpus callosum and centrum semiovale (23). Lesions within the cerebral peduncles, brainstem, and cerebellum are also common. They tend to be of high-signal intensity on T2-weighted scans with normal-to-low signals on T1-weighted images. Gadolinium-enhancement occurs in the early stages of lesion development, coinciding with blood–brain barrier disruption. Although white matter abnormalities similar to those seen in MS can be found in other conditions, the finding of typical lesions, with a periventricular predominance in the appropriate clinical setting, allows a confident diagnosis to be made.

Spinal cord MRI reveals regions of demyelination, but these are usually more difficult to image due to technical reasons. Altogether, 75% of MS lesions occur in the cervical region. They are generally one to two vertebral segments in length; however, longer plaques are more likely to be associated with swelling or atrophy of the cord. Most occupy less than half of the cross-sectional area of the cord, centering on the lateral or posterior funiculi. As with brain MRI, gadolinium-enhancement may occur within regions of T2-weighted signal abnormality (24).

Several MRI studies have demonstrated that cerebral demyelination is a more dynamic process than clinical changes in relapsing-remitting or progressive disease would suggest (25). During periods of apparent clinical stability, new and enlarging lesions are frequently seen on serial imaging and correlate with clinical activity and worsening disability over time. Associations with serial spinal MRI have been more difficult to demonstrate. The discrepancy may be partly related to technical limitations in spinal MRI, because more recent studies have found a strong correlation between spinal cord cross-sectional area and disability (26).

Evoked responses are useful in detecting subclinical lesions and in confirming the relation of questionable symptoms and signs to a CNS process (27). Three types of studies are commonly used in clinical practice: visual evoked responses (VER), brainstem auditory evoked responses (BAER), and somatosensory evoked potentials (SSER). VER have the most clinical utility in confirming optic nerve demyelination in patients with visual symptoms and in detecting subclinical lesions. A prolonged P100 latency and intereye latency difference with preserved amplitude is seen in 80 to 95% of patients with optic neuritis; others have a reduced amplitude, but these are less specific for demyelination. Thirty percent of MS patients without a history of visual complaints or signs on examination have abnormal VER. Although prolonged latencies suggest the presence of prechiasmal optic nerve demyelination, up to a 30% incidence of false positives has been reported, often related to opaque media, severe glaucoma, or uncorrected refractive errors.

BAER reveal prolonged interpeak latencies in 65% of patients with clinically definite lesions. The typical abnormalities found in MS patients include prolonged wave III to IV interpeak latencies and disappearance of wave V. These abnormalities are not specific for MS but are more sensitive for brainstem lesions than MRI.

SSER are considered definitely abnormal when the potential is absent, not just prolonged. The sensitivity in clinically definite MS is 86%, but only 40 to 50% in cases without proven dissemination. When patients present with sensory complaints that do not conform to a radicular or peripheral nerve distribution, abnormal SSER may confirm CNS pathology. However, they can rarely be considered a clear indicator of subclinical disease because of the high false positive rate.

Motor evoked responses (MER), obtained using transcranial magnetic stimulation, may also be obtained, although their clinical utility remains uncertain. Patients with MS have significantly delayed central motor conduction, reduced motor amplitudes, and increased dispersion of MER (28). Conduction to the lower extremities is more likely to be abnormal than to the upper extremities because pathways to the lower extremities are longer. Sensitivity can be enhanced by considering interside differences, although this may increase the incidence of false-positive abnormalities (29). The overall utility of this technique for detecting subclinical motor deficits appears to be relatively low compared with VER. MER are potentially useful in the evaluation of vague symptoms and corroborate objective signs; they also prove useful as secondary measures of efficacy in the evaluation of new treatments. MER are better suited for this purpose than VER because they improve with symptomatic treatments such as corticosteroid pulses, whereas VER do not change (30); in addition, central motor conduction time correlates well with strength. Signals may be difficult to obtain in the lower extremities, but the absence of a signal is clearly associated with more impaired strength and ambulation (31).

Although MRI and evoked potentials may be helpful for verifying the presence of multiple CNS lesions, abnormalities on these tests are not specific for MS; therefore, proof of an inflammatory process in the CNS provides further diagnostic certainty. CSF pleocytosis, increased IgG production, elevated myelin basic protein, and oligoclonal bands on CSF electrophoresis are all suggestive of MS but are not specific. A lymphocytic pleocytosis of 5 to 50 cells/mm^3 is seen in about 65% of patients. Tourtellotte (32) calculated a CSF IgG synthesis rate and showed that it could be reduced with corticosteroids and other immunosuppressants. CSF oligoclonal bands are detected in over 90% of patients (33). They may not be present during the first few years of the disease, but once present they persist, and therefore are not indicative of disease activity. They are also commonly detected in patients with other inflammatory CNS disorders such as encephalitis, meningitis, Guillain-Barré syndrome, and even cerebral infarction (34).

Because none of these tests is perfectly sensitive or specific for MS, false-positive diagnoses can occur in up to 12% of patients. The most commonly misdiagnosed lesions are spinal tumors presenting as a chronic progressive myelopathy. "Red flags" in making the diagnosis of MS include a progressive course before age 35, localized pain, normal CSF, absence of bowel or bladder symptoms, a strongly positive family history, and peripheral neuropathy. The absence of ocular signs, normal vibratory sensation, and retained abdominal reflexes should also raise concern about the diagnosis (35).

DIFFERENTIAL DIAGNOSIS

The differential diagnosis of MS includes a variety of disorders affecting the CNS in young adults. In patients with isolated optic neuritis or transverse myelitis, debate continues about whether these constitute mild or localized forms of MS or distinct disease entities. Although there is no demonstrable pathologic difference between the two, there is clearly a subset of patients with these disorders that never develop further demyelinating events. Several studies have shown that patients presenting with a monophasic demyelinating event who have abnormal brain MRI or oligoclonal banding in the CSF are much more likely to experience MS-defining attacks in the next 5 to 10 years (36,37).

Acute disseminated encephalomyelitis may also be considered a monophasic demyelinating event but with multifocal lesions. There is typically acute and rapidly progressive demyelination involving the cerebrum, spinal cord, and occasionally the peripheral nervous system (38,39). Acute disseminated encephalomyelitis is most often encountered in children after infection or immunization; it carries a high rate of morbidity and mortality. Milder versions in adults have been described, including relapsing-remitting cases that may be impossible to distinguish from typical MS and some with full recovery. A fulminant fatal course, often associated with widespread cerebral hemorrhage and necrosis, is intentionally excluded from the diagnostic criteria for MS but is most likely an extreme variant of the same disease process.

Neuromyelitis optica, or Devic syndrome, with CNS involvement isolated to the optic nerves and spinal cord, may also be a variant of MS. Classically, patients present with acute transverse myelitis in association with bilateral optic or retrobulbar neuritis, but incomplete syndromes have also been described. Although this may simply be a subset of MS, published reports cite several key differences, including a higher percentage of patients of Asian descent and a lower percentage of patients with abnormal brain MRI and CSF oligoclonal bands. The disease may be monophasic, relapsing, or progressive but tends to have a poorer prognosis and response to immunomodulation than straightforward cases of MS (40).

CNS inflammation may also be associated with a systemic collagen vascular disorder (41). Systemic lupus erythematosus typically presents with systemic involvement, but mild proteinuria, rash, or pulmonary symptoms may be initially overlooked. Rarely, patients may present with isolated CNS involvement followed years later by a more typical disease patterns. Various types of neurologic presentations exist, including myelopathy, which may be acute, relapsing, or progressive; seizures; psychiatric disease; and strokes (42). The diagnosis is suggested by an unusually elevated erythrocyte sedimentation rate and renal, pulmonary, or dermatologic disease. An antinuclear antibody may be present in up to 40% of patients with MS (13); anti-double-stranded DNA antibodies or hypocomplementemia should be preferably obtained. Sjögren syndrome is characterized by the insidious development of dry eyes or keratoconjunctivitis sicca and dry mouth or xerostomia, often in conjunction with episodic parotitis. CNS manifestations are uncommon but include myelopathic, cerebellar, and visual presentations (43). The manifestations of Behçet syndrome are headache, fever, and mucocutaneous ulcers, but they rarely present with a progressive myelopathy and retrobulbar neuritis (44). Sarcoidosis involves the nervous system in 5 to 10% of all cases. Most of these cases manifest with cranial neuropathies and meningoencephalitis, but progressive myelopathy and ataxia have also been reported (45,46).

CNS vasculitis can mimic MS but is usually associated with a collagen-vascular disorder such as polyarteritis nodosa or another systemic vasculitis. Rarely, isolated CNS vasculitis occurs, causing headache, mental change, and strokelike episodes, without systemic involvement. CSF typically reveals pleocytosis and elevation of the protein content. Cerebral angiography and meningeal and cortical biopsy are essential in establishing the diagnosis (47).

Infectious disorders such as syphilis, tuberculosis, and Lyme disease should be considered in the differential diagnosis of chronic meningoencephalitis due to MS, but generally they show other systemic signs and symptoms (48). Progressive myelopathy may also be caused by these agents and by human T-lymphotropic virus type I, the agent of tropical spastic paraparesis. This disease is transmitted through blood and sexual contact and is endemic in the Caribbean and several other regions throughout the world, as well as the southeastern United States. Why some of those infected develop paraparesis and others remain asymptomatic remains to be determined. Other than the presence of antiviral antibodies, the disease is indistinguishable from the progressive myelopathy related to MS (49,50).

Human immunodeficiency virus infection causes progressive myelopathy, multiple cranial neuropathies, chronic meningoencephalitis, and subacute subcortical dementia (51,52). Cytomegalovirus, herpes simplex virus, and varicella zoster virus also cause myelopathy, particularly in immunosuppressed patients, but they are usually acute and necrotizing (53–55).

Common metabolic causes of progressive leukodystrophy and myelopathy in adults include hereditary disorders, such as adrenoleukodystrophy and Refsum disease, and acquired disorders, such as subacute combined degeneration due to vitamin B_{12} deficiency, with or without demyelinating neuropathy (56). Degenerative disorders of unknown etiology that should also be considered include primary lateral sclerosis and the several types of spinocerebellar degeneration. Clues to the presence of an inherited degenerative process are an informative pedigree, symmetry of disease, lack of sensory involvement, early severe optic atrophy, skeletal deformities such as scoliosis or pes cavus, neuropathy, and normal CSF profile (57).

Cerebrovascular disease is sometimes difficult to distinguish from MS, particularly in older hypertensive patients that present with progressive subcortical disease; generally, stepwise progression is more suggestive of vascular disease. Cerebral autosomal dominant arteriopathy with subcortical infarcts and leukoencephalopathy is a cause of progressive white matter degeneration that may be difficult to distinguish from MS. At present, however, the incidence of this disease remains uncertain, and there is no known test to make the diagnosis certain in life (58,59).

A CNS tumor, arteriovenous malformation, spondylosis, Chiari malformation, and syringomyelia may all mimic MS clinically and should be considered, especially when all signs and symptoms are referable to a single lesion on neuroimaging. Even in a patient with established MS, these conditions may require further consideration when relatively uncommon symptoms occur, such as aphasia, hemianopia, cervical radicular pain, weakness, and sensory loss.

CLINICAL COURSE AND PROGNOSIS

The course of MS is quite variable but can be divided into a relapsing-remitting pattern of distinct attacks and relatively symptom-free or stable periods and a chronic progressive pattern of steadily worsening symptoms without clear attacks. At least half of patients that start with a relapsing-remitting pattern will subsequently develop a progressive course (60). This is termed secondary progressive MS to distinguish it from primary progressive MS, which is progressive from the onset (61). Regardless of the clinical course, however, serial MRI indicates that the underlying disease process is more dynamic, with new lesions occurring and old lesions enlarging in relapsing, progressing, and even clinically stable patients.

Prognostic indicators have been extensively studied. Although conflicting reports exist (62), it has been suggested that sensory symptoms at the onset correlate with a benign illness (63), whereas motor or cerebellar signs, early relapse, and onset after age 40 predict an aggressive course (64–66). Gender, relapse rate, monosymptomatic onset, and laboratory data have not been consistently shown to carry prognostic value. Motor symptoms from corticospinal tract involvement occurs with the initial attack of MS in 32 to 41% of patients and eventually affects nearly all patients to an extent. Men presenting after age 40 with progressive myelopathy tend to have steadily worsening paraparesis with variable involvement of the upper extremities and few deficits related to the cerebral white matter. Overall survival is minimally altered, and the median time to reach a moderate level of disability requiring unilateral assistance to walk 100 meters is approximately 10 years from the onset (67).

CLINICAL MANIFESTATIONS

Symptoms and signs in MS are dependent on the location of demyelinating CNS lesions. Optic neuritis due to optic nerve lesions; diplopia, internuclear ophthalmoplegia, facial weakness and numbness, and vertigo resulting from brainstem lesions; ataxia from cerebellar lesions; bowel and bladder urgency, frequency, and retention due to autonomic lesions; and paresthesias and hypesthesia due to sensory tract lesions are particularly common. Cognitive deficits, including slowed information processing, loss of executive function, and impaired short-term memory, appear to be related to the overall burden of subcortical white matter lesions. Seizures occur in up to 5% of patients, usually coinciding with an active lesion near the cerebral cortex. Fatigue and depression are common throughout the disease course but do not clearly relate to specific CNS lesions.

Spastic paraparesis is the most common motor abnormality, with signs and symptoms of UMN dysfunction. Patients generally complain of stiffness, cramps, weakness, and motor fatigability. Flexor, extensor, and adductor spasms occur with more severe dysfunction. These tend to be provoked by active or passive movements and are often painful. Ambulatory impairment is the usual result of lower extremity involvement, whereas loss of fine motor control is more common in the upper extremities. Presumably, the lower extremities are most affected because the longest tracts have more regions of demyelination, both in the periventricular white matter and spinal cord tracts. Motor deficits may also be quite asymmetric, with isolated monoparesis or hemiparesis related to more focal lesions.

On examination, patients have spasticity, extensor plantar responses, hyperreflexia, clonus, weakness, and loss of fine motor control. As in other UMN disorders, power in the hip flexors and ankle dorsiflexors is most severely affected, whereas knee extensors and upper extremity power is often relatively spared. Absence of cutaneous reflexes such as the superficial abdominal reflexes may be the only early sign in spinal cord disease. Loss of muscle stretch reflexes is usually a late sign and may occur from demyelination at the dorsal root entry zone, antispasticity medication, or extreme spasticity with associated contractures.

Impaired ambulation is one of the most obvious and disabling consequences of motor dysfunction in MS patients. Quantitative assessment reveals that patients have measurable deficits in their walking speed and endurance. In a sample of 237 ambulatory MS patients, 78% took more than 5 seconds to walk 8 m (range, 2.6 to 185.1 seconds), whereas all healthy control subjects tested walk faster (range, 2.9 to 5.0 seconds). Half of these patients were unable to walk 500 m, even with support, and 16% were unable to walk 100 m. Nineteen percent used unilateral assistive devices to walk, and 13% used them bilaterally (68). Because this pattern of gait deficits is so characteristic, the main scale used to measure overall disability in MS patients, the Expanded Disability Status Scale (EDSS), is based largely on ambulatory impairment (69).

Motor symptoms and signs typically worsen with elevations in body temperature. A similar phenomenon was originally described by Uhthoff in 1890 (69a) including noted visual failure in association with exercise. Motor function may also worsen during exercise, fever, hot showers, and sun exposure. This has been considered characteristic enough of MS that the hot bath test has been used as a diagnostic tool. The underlying mechanism involves variable conduction block in partially demyelinated pathways (70).

Fatigue is another extremely common complaint in MS patients, often described as an inability to sustain motor activity during routine tasks. Although subjective aspects of fatigue have been characterized using questionnaires, we have also observed objective evidence for pathologic motor fatigue during sustained motor activity. For example, MS patients experience a 40% greater decline in motor output during a 30-second continuous contraction of the elbow extensor than healthy control subjects, even though the maximum isometric contraction force in this muscle is normal. Weak muscles, such as the ankle dorsiflexors, are even more fatigable, show a 256% greater decline than control subjects. Pathologic decay in motor output also occurs during repetitive tasks, such as repeated maximal isometric contractions or ambulation. When walking up to 500 m, speed declined by 17% for MS patients by the end of the test, whereas healthy control subjects walked above 2% faster (70a). Others have found similar objective evidence for motor fatigability in MS patients but not in patients with chronic fatigue syndrome, further supporting the contention that neurologic dysfunction is the etiology (71).

TREATMENT

Treatments for MS may be divided into four categories: those agents that alter the course of the underlying disease process by modulating the immune system; those that improve conduction through demyelinated pathways; those that enhance remyelination, and those agents that treat symptoms without directly affecting the underlying pathological process. Although the pathogenesis of MS remains uncertain, immune-mediated processes are clearly involved. Therefore, treatments attempting to alter the course of MS generally focus on modulation of the immune system. They include: medications that interfere with activation and proliferation of immune cells; reduce migration of immune cells into the CNS; enhance suppressor activity within the immune system; or limit the destruction caused by activated immune cells and their inflammatory mediators.

Evidence to date suggests that the immune process in MS is fairly constant in nature and similar in various stages of the disease; therefore, more than one type of immunosuppressive agent can be used, each with a unique mode of action. Corticosteroids, for example, are commonly prescribed at the time of an acute exacerbation. Studies show that corticosteroids help signs and symptoms resolve more quickly, without significantly affecting the ultimate outcome of an exacerbation (72). The optimal dose and dosing regimen for a corticosteroid pulse remains uncertain (73), but general consensus exists against the long-term use of daily corticosteroids, which have no established efficacy in MS and cause a myriad of serious side effects (74). Corticosteroid pulses may be associated with temporary insomnia, irritability,

fluid retention, increased appetite, weight gain, hyperglycemia, hypertension, dyspepsia, and depression on withdrawal but rarely cause more serious side effects such as glaucoma, cataracts, femoral avascular necrosis, and psychosis. The main concern with repeated corticosteroid pulses is a possible contribution to the development of osteoporosis. Retrospective studies found no association between prior corticosteroid exposure and bone density in MS patients, and prospective studies have found no change in bone density after sporadic corticosteroid pulses (75).

Interferon β-1b (Betaseron, Berlex) and interferon β-1a (Avonex, Biogen) have been reported to reduce the number of exacerbations occurring in patients prone to relatively frequent exacerbations (76–78); they may also help to prevent worsening disability. Serial MRIs show a dramatic decrease in the incidence of new lesions and less increase in overall lesion burden during treatment (79,80). Efficacy has not been established in patients with early or mild relapsing disease or in those with progressive disease, but studies addressing these indications are currently underway. Side effects include flulike symptoms, injection site reactions, leukopenia, elevated liver function studies, thrombocytopenia, headache, and depression. Neutralizing antibodies to these medications develop in 38% of patients taking interferon β-1b and 10% taking β-1a (81). The clinical significance of these antibodies remains uncertain, but experience suggests that they may seriously compromise efficacy. Glatiramer acetate, formerly known as copolymer-1 (Copaxone, Teva), was equally efficacious in a similar patient population (82). There has not been a direct comparison of these agents, but treatment with any one of them appears to be beneficial in those with actively relapsing MS to reduce the relapse rate and the development of worsening disability over time. Studies now underway suggest a role for them in the treatment of patients with progressive symptoms without exacerbations, but they have not yet been approved for this purpose.

Nonspecific immunosuppressants have been used in MS with variable results (83). The efficacy of azathioprine and cyclophosphamide has never truly been clearly established, although they continue to be administered on occasion (84–86). Weekly oral methotrexate showed less progression of deficits after treatment for 2 years (87); however, it can cause stomatitis, diarrhea, nausea, anemia, transaminitis, and rash, and the poorly quantified risk of malignancy limits the use of this treatment to more severely affected patients.

Cladribine, mitoxantrone, antilymphocyte globulins, cyclosporine, and tacrolimus are chemotherapeutic agents with use as semispecific suppressors of MS disease activity (88). Plasmapheresis (89), total lymphoid irradiation (90), and intravenous immunoglubulin (IVIg) infusions (91) have also been studied in MS, although their proposed mechanisms of action in MS are uncertain.

More specific strategies that have been used successfully in animal models of MS are beginning preliminary assessment in human disease, including agents that block proinflammatory cytokines such as interleukin-2, tumor necrosis factor-α, and interferon-β, and others that supplement the antiinflammatory cytokines interleukin-10 and transforming growth factor-β. Other agents have been envisioned with the potential to interfere with the influx of immune cells across the blood–brain barrier, including antibodies against several adhesion molecules and metalloproteinase inhibitors. Several peptides have been developed to interfere with binding in the trimolecular complex, comprised of the T-cell receptor, antigen, and an MHC class II molecule (92). These strategies should lead to more specific agents to decrease the activity of the disease and prevent further CNS damage with minimal systemic immunosuppression.

Other therapies are also under study to improve conduction through demyelinated pathways or enhance remyelination. Two agents, 4-aminopyridine (4-AP) and 3,4-diaminopyridine (3,4-DAP) are potassium channel blockers that increase the amplitude and duration of action potentials. Preliminary in vitro studies suggest a benefit in enhancing conduction through partially demyelinated axons (93–95). Clinical studies, on the other hand, have had mixed results. Preliminary studies using 4-AP found improvement in a variety of subjective and semiquantitative measures of neurologic function (96–98), but a multicenter, double-blind, placebo-controlled, parallel study using in 161 patients with MS and stable deficits failed to show an effect on EDSS. This may have been an inadequate outcome variable because of poor responsiveness for clinically significant changes. Other studies using quantitative outcome measures of motor function found beneficial therapeutic effects of 4-AP and 3,4-DAP (99,100). Optimal administration of these agents requires further study because they can cause seizures and encephalopathy with high peak serum levels (101).

In animal models of MS, IVIg has the potential to enhance remyelination; however, it is not clear whether a significant effect occurs in patients with MS (102). Fixed motor deficits did not improve with IVIg treatment, but studies of visual deficits are continuing. Other strategies to enhance remyelination are also being considered, including myelin transplantation and manipulation of oligodendrocyte growth factors yet to be identified, but these are not yet ready for trials in MS patients.

Most patients receive medication for the management of residual symptoms with agents that do not directly affect the underlying disease process. For example, antidepressants and anticonvulsants reduce paresthesias, anticholinergics and β-blockers improve bladder function, and amantadine and CNS stimulants minimize fatigue (103).

Motor symptoms tend to be the most debilitating. With the possible exception of 4-AP, there are no available treatments to improve strength. Weakness requires physical therapy to minimize the component related to disuse; adaptive equipment such as ankle-foot orthoses for weakness of the ankle dorsiflexors; and canes, walkers, and wheelchairs to foster mobility. Spasticity, muscle cramps, and spasms generally respond to regular stretching or pharmacologic agents. Baclofen, a GABA agonist, can be gradually increased for optimal effect, beginning with 5 mg every 4 to 6 hours to 40 mg or more every 3 hours (104). The limiting side effects are sedation and dizziness, and if spasticity is relieved excessively, the resultant lack of tone may interfere with ambulation. Tizanidine, β-2-adrenergic agonist, can also be used to relieve spasticity (105). The most common side effects are drowsiness, dry mouth, dizziness, and orthostatic hypotension. Although baclofen and tizanidine act by different mechanisms, they can theoretically be used together for a synergistic effect with fewer side effects. Commonly used alternatives include benzodiazepines and dantrolene, which acts peripherally as a muscle relaxant. Refractory cases may respond to botulinum toxin, but injection into very large muscles is impractical. Alcohol blocks and dorsal root rhizotomies have also been attempted with variable results. Intrathecal baclofen by an implantable subcutaneous pump is the most appropriate alternative for patients not well managed with oral medications, allowing more precise titration of spinal cord dosage without a similar delivery to the brain and cervical spinal cord. Although this treatment has been used most extensively in patients who are nonambulatory, there are reports of dosages titrated to reduce spasticity without secondary weakness to compromise ambulation (106–108).

Tremor is a disabling symptom that is also often refractory to therapy. Numerous drugs have been tried including benzodiazepines, propranolol, primidone, isoniazid, buspirone, trazadone, baclofen, carbamazepine, gabapentin, and ondansetron, but their therapeutic effect is questionable, and treatment is often limited by adverse effects (109). A poor understanding of the pathogenesis of this symptom remains a significant impediment to the development of effective agents for this symptom. Unilateral thalamotomy has been used with some success but is unpredictable and potentially dangerous (18).

Finally, in conjunction with these efforts to minimize motor impairment, rehabilitation may be attempted to reduce disability and handicap associated with impairment due to MS. Although passive and active stretching programs may lead to symptomatic relief of spasticity, the effects of routine physical therapy have not been clearly demonstrated. Participation in a comprehensive inpatient rehabilitation program, including a multidisciplinary individualized goal-setting approach, does not appear to change the level of neurologic impairment as measured by the EDSS. Disability and handicap, on the other hand, improved significantly during rehabilitation

(110). This occurred with minimal changes in medications, further emphasizing the need for a comprehensive approach to the treatment of motor dysfunction in MS.

REFERENCES

1. Baum HM, Rothschild BB. The incidence and prevalence of reported MS. *Ann Neurol* 1981;10:420–428.
2. Rosati G. Descriptive epidemiology of multiple sclerosis in Europe in the 1980s: a critical overview. *Ann Neurol* 1994;36:S164–174.
3. Kurtzke JF, Beebe GW, Norman JE. Epidemiology of multiple sclerosis in U.S. veterans. 1. Race, sex, and geographic distribution. *Neurology* 1979;29:1228–1235.
4. Kurtzke JF, Beebe GW, Norman JE. Epidemiology of multiple sclerosis in U.S. veterans. 3. Migration and the risk of MS. *Neurology* 1985;35:672–678.
5. Smith CR, Scheinberg LC. Clinical features of multiple sclerosis. *Semin Neurol* 1985;5:85–93.
6. McFarland HF, Greenstein F, McFarlin DE, et al. Family and twin studies in multiple sclerosis. *Ann NY Acad Sci* 1985;436:118–124.
7. Ebers GC, Bulman DE, Sadovnick AD, et al. A population based study of multiple sclerosis in twins. *N Engl J Med* 1986;315:1638–1642.
8. Ebers GC. Genetics and multiple sclerosis: an overview. *Ann Neurol* 1994;36:S12–14.
9. Hillert J. Human leukocyte antigen studies in multiple sclerosis. *Ann Neurol* 1994;36:S15–17.
10. Kira J, Kanai T, Nishimura Y, et al. Western versus Asian types of multiple sclerosis: immunogenetically and clinically distinct disorders. *Ann Neurol* 1996;40:569–574.
11. Cannella B, Raine CS. The adhesion molecule and cytokine profile of multiple sclerosis lesions. *Ann Neurol* 1995;37:424–435.
12. Hintzen RQ, Polman CH, Lucas CJ, et al. Multiple sclerosis: immunological findings and possible implications for therapy. *J Neuroimmunol* 1992;39:1–10.
13. Collard RC, Koehler RPM, Mattson DH. Frequency and significance of antinuclear antibodies in multiple sclerosis. *Neurology* 1997;49:857–861.
14. Waxman SG. Membranes, myelin, and the pathophysiology of multiple sclerosis. *N Engl J Med* 1982;306:1529–1533.
15. Brinkmeier H, Wolinsky KH, Seewald MJ, et al. Factors in the cerebrospinal fluid of multiple sclerosis interfering with voltage-dependent sodium channels. *Neurosci Lett* 1993;156:172–175.
16. Young RR. Spasticity: a review. *Neurology* 1994;44:S12–S20.
17. Hassler R, Bronisch F, Mundinger F, Riechert T. Intention myoclonus of multiple sclerosis: its patho-anatomical basis and its stereotactic relief. *Neurochirurgie* 1975;18:90–106.
18. Whittle IR, Haddow LJ. CT guided thalamotomy for movement disorders in multiple sclerosis: problems and paradoxes. *Acta Neurochir* 1995;64:S13–16.
19. McDonald WI, Sears TA. The effects of experimental demyelination on conduction in the central nervous system. *Brain* 1970;93:583–598.
20. Sheean GL, Murray NMF, Rothwell JC, et al. An electrophysiological study of the mechanism of fatigue in multiple sclerosis. *Brain* 1997;120:299–315.
21. Poser CM, Paty DW, Scheinberg L, et al. New diagnostic criteria for multiple sclerosis: guidelines for research protocols. *Ann Neurol* 1983;13: 227–231.
22. Giang DW, Grow VM, Mooney C, et al. Clinical diagnosis of multiple sclerosis. The impact of magnetic resonance imaging and ancillary testing. Rochester-Toronto Magnetic Resonance Study Group. *Arch Neurol* 1994;51:61–66.
23. Koopmans RA, Li DKB, Oger JJF, et al. The lesion of multiple sclerosis: imaging of acute and chronic stages. *Neurology* 1989;39:959–963.
24. Tartaglino LM, Friedman DP, Flanders AE, et al. Multiple sclerosis in the spinal cord: MR appearance and correlation with clinical parameters. *Radiology* 1995;195:725–732.
25. McFarland HF, Frank JA, Albert PS, et al. Using gadolinium-enhanced magnetic resonance imaging lesions to monitor disease activity in multiple sclerosis. *Ann Neurol* 1992;32:758–766.
26. Losseff NA, Webb SL, O'Riordan JI, et al. Spinal cord atrophy and disability in multiple sclerosis: a new reproducible and sensitive MRI method with potential to monitor disease progression. *Brain* 1996; 119:701–708.
27. Hume AL, Waxman SG. Evoked potentials in suspected multiple sclerosis: diagnostic value and prediction of clinical course. *J Neurol Sci* 1988;83:191–210.
28. Ingram DA, Thompson AJ, Swash M. Central motor conduction in multiple sclerosis: evaluation of abnormalities revealed by transcutaneous magnetic stimulation of the brain. *J Neurol Neurosurg Psychiatry* 1988;51:487–494.
29. Kandler RH, Jarrett JA, Gumpert EJW, et al. The role of magnetic stimulation in the diagnosis of multiple sclerosis. *J Neurol Sci* 1991;106:25–30.
30. Kandler RH, Jarrett JA, Davies-Jones, et al. The role of magnetic stimulation as a quantifier of motor disability in patients with multiple sclerosis. *J Neurol Sci* 1991;106:31–34.
31. Tan G, Schwid SR, Goodman AD, et al. Central motor conduction time is related to quantitative measures of motor function in multiple sclerosis. *Muscle Nerve* 1996;19:1204.
32. Tourtellotte WW, Potvin AR, Fleming JO, et al. Multiple sclerosis: measurement and validation of central nervous system IgG synthesis rate. *Neurology* 1980;30:1155–1162.
33. Thompson AJ, Kaufman P, Shortman RC, et al. Oligoclonal immunoglobulins and plasma cells in spinal fluid of patients with multiple sclerosis. *Br Med J* 1979;1:16–17.
34. Kostulas VK, Link H, Lefvert AK. Oligoclonal IgG bands in cerebrospinal fluid. Principles for demonstration and interpretation based on findings in 1114 neurological patients. *Arch Neurol* 1987;44: 1041–1044.
35. Rudick RA, Schiffer RB, Schwetz KM, Herndon RM. Multiple sclerosis: the problem of incorrect diagnosis. *Arch Neurol* 1986;43:578–583.
36. Morrissey SP, Miller DH, Kendall BE, et al. The significance of brain magnetic resonance imaging abnormalities at presentation with clinically isolated syndromes suggestive of multiple sclerosis: a 5-year follow-up study. *Brain* 1993;116:135–146.
37. Filippi M, Horsfield MA, Morrissey SP, et al. Quantitative brain MRI lesion load predicts the course of clinically isolated syndromes suggestive of multiple sclerosis. *Neurology* 1994;44:635–641.
38. Orrell RW. Distinguishing acute disseminated encephalomyelitis from multiple sclerosis. *Br Med J* 1996;313:802–804.
39. Kesselring J, Miller DH, Robb SA, et al. Acute disseminated encephalomyelitis. MRI findings and the distinction from multiple sclerosis. *Brain* 1990;113:291–302.
40. O Riordan JI, Gallagher HL, Thompson AJ, et al. Clinical, CSF, and MRI findings in Devic's neuromyelitis optica. *J Neurol Neurosurg Psychiatry* 1996;60:382–387.
41. Pender MP, Chalk JB. Connective tissue disease mimicking MS. *Aust NZ J Med* 1989;19:469–472.
42. Andrianakos AA, Duffy J, Suzuki M, Sharp JT. Transverse myelopathy in systemic lupus erythematosus: report of three cases and review of the literature. *Ann Intern Med* 1975;83:616–624.
43. Alexander EL, Malinow K, Lejewski JE, et al. Primary Sjögren's syndrome with central nervous system disease mimicking multiple sclerosis. *Ann Intern Med* 1986;104:323–330.
44. Motomura S, Tabira T, Kuroiwa Y. A clinical comparative study of multiple sclerosis and neuro-Behcet's syndrome. *J Neurol Neurosurg Psychiatry* 1980;43:210–213.
45. Stern BJ, Krumholz A, Johns C, et al. Sarcoidosis and its neurological manifestations. *Arch Neurol* 1985;42:909–917.
46. Sharma OP, Sharma AM. Sarcoidosis of the nervous system. A clinical approach. *Arch Intern Med* 1991;151:1317–1321.
47. Moore PM. Neurological manifestations of vasculitis: update on immunopathogenic mechanisms and clinical features. *Ann Neurol* 1995;37:S131–141.
48. Reik L, Burgdorfer W, Donaldson JO. Neurologic abnormalities in Lyme disease without erythema chronicum migrans. *Am J Med* 1986; 81:73–78.
49. Poser CM, Roman GC, Vernant JC. Multiple sclerosis or HTLV-1 myelitis? *Neurology* 1990;40:1020–1022.
50. Gessain A, Gout O. Chronic myelopathy associated with human T-lymphotropic virus type I (HTLV-1). *Ann Intern Med* 1992;117: 933–946.
51. McArthur J. Neurologic manifestations of AIDS. *Medicine* 1987;66: 407–437.
52. Berger JR, Sheremata WA, Resnick L, et al. Multiple sclerosis-like ill-

ness occurring with human immunodeficiency virus infection. *Neurology* 1989;39:324–329.

53. Moskowitz LB, Gregorios JB, Hensley GT, Berger JR. Cytomegalovirus: induced demyelination associated with acquired immune deficiency syndrome. *Arch Pathol Lab Med* 1984;108:873–877.

54. Tucker T, Dix RD, Katzen C, et al. Cytomegalovirus and herpes simplex virus ascending myelitis in a patient with acquired immune deficiency syndrome. *Ann Neurol* 1985;18:74–79.

55. Ketonen LM, Schwid SR, Valanne LK, et al. Herpes simplex myelitis simulating neoplasm on MRI. *J Neuroimaging* 1995;5:190–191.

56. Eldridge R, Anayiotos CP, Schlesinger S, et al. Hereditary adult-onset leukodystrophy simulating chronic progressive multiple sclerosis. *N Engl J Med* 1984;311:948–953.

57. Naidu S, Moser HW. Peroxisomal disorders. *Neurol Clin* 1990;8:507–528.

58. Bousser MG, Tournier-Lasserve E. Summary of the proceedings of the first international workshop on CADASIL. *Stroke* 1994;25:704–707.

59. Malandrini A, Carrera P, Ciacci G, et al. Unusual clinical features and early brain MRI lesions in a family with cerebral autosomal dominant arteriopathy. *Neurology* 1997;48:1200–1205.

60. Goodkin DE, Hertsgaard D, Rudick R. Exacerbation rates and adherence to disease type in a prospectively followed-up population with multiple sclerosis: implications for clinical trials. *Arch Neurol* 1989;46:1107–1112.

61. Lublin FD, Reingold SC. Defining the clinical course of multiple sclerosis: results of an international survey. *Neurology* 1996;46:907–911.

62. Kurtzke JF, Beebe GW, Nagler B, et al. Studies on the natural history of multiple sclerosis: early prognostic features of the later course of the illness. *J Chronic Dis* 1977;30:819–830.

63. McAlpine D. The benign form of multiple sclerosis: a study based on 241 cases seen with three years of onset and followed up until the tenth year or more of the disease. *Brain* 1961;84:185–203.

64. Detels R, Clark VA, Valdiviezo NL, et al. Factors associated with a rapid course of multiple sclerosis. *Arch Neurol* 1982;39:337–341.

65. Poser S, Kurtzke JF, Poser W, Sclaf G. Survival in multiple sclerosis. *J Clin Epidemiol* 1989;42:159–168.

66. Runmarker B, Andersen O. Prognostic factors in a multiple sclerosis incidence cohort with twenty-five years of follow-up. *Brain* 1993;116:117–134.

67. Weinshenker BG, Bass B, Rice GPA, et al. The natural history of multiple sclerosis: a geographically based study. 1. Clinical course and disability. *Brain* 1989;112:133–146.

68. Schwid SR, Goodman AD, Mattson DH, et al. The measurement of ambulatory impairment in multiple sclerosis. *Neurology* 1997;49:1419–1424.

69. Kurtzke JF. Rating neurologic impairment in multiple sclerosis: an expanded disability status scale (EDSS). *Neurology* 1983;33:1444–1452.

69a. Uhthoff W. Untersuchungen uber die bei der multiplen Herdsklerose vorkommenden Augenstorungen. *Arch Psychiatr Nervenkr* 1890;21:55–116.

70. Rasminsky M. The effects of temperature on conduction in demyelinated single nerve fibers. *Arch Neurol* 1973;28:287–292.

70a. Schwid SR, Thornton CA, Pandya S, et al. Quantitative assessment of motor fatigue and strength in multiple sclerosis. *Neurology*, in press.

71. Djaldetti R, Ziv I, Achiron A, Melamed E. Fatigue in multiple sclerosis compared with chronic fatigue syndrome: a quantitative assessment. *Neurology* 1996;46:632–635.

72. Beck RY, Cleary PA, Anderson MM, et al. A randomized controlled trial of corticosteroids in the treatment of acute optic neuritis. *N Engl J Med* 1992;326:581–588.

73. Barkhof F, Polman C. Oral or intravenous methylprednisolone for acute relapses of MS? *Lancet* 1997;349:893–894.

74. Troiano R, Cook SD, Dowling PC. Steroid therapy in multiple sclerosis: point of view. *Arch Neurol* 1987;44:803–807.

75. Schwid SR, Goodman AG, Puzas JE, et al. Sporadic corticosteroid pulses and osteoporosis in multiple sclerosis. *Arch Neurol* 1996;53:753–757.

76. IFNB Multiple Sclerosis Study Group. Interferon beta-1b is effective in relapsing-remitting multiple sclerosis. *Neurology* 1993;43:655–667.

77. IFNB Multiple Sclerosis Study Group and the University of British Columbia MS/MRI Analysis Group. Neutralizing antibodies during treatment of multiple sclerosis with interferon beta-1b: experience during the first three years. *Neurology* 1996;47:889–894.

78. Jacobs LD, Cookfair DL, Rudick RA, et al. Intramuscular interferon beta 1a for disease progression in relapsing multiple sclerosis. *Ann Neurol* 1996;39:285–294.

79. Paty DW, Li DKB, The UBC MS-MRI Study Group and the IFN-b MS Study Group. Interferon beta-1b is effective in relapsing and remitting multiple sclerosis 2: MRI analysis results of a multi-center, randomized, double-blind, placebo-controlled trial. *Neurology* 1993;43:662–667.

80. Stone LA, Frank JA, Albert PS, et al. Characterization of MRI response to treatment with interferon beta-1b: contrast-enhancing MRI lesion frequency as a primary outcome measure. *Neurology* 1997;49:862–869.

81. Rudick RA, Jones W, Alam J, et al. Significance of serum neutralizing antibodies to Avonex (IFN beta-1a) in multiple sclerosis. *Neurology* 1996;48:A80.

82. Johnson KP, Brooks BR, Cohen JA, et al. Copolymer 1 reduces relapse rate and improves disability in relapsing-remitting multiple sclerosis: results of a phase III multicenter, double-blind, placebo controlled trial. *Neurology* 1995;45:1268–1276.

83. Carter JL, Rodriguez M. Immunosuppressive treatment of multiple sclerosis. *Mayo Clin Proc* 1989;64:664–669.

84. Yudkin PL, Ellison GW, Ghezzi A, et al. Overview of azathioprine treatment in multiple sclerosis. *Lancet* 1991;338:1051–1055.

85. Canadian Cooperative Multiple Sclerosis Study Group. The Canadian cooperative trial of cyclophosphamide and plasma exchange in progressive multiple sclerosis. *Lancet* 1991;337:441–446.

86. Weiner HL, Mackin GA, Orav EJ, et al. Intermittent cyclophosphamide pulse therapy in progressive multiple sclerosis: final report of the Northeast Cooperative Multiple Sclerosis Treatment Group. *Neurology* 1993;43:910–918.

87. Goodkin DE, Rudick RA, Medendorp S, et al. Low dose oral methotrexate reduces the rate of progression in chronic progressive multiple sclerosis. *Ann Neurol* 1994;37:30–40.

88. Beutler E, Sipe JC, Romine JS, et al. The treatment of chronic progressive multiple sclerosis with cladribine. *Proc Natl Acad Sci USA* 1996;93:1716–1720.

89. Khatri BO, McQuillen MP, Hoffmann RG, et al. Plasma exchange in chronic progressive multiple sclerosis: a long-term study. *Neurology* 1991;41:409–414.

90. Cook SD, Devereux C, Troiano R, et al. Total lymphoid irradiation in MS: blood lymphocytes and clinical course. *Ann Neurol* 1987;22:634–638.

91. Fazekas F, Deisenhammer F, Strasser-Fuchs S, et al. Randomized placebo-controlled trial of monthly intravenous immunoglobulin therapy in relapsing-remitting multiple sclerosis. *Lancet* 1997;349:589–593.

92. Vandenbark AA, Chou YK, Whitham R, et al. Treatment of multiple sclerosis with T-cell receptor peptides: results of a double-blind pilot trial. *Nat Med* 1996;2:1109–1115.

93. Sherrat RM, Bostock H, Sears TA. Effects of 4-aminopyridine on normal and demyelinated mammalian nerve fibers. *Nature* 1980;283:570–572.

94. Bostock H, Sears TA, Sheratt RM. The effects of 4-aminopyridine and tetraethylammonium ions on normal and demyelinated mammalian nerve fibers. *J Physiol* 1981;313:301–315.

95. Targ EF, Kocsis JD. 4-Aminopyridine leads to restoration of conduction in demyelinated rat sciatic nerve. *Brain Res* 1985;328:358–361.

96. Stefoski D, Davis FA, Fitzsimmons WE, et al. 4-Aminopyridine in multiple sclerosis: prolonged administration. *Neurology* 1991;41:1344–1348.

97. van Diemen HAM, Polman CH, van Dongen TMMM, et al. The effect of 4-aminopyridine on clinical signs in multiple sclerosis: a randomized, placebo-controlled, double-blind, cross-over study. *Ann Neurol* 1992;32:123–130.

98. Bever CT. The current status of studies of aminopyridines in patients with multiple sclerosis. *Ann Neurol* 1994;36:S118–121.

99. Bever CT, Anderson PA, Leslie J, et al. Treatment with oral 3,4 diaminopyridine improves leg strength in multiple sclerosis patients: results of a randomized, double-blind, placebo-controlled, crossover trial. *Neurology* 1996;47:1457–1462.

100. Schwid SR, Petrie MD, McDermott MP, et al. Quantitative assessment of sustained-release 4-aminopyridine for symptomatic treatment of multiple sclerosis. *Neurology* 1997;48:817–821.

101. Bever CT, Young D, Anderson PA, et al. The effects of 4-aminopyridine in multiple sclerosis patients: Results of a randomized, placebo-controlled, double-blind, concentration-controlled, crossover trial. *Neurology* 1994;44:1054–1059.

102. Noseworthy JH, O Brien PC, Van Engelen BGM, Rodriguez M. Intravenous immunoglobulin therapy in multiple sclerosis: progress from remyelination in Theiler's virus model to a randomized, double blind, placebo-controlled clinical trial. *J Neurol Neurosurg Psychiatry* 1996; 57:11–14.

103. Schapiro RT. Symptom management in multiple sclerosis. *Ann Neurol* 1994;36:S123–124.

104. From A, Heltberg A. A double-blind trial with baclofen (Lioresal) and diazepam in spasticity due to multiple sclerosis. *Acta Neurol Scand* 1975;51:158–166.

105. Nance PW, Sheremata WA, Lynch SG, et al. Relationship of the anti-spasticity effect of tizanidine to plasma concentration in patients with multiple sclerosis. *Arch Neurol* 1997;54:731–736.

106. Penn RD, Savoy SM, Corcos D, et al. Intrathecal baclofen for severe spinal spasticity. *N Engl J Med* 1989;320:1517–1521.

107. Becker WJ, Harris CJ, Long ML, et al. Long term intrathecal baclofen therapy in patients with intractable spasticity. *Can J Neurol Sci* 1995;22:208–217.

108. Azouvi P, Mane M, Thiebaut J-B, et al. Intrathecal baclofen administration for control of severe spinal spasticity: functional improvement and long term follow up. *Arch Phys Med Rehabil* 1996;77:35–39.

109. Rice G, Dickey C, Lesaux J, et al. Ondansetron for disabling cerebellar tremor. *Ann Neurol* 1995;38:973.

110. Freeman JA, Langdon DW, Hobart JC, Thompson AJ. The impact of inpatient rehabilitation on progressive multiple sclerosis. *Ann Neurol* 1997;42:236–244.

Motor Disorders,
edited by David S. Younger.
Lippincott Williams & Wilkins, Philadelphia © 1999.

CHAPTER 25

Hereditary Ataxias

Timothy Lynch and Susan Bressman

ATAXIA

The current genetic classification of inherited ataxia, shown in Table 1, has replaced pathology-based nosology that was plagued by overlapping features both within and between families. Although further progress in the classification of the hereditary ataxias will be based on the combination of genotype and phenotype descriptions, clinicians will continue to be challenged to arrive at a provisional clinical-genetic diagnosis, because the different ataxia genes may be expressed as similar phenotypes. Formulating a logical differential diagnosis now and in the future requires consideration of a growing list of gene loci that expands almost each week. This chapter is an introduction and guide to the hereditary ataxias.

Early-Onset Ataxias

Friedreich Ataxia

Friedreich's ataxia (FRDA), described by Friedreich in 1863 (1), is an autosomal recessive (AR) disorder and the most common form of early-onset ataxia. The prevalence is 1 per 50,000 with a carrier rate of 1 in 120 in the United States. The clinical features include onset of symptoms in childhood, usually before 25 years; progressive ataxia of the gait and limbs; and areflexia of the legs (2–5). Other common features include Babinski signs, dysarthria, pyramidal weakness and proprioceptive loss in the legs, scoliosis, and cardiomyopathy (Table 2). All races are affected, and boys and girls are equally affected. Because the disorder is inherited in an AR fashion, parents are asymptomatic and consanguinity is high (5.6 to 28%). The risks for siblings is 25%; therefore, in small families, the patient may be the only affected member of a family.

T. Lynch: Department of Neurology, Neurological Institute, New York Presbyterian Hospital, New York, NY 10032.
S. Bressman: Department of Neurology, Beth Israel Medical Center, Phillips Ambulatory Care Center, New York, New York 10003.

Harding (3–5) proposed that early-onset cerebellar ataxia (EOCA) with retained tendon reflexes constituted an etiologically distinct FRDA-like clinical subgroup. The features distinguishing EOCA from FRDA include preservation of tendon reflexes, better prognosis, absence of optic atrophy, hypertrophic cardiomyopathy, diabetes mellitus, and severe skeletal deformities. The findings of magnetic resonance imaging differs in FRDA and EOCA; cerebellar atrophy was more common in EOCA and spinal atrophy is more common in FRDA (7). Recent genetic analysis indicates that some cases of EOCA actually have FRDA demonstrated by linkage studies at the FRDA locus (8) or by gene mutation analysis (9). Age at onset, rate of progression, and associated signs vary both within and between families. Specifically, linkage studies at the FRDA locus and subsequent mutation analysis have revealed families with atypical features of late-onset (ages 25 to 36 years) and others with retained or increased lower limb reflexes (8,10–12). Some families appear to breed true with late-onset or retained reflexes and others have variable phenotypes. Such intrafamilial variation may be secondary to variable GAA repeat length in the FRDA gene, other modifying genes, or environmental factors.

The FRDA gene maps to the proximal long arm of chromosome 9 and underlies the disorder in all families with strictly defined disease (13–17). There is linkage disequilibrium in different populations, including French (14), Spanish (18), and Acadian families (19). The gene was recently identified and named *X25*. It contains five exons and encodes a 210-amino acid protein named frataxin (20). Most FRDA patients are homozygous for an unstable GAA trinucleotide expansion in the first intron of *X25*, a noncoding region. There are 10 to 36 copies of the GAA repeat in normal chromosomes, but between 120 and 1,700 or more GAA repeats are present in greater than 95% of FRDA chromosomes (Table 3). The longer normal alleles of greater than 27 GAA repeats are interrupted by the hexanucleotide repeat GAGAA

TABLE 1. *Inherited ataxias*

Early-onset ataxias (usually before 20 years) without a known biochemical defect
Autosomal recessive
  Friedreich ataxia
  Other recessive ataxias
    Resembling Friedreich but with retained tendon reflexes/no cardiomyopathy
    With hypogonadism
    With myoclonus
    With optic atrophy and mental retardation
    With deafness
    With cataracts and mental retardation (Marinesco-Sjögren)
  X-Linked
Late-onset ataxias without a known biochemical defect
Autosomal dominant cerebellar ataxia
  Without retinal degeneration (ADCAI)
    SCA 1
    SCA 2
    SCA 3/MJD
    SCA 4
    SCA 5
    Other unidentified SCA loci-SCA 6
  DRPLA
  With retinal degeneration (ADCAII)-SCA 7
  Paroxysmal ataxia
    With interictal myokymia
    With interictal nystagmus
Ataxias with identified biochemical defects
Ataxia/vitamin E deficiency
Abeta- and hypobetalipoproteinemia
Mitochondrial encephalomyopathies (MERFF, NARP, KS)
Leigh's syndrome
Carboxylase deficiencies
Urea cycle defects
Aminoacidurias
Wilson's disease
Prion disease (Gerstmann-Straussler-Scheinker disease)
Sialidosis
Refsum's
Ceroid lipofuscinosis
Leukodystrophies
Cholestanolosis (cerebrotendinous xanthomatosis)
Sphingomyelin storage disorders
Gangliosidosis (e.g., hexosaminidase deficiency)
Ataxia telangiectasia
Xeroderma pigmentosum
Cockayne's syndrome

ity. The smaller of the two GAA expansions correlates with an increased frequency of cardiomyopathy, diabetes mellitus, and areflexia (9,23–25). Meiotic instability shows a sex bias; paternally transmitted alleles tend to decrease, whereas maternal alleles can either increase or decrease (24). DNA and prenatal diagnosis is based on detection of homozygous GAA expansions in the patient or fetus or a point mutation on one allele and a GAA expansion on the other.

The expression of *X25* is highest in the primary sites of degeneration in FRDA including heart, liver, skeletal muscle, pancreas, spinal cord, cerebellum, and cerebrum. There is germline and somatic instability with varied GAA lengths in different tissues. The expanded GAA repeat results in a massive number of consecutive AG splice acceptor sites and a consequent loss of function. It can interfere in frataxin nuclear RNA processing and cause an absence of a mature message in the cytoplasm (20). Patients with FRDA have undetectable or extremely low levels of *X25* mRNA; thus, the disease is probably caused by a loss of function of frataxin. Frataxin localizes to mitochondria and is associated with mitochondrial membranes and crests (21,26,27). It has homology to genes in distant species such as *Caenorhabiditis elegans* and *Saccharomyces cerevisiae*. A yeast homolog of frataxin is involved in iron homeostasis and respiratory function. This raises the intriguing possibility that abnormal iron mitochondrial metabolism in FRDA produces toxic free radical via the Fenton reaction and ultimately oxidative damage (27,28). Thus, FRDA is a mitochondrial disease caused by loss of function of a nuclear-encoded protein. FRDA differs from the other triplet repeat ataxic disorders in the following ways: it is an AR disorder, it results from GAA repeats as compared to GC rich repeats found in the spinocerebellar ataxias (SCAs), and the GAA expansion is intronic and results in a loss of function as compared to gain of function seen in the SCAs (29).

Other Early-Onset Ataxias

EOCA with retained reflexes is the most common other AR ataxia (Table 1). One other early-onset recessive ataxia is the Marinesco-Sjögren syndrome characterized by ataxia, bilateral cataracts, mental retardation, and short stature. Other rare AR subtypes include ataxia with pigmentary retinopathy, ataxia with deafness, and ataxia with hypogonadism. One rare infantile-onset AR disorder restricted to Finnish families mapped to chromosome 10q23 (6). These children developed ataxia, athetosis, and areflexia in the second year of life, followed by hypotonia, optic atrophy, ophthalmoplegia, deafness, and sensory neuropathy.

One early-onset ataxia, the Ramsay-Hunt syndrome, has been the subject of controversy because of its etiologic heterogeneity. The syndrome, which consists of

(21). Less than 5% of FRDA patients are compound heterozygotes, with a GAA expansion of one allele and a missense or nonsense point mutation in the other allele (20). Compound heterozygotes tend to have atypical clinical findings. Surprisingly, about 20% of patients with homozygous GAA expansions, especially the Acadian variant, have atypical FRDA characterized by an older age at presentation, usually up to age 51, and elicitable tendon reflexes (12,22). Larger GAA expansions correlate with earlier age at onset and shorter time to immobility. The smaller GAA expansion of each pair of alleles is the main determinant of disease phenotype and sever-

TABLE 2. *Clinical features of the hereditary ataxias*

Name	Inheritance	Onset (yr)	Duration	Phenotype	Gene identified
SCA-1	AD	Adult/child (6–60)	10–20 yr	Ataxia, bulbar symptoms, pyramidal and extrapyramidal signs, ophthalmoparesis	Yes
SCA-2	AD	Adult/child (2–67)	10–25 yr	Ataxia, neuropathy, slow saccades	Yes
SCA-3/MJD	AD	Adult/child (6–70)	20 yr	Ataxia, ophthalmoparesis, pyramidal and extrapyramidal signs, amyotrophy	Yes
SCA-4	AD	Adult (19–59)	>20 yr	Ataxia, normal eye movements, axonal sensory neuropathy, pyramidal signs	No
SCA-5	AD	Adult (10–68)	Decades	Ataxia and dysarthria	No
SCA-6	AD	Adult (28–50)	>20–30 yr	Slowly progressive ataxia, nystagmus, dysarthria, proprioception/vibration loss	Yes
SCA-7	AD	Adult/child (3–58)	10 yr	Ataxia, pigmentary retinopathy	Yes
DRPLA	AD	Adult/child	10 yr	Ataxia, dementia, chorea, myoclonus, epilepsy	Yes
Episodic ataxia-1	AD	Child	Lifelong	Exercise or startle-induced episodic ataxia (minutes), myokymia, contractures, phenytoin responsive	Yes
Episodic ataxia-2	AD	Child	Lifelong	Stress or fatigue-induced episodic ataxia (days), downgaze nystagmus, acetolamide-responsive	Yes
Friedreich ataxia	AR	Child/adult	20+ yr	Ataxia, position sense loss, sensory neuropathy, pyramidal signs, cardiomyopathy, diabetes, scoliosis, pes cavus	Yes
Familial isolated vitamin E deficiency	AR	Adult	20+ yr	Friedreich-like phenotype	Yes
Ataxia telangiectasia	AR	Child (<10)	10+ yr	Ataxia, immune deficiency, developmental delay, telangiectasia	Yes

SCA, spinocerebellar ataxia; MJD, Machado-Joseph disease; DRPLA, dentatorubral pallidal luysian atrophy; AD, autosomal dominant; AR, autosomal recessive.

myoclonus and progressive ataxia, may be produced by a number of diseases, including mitochondrial encephalomyopathy of myoclonic epilepsy and ragged red fibers (MERRF) and the AR condition Unverricht-Lundborg and sialidosis (EPM1). EPM1 maps to chromosome 21q, and the gene encodes cystatin B that acts within cells to block the action of certain cathepsins, protease enzymes that degrade other cell proteins (30). The Ramsay-Hunt syndrome is most commonly caused by MERRF. Clinical features include ataxia, myoclonus, seizures, myopathy, and hearing loss. Maternal relatives may be asymptomatic or have partial syndromes, including the characteristic horse collar distribution of lipomas. Pathogenic mitochondrial DNA mutations have been demonstrated at the nucleotide positions 8433 and 8356 in the transfer RNA[lys] gene (31–34).

X-linked inherited ataxias are rare. Syndromes of pure ataxia and spastic paraparesis beginning in childhood, adolescence, or early adulthood have been reported in several families that display an X-linked recessive pattern of inheritance. There is also an infant-onset X-linked form of ataxia, deafness, optic atrophy, and hypotonia.

The diagnostic workup of a patient with early-onset ataxia will, of course, depend on the constellation of clinical features, including findings in other family members. One biochemical measurement of importance in all suspected FRDA cases is a serum vitamin E level. Except for cases of abetalipoproteinemia (35) and cholestatic liver disease, vitamin E deficiency occurs as an isolated abnormality, not associated with fat malabsorption. This condition, known as familial isolated vitamin deficiency, is AR. Clinical features usually mimic FRDA, but onset in the sixth decade has been encountered, including one family with retinitis pigmentosa (36) (Table 2). The responsible gene, termed ataxia/vitamin E deficiency or AVED, maps to chromosome 8q13 (37). Frame shift mutations (38) and missense point mutations (39) in the α-tocopherol transfer protein gene that maps to the AVED gene-containing region have been demonstrated in patients with this condition (Table 3). The defect involves

TABLE 3. *Genetic aspects of the hereditary ataxias*

Ataxic disorder protein	Inheritance	Chromosome region	Gene	Trinucleotide repeat	Protein
SCA-1	AD	6p22.23	Sca1	CAG (exonic) N = 3–39;A = 42–81	ataxin-1
SCA-2	AD	12q23-21.1	Sca2	CAG (exonic) N = 14–29;A = 34–59	ataxin-2
SCA-3/MJD	AD	14q32.1	MJD1	CAG (exonic) N = 12–40;A = 61–89	ataxin-3
SCA-4	AD	16q22.1	N/I	N/I	N/I
SCA-5	AD	11cent	N/I	N/I	N/I
SCA-6	AD	19p13	Sca6 (CACNA1A)	CAG (exonic) N = 4–20;A = 21–30	CACNA1A P/Q-type Ca channel
SCA-7	AD	3p12-21.1	Sca7	CAG (exonic) N = 7–17;A = 38–130A	ataxin-7
DRPLA	AD	12p12-ter	CTG-B37	CAG (exonic) N = 3–35;A = 49–88	Atrophin
Episodic ataxia-1	AD	12p13	KCNA1	No (point mutations)	Shaker-like K channel
Episodic ataxia-2	AD	19p13	CACNA1A	No (nucleotide deletion)	CACNA1A P/Q-type Ca channel
Friedreich ataxia	AR	9q13-21.1	X25	GAA(intronic) N = 7–36;A = >120–1700	Frataxin
Familial isolated vit E def	AR	8q13.1-13.3	AVED	No (point mutations)	Alpha tocopherol transfer protein
Ataxia Telangiectasia	AR	11p22-23	ATM	No (point mutations)	Phosphatidyl inositol-3 kinase

SCA, spinocerebellar ataxia; MJD, Machado-Joseph disease; DRPLA, dentatorubral pallidal luysian atrophy; AD, autosomal dominant; AR, autosomal recessive; cent, centromere; vit, vitamin; def, deficiency; CAG, cytosine-adenosine-guanine trinucleotide repeat; N, normal; A, affected; KCNA1, potassium voltage-gated channel (Shaker-related subfamily); CACNA1A (previously known as CACNL1A4), alpha$_{1A}$ CA^{2+} channel; AVED, ataxia/vitamin E deficiency; ATM, AT mutated; N/A, not available; N/I, not identified.

impaired incorporation of α-tocopherol into very-low-density lipoprotein, which is needed for efficient vitamin E recycling. The mutated form of the transfer protein decreased transfer activity in cell culture (39).

The genetic basis of another AR early-onset ataxia, termed ataxia telangiectasia, is due to defective DNA repair (40). The clinical features include ataxia, telangiectasia, dystonia, tremor, myoclonus, cellular and humoral immune deficiencies, growth retardation, progeria, high serum alpha-fetoprotein, chromosomal instability, predisposition to lymphoreticular malignancy, and sensitivity to ionizing radiation (Table 2). Heterozygotes are at high risk for cancer, especially breast cancer in carrier women. The gene for ataxia telangiectasia was mapped to chromosome 11 (14), cloned, and named ATM for ataxia telangiectasia mutated (40) (Table 3). The 12-kilobase (kb) transcript was mutated in all ataxia telangiectasia cases so studied, confirming that despite the presence of four different complementation groups, only one gene was responsible for the disease. Mutations include deletions leading to sequence changes with premature truncation and inframe deletions. A partial cDNA clone encoded a protein similar to yeast mammalian phosphatidylinositol-3′ kinases that was involved in mitogenic signal transduction, meiotic recombination, and cell cycle control. Approximately

1% of the population is heterozygous for ATM, and it is estimated that the gene accounts for 8% of breast cancers; however, population screening for the mutation is difficult because the gene is large and there are many different mutations.

Late-Onset Ataxias

In 1893, Marie applied the term hereditary cerebellar ataxia to patients with later-onset symptoms, autosomal dominant (AD) inheritance, hyperreflexia, and oculomotor palsy (4). Before the application of molecular genetics, the classification of the adult-onset hereditary ataxias was the subject of considerable debate, due in part to the wide range of clinical and pathologic findings within families. The multitude of nosologic terms used over the years, including Marie ataxia, Menzel ataxia, cerebellar degeneration of Holmes, olivopontocerebellar atrophy (OPCA), SCA, and AD cerebellar ataxia (ADCA), have not clarified matters. Based on the lack of clinicopathologic specificity, Harding (4) referred to the entire class of disorders as ADCA. The latter was subsequently divided by clinical characteristics into four groups: ADCA without retinal degeneration, ADCA with dentatorubral-pallidoluysian atrophy, ADCA with retinal degeneration, and ADCA with paroxysmal or episodic ataxia (Table 1). Gene loci have been assigned in the various clinical subtypes. To date, six loci (SCA1–6) have been identified for ADCA without retinal degeneration. In addition, one locus, SCA7, was assigned to ADCA with retinal degeneration, one for dentatorubral-pallidoluysian atrophy (DRPLA), and two others for paroxysmal and episodic ataxia (Tables 2 and 3).

Kindreds with ADCA display a shared clinical spectrum, although certain clinical differences exist among the six genetic subtypes. In general, symptoms begin in the third to fourth decade, but the age at onset ranges from childhood to the seventh decade (Table 2). The earliest and generally most prominent sign is gait ataxia, and frequent sudden falls may also occur. Limb ataxia and dysarthria are usually present early in the course of the disease. Hyperreflexia may be present initially, although as the disease progresses there is loss of vibration and proprioception, and tendon reflexes become depressed. Nystagmus and subsequent ophthalmoparesis are common, and dementia, dystonia, facial fasciculations, and distal wasting can occur. Anticipation, an earlier onset, and more severe phenotype in later generations may be observed. Most affected individuals are severely disabled or dead 10 to 20 years after symptom onset (Table 2).

SCA1

The first ADCA locus, SCA1, was mapped to the short arm of chromosome 6 based on linkage to human leukocyte antigen (42,43). Subsequently, the highly polymorphic DNA markers D6S89 and D6S274 flanking the *Sca1* gene were identified. Orr et al. (44) assessed the SCA1 gene-containing region for trinucleotide repeats because of the presence of anticipation in SCA1 families and the previous finding of expanded trinucleotide repeats in other disorders displaying anticipation. They identified an unstable CAG repeat within a 10-kb MRNA transcript in the SCA1 locus.

Abnormal alleles have 40 or more repeats (45), whereas normal alleles have less than 36. Intermediate ranges are rarely found (37–39), and based on analyses of family members and clinical data, they are considered normal (45,46) (Table 3). There is an inverse relation between age at onset and repeat length (44,47,48), with the longest repeats associated with the earliest onset and most progressive course (44,49). Repeat size accounts for 60 to 70% of the variation in age at onset. Even after correcting for repeat size, interfamilial differences in age at onset persist, suggesting that additional genetic factors can affect expression (50,51). In one large family, a possible sex effect was suggested for the same number of repeats, and disease-onset was earlier in men (46). Several groups found that the sex of the transmitting parent influences repeat size (48,49); the repeat is more unstable and larger when transmitted paternally. Instability with a

wide range of the expanded repeat size is present in sperm (52); a narrower range of instability is observed in DNA extracted from leukocytes. This suggests that both meiotic and mitotic instability may contribute to the intergenerational expansion, although expansion during meiosis probably accounts for the greater instability seen in sperm. It is postulated that the trinucleotide repeat can assume a hairpin or triple helical structure possibly related to its instability. CAG tracts in the normal gene are interrupted by 1-3 CAT trinucleotides; in SCA1 alleles, however, there is no interruption of the CAG stretch. These CAT interruptions may help maintain intergenerational stability (52,53).

The protein encoded by *Sca1* has been named ataxin-1 and has between 792 and 825 amino acids, depending on the length of the polyglutamine stretch encoded by the CAG repeat (Table 3). It is a novel protein, not known to share homologies with other proteins, and its function is unknown (54). The murine homolog is highly homologous to the human ataxin-1 except that the CAG repeat is virtually absent, suggesting the polyglutamine stretch is not essential for the normal function of ataxin-1 in mice (55). Ataxin-1 was recently characterized by immunoblot and immunohistochemistry in brain and also in nonneural tissue (56). The wild-type protein is detected in both normal and affected individuals, and the mutant protein is detected in both neural and nonneural tissues of SCA1 individuals. The mutant and wild-type proteins are localized to nuclei of neurons throughout various brain regions except in Purkinje cells, where it is present in both the nucleus and cytoplasm (56).

The pathogenic mechanism of the mutant protein, with its expanded polyglutamine stretch, is unknown. It is hypothesized that the mutant expanded protein gains a function perhaps to stimulate or inhibit an unrelated target and that the effectiveness of this function is proportional to the length of the glutamine stretch (56). This proposed gain of function may be due to a variety of factors: overexpression of the glutamine tract, a toxic effect of the free intracellular glutamine tract, altered protein–protein interactions, or possible aggregation of protein. The glycolytic enzyme glyceraldehyde-3-phosphate dehydrogenase (GADPH) interacts with the polyglutamine tract of SCA1, SCA2, SCA3, DRPLA, and Huntington disease (HD) (57). Thus, it is possible that the polyglutamine tract interferes with cell energy metabolism indirectly via associated proteins, resulting in cell dysfunction and ultimately cell death. The mechanism is unclear, although the polyglutamine tract may result in apoptotic cell death in polyglutamine expansion disorders (58,59). Neuronal intranuclear inclusions containing the proteins huntintin and ubiquitin occur in transgenic mice harboring the human HD gene with expanded CAG repeats (60,61). In SCA3, similar excessive encoding of the amino acid glutamine occurs in the nuclei of selected neurons in affected regions of the human brain and fragments of the expanded glutamine-containing protein form insoluble aggregates that may disrupt critical nuclear processes (62). In addition, insoluble high-molecular-weight protein aggregates were found in vitro only when the HD polyglutamine expansion was in the pathogenic range (61).

Homozygous null *Sca1* knockout mice in which exon 8 of the SCA1 gene is deleted are viable and have normal brain morphology, but they are less likely to explore their environment. A transgenic mouse model for SCA1 has been developed. When mutant repeat-bearing ataxin-1 was overexpressed in six lines of transgenic mice, five lines demonstrated spontaneous ataxia and Purkinje cell degeneration at about 3 months of age (63). Thus, expanded CAG repeats expressed in Purkinje cells are sufficient to produce degeneration and ataxia. The transgenic CAG repeats were stable, raising the possibility that trinucleotide repeat instability was peculiar to human disease. However, in subsequent studies by three groups, intergenerational and somatic cell instability of the trinucleotide repeat in the mouse was demonstrated (64–66). The mechanism of how mutant repeat-bearing ataxin-1 kills neurons remains unknown; however, the successful transfer of human disease to mouse will enable detailed molecular investigation to be performed.

The worldwide frequency of SCA1 as determined by the CAG repeat has been assessed. The proportion of AD ataxia cases that are SCA1 varies from 3 to 50%, depending on geographic and ethnic background and clinical and familial criteria for inclusion (45,48,67–70). The largest U.S. series reported that only 3% of 149 dominant kindreds were SCA1 (45). SCA1 rarely, if ever, underlies ataxia in singular cases or in those that appear to be AR. Most analyses confirm onset in the fourth decade (6–60). Gait ataxia predominates and is often the first sign accompanied by nystagmus, whereas hyperreflexia, Babinski signs, upgaze ophthalmoparesis, dysarthria, dysphagia, and sensory loss appear with disease progression (Table 2). Sphincter disturbances; dementia and personality change; dystonia, especially torticollis; chorea; and fasciculation are less common findings (46,48,69). Histopathology shows loss of Purkinje cells and neurons in the inferior olives, cranial nerve nuclei restiform body, and occasionally anterior horn cells of the spinal cord and degeneration in the spinocerebellar tracts, dorsal columns, brachium conjunctivum, dorsal and ventral spinocerebellar tracts, posterior columns (71), and sparing the substantia nigra and basal ganglia.

SCA2

This locus was mapped to chromosome 12q23-24 in 1993 (72). SCA2 was first localized in a population of AD ataxic patients originating from the Holguin province of Cuba and descended from an Iberian founder. The age at onset ranged from 2 to 65 years and averaged 32 years. The clinical features in this population included limb ataxia, gait ataxia, and dysarthria in all. Other common features included action tremor, cramps, ophthalmoparesis, slowed saccades, hypotonia, decreased upper limb reflexes, and either increased or decreased lower limb reflexes. Myoclonus and nystagmus were uncommon, and only 1 of 263 individuals was demented (73). Several additional SCA2 pedigrees of Italian-American (75), Italian (76), Austrian-Canadian, French-Canadian (77), and Tunisian ancestry were subsequently identified (74). Clinically, it expresses itself somewhat distinctly from the other ADCA gene disorders. Pyramidal signs are uncommon, but axonal sensory neuropathy with loss of arm reflexes occurs in about 60% and slow saccades in about 55% of cases; tremor is almost always present (78,79). Pathology reveals a pattern of OPCA with severe neuronal loss in the inferior olive, pons, cerebellum and to a limited degree the anterior horn cells, with degeneration of the substantia nigra and the dorsal columns (73).

A CAG expansion at the SCA2 locus on chromosome 12q was identified independently by three research groups using three different techniques: positional cloning (80), a specific antibody for polyglutamine repeats (81), and by direct identification using the repeat expansion and cloning technique (DIRECT) (82). Normal individuals have 14 to 31 CAG repeats in the open reading frame, and there are one to three CAAs within the CAG repeat (79,83). SCA2 patients have CAG expansions of 34 to 59 and no CAAs within the repeat (Table 3). There is an inverse correlation between age at onset and CAG number, as in the other CAG repeat disorders. Myoclonus, dystonia, chorea, and dementia are more likely to occur when the CAG expansion is large (70,78,83). The CAG expansion is unstable in both paternal and maternal transmission. There is evidence for anticipation, but the influence of the transmitting parent's gender on age at onset is not clear; anticipation has been reported with paternal transmission in one study (79) but not in others (74,83). The gene contains 16 exons, with the CAG expansion present in exon 1. It encodes a 1,313 amino acid protein of molecular weight 140 kDa, termed ataxin-2 (81). The gene has no homology with *Sca1* or *Sca3* genes; it is expressed ubiquitously, and its function is unknown. Although the mouse *Sca2* homologue has 90% amino acid sequence identity, it does not contain the polyglutamine repeat. This suggests that the ataxin-2 repeat, like ataxin-1, is not necessary for normal function (84).

SCA3/Machado-Joseph Disease

This ADCA gene has a particularly wide range of clinical expression. Machado-Joseph disease (MJD) was first described in patients of Azorean-Portuguese descent (85–87). Over the past 20 years, the broad spectrum of clinical features in this disease has been delineated. There is clustering of features related to age at onset and duration of disease. Gait and limb ataxia, dysarthria, and progressive ophthalmoplegia are commonly observed regardless of age at onset (Table 2), whereas pyramidal signs, dystonia and rigidity, peripheral amyotrophy, facial and lingual fasciculation, and bulging eyes occur with younger age at onset. Clinical subclasses of MJD have been proposed, including adolescent/young adulthood onset with a rapidly progressive course that includes spasticity, rigidity, bradykinesia, weakness, dystonia, and ataxia; mid-adulthood onset in the fourth and fifth decades, with moderate progression of ataxia; late-adulthood onset in the fifth to seventh decades with slower progression of ataxia and prominent peripheral signs without long tract or extrapyramidal findings; and adulthood type with parkinsonism and peripheral neuropathy. Saccades are slow and there is nystagmus and ocular dysmetria, followed by supranuclear ophthalmoparesis that spares downgaze until the late stages. Lid retraction and decreased blinking produces bulging of the eyes in about a third of cases. The pathologic findings distinguish MJD from other AD forms of cerebellar ataxia. The pathologic changes in MJD are extensive, involving the dentate, spinocerebellar tracts, anterior horn cells, and neurons in the pons, nigra, oculomotor nucleii, and basal ganglia, with sparing of the olives and cerebellar cortex. One case, diagnosed clinically and pathologically as DRPLA, was subsequently found to have the MJD CAG repeat (88).

A disorder similar to MJD was reported in families not clearly of Portuguese descent, including German, Dutch, Japanese, and African-American families (89,90). We identified three additional affected individuals in the next generation of the African-American family described by Healton et al. (90). Their phenotype varied from predominant pure cerebellar ataxia to a combination of ataxia, fasciculations, ophthalmoparesis, pyramidal, and extrapyramidal symptoms and signs. One patient developed autonomic dysfunction characterized by persistent tachycardia, hypertension, sweating, and fluctuating burning neuropathic leg pain.

In 1993 Takiyama et al. (91) mapped the gene for MJD in several Japanese families to chromosome 14q24.3-32. This locus was confirmed in MJD families of Azorean descent (92), including Azorean families with the unusual phenotype (type 4) of dopa-responsive parkinsonism (93). In 1994, a linkage study of French families implicated the same region, and the locus was numbered SCA3 (94). Because the families were not of Azorean descent and because of several clinical differences, including the lack of dystonia and facial fasciculation, the question remained as to whether MJD and SCA3 were disorders due to different genes, different mutations in the same gene, or in the phenotypic spectrum of the same mutation in individuals with differing ancestry. However, in 1994 an expanded and unstable CAG repeat in the coding region of the MJD gene (*MJD1*) was identified (95). Subsequent studies of ataxia patients have confirmed that all 14q linked families have the same unstable CAG repeat within the MJD gene (45,89,96).

Unlike SCA1 and SCA2, there appears to be a wide difference between normal subjects and affected subjects in the number of repeats, with normal ranging from 12 to 40 and in disease alleles from 61 to 89 (45,88,96,97) (Table 3). Like other CAG repeat diseases, there is an inverse relation between the length of the repeat and the age at onset, and unlike these disorders, there is no difference in the number of expanded repeats whether inherited from mothers or fathers (88,97). A current controversy is whether gender affects expression. Japanese investigators (98) found that for the same number of repeats, brothers developed signs earlier than sisters; however, others (99,100) failed to confirm this. Further, there may be a dosage effect with some homozygous individuals for the CAG expansion manifesting an onset earlier than expected (98,101). Finally, analyses of families from Japan, the United States, and Europe indicate that the MJD expansion is responsible for a sizable proportion of ADCA cases, including 21% of one U.S. sample compared with 3% for SCA1 (45) and up to 40% of European cases, including Portuguese patients, (67) compared with 15% for SCA1 and SCA2 (78). Almost all cases with the MJD CAG expansion have a familial pattern consistent with AD inheritance and only rarely are MJD expansions found in sporadic ataxia cases (45). Assessment of ethnic background in U.S. MJD cases indicates that most are of German and not Portuguese extraction (45). With the localization of the MJD/SCA3 gene, linkage disequilibrium studies suggest that a single founder may account for the French and Brazilian MJD kindreds. At least two different founders may account for the Portuguese families, and other mutations probably account for MJD kindreds in Algeria, French-Guiana, and Belgium (102). Haplotype studies show certain alleles predispose to the expansion of the CAG repeat (102,103).

The disease gene *MJD1* encodes for an intracellular protein, ataxin-3, of unknown function (Table 3). Ataxin-3 has a predicted molecular weight of 42 kDa and is ubiquitously expressed in the cytoplasm of cell bodies and their processes (95). However, in MJD brain there is aberrant nuclear localization and accumulation of ubiquitinated nuclear inclusions (62). As with the other CAG expansion disorders, the mechanism of cell death in MJD is not known.

SCA4

Linkage to chromosome 16q24-qter was found in one five-generational Utah family with AD late-onset ataxia, prominent sensory axonal neuropathy, pyramidal tract signs, and normal eye movements (104). Subsequent genetic localization reassigned the locus to 16q22.1, but the gene itself remains to be identified (Table 3) (105). Age at onset was in the fourth or fifth decade, with a range of age at onset of 19 to 59 years (Table 2). The earliest symptom was unsteadiness of gait. Absent ankle jerks and decreased sensation was present in all cases; dysarthria was present in one half of patients, extensor plantar responses were present in 20%, and saccadic pursuit eye movements in only 15% so studied (104,105). Nerve conduction studies confirmed an axonal sensory neuropathy. Some branches of the pedigree appeared to display anticipation, although ascertainment bias could account for the earlier age at onset in the later generations. The Utah family bears strong resemblance to a small French-German family with late-onset ataxia, areflexia, and dorsal column sensory loss (106).

SCA5

This locus mapped to the centromeric region of chromosome 11q13 in a large kindred that descended from the paternal grandparents of President Lincoln (107). The primary feature in this family was a relatively benign, slowly progressive, cerebellar syndrome. The age at onset was in the third to fourth decade, but varied from 10 to 68 years, and there was evidence of anticipation (Table 2). All four juvenile-onset patients of age 10 to 18 years resulted from maternal transmission, suggesting maternal anticipation bias for SCA5 rather than the paternal type seen in SCA1. The juvenile-onset patients presented with cerebellar dysfunction, pyramidal tract signs, and bulbar dysfunction. The role of this gene in other families with late-onset and benign cerebellar ataxias, often classified separately as ADCAIII/Holmes ataxia/familial pure cerebellar degeneration, remains to be established.

SCA6

The SCA6 locus maps to chromosome 19p13 and encodes the α 1A voltage-dependent calcium subunit *CACNA1A*, previously named *CACNL1A4* (108). A polymorphic CAG repeat was identified at the 3′ end of *CACNA1A* in eight American families of European, African-American, Hispanic, and Asian origin with a late insidious onset of ataxia (109). The patients developed slowly progressive ataxia, dysarthria, nystagmus, and mild vibratory and proprioceptive sensory loss (Table 2). They have 21 to 30 repeats, whereas normal individuals have 4 to 20 repeats (Table 3) (109–112). As in other CAG repeat disorders, there is an inverse correlation between age at onset and CAG number. The SCA6 mutation causes disease in about 10% of AD SCA cases in Germany and also sporadic ataxia (111). Repeat instability in parental transmission has not been noted, although anticipation was reported in some, but not all, Japanese and German families (110,111,112). The CAG repeat lies within the open reading frame and encodes for a polyglu-

tamine stretch. There are no interrupting sequences within the expansion (109). There are differences between the mutation in SCA6 and those responsible for SCA1, SCA2, SCA3, Huntington disease, DRPLA, and spinobulbar muscular atrophy. First, the expanded mutant alleles in SCA6 (21–30) are smaller than in any of the other neurodegenerative diseases (36–121) and are within the normal range of polyglutamine tracts at other SCA loci. Second, the size of normal alleles is continuous, up to 20 repeats, with no gap between the distribution of CAG-repeat numbers on the normal and SCA6 chromosome. Third, the CAG expansion occurs in a gene known to be important for normal Purkinje cell function and survival. Thus, the CAG repeat may result in a loss of function or a dominant negative effect. For example, the transcribed abnormal allele could interfere with transcription and translation of the normal allele rather than the gain of function seen with the polyglutamine stretches in SCA1, SCA2, SCA3, Huntington disease, DRPLA, and spinobulbar muscular atrophy (109).

Notably, a single nucleotide deletion in CACNA1A, disrupting the reading frame, results in protein truncation and underlies episodic paroxysmal ataxia and myokymia (EP-2) (18). In contrast, missense point mutations, in conserved functional domains resulting in amino acid substitution, result in ataxic hemiplegic migraine (Table 3) (113). Interestingly, one report demonstrated that CAG expansions of 23 CAGs in the CACNA1A gene caused both an intermittent and a progressive cerebellar dysfunction within the same family, thus blurring the distinction between SCA6 and EA2 (114).

Autosomal Dominant Cerebellar Ataxia with Retinal Degeneration/SCA7

This ADCA subtype was first distinguished from other forms of ADCA in 1937. Age at onset ranges from childhood to the seventh decade and averages about 30 years. The clinical course varies with age at onset. The duration of the disease to death averages 6 years in those with onset before age 6, and in those with onset after age 10, the average duration of disease was 20 years. There is anticipation that is significantly greater with male transmission (115–117). The typical clinical picture is early and progressive deterioration of vision and limb and gait ataxia. In cases with onset in the fourth to sixth decade, ataxia can occur in isolation or precede visual complaints (Table 2). Affected individuals all have abnormal yellow-blue color discrimination, which in the earliest or mildest forms may be asymptomatic. Clinical signs include optic disc pallor, granular and atrophic changes in the macula, slow saccades and ophthalmoparesis especially in upgaze, gait and limb ataxia, dysarthria, and pyramidal signs. Parkinsonism and decreased vibration sense may also occur (115,116). There is atrophy of posterior fossa structures on magnetic resonance imaging, and pathologically, there is degeneration of the cerebellum, basis pontis, inferior olive, and retinal ganglion cells.

After excluding known ADCA loci and the genes for AD retinitis pigmentosa, two groups mapped the gene for this disorder to chromosome 3p14-21.1 (117,118). There is evidence for genetic homogeneity among families of diverse geographic origin because all families with this clinical subtype map to the same locus (119–122). Because anticipation was present in SCA7 cases, an unstable CAG expansion was sought and the CAG-containing gene (*Sca* 7) was later found using a monoclonal antibody raised against the polyglutamine-containing TATA binding protein (123,124). Moreover, a CAG expansion was seen using the repeat-expansion detection technique (125), and a gene of unknown function was identified by positional cloning (126). An expanded CAG repeat of 38 to 130 was present in SCA7 patients compared with CAG repeat lengths of 7 to 17 in normal subjects (Table 3). Gonadal instability is associated with paternal transmission and is greater than in any of the seven neurodegenerative diseases caused by translated CAG repeat expansions (126). Ataxin-7 has a molecular weight of 130 kDa and is expressed ubiquitously; there is no correlation between expression within the CNS and neurodegeneration (126). Ataxin-7 is present in the nuclear fraction of lymphoblasts and contains a nuclear localization signal, suggesting it may be a transcription factor.

Dentatorubral-Pallidoluysian Atrophy

This condition was first described in 1946 (127) and is more common in Japan, although African-American, North American white, and European cases are described (8,128–133). Pathology is distinguished by involvement of the dentate, red nucleus, subthalamic nucleus, and the external globus pallidus. The posterior columns may also be involved, and in one case was the primary abnormality (131). The phenotype is quite varied, even within families, and depends to some extent on the age at onset. Early-onset cases generally show severe and rapid progression of myoclonus, myoclonic epilepsy, and cognitive decline, whereas late-onset cases display ataxia, chorea, and dementia, with the major differential diagnosis of Huntington's disease (Table 2). There is anticipation, and paternal transmission is associated with more severe early-onset disease (134). A clinical variant, The Haw River syndrome, was described in one African-American family from the Haw River area of North Carolina (135). This variant shares all the above symptoms except myoclonic seizures, and in addition, basal ganglia calcification, neuroaxonal dystrophy, and demyelination of the central white matter are found (135).

The disorder is due to an expansion of a CAG repeat in a DRPLA candidate gene (*CTG-B37*) that maps to chromosome 12p12-ter (136,137). An expanded CAG repeat

at the same locus was also found in the Haw River syndrome (132). There is an inverse relationship between repeat size and age at onset, with control subjects having up to 35 repeats and disease alleles having 49 or more (Table 3). The gene has been sequenced, and the cDNA is composed of 4,294 bases and encodes a protein of 1,184 amino acids (137,138). The gene is expressed in all tissues, including brain, and recent immunohistochemical studies indicate that the DRPLA gene product is observed mainly in neuronal cytoplasm (139). Both the function of the gene and the role of the polyglutamine stretch in pathogenesis remains to be elucidated. Both atrophin and huntingtin selectively interact through their polyglutamine tracts with the enzyme GADPH (57). It is possible that inhibition of GADPH results in loss of energy metabolism and selective neuronal loss.

Other Unmapped Autosomal Dominant Cerebellar Ataxias

Other loci for ADCAs remain to be identified because the known seven loci for SCAs and DRPLA do not account for all ADCA families (112). Linkage to the known SCA loci was excluded in seven Japanese families with late-onset pure cerebellar ataxia. Anticipation was noted in these families, suggesting the responsible gene or genes contain repeat expansions (112). In addition, all SCA loci were excluded, except the SCA6 locus, in an American-British family with cerebellar ataxia, ophthalmoplegia, parkinsonism, posterior column signs, and a relapsing course, in some similar to multiple sclerosis (140). It is unlikely that an SCA6 CAG expansion is responsible for this disorder because the phenotype is unlike that found in SCA6 (140).

Episodic or Paroxysmal Ataxias

Episodes of ataxia can be the initial sign of metabolic disorders such as multiple carboxylase deficiencies and the aminoacidurias. However, the term episodic or paroxysmal ataxia is generally applied to a condition in which the major finding is self-limited episodes of cerebellar dysfunction with little fixed or progressive neurologic dysfunction. The two major clinical-genetic subtypes of this rare condition are episodic ataxia with myokymia (EA1/myokymia) and episodic ataxia with nystagmus (EA2/nystagmus) (Table 2).

EA1/myokymia attacks are brief, usually lasting minutes, and are provoked by startle, sudden movements, or changes in posture and exercise, especially if excited or fatigued. They can occur 1 to 15 times per day. Onset is in childhood and adolescence. The disorder is not associated with neurologic deterioration, but subtle myokymia around the eyes and in the hands can occur. The Achilles tendons may be shortened, and there may be tremor of the hands. The attacks are often heralded by an aura of weightlessness or weakness, and during attacks there is ataxia, dysarthria, shaking or tremor, and twitching (141–143). In some families, acetazolamide reduces attack frequency, and anticonvulsants may reduce the myokymia (144). The cause of this disorder is missense point mutations in the potassium voltage-gated channel gene *KCNA1* on chromosome 12p (145). *KCNA1* is a member of the Shaker-related subfamily of potassium channel genes (Table 3).

EA2/nystagmus attacks last longer, usually hours to days. Attacks are provoked by stress, exercise, fatigue, and alcohol and, at most, occur once per day. Age at onset varies from infancy to 40 years, and unlike EA/ myokymia, there can be mild but progressive cerebellar degeneration with ataxia and dysarthria. Frequently, there is interictal nystagmus (Table 2). During the attacks, headache, diaphoresis, nausea, vertigo, ataxia, dysarthria, ptosis, and ocular palsy can occur (141,146–150). Acetazolamide is effective in reducing the frequency of attacks. Several different clinical profiles can exist and tend to run true within a family, although there is phenotypic variation within the same family (149). The gene for this disorder maps to chromosome 19p (134,149,151–153). The gene is a brain-specific P/Q-type encoding *CACNA1A* (Table 3). Several different point mutations that disrupt the reading frame have been identified (113). CAG repeat expansion in this gene is responsible for SCA6 and raises the intriguing question of a continuum between paroxysmal and progressive forms of ataxia (114).

A third form of acetazolamide-responsive episodic ataxia associated with spasticity and kinesigenic chreoathetosis mapped to chromosome 1p; no mutation has yet been detected in the nearby potassium channel genes (154).

Management of Hereditary Ataxias

No specific treatments influence the course of most hereditary ataxias. Vitamin E replacement can prevent or improve the cerebellar ataxia found in familial isolated vitamin E deficiency. In Friedreich ataxia, orthopedic procedures are indicated for the relief of foot deformity. In the SCAs, especially MJD/SCA3, levodopa may be of benefit for symptomatic relief of rigidity or other parkinsonian features; antispasmodics may be of benefit for spasticity. Acetazolamide controls the attacks of the episodic paroxysmal cerebellar ataxias (EA1 and EA2) and phenytoin benefits the facial and hand myokymia associated with EA1. Amantadine and buspirone have been reported to improve different forms of cerebellar ataxia, although the effect is moderate (155). Genetic counseling should be offered to patients and families with these disorders and should always accompany genetic testing. Finally, in the near future we can expect novel specific therapies based on our increasing knowledge of the molecular mechanism underlying the hereditary ataxias.

APPENDIX

Internet Address for information regarding hereditary ataxia:

INTERNAF: International Network of Ataxia Friends is a mailing list for ataxia patients and family that serves as a support group and information exchange vehicle. To subscribe to INTERNAF, send an e-mail to Major-domo@connect.org.uk with a two-word message: subscribe InterNAF.

INTER-PRO: International Network of Ataxia is a list for professionals only and can be subscribed to by sending an e-mail to pbower@inforamp.net.

ACKNOWLEDGMENTS

T.L. is supported by NINDS K08 MS01966, an Irving Scholar award, NARSAD award, The Parkinson's Disease Foundation (Merrill Young Investigator award), and The Lowenstein Foundation. S.B. is supported by grant RO1-NS266656 and The Parkinson's Disease Foundation and The Lowenstein Foundation. We thank Pat White and Arnold Lee for assistance with compiling the manuscript.

REFERENCES

1. Friedreich N. Uber Ataxie mit besonderer Berucksichtigung der hereditaren Formen. *Virchows Arch Pathol Anat* 1863;26:391–419, 433–459, and 27:1–26.
2. Geoffroy G, Barbeau A, Breton A, et al. Clinical description and roentgenologic evaluation of patients with Friedreich's ataxia. *Can J Neurol Sci* 1976;3:278–286.
3. Harding AE. Friedreich's ataxia: a clinical and genetic study of 90 families with an analysis of early diagnostic criteria and intrafamilial clustering of clinical features. *Brain* 1981;104:589–602.
4. Harding AE. *The hereditary ataxias and related disorders.* Edinburgh: Churchill Livingstone, 1984.
5. Harding AE. Clinical features and classification of inherited ataxias. *Adv Neurol* 1993;61:1–14.
6. Nikali K, Suomalainen A, Terwilliger J, Koskinen T, Weissenbach J, Peltonen L. Random search for shared chromosomal regions in four affected individuals: the assignment of a new hereditary ataxia locus. *Am J Hum Genet* 1995;56:1088–1095.
7. Wullner U, Klockgether T, Petersen D, Naegele T, Dichgans J. Magnetic resonance imaging in hereditary and idiopathic ataxia. *Neurology* 1993;43:318–323.
8. Palau F, DeMichele G, Vilchez J, et al. Early-onset ataxia with cardiomyopathy and retained tendon reflexes maps to the Friedreich's ataxia locus on chromosome 9q. *Ann Neurol* 1995;37:359–362.
9. Durr A, Cossee M, Agid Y, et al. Clinical and genetic abnormalities in patients with Friedreich's ataxia. *N Engl J Med* 1996;335:1222–1224.
10. Klockgether T, Chamberlain S, Wullner V, et al. Late onset Friedreich's ataxia: molecular genetics, clinical neurophysiology and magnetic resonance imaging. *Arch Neurol* 1993;50:802–806.
11. DeMichele G, Filla A, Cavalcanti F, et al. Late onset Friedreich's disease: clinical features and mapping of mutation to FRDA locus. *J Neurol Neurosurg Psych* 1994;57:977–979.
12. Pandolfo M. The effect of molecular testing on the diagnostic criteria for Friedreich ataxia. *Neurology* 1997;48:A211.
13. Chamberlain S, Shaw S, Rowland S, et al. Mapping of the mutation causing Friedreich's ataxia to human chromosome 9. *Nature* 1988;334:248–250.
14. Hanauer A, Chery M, Fujita R, Driesel R, Gilgenkrantz S, Mandek J. The Friedreich ataxia gene is assigned to chromosome 9q13-q21 by mapping of the tightly linked markers and shows linkage disequilibrium with D9S15. *Am J Hum Genet* 1990;46:133–137.

15. Chamberlain S, Shaw J, Wallis J, et al. Genetic homogeneity at Friedreich's ataxia locus on Chromosome 9. *Am J Hum Genet* 1989; 44:518–521.

16. Pandolfo M, Sirugo G, Antonelli A, et al. Friedreich's ataxia in Italian families: genetic homogeneity and linkage disequilibrium with the marker loci D9S5 and D9S15. *Am J Hum Genet* 1990;47:228–235.

17. Richter A, Melancon S, Farrall M, Chamberlain S. Friedreich's ataxia: confirmation of gene localization to chromosome 9 in the Quebec French-Canadian population. *Cytogenet Cell Genet* 1980;51:A1066.

18. Monros E, Canizares J, Molto MD, et al. Evidence for a common origin of most Friedreich ataxia chromosomes in the Spanish population. *Eur J Hum Genet* 1996;4:191–198.

19. Sirugo G, Keats B, Fujita R, et al. Friedreich ataxia in Louisiana Acadians: demonstration of a founder by analysis of microsatellite generated haplotypes. *Am J Hum Genet* 1992;50:559–566.

20. Campuzano V, Montermini L, Molto MD, et al. Friedreich's ataxia: autosomal recessive disease caused by an intronic triplet repeat expansion. *Science* 1996;271:1374–1375.

21. Montermini L, Andermann E, Labuda M, et al. The Friedreich ataxia GAA triplet repeat: premutation and normal alleles. *Hum Mol Genet* 1997;6:1261–1266.

22. Campuzano V, Montermini L, Lutz Y, et al. Frataxin is reduced in Friedreich ataxia patients and is associated with mitochondrial membranes. *Hum Mol Genet* 1997;6:1771–1780.

23. Filla A, De Michele G, Cavalcanti F, et al. The relationship between trinucleotide (GAA) repeat length and clinical features in Friedreich ataxia. *Am J Hum Genet* 1996;59:554–560.

24. Monros E, Molto MD, Martinez F, et al. Phenotype correlation and intergenerational dynamics of the Friedreich ataxia GAA trinucleotide repeat. *Am J Hum Genet* 1997;61:101–110.

25. Lamont PJ, David MB, Wood NW. Identification and sizing of the GAA trinucleotide repeat expansion of Friedreich's ataxia in 56 patients. Clinical and genetic correlates. *Brain* 1997;120:673–680.

26. Priller J, Scherzer CR, Faber PW, MacDonald ME, Young AB. Frataxin gene of Friedreich's ataxia is targeted to mitochondria. *Ann Neurol* 1997;42:265–269.

27. Kounikova H, Campuzano V, Foury F, Dolle P, Cazzalini O, Koenig M. Studies of human, mouse and yeast homologues indicate a mitochondrial function for frataxin. *Nat Genet* 1997;16:345–351.

28. Babcock M, de Silva D, Oaks R, et al. Regulation of mitochondrial iron accumulation by Yfh 1 p, a putative homolog of frataxin. *Science* 1997;276:1709–1712.

29. Warren ST. The expanding world of trinucleotide repeats. *Science* 1996;271:1374–1375.

30. Pennacchio LA, Lehesjoki AE, Stone NE, et al. Mutations in the gene encoding cystatin B in progressive myoclonus epilepsy (EPM1). *Science* 1996;271:1731–1734.

31. Silvestri G, Ciafoni E, Santorelli FM, et al. Clinical features associated with the A-G transition at nucleotide 8344 of mtDNA ("MERRF mutation"). *Neurology* 1993;43:1200–1206.

32. Johns DR. Seminars in medicine of the Beth Israel Hospital, Boston: mitochondrial DNA and disease. *N Engl J Med* 1995;333:638–644.

33. DiMauro S, Moraes CT. Mitochondrial encephalomyopathies. *Arch Neurol* 1993;50:1197–1208.

34. Schon EA, Hirano M, DiMauro S. Mitochondrial encephalomyopathies: clinical and molecular analysis. *J Bioenerg Biomembr* 1944; 26:291–299.

35. Sharp D, Blinderman L, Combs KA, et al. Cloning and gene defects in microsomal triglyceride transfer protein associated with abetalipoproteinaemia. *Nature* 1993;365:65–69.

36. Yokota T, Shiojiri T, Gotoda T, et al. Friedreich-like ataxia with retinitis pigmentosa caused by the His[101] Gln mutation of the alpha-tocopherol transfer protein gene. *Ann Neurol* 1997;41:826–832.

37. Ben Hamida C, Doerflinaer N, Belal S, et al. Localization of Friedreich ataxia phenotype with selective vitamin E deficiency to chromosome 8q by homozygosity mapping. *Nat Genet* 1993;5:195–200.

38. Ouahchi K, Arita M, Kayden H, et al. Ataxia with isolated vitamin E deficiency is caused by mutations in the alpha tocopherol transfer protein. *Nat Genet* 1995;9:141–145.

39. Gotoda T, Arita M, Arai H, et al. Adult-onset spinocerebellar dysfunction caused by a mutation in the gene for the alpha tocopheral transfer protein. *N Engl J Med* 1995;333:1313–1318.

40. Savitsky K, Bar-Shira A, Gilad S, et al. A single ataxia telangiectasia gene with a product similar to PI-3 kinase. *Science* 1995;268: 1749–1753.

41. Gatti RA, Berkel I, Boder E, et al. Localization of an ataxia-telangiectasia gene to chromosome 11q22-23. *Nature* 1988;336:577–580.

42. Yakura H, Nakisaka A, Fujimoto S, Itakura K. Hereditary ataxia and HLA genotypes. *N Engl J Med* 1974;291:154–155.

43. Jackson JF, Currier RD, Terasaki PL, Morton NE. Spinocerebellar ataxia and HLA linkage: Risk prediction by HLA typing. *N Engl J Med* 1977;296:1138–1141.

44. Orr Ht, Chung M-Y, Banfi S, et al. Expansion of an unstable trinucleotide (CAG) repeat in spinocerebellar ataxia type I. *Nat Genet* 1993;4:221–226.

45. Ranum LPW, Lundgren JK, Schut LJ, et al. Spinocerebellar ataxia type I and Machado-Joseph disease: incidence of CAG expansions among adult-onset ataxia patients from 311 families with dominant, recessive, and sporadic ataxia. *Am J Hum Genet* 1995;57:603–668.

46. Genis D, Matilla T, Volpini V, et al. Clinical, neuropathologic, and genetic studies of a large spinocerebellar ataxia type I (SCA1) kindred: (CAG)n expansion and early premonitory signs and symptoms. *Neurology* 1995;45:24–30.

47. Matilla T, Volpini V, Genis D, et al. Presymptomatic analysis of spinocerebellar ataxia type I (SCAI) via the expansion of the SCAI CAG repeat in a large pedigree displaying anticipation and parental male bias. *Hum Mol Genet* 1997;6:1283–1287.

48. Dubourg O, Durr A, Cancel G, et al. Analysis of the SCA1 CAG repeat in a large number of families with dominant ataxia: clinical and molecular correlation. *Ann Neurol* 1995;37:176–188.

49. Jodice C, Malaspina P, Persichetti F, et al. Effect of trinucleotide repeat length and parental sex on phenotypic variation in spinocerebellar ataxia I. *Am J Hum Genet* 1994;54:959–964.

50. Ranum LP, Chung M, Banfi S, et al. Molecular and clinical correlations in spinocerebellar ataxia type I: evidence for familial effects on the age at onset. *Am J Hum Genet* 1994;55:244–252.

51. Quan F, Janas J, Popovich BW. A novel CAG repeat configuration in the SCA1 gene: implications for the molecular diagnostics of spinocerebellar ataxia type 1. *Hum Mol Genet* 1995;4:2411–2413.

52. Chong SS, McCall AE, Cota J, et al. Gametic and somatic tissue specific heterogeneity of the expanded SCA1 CAG repeat in spinocerebellar ataxia type I. *Nat Genet* 1995;10:344–350.

53. Chung M, Ranum LPW, Duvick LA, Servadio A, Zoghbi HY, Orr HT. Evidence for a mechanism predisposing to intergenerational CAG repeat instability in spinocerebellar ataxia type I. *Nat Genet* 1993; 5:254–258.

54. Banfi S, Servadio A, Chung MY, et al. Identification and characterization of the gene causing type I spinocerebellar ataxia. *Nat Genet* 1994;7:513–520.

55. Banfi S, Servadio A, Chung M, et al. Cloning and developmental expression analysis of the murine homolog of the spinocerebellar ataxia type I gene (SCA1). *Hum Mol Genet* 1996;5:33–40.

56. Servadio A, Koshy B, Armstrong D, Antalffy B, Orr H, Zoghbi HY. Expression analysis of the ataxin-I protein in tissues from normal and spinocerebellar ataxia type I individuals. *Nat Genet* 1995;10:94–98.

57. Koshy G, Matilla EN, Merry DE, Fischbeck KH, Orr HT, Zoghbi HY. Spinocerebellar ataxia type-1 and spinocerebellar muscular atrophy gene products interact with glyceraldehyde-3-phosphate dehydrogenase. *Hum Mol Genet* 1996;9:1311–1318.

58. Goldberg YP, Nicholson DW, Rasper DM, et al. Cleavage of huntingtin by apopain, a proapoptotic cysteine protease, is modulated by the polyglutamine tract. *Nat Genet* 1996;13:442–449.

59. Ikeda H, Yamaguchi M, Sugai S, Aze Y, Narumiya S, Kakizuka A. Expanded polyglutamine in the Machado-Joseph disease protein induces cell death in vitro and in vivo. *Nat Genet* 1996;13:196–202.

60. Davies SW, Turamine M, Cozens BA, et al. Formation of neuronal intranuclear inclusions underlies the neurological dysfunction in mice transgenic for the HD mutation. *Cell* 1997;90:537–548.

61. Scherzinger E, Lurz R, Turmaine M, et al. Huntingtin-encoded polyglutamine expansions form amyloid-like protein aggregates in vitro and in vivo. *Cell* 1997;90:549–558.

62. Paulson HL, Perez MK, Trottier PY, et al. Intranuclear inclusions of expanded polyglutamine protein in spinocerebellar ataxia type 3. *Neuron* 1997;19:333–344.

63. Burright EN, Clark HB, Servadio A, et al. SCA1 transgenic mice: a model for neurodegeneration caused by an expanded CAG trinucleotide repeat. *Cell* 1995;82:937–948.

64. Monckton DG, Coolbaugh MI, Ashizawa KT, Siciliano MJ, Caskey CT. Hypermutable myotonic dystrophy CTG repeats in transgenic mice. *Nat Genet* 1997;15:193–196.

65. Gourdon G, Radvanyi F, Lia A-S, et al. Moderate intergenerational and somatic instability of a 55-CTG repeat in transgenic mice. *Nat Genet* 1997;15:190–193.

66. Mangiarini L, Sathasivam K, Mahal A, Mott R, Seller M, Bates GP. Instability of highly expanded CAG repeats in mice transgenic for the Huntington's disease mutation. *Nat Genet* 1997;54:197–200.

67. Silveira I, Lopes-Cendes I, Sequeiros J, Rouleau GA. Molecular diagnosis of SCAI, DRPLA, and MJD mutations in a large group of ataxia patients. *Am J Hum Genet* 1995;57[Suppl]:A228.

68. Giunti P, Sweeny MG, Spadaro M, et al. The trinucleotide repeat expansion on chromosome 6p (SCA1) in autosomal dominant cerebellar ataxias. *Brain* 1994;117:645–649.

69. Kameya T, Abe K, Aoki M, et al. Analysis of spinocerebellar ataxia type I (SCAI) related CAG trinucleotide expansion in Japan. *Neurology* 1995;45:1587–1593.

70. Takano H, Ikeuchi T, Igarashi I, et al. A molecular genetic study on autosomal dominant ataxias in Japanese. Comparison of the prevalences and CAG repeat expansions among spinocerebellar ataxia (SCA1), spinocerebellar ataxia type 2 (SCA2), Machado-Joseph disease (MJD) and dentatorubral-pallidoluysian atrophy (DRPLA). *Neurology* 1997;48:A209.

71. Zoghbi HY. Spinocerebellar ataxia type 1. *Clin Neurosci* 1995;3:5–11.

72. Gispert S, Twells R, Orozco G, et al. Chromosomal assignment of the second locus for autosomal dominant cerebellar ataxia (SCA2) to human chromosome 12q23-24.1. *Nat Genet* 1993;4:295–298.

73. Orozco-Diaz G, Nodarse-Fleites A, Cordoves-Sagaz R, Auburger G. Autosomal dominant cerebellar ataxia: clinical analysis of 263 patients from a homogenous population in Holquin, Cuba. *Neurology* 1990;40:1369–1375.

74. Pulst SM, Nechiporuk A, Starkuan S. Anticipation in spinocerebellar ataxia type 2. *Nat Genet* 1933;5:8–10.

75. Filla A, DeMichele G, Banfi S, et al. Has spinocerebellar ataxia type 2 a distinct phenotype: Genetic and clinical study of an Italian family. *Neurology* 1995;45:793–796.

76. Lopes-Cendes I, Andermann E, Attiq E, et al. Confirmation of the SCA-2 locus as an alternative locus for dominating inherited spinocerebellar ataxias and refinement of the candidate region. *Am J Hum Genet* 1994;54:774–781.

77. Belal S, Cancel G, Stevanin G, et al. Clinical and genetic analysis of a Tunisian family with autosomal dominant cerebellar ataxia type I linked to the SCA2 locus. *Neurology* 1994;44:1423–1426.

78. Brice A, Cancel G, Durr A, et al. SCA2 (spinocerebellar ataxia): another unstable CAG expansion. Molecular and clinical analysis of 101 patients. *Neurology* 1997;48:A201.

79. Schols L, Gispert S, Vorgerd M, et al. Spinocerebellar ataxia type 2. *Arch Neurol* 1997;54:1073–1080.

80. Pulst SM, Nechiporuk A, Nechiporuk T, et al. Moderate expansion of a normally biallelic trinucleotide repeat in spinocerebellar ataxia type 2. *Nat Genet* 1996;14:269–284.

81. Imbert G, Saudou F, Devys D, et al. Cloning of the gene for spinocerebellar ataxia 2 reveals a locus with high sensitivity to expanded CAG/glutamine repeats. *Nat Genet* 1998;14:237–238.

82. Sanpei K, Takano H, Igarashi S, et al. Identification of the spinocerebellar ataxia type 2 gene using a direct identification of repeat expansion and cloning technique, DIRECT. *Nat Genet* 1996;14:277–284.

83. Cancel G, Durr A, Didierjean O, et al. Molecular and clinical correlations in spinocebellar ataxia 2: a study of 32 families. *Hum Mol Genet* 1997;6:709–715.

84. Pulst SM, Nechiporuk T, Nechiporuk A. Characterization of the spinocerebellar ataxia type 2 (SCA2) gene. *Neurology* 1997;48:A209.

85. Nakano K, Dawson D, Spence A. Machado disease: hereditary ataxia in Portuguese immigrants to Massachusetts. *Neurology* 1972;22:49–59.

86. Woods BT, Schaumburg HH. Nigro-spinodentatal degeneration with nuclear ophthalmoplegia. A unique and partially treated clinico-pathologic entity. *J Neurol Sci* 1972;17:149–166.

87. Rosenbert RN, Nyhan WL, Bay C, Shore P. Autosomal dominant striatonigral degeneration: a clinical, pathologic and biochemical study of a new genetic disorder. *Neurology* 1976;26:703–714.

88. Cancel G, Abbas N, Stevanin G, et al. Marked phenotypic heterogeneity associated with expansion of a CAG repeat sequence at the spinocerebellar ataxia 3/Machado Joseph locus. *Am J Hum Genet* 1995;57:809–816.

89. Brunt ERP, Verschuuren CC, Joosten AAJ, Stolte F, Scheffer H. Confirmation of spinocerebellar ataxia (SCA) 3 locus in a Dutch family showing anticipation in male offspring. *Neurology* 1995;45[Suppl 4]:A453.

90. Healton EB, Brust JCM, Kerr D. Presumably Azorean disease in a presumably non-Portuguese family. *Neurology* 1980;30:1084–1089.

91. Takiyama Y, Nishizawa M, Tanaka H, et al. The gene for Machado-Joseph disease maps to human chromosome 14q. *Nat Genet* 1993;4:300–303.

92. St. George-Hyslop PH, Rogaeva E, Hutterer J, et al. Machado-Joseph disease in pedigrees of Azorean descent is linked to chromosome 14. *Am J Hum Genet* 1994;55:120–125.

93. Tuite PJ, Rogaeva EA, St. George-Hyslop PH, Lang AE. Dopa-responsive parkinsonism phenotype of Machado-Joseph disease: confirmation of 14q CAG expansion. *Ann Neurol* 1995;38:684–687.

94. Stevanin G, LeGuern E, Ravise N, et al. A third locus for autosomal dominant cerebellar ataxia type I maps to chromosome 14q24-3-qter: evidence for the existence of a fourth locus. *Am J Hum Genet* 1994;54:11–30.

95. Kawaguchi Y, Okamoto T, Taniwaki M, et al. CAG expansions in a novel gene from Machado-Joseph disease at chromosome 14q32.1. *Nat Genet* 1994;8:221–228.

96. Matilla T, McCall A, Subramory SH, Zoghbi HY. Molecular and clinical correlations in spinocerebellar ataxia type 3 and Machado-Joseph disease. *Ann Neurol* 1995;38:68–72.

97. Maryuama H, Nakcamura S, Matsuyama Z, et al. Molecular features of the CAG repeats and clinical manifestations of Machado-Joseph disease. *Hum Mol Genet* 1995;4:807–812.

98. Kawakami H, Maruyama H, Nakamura S, Kawaguchi A, Doyu M, Sobue G. Unique features of the CAG repeats in Machado-Joseph disease. *Nat Genet* 1995;9:344–345.

99. Durr A, Stevanin G, Cancel G, et al. Gender equality in Machado-Joseph disease. *Nat Genet* 1995;11:118–119.

100. DeStefano A, Farrer L, Maciel P, et al. Gender equality in Machado-Joseph disease. *Nat Genet* 1995;11:119.

101. Lang AE, Rogaeva EA, Tsuda T, Hutterer J, St. George-Hyslop PH. Homozygous inheritance of the Machado-Joseph disease gene. *Ann Neurol* 1994;36:443–447.

102. Stevanin G, Cancel G, Didierjean O, et al. Linkage disequilibrium at the Machado-Joseph disease/spinal cerebellar ataxia 3 locus: evidence for a common founder effect in French and Portuguese-Brazilian families as well as a second ancestral Portuguese-Azorean mutation. *Am J Hum Genet* 1995;57:1247–1250.

103. Igarashi S, Takiyama Y, Cancel G, et al. Intergenerational instability of the CAG repeat of the gene for Machado-Joseph disease (MJD1) is affected by the genotype of the normal chromosome: Implications for the molecular mechanisms of the instability of the CAG repeat. *Hum Mol Genet* 1996;5:923–932.

104. Gardner K, Alderson K, Galster B, Kaplan C, Leppert M, Ptacek L. Autosomal dominant spinocerebellar ataxia: clinical description of a distinct hereditary ataxia and genetic localization to chromosome 16 (SCA4) in a Utah kindred. *Neurology* 1994;44[Suppl 2]:A361.

105. Flanigan K, Gardner K, Alderson K, et al. Autosomal dominant spinocerebellar ataxia with sensory axonal neuropathy (SCA4): clinical description and genetic localization to chromosome 16q22.1. *Am J Hum Genet* 1996;59:392–399.

106. Biemond A. LaForme radiculo-cordonnale postérieure des dégénéresces spinocérébelleuses. *Rev Neurol* 1954;91:3–21.

107. Ranum LP, Schut LJ, Lundgren JK, Orr HT, Livingston PM. Spinocerebellar ataxia type 5 in a family descended from the grandparents of President Lincoln maps to chromosome 11. *Nat Genet* 1994;8:280–284.

108. Lory P, Ophoff RA, Nahmias J. Toward a unified nomenclature describing voltage-gated calcium channel genes. *Hum Genet* 1997;100:149–150.

109. Zhuchenko O, Bailey J, Bonnen P, et al. Autosomal dominant cerebellar ataxia (SCA6) associated with small polyglutamine expansions in the alpha 1A-voltage-dependent calcium channel. *Nat Genet* 1997;15:62–69.

110. Matsuyama Z, Kawakami H, Maruyama H, et al. Molecular features of the CAG repeats of spinocerebellar ataxia 6 (SCA6). *Hum Mol Genet* 1997;6:1283–1287.

111. Riess O, Schols L, Bottger H, et al. SCA6 is caused by moderate CAG expansion in the alpha 1A-voltage-dependent calcium channel gene. *Hum Mol Genet* 1997;6:1289–1293.

112. Ishikawa K, Tanaka H, Saito M, et al. Japanese families with autosomal dominant pure cerebellar ataxia map to chromosome 19p13.1-

p13.2 and are strongly associated with mild CAG expansions in the spinocerebellar ataxia type 6 gene in chromosome 19p13.1. *Am J Hum Genet* 1997;61:336–346.

113. Ophoff RA, Terwindt GM, Vergouwe MN, et al. Familial hemiplegic migraine and episodic ataxia type 2 are caused by mutations in the CA2- channel gene CACNL1A4. *Cell* 1996;87:543–552.

114. Jodice C, Mantuano E, Veneziano L, et al. Episodic ataxia type 2 (EA2) and spinocerebellar ataxia type 6 (SCA6) due to CAG repeat expansion in the CACNA1A gene on chromosome 19p. *Hum Mol Genet* 1997;11:1973–1978.

115. Gouw LG, Digre KB, Harris CP, Haines JH, Ptacek LJ. Autosomal dominant cerebellar ataxia with retinal degeneration: clinical, neuropathologic, and genetic analysis of a large kindred. *Neurology* 1994;44:1441–1447.

116. Benomar A, Le Guern E, Durr A, et al. Autosomal dominant cerebellar ataxia with retinal degeneration (ADCA type II) is genetically different from ADCA type I. *Ann Neurol* 1994;35:439–444.

117. Benomar A, Krols L, Stevanin G, et al. The gene for autosomal dominant cerebellar ataxia with pigmentary macular dystrophy maps to chromosome 3p12-p21.1. *Nat Genet* 1995;10:84–88.

118. Gouw LG, Kaplan CD, Haines JH, et al. Retinal degeneration characterizes a spinocerebellar ataxia mapping to chromosome 3p. *Nat Genet* 1995;10:89–93.

119. David G, Giunti P, Abbas N, et al. The gene for autosomal dominant cerebellar ataxia type II is located in a 5-cM region in 3p12-p13: Genetic and physical mapping of the SCA7 locus. *Am J Hum Genet* 1996;59:1328–1336.

120. Holmberg M, Johansson J, Forsgren L, Heijbel J, Sangren O, Holmgren G. Localization of autosomal dominant cerebellar ataxia associated with retinal degeneration and anticipation to chromosome 3p12-p21.1. *Hum Mol Genet* 1995;4:1441–1445.

121. Krols L, Martin JJ, David G, et al. Refinement of the locus for autosomal dominant cerebellar ataxia type II to chromosome 3p21.1-14.1. *Hum Genet* 1997;99:225–232.

122. Jobsis GJ, Weber JW, Barth PG, et al. Autosomal dominant cerebellar ataxia with retinal degeneration (ADCAII): clinical and neuropathological findings in two pedigrees and genetic linkage to 3p21.1-14.1. *J Neurol Neurosurg Psychiatry* 1997;62:367–371.

123. Trottier Y, Lutz Y, Stevanin G, et al. Polyglutamine expansion as a pathological epitope in Huntington's disease and four dominant cerebellar ataxias. *Nature* 1995;378:403–406.

124. Stevanin G, Trottier Y, Cancel G, et al. Screening for proteins with polyglutamine expansions in autosomal dominant cerebellar ataxias. *Hum Mol Genet* 1996;5:1887–1892.

125. Lindblad K, Savontaus ML, Stevanin G, et al. An expanded CAG repeat sequence in spinocerebellar ataxia type 7. *Genome Res* 1996;6: 965–971.

126. David G, Abbas N, Stevanin G, et al. Cloning of the SCA7 gene reveals a highly unstable CAG repeat expansion. *Nat Genet* 1997;17: 65–70.

127. Smith JK, Gonda VE, Malamud N. Unusual form of cerebellar ataxia: combined dentatorubral and pallidolysian degeneration. *Neurology* 1958;13:266–269.

128. Titica J, Van Bogaert L. Heredodegenerative hemiballismus: a contribution to the question of primary atrophy of the corpus luysii. *Brain* 1946;69:251–263.

129. Naito H, Oyanagi S. Familial myoclonus epilepsy and choreoathetosis: hereditary dentatorubral-pallidoluysian atrophy. *Neurology* 1982; 32:798–802.

130. Takahashi H, Ohama E, Naito H, et al. Hereditary dentatorubral-pallidoluysian atrophy in clinical and pathologic variants in a family. *Neurology* 1988;38:1063–1070.

131. Warner TT, Williams ID, Walker WH, et al. A clinical and molecular genetic study of dentatorubropallidoluysian atrophy in four European families. *Ann Neurol* 1995;37:452–459.

132. Burke JR, Wingfield MS, Lewis KE, et al. The Haw River syndrome: dentatorubropallidoluysian atrophy in an African-American family. *Nat Genet* 1994;7:521–524.

133. Ikeuchi T, Koide R, Onodera O, et al. Dentatorubral-pallidoluysian atrophy (DRPLA). *Clin Neurosci* 1995;3:23–27.

134. Komure O, Sano A, Nishino N, et al. DNA analysis in hereditary dentatorubral-pallidoluyrian atrophy: correlation between CAG repeat length and phenotypic variation and the molecular basis of anticipation. *Neurology* 1995;45:143–149.

135. Farmer TW, Windfield MS, Lynch SA, et al. Ataxia, chorea, seizures and dementia. Pathologic features of a newly defined familial disorder. *Arch Neurol* 1989;46:774–779.

136. Koide R, Ikeuchi T, Tanaka H, et al. Unstable expansion of CAG repeat in hereditary dentatorubral-pallidoluysian atrophy (DRPLA). *Nat Genet* 1994;6:9–13.

137. Nagafuchi S, Yanagisawa H, Satok, et al. Dentatorubral and pallidoluysian atrophy expansion of an unstable CAG trinucleotide on chromosome 12. *Nat Genet* 1994;6:14–18.

138. Nagafuchi S, Yanagisawa H, Ohsaki E, et al. Structure and expression of the gene responsible for the triplet repeat disorder, dentatorubral and pallidoluysian atrophy (DRPLA). *Nat Genet* 1994;8:177–182.

139. Yazawa I, Nukina N, Hashida H, Goto J, Yamada M, Kanazawa I. Abnormal gene product identified in hereditary dentatorubral pallidoluysian atrophy (DRPLA) brain. *Nat Genet* 1995;10:99–103.

140. Higgins JJ, Pho LT, Ide SE, Nee LE, Polymeropoulos M. Evidence of a new spinocerebellar ataxia locus. *Mov Disord* 1997;12:412–417.

141. Gancher ST, Nutt JC. Autosomal dominant episodic ataxia: a heterogenous syndrome. *Mov Disord* 1986;1:239–253.

142. Brunt EP, Van Weerden TW. Familial paroxysmal kinesigenic ataxia and continuous myokymia. *Brain* 1990;113:1361–1382.

143. Vaamond J, Artieda J, Obeso JA. Hereditary paroxysmal ataxia with neuromyotonia. *Mov Disord* 1991;6:180–182.

144. LaFrance R, Giggs R, Moxley R, McQuillen J. Hereditary paroxysmal ataxia responsive to acetazolamide. *Neurology* 1977;23:310.

145. Browne DL, Gancher ST, Nutt JG, et al. Episodic ataxia-myokimia syndrome is associated with point mutations in the human potassium channel gene, KCNA1. *Nat Genet* 1994;8:136–140.

146. Griggs RC, Nutt JG. Episodic ataxias as channelopathies. *Ann Neurol* 1995;37:285–286.

147. Griggs RC, Moxley RT, LaFrance RA, McQuillen J. Hereditary paroxysmal ataxia: responsive to acetazolamide. *Neurology* 1978; 28:1259–1264.

148. Baloh RW, Winder A. Acetazolamide-responsive vestibulocerebellar syndrome: clinical and oculographic feature. *Neurology* 1991;41: 429–432.

149. Baloh RW, Qing Y, Furman JM, Nelson SF. Familial episodic ataxia: Clinical heterogeneity in four families linked to chromosome 19p. *Ann Neurol* 1997;41:8–16.

150. Bain PG, Larkin GBR, Calver DM, O'Brien MD. Persistent superior oblique paresis as a manifestation of familial periodic cerebellar ataxia. *Br J Ophthalmol* 1991;75:619–621.

151. The BT, Silburn P, Betz R, Boyle R, Schalling M, Larsson C. Familial periodic cerebellar ataxia without myokymia maps to a 19-cM region on 19p13. *Am J Hum Genet* 1995;56:1443–1449.

152. Von Brederlow B, Hahn AF, Koopman WJ, Ebers GC, Bulman DE. Mapping the gene for acetazolamide responsive hereditary paroxysmal ataxia to chromosome 19p. *Hum Mol Genet* 1995;4:279–284.

153. Vahedi K, Joutel A, Van Bogaert P, et al. A gene for hereditary paroxysmal cerebellar ataxia maps to chromosome 19p. *Ann Neurol* 1995; 37:289–293.

154. Aurburger G, Ratzlaff T, Lunkes A, et al. A gene for autosomal dominant paroxysmal choreoathetosis/spasticity (CSE) maps to the vicinity of a potassium gene cluster on chromosome 1p, probably within 2cM between D1S443 and D1S197. *Genomics* 1996;31:90–94.

155. Trouillas P, Jing X, Adeleine P, et al. Buspirone, a 5-hydroxytryptamine 1A agonist, is active in cerebellar ataxia. *Arch Neurol* 1997; 54:749–752.

Motor Disorders,
edited by David S. Younger.
Lippincott Williams & Wilkins, Philadelphia © 1999.

CHAPTER 26

Cervical Spondylotic Myelopathy

Amory J. Fiore, William E. Krauss, and Paul C. McCormick

Cervical spondylotic myelopathy (CSM) is the most common myelopathic disorder of adults over the age of 55 years. It results from the progression of severe degenerative changes occurring in the cervical spine, leading to spinal cord compression. Like cervical spondylosis, it results from intervertebral disc degeneration, osteophytic spur formation, and hypertrophy of joints and ligaments. Our understanding of CSM has evolved considerably in the past several decades. A variety of operative approaches has been developed to forestall its progression, although there is still a lack of unified consensus regarding its natural history and optimum treatment. This chapter reviews the natural history, clinical and laboratory diagnosis, and treatment of CSM.

PATHOPHYSIOLOGY

The bony and ligamentous degenerative changes that are the hallmarks of cervical spondylosis are thought to be the primary causative factors underlying CSM. Multiple types of degenerative change may be present in varying combinations, with the principal spinal column pathology located anteriorly, posteriorly, or laterally. Because almost 90% of people have cervical osteophytes by age 60 (1), other factors appear to predispose certain individuals to the development of myelopathy.

Cervical disc dehydration occurs with advancing age, leading to loss of disc height and disc bulging and predisposing to osteophytic spur formation at disc space margins (2). These changes may be exacerbated by trauma or chronic heavy use. Disc degeneration may result in increased segmental motion or subluxation that can further exacerbate disc breakdown and lead to annulus rupture and herniation (3). Herniated discs may calcify, further contributing to osteophytic bar formation (4). Bony fusion may occur between segments, increasing segmental motion at adjacent levels. Subluxation and translation of motion segments can lead to degenerative change in the facet joints and posterior elements, resulting in facet hypertrophy and hypertrophy of the ligamentum flavum (5). The result of these anterior and posterior processes is reduction of the cross-sectional area of the spinal canal (6). Another important factor contributing to development of CSM is a congenitally decreased spinal canal diameter (7–10). Patients with CSM have been shown to have smaller canal diameters than age-matched control subjects; symptomatic disease is also rare in patients with a diameter greater than 13 mm (11,12). Patients with congenital nonspondylotic canal stenosis have an increased risk of developing myelopathy compared with those with normal canal diameter, and the clinical course is similar to CSM (13). Thickening and ossification of the posterior longitudinal ligament has also been implicated in the development of CSM. This finding is more prevalent in Asians, in whom the more typical findings of CSM are often absent (14).

In the severely spondylotic spine, the dynamic factors of flexion and extension appear to play a significant role in the development of canal narrowing and static cord compression. During flexion, the spinal cord assumes a more anterior position in the spinal canal, and in the presence of anterior disease, the cord may be draped over anterior osteophytes (15). During extension, the cord shortens and its cross-sectional area increases. At the same time, the ligamentum flavum buckles inward, so that hypertrophied posterior elements may cause dynamic compression (11). Flexion or extension of the compromised canal may result in repetitive subclinical cord injuries with cumulative effects. Myelopathy can also result from vascular compromise and ischemia in the affected segments. This probably results from shearing of intramedullary arteries during flexion and extension (16),

A. J. Fiore and W. E. Krauss: Department of Neurosurgery, Neurological Institute, New York Presbyterian Hospital, New York, New York 10032.

P. C. McCormick: Department of Neurosurgery, Columbia University College of Physicians and Surgeons and New York Presbyterian Hospital, New York, New York 10032.

with a lesser contribution of occlusion of anterior spinal or radicular arteries. Venous compromise is also likely to have significant impact. Postmortem studies demonstrate a combination of focal demyelination, cord atrophy, gray matter degeneration, and nerve root scarring along involved segments (6,10,17).

CLINICAL FEATURES

CSM presents primarily in the middle-aged and elderly without sex predilection. There may be a stepwise or slow steady progression of symptoms (12,18) or an initial phase of deterioration followed by stabilization lasting for years (19–21). The classically described clinical picture is that of a spastic paraparesis, with neck pain and cervical radiculopathy; however, transverse myelitis, pure paraparesis, Brown-Sequard and central cord syndromes, and brachialgia have been reported (22).

Motor deficits include arm weakness, hemiparesis, quadriparesis, muscle wasting, and fasciculation. Sensory findings may include paresthesia of the hands and a sensory level. Impairment of posterior column function, especially vibratory sensory loss in the legs, and a positive Romberg sign are all common. Ataxic gait may result from spinocerebellar tract compression. A combined sensory and motor deficit due to a central cord lesion results in the syndrome of "numb and clumsy hands" (22).

Radicular arm symptoms occur in up to 41% of patients, whereas radicular leg symptoms frequently result from tandem lumbar stenosis or disc disease (23,24). Hyperreflexia below the level of myelopathy occurs in up to 87% of patients. Babinski signs and clonus are frequently detectable, whereas Hoffman's sign is seen infrequently. Urinary urgency or hesitancy is relatively common, often without anal sphincter disturbance.

DIFFERENTIAL DIAGNOSIS

The diagnosis of CSM can be troublesome for two reasons. First, spondylotic change with associated cord compression is found radiographically and at autopsy among asymptomatic patients. Second, the associated myelopathy is not clinically distinctive and shares many signs and symptoms with other progressive neurologic disorders. These facts make a careful history and physical examination, in conjunction with relevant imaging studies and other diagnostic tests, essential in arriving at a proper diagnosis. The clinician should take great care to carefully consider all other diagnostic alternatives. There are three broad categories of lesions that mimic CSM: (i) extramedullary spinal tumors, epidural metastases, epidural abscesses, nerve sheath tumors, spinal cysts, dural vascular malformations, and congenital causes of stenosis that are the proximate cause of cord compression; (ii) intramedullary spinal cord tumors, syrinxes, and arteriovenous malformations; and (iii) amyotrophic lat-

eral sclerosis, multiple sclerosis, neurosyphilis, and B_{12} deficiency (25). Radiographic studies, especially magnetic resonance imaging (MRI), can usually easily identify extramedullary and intramedullary mass lesions and demyelinating plaques. The diagnosis of neurosyphilis and B_{12} deficiency is aided by serologic testing of B_{12}, homocysteine, and methylmalonic acid levels in the blood. The presence of sensory deficits makes amyotrophic lateral sclerosis highly unlikely, and lower motor neuron bulbar involvement, including tongue atrophy, fasciculation, and dysarthria, are incompatible with CSM and more typical of amyotrophic lateral sclerosis.

DIAGNOSTIC TECHNIQUES

Before the advent of computed tomography (CT) and MRI, plain cervical spine films were the mainstay of radiologic diagnosis of cervical spondylosis. Lateral views delineate bony changes such as osteophyte formation, loss of disc height, laminar shingling, and congenital block vertebrae (12). The anteroposterior canal diameter can be visualized, although laterally placed osteophytes may falsely exaggerate the degree of stenosis. Flexion-extension views may demonstrate segmental instability.

Myelography can provide considerable anatomic detail of spondylotic deformities and is particularly useful for visualizing nerve root take-off. Myelography was commonly used to provide dynamic information before the introduction of flexion-extension MRI. When combined with CT, anatomic detail of the canal is greatly improved. CT-myelography provides the most accurate estimate of canal diameter and can clearly delineate cord compression and spinal cord atrophy. Compressive lesions, including anterior and lateral osteophytes and hypertrophied ligaments, are well visualized. A small risk of neurologic deterioration from myelography exists, although this has been reduced with the introduction of non-ionic contrast media (26).

MRI is the test of choice for the initial evaluation of CSM. It offers multiplanar imaging and detailed imaging of spinal cord and nerve roots and does not subject the patient to myelography or its attendant risks (23,27). T2-weighted images may demonstrate intrinsic cord changes such as atrophy, demyelination, syrinx, and edema. High signal lesions adjacent to areas of spondylotic compression may correlate with a poor outcome. T2-weighted images may also demonstrate attenuation of cerebrospinal fluid spaces surrounding the cord, indicative of extradural compression. MRI offers the best means for delineating other spinal lesions, including intramedullary and extramedullary tumors, epidural abscesses, vascular malformations, and chiari malformations. The principal shortcomings of MRI include reduced detail of bony structures and inability to clearly delineate soft disc from osteophytic spurs. In addition, T1-weighted images may exaggerate spinal cord compression by osteophytes. Correlation with plain films may be useful in these instances.

TREATMENT

Treatment of CSM remains a controversial issue for several reasons. First, confounding variables can lead to a mistaken diagnosis of CSM in the presence of another neurologic disorder. Second, the natural history of CSM as described in the literature can be extremely variable, with some patients demonstrating a relentless progression of disability and others reaching a plateau where their disease seems to stabilize. Third, results of therapeutic trials, both conservative and surgical, have been inconsistent. Most series have been poorly controlled, uncontrolled, or retrospective.

Conservative management includes various methods aimed at immobilization of the cervical spine to reduce the excessive motion thought to contribute to CSM. Immobilization devices used include the soft cervical collar, Philadelphia collar, and minerva jacket. Physical therapy and nonsteroidal anti-inflammatory drugs have also been used. The high rate of noncompliance with immobilization therapy and the inability of many devices to effectively immobilize the spine have cast doubt on the validity of conservative therapy. The results of conservative trials have been mixed, with reported improvement rates of 29 to 55% (12,19). These reports of stabilization of symptoms with conservative therapy should be considered in light of the natural history of CSM, which may stabilize without intervention in certain instances.

When surgery has been established as the appropriate management for CSM, then the most appropriate procedure is chosen. Its goals are twofold: to decompress the spinal cord and nerve roots and to slow disease progression by reducing hypermobility of the spine. Selection of the proper surgical approach is critical to maximize beneficial outcome. The surgical approaches to CSM include anterior and posterior approaches. Factors influencing the choice of approach depend on cervical spine curvature, location of predominant compression, and rostrocaudal extent of involvement.

Posterior Decompression

Historically, the most widely used surgical treatment for CSM consisted primarily of posterior decompression via laminectomy (28,29). This entails removal of the lamina, spinous processes, medial facet joints, and ligamentum flavum. Modifications were subsequently described that included sectioning of the dentate ligament, decompression of nerve roots by foraminotomies, and removal of anterior osteophytes. The aim was to safely remove as much of the compressive pathology as possible, allowing the cord to expand posteriorly.

Posterior laminectomy has the primary advantage of relative ease of performance. The wide visualization of the nerve roots and cord allows direct assessment of adequacy of decompression. It is indicated in patients with posteriorly located compressive elements, those with exaggerated cervical lordosis that accentuates draping of the cord over posterior elements, and patients with congenital cervical stenosis. The posterior approach also allows multiple segments to be decompressed without need for complicated reconstruction procedures.

The disadvantages of the posterior approach include inability to adequately treat anterior compression when it is the predominating pathologic process. Another serious problem is destabilization of the cervical spine which may occur after extensive laminectomies. Utilization of lateral mass plates for fusion of decompressed levels provides adequate postoperative stabilization, especially in those with radiographic evidence of subluxation. Some patients may deteriorate after posterior decompression due to dorsal kinking of the cord after inadequate decompression in the presence of prominent ventral osteophytes. Postoperative scar formation can cause further compression. Many variants of laminoplasty with preservation and hinging of posterior elements have been proposed to remedy this problem, but results have been equivocal (30).

Anterior Decompression

The anterior approach (31) has only recently come into widespread acceptance for treatment of CSM (32–36). This procedure entails resection of the median portion of vertebral bodies at the most severely compressed levels, along with resection of intervertebral discs and osteophytes. It has the clear advantage of directly decompressing the anterior cord, the most common site of significant compressive pathology in CSM. It is indicated in those with normal cervical curvature, which predisposes to draping of the cord over the anterior spinal elements. Anterior corpectomy is accompanied by intervertebral fusion with either an allograft, harvested iliac crest, or fibular strut. An effective anterior approach establishes the goals of decompression via anterior osteophyte removal and stabilization of excessively mobile segments by interbody graft fusion.

The most widely cited disadvantages of the anterior approach are increased operative time and complexity and a higher incidence of operative complications (35,36). In addition, technical and biomechanical considerations preclude anterior decompression of disease that extends beyond three spinal segments. Complications are typically related to injury of the various vascular, neural, and visceral structures in the anterior neck. One of the most common complications is C-5 radiculitis. Other complications may include hoarseness due to recurrent laryngeal nerve injury, dysphagia, wound infection, and hematoma in addition to worsening of the myelopathy. Complications related to fusion include bleeding and infection at the graft donor site and graft extrusion; these may occur in 3 to 10% of patients.

RECOMMENDATIONS

Analysis of the results reported for anterior and posterior decompressive approaches to CSM provides no clear consensus as to which approach provides optimal results. However, among 84 patients treated with anterior corpectomy or posterior laminectomy and followed a mean of 7.35 years (37), initial improvement was seen in about 70% of patients operated by either approach. Long-term follow-up revealed sustained improvement in 54% of anterior operated cases and 37% of posterior approaches. At follow-up, 18% of anterior patients and 37% of posterior patients had deteriorated. Posterior approaches were not combined with fusion in this series, and the issue of postoperative instability was not addressed. The risk of late decline strongly correlated with duration of preoperative symptoms, so suggesting that some patients with CSM have sustained irreversible cord damage before surgery, a supposition supported by pathologic cord studies. The vascular pathology associated with CSM may be a contributing factor in late deterioration. When evaluating approaches to CSM, a complete evaluation of potential morbidity and mortality must be undertaken. The incidence of reported complications from anterior approaches is extremely variable, ranging from 3 to 48%. Complications are somewhat less frequent in posterior decompressive surgery, but the incidence of postoperative deformity is as high as 25 to 42%. Mortality for both approaches ranges from zero to 2%.

It is our practice to use the approach that allows us to remove the compressive elements most directly, taking into consideration the curvature of the cervical spine, whether lordotic or kyphotic, and the location and extent of compression. For segmental disease over one to three spinal levels, this usually entails anterior discectomy or corpectomy with interbody fusion. For posteriorly located compressive elements or diffuse disease that extends over more than three levels, we prefer a posterior approach. Additionally, posterior fusion and instrumentation may be required to avoid postoperative instability. In some instances, a combined anterior and posterior approach may be necessary. It is our position that in the hands of the experienced surgeon, good outcome and minimal morbidity may be achieved with either approach. As our understanding of CSM and the biomechanics of the spondylotic cervical spine evolves, it is our expectation that even more favorable outcomes will be achieved.

REFERENCES

1. Schmorl G, Junghanns H. Gesunde und kranke Wirbelsaule, [etc.]. In: Schmorl G, Junghanns H, eds. *Pathologische-anatomische untersuchungen*. Leipzig: Georg Thieme, 1932.
2. McNab I. The traction spur. *J Bone Joint Surg* 1971;53A:663–670.
3. Payne EE, Spillane JD. The cervical spine: an anatomicopathologic study of 70 patients. *Brain* 1957;70:557–596.
4. Wilkinson M. The morbid anatomy of cervical spondylosis and myelopathy. *Brain* 1960;83:589–616.
5. Barnes MP, Saunders M. The effect of cervical mobility on the natural history of cervical spondylotic myelopathy. *J Neurol Neurosurg Psychiatry* 1984;47:17–20.
6. Nurick S. The pathogenesis of the spinal cord disorder associated with cervical spondylosis. *Brain* 1972;95:87–100.
7. Adams CBT, Logue V. Studies in cervical spondylotic myelopathy. II. The movement and contour of the spine in relation to the neural complications of cervical spondylosis. *Brain* 1957;94:569–586.
8. Cusick JF. Pathophysiology and treatment of cervical spondylotic myelopathy. *Clin Neurosurg* 1991;37:661–681.
9. Epstein JA, Epstein NE. The surgical management of cervical spinal stenosis, spondylosis, and myeloradiculopathy by means of the posterior approach. In: Sherk HH, Dunn EJ, Eismont FJ, et al., eds. *The cervical spine*. Philadelphia: J.B. Lippincott, 1989;625–643.
10. Ogino H, Tada K, Okada K, et al. Canal diameter, anteroposterior compression ratio, and spondylotic myelopathy of the cervical spine. *Spine* 1983;8:1–15.
11. Parke WW. Correlative anatomy of cervical spondylotic myelopathy. *Spine* 1988;13:831–837.
12. Symon L, Lavender P. The surgical treatment of cervical spondylotic myelopathy. *Neurology* 1967;17:117–127.
13. Epstein JA, Carras R, Hyman RA, et al. Cervical myelopathy caused by developmental stenosis of the spinal canal. *J Neurosurg* 1979;51:362–367.
14. Nagashima C. Cervical myelopathy due to ossification of the posterior longitudinal ligament. *J Neurosurg* 1972;37:653–660.
15. Panjabi MM, White AA. Biomechanics of nonacute cervical spinal cord trauma. *Spine* 1988;13:838–842.
16. Doppman JL. The mechanism of ischemia in anteroposterior compression of the spinal cord. *Invest Radiol* 1975;10:543–554.
17. Ono K, Ota H, Tada K, et al. Cervical myelopathy secondary to multiple spondylotic protrusions: a clinicopathologic study. *Spine* 1977;2:109–125.
18. Phillips DG. Surgical treatment of myelopathy with cervical spondylosis. *J Neurol Neurosurg Psychiatry* 1973;36:879–884.
19. Lees F, Aldren-Turner JWA. Natural history and prognosis of cervical spondylosis. *Br Med J* 1963;2:1607–1610.
20. Nurick S. The natural history and the results of surgical treatment of the spinal cord disorder associated with cervical spondylosis. *Brain* 1972;95:101–108.
21. Roberts AH. Myelopathy due to cervical spondylosis treated by collar immobilization. *Neurology* 1966;16:951–954.
22. Crandall PH, Batzdorf U. Cervical spondylotic myelopathy. *J Neurosurg* 1966;25:57–66.
23. Dagi TF, Tarkington MA, Leech JJ. Tandem lumbar and cervical spinal stenosis. Natural history, prognostic indices, and results after surgical decompression. *J Neurosurg* 1987;66:842–849.
24. Epstein NE, Epstein JA, Carras R, et al. Coexisting cervical and lumbar spinal stenosis: diagnosis and management. *Neurosurgery* 1984;15:489–496.
25. Rowland LP. Surgical treatment of cervical spondylotic myelopathy: time for a controlled trial. *Neurology* 1992;42:5–13.
26. Robertson HJ, Smith RD. Cervical myelography: survey of modes of practice and major complications. *Radiology* 1990;174:79–83.
27. Nagata K, Kiyonaga K, Ohashi T, et al. Clinical value of magnetic resonance imaging for cervical myelopathy. *Spine* 1990;15:1088–1096.
28. Brain WR. Spondylosis: the known and the unknown. *Lancet* 1953;1:687–693.
29. Frykholm R. Cervical root compression resulting from disc degeneration and root-sleeve fibrosis. A clinical investigation. *Acta Chir Scand* 1951;160:1–149.
30. Lee TT, Manzano GR, Green BA. Modified open-door cervical expan-

sive laminoplasty for spondylotic myelopathy: operative technique, outcome, and predictors for gait improvement. *J Neurosurg* 1997;86:64–68.

31. Cloward R. The anterior approach for the removal of ruptured cervical discs. *J Neurosurg* 1958;14:602–607.

32. Bohlman HH. Cervical spondylosis with moderate to severe myelopathy: a report of seventeen cases treated by Robinson anterior cervical discectomy and fusion. *Spine* 1977;2:151–161.

33. Herkowitz HN. A comparison of anterior cervical fusion, cervical laminectomy, and cervical laminoplasty for the surgical management of multiple level spondylotic radiculopathy. *Spine* 1988;13:774–780.

34. Robinson RA, Walker AE, Ferlic DC. The result of an anterior interbody fusion of the cervical spine. *J Bone Joint Surg* 1969;44A:1959.

35. Saunders RL, Bernini PM, Shirreffs TG Jr, et al. Central corpectomy for cervical spondylotic myelopathy: a consecutive series with long-term follow-up evaluation. *J Neurosurg* 1991;74:163–170.

36. Whitecloud TS. Anterior surgery for cervical spondylotic myelopathy. Smith-Robinson, Cloward, and vertebrectomy. *Spine* 1988;13:861–863.

37. Ebersold MJ, Pare MC, Quast LM. Surgical treatment for cervical spondylotic myelopathy. *J Neurosurg* 1995;82:745–751.

Motor Disorders,
edited by David S. Younger.
Lippincott Williams & Wilkins, Philadelphia © 1999.

CHAPTER 27

Spinal Cord and Foramen Magnum Tumors

Gerald W. Honch and James M. Powers

The accurate diagnosis of masses in the spinal cord and foramen magnum remains a challenge for clinicians. An elusive history, poorly localized signs, and problems with laboratory studies all contribute to this frustration. In the past, the radiologic workup has been tedious, nonspecific, and invasive. The advent of magnetic resonance imaging (MRI) has had a great impact on these problems. MRI allows great precision in evaluating the spinal cord, meningeal and epidural regions, the vertebrae, and paravertebral spaces.

STATISTICAL DATA

Primary spinal cord tumors are uncommon. In the series by Percy et al. (1) in Rochester, Minnesota, the rate was 1.3 per 100,000 population. This figure contrasts with the rate for primary brain tumors of 12.5 per 100,000 population. There was no sex predominance, except for meningioma in which a clear predominance in women was noted. Elsberg (2) found primary intraspinal tumors to be less common in younger age groups; 90% of the tumors were found in patients 20 years of age or older.

The histologic classification of these tumors is interesting. Sloof et al. (3) (Table 1) noted nearly equal percentages for three main types of spinal tumors: schwannoma, meningioma, and glioma (29%, 25.5%, and 22.0%, respectively). Sarcomas, vascular tumors, chordomas, and epidermoid tumors comprise the remaining 23.5%. Thus, in contrast to intracranial tumors, spinal tumors are predominantly extra-axial. In this series, the distribution by vertebral level gave a clearly predictable

site only for meningiomas (Table 2). Eighty-one percent of the spinal meningiomas occurred at the thoracic level.

CLINICAL FEATURES

The symptoms produced by spinal tumors are related to the site of origin and the dynamics of their growth. Many are histologically benign and are slow growing. They occur in three main groups: intramedullary, extramedullary, and extradural. A summary of clinical findings was suggested by Schliack and Stille (4):

1. Intramedullary tumors cause direct interference with the intrinsic structures of the spinal cord. There is an absence of root symptoms. Pain is dull and poorly localized.
2. Extramedullary intradural tumors cause symptoms by involving the nerve roots, compressing the spinal cord, or occluding the spinal blood vessels. The Brown-Séquard syndrome is not uncommon and includes ipsilateral involvement of pyramidal and posterior column tracts and contralateral spinothalamic tract and root involvement, the latter at the site of the cord injury.

TABLE 1. *Histologic classification of 1,322 tumors of the spinal canal*

Type	No.	%
Neurilemoma	383	29.0
Meningioma	338	25.5
Glioma (18 extramedullary)	291	22.0
"Sarcoma" (7 intramedullary)	157	11.9
Vascular tumor (10 intramedullary)	82	6.2
Chordoma	53	4.0
Epidermoid, and others (10 intramedullary)	18	1.4
Total	1,322	100

From Ref. 3, with permission.

G. W. Honch: Department of Neurology, University of Rochester and Rochester General Hospital, Rochester, New York 14621.

J. M. Powers: Department of Pathology and Laboratory Medicine, University of Rochester, Rochester, New York 14642.

TABLE 2. *Distribution of neurilemomas, meningiomas, and gliomas by vertebral level*

Lesion	Cervical		Cervicothoracic		Thoracic		Thoracolumbar		Lumbar	
	No.	%	No.	%	No.	%	No.	%	No.	%
Neurilemoma	88	23.3	3	0.7	125	33.4	9	2.3	152	40.3
Meningioma	43	13.4	10	3.1	261	81.0	2	0.6	6	1.9
Glioma	34	13.9	20	8.2	63	25.7	63	25.7	65	26.5
Total	165	17.5	33	3.5	449	47.6	74	7.8	223	23.6

From Ref. 3, with permission.

3. Extradural lesions cause bony symptoms, spinal cord compression, and compromise of spinal blood vessels. The site of the lesion is made obvious by motor, sensory, and reflex levels after functional transection of the spinal cord has occurred. Babinski signs are elicited in lesions of the 11th thoracic vertebra. Bladder, bowel, and sexual dysfunction are common presenting complaints in all spinal cord tumors. The type of bladder abnormality, whether spastic or flaccid, relates to the level and chronicity of the lesion.

Lower cranial nerve involvement may be seen in lesions involving the upper cervical spinal cord, often with Lhermitte sign and unusual or abnormal postures of the head. Painful, forced-flexion, and stiffness of the neck are important signs that may be overlooked. With lesions in the middle and lower cervical spine, reflex changes, segmental weakness, and atrophy occur. When there is involvement at the thoracic level, there may be persistent intercostal neuralgia and disturbances of sweating and piloerection. In lumbosacral lesions, root pain is the predominant symptom, often with flaccid paralysis and bowel, bladder, and sexual dysfunction. Pain can assist in establishing the level of the lesion when there is destruction of bone and root symptomatology. The level is often higher by one or two spinal vertebrae than the segmental level indicated by the clinical examination with extramedullary lesions that compress the spinal cord. The explanation for this relates to the orderly lamination of the long tracts, with the more peripherally located tracts affected first. With intramedullary processes, there is a tendency for extension over multiple segments and a dissociated sensory disturbance, muscle atrophy, and reflex changes.

LABORATORY STUDIES

Electromyography can help determine the spinal level of a lesion by revealing fibrillation or denervation potentials in muscles that receive their innervation from a specific nerve root. Examination of the cerebrospinal fluid for increased protein content, pleocytosis, and cytology provides essential supportive data of a tumor. In the past, measuring the opening pressure, sometimes with an observation of pressure dynamics to jugular compression, that is, the Queckenstedt test, was routinely performed.

Lumbar puncture may aggravate the patient's symptoms if a partial block is converted to a total block of the subarachnoid space in the presence of a mass lesion. Myelography of the entire spinal subarachnoid space was previously necessary to survey and evaluate the contents of the spinal canal, but that has changed because of the utility of noninvasive neuroimaging studies discussed below.

RADIOGRAPHIC STUDIES

Plain radiographs of the spine remain useful in imaging the bones and their margins, contours, density, alignment, and integrity; however, soft tissues are less well seen. Areas of bony destruction and foraminal alterations can be useful clues to an underlying tumor even before proceeding to more sophisticated imaging modalities. Radioisotope bone scans can show increased activity in a lesioned area, but the cause generally requires further analysis. Radionuclide bone scans are more sensitive than plain radiographs in detecting vertebral metastases, except in multiple myeloma, but are nonspecific (5).

Myelography is used to show the patency of the spinal canal and define its contents. In recent years, high-density oil contrast has been replaced by water (cerebrospinal fluid)-soluble contrast agents. It can answer the question of spinal cord compression, define the limits of the lesion in the cord or canal, demonstrate multiple lesions, and contribute to the planning of radiotherapy. An advantage of myelography is its ability to examine the *length* of the spinal canal. The disadvantages are invasiveness, the tedious positioning required with contrast agents, and the dilution of water-soluble agents, particularly in the cervical and foramen magnum regions. Computed tomography (CT) should be used in conjunction with myelography, although it is limited in its ability to cover large areas of interest (6,7). Water-soluble contrast introduced by lumbar puncture provides an outline of the bony spine and its relationship to neural elements.

MRI combines the best of available modalities with few, if any, disadvantages (8). It is noninvasive and multiplanar, and lesions can be characterized on the basis of their structure and location with respect to the spinal cord. In addition, signal intensity characteristics that reflect tissue T1, T2, and spin density and paramagnetic, chemical shift, or susceptibility effects and motion add useful information in the analysis of a particular lesion. The technology and its refinements of MRI are, however, changing rapidly. Experience with intravenous gadolinium diethylenetriamine pentaacetic acid (Gd-DTPA) continues to refine workup protocols for these spinal cord lesions. In summary, CT provides better evaluation of bony destruction, whereas MRI is better for delineation of the exact extent of the tumor. The clinical signs and symptoms provide localization for investigative modalities.

TUMOR TYPES

Meningiomas, schwannomas (neurilemoma, neurinoma), and *neurofibromas* account for over half of all spinal cord tumors (9). Table 3 summarizes spinal cord tumor types and their characteristics.

Schwannomas are the most common primary tumors of the spinal canal. In the series by Sloof et al. (3), most of these nerve sheath tumors were intradural. About a third were extradural, and a few were both intradural and extradural, bridging that span in an hourglass or dumbbell fashion. The bony foramen is usually enlarged with hourglass tumors and is a helpful finding on plain radiographs. The tumor arises on the segment of the root, usually posterior, after it has penetrated the pia mater. These tumors are firm, circumscribed, and encapsulated. In most instances they are solitary. Microscopically, the appearance is one of interwoven bundles of long bipolar cells, the Antoni A pattern, or admixed with looser areas of irregular nuclei in an Antoni B pattern. The parallel alignment of spindle nuclei separated by an eosinophilic matrix, the Verocay body, is a modification of the Antoni A pattern that is of diagnostic value (Fig. 1). The presenting symptoms are most often of posterior nerve root origin. The lumbar region is a common site of these tumors because of the multiplicity of nerve roots in the cauda equina, but schwannomas occur at any location in the spinal canal.

Many nerves are usually involved in neurofibromas. Nerve root symptoms predominate in the dominantly inherited disorder von Recklinghausen disease or neurofibromatosis type I. A family history is usually informative. Stigmata of the disorder include cafe au lait spots, neurocutaneous tumors or neurofibromas, multiple nodules within the iris, skeletal abnormalities, and involvement of visceral organs, as for example, pheochromocytoma. These tumors, in contrast to schwannomas, have a loose and more haphazard arrangement of fewer nuclei in a more collagenous matrix (Fig. 2). These usually distinct histologic patterns may be admixed, especially in neurofibromatosis. There is a greater risk of malignant transformation with neurofibromas. Clinically, the diagnosis is often accomplished at the bedside because of the cutaneous stigmata. The therapeutic dilemma is when to treat the lesion responsible for the symptoms without adding to the burden of disability.

Both schwannomas and neurofibromas can open or widen the adjacent neural foramen. In the past, myelography was necessary to outline these masses. MRI demonstrates both types of tumor well. The nerve sheath tumors can be seen beyond the limit of the dura in distinction to myelography. T1-weighted images demonstrate these lesions as high signal intensity masses outlined by lower signal spinal and paraspinal soft tissues. Intravenous paramagnetic contrast (Gd-DTPA) enhances these tumors on T1-weighted images (10).

Meningiomas comprised about 25% of the intraspinal tumors in the series of Sloof et al. (3) (Table 1); about 85% were both intradural and extramedullary, and the thoracic region was the most commonly involved area (Table 2). Clinical signs are usually nonspecific until insidious progression leads to spinal cord compression. Meningiomas of the spinal cord favor women (10:1) over men (11). Most lesions become apparent after age 40. With MRI, the T1-weighted images demonstrate a soft tissue mass within the spinal canal that is isointense to the spinal cord and may displace it (12). Meningiomas show marked enhancement with paramagnetic contrast agents on T1-weighted images.

Tumors of the region of the foramen magnum are a special case (13,14). Meningiomas constitute the most common benign extramedullary tumor in this area. Neurofibromas in this area may be of even greater frequency if one includes the upper cervical segments as well. The commonest early clinical complaints are headache and pain in the head, neck, or upper back. The patient may assume bizarre head and neck postures. Progressive weakness is often followed by atrophy, first in one arm and then in the ipsilateral leg, followed by involvement of the other leg and then finally the opposite arm; sensory progression parallels that of the motor findings. Lower cranial nerve involvement is rare. The neurologic disorder evolves over months to years, sometimes with fluctuations, relapses, and remissions so much so that the clinical picture may be confused with that of multiple sclerosis. Myelography with attention to the foramen magnum is a tedious procedure, partly because of the need of special positioning to visualize this region without loss of contrast into the basilar cisterns. MRI evaluation of the foramen magnum tumors is simpler and more accurate (12).

Astrocytomas are the most common spinal cord tumors arising from the spinal cord itself and are more typically found in the upper cord (3,15). They are usually diffuse and infiltrative in contrast to well-demarcated *ependymomas*. *Oligodendrogliomas* are rare but resemble astrocytomas clinically. Both are intramedullary or intraaxial and hence appear as a fusiform swelling on neuroimaging studies. Classically, back pain is the initial symptom in most patients. With progression, motor and sensory findings occur. The fusiform enlargement of the spinal cord on MRI spreads out over one or more segments, suggesting a soft tissue mass of normal of slightly decreased signal

TABLE 3. *Spinal tumor types and their characteristics*

Tumor type	Location	Characteristic	Cellular composition	MRI characteristics	Gd-DTPA properties
Schwannomas	Extramedullary intradural and extradural dumbbell	Single	Schwann cells	T1 soft tissue outlined by CSF; T2 high signal	Improves T1 image
Neurofibromas	Same	Multiple	Schwann cells; fibroblasts and perineural cells	Same	Same
Meningiomas	Intradural extramedullary; rarely dumbbell	Thoracic preference, female predominance, most common tumor of foramen magnum	Arachnoid cells with variable patterns	T1 is isointense with spinal cord; T2 is isointense with spinal cord	Enhances T1
Astrocytomas	Intramedullary	Fusiform enlargement of spinal cord	Astrocytomas	T1 shows fusiform enlargement of spinal cord; T2 shows focal areas of increased signal. Cysts or cavities occur	Enhances T1, delineates margins
Ependymomas	Intramedullary or extramedullary	As fusiform enlargement of spinal cord or in filum terminale and cauda equina, encapsulated	Ependymal cells	Similar to astrocytomas	Enhances T1, delineates margins
Vascular tumors—hemangioblastomas	Intramedullary	Single of multiple	Pericyte	Flow void; T1 has low signal; T2 has high signal	Enhances
Lipomas	Extramedullary intradural	Often associated with developmental tumors (epidermoid, dermoid, and teratoma) or with spinal dysraphic states	Relates to character of tumor	T1 has high signal intensity; T2 has less intense signal	
Chordomas	Extradural either end of vertebral column	50% in sacrococcygeal area, 30–40% in basisphenoid area	Expanding and destructive of bone	T1 is isointense or hypointense	
Metastases	Extradural, uncommonly intramedullary	Bony involvement	Similar to primary	One or more vertebrae involved; T1 has decreased signal intensity; T2 is variable	May accentual soft tissue and dural metastases, enhance pial lining

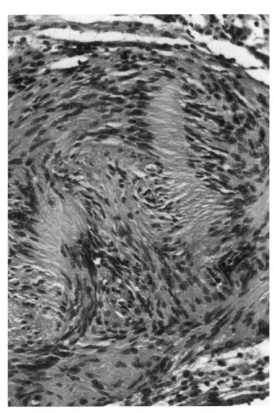

FIG. 1. Schwannoma: demonstrating a Verocay body. The parallel alignment of spindle nuclei separated by an eosinophilic matrix is a modification of the Antoni A pattern.

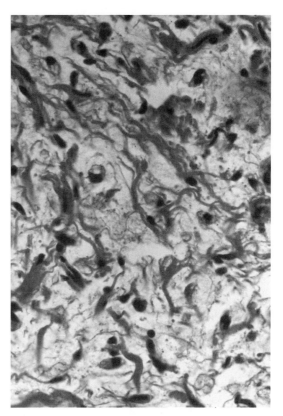

FIG. 2. Neurofibroma: demonstrating a loose and haphazard arrangement of nuclei within a collagenous matrix.

intensity on T1-weighted studies. However, T2-weighted images show an increased signal within the enlarged cord; often cysts or cavities can be demonstrated. Gd-DTPA enhances the T1 images (8) and correlates with neoplastic changes, aiding in the guidance of biopsy.

Ependymomas originate from the ependymal lining or ependymal cell rests and present either as intramedullary spinal cord tumors or as tumors of the conus medullaris or cauda equina (16). They are more common in males; however, both children and adults are affected. Pain is the most common complaint in this slowly evolving tumor. In 50% of cases, tumors occur as a fusiform intradural enlargement of the spinal cord. The other 50% occur in the cauda equina. Most are composed of elongated to polygonal cells with nuclear fibrillated perivascular rosettes. A small percentage are heavily fibrillated and mimic an astrocytoma (Fig. 3). This variant has been referred to as tanycytic and may lead to an error in the intraoperative pathologic diagnosis. The cauda equina lesions can be surgically removed with greater ease than the intramedullary variety and almost always are of the myxopapillary type in which the perivascular fibrillary areas exhibit a mucinous degeneration (Fig. 4). The MRI appearance is similar to gliomas with enhancement on T1-weighted study. Often, the location provides the most important clue to diagnosis (8).

Vascular tumors of the spinal cord are relatively rare, accounting for only 6.2% in the series by Sloof et al. (3). *Vascular malformations* are discussed in a separate chapter. In the review by Umbach and Kunft (17), *hemangioblastomas* were described as dysontogenetic tumorlike malformations of the embryonic mesoderm. These tumors are associated with angiomatous changes in the retina in von Hippel-Lindau syndrome and hemangioblastomas of the cerebellum. They are considered to be intramedullary tumors but may extend outside neural tissue. They occur over the length of the spinal cord but are most common in the cervical region. MRI (18) may demonstrate intramedullary cysts containing a vascular nodule. Their cystic component has a low signal intensity on T1-weighted images that changes to a high signal intensity on T2-weighted images. Hemangioblastomas enhance intensely with paramagnetic contrast medium. Flow void defects may be demonstrated with enlarged feeding vessels.

Lipomas of the spinal cord are infrequent; they occurred in 0.45% of 1,322 tumors so studied (3). They are congenital tumors, which are generally intradural and extramedullary in location and associated with spinal dysraphic states, but they may also be intramedullary or extradural (19). The clinical presentation is quite variable. There may be cutaneous clues in the form of subcutaneous lipoma, a hairy patch, sacral dimple, sinus tract, or unusual pigmentation. Bony changes such as spina bifida may be seen on

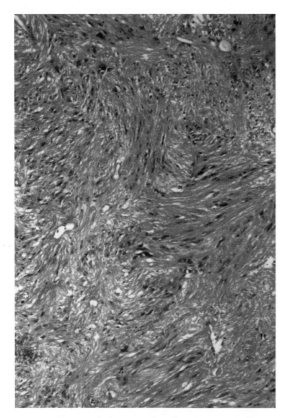

FIG. 3. Tanycytic ependymoma: note the elongated and polygonal cells with nuclear fibrillated perivascular rosettes. In this illustration, heavy fibrillation is noted, mimicking an astrocytoma.

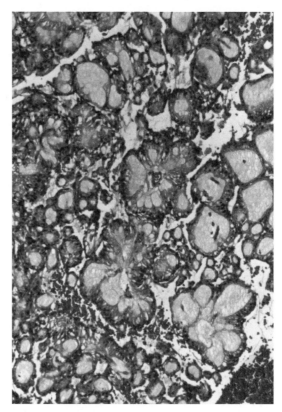

FIG. 4. Myxopapillar ependymoma: perivascular fibrillary areas exhibiting a mucinous degeneration.

plain radiographs. The MRI characteristics are high signal intensity on T1-weighted images and less intense signal on T2-weighted images. There may be other developmental defects in the form of epidermoid or dermoid tumors or teratomas accompanying lipomas.

Chordomas are uncommon tumors of the spinal canal occurring in about 4% of cases according to Sloof et al. (3). They are extradural lesions of the bony spine. They have a variable microscopic appearance but usually are seen as epithelial lobules of cells that express both S-100 and epithelial or cytokeratin epitopes. They arise from remnants of the embryonic notochord (20). About 40% of chordomas occur in the clivus; the remainder are distributed in the cervical, thoracic, lumbar, and sacral regions in a ratio of 5:1:1:20 (11). These are aggressive destructive tumors that generally present with pain. Plain radiographs may show a nonspecific osteolytic lesion associated with a soft tissue mass (21). Sze et al. (22) compared CT with MRI in 20 cases of chordoma. CT was superior in the demonstration of bony destruction, but MRI was better in delineating the exact extent of the tumor. The lesions are isointense or hypointense on T1-weighted study and of high signal intensity on T2-weighted images. They are malignant tumors biologically and commonly metastasize in patients with long survival.

Metastatic tumors of the spine account for most cases of epidural spinal cord compression. The metastases occur in the vertebral column or paravertebral spaces but rarely the epidural space itself. In 96% of cases, the initial symptom was pain (23), which may be local or radicular. Weakness in 76%, autonomic dysfunction in 57%, and sensory loss in 51% of cases were prominent clinical findings. The primary responsible neoplasms in the order of decreasing frequency are lung, breast, lymphoma, prostate, kidney, myeloma, thyroid, uterus, rectum, and sarcoma. Bony changes help localize a site of interest for myelographic block, with or without CT. MRI is useful in demonstrating bony changes in multiple vertebrae. The T1-weighted images often show a decreased signal intensity, whereas T2-weighted images are variable. Paramagnetic contrast medium helps enhance the mass and the pial lining with meningeal metastases (24).

TREATMENT

Benign tumors of the spine are generally slow growing and present after years of slowly progressive symptoms. Malignant tumors usually present with a more dramatic acute course measured in days or weeks.

Once the diagnosis of a spinal tumor has been made, surgical intervention should be considered. External compression of the spinal cord caused by meningiomas, neurofibromas, or other benign encapsulated tumors should be treated surgically because they are radioresistant. Ependymomas and astrocytomas, the most common intramedullary tumors, are treated by myelotomy, biopsy, and microsurgical removal. Radiation therapy may be useful. Similar practices are useful for hemangioblastomas, teratomas, and dermoids.

Extradural metastatic lesions are a special case. Corticosteroids and radiation therapy are the mainstays of treatment. A loading dose of dexamethasone of 10 to 100 mg IV followed by 4 to 24 mg four times daily improves neurologic function and alleviates pain short term (25). Corticosteroids are tapered during the course of radiation therapy. In patients so treated, surgical intervention has been associated with increased morbidity and spinal instability (26). There is renewed interest in anterior decompression or vertebral-body resection and stabilization, but these are difficult lengthy procedures in a debilitated patient. Surgery is useful for tissue diagnosis, to correct or benefit spinal instability, to rescue progressive deterioration during chemotherapy or radiation therapy, for recurrent disease at a previously radiated site, and for radioresistant tumors. Overall, outcome is closely linked to the best neurologic function at the time of radiation therapy. The proportion of patients who are ambulatory after radiation therapy declines from more than 80% at the initiation of treatment to less than 50% for those who were paraparetic and to less than 10% for patients who were paraplegic (22,27,28).

CONCLUSION

Clinical difficulties in recognizing and localizing the symptoms of tumors of the spinal cord and foramen magnum are significant challenges for the clinician. The radiologic evaluation has dramatically changed in the past two decades. CT provides the best means of examining both the intradural and extradural spaces and bony changes; however, water-soluble contrast by intrathecal injection is necessary to image the spinal cord. MRI provides a noninvasive method of evaluating the spine and the contents of the spinal canal. MRI characteristics, including enhancement, add a remarkable dynamic dimension to a current workup.

REFERENCES

1. Percy AK, Elveback LR, Okazaki H, Kurland LT. Neoplasms of the central nervous system: epidemiologic considerations. *Neurology* 1972;22:40–48.
2. Elsberg CA. *Surgical diseases of the spinal cord, membranes and nerve roots: symptoms, diagnosis and treatment.* New York: Paul Hoeber, 1941:209.
3. Sloof JL, Kernohan JW, MacCarty CS. *Primary intramedullary tumors of the spinal cord and filum terminale.* Philadelphia: W.B. Saunders, 1964:11.
4. Schliack H, Stille D. Clinical symptomatology of intraspinal tumors. In: Vinken PJ, Bruyn GW, eds. *Handbook of clinical neurology.* New York: Elsevier, 1975:23–49.
5. Portenoy RK, Galer BS, Salamen O, et al. Identification of epidural neoplasm: radiography and bone scintigraphy in the symptomatic and asymptomatic spine. *Cancer* 1989;64:2207–2213.
6. Aubin ML, Jardin C, Bar D. Computed tomography in 32 cases of intraspinal tumor. *J Neuroradiol* 1979;6:81–92.
7. Hammerschlag SB, Wolpert SM, Carter BL. Computed tomography of the spinal cord. *Radiology* 1976;121:361–367.
8. Masaryk TJ. Neoplastic diseases of the spine. *Radiol Clin North Am* 1991;29:928–945.
9. Nittner K. Spinal meningiomas, neurinomas, and neurofibromas and hourglass tumours. In: Vinken PJ, Bruyn GW, eds. *Handbook of clinical neurology.* New York: Elsevier, 1976:177–322.
10. Levine E, Huntrakoon M, Wetzel LH. Spinal and paraspinal neurofibromatosis distinctions from benign tumors using imaging techniques. *AJR Am J Roentgenol* 1987;149:1059–1064.
11. Burger PC, Scheithauer BW, Vogel FS. *Surgical pathology of the nervous system and its coverings.* New York: Churchill Livingstone, 1991.
12. Schroth G, Thron A, Guhl L, et al. Imaging of spinal meningiomas and neurinomas: improvement of imaging by paramagnetic contrast enhancement. *J Neurosurg* 1987;66:695–700.
13. Cohen L. Tumors in the region of the foramen magnum. In: Vinken PJ, Bruyn GW, eds. *Handbook of clinical neurology.* New York: Elsevier, 1974:719–730.
14. Meyer FB, Ebersold MJ, Reese DF. Benign tumors of the foramen magnum. *J Neurosurg* 1984;61:136–142.
15. Russell DS, Rubinstein LJ. *Pathology of tumors of the nervous system.* Baltimore: Williams & Wilkins, 1989.
16. Fischer G, Tommasi M. Spinal ependymomas. In: Vinken PJ, Bruyn GW, eds. *Handbook of clinical neurology.* New York: Elsevier, 1976: 353–387.
17. Umbach W, Kunft J. Vascular tumors of the spinal cord. In: Vinken PJ, Bruyn GW, eds. *Handbook of clinical neurology.* New York: Elsevier, 1976:435–480.
18. Sato U, Waziri M, Smith W, Von Hippel-Lindau disease: MR imaging. *Radiology* 1988;166:241–246.
19. Giuffre R. Spinal lipomas. In: Vinken PJ, Bruyn GW, eds. *Handbook of clinical neurology.* New York: Elsevier, 1976:389–414.
20. Dahlin DS. *Bone tumors: general aspects and data on 3,987 cases.* Springfield, IL: Charles C Thomas, 1967:222–233.
21. Firoozia H, Pinto RS, Lin JP, et al. Chordoma: radiologic evaluation in 20 cases. *AJR Am J Roentgenol* 1976;127:797–805.
22. Sze G, Vichanco LS, Brant-Zawadzki MN, et al. Chordomas: MR imaging. *Radiology* 1988;166:187–191.
23. Gilbert RW, Kim JH, Posner JB. Epidural spinal cord compression from metastatic tumor. *Ann Neurol* 1978;3:40–51.
24. Lim V, Sobel DF, Zyroff J. Spinal cord pial metastasis: MR imaging with gadopentetate dimeglumine. *Am J Radiol* 1990;155:1077–1084.
25. Byrne TN. Spinal cord compression from epidural metastases. *N Engl J Med* 1993;327:614–619.
26. Argnello F, Baggs RB, Duerst RE, Johnstone L, McQueen K, Frantz CN. Pathogenesis of vertebral metastasis and epidural spinal cord compression. *Cancer* 1990;65:98–106.
27. Findlay GFG. Adverse effects of the management of malignant spinal cord compression. *J Neurol Neurosurg Psychiatry* 1984;47:761–768.
28. Greenbery HS, Kim J-H, Posner JB. Episural spinal cord compression from metastatic tumor: results with a new treatment protocol. *Ann Neurol* 1980;8:361–366.

Motor Disorders,
edited by David S. Younger.
Lippincott Williams & Wilkins, Philadelphia © 1999.

CHAPTER 28

Spinal Vascular Malformations

Michael G. Kaiser and Paul C. McCormick

Spinal vascular malformations comprise 2 to 11.5% of primary intraspinal lesions (1) and are a rare but treatable cause of acute, subacute, episodic, and progressive myelopathy. These lesions are appropriately termed "malformation" as opposed to "angioma" because of their nontumorous origin. Spinal vascular malformations typically produce a myeloradiculopathy through various pathophysiologic mechanisms, including ischemia secondary to venous hypertension or vascular steal, compression, hemorrhage, or thrombosis. The exact nature of the signs and symptoms depends on the location of the lesion but typically includes paresis, sensory loss, sphincter dysfunction, and pain.

In 1888, Gaupp (2) first described spinal vascular malformations as "hemorrhoids of the pia mater." In 1943 Wyburn-Mason (3) divided spinal vascular malformations into parenchymal lesions, termed *angioma arteriovenosum*, and dural lesions, termed *angioma racemosum venosum,* based on the clinical data obtained from 80 patients. McCormick (4) divided them into five categories based on distinct histopathologic characteristics: arteriovenous malformations (AVM), cavernous malformations, venous malformations, capillary telangiectasias, and the venous varices. Cavernous malformation and capillary telangiectasia belong to a single pathologic entity (5). AVM and cavernous malformations are of clinical significance in the spinal cord. Although vascular malformations of the spinal cord are commonly grouped under the heading of AVM, a more accurate and precise classification scheme has been developed (Table 1). However, it differs in the inclusion of the dural fistula, which although not a true AVM is nonetheless the most common symptomatic vascular malformation of the spinal cord.

The current understanding and management of spinal vascular malformations has depended on improvements in neuroradiology, especially spinal angiography. Initially introduced in the 1960s, spinal angiography has rapidly evolved over the past decade with the introduction of microcatheters and advanced imaging techniques. Current neuroangiography has allowed an increased understanding of the pathophysiology and anatomy of spinal vascular malformations, leading to a more accurate classification scheme. These advancements have also led to the development of more sophisticated endovascular techniques in the treatment of these lesions. Along with improvements in microsurgical techniques and intraoperative spinal monitoring, spinal vascular malformations are now effectively treated in a growing percentage of cases. A comparison of various clinical characteristics of the three major types of spinal vascular malformations is shown in Table 2.

DURAL FISTULA

The most common spinal vascular malformation is the dural arteriovenous fistula, also known as a type I vascular malformation (Table 1). Previously known as the *long dorsal AVM, dorsal extramedullary AVM, angioma racemosum venosum,* or *angioma racemosum* (3,6,7), they comprise 75 to 90% of spinal vascular malformations (8–10). It consists of an abnormal communication between a radicular artery in the dural nerve root sleeve and an intradural vein located along the dorsal surface of

M. G. Kaiser: Neurological Institute, New York Presbyterian Hospital, New York, New York 10032.

P. C. McCormick: Department of Neurosurgery, Columbia University College of Physicians and Surgeons and New York Presbyterian Hospital, New York, New York 10032.

TABLE 1. *Classification of spinal vascular malformations*

Dural fistula (type I)
Intradural (true) AVMs
Glomus (type II)
Juvenile (type III)
Intradural arteriovenous fistula (type IV)
Cavernous malformation

TABLE 2. *Characteristics of spinal vascular malformations*

	Dural fistula	Intradural AVM	Cavernous malformation
Percentage	75–85%	10–20%	5%
Age of presentation	40–50 yr	10–30 yr (older with type IV)	40 yr
Gender	Male	Equal	Female
Common location	Lower thoracic-lumbar levels	Cervical and lumbar enlargements	Entire spinal axis
Origin	Acquired	Congenital (? type IV)	Congenital
Timing of presentation	Progressive	Acute-progressive	Acute-progressive

AVM, arteriovenous malformations.

the spinal cord. Unlike a true AVM, this venous plexus is part of the normal drainage pattern of the spinal cord and appears aberrant as the result of increased flow from the fistula. Dural fistulas typically contain one feeding artery (type I-A); however, multiple arterial feeders can occur (type I-B). This distinction is critical for the appropriate treatment of these lesions. Dural fistulas affect men four times as often as women and are most often located in the lower thoracic or lumbar spinal cord. The onset of symptoms usually occurs during the fifth and sixth decades of life (9,11). Because of the later-life presentation and a limited anatomic location, they are considered acquired, not congenital, lesions (11,12), another distinction from true AVM.

The dural location of this lesion was identified in 1977 by Kendall and Logue (13). Because of the lack of valves in intradural veins, the increased pressure within the radicular vein produces a retrograde flow within the intradural venous system. Direct measurements of the intradural venous pressure is markedly elevated compared with the central venous pressure, 44.1 ± 17.7 mm Hg compared with 6.4 ± 2.3 mm Hg (9). The resulting venous hypertension produces a reduction in spinal cord perfusion pressure that leads to chronic spinal cord ischemia and progressive myelopathy. Clinical symptoms are acutely exacerbated by maneuvers that increase venous pressure, such as exercise or Valsalva, and by venous thrombi. These ischemic changes were clearly illustrated by the autopsy studies performed by Wyburn-Mason (3).

The venous engorgement produced by a dural fistula is restricted to the dorsal venous plexus for unknown reasons and has a predilection for rostral drainage. It is possible that a preexisting venous abnormality contributes to, or is required for, symptoms to develop. It has been hypothesized that these lesions therefore share a common pathophysiology with intracranial dural malformations, which are frequently associated with a dural sinus thrombosis.

Dural fistula should be considered in the differential diagnosis of a patient with progressive myelopathy. Early diagnosis is critical in these patients because deficits resulting from the ischemic changes are often irreversible.

Myelography has typically been used in the past, with the dorsal venous engorgement demonstrating a characteristic serpentine filling defect. Magnetic resonance imaging (MRI) has replaced myelography as the screening test of choice because of the increased sensitivity and specificity, increased accuracy in locating the lesion nidus, and the ease of performance. Despite the advantages of MRI, false-positive tests may result from arachnoid bands simulating flow defects. A definitive diagnosis of a dural fistula or another spinal vascular malformation can only be achieved with spinal angiography that typically shows a dorsal rostrally draining serpentine vein. Once the location is demonstrated by angiography, individual segmental vessels can be catheterized from the lower thoracic through all the lumbar levels. A small percentage of lesions may be supplied by lower lumbar or sacral vessels. The importance of somatosensory evoked potential monitoring to demonstrate dorsal column activity and spinal cord function is reviewed elsewhere (14,15,16).

The treatment of a dural fistula is surgical ligation. Endovascular occlusion alone is often ineffective as suggested by the high recanalization rate (17) and the presence of a radicular artery in about 10% of patients that arises from a segmental branch and gives rise to the medullary artery supplying the spinal cord; embolization of this common trunk can lead to infarction. Endovascular therapy is generally reserved for patients who are not surgical candidates.

Surgical treatment involves ligation of the intradural segment of the fistula (Fig. 1A and B). The identification of all feeding arteries and fistulas, because incomplete ligation will lead to recurrence, emphasizes the importance of the preoperative distinction between type I-A and I-B dural fistulas. Because the engorged vessels along the dorsal surface of the spinal cord are part of the normal drainage pattern, it is contraindicated to resect these vessels. A favorable outcome with this approach is seen in 65 to 72% of cases (18,19). Unlike motor function, which shows a direct correlation to outcome (18), preoperative sensory loss and rate of neurologic decline is not generally related to outcome. Because long-standing deficits are unlikely to resolve, early diagnosis and treatment are essential in the management of these lesions.

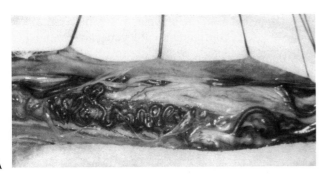
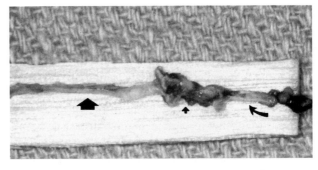

A   B

FIG. 1. A: Intraoperative photograph of a dural fistula demonstrates the tortuous draining vein located along the dorsal surface of the spinal cord. B: Photograph of an excised specimen with feeding artery (*curved arrow*), draining vein (*large arrow*), and intervening dural fistula (*small arrow*).

INTRADURAL ARTERIOVENOUS MALFORMATIONS

Intradural spinal vascular malformations are divided into three major types: the glomus and juvenile malformations and the intradural arteriovenous fistula (Table 2). These lesions are typically found in regions of dense spinal cord vasculature, such as the cervical and lumbar enlargements, and to a lesser degree in the thoracic spinal cord.

Glomus Arteriovenous Malformations

Glomus malformations, or type II spinal vascular malformations, previously known as *angioma racemosum arteriovenosum or angioma arteriovenosum* (3), comprise greater than 90% of intradural AVM (11) and, like their intracranial counterparts, usually consist of a compact definable nidus with arterial feeders derived from medullary vessels. In most cases the nidus of the glomus AVM is present either on the pial surface, within the parenchyma, or both. The intraparenchymal nidus is usually in the anterior portion of the spinal cord and is typically fed by branches from an enlarged anterior spinal artery. Drainage of the glomus AVM into the coronal venous plexus leads to marked engorgement of these vessels. Flow through a glomus AVM is usually greater than observed through a dural fistula, and those occurring within the cervical spinal cord may have marked increased flow.

Cervical glomus malformations receive multiple feeding vessels from several arterial sources, including vertebral, thyrocervical, costocervical, cervical, deep cervical, supreme intercostal, and from the descending limb of the anterior spinal artery. The high flow observed in these lesions is likely a reflection of the abundant vascularity and anastomotic channels present in the cervical spinal cord. Those occurring below the cervical cord usually have lower flow and demonstrate only one or two feeding vessels by angiography. This appearance is misleading,

however, and is likely due to a flow-related phenomenon. If flow through a major feeding vessel is obstructed, smaller vessels are recruited.

A glomus AVM in the pia may occur anywhere but is typically found along the lateral or dorsolateral surface of the spinal cord. Pure dorsal lesions are located with increased frequency at the cervicomedullary junction (see Fig. 4). The blood supply for the pial lesions is typically derived form both the anterior and posterior spinal arteries via circumferential branches. An occasional branch originates directly from a medullary artery. If there is an intraparenchymal component to the AVM, deep penetrating branches are encountered from the anterior spinal artery.

Glomus malformations typically present at a younger age with signs and symptoms of subarachnoid hemorrhage, such as meningismus, headache, photophobia, and even hydrocephalus, or those of intramedullary hemorrhage or hematomyelia, with about two thirds of symptomatic lesions in adolescence or early adulthood (18). The acute onset of symptoms is usually due to subarachnoid or intraparenchymal hemorrhage or venous thrombosis. About a third harbor an aneurysmal dilatation, typically in the venous system, which increases the risk of hemorrhage. Once a hemorrhage is identified, the risk of subsequent hemorrhages increases. Additional causes of neurologic deficit with glomus malformations include arterial steal and mechanical compression.

Because the location of the glomus AVM is variable, the upper and lower extremities are affected equally. Unlike the dural fistula, symptoms related to the glomus malformation are not exacerbated with maneuvers increasing intraabdominal pressure. The hereditary nature of these lesions is reflected in epidemiologic data and the occasional association with metameric skin, bone, and mesenchymal anomalies (12).

The standard treatment of glomus malformation is difficult to formulate for three reasons. First, they are rare, and their natural history is not well known. Second, studies of their natural history have often included the more common dural fistula (8,10). Third, treatments, both surgical and endovascular, carry a significant risk of neurologic morbidity.

MRI is the screening test of choice for intradural AVM (Fig. 2A). Axial and sagittal views allow precise localization of its nidus and its relationship to the surrounding structures. Magnetic resonance angiography has been shown to be a useful adjunct to MRI in the evaluation of an intradural AVM but does not define the vascular anatomy as well as spinal angiography (Fig. 2B) (20). The latter is essential in the preoperative evaluation to determine the exact configuration of feeding and draining vessels, whether feeding vessels are involved in the normal blood supply, and the presence of venous or arterial aneurysms essential to the formulation of the operative strategy.

Glomus malformations are typically amenable to surgical resection. Preoperative embolization is helpful in high flow lesions but should not be considered definitive treatment. Vessels supplying the AVM are only sacrificed when it is certain that they do not supply the normal parenchyma.

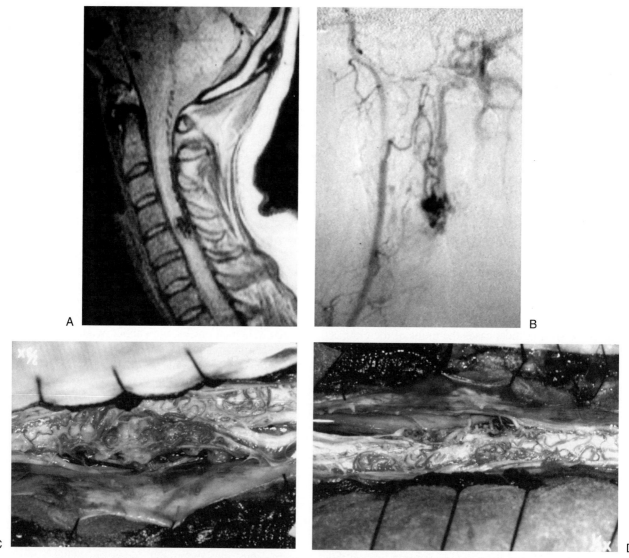

FIG. 2. A: T2-weighted sagittal magnetic resonance image (MRI) of the cervical spinal cord demonstrates a flow void signal at C4-5, which is characteristic of a glomus arteriovenous malformation (AVM). A large linear flow void signal is also present along the dorsal surface of the spinal cord running cephalad from the AVM, most likely a draining vein. **B:** Selective angiogram demonstrates the vascular architecture of this spinal AVM, and two medullary feeding arteries supply the AVM that is drained by a single draining vein coursing cephalad. Note that this draining vein is also identified on the MRI. **C:** Intraoperative photograph of a glomus AVM located at the thoracic spinal cord protruding form the pial surface. **D:** Photograph after the complete resection of the lesion demonstrates the gross myelopathic changes that have occurred at the level of the lesion; however, the normal vasculature has been left intact.

Resection of these lesions requires microsurgical techniques along a plane of gliotic tissue that separates the AVM from normal tissue (Fig. 2C and D). The surgical outcome depends on the level of the spinal cord and whether there is increased compensatory blood flow. Accordingly, the most favorable outcomes were observed in the cervical and lumbar enlargements, less so in the thoracic cord, with an overall improvement in 80 to 90% of cases (21).

Juvenile Malformations

Juvenile, or type III spinal malformation, another true AVM, occurs less frequently than either the dural fistula and glomus AVM. In contrast to the latter, the juvenile AVM contains extramedullary and extraspinal components and numerous feeding arteries, often over multiple vertebral segments. They present in childhood or adolescence with equal frequency among boys and girls (18). The symptoms may be abrupt in onset due to hemorrhage or progressive due to vascular steal or mechanical compression. Cardiovascular abnormalities can occur because of the large volume of blood shunted through the lesion. Similar to the glomus AVM, the juvenile AVM is also thought to be heritable (12).

Because of the extensive nature of these lesions, definitive treatment is often unobtainable, and the prognosis is often much worse than with the glomus AVM. Unless a discrete nidus is identified (22), complete surgical resection is impossible, especially because most occupy the entire transverse area of the spinal cord. Endovascular techniques are essential in their preoperative management and may even be the only intervention indicated. If embolization and surgery are chosen, multiple staged procedures invariably are required to obtain the best possible results. The rarity of juvenile AVMs makes it difficult to determine treatment outcomes; however, various case reports of lesions treated in multiple stages with both surgery and embolization indicate satisfactory outcomes in most cases (22,23).

Arteriovenous Fistula

Also known as type IV spinal vascular malformation, these lesions are usually located on the anterior surface of the spinal cord, where the anterior spinal artery directly communicates with an enlarged tortuous vein through single or multiple abnormal connections (Fig. 3A and B). Based on the number of fistulas, their size, and the amount of blood flow, they are further subdivided into type IV-A lesions, which contain a single fistula with slow flow, and types IV-B and IV-C, which are increasingly complex. Intradural arteriovenous fistulas usually present clinically with slowly progressive myelopathy; however, subarachnoid or intraparenchymal hemorrhage also occurs. Onset of symptoms typically occurs in the third to sixth decade, with an equal distribution between men and women. Because these lesions can occur anywhere along the spinal cord, variable neurologic deficits are observed. Although not clear, a congenital origin is hypothesized (12,18).

In general, treatment of intradural arteriovenous fistulas is directed at interrupting flow through the fistula between the anterior spinal artery and the dilated draining vein, without affecting normal spinal cord channels. Surgery is the treatment of choice for type IV-A malformations via an anterior approach because they are commonly located on the ventral aspect of the spinal cord. Treatment of type IV-B lesions is determined by the individual characteristics of the lesion and may consist of surgery, embolization, or both. Type IV-C lesions are best treated by endovascular occlusion because the size and flow through the fistula increases the surgical risk (24).

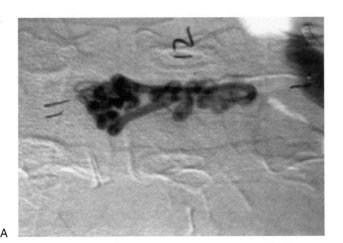
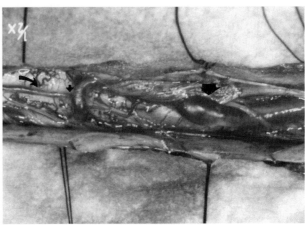

A   B

FIG. 3. A: Spinal angiogram demonstrates a type IV lesion, or intradural arteriovenous fistula, located at the T11-12 level. **B:** Intraoperative photograph demonstrates the direct connection (*small arrow*) between an enlarged feeding artery (*curved arrow*) to a massively engorged surface vein (*large arrow*).

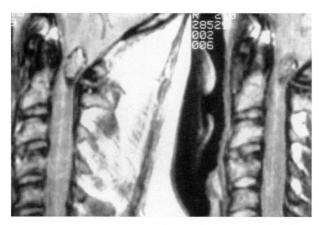 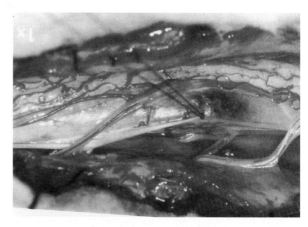

A   B

FIG. 4. A: T2-weighted sagittal magnetic resonance images of the cervical spinal cord demonstrate an intramedullary mass at the cervicomedullary junction. The heterogeneous signal intensity with a surrounding rim of hypointensity is the characteristic radiographic finding for a cavernous malformation. **B:** Intraoperative photograph demonstrates the typical mulberry appearance of a cavernous malformation at the dorsolateral surface of the spinal cord.

CAVERNOUS MALFORMATIONS

Cavernous malformations are rare congenital lesions that consist of irregular sinusoidal vascular channels without intervening neural tissue (25–27) that are typically lined with endothelium and contain thrombus of varying age. They are typically isolated lesions but can occasionally be multiple and familial (28). They have been identified with increased frequency due to the increased sensitivity of MRI (26). Nonetheless, only 10% of central nervous system cavernous malformations occur in the spinal cord (11).

They present with acute or progressive myelopathy; relapsing symptoms are commonly due to recurrent hemorrhage. Although it is rare for a cavernous malformation to produce a catastrophic event, such cases have been described (26). A progressive course is likely due to enlargement of the lesion with repeated internal hemorrhage, vessel dilatation, and capillary budding; however, the neurotoxic effects of hemosiderin and mechanical compression are possible contributing factors. Cavernous malformations can be located anywhere along the neuraxis but are most commonly found in the thoracic cord. The highest incidence of presentation occurs in the fourth decade with a slight predominance in women (27).

The typical MRI appearance of a cavernous malformation is a central area of heterogeneous signal intensity, representing thrombi of varying age, surrounded by a rim of hypointensity due to the deposition of hemosiderin (Fig. 4A). These findings can be obscured by the small size of the spinal cord, surrounding edema, and cyst formation. Both myelography and angiography are usually normal with cavernous malformations.

Surgical resection is reserved for lesions that are symptomatic (26,28). Appropriate candidates have lesions that

are well circumscribed and amenable to complete resection (Fig. 4B). The outcome after surgery is generally favorable; however, there are instances in which the lesion is infiltrative and unresectable. Stereotactic radiosurgery is a promising technique for inaccessible lesions, but the outcome of this treatment modality is still unknown.

SUMMARY

Spinal vascular malformations consist of a heterogeneous group of lesions responsible for a rare but treatable cause of myelopathy. Improvements in diagnosis, classification, and treatment planning have essentially occurred through the advancements made in modern neuroradiologic techniques, namely MRI and spinal angiography. Surgical intervention is the favored treatment for the dural fistula but should be limited to ligation of the fistula without disturbing the surface venous plexus. Intradural AVMs are best treated on an individual basis combining both surgical and endovascular techniques. The role of embolization as the sole treatment modality is still questionable. Cavernous malformations are usually amenable to surgical resection; however, the role of stereotactic radiosurgery for inaccessible lesions requires further investigation. The prognosis of most spinal vascular malformations is generally favorable provided that an early diagnosis is made and an appropriate treatment plan is constructed from high-quality diagnostic imaging.

REFERENCES

1. Grote E, Bien S. Arteriovenous malformations of the spinal cord. In: Youmans J, ed. *Neurological surgery. A comprehensive reference guide to the diagnosis and management of neurosurgical problems.* Philadelphia: W.B. Saunders, 1996:1511–1530.
2. Gaupp J. Hamorrhoiden der Pia mater spinalis im Gebiet des Lendenmarks. *Beitr Pathol* 1888;2:516–518.

3. Wyburn-Mason R. *The vascular abnormalities and tumors of the spinal cord and its membranes.* London: Henry Kingston, 1943.
4. McCormick W. Pathology of vascular malformations of the brain. In: Wilson C, Stein B, eds. *Intracranial arteriovenous malformations.* Baltimore: Williams & Wilkins, 1984:44–63.
5. Rigamont D, Spetzler R, Johnson P. Cerebral vascular malformations. *Barrow Neurol Inst Q* 1987;3:18–28.
6. Krayenbuhl H, Yasargil M, McClintock H. Treatment of spinal cord vascular malformations by surgical excision. *J Neurosurg* 1969;30:427–435.
7. Malis L. Arteriovenous malformations of the spinal cord. In: Youmans J, ed. *Neurological surgery. A comprehensive reference guide to the diagnosis and management of neurological problems.* Philadelphia: W.B. Saunders, 1982:1850–1874.
8. Aminoff M, Logue V. Clinical features of spinal vascular malformations. *Brain* 1974;97:211–218.
9. Hamilton M, Anson J, Spetzler R. Spinal vascular malformations. In: Tindall G, Cooper P, Barrow D, eds. *The practice of neurosurgery.* Baltimore: Williams & Wilkins, 1996:2271–2293.
10. Tobin W, Layton D. The diagnosis and natural history of spinal arteriovenous malformations. *Mayo Clin Proc* 1976;51:637–646.
11. McCormick P. Spinal vascular malformations. *Semin Neurol* 1993;13:349–358.
12. Oldfield E, Doppman J. Spinal arteriovenous malformations. *Clin Neurosurg* 1988;34:161–183.
13. Kendall B, Logue V. Spinal epidural angiomatous malformations draining into intrathecal veins. *Neuroradiology* 1977;13:181–189.
14. Berenstein A, Young W, Ransohoff J, Benjamin V, Merkin H. Somatosensory evoked potentials during spinal angiography and therapeutic transvascular embolization. *J Neurosurg* 1984;60:777–785.
15. Greenberg R, Ducker T: Evoked potential in the clinical neurosciences. *J Neurosurg* 1982;56:1–18.
16. Grundy B. Monitoring of sensory evoked potentials during neurosurgical operations: methods and applications. *Neurosurgery* 1982;11:556–575.
17. Hall W, Oldfield E, Doppman J. Recanalization of spinal arteriovenous malformations following embolization. *J Neurosurg* 1989;70:714–720.
18. Rosenblum B, Oldfield E, Doppman J, Di Chiro G. Spinal arteriovenous malformations: a comparison of dural fistulas and intradural AVM's in 81 patients. *J Neurosurg* 1987;70:795–802.
19. Symon L, Kuyama H, Kendall B. Dural arteriovenous malformations of the spine. Clinical features and surgical results in 55 cases. *J Neurosurg* 1984;60:238–247.
20. Mascalchi M, Bianchi M, Quilici N, et al. MR angiography of spinal vascular malformations. *Am J Neuroradiol* 1995;16:289–297.
21. Cogen P, Stein B. Spinal cord arteriovenous malformations with significant intramedullary components. *J Neurosurg* 1983;59:471–478.
22. Spetzler R, Zabramski J, Flom R. Management of juvenile spinal AVM's by embolization and operative excision. *J Neurosurg* 1989;70:628–632.
23. Touho H, Karasawa J, Shishido H, Yamada K, Shibamoto K. Successful excision of a juvenile-type spinal arteriovenous malformation following intraoperative embolization. Case report. *J Neurosurg* 1991;75:647–651.
24. Heros R, Debrun G, Ojemann R, Lasjaunias P, Naessens P. Direct spinal arteriovenous fistula: a new type of spinal AVM. Case report. *J Neurosurg* 1986;64:134–139.
25. Anson J, Spetzler R. Surgical resection of intramedullary spinal cord cavernous malformations. *J Neurosurg* 1993;78:446–451.
26. McCormick P, Michelson W, Post K, et al. Cavernous malformations of the spinal cord. *Neurosurgery* 1988;23:459–463.
27. Ogilvy C, Louis D, Ojemann R. Intramedullary cavernous angiomas of the spinal cord: clinical presentation, pathological features, and surgical management. *Neurosurgery* 1992;59:1019–1030.
28. Lee K, Spetzler R. Spinal cord cavernous malformation in a patient with familial intracranial cavernous malformations. *Neurosurgery* 1990;26:877–880.

Motor Disorders,
edited by David S. Younger.
Lippincott Williams & Wilkins, Philadelphia © 1999.

CHAPTER 29

Syringomyelia

Robert N. N. Holtzman

HISTORICAL CONSIDERATIONS

The derivation of syringomyelia, from the Greek words *syrinx* for channel or tube and *myelos* for marrow, serves well as the title for pathologic conditions characterized by the presence of fluid-filled cavities of the spinal cord. The term was contributed by d'Angers in 1827 (1), although others had recognized its existence. The first recorded description of syringomyelia was provided by Estienne in 1546 (2). Morgagni noted its association with spina bifida in 1761 (3). The first description of the symptoms and signs of a cervicothoracic syrinx was provided by Portal in 1803 (4).

The initial stages in syrinx formation are not well understood (5,6). When a cavity develops, progressive enlargement occurs by one of several mechanisms. There can be downward flow of cerebrospinal fluid (CSF) into the central canal through a patent obex (7–9). Repetitive cerebellar tonsillar impaction of the foramen magnum can act as a water hammer, generating pulsatile pressure gradients that pass downward along the pial surface, exerting pressure differentials that compress and "milk" (10) the spinal cord, actively driving fluid into the Virchow-Robin spaces (11,12). CSF, propelled by penetrating arterial pulsations (13,14), can cross the perivascular spaces, parenchyma, and ependyma and enter into a cavity. Syringomyelic cavities can also expand from intracavitary hydrodynamic forces driving CSF due to the failure of instantaneous spinal compartment pressure equilibration. Similar local influences are thought to be exerted on the spinal cord at sites of focal arachnoiditis (15) and tethering (16–18). Finally, ependymal secretion and absorption of CSF may be contributing factors (19,20).

The spinal cord central canal of the fetus and newborn persists, often in a discontinuous pattern (21) with stenoses

(22), into adulthood. In the presence of hydrocephalus it can undergo progressive concentric dilation, communicating with the IVth ventricle through the obex, keeping its ependymal lining intact (8). Still referred to as hydromyelia (23), in the setting of a variety of obstructions along the foramen magnum and vertebral canal, a cavity can develop in the spinal cord parenchyma, maintaining its continuity with the dilated central canal. These have been described as paracentral dissections (24), but in some instances, they may be enlarging diverticuli of the central canal (8,25). Posttraumatic cavities as well may form apart from the central canal (22) as in the case of intramedullary tumors (26).

Early investigators recognized the importance of the cerebellar tonsils in the evolution of spinal cord cavities containing clear CSF (27,28); however, hydrocephalus (29), basilar arachnoiditis (30), posterior fossa arachnoid cysts (31), Dandy-Walker cysts (32), spinal cord trauma (33,34), tethering and retethering (18,35–37), diastematomyelia (38,39), and diplomyelia or the split spinal cord (39) can also be contributing factors. Neoplastic syringomyelic cavities associated with intramedullary ependymomas, astrocytomas, and hemangioblastomas (26) contain proteinaceous xanthochromic fluid.

Syringomyelia causes amyotrophy of the arms and dissociated sensory loss, with or without spastic myelopathy. The sensory disturbance is painless or painful and segmental, affecting pain and temperature sensation with preserved tactile sensation—and one explanation for the apparent "fearless" demonstration of the Roman hero, Gaius Mucius Scaevola, who put his right hand into a blazing fire until it was consumed, stunning the King of the Etruscans (40,41).

There can be confusion with cervical radiculopathy (42), ulnar and median neuropathies (43), amyotrophic lateral sclerosis (44), and multiple sclerosis (45,46). Signs and symptoms appear slowly, reach a plateau, and then worsen frequently without warning, typically after attacks of sneezing or coughing accompanied by "searing pain" (15,47). There are five hydrodynamic theories: the *water-hammer*

R. N. N. Holtzman: Department of Neurological Surgery, Columbia University School of Medicine and Neurological Institute, New York Presbyterian Hospital, New York, New York 10032.

pulsation theory of Gardner (48); the *craniospinal pressure dissociation theory with CSF "sucking" and "sloshing"* of Williams (49); the *craniospinal pressure dissociation, CSF hypertension, and dorsal root zone entry theory* of Aboulker (50); the *CSF systolic "pistonlike" pressure wave theory* of Oldfield et al. (12); and *the theory of arterial pulsation-driven perivascular CSF flow into the central canal* of Rennels et al. (13) and Stoodley et al. (14).

EPIDEMIOLOGY

Syringomyelia is a disease of young adults, with the onset of symptoms before the fifth decade in 80% of patients (51). It may rarely occur in utero (52) or infancy (53). At the National Hospital in London, syringomyelia accounted for 1.6% of admissions from 1909 to 1925 (54). Brewis et al. (55) reported a prevalence of 8.4 per 100,000 inhabitants in an English city. Schliep (56) identified 149 patients with syringomyelia of 35,588 admissions (0.42%) over the period 1956 to 1973 that consisted of 100 men and 49 women, with an age of less than 40 years in two thirds. In Japan the prevalence was 1 per 101,270 among 1,243 cases in 1995 with equal sex predilection and mean age at onset of 28 years; overall, 51.2% occurred with a Chiari malformation, 3.7% with dysraphism, 11% posttraumatic, 6% with spinal arachnoiditis, and 10.5% with spinal cord tumor (57). Williams (58) estimated a prevalence of 10 per 100,000 among 862 cases of which 32% had a Chiari I malformation, 10% had hydrocephalus, 4% had an intramedullary spinal cord tumor, and 11% were posttraumatic.

The reported incidence of posttraumatic syringomyelia is 1% to 4.5% (59) but is higher in paraplegia (2.3%) than tetraplegia (0.3%), especially with lesions above T-2 (60). Intramedullary spinal cord tumors have an incidence of associated syringomyelia of 25% to 58% (61,62) with a cystic yellow proteinaceous appearance characteristic of an exudate (63).

Syringomyelia occurs sporadically in about 2% of cases, usually in an autosomal dominant or recessive pattern (64). The statistically significant frequency of HLA-A9 in patients with syringomyelia suggests that genetic factors influence its development (64,64). The occurrence of monozygotic twins with syringomyelia and basilar impression (66,67), dizygotic twins (68), and a higher incidence in certain stable regions of Germany (69) and the Tater Republic (70) make it important to consider neurologic and radiologic evaluations in family members of affected patients (64).

CLINICAL PROFILE

The course of syringomyelia can be chronic, stationary, progressive, nonprogressive, or partially remitting. Besides the classic dissociated sensory loss, there may also be patterns of loss involving the torso or arms alone, called a *suspended sensory level*; those involving the shoulders and upper torso, extending up to the occiput, called *en cuirasse*; and those involving the face in an *onion-skin* pattern. Other sensory symptoms include paraesthesias and dysaesthetic pain in affected zones or in more remote locations (71,72). Intense dysaesthetic pain below the level of the syrinx can be seen postoperatively with cavity collapses. Muscle wasting of the arms and hands, often with fasciculations and absent reflexes, results from anterior horn cell involvement in the cervical cord. This produces a *main en griffe* or claw deformity (Fig. 1). A lumbar syringomyelic cavity can sometimes mimic that of a cervical syrinx (73).

Autonomic involvement leads to altered sweating patterns, a Bernard-Horner syndrome, abnormal micturition, defecation (74), swallowing (75), and orthostasis (76).

Trophic skin changes can occur, leading to cyanosis and hypothermia and progressing to subcutaneous edema and hyperhidrosis, the *main succulente* of Marinesco. Phalangeal absorption or acrodystrophy, the Morvan's syndrome, is its most severe expression. Secondary disturbances to skeletal structures result from neurogenic arthropathy or *Charcot joint* of the shoulder (Fig. 2), elbow, and wrist (77) seen in 25% of cases and *cheiromegaly* (78) due to overgrowth of the distal extremities. There may be associated scoliosis, and kyphosis has been reported (Fig. 3), but these symptoms alone are rarely the reason to screen for a syrinx (79). Syringomyelia and syringobulbia can be associated with acute respiratory disturbances (48,80,81). The latter is due to upward extension of the syrinx (Fig. 4A–C) (82). There may be one or more cranial nerve signs such as lingual wasting and fasciculations of the tongue, sternocleidomastoid weakness, pharyngeal or palatal weakness with dysphagia, trigeminal nucleus sensory loss, diplopia, nys-

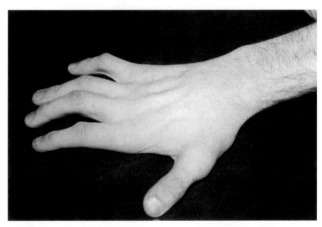

FIG. 1. Typical claw hand.

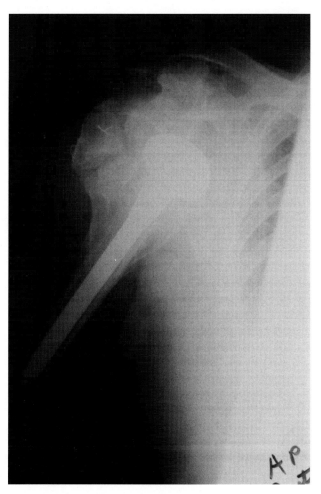

FIG. 2. Charcot joint with syringomyelic cavity.

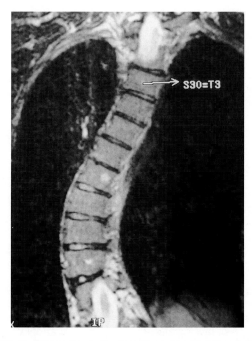

FIG. 3. Thoracic scoliosis with syringomyelic cavity.

tagmus, or labyrinthine disturbances. Higher dissection of the cavity results in syringopontis (83) or syringocephalus (84,85).

CLASSIFICATION AND CATEGORIZATION

Syringomyelia can be classified by the underlying anatomic structure, location, and associated clinical and pathologic findings (Tables 1–3). Primary and secondary syringomyelia have been recognized (5) as well as communicating and noncommunicating forms (86–90) (Table 1). In neural tube embryogenesis, focal occlusions at stages 9–15 have been considered common (91). Reopening in infancy is suggested by patent central canals and later by regions of stenosis (22). If the neural tube is dilated embryonically, later growth and development leads to *primary hydromyelia*. Most syringomyelia cavities that develop after the initial transient collapse, and reopening of the neural tube, showing either concentric enlargement of the central canal, an associated diverticulum, or extension of a parenchymal dissection, can be considered *secondary hydromyelia or syringomyelia*.

The term *communicating* syringomyelia originally distinguished those cavities that contained clear CSF-like fluid and were in continuity with the IVth ventricle from the noncommunicating forms that contained proteinaceous xanthochromic fluid; however, later investigators questioned this distinction (92). Communicating syringomyelia was also applied to those cavities capable of exchanging fluid with the IVth ventricle via the obex, as compared with the noncommunicating types with a "syrinx-free" segment between their upper poles and the IVth ventricle (24).

The recent observations of the rapid entrance of water-soluble myelographic dye into syringomyelic cavities and its rapid clearance confirms the importance of these descriptive terms. A cavity with clear fluid must experience a continuous turnover or washout. It can communicate with the IVth ventricle via the obex, Virchow-Robin, or interstitial spaces or other undescribed "pores" in the pia, parenchyma, and ependyma. Those cavities with mildly elevated protein and mildly xanthochromic fluid should be considered communicating but to a lesser extent in the sense that they cannot as efficiently irrigate their contents. The noncommunicating cavities with highly proteinaceous fluid and a thick gliotic lining certainly do not have an equivalent ability to irrigate their contents. Dye may enter posttraumatic syrinxes through "fistulous ruptures" (see Fig. 13). The entrance of dye into highly proteinaceous syringes associated with tumors and areas of myelomalacia (93) is not as readily explained but may be due to absorption and exudation or direct penetration though perivascular spaces.

The three methods of classifying syringomyelia and its variants, anatomic, pathologic, and clinical classifications, are presented in Tables 1–3, respectively.

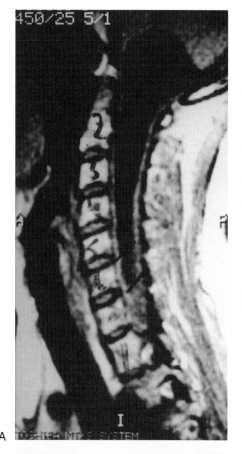

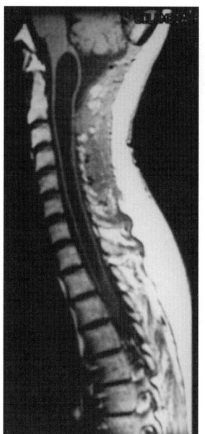

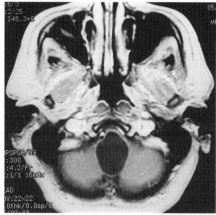

FIG. 4. Syringobulbia and syringomyelia in a 58-year-old woman without an Arnold-Chiari malformation. Preoperative computed tomographies **(A)** and T1-weighted magnetic resonance images **(B and C)** after suboccipital craniectomy and aspiration of the cavity. (Courtesy of Dr. Ronald Brisman.)

TABLE 1. *Anatomic classification*

Hydromyelia
Syringomyelia
Cervicothoracic syringomyelia—
  most often associated with the Chiari I malformation, obstruction at the foramen magnum, but also occurs with trauma or spinal cord tumors.
Lumbar syringomyelia—
  often associated with myelomeningocoele, spinal cord tethering, and focal arachnoiditis.
Syringobulbia, syringopontis, and syringocephalus—
  often occurring in continuity with syringomyelia.

TABLE 2. *Pathologic classification*[a]

Central canal syrinx—
  communicating form seen primarily in children.
Central canal syrinx—
  noncommunicating by a "syrinx-free" segment in adults (often in association with Chiari I malformation, cervical spinal stenosis, and basilar impression).
Extracanalicular syrinx—in adults (this cavitation is often seen in association with spinal cord injury, ischemic infarction, and intramedullary hemorrhage, with varying degrees of myelomalacia and spinal cord atrophy).

[a]Based on 105 cases studied by Milhorat (24).

TABLE 3. *Clinical classification**

Syringomyelia communicating with IVth ventricle and hydrocephalus
Syringomyelia without IVth ventricular communication with the Chiari I malformation or other compressive or inflammatory processes
Posttraumatic syringomyelia
Syringomyelia and spinal dysraphism often accompanied by Chiari II malformation
Syringomyelic with intramedullary and extramedullar tumors, mainly ependymomas, astrocytomas, and hemangioblastomas

*Adapted from ref. 94.

PATHOLOGY

The pathology of syringomyelia can be approached from several perspectives. The first concerns the vulnerable parenchymal sites. The second concerns the initial changes in the spinal cord that precede formation of a syringomyelic cavity. The third relates to the concentric enlargement of the central canal or in conjunction with an enlarging diverticulum or paracentral dissection. The fourth is the development of a cavity unassociated with the central canal. There may be other evolutionary factors, including spontaneous rupture (95), spinal cord atrophy (96) with associated neuronal drop-out, loss of the ependymal lining, demyelination of long tracts, gliosis, proliferation of a vascular matrix subadjacent to the gliotic changes surrounding the cavity, and enlargement of the Virchow-Robin spaces.

Little is known about the early phases of syrinx formation, and most of the ideas advanced are speculative. Greenfield (97) suggested instability in the lines of junction of the alar and basal laminae, particularly in the medulla, and small parenchymal "tears" caused by neck flexion and torsion. Tissue slits or clefts may exist in the spinal cord parenchyma (98,99) similar to those documented in the medulla in syringobulbia (100). Similarly, small ependymal diverticuli of the central canal have been described as well as small breaches in the ependymal lining of the central canal communicating with syrinxes (101), all of which may represent potential sites of syrinx origin.

Once a syringomyelic cavity starts to develop, it is presumed that certain architectural limitations are imposed, restricting its shape. The variations in appearance, including spherical, cigar-shaped, and spindle-shaped cavities with smooth or irregularly constricted walls (Figs. 5–8), are not easily explained. Some constraints relate to the stenoses described by Milhorat et al. (22) and others to processes not well understood exemplified by the relatively few cavities extending through the upper cervical segments to the obex, "concentrically constructed walls" of lengthy cavities that have been likened to "haustrations" (102) or a metameric pattern (103), and septations (Fig. 9) that are also often evident in posttraumatic syrinxes (104).

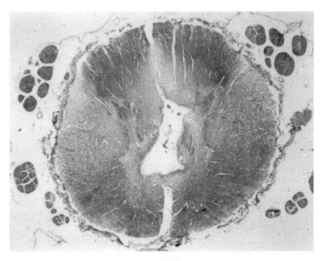

FIG. 5. Syringomyelic cavity occupying the central gray area with disrupted ependymal lining. (Courtesy of James Goldman, M.D., Ph.D.)

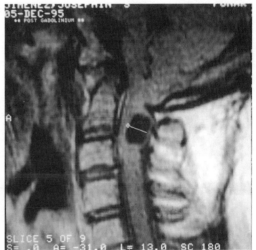

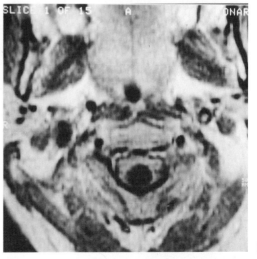

FIG. 6. Spherical-shaped syringomyelic cavity is seen on T1-weighted sagittal **(A)** and axial **(B)** images. It was associated with the Chiari I malformation in a 60-year-old woman presenting with 8 years of ataxia with recent worsening and inability to swallow her saliva.

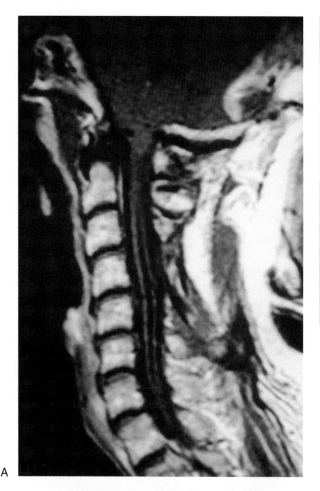

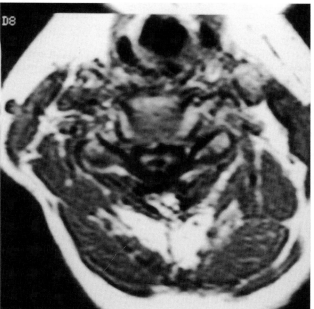

A

B

FIG. 7. Spindle or fusiform syringomyelic cavity is seen on T1-weighted sagittal **(A)** and axial **(B)** images. It was associated with a Chiari I malformation and spinal cord atrophy in a 64-year-old woman who 10 years previously underwent cervical laminectomy myelotomy and placement of a shunt. The Chiari malformation was not addressed initially. When her gait deteriorated she underwent suboccipital craniectomy with significant return of function.

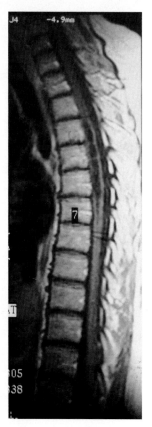

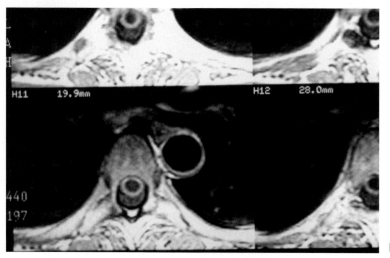

A

B

FIG. 8. Tapered cigar-shaped thoracic syringomyelic cavity seen on T1-weighted sagittal **(A)** and axial **(B)** images. It was associated with the Chiari I malformation in a 52-year-old woman presenting with right arm dissociated sensory loss and right thoracic cage pain.

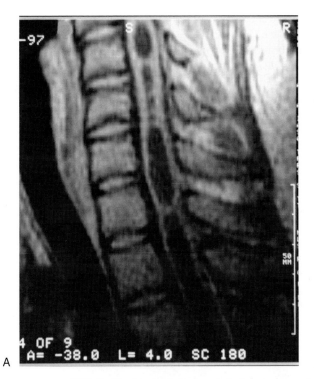

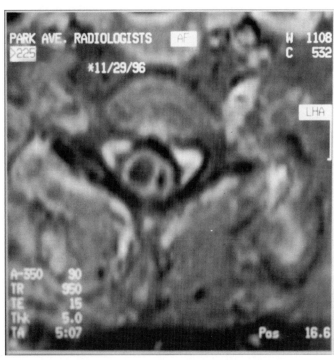

FIG. 9. Double-barreled septated syringomyelic cavity is seen on T1-weighted sagittal **(A)** and axial **(B)** images. It was associated with a Chiari I malformation in a 16-year-old boy who presented with left arm dissociated sensory loss and early clawing. "Haustral pattern" is suggested.

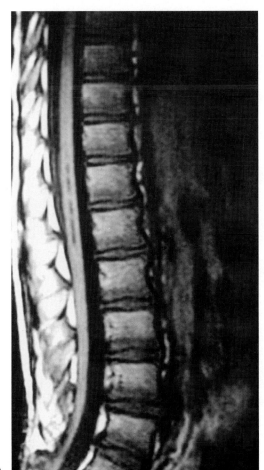

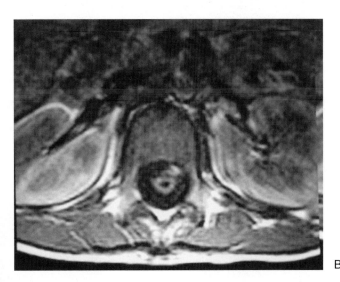

FIG. 10. Thoracolumbar syringomyelic cavity is seen on T1-weighted sagittal **(A)** and axial **(B)** magnetic resonance images. It was associated with tethered cord syndrome after myelomeningocoele repair in a 7-year-old boy who underwent surgical closure of his myelomeningocoele at birth and dramatically regained lower extremity function so that he could run. Neurogenic bladder persisted. Syrinx was initially identified at 6 years of age and has been followed for 4 years without change.

Cavities can exist in a particular area and extend cephalad and caudad along the entire spinal cord. Cervical syrinxes occur in approximately 30 to 50% of patients with a Chiari type I malformation and in 45 to 90% of those with a Chiari type II (104). Lumbar syringes alone can occur with tethering (Figs. 10 and 11) and focal tumors. Syringobulbia is often associated with, and extends cephalad from, a syringomyelic cavity (44,66) (Fig. 4).

On gross inspection, the spinal cord surface may appear swollen and tense or normal (5). Cavities usually occupy the central gray and are of varying size and shape (Fig. 5). Schliep (98) described their extension to the anterior horns with the destruction of anterior and posterior commissures. They may be unilateral or bilateral and separate or unite at higher or lower levels. Slitlike cavities may rarely occupy one (98) or both dorsal horns and extend into the white matter or occupy the entire spinal cord, leaving only a pial membrane with islands of atten-uated parenchyma (105) with the appearance of a myelo-cystocoele (Fig. 12).

Milhorat et al. (24) demonstrated that *communicating syringomyelic cavities* appeared as simple dilations of the central canal that largely retained their ependymal lining. They were associated with hydrocephalus and possessed a dilated opening at the obex that communicated with the IVth ventricle. *Noncommunicating syringomyelic cavi-ties* were characterized by a focal dilation of the central canal that was separated from the IVth ventricle by a syrinx-free segment. These were noted to be associated with Chiari I malformation, cervical spinal stenosis, arachnoiditis, basilar impression, and occipital enceph-alocoele. The cavities were complex and associated with extensive loss of ependymal lining, paracentral dissec-tion, and intracavitary septations admixed with gliotic tis-sue; 10 of 23 (43%) so studied showed evidence of rup-ture into the parenchyma, forming glial-lined cavities or fibroglia in the more extreme instances. Rostral dissec-

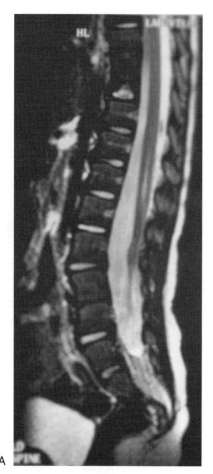

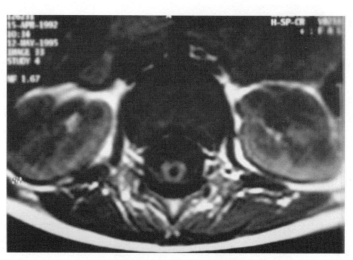

FIG. 11. Syringomyelic cavity is seen on T2-weighted sagittal **(A)** and T1-weighted axial **(B)** magnetic resonance images. It was found incidentally and demonstrates a primary tethered spinal cord syndrome associated with lipomyelomeningocoele in a 4-year-old boy.

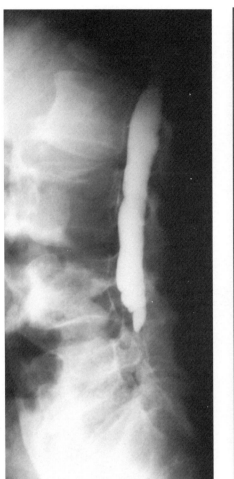 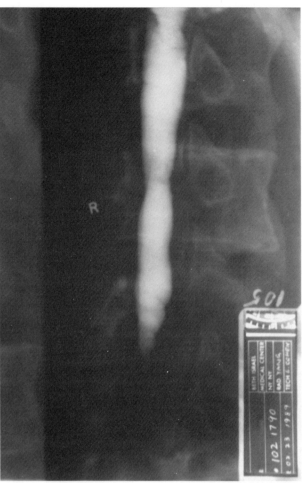

A

B

FIG. 12. Syringography with Omnipaque in a 60-year-old deeply paretic man originally misdiagnosed with sarcoidosis. Lateral and oblique views at lumbar levels (cf. Fig. 16).

tion into the lower pons was seen in one. *Extracanalicular* syrinxes described tubular cavities in the spinal parenchyma that did not communicate with the central canal. They were unique in their association with conditions producing spinal cord injury.

Posttraumatic cavities were derived from cystic myelopathy and dissected rostrally to the brainstem (106) from the site of trauma. They were characterized by lack of communication with the central canal or subarachnoid space. On occasion, there were double cavities (Fig. 9) variably lined by glia and collagen but usually devoid of ependyma. Bridges of glial fibers and vascular tissue have been described passing across the syringomyelic cavity (107). They may be the source of bleeding referred to as "Gowers' syringal hemorrhage" (108). Some of these cavities remain distended despite the fact that they have a fistulous connection to the subarachnoid space (Fig. 13), whereas others spontaneously collapse (95).

Syringomyelic cysts that accompany intramedullary tumors have thicker gliotic walls and a higher incidence of Rosenthal fibers (109). The thickened gliotic walls and the intracavitary highly proteinaceous fluid imply a relative imperviousness of those walls to washout and exchange.

Magnetic resonance (MR) microscopy was recently used in an anatomicopathologic study (110); signals of high intensity in the central gray reflected the syrinx contents and fluid within the central canal. Low signal intensity signals correlated with histopathologically normal ependymal lining. Increased signal intensity also described demyelination and gliosis. Densely packed abnormal microvessels surrounded syringomyelia cavities in areas of adjacent gliosis. They may represent a form of luxury perfusion in areas of ischemia and gliosis. Utilizing this technology, the "T" arm of a syringopleural shunt could be well visualized and was seen to be penetrating into the ventral horn of the central gray matter (110), clearly in an aberrant location.

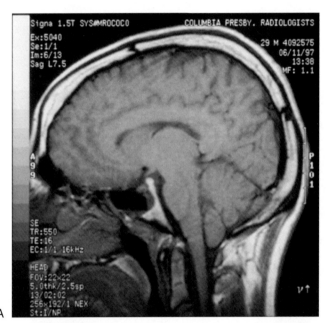

A

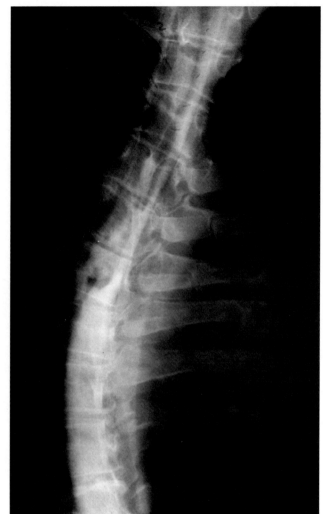

B

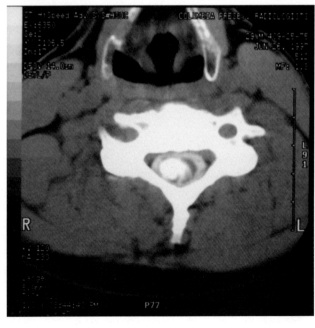

C

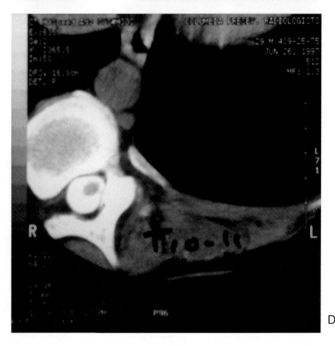

D

PATHOGENESIS

The single common element in the development of a nontumorous syringomyelia is a complete or partial obstruction to CSF flow resulting from pulsatile craniospinal and spino-spinal compartmental pressure dissociation. The outcome is a disturbance in the pressure equilibrium and equilibrium required for normal fluid transfer across compartmental environments of the spinal cord.

Syringomyelia formation de novo from an embryonic central canal and the subsequent enlargement of the syrinx probably entails two entirely different processes. CSF migrates along vascular channels and interstitial spaces and may encounter microscopic parenchymal slits, clefts, and diverticuli of the central canal that may serve as the anatomic substrate for the formation of cavities (111,112). The cause for the existence of these clefts and diverticuli is unknown, although microtrauma may be suspected in cleft formation (97), but these factors are still too inconsequential to provide an adequate pulse pressure to create a syringomyelic cavity (113). The central canal itself could act as a sink for fluid entering via the Virchow-Robin perivascular spaces and pores that could communicate across the anterior and posterior commissures via the posterior median sulcus and the anterior median fissure. India ink injected into the central canal in a postmortem case rapidly diffused through the parenchyma and Virchow-Robin spaces to the subarachnoid space (11). Evans blue and horseradish peroxidase injected into the spinal parenchyma was cleared by the central canal in the direction of the IVth ventricle (112,114). These studies support the contention that both active and passive mechanisms for fluid transport exist. Five possible routes of CSF entry into the spinal cord's central canal include the obex, the spinal subarachnoid space through Virchow-Robin perivascular spaces, through attenuated "weeping" spinal parenchyma where areas of pial/ependymal apposition may exist similar to that seen in schizencephaly, as yet ill-defined pores in the region of the dorsal root entry zones or fistulous rupture (24,50) (Fig. 13), and the secretion and absorption of the glial and ependymal cells lining the cavity (19,20,115).

From the standpoint of fluid mechanics, the CSF exerts pressure against the thin-walled syringomyelic cavity. If the intracavitary pressure is greater than the subarachnoid pressure, then the cavity should expand horizontally and especially vertically. Simply raising the environmental pressure on the spinal cord continuously will in general not develop a syrinx (116,117). Therefore, it appears that a deeper understanding of compartmental pressures and their gradients is necessary to come to terms with this problem. One particular difficulty is understanding how the spinal fluid functions as an architectural component in sustaining a cavity which would collapse immediately during air myelography (118,119) or upon autopsy examination (5). This is made even more conceptually difficult when there is a direct fistula to the syrinx from the subarachnoid space (Fig. 13).

These factors point to the need to substantially reduce the forces maintaining compartmental pressure gradients, thereby permitting the syrinx to collapse. Evidently, this is accomplished with surgical decompressions. LaPlace's equations for a sphere (120), perhaps not entirely applicable to a cylindrical cavity, suggest that there is a force tending to "blow a sphere apart" expressed as $F_1 = \pi R^2 P$ and a containing force expressed as $F_2 = 2\pi R S_L t$, where P is transmural pressure, R is the radius, and S_L is the stress along the equatorial circle and t is the thickness of the wall. For the sphere to either expand or contract, $F_1 = F_2$. Following this reasoning, it is possible to begin to extrapolate mathematically to the syringomyelic cavity where compliance, tensile strength, and elasticity of the walls must be taken into account. The LaPlace equations do suggest that the larger the cavity, the less pressure is necessary to maintain an equal stress; therefore, less pressure is required to maintain progressive enlargement (120). If a given cavity is to be decompressed, then a lowering of the intracavitary pressure must be accomplished to a point below that required to support the cavity walls. This demonstrates that CSF and its fluid pressure are architectural components involved in maintaining the configuration of a syringomyelic cavity and spinal cord.

The anatomy for fluid communication between the perivascular spaces and the central canal has been

FIG. 13. Posttraumatic syringomyelia with ascending cavitation and associated Chiari I malformation in a 13-year-old boy who suffered a through and through stab wound to the right chest in 1981. He was immediately unable to stand. After thoracotomy for repair of the right mainstem bronchus, a cerebrospinal fluid (CSF) pleural fistula was observed. Substantial recovery to severe spasticity with voluntary motion in his lower extremities occurred in the first month. Weakness and claw hands were noted 8 years later but were confused for median/ulnar palsies. Recent magnetic resonance imaging suggested Chiari I malformation without hydrocephalus **(A)**. Lumber puncture revealed clear normal CSF. Myelogram/computed tomography demonstrated an immediate entry of dye at T6-7 through a fistulous myelotomy into the syrinx cavity **(B)**. The dye rapidly ascended to the top of the syrinx at C3-4 **(C)**. Spinal cord atrophy was present below T6-7 **(D)**.

demonstrated in the rat (121). Subependymal labyrinths around the central canal represent differentiation of the basement membrane of subependymal vessels, which in turn are in communication with the ependymal intercellular space and the central canal. Horseradish peroxidase moved freely from the subarachnoid space along the perivascular spaces of vessels entering the spinal cord from the ventral median fissure and joining the subependymal labyrinth. Rennels et al. (13) showed that the flow along the perivascular space was dependent on arterial pulsations. Horseradish peroxidase injected into the subarachnoid space rapidly outlined the vessels of the spinal cord, but this does not occur if arterial pulsations are diminished by ligating the aorta without reducing mean arterial pressure, suggesting that rather than a "free transfer," there is a net unidirectional flow of fluid driven by arterial pulsations (14,122). Perivascular spaces in the spinal cord are covered at the surface by pia mater and are lined by basement membrane of the glia limitans extending as far as capillaries. Capillaries have a sleevelike basal lamina composed of a macromolecular meshword that communicates with the extracellular space via gaps between adjacent astrocytic endfeet (122).

The implication of this is that systolic expansion of arteries in the perivascular space may force fluid through the surrounding basement membrane, whereas in diastole fluid may enter the perivascular space from the subarachnoid space and through gap junctions in the covering pia. This could easily account for the rapid accumulation of contrast material in what are described as noncommunicating cavities that develop with caudal and cephalic stenoses (22,24,112) (see Fig. 19c and d), but it does not explain the outflow or washout of dye or CSF from a syringomyelic cavity.

NEUROIMAGING

Plain radiography has a limited usefulness in the diagnosis of syringomyelia; nonetheless, there may be a small posterior fossa (123), widening of the vertebral canal, thinning of the pedicles (124), and various skull base abnormalities such as platybasia, basilar impression, or invagination accompanied by spina bifida with assimilation or absence of the posterior arch of the atlas.

Years ago the presence of syringomyelia was inferred by a widened cervical spinal cord on pantopaque myelography. Ventricular puncture and ventricular installation of pantopaque facilitated the diagnosis by observing opacification of the cavity after transiting the obex, and air myelography demonstrated a fluctuation in the size of syringomyelic cavities presumably by the exchange of air for CSF during the procedure (118,119,125). Direct-puncture syringography demonstrated cavities with "constrictions" that were likened to a metameric pattern (124). Computed tomography myelography remains the definitive procedure for demonstrating instantaneous and delayed filling of syringomyelic cavities. It is also useful for demonstrating obstructions at spinal levels and at the foramen magnum due to arachnoiditis.

MR imaging (MRI) is now the standard examination for syringomyelia. It shows the detailed configuration of the cavity such as in single cigar-shaped (Fig. 8),

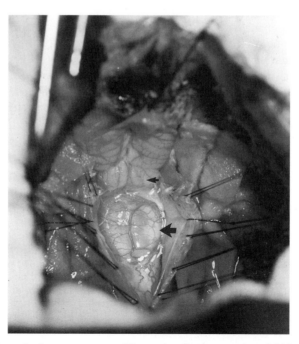

FIG. 14. Suboccipital craniectomy exposure of the syrinx (*large arrow*) and Chiari I malformation (*small arrow*).

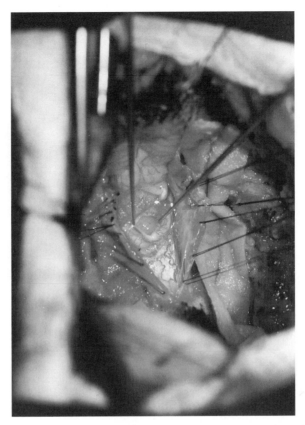

FIG. 15. Opening of the syringomyelic cavity (syringostomy) after aspiration of clear cerebrospinal

spherical (Fig. 6), and "double-barreled" cavities (Fig. 9); associated spinal cord atrophy is also readily observed (Figs. 7 and 13). It is also useful for following their status after surgical decompression (Figs. 17–19). Lumbar syringomyelic cavities have been seen with tethering and a thickened filum terminale (Figs. 10 and 11). Possible tumors can be studied by the contrast agent gadolinium-diethylenetriamine pentaacetic acid. MRI can be used as a dynamic test to show CSF flow in the region of the aqueduct of Sylvius and to exclude aqueductal stenosis and basilar arachnoiditis. Phase contrast-cine MRI can demonstrate CSF subarachnoid flow

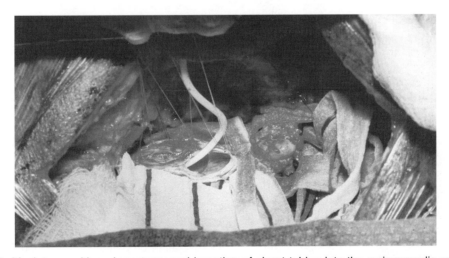

FIG. 16. Myelotomy with syringostomy and insertion of shunt tubing into the syringomyelic cavity (cf. Fig. 12) that was then implanted into the peritoneal cavity. The parenchyma was so attenuated that in places only a pial layer was evident (viz. schizencephaly).

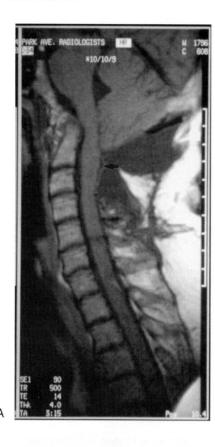

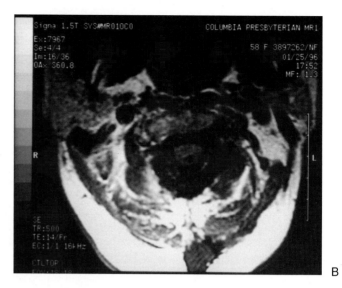

FIG. 17. (A and B) T1-weighted axial magnetic resonance images show collapse of the syrinx seen in Fig. 6A (*small arrow*) and B at 3 months. Pseudomeningocoele is evident (cf. Fig. 20).

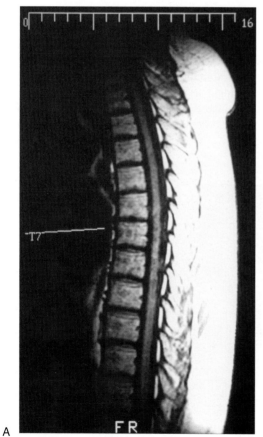

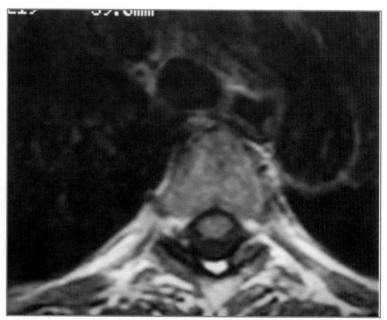

FIG. 18. T1-weighted sagittal (A) and T1-weighted axial (B) magnetic resonance images show collapse of the syrinx seen in Fig. 8A and B after suboccipital craniectomy with dural patching that was maintained at 4 years.

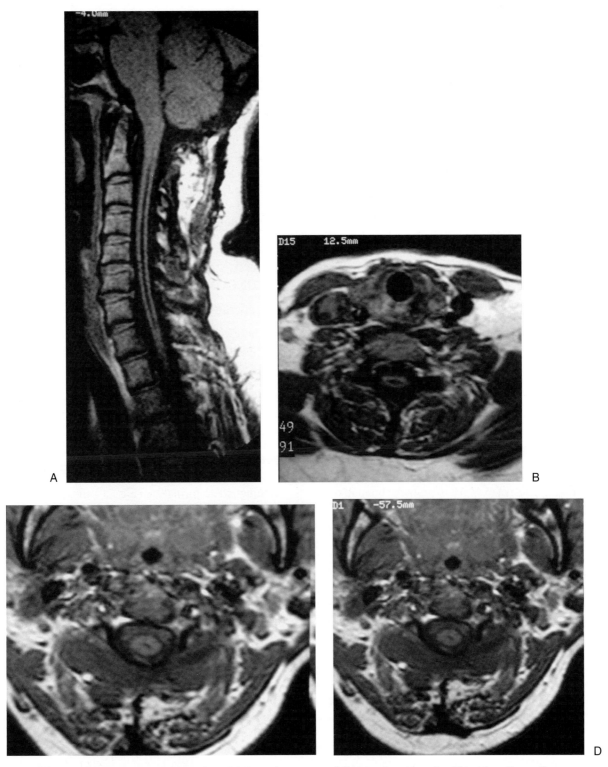

FIG. 19. Eighteen years after suboccipial craniectomy and C-1 laminectomy for Chiari I malformation with syringomyelia in a 29-year-old woman with claw hands, main succulente and no evident postoperative clinical progression. The T1-weighted magnetic resonance images show remission of the Chiari I malformation and cyst collapse with cord atrophy. This cyst appears to be in continuity with the central canal on axial views at its upper and lower poles with a syrinx-free segment and would be called non-communicating according to Milhorat (24). It seems to have achieved a stable balance and is at this time not expanding due to ingress of cerebrospinal fluid. The spinal cord atrophic process may be the major determinant of her clinical course in the future.

across the foramen magnum and in syringomyelic cavities (12).

SURGICAL EXPERIENCE WITH SYRINGOMYELIA, OPERATIVE TECHNIQUES, OUTCOMES, AND COMPLICATIONS

Wide decompression of the cerebellar tonsillar–cervicomedullary junction is achieved by suboccipital craniectomy combined with opening of the foramen magnum and cervical laminectomy exposing the Chiari malformation and upper cervical spinal cord. Preservation of the cisterna magna arachnoid layer followed by a watertight duroplasty is the optimum treatment for cervical syringomyelic cavities associated with the Arnold Chiari I malformation (Figs. 6 and 17) and even some thoracic syringomyelic cavities that have a syrinx-free interval between the obex and the upper end of the cavity (Figs. 8 and 18). Plugging the obex and opening and resuturing the arachnoid overlying the tonsils are techniques that are no longer used. Careful tonsillar reduction has its proponents but carries the risk of medullary vascular injury (127). Odontoid peg resection may be a useful adjunct in cases with basilar invagination (125).

Ventriculoperitoneal shunting of symptomatic syringomyelia and with hydrocephalus has been successfully accomplished (128). Cyst/subarachnoid, cyst/pleural, and cyst/peritoneal shunts from the syrinx cavity to the pleural, peritoneal, and subarachnoid space have been successfully performed. These may be used initially with a suboccipital craniectomy or at a later date in the event that the cyst collapse is incomplete. An example of primary shunting of the lumbar syringomyelic cavity (Fig. 12) is shown in Fig. 16. The technique involves placement of either a silastic tube or a myringostomy tube (129) attached to the pia by 8-0 suture or alternatively a T tube, which may obviate the need for suturing.

Myelotomy and syringostomy are not always sufficient to promote adequate drainage and cyst collapse but may be successful (Figs. 6,14,15,17). Percutaneous aspiration has been virtually abandoned as a therapeutic modality. Terminal ventriculostomy has not been universally in use (130) because of its failure to reestablish an improved pressure relationship between the intracavitary environment and the surrounding subarachnoid space to promote the egress of fluid from the syrinx. Spinal cordectomy with drainage was effective in paraplegic patients with ascending syringomyelic cavities but may cease due to intense arachnoiditis (131) or dysfunction of the shunt tubing (58). Williams (132) suggested performing a wide laminectomy, leaving the dura open by using temporary stents to bring about a lower environmental CSF pressure, favoring drainage from the cavity.

Future work should involve syringoscopy for exploration of these cavities to obliterate septations (133), communicate dissections and diverticuli, and remove clotted blood. These maneuvers may enhance intracavitary flow and facilitate collapse of a syrinx. Recent success with flexible endoscopic third ventriculostomy in treating hydrocephalus and reducing the size of a syrinx in instances of communicating syringomyelia can dramatically improve the clinical disorder (134).

Full collapse of a syringomyelic cavity may not be necessary to achieve a good and stable long-term clinical result (Figs. 4 and 13). A too rapid collapse of a large cavity may be dangerous and lead to paralysis. Incompletely collapsed syringes may reflect spinal cord atrophy and hydromyelia ex vacuo or a stabilized intracavitary and subarachnoid pressure relationship.

POSTOPERATIVE COLLAPSE OF SYRINGOMYELIC CAVITIES

Postoperative Complications

There can be persistence of the syringomyelic cavity due to an insufficient suboccipital craniectomy or inadequate space for CSF communication. Some authors believe that reoperation and tonsillar resection may be a solution (127). This decision should be based on clinical and radiographic data. The posterior fossa syndrome or aseptic meningitis should be distinguished from a bacterial meningitis; it often responds to cortisone. Persisting dysaesthetic pain and dysaesthetic pain associated with cyst collapse has been transient (71,72). Pseudomeningocoele formation (Fig. 20) should be treated with reoperation and closure of the fistula in most cases. Unilateral blindness due to positioning at surgery (135) can be avoided by careful monitoring during preoperative positioning and frequent intraoperative evaluations. Obstruction of a syringoperitoneal or a syringopleural shunt (58) may require revision; dislocation of the shunt tube from the syringomyelic cavity may require reoperation and replacement if collapse has not occurred; and shunt infection is generally managed with antibiotic therapy or shunt replacement. Tethering of the spinal cord due to arachnoiditis may require reoperation to achieve release. Penetration of a T tube arm into the spinal cord parenchyma (110) may require revision if it can be identified. Acute and delayed neurologic deterioration sometimes associated with too rapid cyst collapse may be irreversible if full decompression has already been achieved. Postoperative basilar arachnoiditis with subsequent hydrocephalus can occur and is managed with third ventriculostomy. Acute enlargement of a syringomyelic cavity after shunting may require reoperation (136). Low CSF pressure headache related to overshunting or leakage occurs if the dura is left open and may last for the period required for its closure.

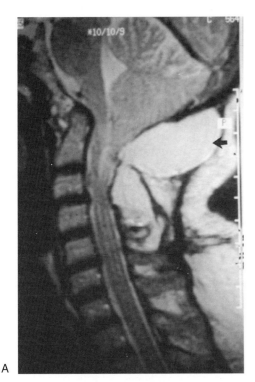
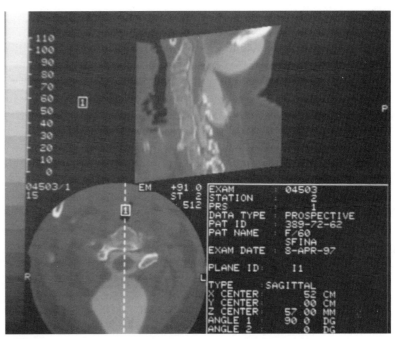

FIG. 20. T2-weighted magnetic resonance image **(A)** and a postmyelogram computed tomography **(B)** demonstrate the pseudomeningocoele collection and its communication with the subarachnoid space.

CONCLUSION

The history, classification, anatomy, clinical and laboratory diagnosis, pathophysiology, and surgical treatment of syringomyelia have been described. The fundamental anomaly appears to be systolic pressure waves traversing the spinal subarachnoid space, impelling CSF into the central canal or associated diverticuli. Hydrocephalus, Chiari malformations, arachnoiditis, and lumbosacral tether facilitate these systolic pressure waves along the pial surface of the spinal cord, and local pulsations of vessels along the Virchow-Robin spaces further contribute to the influx of fluid into syrinx cavities, which most often has a normal CSF composition.

Slits, clefts, and microdiverticuli acting as sinks or sump pits for the accumulation of CSF represent vulnerable primary sites later leading to their steady enlargement. There is then a steady loss of existing ependymal lining with the exception of some cavities that are concentric dilations of the central canal. Gliosis occurs later with fluid accumulation. Gliosis induces a mural ischemia leading to the proliferation of a vascular matrix that may in fact be a form of luxury perfusion permitting ever larger amounts of fluid to accumulate. Dissection into parenchyma to varying degrees becomes more noticeable, and fluid accumulates at the expense of the spinal cord parenchyma, leading to further parenchymal disruption, progressive neurologic symptomatology, and ultimately spinal cord atrophy.

Surgery is directed at reversing the mechanical disturbance underlying the syringomyelic cavity. The ischemic changes and gliotic reparative processes will in all probability not be affected by any surgical procedure. Neuronal loss will not be replaced nor will demyelination be significantly reversed. Recoveries that are seen probably speak to the phenomenon of neurapraxia rather than actual cellular and axonal destruction. Certainly regeneration and phenomena, such as "unmasking" of existing but previously unrecognized pathways, could play a part in recoveries (137). Efforts have recently been made to transplant embryonic nerve tissue into syringomyelic cavities (138).

Posttraumatic cysts whether they involve focal myelomalacia and cystic degeneration as the precursor to syrinx formation may also use some mechanisms of transparenchymal and transependymal diffusion to maintain themselves and to enlarge. They may be accompanied by diapedesis of erythrocytes or exudation of fluid that may explain some of the cysts having higher protein fluid contents. Periependymitis, either viral (137) or inflammatory, may also contribute to high protein fluid cavities with septations and stenoses (22,24).

Neoplastic syringomyelic cavities are typically noncommunicating, although this designation need not be considered in absolute terms. They are seen to resolve with excision of the tumor.

The areas of cystic enlargement are subject to developing spinal cord atrophy. This clearly can become part of the evolving clinical picture or part of progressive neurologic deteriorations that may occur on a delayed basis (94). It may also account for some of the failures of recovery.

ACKNOWLEDGMENT

I thank Mr. Ronald H. Winston, President of the Harry Winston Research Foundation, Inc., for his invaluable assistance with this manuscript.

NOTE ADDED IN PROOF

The author has made a theoretical assumption that spinal compartments exist and that passive fluid transfer by differential pressure can occur from one to another. For the sake of this argument it may be considered that the epidural, subdural, subarchnoid, parenchymal, and central canal spaces, in a gross sense, are such compartments and that differences in pressure can occur in these compartments which instantaneously equilibrate with the other compartments in the normal setting to maintain pressure homeostasis and the architectural integrity of the spinal cord. Failure of instantaneous compartment pressure equilibration may lead to the preferential fluid accumulation in one or another of the compartments—viz. the central canal—due in part to pressure-directed diffusion and in part to cerebrospinal fluid (CSF) oscillations with net bulk flow.

REFERENCES

1. Ollivier d'Angers CP. *Traite de la moelle epiniere et de ses malades.* Paris: Chez Crevot, 1827:173–181.
2. Estienne C. *La dissection des parties du corps humaine divisee en trois livres.* Paris: Simon de Collines, 1546.
3. Morgagni GB [Alexander B, trans.]. *The seats and causes of disease.* London: Millar and Cadel, 1769 (Letter XII, Article 9:370).
4. Portal A. *Cours d'anatomie medicale.* Vol. 4. Paris: Beaudoin, 1803: 117–118.
5. Graham DI, Lantos PL, eds. *Greenfield's neuropathology,* 6th ed. London: Arnold, 1997:486–492.
6. Schliep G. Syringomyelia and syringobulbia. In: Vinken PJ, Bruyn GW, eds. *Handbook of clinical neurology.* Amsterdam: Elsevier/North-Holland Biomedical Press, 1978:300–315.
7. Gardner WJ, Angel J. The mechanism of syringomyelia and its surgical corrections. *Clin Neurosurg* 1959;6:131–140.
8. Foster JB, Hudgson P. The pathology of communicating syringomyelia. In: Barnett HJM, Foster JB, Hudgson P, eds. *Syringomyelia.* London: W.B. Saunders, 1973:97–98.
9. Lichtenstein BW. Cervical syringomyelia and syringomyelia-like states associated with Arnold-Chiari deformity and platybasia. *Arch Neurol Psychiatry* 1943;49:881–894.
10. DuBoulay G, Shah SH, Currie JC, Logue V. The mechanism of hydromyelia in Chiari type I malformations. *Br J Radiol* 1974;47:579–587.
11. Ball BJ, Dayan AD. Pathogenesis of syringomyelia. *Lancet* 1972;2:799–801.
12. Oldfield EH, Muraszko K, Shawker TH, Patronas NJ. Pathophysiology of syringomyelia associated with Chiari I malformation of the cerebellar tonsils. *J Neurosurg* 1994;80:3–15.
13. Rennels ML, Gregory TF, Blaumanis OR, Fujimoto K, Grady PA. Evidence for a 'paravascular' fluid circulation in the mammalian central nervous system provided by the rapid distribution of tracer protein throughout the brain from the subarachnoid space. *Brain Res* 1985; 326:47–63.
14. Stoodley MA, Brown SA, Brown CJ, Jones NR. Arterial pulsation-dependent perivascular cerebrospinal fluid flow into the central canal in the sheep spinal cord. *J Neurosurg* 1997;86:686–693.
15. Bertrand G. Dynamic factors in the evolution of syringomyelia and syringobulbia. *Clin Neurosurg* 1973;20:322–333.
16. Cho KH, Iwasaki Y, Imamura H, Kazutoshi H, Abe H. Experimental model of posttraumatic syringomyelia: the role of adhesive arachnoiditis in syrinx formation. *J Neurosurg* 1994;80:133–139.
17. Baldwin NG, Malone DG. Posttraumatic syringomyelia. In: Anson JA, Benzel EC, Awad IA, eds. *Syringomyelia and the Chiari malformations.* Park Ridge, IL: American Association of Neurological Surgeons, 1997:106.
18. Hinshaw DB Jr, Engelhart JA, Kaminsky CK. Imaging of the tethered spinal cord. In: Yamada S, ed. *Tethered cord syndrome.* Park Ridge, IL: American Association of Neurological Surgeons, 1996:60–61.
19. Barnett HJM. The epilogue. In: Barnett HJM, Foster JP, Hudgson P, eds. *Syringomyelia.* London: W.B. Saunders, 1973:310.
20. Stammler A. Chronaxieveranderungen bei Erkrankungen des peripheren motorischen Neurons. *Wien Z Nervenheilk* 1952;5:41–80.
21. Carpenter MB. *Human neuroanatomy,* 7th ed. Baltimore: Williams & Wilkins, 1976:215.
22. Milhorat TH, Kotzen RM, Anzil AP. Stenosis of central canal of spinal cord in man: incidence and pathological findings in 232 autopsy cases. *J Neurosurg* 1994;80:716–722.
23. Foster JB. Hydromyelia. In: Myrianthopoulos NC, ed. *Handbook of clinical neurology.* Amsterdam: Elsevier Scientific Publishers B.V., 1987:425–433.
24. Milhorat TH, Capocelli AL Jr, Anzil AP, Kotzen RM, Milhorat RH. Pathological basis of spinal cord cavitation in syringomyelia: analysis of 105 autopsy cases. *J Neurosurg* 1995;82:802–812.
25. Williams B. Current concepts of syringomyelia. *Br J Hosp Med* 1970; 4:331.
26. Zeidman SM, McCormick PC, Ellenbogen RG. Syringomyelia associated with intraspinal neoplasms. In: Anson JA, Benzel EC, Awad IA, eds. *Syringomyelia and the Chiari malformations.* Park Ridge, IL: American Association of Neurological Surgeons, 1997:115.
27. Cleland J. Contribution to the study of spina bifida, encephalocele and anencephalus. *J Anat Physiol* 1883;17:257–291.
28. Russell DS, Donald C. Mechanism of internal hydrocephalus in spina bifida. *Brain* 1935;58:203–215.
29. Antunes JL. Syringomyelia. In: Holtzman RNN, Stein BM, eds. *Surgery of the spinal cord potential for regeneration and recovery.* New York: Springer-Verlag, 1992:326.
30. Foster JB, Hudgson P. Basal arachnoiditis. In: Barnett HJM, Foster JB, Hudgson P, eds. *Syringomyelia.* London: W.B. Saunders, 1973:30–49.
31. Tokime T, Okamoto S, Yamagata S, Konishi T. Syringomyelia associated with a posterior fossa cyst. *J Neurosurg* 1997;86:907.
32. Cinnalli G, Vinikoff L, Zerah M, Rrenier D, Pierre-Kahn A. Dandy-Walker malformation associated with syringomyelia. *J Neurosurg* 1997;86:571.
33. Klekamp J, Batzdorf U, Samii M, Bothe HW. Treatment of syringomyelia associated with arachnoid scarring caused by arachnoiditis or trauma. *J Neurosurg* 1997;86:233–240.
34. Williams B. Surgical management of non-hindbrain-related and posttraumatic syringomyelia. In: Schmidek HH, Sweet WH, eds. *Operative neurosurgical techniques,* 3rd ed. Vol. 2. Philadelphia: W.B. Saunders, 1995:2119–2138.
35. Naidich TP, McClone DG. Ultrasonography versus computed tomography. In: Holtzman RNN, Stein BM, eds. *The tethered spinal cord.* New York: Thieme-Stratton, 1985:55–56.
36. Chapman PH, Frim DM. Symptomatic syringomyelia following surgery to treat retethering of lipomyelomeningocoeles. *J Neurosurg* 1995;82:752–755.
37. McClone DG, Naidich TP. Spinal dysraphism: experimental and clinical. In: Holtzman RNN, Stein BM, eds. *The tethered spinal cord.* New York: Thieme-Stratton, 1985:25–26.
38. Schlesinger AE, Naidich TP, Quencer RM. Concurrent hydromyelia and diastematomyelia. *AJNR* 1986;7:473–477.
39. Yamada S, Yamada SM, Mandybur GT, Yamada BS. Conservative versus surgical treatment and tethered cord syndrome prognosis. In:

Yamada S, ed. *Tethered cord syndrome*. Park Ridge, IL: American Association of Neurological Surgeons, 1996:196–197.

40. Schliep G. Syringomyelia and syringobulbia. In: Vinken PJ, Bruyn GW, eds. *Handbook of clinical neurology*. Amsterdam: Elsevier/North-Holland Biomedical Press, 1978:255.

41. *The new encyclopedia Britannica micropaedia ready reference*. Vol. 10. Chicago, IL: Encyclopedia Britannica, Inc., 495.

42. Kaar GF, N'Dow JM, Bashir SH. Cervical spondylotic myelopathy with syringomyelia. *Br J Neurosurg* 1996;10:413–415.

43. Kline DG, Hudson AR. *Nerve injuries operative results for major nerve injuries, entrapments, and tumors*. Philadelphia: W.B. Saunders, 1995:258.

44. Nogués MA. Syringomyelia and syringobulbia. In: Myrianthopoulos NC, ed. *Handbook of clinical neurology malformations*. Amsterdam: Elsevier Science Publishers, 1987:452.

45. Peres Serra J, MartInez Yielamos S, Ballabriga Planas J, Basart Tarrats E, Arbizu Urdiain T. Dissociated sensory loss in multiple sclerosis. *Neurologia* 1994;9:233–237.

46. Tomida M, Yamamoto T, Matsuzawa Y, Nakazima S, Uemura K. Multiple sclerosis with syrinx formation in the spinal cord: a case report. *No Shinkei Geka* 1994;22:589–592.

47. Barnett HJM, Jousse AT. Syringomyelia as a late sequel to traumatic paraplegia and quadriplegia—clinical features. In: Barnett HJM, Foster JB, Hudgson P, eds. *Syringomyelia*. London: W.B. Saunders, 1973:133–134.

48. Gardner WJ. Hydrodynamic mechanism of syringomyelia: its relationship to myelocoele. *J Neurol Neurosurg Psychiatry* 1965;28:247–259.

49. Williams B. Simultaneous cerebral and spinal fluid pressure recordings. 2. Cerebrospinal dissociation with lesions at the foramen magnum. *Acta Neurochir* 1981;59:123–142.

50. Aboulker J. La syringomyelie et les liquordes intrarachidiens. *Neurochirurgie* 1979;25[Suppl 1]:1–144.

51. Boman K, Ilvanainen M. Prognosis of syringomyelia. *Acta Neurol Scand* 1967;43:61–68.

52. Fischel A. *Uber Anomalieen des zentral Nervensystems bei jungen menschlichen Embryonen. Beitrage zur pathologischen Anatomie und zur Allgemeinen Pathologie*. Jena: Verlag von Gustav Fisher, 1907:553–564.

53. Duffy PE, Ziter FA. Infantile syringobulbia. *Neurology* 1964;14:500–509.

54. Wilson SAK. Syringomyelia: syringobulbia. In: Bruce AN, ed. *Neurology*. Vol. II [Facsimile of the 1940 Edition]. New York: Hafner, 1970:1389–1405.

55. Brewis M, Poskanzer DC, Roland C, Miller H. Neurological disease in an English city. *Acta Neurol Scand* 1966;42[Suppl 24]:9.

56. Schliep G. Syringomyelia and syringobulbia. In: Vinken PJ, Bruyn GW, eds. *Handbook of clinical neurology*. Amsterdam: North-Holland Publishing Co., 1978:256–257.

57. Moriwaka F, Tashiro K, Tachibana S, Yada K. Epidemiology of syringomyelia in Japan—the nationwide survey. *Rinsho Shinkeigaku* 1995;35:1395–1397.

58. Williams B. Surgical management of non-hindbrain-related and posttraumatic syringomyelia. In: Schmidek HH, Sweet WH, eds. *Operative neurosurgical techniques*, 3rd ed. Vol. 2. Philadelphia: W.B. Saunders, 1995:2119–2120.

59. Baldwin NG, Malone DG. Posttraumatic syringomyelia. In: Anson JA, Benzel EC, Awad IA, eds. *Syringomyelia and the Chiari malformations*. Park Ridge, IL: The American Association of Neurological Surgeons, 1997:105.

60. Barnett HJM, Jousse AT. Posttraumatic syringomyelia. In: Vinken PJ, Bruyn GW, eds. *Handbook of clinical neurology*. Vol. 26. Amsterdam: North-Holland Publishing Co., 1976:122–123.

61. Zeidman SM, McCormick PC, Ellenbogen RG. Syringomyelia associated with intraspinal neoplasms. In: Anson JA, Benzel EC, Awad IA, eds. *Syringomyelia and the Chiari malformations*. Park Ridge, IL: American Association of Neurological Surgeons, 1997:113.

62. Samii M, Klekamp J. Surgical results of 100 intramedullary tumors in relation to accompanying syringomyelia. *Neurosurgery* 1994;35:865–873.

63. Zeidman SM, McCormick PC, Ellenbogen RG. Syringomyelia associated with intraspinal neoplasms. In: Anson JA, Benzel EC, Awad LA, eds. *Syringomyelia and the Chiari malformations*. Park Ridge, IL: American Association of Neurological Surgeons, 1997:115.

64. Zakeri A, Glasauer FE, Egnatchik JG. Familial syringomyelia: case report and review of the literature. *Surg Neurol* 1995;44:48–53.

65. Newman PK, Wentzel J, Foster JB. HLA and syringomyelia. *J Neuroimmunol* 1982;3:23–26.

66. Wild H, Behnert J. Konkordante Syringomyelie mit okzipito-zervikaler Dysplasie bei eineiigem Zwillingspaar. *Munch Med Wochenschr* 1964;106:1421–1428.

67. Malessa R, Jorg J. Discordant syringomyelia twins in familial syringomyelia. *Nervenarzt* 1986;57:522–526.

68. Krabbe KH. Syringomyelie et cotes cervicales chez des jumeaux heterozygotes. *Acta Psychiatr* 1939;14:489–508.

69. Ishchenko MM, Degtiar VV, Komorovskaia IAM. Four cases of familial syringomyelia in a single generation. *Zh Nevropatol Psikhiatr Im S S Korsakova* 1976;76:662–665.

70. Sirotkin BM. Regional peculiarities of syringomyelia. *Genetica* 1970;6:166–178.

71. Milhorat TH, Kotzen RM, Mu HTM, Capocelli AL Jr. Dysaesthetic pain in patients with syringomyelia. *Neurosurgery* 1996;38:940–947.

72. Milhorat TH, Mu HTM, LaMotte CC, Milhorat AT. Distribution of substance P in the spinal cord of patients with syringomyelia. *J Neurosurg* 1996;84:992–998.

73. Fujimura Y, Kimura F, Ishida S, Shinoda K, Ohsawa N. An adult case of tethered cord syndrome with lipoma and thoraco-lumbar syringomyelia presenting slow progressive muscular atrophy in the lower limbs. *Rinsho Shinkeigaku* 1994;34:918–921.

74. Schliep G. Syringomyelia and syringobulbia. In: Vinken PJ, Bruyn GW, eds. *Handbook of clinical neurology*. Amsterdam: Elsevier/North-Holland Biomedical Press, 1978:268–269.

75. Bleck TP, Shannon KM. Disordered swallowing due to a syrinx: correction by shunting. *Neurology* 1984;34:1497–1498.

76. Aminoff MJ, Wilcox CS. Autonomic dysfunction in syringomyelia. *Postgrad Med J* 1972;48:113–115.

77. Schliep G. Syringomyelia and syringobulbia. In: Vinken PJ, Bruyn GW, eds. *Handbook of clinical neurology*. Amsterdam: Elsevier/North-Holland Biomedical Press, 1978:272–273.

78. Kita K, Hirayama K, Tokumara Y, Kijima M. Chiromegaly in syringomyelia—radiologic studies of hand bones. *Rinsho Shinkeigaku* 1994;34:1089–1092.

79. Charry O, Koop S, Winter R, Lonstein J, Denis F, Bailey W. Syringomyelia and scoliosis: a review of twenty-five pediatric patients. *J Pediatr Orthop* 1994;14:309–317.

80. Kabinoff G, Sharma KC, Brandstetter RD. Death by syrinx: worse than Ondine's curse [Editorial]? *Chest* 1996;109:598–599.

81. Shiihara T. Isolated sleep apnea due to Chiari type I malformation and syringomyelia. *Pediatr Neurol* 1995;13:266–267.

82. Schliep G. Syringomyelia and syringobulbia. In: Vinken PJ, Bruyn GW, eds. *Handbook of clinical neurology*. Amsterdam: North-Holland Publishing Co., 1978:273.

83. Ostertag B. Dysraphie und Syringomyelie. In: Scholz W, ed. *Handbuch deer Speziellen Pathologischen Anatomie und Histologie*. Vol. 13, Part IV. Berlin: Springer, 1965:427–491.

84. Berry RG, Chambers RA. Syringoencephalomyelia. *J Neuropathol Exp Neurol* 1981;40:633–644.

85. Foster JB, Hudgson P. The pathology of communicating syringomyelia. In: Barnett HJM, Foster JB, Hudgson P, eds. *Syringomyelia*. London: W.B. Saunders, 1973:100.

86. Graham DI, Lamtos PL, eds. *Greenfield's neuropathology*, 6th ed. London: Arnold 1997:486–491.

87. Gardner WJ. *The dysraphic states—from syringomyelia to anencephaly*. Amsterdam: Exerpta Medica, 1973.

88. Williams B. The distending force in the production of communicating syringomyelia [letter]. *Lancet* 1970;2:41–42.

89. Foster JB, Hudgson P. The clinical features of communicating syringomyelia. In: Barnett HJM, Foster JB, Hudgson P, eds. *Syringomyelia*. London: W.B. Saunders, 1973:16–29.

90. Barnett HJM, Jousse AT. Syringomyelia as a late sequel to traumatic paraplegia and quadriplegia—clinical features. In: Barnett HJM, Foster JB, Hudgson P, eds. *Syringomyelia*. London: W.B. Saunders, 1973:129–153.

91. Desmond ME. Description of the occlusion of the spinal cord lumen in early human embryos. *The Anatomical Record* 1982;204:89–93.

92. Gardner WJ, McMurry FG. "Non-communicating" syringomyelia: a non-existent entity. *Surg Neurol* 1976;6:251–256.

93. Kochana JP, Quencer RM. Imaging of cystic and cavitary lesions of the spinal cord and canal. In: Modic MT, ed. *The radiologic clinics of North America*. Philadelphia: W.B. Saunders, 1974:457–472.

94. Moufarrij N, Awad IA. Classification of the Chiari malformations and syringomyelia. In: Anson JA, Benzel EC, Awad IA, eds. *Syringomyelia and the Chiari malformations*. Park Ridge, IL: The American Association of Neurological Surgeons, 1997:27–34.

95. Santoro A, Delfini R, Innocenzi G, et al. Spontaneous drainage of syringomyelia. Report of two cases. *J Neurosurg* 1993;79:132–134.

96. Holtzmann RNN, Yang WC. Spinal cord atrophy. In: Holtzman RNN, Stein BM, eds. *Surgery of the spinal cord potential for regeneration and recovery*. New York: Springer-Verlag, 1992:165–196.

97. Graham DI, Lantos PL, eds. *Greenfield's neuropathology*, 6th ed. London: Arnold, 1997:491–492.

98. Schliep G. Syringomyelia and syringobulbia. In: Vinken PJ, Bruyn GW, eds. *Handbook of clinical neurology*. Amsterdam; Elsevier/North-Holland Biomedical Press, 1978:295.

99. Padget DH. Neuroschisis and human embryonic maldevelopment. *J Neuropathol Exp Neurol* 1970;29:192–216.

100. Graham DI, Lantos PL, eds. *Greenfield's neuropathology*. 6th ed. London: Arnold, 1997:488–490.

101. Foster JB, Hudgson P. The pathology of communicating syringomyelia. In: Barnet HJM, Foster JB, Hudgson P, eds. *Syringomyelia*. London: W.B. Saunders, 1973:96–97.

102. McClone DG. The Chiari II malformation of the hindbrain and the associated hydromyelia. In: Anson JA, Benzel EC, Awad IA, eds. *Syringomyelia and the Chiari malformations*. Park Ridge, IL: The American Association of Neurological Surgeons, 1997:77.

103. Williams B. Post-traumatic syringomyelia (cystic myelopathy). In: Frankel HL, ed. *Handbook of clinical neurology spinal cord trauma*. Vol. 17. Amsterdam: Elsevier Science Publishers B.V., 1992:378.

104. Barnett HJM, Jousse AT. Syringomyelia as a late sequel to traumatic paraplegia and quadriplegia—clinical features. In: Barnett HJM, Foster JB, Hudgson P, eds. *Syringomyelia*. London: W.B. Saunders, 1973:144.

105. Emery JL, Lendon RG. The local cord lesion in neurospinal dysraphism (meningomyelocele). *J Pathol* 1973;110:83–96.

106. Barnett HJM, Jousse AT. Posttraumatic syringomyelia. In: Vinken PJ, Bruyn GW, eds. *Injuries of the spine and spinal cord. Part II. Handbook of clinical neurology*. Amsterdam: North-Holland Publishing Co., 1976:126.

107. Barnett HJM, Jousse AT. Posttraumatic syringomyelia. In: Vinken PJ, Bruyn GW, eds. *Injuries of the spine and spinal cord. Part II. Handbook of clinical neurology*. Amsterdam: North-Holland Publishing Co., 1976:116.

108. Barnett HJM. The epilogue. In: Barnett HJM, Foster JP, Hudgson P, eds. *Syringomyelia*. London: W.B. Saunders, 1973:310.

109. Barnett HJM, Newcastle NB. Syringomyelia and tumours of the nervous system. In: Barnett HJM, Foster JB, Hudgson P, eds. *Syringomyelia*. London: W.B. Saunders, 1973:279.

110. Beuls EAM, Vandersteen MAM, Vanormelingen LM, et al. Deformation of the cervicomedullary junction and spinal cord in a surgically treated adult Chiari I hindbrain hernia associated with syringomyelia: a magnetic resonance microscopic and neuropathological study. *J Neurosurg* 1996;85:701–708.

111. Barnett HJM. Epilogue. In: Barnett HJM, Foster PJ, Hodgson P, eds. *Syringomyelia*. London: W.B. Saunders, 1973:306–309.

112. Milhorat TH, Miller JI, Johnson WD, Adler DE, Heger IM. Anatomical basis of syringomyelia occurring with hindbrain lesions. *Neurosurgery* 1993;32:748–785.

113. Ball MJ, Roach M. Syringomyelia—is Gardner correct? Presented to 7th Canadian Congress of Neurological Sciences, Banff, June 1972 cited by Barnett HJM. Epilogue. In: Barnett HJM, Foster PJ, Hodgson P, eds. *Syringomyelia*. London: W.B. Saunders, 1973:311.

114. Milhorat TH, Johnson RW, Johnson WD. Evidence of CSF flow in rostral direction through the central canal of spinal cord in rats. In: Matsumoto S, Tamaki N, eds. *Hydrocephalus, pathogenesis and treatment*. Tokyo: Springer-Verlag, 1991:207–217.

115. Pollay M, Curl F. Secretion of cerebrospinal fluid by the ventricular ependyma of the rabbit. *Am J Physiol* 1967;213:1031–1038.

116. Sullivan LP, Stears JC, Ringel SP. Resolution of syringomyelia and Chiari I malformation by ventriculoatrial shunting in a patient with pseudotumor cerebri and a lumboperitoneal shunt. *Neurosurgery* 1988;22:744–747.

117. Ashraf R, Sostre S. Differing scintigraphic patterns of lumboperitoneal shunt dysfunction in patients with normal pressure hydrocephalus and pseudotumor cerebri. *Clin Nucl Med* 1995;20:140–146.

118. Conway LW. Hydrodynamic studies in syringomyelia. *J Neurosurg* 1967;27:501.

119. Ellertson AB, Greitz T. Myelocystographic and fluorescein studies to demonstrate communication between intramedullary cysts and the cerebrospinal fluid space. *Acta Neurol Scand* 1969;45:418.

120. Early CB, Fink LH. Some fundamental applications of the law of La Place in neurosurgery. *Surg Neurol* 1976;3:185–189.

121. Cifuentes M, Fernandez LL, Perez J, Perez Figares JM, Rodriguez EM. Distribution of intraventricularly injected horseradish peroxidase in cerebrospinal fluid compartments of the rat spinal cord. *Cell Tissue Res* 1992;270:485–494.

122. Stoodley MA, Jones NR, Brown CJ. Evidence for rapid fluid flow from the subarachnoid space into the spinal cord central canal in the rat. *Brain Res* 1996;707:155–164.

123. Marin-Padilla M. The tethered cord syndrome: developmental considerations. In: Holtzman RNN, Stein BM, eds. *The tethered spinal cord*. New York: Thieme-Stratton, 1985:3–13.

124. Tavares JM, Wood EH. *Diagnostic neuroradiology*, 2nd ed. Baltimore: Williams & Wilkins, 1976.

125. Rhoton AL Jr. Microsurgery of syringomyelia and syringomyelic cord syndrome. In: Schmidek HH, Sweet WH, eds. *Operative neurosurgical techniques*, 3rd ed. Philadelphia: W.B. Saunders, 1995:1754.

126. Schlesinger EB, Antunes JL, Michelsen WJ, Louis KM. Hydromyelia. Clinical presentation and comparison of modalities of treatment. *Neurosurgery* 1981;9:356–365.

127. Williams B. Management schemes for syringomyelia: surgical indications and nonsurgical management. In: Anson JA, Benzel EC, Awad IA, eds. *Syringomyelia and the Chiari malformations*. Park Ridge, IL: American Association of Neurological Surgeons, 1997:125–133.

128. Ogilvy CS, Borges LF. Treatment of symptomatic syringomyelia with a ventriculo-peritoneal shunt: a case report with magnetic resonance scan correlation. *Neurosurgery* 1988;22:748–750.

129. Ventureyra ECG, Tekkok IH. Syringostomy using myringostomy tube: technical note. *Neurosurgery* 1997;41:495–497.

130. Williams B, Fahy G. A critical appraisal of "terminal ventriculostomy" for the treatment of syringomyelia. *J Neurosurg* 1983;58:188–197.

131. Nogués MA. Syringomyelia and syringobulbia. In: Myrianthopoulos NC, ed. *Handbook of clinical neurology malformations*. Amsterdam: Elsevier Science Publishers, 1987:459–460.

132. Williams B. Surgical management of non-hindbrain-related and posttraumatic syringomyelia. In: Schmidek HH, Sweet WH, eds. *Operative neurosurgical techniques*, 3rd ed. Philadelphia: W.B. Saunders, 1995:2126–2127.

133. Huewel ER, Perneczky A, Urban V, Fries G. Neuroendoscopic technique for the operative treatment of septated syringomyelia. *Acta Neurochir Suppl (Wien)* 1992;54:59–62.

134. Nishihara T, Hara T, Suzuki I, Kirino T, Yamakawa K. Third ventriculostomy for symptomatic syringomyelia using flexible endoscope: case report. *Minim Invasive Neurosurg* 1996;39:130–132.

135. Bekar A, Tureyen K, Aksoy K. Unilateral blindness due to patient positioning during cervical syringomyelic surgery: unilateral blindness after prone position. *J Neurosurg Anesthesiol* 1996;8:227–229.

136. Takayasu M, Shubuya M, Kouketsu N, Suzuki Y. Rapid enlargement of a syringomyelic cavity following syringo-subarachnoid shunt: case report. *Surg Neurol* 1996;45:366–369.

137. Friedman ED. The exuberance of youth: application of the Kennard principle to studies on spinal cord plasticity. In: Holtzman RNN, Stein BM, eds. *Surgery of the spinal cord potential for regeneration and recovery*. New York: Springer-Verlag, 1992:53–70.

138. Blagodatskili MD, Sufianov AA, Larionov SN, Kibbort RV, Seminskili IZh, Manokhin PA. The transplantation of embryonic nerve tissue in syringomyelia: initial clinical experience. *Zh Vopr Neirokhir Im N N Burdenko* 1994;3:27–29.

139. Milhorat TH, Kotzen RM. Stenosis of the central canal of the spinal cord following inoculation of suckling hamsters with reovirus type I. *J Neurosurg* 1994;81:103–106.

Motor Disorders,
edited by David S. Younger.
Lippincott Williams & Wilkins, Philadelphia © 1999.

CHAPTER 30

Childhood Spinal Muscular Atrophy

Susan T. Iannaccone

HISTORY

Werdnig and Hoffmann were working in the tradition of German neurology of the late 19th century when they conducted autopsies on their patients who had a new form of infantile paralysis. They described a striking atrophy of the ventral nerve roots of the spinal cord on gross examination and correlated this finding with the histologic appearance of the anterior horns that showed a decreased number of motor neurons. Moreover, a pattern of atrophy in muscle fibers was consistent with loss of innervation (1). In the 1890s, Guido Werdnig was a retired battalion physician working at the Institute of Anatomy and Physiology of the Central Nervous System at the University of Vienna. His lecture, entitled "On a case of muscular dystrophy with positive spinal cord findings" (2), was probably the first full description of spinal muscular atrophy (SMA). In 1891, he published a paper describing two infantile hereditary cases of progressive muscular atrophy. The following year, Professor Johann Hoffmann of Heidelberg University used the term, in German, "spinale muskelatrophie," in English, "spinal muscular atrophy" (3). Together, their papers presented the clinical and pathologic aspects of infantile SMA: onset during the first year of life, occurrence in siblings with normal parents, progressive hypotonia and weakness, hand tremor, and death from pneumonia in early childhood. Moreover, Hoffmann talked about progressive and chronic types of SMA (4,5).

CLASSIFICATION

The classification of SMA has always been controversial. The work of Hoffmann and Werdnig immediately suggested some biologic difference between those

infants with a severe fatal form of the disease and those with the chronic form. Beginning with Byers and Banker (6), a classification of SMA according to severity was thought to facilitate prognostication. The relationship between age at onset and severity was supported by the observations of Dubowitz (7). Based on the work of an international collaboration (8,9), most pediatric neurologists now use the following nomenclature: SMA type 1 (or I) for onset of symptoms before age 6 months, SMA type 2 (II) for onset between 6 and 18 months, and SMA type 3 (III) for onset after age 18 months (Table 1). The three types may be subdivided on the basis of mortality or highest motor milestone achieved. For example, SMA1 patients almost never sit without support when placed (10). In fact, most SMA patients of all types can never pull themselves to sitting position or roll over at any age. SMA1 patients with onset before 3 months of age have the highest mortality rate (90%), whereas those with onset after age 3 months may survive to adulthood, albeit with severe motor handicap. SMA3 patients often are independently ambulatory at least for part of their life and may have a normal life expectancy (11). Most SMA patients have type 1, with decreasing incidence for types 2 and 3, respectively. In other words, the incidence is highest for type 1, then 2, and type 3 has the lowest incidence. Considering the relative mortality rates, it is not surprising that the highest prevalence is for SMA types 2 and 3.

Spinal Muscular Atrophy Type 1

One of the difficulties with previous classification systems has been the inconsistent use of eponyms. Synonyms for SMA type 1 are "infantile onset SMA" and "Werdnig-Hoffmann disease." SMA1 is the most severe form of the disease beginning at birth or in the first few months of life and frequently resulting in death from respiratory failure before 2 years of age. On physical exam-

S. T. Iannaccone: University of Texas Southwestern Medical Center at Dallas and Department of Neurology, Texas Scottish Rite Hospital for Children, Dallas, Texas 75235.

TABLE 1. *Classification of SMA*

	Onset of weakness (mo)	Highest function	Mortality
SMA1	<6	Most nonsitters; few sitters	90%; a few survive to 2nd decade
SMA2	6–18	Most sitters; few walkers	Variable; most survive to 2nd or 3rd decade
SMA3	>18	Many walkers	Many with normal life expectancy

SMA, spinal muscular atrophy.

ination, these infants have severe weakness and profound hypotonia. There is a striking discrepancy between the infant's level of social interaction and lack of motor skills. There may be no spontaneous movement except in the hands and feet. The infant lies in the frog-leg position. There is often a fine tremor in the fingers called polyminimyoclonus. Deep tendon reflexes are usually absent, whereas sphincter tone and sensation remain intact. Tongue fasciculations are common. Atrophy of the tongue may be manifest as scalloping of the border. Weak intercostal muscles countered by diaphragmatic breathing result in inefficient respiration, the pectus excavatum deformity, and flaring of the lower ribs (bell-shaped deformity) (Fig. 1). Bilateral eventration or paralysis of the diaphragm may be a presenting manifestation (12).

The most common cause of death is respiratory failure, although it may be preceded by several months of subtle changes due to complications of weakness. SMA1 babies tire quickly during feeding and, if breast fed, may begin to lose weight before it is evident that they are not taking in appropriate calories. Malnutrition and respiratory insufficiency exacerbate fatigue and cause susceptibility to aspiration. Any minor upper respiratory infection may quickly become a life-threatening crisis.

Spinal Muscular Atrophy Type 2

Synonyms for SMA2 include "juvenile SMA," "intermediate SMA," or "chronic SMA" (13,14). Patients usually achieve normal milestones up to 6 to 8 months of age, although they are hypotonic. The legs tend to be more involved than the arms so that failure to walk is a typical chief complaint (Fig. 2). Patients may be thought to have a paraparesis and occasionally are born with club foot deformity. The pattern of deep tendon reflexes may be variable with preservation in muscle groups that are fairly strong. Minipolymyoclonus may be prominent in these infants. The pathophysiologic origin of these movements is not known, although fasciculations of the intrinsic hand muscles may contribute.

Many patients with type 2 are able to sit without support if placed in position during all or some of their life; rarely, some are able to stand or walk with aid. The age for sitting or walking is nearly always delayed, and walking, whether with or without assist, is usually temporary. The age at death is quite variable, from 7 months to 7 years (6). Many survive to the third or the fourth decade; the eldest patient in one prospective study died at age 72

years (15). The difference between survivors and nonsurvivors seems to be good pulmonary function.

Spinal Muscular Atrophy Type 3

"Wohlfart-Kugelberg-Welander syndrome" is the eponym for mild SMA or SMA type 3 (16,17) when onset may be any time after age 18 months. SMA3 usually presents in late childhood or adolescence as a proximal neurogenic muscular atrophy that may be confused with limb girdle muscular dystrophy (18–21). Patients frequently have elevated serum creatine kinase levels (22), although the mechanism is poorly under-

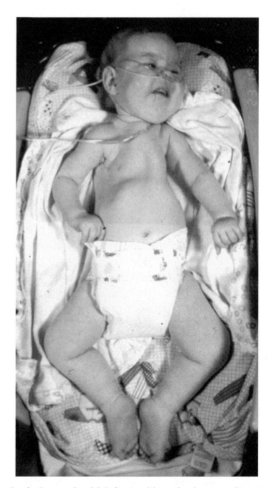

FIG. 1. A 3-month-old infant with spinal muscular atrophy type 1 who has a bell-shaped chest. She died of respiratory failure soon afterward.

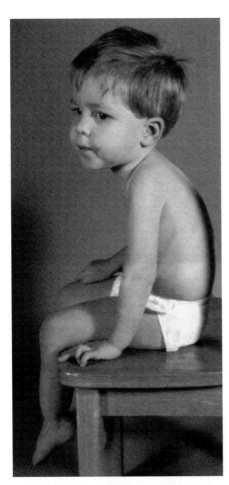

FIG. 2. This 11-month-old boy was diagnosed with spinal muscular atrophy type 2. He learned to sit without support at 12 months of age.

stood. This syndrome is distinguished from Werdnig-Hoffmann disease by later onset and long survival. It is distinguished from amyotrophic lateral sclerosis by the benign course and the absence of any clinical evidence of corticospinal dysfunction. Some authors have called adult-onset SMA (i.e., after age 21) type 4; however, this designation is not consistently used in current literature.

SMA3 patients who are ambulatory have a waddling gait, with lumbar lordosis, genu recurvatum, and a protuberant abdomen or may appear very thin, like a "stick man." Deep tendon reflexes may be or may not be elicited but are never pathologically hyperactive. Byers and Banker (6) reported on six of eight children who were able to stand without aid between 1 and 2 years of age, whereas only two of eight were eventually able to walk without assistance. The prognosis for continued independent ambulation can be correlated with age at onset of weakness (23). If onset is before 2 years of age, the patient is likely to stop walking by age 15, whereas if onset occurs later than 2 years, it is highly likely that ambulation will be possible into the fifth decade (15). A large prospective clinical study showed little or no pro-

gression of weakness over several years in patients with type 2 or 3 (11). The authors suggested that SMA may not be a neurodegenerative disease.

The classification of SMA into three types is an artificial representation of a biologic spectrum of disease. However, understanding the underlying mechanisms that result in mild or severe disease may contribute toward finding effective treatment.

LABORATORY EVALUATION

The diagnostic workup for SMA has changed since the discovery of the *SMN* gene. The diagnosis now can begin with blood DNA for direct mutation analysis of the gene (24,25). For infants who have deletions of exons 7 and 8, no further workup is necessary. Although most patients have deletions in *SMN*, rare patients with duplication have been described. If DNA analysis is normal, then a more traditional approach may be necessary for diagnosis.

This traditional approach includes measurement of serum creatine kinase; electrodiagnostic studies, including nerve conduction velocities (NCV) and needle electromyography; and muscle biopsy. As already stated, the creatine kinase may or may not be elevated, although it usually is normal in SMA types 1 and 2.

Measurement of motor NCV in infants may be difficult because of the small-sized limbs and short distance between stimulus and recording electrodes. Examination usually documents either normal NCV or, occasionally, faster conduction velocities than expected. If there is profound muscle atrophy, it may be difficult to interpret responses to nerve stimulus (26). International diagnostic criteria mandate that motor and sensory NCV be normal. The occasional case of typical SMA in which NCV or amplitudes are abnormal may be explained as a technical artifact, but not always. Axonal dysfunction can theoretically result in abnormal electrodiagnostic studies. Needle electromyography usually shows evidence of acute denervation including fibrillation potentials and reinnervation in the form of large polyphasic motor units and reduced recruitment. In infants, electromyography may be normal or suggestive of a myopathic process because of small amplitude, short duration, polyphasic motor units.

Muscle biopsy should show neurogenic atrophy and/or evidence of reinnervation. Preservation of large round fibers in the denervated fasciculi is common (6). This is frequently called the "infantile pattern of neurogenic atrophy." From mid-childhood, one may see angular fibers indicating acute denervation and type grouping indicating reinnervation. Nonspecific changes such as fiber size disproportion may occur, possibly as a result of sampling error (12) or developmental variations. In such a case, repeat biopsy of another muscle or at a later age may show more typical evidence of neurogenic atrophy.

GENETICS

Epidemiologic studies indicate an autosomal recessive mode of inheritance (27) and nearly equal sex distribution with a slight predominance in males (28), but autosomal dominant transmission is a rare occurrence (29). Several families have been described in which the co-occurrence of SMA and amyotrophic lateral sclerosis was documented (30,31). Molecular testing is required to determine whether such occurrences are merely coincidental.

A rare form of severe SMA with arthrogryposis occurs in an X-linked inheritance pattern. Symptoms are apparent at birth or shortly after birth (32,33). Death usually occurs from respiratory failure within the first few months of life. Male infants are exclusively affected, whereas carriers are asymptomatic. Only a few families with this entity have been identified worldwide, but linkage analysis has shown that all map to the same locus.

Linkage of autosomal recessive SMA to chromosome 5q11.2-13.3 was reported by Gilliam et al. in 1990 (34). An international consortium studied families with evidence of recessive transmission only, although they were able to document phenotypic heterogeneity within families (35–37). In 1994, Melki et al. (38) reported the occurrence of major deletions at 5q11.2-13.3 in patients with severe SMA (Werdnig-Hoffmann phenotype) as compared with patients with mild SMA (Kugelberg-Welander phenotype) who had none or smaller deletions. Clinical evidence suggests that early-onset SMA represents a spectrum of disease, a finding that would be consistent with a single gene locus (39,40).

Two genes were found at the 5q locus. The gene for neuronal apoptosis inhibitory protein (*NAIP*) maps to the 5q13 region and 67% of SMA patients were shown to have deletions in this gene, whereas only 2% of control subjects had deletions (41). A novel gene, whose function remains unknown, called the survival motor neuron gene (*SMN*), also at 5q13, was found to contain deletions in 229 (>98%) SMA patients (42,43). Furthermore, at least two patients with duplications of *SMN* have now been reported, providing more evidence that *SMN* is the correct gene. The presence of multiple copies of *SMN* (telomeric, SMN_t, and centromeric, SMN_c) and of heterogeneity in deletions of various exons has been a challenge for investigators (44). A role for gene dosage in clinical severity is under investigation (45). Normal individuals have two alleles each of SMN_t and SMN_c. The disease appears to be caused by mutations in both alleles of SMN_t, whereas there may be some or none of SMN_c present. Recent work has shown that in some cases of SMA2 or 3, SMN_t is converted to SMN_c. It appears that SMA disease is caused by mutation of both telomeric alleles of *SMN*, whereas increasing the number of SMN_c copies may ameliorate the severity of the phenotype. (46) The addition of muta-

tions in *NAIP* may increase the severity of the clinical phenotype.

The protein product of *SMN* is known to interact with RNA-binding proteins and may actually be a spliceosome. Immunohistochemistry of tissues from control individuals has shown normal *SMN* activity in both nuclei and cytoplasm of motor neurons (47). Nuclear activity occurs in structures called gems that are closely related to chromosome activity during mitosis. Reaction product was absent from neurons of SMA1 patients and reduced in neurons of SMA2 and SMA3 patients compared with motor neurons from control subjects. Thus, it seems that the amount of gene product may be inversely proportional to the severity of the clinical phenotype. Loss of spliceosomes could theoretically affect the production of mRNA, but there is no clear indication as to why only motor neurons are affected. A knockout mouse model was nonviable past the blastocyst stage of embryo development.

MANAGEMENT

Because there is no effective therapy for SMA, management consists of preventing or treating the complications (48). Complications of severe weakness include restrictive lung disease, poor nutrition, orthopedic deformities, immobility, and psychosocial problems (Table 2). Restrictive lung disease results from weakness of intercostal muscles and diaphragm, causing hypoventilation and weak cough (Fig. 3). Aggressive prophylaxis against pneumonia and atelectasis may include assisted cough, chest percussion therapy, and intermittent positive pressure breathing. Some clinics recommend ambu-bagging, in/exsufflation, and night-time mask ventilation to prevent or reverse microatelectasis. Patients require assistance to maintain good pulmonary toilet even when not experiencing an acute infection and may require intervention to prevent progressive atelectasis (49–52).

Risk for pneumonia increases as forced vital capacity (FVC) decreases, which may occur even without significant change in limb or trunk strength. Some clinicians begin prophylaxis before the FVC reaches 50% of expected. A few clinics monitor maximum inspiratory pressure, which has been shown to be an early indicator of restrictive disease. Oxygen therapy should be contraindicated except with the use of assisted ventilation. Patients with restrictive lung disease develop retention of CO_2 before hypoxia, and administration of oxygen may cause death from apnea secondary to suppression of the respiratory drive. It is helpful to monitor blood gases on a regular basis along with the FVC. When CO_2 retention occurs, then noninvasive ventilation, either positive or negative pressure, during acute infection or at night as prophylaxis may be helpful and restorative.

Poor nutrition with failure to thrive often occurs as a result of a weak suck, unprotected airway, or easy fatiga-

TABLE 2. *Complications of SMA*

Complication	Characteristics
Respiratory insufficiency	Proportional to general weakness
	May occur during sleep before clinically apparent
	Responds well to noninvasive ventilation
FTT	Particularly infants
	Exacerbates weakness, fatigue
	Reduce reserves
Constipation	Very common
	Responds to dietary management
Orthopedic deformities	Club foot
	Scoliosis, kyphosis
	Flexion contractures
Psychosocial dysfunction	Inadequate intellectual challenge
	Depression rare in patients, common in siblings
	Marital discord

SMA, spinal muscular atrophy; FTT, failure to thrive.

bility. Particularly in infants, but also older children, there may be an exacerbation of weakness and fatigue secondary to negative nitrogen balance. The mechanism for this effect is not well understood. At least some SMA patients suffer from chronic malnutrition that may manifest as easy fatigability and reduced reserve. Some cases of organic aciduria in SMA may have been caused by inadequate nutrition.

A feeding evaluation should be done by a team of occupational and speech therapists and dieticians. Such professionals can adjust the feeding schedule, positioning during feeding, or food textures to maximize caloric intake. If necessary, the child should be examined during a modified barium swallow using several food textures, including liquid, semiliquid, soft, and solid food. If aspi-

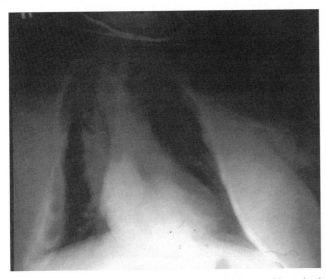

FIG. 3. A chest x-ray from a 14-year-old boy with spinal muscular atrophy type 2. The lung volume is markedly decreased, and the rib cage has collapsed into a bell-shape.

ration occurs, a gastrostomy should be recommended. In some cases, supplemental gastrostomy feedings may be indicated in the absence of aspiration because the child cannot take in enough by mouth before fatiguing. Constipation is nearly universal in such patients because of immobility, but it responds easily to increasing fluid and fiber intake.

Scoliosis is the most serious orthopedic problem among patients with SMA (53). Nonwalkers tend to develop spinal deformities earlier than walkers. Most curves are thoracolumbar in location. Spinal orthoses usually do not prevent or retard scoliosis; they may, however, help the patients to sit. Pulmonary function tests (PFTs) should be monitored with the child wearing the orthosis and without it. Frequently, it is necessary to cut a window in the front to allow for movement of the abdominal wall with breathing. If the orthosis limits breathing, its use should be discontinued. The timing of spine surgery is crucial, because one would maximize the child's growth and so wait until the curve is severe while wanting to do surgery when PFTs are relatively normal. Vigorous preoperative and postoperative physical therapy is required to prevent loss of strength or function after spinal fusion and to prevent respiratory complications. Marked improvement in the degree of scoliosis is often possible after fusion or instrumentation, with associated improvement in vital capacity, sitting, balance, and comfort (54–56). Patients who do not undergo correction of scoliosis will experience progressive deformity with discomfort, inability to position, and further decompensation of PFTs.

Club foot deformity, although not common, may be a presenting complaint for SMA during infancy. It is usually flexible and may not require surgical correction. More common deformities include flexion contractures secondary to immobility. They affect hips, knees, and ankles very quickly. Range of motion exercises are used to prevent such contractures, but they must be done daily and consistently, a feat most patients and families find impossible to accomplish. Splints and braces have been of little help in preventing deformities because of lack of compliance as well.

Walking may occasionally be facilitated by lightweight orthoses for the legs, although for SMA1 or 2 patients, it will likely be a temporary skill (15). Power chairs should be prescribed as close to the second birthday as possible to provide some independent mobility at an appropriate developmental age (57). Because SMA children have high cognitive function (58), they easily learn how to maneuver a joy stick. The motor speed can be adjusted as needed, and the parents should be encouraged to set consistent limits for behavior. As the child grows, pneumatic lifts, special mattresses, and bath accessories will be beneficial for many patients. An in-home occupational therapy consult will ensure that the patient receives appropriate equipment.

School-aged children may benefit from a full-time aid who can help with toileting and feeding and maintain the respiratory and physical therapy regimens during the school day. Parents can be encouraged to seek resources for such help and to communicate freely with school district officials to provide their child with an education that will maximize his or her abilities. A common hurdle for parents is a lack of adequate intellectual challenge for their child. Because of the structure of special education programs, many educators fail to recognize that the SMA child is actually gifted intellectually. It can be helpful to perform psychometric testing at age 4 years to document the level of functioning before entering school.

Families of SMA children suffer from all the common complications seen with chronic disease in childhood: financial stress, marital discord, and depression among siblings. The SMA child is rarely depressed, presumably because there is usually no discernible loss of function after mid-childhood. However, it is advisable to encourage the families to participate in formal counseling and support group activities soon after diagnosis.

REFERENCES

1. Iannaccone ST, Caneris O. Johann Hoffmann. In: Ashwal S, ed. *Founders of child neurology*. San Francisco: Norman Publishing, 1990:278–284.
2. Groger H. Guido Werdnig. In: Ashwal S, ed. *The Founders of child neurology*. San Francisco: Norman Publishing, 1990:383–388.
3. Hoffmann J. Ueber familiäre progressive spinale muskelatrophie. *Arch Psych (Berlin)* 1892;24:644–646.
4. Hoffmann J. Ueber chronische spinale muskelatrophieim kindesalter auf familiärer basis. *Dtsch Zeit Nervenheilk* 1892;3:427–470.
5. Hoffmann J. Weiterer beitrag zur lehre von der hereditaren progressiven spinalen muskelatrophie im kindesalter nebst bemerkungen über den fortschreitenden muskelschwund im Allgemeinen. *Dtsch Zeit Nervenheilk* 1896;10:292–320.
6. Byers RK, Banker BQ. Infantile muscular atrophy. *Arch Neurol* 1961; 5:140–164.
7. Dubowitz V. Infantile muscular atrophy A prospective study with particular reference to a slowly progressive variety. *Brain* 1964;87: 707–718.
8. Munsat TL. Workshop report: international SMA collaboration. *Neuromusc Disord* 1991;1:81.
9. Dubowitz V. Chaos in the classification of SMA: a possible resolution. *Neuromusc Disord* 1995;5:3–5.
10. Iannaccone ST, Browne RH, Samaha FJ, Buncher CR, DCN/SMA Group. Prospective study of spinal muscular atrophy before age 6 years. *J Child Neurol* 1993;9:187–193.
11. Russman BS, Iannaccone ST, Buncher CR, et al. Spinal muscular atrophy: new thoughts on the pathogenesis and classification schema. *J Child Neurol* 1992;7:347–353.
12. Bove KE, Iannaccone ST. Atypical infantile spinomuscular atrophy presenting as acute diaphragmatic paralysis. *Pediatr Pathol* 1988;8: 95–107.
13. Hausmanowa-Petrusewicz I. *Spinal muscular atrophy infantile and juvenile type*. Springfield: National Technical Information Service, 1978:1.
14. Dubowitz V. 38th ENMC International Workshop Spinal Muscular Atrophy Trial Group. *Neuromusc Disord* 1996;6:293–294.
15. Russman BS, Buncher CR, White M, Samaha FJ, Iannaccone ST, DCN/SMA Group. Function changes in spinal muscular atrophy II and III. *Neurology* 1996;47:973–976.
16. Kugelberg E, Welander L. Familial neurogenic (spinal?) muscular atrophy simulating ordinary proximal dystrophy. *Acta Psychiatr Scand* 1954;29:42–53.
17. Kugelberg E, Welander L. Heredofamilial juvenile muscular atrophy simulating muscular dystrophy. *Arch Neurol Psychiatry* 1956;75: 500–509.
18. Lunt PW, Cumming WJK, Kingston H, et al. DNA probes in differential diagnosis of Becker muscular dystrophy and spinal muscular atrophy. *Lancet* 1989;1:46–47.
19. Topaloglu H, Renda Y, Kale G, Gucuyener K. Muscular dystrophy or spinal muscular atrophy? *Lancet* 1989;1:960–961.
20. Furukawa T, Nakao K, Sugita H, Tsukagoshi H. Kugelberg-Welander disease with particular reference to sex-influenced manifestations. *Arch Neurol* 1968;19:156–162.
21. Zerres K, Rudnik-Schoneborn S. Natural history in proximal spinal muscular atrophy. *Arch Neurol* 1995;52:518–523.
22. Kugelberg E. Chronic proximal (pseudomyopathic) spinal muscular atrophy. In: Vinkyn PJ, Bruyn GW, eds. *Handbook of clinical neurology*. Amsterdam: North-Holland Publishing Co., 1975:67–80.
23. Zerres K, Rudnik-Schoneborn S, Forrest E, Lusakowska A, Borkowska J, Hausmanowa-Petrusewicz I. A collaborative study on the natural history of childhood and juvenile onset proximal spinal muscular atrophy (type II and III SMA): 569 patients. *J Neurol Sci* 1997;146:67–72.
24. Rudnik-Schoneborn S, Forkert R, Hahnen E, Wirth B, Zerres K. Clinical spectrum and diagnostic criteria of infantile spinal muscular atrophy: further delineation on the basis of SMN gene deletion findings. *Neuropaediatrie* 1996;27:8–15.
25. Parano E, Pavone L, Falsaperla R, Trifiletti R, Wang C. Molecular basis of phenotypic heterogeneity in siblings with spinal muscular atrophy. *Ann Neurol* 1996;40:247–251.
26. Iijama M, Arasaki K, Iwamoto H, Nakanishi T. Maximal and minimal motor nerve conduction velocities in patients with motor neuron disease: correlation with age of onset and duration of illness. *Muscle Nerve* 1991;14:1110–1115.
27. Zellweger H, Schneider HJ, Schuldt DR. A new genetic variant of spinal muscular atrophy. *Neurology* 1969;19:865–869.
28. Hausmanowa-Petrusewicz I, Zaremba J, Borkowska J, Szirkowiec W. Chronic proximal spinal muscular atrophy of childhood and adolescence: sex influence. *J Med Genet* 1984;21:447–450.
29. Jansen PHP, Joosten EMG, Jaspar HHJ, Vingerhoets HM. A rapidly progressive autosomal dominant scapulohumeral form of spinal muscular atrophy. *Ann Neurol* 1986;20:538–540.
30. Shaw PJ, Ince PG, Goodship J, et al. Adult-onset motor neuron disease and infantile Werdnig-Hoffmann disease (spinal muscular atrophy type 1) in the same family. *Neurology* 1992;42:1477–1480.
31. Appelbaum JS, Roos RP, Salazar-Grueso EF, et al. Intrafamilial heterogeneity in hereditary motor neuron disease. *Neurology* 1992;42: 1488–1492.
32. Greenberg F, Fenolio KR, Hejtmaneik JF, et al. X-linked infantile spinal muscular atrophy. *Am J Dis Child* 1988;142:217–219.
33. Kobayashi H, Baumbach L, Matise TC, Schlavi A, Greenberg F, Hoffman EP. A gene for a severe lethal form of X-linked arthrogryposis (X-linked infantile spinal muscular atrophy) maps to human chromosome Xp11.3-q11.2. *Hum Mol Genet* 1995;4:1213–1216.
34. Gilliam TC, Brzustowicz LM, Castilla LH, et al. Genetic homogeneity between acute (SMA I) and chronic (SMA II & III) forms of spinal muscular atrophy. *Nature* 1990;345:823–825.
35. Muller B, Melki J, Burlet P, Clerget-Darpoux F. Proximal spinal muscular atrophy (SMA) types II and III in the same sibship are not caused by different alleles at the SMA locus on 5q. *Am J Hum Genet* 1992;50: 892–895.
36. Munsat TL, Skerry L, Korf B, et al. Phenotypic heterogeneity of spinal muscular atrophy mapping to chromosome 5q11.2-13.3 (SMA 5q). *Neurology* 1990;40:1831–1836.
37. Brzustowicz LM, Lehner T, Castilla LH, et al. Genetic mapping of chronic childhood-onset spinal muscular atrophy to chromosome 5q11.2-13.3. *Nature* 1990;344:540–541.
38. Melki J, Lefebvre S, Burglen L, et al. De novo and inherited deletions of the 5q13 region in spinal muscular atrophies. *Science* 1994;264: 1474–1477.
39. Iannaccone ST, Russman BS, Samaha F, White MS, Buncher CR. Spinal muscular atrophy: functional testing before age 5. *Ann Neurol* 1991;30:502.
40. Melki J, Abdelhak S, Sheth P, et al. Gene for chronic proximal spinal muscular atrophies maps to chromosome 5q. *Nature* 1990;344: 767–768.
41. Roy N, Mahadevan MS, McLean M, et al. The gene for neuronal apop-

tosis inhibitory protein is partially deleted in individuals with spinal muscular atrophy. *Cell* 1995;80:167–178.

42. Lefebvre S, Burglen L, Reboullet S, et al. Identification and characterization of a spinal muscular atrophy-determining gene. *Cell* 1995;80:155–165.

43. Gilliam TC. Is the spinal muscular atrophy gene found? *Nat Med* 1995;1:124–127.

44. Crawford TU. From enigmatic to problematic: the new molecular genetics of childhood spinal muscular atrophy. *Neurology* 1996;46:335–340.

45. Zerres K, Wirth B, Rudnik-Schoneborn S. Spinal muscular atrophy—clinical and genetic correlations. *Neuromusc Disord* 1997;7:202–207.

46. Talbot K. What's new in the molecular genetics of spinal muscular atrophy? *Eur J Pediatr Neurol* 1997;5:149–155.

47. Lefebvre S, Burlet P, Liu Q, et al. Correlation between severity and SMN protein level in spinal muscular atrophy. *Nat Genet* 1997;16:265–269.

48. Eng GD, Binder H, Koch B. Spinal muscular atrophy: experience in diagnosis and rehabilitation management of 60 patients. *Arch Phys Med Rehabil* 1984;65:549–553.

49. Bach JR. Update and perspective on noninvasive respiratory muscle aids. *Chest* 1994;105:1538–1544.

50. Bach JR. Management of chronic alveolar hypoventilation by nasal ventilation. *Chest* 1990;97:52–57.

51. Bach JR, Alba AS. Intermittent abdominal pressure ventilator in a regimen of noninvasive ventilatory support. *Chest* 1991;99:630–636.

52. Wang T, Bach JR, Avilla C, Alba AS, Yang GW. Survival of individuals with spinal muscular atrophy on ventilatory support. *Am J Phys Med Rehabil* 1994;73:207–211.

53. Shapiro F, Specht L. The diagnosis and orthopaedic treatment of childhood spinal muscular atrophy, peripheral neuropathy, Friedreich ataxia, and arthrogryposis. *J Bone Joint Surg Am* 1993;75:1699–1714.

54. Piasecki JO, Mahinpour S, Levine DB. Long-term follow-up of spinal fusion in Spinal Muscular Atrophy. *Clin Ortho Rel Res* 1986;207:44–54.

55. Aprin H, Bowen JR, MacEwen GD, Hall JE. Spine fusion in patients with spinal muscular atrophy. *J Bone Joint Surg* 1982;64:1179–1187.

56. Daher YH, Lonstein JE, Winter RB, Bradford DS. Spinal surgery in spinal muscular atrophy. *J Pediatr Orthoped* 1985;5:391–395.

57. Siegel IM, Silverman M. Upright mobility system for spinal muscular atrophy patients. *Arch Phys Med Rehabil* 1984;65:418.

58. Whelan TB. Neuropsychological performance of children with Duchenne muscular dystrophy and spinal muscle atrophy. *Dev Med Child Neurol* 1987;29:212–220.

Motor Disorders,
edited by David S. Younger.
Lippincott Williams & Wilkins, Philadelphia © 1999.

CHAPTER 31

Recent Progress in Understanding the Inherited Motor Neuron Diseases

Robert H. Brown, Jr.

Over the last 10 years there has been substantial progress in understanding the genetic and molecular basis for several inherited motor neuron diseases (Table 1). An understanding of the range of genetic defects that cause diverse forms of motor neuron degeneration both illuminates the pathogenesis of the diseases and provides insight into the biologic properties of motor neurons. Ultimately, such studies should lead both to new diagnostic approaches to these diseases and ultimately to suggest new strategies for their treatment. This review briefly summarizes recent research advances in this field.

DOMINANT (ADULT-ONSET) AMYOTROPHIC LATERAL SCLEROSIS

About 10% of amyotrophic lateral sclerosis (ALS) cases are inherited as an autosomal dominant trait (familial ALS–autosomal dominant [FALS-AD]). FALS-AD is clinically and pathologically indistinguishable from sporadic and thus appears to share important pathogenic mechanisms with sporadic ALS. Both sporadic and FALS are almost invariably lethal, with a median survival of less than 5 years (1). Pathologic findings in FALS include degeneration and loss of large motor neurons in the cerebral cortex, brainstem, and cervical and lumbar spinal cord. Occasionally, there is subclinical involvement of nonmotor cells and tracts in the central nervous system. These include the posterior columns, Clarke's column, and the spinocerebellar tracts (2–4). In 1993, a multicenter collaborative study identified several mutations in the gene for Cu/Zn superoxide dismutase in FALS-AD (5).

R.H. Brown: Department of Neurology, Harvard Medical School, Boston Massachusetts 02115 and Massachusetts General Hospital, Charlestown, Massachusetts 02129.

Cu/Zn superoxide dismutase 1 (SOD1) is a protein of 153 amino acids encoded by five exons within the SOD1 locus (6). The *SOD1* gene has been highly conserved during evolution; it is expressed in multiple cell types in many species (7). Its primary function is to detoxify the superoxide free radical O_2^-, converting it to H_2O_2. In turn, peroxide is converted to water through the action of either catalase or glutathione peroxidase (7,8). As a free radical, the superoxide anion can interact with numerous cellular constituents (e.g., DNA, lipid, carbohydrate, protein) to be cytotoxic. It is important to note that there are mechanisms whereby H_2O_2 can also generate free radicals. For example, in the Fenton reaction, transition metals such as iron or copper interact with superoxide anion to form the hydroxyl radical OH^-. This species of free radical interacts on formation with any cellular constituent at hand (9,10). Taken broadly, these data suggest that FALS-AD occurs because motor neurons are unusually sensitive to disturbances of free radical homeostasis. A corollary premise is that sporadic ALS is also a free radical disorder. Indeed, experimental studies of ALS tissues support this contention; levels of two markers of oxidative molecular injury, carbonyl proteins and oxidatively modified DNA, are abundant in ALS spinal cord (11).

The mechanisms whereby mutations in the *SOD1* gene trigger ALS are not clear. Some ALS tissues bearing some mutant forms of ALS have reduced SOD1 activity, as do the red cell lysates in some cases (12,13). However, this loss of activity is not uniform. Especially in light of the dominant mode of inheritance of FALS, these facts argue strongly that the neurotoxic properties of mutant SOD1 protein are acquired, adverse, and directly a consequence of the mutation. Two additional findings corroborate this view. First, mice generated with inactivation of the *SOD1* gene do not demonstrate exaggerated motor neuronal cell death, although their neurons have a sub-

TABLE 1. *Inherited motor neuron disorders*

Disease	Defect	Locus	Reference
Lower motor neurons			
Spinal muscular atrophy	Spinal motor neuron (SMN)	5q11,2-13.3	72
GM2 gangliosidoses			
Late onset Tay-Sachs disease	Hex A deficiency (alpha subunit)	15q23-24	50
Sandhoff disease	Hex A + B deficiency (beta subunit)	5q11.2-13.6	51
AB variant	GM2 activator protein	5q	51
X-linked spinal bulbar	Androgen receptor	Xq11	55
Other			
Scapuloperoneal SMA			41, 73, 74
Facioscapulohumeral SMA			
Fazio-Londe disease			
Upper and lower motor neurons			
(amyotrophic lateral sclerosis)			
Dominant ALS, adult onset	Superoxide dismutase	21q	5
	Neurofilament, heavy subunit	11	75
Dominant ALS, juvenile onset		9q	76
Recessive ALS, juvenile onset		2q33	77
ALS with dementia and Parkinsonism		17q	78
ALS with Pick disease			79
Upper motor neurons (familial spastic paraplegia)			
Dominant		2p	64
		14q	65
		15q	66
Recessive	Proteolipid myelin protein	Xq22	68
	LICAM	Xq28	69
Adrenoleukodystrophy	ATP binding protein	Xq28	80

SMA, spinal muscular atrophy.

normal capacity to resist physical and metabolic stress (14). Second, it is striking that mice expressing high levels of mutant SOD1, with normal or greater than normal total SOD1 activity, develop a phenotype that is clinically and pathologically stunningly like human FALS (15).

The nature of the adverse property of the mutant SOD1 protein has been elusive, although possible explanations arise. Several are predicated on the observation that the mutations seem to diminish the stability of the SOD1 protein, shortening its half-life (16,17) and potentially opening up the folded structure of the protein. One consequence of this change might be either release of copper and zinc into the cytosol or enhanced exposure of molecules in the cytosol to the bound copper and zinc. Another consequence of aberrant SOD1 folding might be enhanced access of atypical substrates to the active channel of the protein. Thus, it has been proposed that the mutations enhance the interaction of peroxynitrite with SOD1, increasing formation of nitrotyrosine groups (18–20). Depending on the particular tyrosine residues that are nitrated, this process may be injurious. Examples might include tyrosines in neurotrophic factor receptors functioning as tyrosine kinases. Recent studies document that nitration of tyrosines on neurofilament subunits can impair neurofilament maturation (21). Over the last year, reports have documented that free nitrotyrosine levels are increased in both human and murine ALS (22–24). The significance of these findings has not been defined.

Another proposed mechanism for neurotoxicity of mutant SOD1 invokes enhanced ability of the mutant protein to act as a peroxidase, using substrates like H_2O_2 to generate hyrdoxyl radicals (25–27). Yet another mechanism invokes abnormal protein binding and aggregation as the primary source of toxicity. Thus, one report indicates that mutant SOD1 protein binds proteins not normally bound by wild-type SOD1 (28); an alternate possibility is that SOD1 itself may aggregate and precipitate (29). Consistent with this is the finding that cytoskeletal aggregates in motor neurons in ALS may contain SOD1 protein (30–33). However, the specificity of this finding is unclear because such SOD1-positive deposits are seen in both sporadic and FALS.

Regardless of the specific chemistry implicated, several lines of inquiry demonstrate that one consequence of the presence of mutant SOD1 protein is activation of one or more apoptotic cell death pathways. In neurons in vitro, forced expression of mutant SOD1 is clearly proapoptotic (34–36), whereas the wild-type SOD1 molecule is distinctly antiapoptotic (37–40). In the ALS mice in vivo, inactivation of caspase 1 (interleukin-converting enzyme 1) produces a modest but statistically significant increase in disease duration (41); overexpression of Bcl-2 significantly delays disease onset (42). These observations are consistent with a role for apoptotic death as one element in the pathogenesis of motor neuron degeneration in these mice but by no means can be interpreted to exclude neuronal death via other nonapoptotic pathways. Clear data have not emerged confirming evidence of apoptosis in ALS autopsy tissues, although two initial reports are consistent with this possibility (43,44).

RECESSIVE (JUVENILE-ONSET) AMYOTROPHIC LATERAL SCLEROSIS

Ben Hamida et al. (45) described a form of motor neuron disease characterized by chronic slow degeneration of both upper and lower motor neurons. This juvenile-onset disease is inherited as an autosomal recessive trait; survival may be decades. Clinically, the lower motor neuron findings resemble those in denervating polyneuropathy. Nonetheless, some affected individuals are also markedly spastic and may demonstrate pseudobulbar disturbances of affect. Cognition is normal in affected individuals. Autopsy tissue has not yet been examined in these cases. A genetic locus for a form of this disease has been defined, but the underlying gene defect is not yet known (46).

ADULT-ONSET TAY-SACHS DISEASE

Although GM2 gangliosidosis usually is evident in early childhood, there are variant forms (adult-onset Tay-Sachs disease) that have a clinical phenotype resembling a lower motor neuropathy (47). Patients with this illness usually offer a history of lifelong motor incoordination. As young adults, they note the subtle onset of progressive proximal muscle weakness with features indicating lower motor neuron dysfunction (fasciculations, mild denervation atrophy, and electromyographic abnormalities). This may then evolve to frank leg weakness, sometimes with dysarthria. Some patients also show psychiatric manifestations (e.g., anxiety, subnormal attention span, or even psychotic episodes) (48). Some patients may reveal spasticity and Babinski signs as the illness progresses. Involvement of the central nervous system is indicated not only by the corticospinal signs but also some atrophy, particularly in the cerebellum. A salient pathologic finding is the presence of distended neurons with periodic acid-Schiff–positive inclusions (49).

The underlining defect in this disease is an accumulation of GM2 ganglioside, which is normally metabolized by N-acetyl-hexosaminidases A and B (Hex A and B); these are dimeric enzymes made up of two polypeptides. An alpha and beta subunit are combined in HEX A, and HEX B has two beta subunits. The activity of both enzymes is augmented by GM2 activator protein, which enhances access of substrate to the enzyme. The genes for the alpha and beta subunits are encoded on chromosomes l5q and 5q (50). The GM2 activator protein may be encoded on chromosome 5 (51). Patient DNA analysis reveals mutations in the alpha and beta subunits and the GM2 activator protein (52,53).

X-LINKED SPINAL BULBAR ATROPHY

The hallmark of this disorder is a slowly progressive lower motor neuropathy arising in adult males (54). Unlike the situation in ALS, pathology in X-linked spinal bulbar atrophy is confined to lower motor neurons. Moreover, the time course is slower than in ALS. In X-linked spinal bulbar atrophy, there may be gynecomastia and testicular atrophy with reduced fertility. LaSpada et al. (55) discovered that the molecular defect in X-linked spinal bulbar atrophy is an expansion of a CAG repeat in the first exon of the androgen receptor gene. This expands a polyglutamine tract within the receptor. It is apparent that as the length of the tract of CAGs increases, the illness becomes more severe (56). It is not clear how this molecular lesion causes motor neuron disease. However, important insights have come from the discoveries that there are diverse inherited neurodegenerative diseases associated with CAG repeat expansions, including Huntington's disease and several of the spinocerebellar ataxias; in each of these, there is a predicted polyglutamine expansion; and in each, careful ultramicroscopy and analysis with antibodies to expanded glutamine tracts document the presence of intranuclear inclusions of protein consisting in part of polyglutamine (57). That these are abnormal is indicated in part by their aggregation within nuclei and in part by the fact that they are ubiquitinated (57).

SPINAL MUSCULAR ATROPHY

The spinal muscular atrophies are discussed in detail in Chapter 30. Briefly, this family of disorders characterized by progressive degeneration of motor neurons in the brainstem and spinal cord is caused by deficiencies of a survival motor neuron or SMN protein. Recent studies indicate that SMN is important in the formation and function of spliceosomes and thus is important in the processes of splicing of nuclear and nucleolar RNA (58,59).

FAMILIAL SPASTIC PARAPLEGIA

Familial spastic paraplegia (FSP) is an autosomal dominant disorder characterized by slowly worsening spastic weakness that typically starts in the distal legs (60,61). Although the age at onset is variable, in a large preponderance of families the disease begins in the third or fourth decade. Many patients live several decades with this illness. Sphincter disturbance and weakness of the upper extremities are uncommon but may be seen late in the course. By the same token, minor sensory loss may be evident in late-stage FSP. The most prominent pathologic feature in FSP is degeneration of the corticospinal tracts (62). Rarely, FSP is associated with involvement of other regions of the nervous system (63) and thus may entail amytrophy, mental retardation, optic atrophy, and sensory neuropathy. Although these complex forms of the disease attest to the difficulty in classifying subtypes of FSP, it seems likely that genetic and molecular studies will clarify these nosologic issues. For example, in only the last 5 years, loci for FSP have been identified on chromosomes 2p (64), 14q (65), and 15q (66). X-linked and recessive forms of FSP are also encountered; the latter is more common in regions with consanguinity (67). Atypical FSP has been associated with mutations in genes encoding the proteolipid protein (68) and the cell adhesion protein L1CAM (69). A form of adrenoleukodystrophy (adrenomyeloneuropathy) can resemble FSP (70,71).

REFERENCES

1. Mulder D, Kurland L, Offord K, Beard C. Familial adult motor neuron disease: amyotrophic lateral sclerosis. *Neurology* 1986;36:511–517.
2. Tanaka J, Nakamura H, Tabuchi Y, Takahasi K. Familial amyotrophic lateral sclerosis: features of multi-system degeneration. *Acta Neuropathol* 1984;64:22–29.
3. Horton WA, Eldridge R, Brody JA. Familial motor neuron disease: evidence for at least three different types. *Neurology* 1976;26:460–465.
4. Hirano A, Kurland L, Sayre G. Familial amyotrophic lateral sclerosis. A subgroup characterized by posterior and spinocerebellar tract involvement and hyaline inclusions in the anterior horn cells. *Arch Neurol* 1967;16:232–243.
5. Rosen DR, Siddique T, Patterson D, et al. Mutations in Cu/Zn superoxide dismutase gene are associated with familial amyotrophic lateral sclerosis. *Nature* 1993;362:59–62.
6. Levanon D, Lieman-Hurwitz J, Dafni N, et al. Architecture and anatomy of the chromosomal locus in human chromosome 21 encoding the Cu/Zn superoxide dismutase. *EMBO J* 1985;4:77–84.
7. Fridovich I. Superoxide radical and superoxide dismutases. *Annu Rev Biochem* 1995;64:97–112.
8. Fridovich I. Superoxide anion radical ($O_2^{-\cdot}$), superoxide dismutases and related matters. *J Biol Chem* 1997;272:18515–18517.
9. Halliwell B, Gutteridge JM. Role of free radicals and catalytic metal ions in human disease: an overview. *Methods Enzymol* 1990;186:1–85.
10. Halliwell B, Aruoma OI. Molecular biology of free radical scavenging systems. Cold Spring Harbor, NY: Cold Spring Harbor Laboratory Press, 1992:47–67.
11. Ferrante R, Browne S, Shinobu L, et al. Evidence of increased oxidative damage in both sporadic and familial amyotrophic lateral sclerosis. *J Neurochem* 1997;69:2064–2074.
12. Bowling AC, Schulz JB, Brown RHJ, Beal MF. Superoxide dismutase activity, oxidative damage and mitochondrial energy metabolism in familial and sporadic amyotrophic lateral sclerosis. *J Neurochem* 1993;61:2322–2325.
13. Bowling A, Barkowski E, McKenna-Yasek D, et al. Superoxide dismutase concentration and activity in familial amyotrophic lateral sclerosis. *J Neurochem* 1995;64:2366–2369.
14. Reaume A, Elliott J, Hoffman E, et al. Motor neurons in Cu/Zn superoxide dismutase-deficient mice develop normally but exhibit enhanced cell death after axonal injury. *Nat Genet* 1996;13:43–47.
15. Gurney ME, Pu H, Chiu AY, et al. Motor neuron degeneration in mice that express a human Cu,Zn superoxide dismutase mutation. *Science* 1994;264:1772–1775.
16. Borchelt DR, Lee MK, Slunt HS, et al. Superoxide dismutase 1 with mutations linked to familial amyotrophic lateral sclerosis possesses significant activity. *Proc Natl Acad Sci USA* 1994;91:8292–8296.
17. Borchelt DR, Guarnieri M, Wong P-C, et al. Superoxide dismutase 1 subunits with mutations linked to familial amyotrophic lateral sclerosis do not affect wild-type subunit function. *J Biol Chem* 1995;270:1–5.
18. Ischiropoulos H, Zhu L, Chen J, et al. Peroxynitrite-mediated tyrosine nitration catalyzed by superoxide dismutase. *Arch Biochem Biophys* 1992;298:431–437.
19. Beckman JS, Carson M, Smith CD, Kuppenol WH. ALS, SOD, and peroxynitrite. *Nature* 1993;364:584.
20. Crow J, Sampson J, Zhuang Y, Thompson J, Beckman J. Decreased zinc affinity of amyotrophic lateral sclerosis—associated superoxide dismutase mutants leads to enhanced catalysis of tyrosine nitration by peroxynitrite. *J Neurochem* 1997;69:1936–1944.
21. Crow J, Ye Y, Strong M, Kirk M, Barnes S, Beckman J. Superoxide dismutase catalyzes nitration of tyrosines by peroxynitrite in the rod and head domains of neurofilament-L. *J Neurochem* 1997;69:1945–1953.
22. Bruijn L, Beal M, Becher M, et al. Elevated free nitrotyrosine levels but not protein-bound nitrotyrosine or hydroxyl radicals, throughout amyotrophic lateral sclerosis (ALS)-like disease implicate tyrosine nitration as an aberrant in vivo property of one familial ALS-liked superoxide dismutase 1 mutant. *Proc Natl Acad Sci USA* 1997;94:7606–7611.
23. Beal M, Ferrante R, Browne S, Matthews R, Kowall N, Brown R Jr. Increased 3-nitrotyrosine in both sporadic and familial amyotrophic lateral sclerosis. *Ann Neurol* 1997;42:644–654.
24. Ferrante R, Shinobu L, Schultz J, et al. Increased 3-nitrotyrosine and oxidative damage in mice with human copper zinc superoxide dismutase mutations. *Ann Neurol* 1997;42:326–334.
25. Wiedau-Pazos M, Goto J, Rabizadeh S, et al. Altered reactivity of superoxide dismutase in familial amyotrophic lateral sclerosis. *Science* 1996;271:515–518.
26. Yim M, Kang J, Yim H, Kwak H, Chock P, Stadtman E. A gain-of-function mutation of an amyotrophic lateral sclerosis-associated Cu,Zn-superoxide dismutase mutant: an enhancement of free radical formation due to a decrease in Km for hydrogen peroxide. *Proc Natl Acad Sci USA* 1996;93:5709–5714.
27. Yim H, Kang J, Chock P, Stadtman E, Yim M. A familial amyotrophic lateral sclerosis-associated A4V Cu,Zn superoxide dismutase mutant has a lower Km for hydrogen peroxide. Correlation between severity and the Km value. *J Biol Chem* 1997;272:8861–8863.
28. Kunst C, Mezey E, Brownstein M, Patterson D. Mutations in SOD1 associated with familial ALS cause novel protein interactions. *Nat Genet* 1997;15:91–94.
29. Brown RH Jr. Amyotrophic lateral sclerosis: recent insights from genetics and transgenic mice. *Cell* 1995;80.867–892.
30. Shibata N, Hirano A, Kobayashi A, et al. Immunohistochemical demonstration of Cu/Zn superoxide dismutase in the spinal cord of patients with familial amyotrophic lateral sclerosis. *Acta Histochem Cytochem* 1993;26:619–622.
31. Shibata N, Hirano A, Kobayashi M, et al. Cu/Zn superoxide dismutase-like immunoreactivity in Lewy body-like inclusions of sporadic amyotrophic lateral sclerosis. *Neurosci Lett* 1994;179:149–152.
32. Shibata N, Hirano A, Kobayashi M, et al. Intense superoxide dismutase-1 immunoreactivity in intracytoplasmic hyaline inclusions of familial amyotrophic lateral sclerosis with posterior column involvement. *J Neuropathol Exp Neurol* 1996;4:481–490.
33. Chou S, Wang H, Komai K. Colocalization of NOS and SOD1 in neurofilament accumulations within motor neurons of amyotrophic lateral sclerosis: an immunohistochemical study. *J Chem Neuroanat* 1996;10:249–258.
34. Durham H, Roy J, Dong L, Figlewicz D. Aggregation of mutant Cu/Zn superoxide dismutase proteins in a culture model of ALS. *J Neuropathol Exp Neurol* 1997;56:523–530.
35. Ghadge G, Lee J, Bindokas V, et al. Mutant superoxide dismutase-1-linked familial amyotrophic lateral sclerosis: molecular mechanisms of neuronal death and protection. *J Neurosci* 1997;17:8756–8766.
36. Rabizadeh S, Gralla E, Borchelt D, et al. Mutations associated with amyotrophic lateral sclerosis convert superoxide dismutase from an antiapoptotic gene to a proapoptotic gene: studies in yeast and neural cells. *Proc Natl Acad Sci USA* 1995;92:3024–3028.
37. Greenlund L, Deckwerth T, Johnson E. Superoxide dismutase delays neuronal apoptosis: a role for reactive oxygen species in programmed neuronal death. *Neuron* 1995;14:303–315.
38. Rothstein JD, Bristol LA, Hosler BA, Brown RH Jr, Kuncl RW. Chronic inhibition of superoxide dismutase produces apoptotic death of spinal neurons. *Proc Natl Acad Sci USA* 1994;91:4155–4159.
39. Troy CM, Shelanski M. Down-regulation of copper/zinc superoxide dismutase causes apoptotic death in PC12 neuronal cells. *Proc Natl Acad Sci USA* 1994;91:6384–6387.
40. Troy C, Derossi D, Prochiantz A, Greene L, Shelanski M. Downregulation of Cu/Zn superoxide dismutase leads to cell death via the nitric oxide-peroxynitrite pathway. *J Neurosci* 1996;16:253–261.
41. Friedlander R, Brown RH Jr J, Gagliardini V, Wang J, Wang J. Inhibition of ICE slows ALS in mice. *Nature* 1997;388:31.

42. Kostic V, Jackson-Lewis V, Bilbao FD, Dubois-Dauphin M, Przedborski S. Bcl-2: prolonging life in a transgenic mouse model of familial amyotrophic lateral sclerosis. *Science* 1997;277:559–562.

43. Mu X, He J, Anderson D, Trojanowski J, Springer J. Altered expression of bcl-2 and bax mRNA in amyotrophic lateral sclerosis spinal cord motor neurons. *Ann Neurol* 1996;40:379–386.

44. Troost D, Aten J, Morsink F, Jong JD. Apoptosis in not restricted to motoneurons: Bcl-2 expression is increased in post-central cortex, adjacent to affected motor cortex. *J Neurol Sci* 1995;129[Suppl]:79–80.

45. Ben Hamida M, Hentati F, Ben Hamida C. Hereditary motor system diseases (chronic juvenile amyotrophic lateral sclerosis). Conditions combining a bilateral pyramidal syndrome with limb and bulbar atrophy. *Brain* 1990;113:347–363.

46. Hentati A, Bejaoui K, Pericak-Vance MA, et al. Linkage of recessive familial amyotrophic lateral sclerosis to chromosome 2q33-35. *Nat Genet* 1994;7:425–428.

47. Kolodny EH. The GM2 gangliosidoses. In: Rosenberg RN, et al., eds. *The molecular and genetic basis of neurological disease.* Oxford: Butterworth-Heinemann, 1992:531–540.

48. Streifler H, Golomb M, Gadoth N. Psychiatric features of adult GM2 gangliosidosis. *Br J Psych* 1989;155:410–413.

49. Klenk E. On gangliosides. *Am J Child Dis* 1959;9:711–714.

50. Takeda K, Nakai H, Hagiwara H, et al. Fine assignment of beta-hexosaminidase A alpha subunit on 15q23-24 by high resolution in situ hybridization. *Tohoku J Exp Med* 1990;160:203–211.

51. Burg J, Conzelmann E, Sandhoff K, Solomon E, Swallow D. Mapping of the gene coding for the human GM2-activator protein to chromosome 5. *Ann Hum Genet* 1985;49:41–45.

52. Myerowitz R. Tay-Sachs disease-causing mutations and neutral polymorphisms and neutral polymorphisms in the Hex A gene. *Hum Mutat* 1997;9:195–208.

53. Natowicz M, Prence E. Heterozygote screening for Tay-Sachs disease: past successes and future challenges. *Curr Opin Pediatr* 1996;8:625–629.

54. Kennedy WB, Alter M, Sung JG. Report of an X-linked form of spinal muscular atrophy. *Neurology* 1968;18:671–680.

55. LaSpada AR, Wilson EM, Lubahn DB, Harding AE, Fischbeck KH. Androgen receptor gene mutations in X-linked spinal and bulbar muscular atrophy. *Nature* 1991;352:77–79.

56. LaSpada AR, Roling DB, Harding AE, et al. Meiotic instability and genotype-phenotype correlation of the trinucleotide repeat in X-linked spinal and bulbar muscular atrophy. *Nat Genet* 1992;2:301–304.

57. Davies S, Turmaine M, Cozens B, et al. Formation of neuronal intranuclear inclusions underlies the neurological dysfunction in mice transgenic for the HD mutation. *Cell* 1997;90:537–548.

58. Fischer U, Liu Q, Dreyfuss G. The SMN-SIP1 complex has an essential role in spliceosomal snRNP biogenesis. *Cell* 1997;90:1023–1029.

59. Liu Q, Fischer U, Wang F, Dreyfuss G. The spinal muscular atrophy disease gene product, SMN, and its associated protein SIP-1 are in a complex with spliceosomal snRNP proteins. *Cell* 1997;90:1013–1021.

60. Harding AE. Hereditary "pure" spastic paraplegia: a clinical and genetic study of 22 families. *J Neurol Neurosurg Psychiatry* 1981;44:871–883.

61. Harding AE. Hereditary "pure" spastic paraplegia. In: *The hereditary ataxias and related disorders.* London: Churchill Livingstone, 1984:174–190.

62. Behan WMH, Maia M. Strumpell's familial spastic paraplegia: genetics and neuropathology. *J Neurol Neurosurg Psychiatry* 1974;37:8–20.

63. Harding AE. Complicated forms of hereditary spastic paraplegia. In: *The hereditary ataxias and related disorders.* London: Churchill Livingstone, 1984:191–213.

64. Hazan J, Fontaine B, Bruyn R, et al. Linkage to a new locus for autosomal dominant familial spastic paraplegia to chromosome 2p. *Hum Mol Genet* 1994;3:1569–1573.

65. Hazan J, Lamy C, Melki J, Munnich A, deRecondo J, Weissenbach J. Autosomal dominant familial spastic paraplegia is genetically heterogeneous and one locus maps to chromosome 14q. *Nat Genet* 1993;5:163–167.

66. Fink JK, Wu CT, Jones SM, et al. Autosomal dominant familial spastic paraplegia: tight linkage to chromosome 15q. *Am J Hum Genet* 1995;56:188–192.

67. Hentati A, Pericak-Vance MA, Hung WY, et al. Linkage of "pure" autosomal recessive familial spastic paraplegia to chromosome 8 markers and evidence of genetic locus heterogeneity. *Hum Mol Genet* 1994;3:1263–1267.

68. Saugier-Veber P, Munnich A, Bonneau D, et al. X-linked spastic paraplegia and Pelizaeus-Merzbacher disease are allelic disorders at the proteolipid protein locus. *Nat Genet* 1994;6:257–262.

69. Jouet M, Rosenthal A, Armstrong G, et al. X-linked spastic paraplegia (SPG1) MASA syndrome, and X-linked hydrocephalus result from mutations in the L1 gene. *Nat Genet* 1994;7:402–407.

70. Powers J, Moser H. Peroxisomal disorders: genotype, phenotype, major neuropathologic lesions, and pathogenesis. *Brain Pathol* 1998;8:101–120.

71. Moser H. Clinical and therapeutic aspects of adrenoleukodystrophy and adrenomyeloneuropathy. *J Neuropathol Exp Neurol* 1995;54:740–745.

72. Lefebvre S, Bürglen L, Reboullet S, et al. Identification and characterization of a spinal muscular atrophy-determining gene. *Cell* 1995;80:155–165.

73. Kaeser H. Scapuloperoneal muscular atrophy. *Brain* 1965;88:407–418.

74. DeLong R, Siddique T. A large New England kindred with autosomal dominant neurogenic scapuloperoneal amytrophy with unique features. *Arch Neurol* 1992;49:905–908.

75. Figlewicz DA, Krizus A, Martinoli MG, et al. Variants of the heavy neurofilament subunit are associated with the development of amyotrophic lateral sclerosis. *Hum Mol Genet* 1994;3:1757–1761.

76. Chance P. Linkage of autosomal recessive ALS of childhood onset to chromosome 9. 1996.

77. Hentati A, Pericak-Vance M, Lennon F, et al. Linkage of a locus for autosomal dominant familial spastic paraplegia to chromosome 2p markers. *Hum Mol Genet* 1994;3:1867–1871.

78. Wilhelmsen K, Lynch T, Pavlou E, Higgins M, Nygaard T. Localization of disinhibition-dementia-parkinsonism-amytrophy complex to 17q21-22. *Am J Hum Genet* 1994;55:1159–1165.

79. Constantinidis J. A familial syndrome: a combination of Pick's disease and amyotrophic lateral sclerosis. *Encephale* 1987;13:285–293.

80. Mosser J, Douar A, Sarde C, et al. Putative X-linked adrenoleukodystrophy gene shares unexpected homology with ABC transporters. *Nature* 1993;361:726–730.

Motor Disorders,
edited by David S. Younger.
Lippincott Williams & Wilkins, Philadelphia © 1999.

CHAPTER 32

Amyotrophic Lateral Sclerosis

Dale J. Lange

CLINICAL DEFINITIONS

Amyotrophic lateral sclerosis (ALS) was recognized as a distinct clinical and neuropathologic entity more than a century ago (1). The unique neuropathologic findings include anterior horn cell degeneration producing muscle atrophy or amyotrophy and degeneration and sclerosis of the corticospinal tracts. The clinical lower motor neuron (LMN) manifestations due to anterior horn cell loss include weakness, wasting, and fasciculation, with upper motor neuron (UMN) signs due to corticospinal tract degeneration recognized by hyperreflexia, spasticity, clonus, and Hoffmann and Babinski signs. The clinical spectrum of motor neuron disease (MND) is broad, with some patients manifesting LMN signs alone without signs of corticospinal tract dysfunction, so defining progressive spinal muscular atrophy (PSMA), and others demonstrating UMN without LMN signs in the syndrome of primary lateral sclerosis (PLS) (3). The signs of progressive bulbar palsy and bulbar-onset ALS reflect predominant motor neuron loss in the brainstem, supplying the lingual and pharyngeal muscles that leads to early or predominant dysarthria, dysphagia, and respiratory insufficiency (2). MND localized to a single limb is termed monomelic amyotrophy.

There is no marker that uniquely identifies the process of ALS during life; therefore, the diagnosis is absolutely confirmed at postmortem examination. However, in the presence of the classic clinical syndrome, confidence of the diagnosis probably approaches 98%. It is when portions of the clinical syndrome are missing that confidence decreases and the opportunity for other diseases masquerading as ALS becomes a significant issue. Brisk reflexes in limbs exhibiting weakness, wasting, and twitching are probable UMN signs (2). Patients with probable UMN signs and PSMA have the greatest likeli-

hood of having an alternative diagnosis, for example, multifocal motor neuropathy, lymphoma, paraproteinemia, or endocrinopathy. Patients with UMN signs alone and pseudobulbar palsy probably have PLS (3).

The World Federation of Neurology El Escorial Diagnostic Criteria (Table 1) (4) provide a useful scheme for the clinical classification of ALS. For classification purposes, LMN signs consist of weakness, atrophy, and fasciculation. UMN findings consist of overactive tendon reflexes, spasticity, Hoffmann and Babinski signs, and pseudobulbar features. The regions of the body are classified into bulbar, cervical, thoracic, and lumbosacral. Patients with definite ALS have UMN and LMN signs in

TABLE 1. *El Escorial criteria for the diagnosis of amyotrophic lateral sclerosis (ALS)*

The diagnosis of definite ALS requires
  Signs of lower motor neuron degeneration by clinical, electrophysiologic, or neuropathologic examination
  Signs of upper motor neuron degeneration by clinical examination
  Progressive spread of signs within a region or to other regions
  Bulbar and two body regions affected or three body regions affected
Probable ALS
  At least two regions of the body affected by UMN and LMN signs
Possible ALS
  UMN and LMN signs in one region
  UMN signs alone are present in two or more regions
  UMN signs are above UMN signs
  Monmelic ALS, progressive bulbar palsy without spinal UMN or LMN signs, and primary lateral sclerosis without signs of LMN signs may be classified as probable ALS
Suspected ALS
  Manifested as LMN signs in two or more regions (UMN pathology may be demonstrated at autopsy but there are no clinical signs)

UMN, LMN, upper and lower motor neuron.

D. J. Lange: Neurological Institute, New York Presbyterian Hospital, New York, New York 10032.

three spinal regions or bulbar region and two spinal regions. Those with probable ALS have UMN and LMN signs in at least two regions. Possible ALS patients have UMN and LMN signs in one region and UMN signs alone in two or more regions. Suspected ALS has LMN signs in two or more regions. Prognosis is not clearly related to the particular clinical syndrome; however, long-term survival is best with PSMA followed by PLS, ALS, and bulbar palsy. The shortened survival of progressive bulbar palsy and bulbar-onset ALS is due to prominent involvement of swallowing and breathing.

In 5 to 10% of ALS patients, a genetic basis is demonstrable, so termed familial ALS (FALS). The mode of transmission is usually autosomal dominant. FALS-autosomal dominant behaves in a stereotypic manner in successive generations with similar age at onset and course. In 30 to 40% of patients so studied, there is a mutation in the copper/zinc superoxide dismutase (Cu/ZnSOD) gene located on chromosome 21 (5).

CLINICAL PRESENTATION

The annual incidence of ALS is approximately 1 to 2 per 100,000 in developed countries (range, 0.5 to 2.4 per 100,000) (6). The average age at onset is 56 and is more common in men than women (1.3:1). It is less common below the age of 40 and rare below 30. The youngest patient I encountered was 17 years old. The average duration of illness is 3 to 5 years with a large variation in the duration of disease course (7,8), with some patients expiring weeks to months after diagnosis and others surviving decades. Most patients complain of weakness or some functional impairment that results from weakness, such as difficulty writing, buttoning, or holding onto objects indicative of involvement of the arms and frequent stumbling, tripping, and occasionally falls reflecting involvement of the legs. ALS can be misdiagnosed as painless radiculopathy before electromyography (EMG) studies are performed, especially when the signs and symptoms are restricted to a single limb or adjacent root. Occasional patients have isolated weakness of neck extension muscles leading to forward drooping of the head or floppy head syndrome. Hoarseness, slurred speech, and drooling precedes frank respiratory and pharyngeal muscle involvement in patients with bulbar involvement and can lead to complaints of sleep disruption and easy fatigability. Asymmetry and relentless progression of symptoms is diagnostically important. Although fasciculation is common, seldom is it the presenting complaint; rather, it is usually pointed out by the physician to the astonishment of the patient. Muscle twitching without focal weakness or bulbar complaints at presentation is more likely due to a benign disorder rather than ALS. The neurologic examination provides the foundation for the diagnosis of ALS and should demonstrate

the combination of LMN and UMN signs already described. EMG and nerve conditions should be performed in all patients with suspected ALS to confirm the diagnosis.

DIFFERENTIAL DIAGNOSIS AND DIAGNOSTIC TESTING

The recommended evaluation for suspected patients is summarized in Table 2. The singular role of testing in ALS is to confirm the diagnosis and confidently eliminate other disorders that may bear clinical resemblance to it and identify other potentially serious and treatable disorders toward which therapy might also be directed. Clinically apparent or occult Hodgkin and non-Hodgkin lymphoma or macroglobulinemia may be the cause of a motor neuron syndrome resembling PSMA or ALS. Motor neuropathy may be clinically indistinguishable from PSMA. Patients with multifocal motor neuropathy resembling ALS-probable UMN signs with or without GM1 antibodies may have overactive or retained tendon reflexes despite weakness, wasting, and twitching (9,10). The importance of making the diagnosis of multifocal motor neuropathy is that such patients respond dramatically to intravenous immunoglobulin (11). There is little rationale for the routine evaluation of antibodies to GM1 gangliosides and myelin-associated glycoprotein in otherwise typical cases of ALS, because they are rarely

TABLE 2. *Diagnostic evaluation*

1. Blood: CBC, differential, ESR, chemistries (glucose, NA, K, Cl, CO_2, BUN, creatinine, Ca, PO_4, albumin, bilirubin, AST, ALT, LDH, alkaline phosphatase, CK), quantitative immunoglobulins, immunofixation electrophoresis, T-cell subsets, latex fixation, ANA, lyme, GM1, MAG antibodies.
2. Muscle biopsy if an immunologically mediated disease or inflammatory myopathy is supported or to prove neurogenic abnormalities in an otherwise clinically unaffected limb.
3. Lumbar puncture
4. EMG and nerve conduction studies with proximal stimulation for multifocal conduction block and quantitative EMG if a myopathy (IBM) is suspected.
5. MRI with MR spectroscopy if evidence of cortical cell death is required (especially for diagnosis of PLS or PSMA).
6. Blood for genetic testing when appropriate
7. Video swallowing tests to assess upper pharyngeal muscle strength and function
8. Pulmonary function tests

CBC, complete blood count; ESR, erythrocyte sedimentation rate; BUN, blood urea nitrogen; AST, ALT; aspartate and alanine aminotransferase; LDH, lactate dehydrogenase; CK, creatine kinase; ANA, antinuclear antibodies; EMG, electromyography; IBM, inclusion body myositis; MRI, magnetic resonance imaging; PLS, primary lateral sclerosis; PSMA, progressive spinal muscular atrophy.

detected in significant titer to warrant serious consideration of treatment (12).

Disorders that may sometimes be confused with MND but are obvious after an appropriate history and evaluation include post-polio muscular atrophy, postirradiation atrophy or myelitis, myasthenia gravis, inclusion body myositis, and PLS. Patients with PLS complain of stiffness, diminution in fluidity of movement, and imbalance, without muscle twitching or atrophy. Reflexes are hyperactive with pathologic signs of corticospinal tract dysfunction, including Babinski and Hoffmann signs and abnormally active jaw jerk. Pseudobulbar palsy is typical with accompanying slurred speech, inappropriate affect, and hyperactive jaw jerk. EMG does not reveal denervation or fasciculation. The prognosis is one of continued progression of symptoms, but the rate is generally slow. PLS is a diagnosis of exclusion, but recent studies using magnetic resonance spectroscopy suggest that abnormalities in the NAA/creatine ratio in the frontal motor areas correlate with clinical signs of UMN degeneration and corticospinal tract signs. Nevertheless, until diagnostic specificity is proven, all patients should be screened for other causes, such as Chiari malformations, intrinsic lesions of the spinal cord, extrinsic tumors at the foramen magnum, syringomyelia, multiple sclerosis, and human T-cell lymphotropic virus type 1 infection. Therefore, magnetic resonance imaging of the brain and cervical cord, lumbar puncture, and EMG are necessary before the diagnosis is made. Sometimes separation from familial spastic paraparesis is difficult.

Genetic testing for FALS and Kennedy syndrome is indicated in selected situations. In sporadic ALS, it may be useful to screen for an SOD mutation when the family history is vague or incomplete. Kennedy syndrome should be clinically suspected in men with perioral fasciculation limb girdle and bulbar weakness, wasting, twitching, and gynecomastia. Genetic analysis shows more than 40 CAG repeats in the gene for the androgen receptor (13). Creatine kinase and serum gonadotropins may be elevated; however, serum testosterone levels are normal.

PROGNOSIS

The prognosis for an individual patient with ALS cannot be estimated from population studies. Rare patients have had reversible symptoms (14). Poor vital capacity, dysarthria, dysphagia, and four-limb fasciculation are considered poor prognostic findings. Studies regarding the prognosis of patients with progressive muscular atrophy vary. Some show prognosis to be similar to classic ALS, whereas others show a mean survival of 6.5 years. The variation is due to the fact that patients in this group include those with only anterior horn cell degeneration (spinal muscular atrophy), motor neuropathy, and ALS with pathologic involvement of the corticospinal tract

without clinical expression. Patients with bulbar palsy also have a variable course with some dying shortly after onset and others having a very prolonged course.

SYMPTOMATIC TREATMENT

Fatigue and insomnia are disabling symptoms at any time in the course of the illness. One possible cause of fatigue is inefficient neuromuscular transmission in degenerating neurons, with symptoms reminiscent of myasthenia gravis. For this reason, some clinicians give pyridostigmine. Polysomnography occasionally shows disrupted sleep patterns due to airway obstruction and weak pharyngeal musculature; because of resultant hypoxemia, frequent awakenings and daytime fatigue results. Nocturnal noninvasive respiratory support is often therapeutic (15). As weakness worsens, physical activity decreases. The degree of exhaustion at the day's end may be less, and small naps during the day may detract from ease of entering sleep. Frequent nocturnal awakenings may cause insomnia. Therefore, proper diagnosis is essential. If falling asleep is deemed the problem, medications to facilitate sleep may be necessary, either trihexiphenidyl or triazolam (0.25 mg hs).

Patients with bulbar weakness have particular difficulty controlling secretions, and long-term control is often difficult to achieve. Amitriptyline is often used because of its anticholinergic properties. Atropine has recently returned to the pharmaceutical market and may also be helpful. As a last resort, some patients have opted for radiation of the parotid glands. However, because of totality of destruction of glandular tissue, excessive dryness is a common and troubling side effect because infection becomes a problem under such circumstances.

Cramps and fasciculation can be annoying symptoms but are never disabling. Nocturnal cramps are often the earliest symptom of ALS. Patients with cramps report immediate relief from drinking electrolyte-fortified drinks or use of quinine sulfate, and those with fasciculates generally find clonazepam to be helpful. Spasticity and muscle spasms are most often due to dysfunction of the corticospinal tracts. Therapy is usually through physical therapy and antispasticity agents. These include baclofen and tizanidine. Severely affected patients may require baclofen injected directly into the cerebrospinal fluid, administered through a computer-driven pumping system.

Although formal testing does not reveal excessively prevalent depression, it is a frequent enough complaint that antidepressant therapy is often warranted. It is clear that professional education and emotional support is essential for patients and families affected by ALS.

The natural end point of ALS is pulmonary failure. When breathing becomes sufficiently compromised, noninvasive ventilatory support is becoming increasingly helpful. In severely affected patients, tracheostomy and mechanical ventilatory support is the only alternative. Many patients choose not to pursue this therapy because of its dramatic impact on quality of life.

SPECIFIC MEDICAL THERAPY

No known treatment stops or improves the symptoms of ALS or halts the progression of the classic disease. Recent studies have suggested that some agents may slow the progression of the illness, but this is based on statistical analyses of populations using an agent and comparing them with a placebo-treated population. Nevertheless, for the first time in our study of this illness, there are drugs that have a rational basis for use in this disease and have shown evidence that they do indeed affect the course of the illness. To understand the rationale of the use of these agents, we should review essential aspects of current theories of pathogenesis.

Excitotoxicity Theory and Glutamate Receptor Blockers

The excitotoxicity theory has been reviewed extensively elsewhere (16). Glutamate is an excitotoxic amino acid that when present in the extracellular fluid is potentially toxic to nerve cells. It is increased in the cerebrospinal fluid of patients with ALS (17). Such patients may have a defect in the ability to efficiently clear glutamate released into the extracellular space (18). The use of medications to block receptors for glutamate may interfere with its neurotoxicity. Rilutek (or riluzole) is the only approved medication for the treatment of patients with ALS. It blocks the toxic effect of glutamate in many animal models and has been shown to be effective in two clinical trials in ALS patients. One trial demonstrated an improved survival in patients with bulbar-onset disease but not limb-onset (19). A second trial showed significantly prolonged survival, but its effect was unexplained because there was no significant change in strength, respiratory function, or bulbar function in these patients compared with placebo. The most effective dose was 50 mg by mouth twice daily (20). Gabapentin (Neurontin) is also known to have antiglutamate effects. A recent double-blind placebo-controlled study showed that 2,400 mg of neurontin showed a trend but not statistically significant effect on the rate of deterioration. The drug is usually well tolerated, and a larger study is planned (21).

Neurotrophic Factor Deficiency

Another hypothesis is that patients with ALS have a deficiency of one or more nerve growth factors or neurotrophins critical for neuronal functioning. There are many different types of neurotrophins that support a wide array of function and cell types. These include motor neu-

rons, muscle, sensory neurons, or sympathetic neurons. Adding nerve growth factor to nerve cultures dramatically promotes neuronal survival. In the chick embryo, NCF promotes survival of motor neurons and impedes normal programmed cell death during development by excessive amounts. When nerves are transected, adding nerve growth factors will enhance the rate of regrowth.

There have been several clinical trials of neurotrophic factors, and many are still ongoing. Ciliary neurotrophic factor was found to be ineffective in a large-scale trial (22). Higher doses proved to be too toxic to complete another study. Brain-derived nerve growth factor showed no clinical effect in a large multicenter, double-blind, placebo-controlled trial. Insulin-like growth factor type 1 (IGF-1) has shown conflicting results. One study showed a statistically significant change in the rate of progression in patients receiving high-dose IGF-1 (23), measured by the Appel ALS score (8), and a statistically significant slowing of progression of bulbar and limb weakness was also demonstrated. IGF-1 improved quality of life, but paradoxically, the improvement was not statistically significant in the motor portion of this analysis. A second trial in Europe using IGF-1 showed no effect (24). There was, however, a trend toward slowing in the treated group. An ipso facto survival analysis showed that IGF-1 promoted survival in patients taking this drug. Food and Drug Administration approval of this drug is pending at the time of this manuscript preparation.

Antioxidant Therapy

Because of recent evidence of impaired oxidative processes in FALS, attempts to treat patients with agents that interfere with oxidative processes have been of interest. Most investigators promote the use of high-dose vitamins known for their antioxidative properties, especially vitamin E (2,000 U/day), vitamin C (2,000 mg/day), and beta-carotene (25,000 U/day). Selegiline (Eldepryl) has been found to be ineffective as has N-acetyl cysteine (25–27).

Autoimmunity

There is circumstantial evidence to implicate a role for autoimmune processes in ALS. The apparently excessive prevalence of lymphoma and paraproteinemia in patients with ALS suggests an association. One group has reported lymphocytes and activated macrophages in ALS spinal cord and the presence of IgG within ALS motor neurons. IgG from patients with ALS interact with L-type calcium channels and promote entry of calcium into the cell (28). Increased intracellular calcium may overwhelm the intracellular control systems for oxidative processes and contribute to the process of cellular destruction. However, several therapeutic trials have used immunosuppressant agents, including cyclophosphamide, intravenous immunoglobulin, prednisone, cyclosporin, and total body irradiation. None have proven effective. Calcium channel blockers have also proven to be ineffective (29).

Future advances will continue to make symptomatic care better in ALS and give hope that an understanding of what causes this disease is near, clearing the way for an effective therapy that does not slow progression but stops or reverses the process (30).

REFERENCES

1. Williams DB, Windenbank AJ. Motor neuron disease (amyotrophic lateral sclerosis). *Mayo Clinic Proc* 1991;66:54–82.
2. Younger DS, Rowland LP, Latov N, et al. Motor neuron disease and amyotrophic lateral sclerosis: relation of high CSF protein content to paraproteinemia and clinical syndromes. *Neurology* 1990;40:595–599.
3. Younger DS, Chou S, Hays AP, et al. Primary lateral sclerosis: a clinical diagnosis reemerges. *Ann Neurol* 1988;45:1304–1307.
4. Brooks BR. El Escorial Workshop 1994; World Federation of Neurology criteria for the diagnosis of amyotrophic lateral sclerosis. *J Neurol Sci* 1994;124[Suppl]:96–107.
5. Rosen DR, Siddique T, Patterson D, et al. Mutations in Cu/Zn superoxide dismutase gene are associated with familial amyotrophic lateral sclerosis. *Nature* 1993;362:59–62.
6. Kurtzke JF. Risk factors in amyotrophic lateral sclerosis. *Adv Neurol* 1991;56:245–270.
7. Ringel SP, Murphy JR, Alderson MK, et al. The natural history of amyotrophic lateral sclerosis. *Neurology* 1993;43:1316–1322.
8. Haverkamp L, Appel V, Appel SH. Natural history of ALS in a database population: validation of a scoring system and a model for survival prediction. *Brain* 1995;118:707–719.
9. Lange DJ, Trojaborg WT, Latov N, Hays AP. Multifocal motor neuropathy with conduction block: a distinct clinical entity? *Neurology* 1992;42:497–505.
10. Katz JS, Wolfe GI, Bryan WW, Jackson CE, Amato AA, Barohn RJ. Electrophysiologic findings in multifocal motor neuropathy. *Neurology* 1997;48:700–707.
11. Nobile-Orazio E, Meucci N, Barbieri S, Carpo M, Scarlato G. High-dose intravenous immunoglobulin therapy in multifocal neuropathy. *Neurology* 1993;43:537–544.
12. Kinsella LJ, Lange DJ, Trojaborg W, Sadiq SA, Younger DS, Latov N. The clinical and electrophysiological correlates of elevated ant-GM1 antibody titers. *Neurology* 1994;44:1278–1282.
13. Amato AA, Prior TW, Barohn RJ, et al. Kennedy's disease: a clinico-pathologic correlation with mutations in the androgen receptor gene. *Neurology* 1993;43:791–794.
14. Tucker T, Layzer RB, Miller RG, Chad D. Subacute reversible motor neuron disease. *Neurology* 1991;41:1541–1544.
15. Lange DJ, Murphy PL, Maxfield RA, Skarvala AM, Reidel G. Management of patients with amyotrophic lateral sclerosis. *J Neuro Rehab* 1994;8:75–82.
16. Rothstein JD. Excitotoxicity and neurodegeneration in amyotrophic lateral sclerosis. *Clin Neurosci* 1996;3:348–359.
17. Plaitakis A, Coroscio JT. Abnormal glutamate metabolism in amyotrophic lateral sclerosis. *Ann Neurol* 1987;22:575–579.
18. Rothstein JD, Martin LJ, Kuncl RW. Decreased glutamate transport by the brain and spinal cord in amyotrophic lateral sclerosis. *N Engl J Med* 1992;326:1464–1468.
19. Bensimmon G, Lacomblez L, Meininger V, ALS/Riluzole Study Group I. A controlled trial of riluzole in amyotrophic lateral sclerosis. *N Engl J Med* 1994;330:585–591.
20. Lacomblez L, Bensimon G, Leigh PN, Guillet P, Meininger V. Dose-ranging study of riluzole in amyotrophic lateral sclerosis/Riluzole Study Group II. *Lancet* 1996;347:1425–1431.
21. Miller RG, Moore D, Young BS, et al. Placebo-controlled trial of gabapentin in patients with amyotrophic lateral sclerosis. *Neurology* 1996;47:1383–1388.
22. Miller RG, Armon C, Barohn RJ, et al. A placebo controlled trial of recombinant human ciliary neurotrophic factor (rhCNTF) in amyotrophic lateral sclerosis. *Ann Neurol* 1996;39:256–260.
23. Lai EC, Felice KJ, Festoff BW, et al. Effect of recombinant human insulin-like growth factor-I on progression of ALS. A placebo-controlled study. The North America ALS/IGF-I Study Group. *Neurology* 1997;49:1621–1630.
24. Borasio GC, Lange DJ, Lai EC, et al. A double blind placebo-controlled therapeutic trial to assess the efficacy of recombinant human insulin-like growth factor in the treatment of ALS: a multi-center, double-blind, placebo-controlled clinical study [abstract]. Sixth International Symposium on ALS/MND, Dublin, Ireland, 1995.
25. Lange DJ, Murphy PS, Diamond B, et al. Selegiline is ineffective in a collaborative double-blind, placebo-controlled trial for treatment of amyotrophic latral sclerosis. *Arch Neurol* 1998;55:93–96.
26. Louwerse ES, Weverling GJ, Bossuyt PM, Meyjes FE, de Jong JM. Randomized, double-blind, controlled trial of acetylcysteine in amyotrophic lateral sclerosis. *Arch Neurol* 1995;52:559–564.
27. Mazzini L, Testa D, Balzarini C, Mora G. An open-randomized clinical trial of selegiline in amyotrophic lateral sclerosis. *J Neurol* 1994;241:223–227.
28. Smith RG, Hamilton S, Hoffman F, et al. Serum antibodies to L-type calcium channels in patients with amyotrophic lateral sclerosis. *N Engl J Med* 1992;327:1721–1728.
29. Miller RG, Smith SA, Murphy JR, et al. Verapamil does not slow the progressive weakness of amytrophic lateral sclerosis. *Muscle Nerve* 1996;19:511–515.
30. Mitsumoto H, Norris FH, eds. *Amyotrophic lateral sclerosis: a comprehensive guide to management.* New York: Demos Publications, 1994.

PART IV

The Neuronal Degenerations

Motor Disorders,
edited by David S. Younger.
Lippincott Williams & Wilkins, Philadelphia © 1999.

CHAPTER 33

Parkinsonian Syndromes and Multisystem Atrophies

Elan D. Louis and Louis H. Weimer

Involuntary movement disorders may be classified as hypokinetic or hyperkinetic. The hypokinetic movement disorders include idiopathic Parkinson disease (PD) and other forms of parkinsonism (Table 1). These disorders, the subject of this chapter, are unified by a set of distinct clinical features, including bradykinesia, akinesia, and extrapyramidal rigidity, and pathologic alterations of the striatonigral motor system. Idiopathic PD is considered first and foremost because it is the most prevalent, the best understood, and the most treatable.

IDIOPATHIC PARKINSON'S DISEASE

The syndrome of PD, or "paralysis agitans," was first described by James Parkinson in an 1817 treatise on shaking palsy (1). The resting tremor and other clinical features had been recognized earlier, whereas bradykinesia was not fully elucidated until after Parkinson's time (2–4). The mean age at onset of PD in brain bank series is 62 to 64 years (5–8); a juvenile form with onset before age 21 years and a somewhat older onset form usually between 21 and 39 years have both been described (9), the incidence of which are relatively low. The incidence and the prevalence of PD increase with age (10). Although there are no gender differences in the incidence of PD, the lower prevalence of women suggests that their survival may be decreased relative to men (10–12).

The cardinal clinical features of idiopathic PD are tremor at rest, rigidity, bradykinesia, akinesia, postural instability, and freezing phenomena or motor blockage.

E. D. Louis: Department of Neurology, Gertrude H. Sergievsky Center, Columbia University College of Physicians and Surgeons, New York, New York 10032.

L. H. Weimer: Neurological Institute, Columbia University College of Physicians and Surgeons and Department of Neurology, New York Presbyterian Hospital, New York, NY 10032.

The disease typically begins in a single limb or side of the body and with progression impairs axial and contralateral limb function (8,13). Common presenting complaints include tremor, stiffness, achiness, limb weakness, slowness of movement, difficulty arising from a seated position, difficulty buttoning buttons, difficulty cutting food, an alteration in handwriting (typically micrographia), lack of facial expression, and a bent or stooped posture. About 10 to 40% of patients develop dementia (14–18); however, the prevalence of mild cognitive impairment is more common. Neuroimaging studies can be used to diagnose presymptomatic and early PD and to discriminate idiopathic PD from other forms of parkinsonism. Magnetic resonance imaging (MRI) can reveal foci of decreased signal intensity on T2-weighted images in the substantia nigra, caudate, and putamen, indicative of increased iron deposition (19). However, similar findings may be seen in normal age-matched control subjects (19).

TABLE 1. *Forms of parkinsonism*

Idiopathic Parkinson disease[a]
Multiple system atrophy[a]
Striatonigral degeneration[a]
Olivopontocerebellar atrophy[a]
Shy-Drager syndrome[a]
Progressive supranuclear palsy[a]
Corticobasal ganglionic degeneration[a]
Infectious and postinfectious parkinsonism
Toxin-induced parkinsonism
Vascular parkinsonism
Posttraumatic parkinsonism
Normal pressure hydrocephalus
Parkinsonism secondary to space-occupying lesions
Parkinsonism in other neurodegenerative diseases (e.g., Hallervorden-Spatz disease, Wilson disease)

[a]Covered in this chapter.

Studies using 18F-fluorodeoxyglucose (FDG) positron emission tomography (PET) provide further specificity when they show increased metabolism in the globus pallidus of clinically affected patients with PD, probably related to alterations in striatal dopamine metabolism (20), and [^{18}F]6-fluoro L-dopa PET can be used to detect subclinical dopaminergic deficits and patients with early disease (20–22). A reduction in [^{18}F]6-fluoro L-dopa metabolism in the striatum correlates with the Hoehn and Yahr clinical disease stage (20). Finally, [^{11}C]Raclopride can be used to study striatal dopamine D2 receptor density because it reveals initial receptor upregulation with an increase in receptor density in the putamen contralateral to symptomatology in patients with early PD and a decline toward control values with increasing disease severity (20,23).

The characteristic pathologic findings in PD are neuronal loss with depigmentation and eosinophilic intraneuronal inclusions, or Lewy bodies, in the substantia nigra pars compacta. There is also a loss of cells and pigment in other pigmented nuclei of the brainstem, including the dorsal vagal nucleus and the locus ceruleus (5,8). Postmortem studies also reveal an increase in iron concentration in the substantia nigra (19).

The diagnosis of PD is based on clinical criteria, with most research protocols requiring the presence of at least two of the cardinal features (7,8,24). The proportion of PD patients with rest tremor is 90% in clinical series and 76 to 100% in pathologic series (13,25,26). Response to levodopa is found in 85% carrying the clinical diagnosis of PD, although many of those without a clinical response to levodopa probably carried other pathologic diagnoses (27,28). Therefore, based on clinical criteria alone, the diagnosis of PD is not always certain. In one brain bank series, 24% of those diagnosed clinically had other neurodegenerative disorders, including progressive supranuclear palsy (PSP), multiple system atrophy (MSA), and Alzheimer disease at postmortem examination (26). The clinical course varies considerably between patients, with a mean duration of disease of 13.1 years (8). The mean Hoehn and Yahr score at death is 4.3, indicating a severe stage of disease, and the mean age at death is 75.6 years (8).

Treatment of PD can be neuroprotective or symptomatic (Table 2). The benefit of selegiline, a monoamine oxidase type B inhibitor, in delaying the need for levodopa therapy is still debated (29,30). Other medications provide symptomatic benefit as follows: levodopa in combination with carbidopa; the dopamine agonists pergolide and bromocriptine; amantidine and the anticholinergic agents trihexyphenidyl, biperiden, kemadrin, and cogentin; and the catechol-o-methyltransferase inhibitors tolcapone and entacapone (31–34).

There are surgical treatments for more advanced cases, including pallidotomy, thalamotomy, fetal tissue implants, and implantation of deep brain stimulation

TABLE 2. *Treatment of Parkinson's disease*

Medications
  Neuroprotective: selegiline
  Symptomatic
    Selegiline
    Levodopa
    Dopamine agonists (pergolide, bromocriptine)
    Amantidine
    Anticholinergic agents (trihexyphenidyl,
      biperiden, kemidrin, cogentin)
    Catechol-o-methyltransferase inhibitors
      (tolcapone, entacapone)
Surgical interventions
  Pallidotomy
  Thalamotomy
  Fetal tissue implants
  Implantation of deep brain stimulation electrodes

electrodes. Stereotactic pallidotomy improves bradykinesia, rigidity, rest tremor, impaired balance, and medication-induced dyskinesia in the limbs contralateral to the pallidotomy (35–37), and gamma knife pallidotomy reduces dyskinesias in some patients (38). Stereotactic thalamotomy decreases the severity of tremor and allows for reductions in dosages of levodopa (39,40). Striatal fetal ventral mesencephalic tissue implantation (41–47) improved the Unified Parkinson's Disease Rating Scale (UPDRS) scores, Hoehn and Yahr scores, and Schwab and England disability score (45) improved timed motor tasks, allowed for reduction in the dosages of levodopa, increased the percent of "off" time and percent of "on" time without dyskinesia, and increased walking speed (41–43,45). Although some patients continue to benefit for up to 5 years (45), others revert to their preoperative status up to 18 months after surgery (43). Stereotactic implantation of autologous adrenal medullary tissue into the striatum resulted in initial improvement in parkinsonism; however, it progressively lessened with time in accordance with the nonviability of transplanted tissue (48). Parkinsonian tremor and levodopa-induced dyskinesia may be suppressed by electrical stimulation of the ventral intermediate nucleus of the thalamus with implantation of deep brain stimulation electrodes (49–51).

MULTIPLE SYSTEM ATROPHY

These are a group of related hypokinetic movement disorders that include striatonigral degeneration (SND), olivopontocerebellar atrophy (OPCA), and the Shy-Drager syndrome (SDS) (52). They are less prevalent than idiopathic PD, accounting for 11% of misdiagnosed cases of PD in brain bank series (53). The most common clinical features in all MSA syndromes are parkinsonism and autonomic failure, but cerebellar and pyramidal signs may also be present (54). Two pathologic features are shared in MSA. Like PD, there is neuronal loss in the substantia nigra and the putamen; however, in MSA,

Lewy bodies are rare (54,55). The histologic hallmark of MSA is the presence of argyrophilic cytoplasmic inclusions in oligodendrocytes in cerebral white matter and less often in oligodendroglial nuclei, neuronal cytoplasm, nuclei, and axons (56–58). The mean length of survival in MSA is shorter than in PD (59). Among 35 patients with MSA, the median survival was 7.3 years (54), and in another series of 59 patients, the 6-year survival rate was 54%. In the latter series, the survival in SND and SDS was less favorable than in OPCA (60).

Striatonigral Degeneration

In 1961 and 1964, before introduction of levodopa, Adams et al. (61,62) described four patients diagnosed clinically during life with PD because of bradykinesia and rigidity in all four patients, rest tremor in three, and postural instability and brisk deep tendon reflexes in two. At postmortem examination, the major alterations were neuronal loss and gliosis in the putamen and cell loss in the substantia nigra. In addition, lesions were noted in the cerebellum and spinal cord.

It is estimated that 4 to 8% of patients with parkinsonism have SND (63). It is difficult to distinguish SND from idiopathic PD by clinical signs alone (59) (Table 3); in one series of 10 pathologically proven cases, 5 were diagnosed in life as idiopathic PD (59). However, clinical features that may be useful include severe and atypical parkinsonism, poor or absent response to levodopa, rapidly progressive symptoms, orthostatic hypotension, early gait abnormalities with postural instability, severe dysarthria, snoring with severe laryngeal stridor, brisk deep tendon reflexes with Babinski signs, severe anterocollis or dystonic hand postures, and absence of rest tremor at presentation (59,64,65). Levodopa-induced facial dyskinesia and dystonia with only a modest motor improvement is generally more typical of SND than idiopathic PD (66). However, none of these clinical features is either uniformly present in all cases of SND or pathognomonic for SND. Van Leeuwen and Perquin (63) reviewed 33 reported cases of SND. Although all had rigidity and hypokinesia, less

than half had a tremor. Tremor was the initial symptom in 6% of those with SND compared with 70.5% of those with PD. In SND, 84% presented with rigidity or hypokinesia, compared with 27% of PD cases. Finally, 20% of the SND patients responded to levodopa compared with an 80% response rate in those with PD (63). Like idiopathic PD, cognitive impairment is not uncommon in SND; Van Leeuwen and Perquin (63) reported cognitive impairment in 15% of SND cases.

Neuroimaging may be used to discriminate SND from idiopathic PD. In the former, MRI may reveal signal abnormalities in the putamen, cerebellum, or brainstem (64,66,67). Lang et al. (66) reported three patients with SND that had prominent signal hypointensities (slitlike void signals) in the putamen on MRI, probably a result of increased iron deposition. Although this finding is very distinctive and may be pathognomic for SND, the sensitivity has not yet been established (68). FDG PET may be a useful tool for the early diagnosis of SND; it reveals a consistent and significant reduction in glucose metabolism in the caudate and putamen in patients with SND compared with those with PD (68). Proton MR spectroscopy of the lentiform nucleus reveals significant reduction in the *N*-acetyl aspartate/creatinine ratio and the choline/creatinine ratio in SND compared with PD and normal control subjects (69).

Adams et al. (61,62) originally described neuronal loss and gliosis in the putamen and the pars compacta of the substantia nigra and lesions in the cerebellum and spinal cord. Unlike PD, the nigral degeneration in SND was unaccompanied by Lewy bodies (70), and similar to other forms of MSA, glial cytoplasmic inclusions were present (57,58). A prominent feature of this disorder is the accumulation of granular iron-containing pigments in the putamen, corresponding with hypointense T2 signal in the putamen on MRI (71). Kato et al. (71) studied four patients with SND and age- and gender-matched control subjects and noted a mean putaminal iron content five times higher than control subjects.

The diagnosis of SND in life is suggested by certain clinical and neuroimaging features that are more common in SND than in idiopathic PD, for example, absence of resting tremor, a poor or absent response to levodopa therapy, and differences in caudate and lentiform metabolic rates on FDG PET (68,72). SND is more rapidly progressive than PD (59), with generally a 5- to 7-year survival from the onset of symptoms to death (27). Van Leeuwen and Perquin (63) studied 33 patients with SND reported in the literature and found a mean age of onset of 56.6 years and a mean duration of illness of 4.5 years. Fearnley and Lees (59) reported 10 additional patients and noted a mean age at onset of 62 years with a mean disease duration of 6 years.

Despite the presence of pathology in postsynaptic dopamine receptor-containing cells in the striatum, some patients with SND nonetheless improve with levodopa

TABLE 3. *Clinical features reported to distinguish SND from idiopathic Parkinson disease*

Severe or atypical parkinsonism
Absence of rest tremor at presentation
Rapidly progressive symptoms and signs
Orthostatic hypotension
Early gait abnormalities with postural instability
Severe dysarthria
Snoring with severe laryngeal stridor
Brisk deep tendon reflexes with extensor plantar responses
Severe anterocollis and other dystonic hand postures
Poor or absent response to levodopa
Levodopa-induced facial dyskinesias and dystonia

SND, striatonigral degeneration.

(59). Such was the experience of Parati et al. (73) and Lang et al. (66); four of eight (50%) MSA patients so treated had a moderate response to levodopa therapy (73) and three others had a poor or transient response (66). In general, the response is not as consistently noted as in PD, and some have suggested that SND accounts for up to 15% of levodopa treatment failures in parkinsonian patients (27). Stereotaxic thalamic surgery has also been effective in some instances in treating rigidity and tremor (27,74).

Olivopontocerebellar Atrophy

The term OPCA was proposed in 1900 in the description of two patients with sporadic adult-onset cerebellar disorders (75). Since then, the term has been used for patients with parkinsonism and ataxia clinically and neuronal loss in the pons, inferior olives, and cerebellum (76). Only sporadic nonfamilial forms of OPCA are classified under MSA (76).

OPCA commonly presents with akinesia, bradykinesia, and rigidity and cerebellar signs, including an unsteady wide-based gait, slurring, or scanning of speech. Oculomotor disturbances may also be present. The findings may differ from PSP in the initial involvement of upgaze and convergence and the later limitation of downgaze (77). In a review of 63 patients with sporadic OPCA, Berciano (78) found cerebellar signs in 87%, parkinsonism in 55%, pyramidal signs in 46%, and dementia in 35%.

Brain computed tomography and T2-weighted MRI demonstrate atrophy of the cerebellum and brainstem, with demyelination of decussating cerebellopontine fibers (67,76). PET reveals a reduction in both cerebellar and brainstem metabolic rates (79). Proton MR spectroscopy of the lentiform nucleus reveals significant reductions in the *N*-acetyl aspartate/creatinine ratio in OPCA compared with patients with idiopathic PD and normal control subjects (69).

Postmortem gross examination reveals atrophy of the cerebellum, pons, and middle cerebellar peduncle; the substantia nigra may also show depigmentation. Microscopic examination reveals extensive loss of cerebellar Purkinje cells, especially in the region of the vermis; neuronal loss in brainstem nuclei, especially the pontine nuclei; neuronal loss in the striatum; along with depigmentation in the substantia nigra; and demyelination of corticospinal tracts and posterior columns (80). As in other forms of MSA, oligodendroglial cytoplasmic inclusions are present throughout the white matter (81–83). One morphometric analysis reported a poor correlation between OPCA-type pathology and clinical signs; cerebellar signs were noted during life in 6 of 20 patients with MSA, whereas an OPCA-like pathology was noted in 17 (84).

The diagnosis of OPCA is suggested in a patient with a cerebellar syndrome accompanied by an akinetic form of parkinsonism. Parkinsonism was present in 55% of those with sporadic forms of OPCA (78). As noted above, pronounced cerebellar and brainstem atrophy are apparent on neuroimaging (76). In a review of 63 cases of sporadic OPCA, the mean age at onset was 49 years, considerably younger than that of PD. The mean disease duration was 6 years (78). Response to levodopa therapy has been poor, and dopamine agonists are no more effective than levodopa (85). Sixteen of 19 patients nonetheless had some type of improvement with therapy (27,85).

Shy-Drager Syndrome

In 1960, Shy and Drager (86) described two patients with generalized autonomic failure and additional dysfunction in other systems that differed from pure autonomic failure (PAF) described earlier in 1925 by Bradbury and Eggleston (87). The signs of autonomic failure in their cases (86) included orthostatic hypotension, urinary and rectal incontinence, hypohidrosis, impotence, and bladder atony. There was in addition iris atrophy, external ocular palsies, rigidity, tremor, loss of associated movements, fasciculations, amyotrophy, and neurogenic electromyogramy (EMG) (86). SDS with initial or predominant autonomic failure is considered part of the spectrum of MSA (88,89). Distinguishing this form of MSA clinically from PAF or idiopathic PD can be challenging.

Although autonomic failure is the hallmark of the SDS, evidence of autonomic dysfunction is eventually found in up to 97% of all patients clinically diagnosed with MSA (90). Orthostatic hypotension or syncope is often the initial and most disabling symptom; although, retrospectively, other autonomic symptoms, including male impotence or ejaculatory dysfunction, decreased sweating, urinary incontinence, and, less commonly, fecal incontinence, often predate the orthostatic hypotension. Postprandial hypotension, typically starting 10 to 15 minutes after a meal and peaking at approximately 1 hour, can also be disabling. Dysfunction in other systems, for example, parkinsonism with more rigidity and bradykinesia than tremor, is typical and may be mild or not evident for several years after the onset of autonomic failure. The parkinsonism usually responds poorly to levodopa therapy, although some can have initial symptomatic relief. Levodopa therapy may exacerbate underlying orthostatic hypotension. Cerebellar and corticospinal tract signs may be present. Fasciculations with evidence of chronic partial denervation on EMG, present in one of the original SDS cases (86), may rarely be evident. Peripheral neuropathy (91) and signs of a mild frontal lobe dementia (92) may also occur. Inspiratory stridor is common (93) with evidence of laryngeal muscle denervation. A variety of sleep disturbances and altered respiratory patterns including apnea-producing hypoxemia can be seen and are likely underrecognized.

A multitude of tests are used to assess autonomic reflex function (Table 4). Abnormalities in two or more

TABLE 4. *Selected tests of autonomic function*

Primarily parasympathetic
  Heart rate variability to cyclic deep breathing*
  Valsalva ratio*
  Heart rate response to standing (30:15 ratio)*
  Diving reflex/cold face test
  Heart rate variability at rest
Primarily sympathetic
  Blood pressure response to standing and to tilt
  Blood pressure waveform with Valsalva maneuver*
  Blood pressure response to other provocative measures,
    including sustained handgrip, lower body negative
    pressure, mental stress, squatting test
  Tests of sudomotor function,* including quantitative
    sudomotor axon reflex test, sweat imprint test,
    thermoregulatory sweat test, and sympathetic skin
    response
  Plasma norepinephrine levels (supine and standing)

*Well established measures

tests provide evidence of autonomic failure typical of MSA (91) but are nonetheless nonspecific. Simple bedside screening tests for autonomic failure include measurement of heart rate and blood pressure after 1 minute of standing. Other commonly performed tests in the autonomic battery include measures of heart rate variability at rest and on cyclic deep breathing; heart rate and blood pressure responses to the Valsalva maneuver; and heart rate and blood pressure responses to standing, head-up tilt, sustained hand grip, lower body negative pressure, cold water immersion, and mental stress. Sudomotor sweat function and pupillary function can be useful. Urodynamic studies can show detrusor hyperreflexia or atonic bladder, although some patients with idiopathic PD can also demonstrate detrusor hyperreflexia.

The degenerative process in MSA appears to have a special predilection for Onuf's nucleus, composed of somatic motor neurons serving voluntary urinary and anal sphincter function. Concentric needle EMG of striated sphincters is an important part of the evaluation in all forms of MSA, not simply SDS. It can demonstrate electrophysiologic evidence of anterior horn cell involvement with chronic partial denervation. Neurogenic abnormalities include increased mean motor unit potential duration (94,95). Paradoxically, these sphincter muscles are virtually spared in amyotrophic lateral sclerosis (96), and except in multiparous women (97), these findings are more specific for the diagnosis of MSA than an autonomic battery, but the sensitivity varies with different studies.

Formal sleep studies may demonstrate dangerous nocturnal apneic episodes or other altered sleep or respiratory patterns. Serum norepinephrine levels in patients with MSA show normal or mildly reduced levels at rest, which fail to normally elevate with head-up tilt compared with patients with PAF that have lower rest norepinephrine levels which do not rise with tilting.

Demonstration of the argyrophilic cytoplasmic inclusions in oligodendroglia has refined the pathologic diagnosis of MSA over previous assessments using patterns of neuronal loss and gliosis (98). In addition to the sites described earlier, inclusions are also prominent at vital sites of autonomic control, including in the intermediolateral column of the spinal cord, dorsal vagal nucleus, solitary tract and nucleus, pontobulbar reticular formation, and medullary tegmentum (99). Glial cytoplasmic inclusions also correlate better with clinical findings than areas of neuronal loss (99).

The clinical classification of MSA has been problematic, especially in cases with initial autonomic failure that resemble PAF or atypical idiopathic PD. Frank autonomic failure is rare in typical idiopathic PD; however, autonomic symptoms and lesser degrees of autonomic dysfunction are relatively common (100,101). Symptoms such as dysphagia, constipation, and urinary complaints are common but may not be on an autonomic basis. However, dysautonomic sweat disturbances and orthostatic hypotension may occur (100). Magalhaes et al. (102) retrospectively reviewed autonomic symptoms in 135 autopsy-proven idiopathic PD and MSA cases. A third of the 33 MSA cases were misdiagnosed as idiopathic PD before autopsy. Autonomic symptoms were common in the idiopathic PD patients; however, initial autonomic onset, severe autonomic failure, and inspiratory stridor were all exceedingly rare (102). Finally, because autonomic failure may predate evidence of failure of other neuronal systems, most authorities and academic centers will defer the diagnosis of PAF until there is no evidence of other system failure for at least 3–5 years or more. Recent studies of the prognosis have divided MSA into parkinsonian and cerebellar forms (103), so data on patients with autonomic onset are not well established. In general, however, the prognosis of MSA is worse than for both PAF and idiopathic PD with autonomic features. A small subset of PD cases have noted AF and are designated as PD with autonomic failure.

Therapy is aimed at symptomatic relief and improved quality of life. Orthostatic hypotension is generally the most disabling symptom and can be treated with a high sodium diet, elastic stockings with abdominal compression, fludrocortisone, nocturnal head-up tilt, and the alpha-1 agonist midodrine. Desmopressin can reduce nocturnal diuresis, thereby increasing morning supine blood pressure and lessening orthostatic hypotension (104). The pressor drug phenylephrine minimally raises standing blood pressure but often exacerbates supine hypertension when baroreflexes are depressed. Impotence can be partially helped with intracavernous papaverine injections or penile implants. The treatment of urinary complaints includes anticholinergic agent to reduce incontinence, but they can cause urinary retention in susceptible patients. Intermittent or indwelling catheters may be required. Inspiratory stridor may require tracheostomy, and nocturnal positive pressure ventilation may be needed for sleep apnea.

PROGRESSIVE SUPRANUCLEAR PALSY

In 1964 Steele et al. (105) described nine patients with the entity they termed PSP because of supranuclear ophthalmoplegia predominantly involving vertical gaze, pseudobulbar palsy, dysarthria, dystonic rigidity of the neck and upper trunk, and mild dementia; none had parkinsonian tremor. Neuropathologic studies in seven so studied revealed cell loss, gliosis, neurofibrillary tangles, granulovacuolar degeneration, and demyelination in various regions of the brainstem, basal ganglia, and cerebellum.

PSP comprises 4 to 7.5% of parkinsonian cases at movement disorder clinics (9,106,107) and 4% of misdiagnosed cases of idiopathic PD in brain bank series (108). Perhaps the earliest features of PSP are postural and gait abnormalities (9). Rather than the flexed stooped posture commonly seen in idiopathic PD, patients with PSP tend to extend their knees, trunk, and neck, with a tendency to fall backward, not forward (105), an observation described over 140 years ago by Romberg (109) among several patients "who felt a constant desire to walk or fall backwards." The degree of eye movement abnormalities depends on the stage of the disease. Early findings include mild limitation of voluntary downgaze, inability to converge, multistep hypometric slow saccades of long duration, and low amplitude conjugate saccades that move the eyes away from and then back to a fixed point, termed square wave jerks. With disease progression, vertical and horizontal eye movements become more impaired, and eventually, vestibulo-ocular reflexes are lost, indicative of nuclear and supranuclear pathology (110–112). Other clinical features include emotional incontinence due to pseudobulbar palsy, rigidity, bradykinesia, facial dystonia resulting in deeply lined and prominent nasolabial folds and frontalis muscle contraction, and dysarthria characterized by variably spastic hypokinetic ataxic speech (113,114). Cognitive abnormalities can occur (113). A study of 19 patients with PSP and 42 patients with idiopathic PD noted cognitive impairment measured by a Mini-Mental State Examination score of less than 24 in 52% of the patients with PSP (106). Psychiatric disturbances may also be present in PSP; Menza et al. (106) noted that 42% of those with PSP had formal psychiatric diagnoses, most commonly mild depression or anxiety.

Neuroimaging studies, particularly brain MRI, may reveal putaminal lesions. Sagittal views may show thinning of the quadrigeminal plate, especially in the region of the colliculi (67,115–117). Fluorodopa PET reveals reduced mean caudate tracer uptake in PSP compared with idiopathic PD. In 90% of cases, PSP can be discriminated from idiopathic PD based on different patterns of caudate and putamen tracer uptake (53). In addition, [^{11}C]diprenorphine PET imaging has been used to investigate striatal opioid receptor binding. Four of six patients

with PSP had caudate opioid receptor binding that was greater than 2.5 standard durations (SD) below the normal mean; all six had putamen opioid receptor binding that was greater than 2.5 SD below the mean. In comparison, none of eight patients with idiopathic PD had caudate or putamen opioid receptor binding that was greater than 2.5 SD below the normal mean (108).

The pathologic hallmark of this disorder is the globose neurofibrillary tangle, distinct from that seen in Alzheimer disease and present in the substantia nigra, locus coeruleus, nucleus basalis, and globus pallidus (70). Other findings include neuronal loss and gliosis in the pallidosubthalamic complex, substantia nigra pars compacta, superior colliculus, periaqueductal gray matter, and the pretectal area (70,105). Litvan et al. (118) proposed criteria for the diagnosis of PSP that included vertical supranuclear palsy with downgaze abnormalities, severe postural instability with unexplained falls, and progressive disease course, without hallucinations, early cortical dementia, early or prominent cerebellar signs, noniatrogenic dysautonomia, unilateral dystonia, or automatic behavior involving the upper limb or excursion of the upper limb in space, the so-called alien hand phenomenon. One classification for PSP recognizes probable PSP as the presence of vertical supranuclear gaze palsy and prominent postural instability with falls within the first year of disease onset and definite PSP as pathologically confirmed (119). However, not all pathologically confirmed cases of PSP had vertical supranuclear ophthalmoparesis during life (8,26), and conversely, vertical supranuclear ophthalmoparesis may be a feature of diffuse Lewy body and central nervous system Whipple disease (120–122). In addition, when present, the onset of supranuclear gaze palsy may lag behind other clinical features by years, making early diagnosis more difficult (113). Aside from clinical features, neuroimaging, as noted above, may be used to separate PSP from idiopathic PD. Although patients with idiopathic PD demonstrate abnormalities on the University of Pennsylvania Smell Identification Test, overall the olfactory function in PSP is superior to that in idiopathic PD and olfactory testing may be useful in the differential diagnosis (123). The mean age at onset may be as young as 55 years, which is younger than that of idiopathic PD (113), or as old as 63 years, similar to that of idiopathic PD (124). The median survival in one series was 5.6 years (range, 2 to 16.6 years) (124) with most patients dead 10 years after onset (113). Early postural instability, dysphagia, and incontinence are also predictive of a shorter survival time (124).

Treatment has been partially effective (125,126). In a retrospective study of 87 patients with PSP, 32% benefited from amitriptyline, 28% from imipramine, and 38% from levodopa/carbidopa (127). Some patients respond to dopamine agonists or anticholinergic medications (107,128,129). Idazoxan, an alpha-2 presynaptic inhibitor whose overall effect is to increase norepinephrine transmission, has been tried in PSP (129); 9 of 11 patients so treated improved their motor UPDRS scores by 10 to 30% (130). Electroconvulsive therapy has been of limited benefit and resulted in transient worsening of cognition and UPDRS motor scores in one patient. Transient confusion has been uniformly reported. In three of five others so treated, electroconvulsive therapy resulted in improvements that ranged from mild to dramatic (131,132).

CORTICOBASAL GANGLIONIC DEGENERATION

In 1968, Reibez et al. (133) reported three patients with parkinsonism, supranuclear gaze palsy, myoclonus, and apraxia. At postmortem examination, there was corticodentatonigral degeneration and neuronal achromasia. In addition, to parkinsonism, several distinctive clinical features are generally present as follows: asymmetry, focal dystonia, cortical myoclonus, cortical sensory deficits, apraxias, and the alien limb phenomenon (134–137) (Table 5). In one series of 36 cases followed for a mean period of 5 years, the following signs were noted: apraxia and rigidity in 100%, gait abnormality in 97%, supranuclear gaze palsy in 90%, arm dystonia in 80%, myoclonus in 57%, and alien limb phenomenon in 50% (136). The neuropsychologic profile of corticobasal ganglionic degeneration (CBGD) that may allow separation from other diseases such as PSP (138) generally includes the dysexecutive syndrome, explicit learning deficits, disorders of dynamic motor execution, and asymmetric praxis.

MRI may reveal asymmetric cortical atrophy in the parietal region (67). FDG PET reveals a reduction in glucose consumption with a distinct asymmetry between the two cerebral hemispheres (139). Single-photon emission tomography using 99 technetium hexamethylpropulenamine scan may be used to distinguish CBGD from idiopathic PD because affected patients have reduced uptake in the thalamus, posterior frontal cortex, and inferior and anterior parietal cortex (140). Focal cortical atrophy may be present, particularly asymmetrically, in the posterior frontal and parietal regions (70). There is neuronal loss in the cortex, thalamus, striatum, and substantia nigra pars compacta, with achromatic neuronal inclusions in the cortex, substantia nigra, thalamus, and red nucleus (9,70). Massive argyrophilic threadlike structures have been noted in oligodendroglia in CBGD and in some cases of PSP (141).

TABLE 5. *Clinical features reported to distinguish CBGD from idiopathic Parkinson disease*

Markedly asymmetric onset
Focal dystonia
Cortical myoclonus
Cortical sensory deficits
Apraxias
The "alien limb" phenomenon

CBGD, corticobasal ganglionic degeneration.

On clinical grounds the distinction between PSP and CBGD may be difficult. In one study of 15 patients with rigid-akinetic syndromes, hemineglect in combination with limb apraxia was a feature that distinguished the two, being present in all 4 patients with CBGD and none of the 11 patients with PSP (142). Although supranuclear ophthalmoplegia, neck rigidity, and postural instability may be observed in both disorders, in CBGD these were less severe than in PSP (142). The mean age at onset is 61 years (136). Progression is more rapid than in idiopathic PD, with death occurring 4 to 10 years after onset of symptoms (134,136). Fewer than 100 cases have been reported (136). Response to levodopa is poor. The dystonia may respond to botulinum toxin injections (9).

ACKNOWLEDGMENTS

Supported by National Institutes of Health grant NS01863 and the Paul Beeson Physician Faculty Scholars in Aging Research Award (American Federation for Aging Research).

REFERENCES

1. Parkinson J. *An essay on the shaking palsy.* London: Whittingham and Rowland, 1817.
2. Sanders WR. Case of an unusual form of nervous disease, dystaxia or pseudoparalysis agitans, with remarks. *Edinburgh Med J* 1865;10: 987–997.
3. Charcot JM. *Lectures on diseases of the nervous system.* Philadelphia: H.C. Lea and Company, 1879.
4. Charcot JM. *Charcot the clinician. The Tuesday lessons.* New York: Raven Press, 1987. (Original 1888.)
5. Louis ED, Goldman JE, Powers JM, Fahn S. Parkinsonian features of eight pathologically diagnosed cases of diffuse Lewy body disease. *Mov Disord* 1995;10:188–194.
6. Louis ED, Klatka LA, Lui Y, Fahn S. Comparison of extrapyramidal features in 31 pathologically confirmed cases of diffuse Lewy body disease and 34 pathologically confirmed cases of Parkinson's disease. *Neurology* 1997;48:376–380.
7. Hughes AJ, Ben-Shlomo Y, Daniel SE, Lees AJ. What features improve the accuracy of clinical diagnosis in Parkinson's disease: a clinicopathological study. *Neurology* 1992;42:1142–1146.
8. Hughes AJ, Daniel SE, Blankson S, Lees AJ. A clinicopathological study of 100 cases of Parkinson's disease. *Arch Neurol* 1993;50: 140–148.
9. Stacy M, Jankovic J. Differential diagnosis of Parkinson's disease and parkinsonism plus syndromes. *Neurol Clin* 1992;10:341–359.
10. Mayeux R, Marder K, Cote L, et al. The frequency of idiopathic Parkinson's disease by age, ethnic group, and sex in northern Manhattan, 1988–1993. *Am J Epidemiol* 1995;142:820–827.
11. Rajput AH, Offord KP, Beard CM, Kurland LT. Epidemiology of parkinsonism: incidence, classification and mortality. *Ann Neurol* 1984;16:278–282.
12. Diamond SG, Markham CH, Hoehn MM, McDowell FH, Muenter MD. An examination of male-female differences in progression and mortality of Parkinson's disease. *Neurology* 1990;40:763–766.
13. Hoehn MM, Yahr MD. Parkinsonism: onset, progression and mortality. *Neurology* 1967;17:427–442.
14. Celesia GG, Wanamaker WM. Psychiatric disturbances in Parkinson's disease. *Dis Nerv Syst* 1972;33:577–583.
15. Lieberman A, Dziatolowski M, Kupersmith M, et al. Dementia in Parkinson's disease. *Ann Neurol* 1979;6:355–359.
16. Martilla RJ, Rinne UK. Dementia in Parkinson's disease. *Acta Neurol Scand* 1976;54:431–441.

17. Mayeux R, Stern Y, Rosenstein R, et al. An estimate of the prevalence of dementia in idiopathic Parkinson's disease. *Arch Neurol* 1988;45:260–263.

18. Mayeux R, Chen J, Mirabello E, et al. An estimate of the incidence of dementia in patients with idiopathic Parkinson's disease. *Neurology* 1990;40:1513–1517.

19. Antonini A, Leenders KL, Meier D, Oertel WH, Boesiger P, Anliker M. T2 relaxation time in patients with Parkinson's disease. *Neurology* 1993;43:697–700.

20. Antonini A, Bontobel P, Psylla M, et al. Complementary positron emission tomographic studies of the striatal dopaminergic system in Parkinson's patients. *Arch Neurol* 1995;52:1183–1190.

21. Shinotoh H, Calne DB. The use of PET in Parkinson's disease. *Brain Cogn* 1995;28:297–310.

22. Eidelberg D, Moeller JR, Ishikawa T, et al. Early differential diagnosis of Parkinson's disease with 18F-fluorodeoxyglucose and positron emission tomography. *Neurology* 1995;45:1995–2004.

23. Rinne JO, Laihinen A, Ruottinen H, et al. Increased density of dopamine D2 receptors in the putamen, but not in the caudate nucleus in early Parkinson's disease: a PET study with [¹¹C]raclopride. *J Neurol Sci* 1995;132:156–161.

24. Ward CD, Gibb WR. Research diagnostic criteria for Parkinson's disease. *Adv Neurol* 1990;53:245–248.

25. Rajput AH, Rozdilsky B, Ang L. Occurrence of resting tremor in Parkinson's disease. *Neurology* 1991;41:1298–1299.

26. Hughes AJ, Daniel SE, Kilford L, Lees AJ. Accuracy of clinical diagnosis of idiopathic Parkinson's disease: a clinico-pathological study of 100 cases. *J Neurol Neurosurg Psychiatry* 1992;55:181–184.

27. Weiner W, Lang AE. *Movement disorders. A comprehensive survey.* Mt. Kisco, NY: Futura Publishing Co., 1989.

28. Marsden CD, Parkes JD. Success and problems of long-term levodopa therapy in Parkinson's disease. *Lancet* 1977;1:345–349.

29. Olanow CW. Does selegiline monotherapy in Parkinson's disease act by symptomatic or protective mechanisms? *Neurology* 1992;42[Suppl 4]:13–26.

30. Olanow CW. A rationale for monoamine oxidase inhibition as neuroprotective therapy for Parkinson's disease. *Mov Disord* 1993;8[Suppl 1]:S1–7.

31. Limousin P, Pollack P, Pfefen JP, Tournier-Gervason CL, Dubuis R, Perret JE. Acute administration of levodopa-benserazide and tolcapone, a COMT inhibitor, Parkinson's disease. *Clin Neuropharmacol* 1995;18:258–265.

32. Ruottinen HM, Rinne UK. Entacapone prolongs levodopa response in a one month double blind study in parkinsonian patients with levodopa related fluctuations. *J Neurol Neurosurg Psychiatry* 1996;60:36–40.

33. Merello M, Lees AJ, Webster R, Bovingdon M, Gordin A. Effect of entacapone, a peripherally acting catechol-O-methyltransferase inhibitor, on the motor response to acute treatment with levodopa in patients with Parkinson's disease. *J Neurol Neurosurg Psychiatry* 1994;57:186–189.

34. Kaakkola S, Teravainen H, Ahtila S, Rita H, Gordin A. Effect of entacapone, a COMT inhibitor, on clinical disability and levodopa metabolism in parkinsonian patients. *Neurology* 1994;44:77–80.

35. Dogali M, Fazzini E, Kolodny E, et al. Stereotactic ventral pallidotomy for Parkinson's disease. *Neurology* 1995;45:753–761.

36. Lozano AM, Lang AE, Galvez-Jiminez N, et al. Effect of Gpi pallidotomy on motor function in Parkinson's disease. *Lancet* 1995;346:1383–1387.

37. Laitinen LV. Pallidotomy for Parkinson's disease. *Neurosurg Clin North Am* 1995;6:105–112.

38. Friedman JH, Epstein M, Sames JN, et al. Gamma knife pallidotomy in advanced Parkinson's disease. *Ann Neurol* 1996;39:535–538.

39. Jankovic J, Cardoso F, Grossman RG, Hamilton WJ. Outcome after stereotactic thalamotomy for parkinsonian, essential, and other types of tremor. *Neurosurgery* 1995;37:680–686.

40. Diederich N, Goetz CG, Stebbins GT, et al. Blinded evaluation confirms long-term asymmetric effect of unilateral thalamotomy or subthalamotomy on tremor in Parkinson's disease. *Neurology* 1992;42:1311–1314.

41. Kopyov OV, Jacques D, Lieberman A, Duma CM, Rogers RL. Clinical study of fetal mesencephalic intracerebral transplants for the treatment of Parkinson's disease. *Cell Transplant* 1996;5:327–337.

42. Freeman TB, Olanow CW, Hauser RA, et al. Bilateral fetal nigral transplantation into the postcommissural putamen in Parkinson's disease. *Ann Neurol* 1995;38:379–388.

43. Hoffer BJ, Leenders KL, Young D, et al. Eighteen-month course of two patients with grafts of fetal dopamine neurons for severe Parkinson's disease. *Exp Neurol* 1992;118:243–252.

44. Widner H, Tetrud J, Rehncrona S, et al. Bilateral fetal mesencephalic grafting in two patients with parkinsonism induced by 1-methyl-4-phenyl-1,2,3,-6-tetrahydropyridine (MPTP). *N Engl J Med* 1992;327:1556–1563.

45. Freed CR, Breeze RE, Rosenberg NL, et al. Survival of implanted fetal dopamine cells and neurologic improvement 12 to 46 months after transplantation for Parkinson's disease. *N Engl J Med* 1992;327:1549–1555.

46. Spencer DD, Robbins RJ, Naftolin F, et al. Unilateral transplantation of human fetal mesencephalic tissue into the caudate nucleus of patients with Parkinson's disease. *N Engl J Med* 1992;327:1541–1548.

47. Lindvall O, Widner H, Rehncrona S, et al. Transplantation of fetal dopamine neurons in Parkinson's disease: one-year clinical and neurophysiological observations in two patients with putaminal implants. *Ann Neurol* 1992;31:155–165.

48. Chung SS, Park YG, Chang JW, Cho J. Long-term follow-up results of stereotactic adrenal medullary transplants in Parkinson's disease. *Stereotact Funct Neurosurg* 1994;62:141–147.

49. Dieber MP, Pollack P, Passingham R, et al. Thalamic stimulation and suppression of parkinsonian tremor. Evidence of a cerebellar deactivation using positron emission tomography. *Brain* 1993;116:267–279.

50. Benabid AL, Pollak P, Seigneuret E, Hoffmann D, Gay E, Perret J. Chronic VIM stimulation in Parkinson's disease, essential tremor and extra-pyramidal disorders. *Acta Neurochir Suppl* 1993;58:39–44.

51. Caparros-Lefebvre D, Blond S, Vermersch P, Pecheux N, Guieu JD, Petit H. Chronic thalamic stimulation improves tremor and levodopa induced dyskinesias in Parkinson's disease. *J Neurol Neurosurg Psychiatry* 1993;56:268–273.

52. Graham JG, Oppenheimer DR. Orthostatic hypotension and nicotine sensitivity in a case of multiple system atrophy. *J Neurol Neurosurg Psychiatry* 1969;32:28–34.

53. Burn DJ, Sawle GV, Brooks DJ. Differential diagnosis of Parkinson's disease, multiple system atrophy, and Steele-Richardson-Olszewski syndrome: discriminant analysis of striatal ¹⁸F-dopa PET data. *J Neurol Neurosurg Psychiatry* 1994;57:278–284.

54. Wenning GK, Ben-Shlomo Y, Magalhaes M, Daniel SE, Quinn NP. Clinicopathological study of 35 cases of multiple system atrophy. *J Neurol Neurosurg Psychiatry* 1995;58:160–166.

55. Wenning GK, Quinn N, Magalhaes M, Mathias C, Daniel SE. Minimal change multiple system atrophy. *Mov Disord* 1994;9:161–166.

56. Lantos PL, Papp MI. Cellular pathology of multiple system atrophy: a review. *J Neurol Neurosurg Psychiatry* 1994;57:129–133.

57. Mochizucki A, Mizusawa H, Ohkoshi N, et al. Argentophilic intracytoplasmic inclusions in multiple system atrophy. *J Neurol* 1992;239:311–316.

58. Costa C, Duyckaerts C. Oligodendroglial and neuronal inclusions in multiple system atrophy. *Curr Opin Neurol* 1993; 6:865–871.

59. Fearnley JM, Lees AJ. Striatonigral degeneration. *Brain* 1990;113:1823–1842.

60. Saito Y, Matsuoka Y, Takahashi A, Ohno Y. Survival of patients with multiple system atrophy. *Intern Med* 1994;33:321–325.

61. Adams RD, van Bogaert L, vander Eecken H. Dégénérescences nigro-strieées et cerebello-nigro-strees. *Psychiatr Neurol* 1961;142:219–259.

62. Adams RD, van Bogaert L, vander Eecken H. Striato-nigral degeneration. *J Neuropathol Exp Neurol* 1964;23:584–608.

63. Van Leeuwen RB, Perquin WVM. Striatonigral degeneration. *Clin Neurol Neurosurg* 1988;90:121–124.

64. Gouider-Khouja N, Vidailhet M, Bonnet A-M, Pichon J, Agid Y. "Pure" striatonigral degeneration and Parkinson's disease. A comparative clinical study. *Mov Disord* 1995;10:288–294.

65. Suarez GA, Kelly JJ. The dropped head syndrome. *Neurology* 1992;42:1625–1627.

66. Lang AE, Curran T, Provias J, Bergeron C. Striatonigral degeneration: iron deposition in putamen correlates with the slit-like void signal of magnetic resonance imaging. *Can J Neurol Sci* 1994;21:311–318.

67. Savoiardo M, Girotti F, Strada L, Ciceri E. Magnetic resonance imaging in progressive supranuclear palsy and other parkinsonian disorders. *J Neural Transm Suppl* 1994; 42:93–110.

68. Eidelberg D, Takikawa S, Moeller JR, et al. Striatal hypometabolism

distinguishes striatnigral degeneration from Parkinson's disease. *Ann Neurol* 1993;33:518–527.

69. Davie CA, Wenning GK, Barker GJ, et al. Differentiation of multiple system atrophy from idiopathic Parkinson's disease using proton magnetic resonance spectroscopy. *Ann Neurol* 1995;37:204–210.

70. Gibb WR. Neuropathology of Parkinson's disease and related syndromes. *Neurol Clin* 1992;10:361–376.

71. Kato S, Meshitsuka S, Ohama E, Tanaka J, Llena JF, Hirano A. Increased iron content in the putamen of patients with striatonigral degeneration. *Acta Neuropathol* 1992;84:328–330.

72. Eidelberg D, Moeller JR, Dhawan V, et al. The metabolic topography of parkinsonism. *J Cereb Blood Flow Metab* 1994;14:783–801.

73. Parati EA, Fetoni V, Germiniani GC, et al. Response to L-DOPA in multiple system atrophy. *Clin Neuropharmacol* 1993;16:139–144.

74. Andrews JM, Terry RD, Spataro J. Striatonigral degeneration. Clinical-pathological correlations and response to stereotaxic surgery. *Arch Neurol* 1970;23:319–329.

75. Dejerine J, Thomas A. L atrophie olivo-ponto-cerebelleuse. *Nouv Iconogr Salpet* 1900;13:330–370.

76. Berciano J. Olivopontocerebellar atrophy. In: Jankovic J, Tolosa E, eds. *Parkinson's disease and movement disorders—2*. Baltimore: William & Wilkins, 1993;163–190.

77. Lepore FE. Disorders of ocular motility in the olivopontocerebellar atrophies. In: Duvoisan RC, Plaitakis A, eds. *The olivopontocerebellar atrophies*. New York: Raven Press, 1984:149–177.

78. Berciano J. Olivopontocerebellar atrophy. *J Neurol Sci* 1982;53:253–272.

79. Gilman S, Markel DS, Koeppe RA, et al. Cerebellar and brainstem hypometabolism in olivopontocerebellar atrophy with positron emission tomography. *Ann Neurol* 1988;23:223–230.

80. Koeppen AH, Mitzen EJ, Hans MC, Barron KD. Olivopontocerebellar atrophy: immunocytological and Golgi observations. *Neurology* 1986;36:1478–1488.

81. Kato S, Nakamura H. Cytoplasmic argyophilic inclusions in neurons of pontine nuclei in patients with olivopontocerebellar atrophy: Immunohistochemical and ultrastructural studies. *Acta Neuropathol* 1990;79:584–594.

82. Papp M, Lantos P. Accumulation of tubular structures in oligodendroglial and neuronal cells as the basic alteration in multiple system atrophy. *J Neurol Sci* 1992;107:172–182.

83. Lantos PL. The neuropathology of progressive supranuclear palsy. *J Neural Transm Suppl* 1994;42:137–152.

84. Wenning GK, Tison F, Elliott L, Quinn NP, Daniel SE. Olivopontocerebellar pathology in multiple system atrophy. *Mov Disord* 1996;11:157–162.

85. Goetz CG, Tanner CM, Klawans HL. The pharmacology of olivopontocerebellar atrophy. In: Duvoisin RC, Plaitakis A, eds. *The olivopontocerebellar atrophies*. New York: Raven Press, 1984:143–148.

86. Shy GM, Drager GA. A neurological syndrome associated with orthostatic hypotension: a clinical-pathologic study. *Arch Neurol* 1960;2:511–527.

87. Bradbury S, Eggleston C. Postural hypotension: a report of three cases. *Am Heart J* 1925;1:73–86.

88. The Consensus Committee of the American Autonomic Society and the American Academy of Neurology. Consensus statement on the definition of orthostatic hypotension, pure autonomic failure, and multiple system atrophy. *Neurology* 1996;46:1470.

89. Schatz IJ. Farewell to the Shy-Drager syndrome. *Ann Intern Med* 1996;125:74–75.

90. Sandroni P, Ahlskog JE, Fealey RD, Low PA. Autonomic involvement in extrapyramidal and cerebellar disorders. *Clin Auton Res* 1991;1:147–155.

91. Cohen J, Low P, Fealey R, Sheps S, Jiang N-S. Somatic and autonomic function in progressive autonomic failure and multiple system atrophy. *Ann Neurol* 1987 22:692–699.

92. Robbins TW, James M, Owen AM, et al. Cognitive deficits in progressive supranuclear palsy, Parkinson's disease, and multiple system atrophy in tests sensitive to frontal-lobe dysfunction. *J Neurol Neurosurg Psychiatry* 1994;57:1047–1056.

93. Williams A, Hanson D, Calne DB. Vocal cord paralysis in the Shy-Drager syndrome. *J Neurol Neurosurg Psychiatry* 1979;42:151–153.

94. Beck RO, Betts CD, Fowler CJ. Genitourinary dysfunction in multiple system atrophy: Clinical features and treatment in 62 cases. *J Urol* 1994;151:1336–1341.

95. Eardley I, Quinn NP, Fowler CJ, et al. The value of urethral sphincter electromyography in the differential diagnosis of parkinsonism. *Br J Urol* 1989;64:360–362.

96. Mannen T, Iwata M, Toyokura Y, Nagashima K. The Onuf's nucleus and the external anal sphincter muscles in amyotrophic lateral sclerosis and Shy-Drager syndrome. *Acta Neuropathol* 1982;58:255–260.

97. Ravits J, Hallett M, Nilsson J, Polinsky R, Dambrosia J. Electrophysiological tests of autonomic function in patients with idiopathic autonomic failure syndromes. *Muscle Nerve* 1996;19:758–763.

98. Papp MI, Kahn JE, Lantos PL. Glial cytoplasmic inclusion in the CNS of patients with multiple system atrophy (striatonigral degeneration, olivopontocerebellar atrophy and Shy-Drager syndrome). *J Neurol Sci* 1989;94:79–100.

99. Papp MI, Lantos PL. The distribution of oligodendroglial inclusions in multiple system atrophy and its relevance to clinical symptomatology. *Brain* 1994;117:235–243.

100. Martignoni E, Pacchetti C, Godi L, Micieli G, Nappi G. Autonomic disorders in Parkinson's disease. *J Neurol Transm* 1995;45[Suppl]:11–19.

101. Appenzeller O, Goss JE. Autonomic deficits Parkinson's syndrome. *Arch Neurol* 1971;24:50–57.

102. Magalhaes M, Wenning GK, Daniel SE, Quinn NP. Autonomic dysfunction in pathologically confirmed multiple system atrophy and idiopathic Parkinson's disease : a retrospective comparison. *Acta Neurol Scand* 1995;91:98–102.

103. Wenning GK, Shlomo YB, Magalhaes M, et al. Clinical features and natural history of multiple system atrophy. An analysis of 100 cases. *Brain* 1994;117:835–845.

104. Mathias CJ. Desmopressin reduces nocturnal polyuria, reverses overnight weight loss and improves morning postural hypotension in autonomic failure. *Br Med J* 1986;293:353–354.

105. Steele JC, Richardson JC, Olszewski J. Progressive supranuclear palsy: a heterogeneous degeneration involving the brainstem, basal ganglia and cerebellum with vertical gaze and pseudobulbar palsy, nuchal dystonia and dementia. *Arch Neurol* 1964;10:333–359.

106. Menza MA, Cocchiola J, Golbe LI. Psychiatric symptoms in progressive supranuclear palsy. *Psychosomatics* 1995;36:550–554.

107. Jackson JA, Jankovic J, Ford J. Progressive supranuclear palsy: clinical features and response to treatment in 16 patients. *Ann Neurol* 1983;13:273–278.

108. Burn DJ, Rinne JO, Quinn NP, Lees AJ, Marsden CD, Brooks DJ. Striatal opioid receptor binding in Parkinson's disease, striatonigral degeneration and Steele-Richardson-Olszewski syndrome: a [^{11}C]diprenorphine PET study. *Brain* 1995;118:951–958.

109. Romberg MH. *A manual of the nervous diseases of man*. Vol. II. Birmingham, AL: The Classics of Neurology and Neurosurgery Library, 1983. (Original 1853.)

110. Ishino H, Higashi H, Kuroda S, Yabuki S, Hayahara T. Motor nuclear involvement in progressive supranuclear palsy. *J Neurol Sci* 1974;22:235–241.

111. Troost BT, Daroff RB. The ocular motor defects in progressive supranuclear palsy (PSP). *Ann Neurol* 1977;2:397–403.

112. Vidailhet M, Rivaud S, Gouider-Khouja N, et al. Eye movements in parkinsonian syndromes. *Ann Neurol* 1994;35:420–426.

113. Jankovic J. Progressive supranuclear palsy: clinical and pharmacological update. *Neurol Clin* 1984;2:473–486.

114. Kluin KJ, Foster N, Berent S, Gilman S. Perceptual analysis of speech disorders in progressive supranuclear palsy. *Neurology* 1993;43:563–566.

115. Masucci EF, Borts FT, Perl SM, Wener L, Schwankhaus J, Kurtzke JF. MR vs. CT in progressive supranuclear palsy. *Comput Med Imaging Graph* 1995;19:361–368.

116. Stern MB, Braffman BH, Skolnick BE, Hurtig HI, Grossmi RI. Magnetic resonance imaging in Parkinson's disease and parkinsonian syndromes. *Neurology* 1989;39:1524–1526.

117. Drayer BP, Olanow W, Burger P, Johnson GA, Herfkins R, Riederer S. Parkinson plus syndrome: diagnosis using high field MR imaging of brain iron. *Radiology* 1989;159:493–498.

118. Litvan I, Agid Y, Jankovic J, et al. Accuracy of clinical criteria for the diagnosis of progressive supranuclear palsy (Steele-Richardson-Olszewski syndrome). *Neurology* 1996;46:922–930.

119. Litvan I, Agid Y, Calne D, et al. Clinical research criteria for the diagnosis of progressive supranuclear palsy (Steele-Richardson-Olszewski

syndrome): report of the NINDS-SPSP international workshop. *Neurology* 1996;47:1–9.

120. de-Bruin VM, Lees AJ, Daniel SE. Diffuse Lewy body disease presenting with supranuclear gaze palsy, parkinsonism, and dementia: a case report. *Mov Disord* 1992;7:355–358.

121. Fearnley JM, Revesz T, Brooks DJ, Frackowiak RS, Lees AJ. Diffuse Lewy body disease presenting with a supranuclear gaze palsy. *J Neurol Neurosurg Psychiatry* 1991;54:159–161.

122. Louis ED, Lynch T, Kaufmann P, Fahn S, Odel J. Diagnostic guidelines in central nervous system Whipple's disease. *Ann Neurol* 1996; 40:561–568.

123. Doty RL, Golbe LI, McKeown DA, Stern MB, Lehrach CM, Crawford D. Olfactory testing differentiates between progressive supranuclear palsy and idiopathic Parkinson's disease. *Neurology* 1993;43:962–965.

124. Litvan I, Mangone CA, McKee A, et al. Natural history of progressive supranuclear palsy (Steele-Richardson-Olszewski syndrome) and clinical predictors of survival: a clinicopathological study. *J Neurol Neurosurg Psychiatry* 1996;60:615–620.

125. Paulson GW, Lowery HW, Taylor GC. Progressive supranuclear palsy. *Eur Neurol* 1981;20:13–16.

126. Newman GC. Treatment of progressive supranuclear palsy with tricyclic antidepressants. *Neurology* 1985;35:1189–1193.

127. Nieforth KA, Golbe LI. Retrospective study of drug response in 87 patients with progressive supranuclear palsy. *Clin Neuropharmacol* 1993;16:338–346.

128. Duvoisin RC, Golbe LI, Lepore FE. Progressive supranuclear palsy. *Can J Neurol Sci* 1987;14:547–554.

129. Cole DG, Growdon JH. Therapy for progressive supranuclear palsy: past and future. *J Neural Transm Suppl* 1994;42:283–290.

130. Ghika J, Tennis M, Hoffman E, Schoenfeld D, Growdon J. Idazoxan treatment in progressive supranuclear palsy. *Neurology* 1991;41:986–991.

131. Hauser RA, Trehan R. Initial experience with electroconvulsive therapy for progressive supranuclear palsy [letter]. *Mov Disord* 1994;9:467–479.

132. Barclay CL, Duff J, Sandor P, Lang AE. Limited usefulness of electroconvulsive therapy in progressive supranuclear palsy. *Neurology* 1996;46:1284–1286.

133. Rebeiz JJ, Kolodny EH, Richardson EP. Corticodentatonigral degeneration with neuronal achromasia. *Arch Neurol* 1968;18:20–23.

134. Riley DE, Lang AE, Lewis A, et al. Cortico-basal ganglionic degeneration. *Neurology* 1990;40:1203–1212.

135. Doody RS, Jankovic J. The alien hand and related signs. *J Neurol Neurosurg Psychiatry* 1992;55:806–810.

136. Rinne JO, Lee MS, Thompson PD, Marsden CD. Corticobasal degeneration: A clinical study of 36 cases. *Brain* 1994;117:1183–1196.

137. Leiguarda R, Lees AJ, Merello M, Starkstein S, Marsden CD. The nature of apraxia in corticobasal degeneration. *J Neurol Neurosurg Psychiatry* 1994;57:455–459.

138. Pillon B, Blin J, Vidailhet M, et al. The neuropsychological pattern of corticobasal degeneration: comparison with progressive supranuclear palsy and Alzheimer's disease. *Neurology* 1995;45:1477–1483.

139. Blin J, Vidailhet MJ, Pillon B, Dubois B, Feve JR, Agid Y. Corticobasal degeneration: decreased and asymmetrical glucose consumption as studied with PET. *Mov Disord* 1992;7:348–354.

140. Markus HS, Lees AJ, Lennox G, Marsden CD, Costa DC. Patterns of regional cerebral blood flow in corticobasal degeneration studied using HMPAO SPECT; comparison with Parkinson's disease and normal controls. *Mov Disord* 1995;10:179–187.

141. Ikeda K, Akiyama H, Haga C, Kondo H, Aeima K, Oda T. Argyrophilic thread-like structure in corticobasal degeneration and supranuclear palsy. *Neurosci Lett* 1994;174:157–159.

142. Giminez-Roldan S, Mateo D, Benito C, Grandas F, Perez-Gilabert Y. Progressive supranuclear palsy and corticobasal ganglionic degeneration: differentiation by clinical features and neuroimaging techniques. *J Neural Transm Suppl* 1994;42:79–90.

Motor Disorders,
edited by David S. Younger.
Lippincott Williams & Wilkins, Philadelphia © 1999.

CHAPTER 34

Poliomyelitis and the Post-Polio Syndrome

Burk Jubelt and Judy Drucker

In the first half of the this century, epidemics of poliomyelitis (polio) ravaged the world. In the epidemic of 1952, over 20,000 Americans developed paralytic polio. With the introduction of the Salk inactivated polio vaccine (IPV) in 1954 and the Sabin oral polio vaccine (OPV) in 1961, the number of paralytic cases decreased to a handful per year. Polio had vanished and no longer was on the consciousness of Americans. The elimination of polio was a tremendous achievement for science and American medicine. However, in the late 1970s, survivors of paralytic polio began to notice new health problems that included fatigue, pain, and new weakness, thought not to be "real" by the medical establishment. The term "post-polio syndrome" (PPS) was coined by these patients to emphasize their new health problems.

This chapter reviews acute poliomyelitis and the related PPS.

POLIOMYELITIS

History

Poliomyelitis has occurred sporadically from 1600 to 1300 BC (1); however, epidemic poliomyelitis is a modern disease related to improved sanitation and human hygiene of the Western world (2). The first epidemics occurred in Europe in the mid-1800s and in North America in the 1890s. In 1870, Charcot and Joffroy ascribed flaccid paralysis to anterior horn cell damage. In 1905, Wickman recognized that asymptomatic infection and transmission occurred via the gastrointestinal tract (3). In 1909, Landsteiner and Popper (4) transmitted poliomyelitis to monkeys by the intracerebral inoculation of human brain tissue homogenates. In 1949, Enders et al. (5) cultured poliovirus in nonneural tissues, eliminating

animals for pathogenetic studies, and the three poliovirus serotypes were also recognized (6,7).

The most important development in the history of poliomyelitis was the introduction of polio vaccines. They decreased the incidence of paralytic poliomyelitis in the United States to fewer than 10 cases per year (8,9). Recent developments have included the cloning and sequencing of several strains of the three types of poliovirus (10–17) and the resolution of the viral structure to 29 nm by x-ray crystallography (18). These techniques have made it possible to determine the precise viral coat amino acids that induce antibody responses (19) and the location and the amino acid sequence of the site on the virus for cellular attachment (16,18,20). The poliovirus receptor on the cell membrane has been identified and is a member of the immunoglobulin superfamily (21).

Clinical Manifestations

Definitions and Nomenclature

Poliovirus infections can be divided into minor and major forms (22) (Fig. 1). The minor illnesses occur 1 to 3 days before the onset of paralysis, with gastrointestinal complaints of nausea and vomiting, abdominal cramps and pain, and diarrhea and the systemic manifestations of sore throat, fever, malaise, and headache.

The major illness includes all forms of central nervous system (CNS) disease caused by poliovirus, including aseptic meningitis or nonparalytic polio, polioencephalitis, bulbar polio, and paralytic poliomyelitis, alone or in combination. It can follow the minor illness immediately or more often within 3 to 4 days or occur without the minor illness. It is common for patients to have aseptic meningitis recognized by stiff neck, back pain, photophobia, and headache before the onset of paralytic polio. Polioencephalitis precedes paralysis and rarely occurs alone. It can manifest as tremulousness, obtundation, agitation, and autonomic dysfunction. The latter is recog-

B. Jubelt and J. Drucker: Department of Neurology, State University of New York Health Science Center at Syracuse, Syracuse, New York 13210.

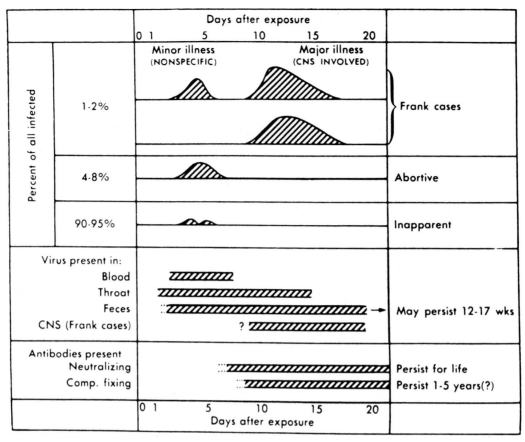

FIG.1. Schematic diagram of the clinical forms of poliomyelitis correlated with the times at which virus is present in various sites and the development of serum antibodies. (From Ref. 22, with permission.)

nized by labile hypertension, hypotension, tachycardia, arrhythmias, and excessive sweating. There may be upper motor neuron (UMN) signs of spasticity and hyper-reflexia and Babinski signs (23). Muscle pains, muscle cramps, fasciculations, and radicular pain rarely occur without paralysis, but when they do, they usually precede paralysis by 24 to 48 hours. Paralytic disease is due to poliovirus infection of the motor neuron. Spinal cord anterior horn cells and other motor neurons are selectively vulnerable to poliovirus infection (24–27). Infection by poliovirus results in a variable distribution and variable extent of paralysis.

Clinical Symptoms and Signs

Paralytic poliomyelitis can be of bulbar, spinal, or bulbospinal types (28). Paralytic disease accounts for 0.1 to 2.0% of all poliovirus infections during an epidemic (22,29). Spinal paralytic poliomyelitis is the most common type. It affects the lower extremities more frequently than the upper, and paralysis is usually asymmetric, flaccid, patchy, and more proximal than distal (30). As paralysis progresses, reflexes are lost. Over several days, the other extremities may become paralyzed, and bulbar involvement may occur. Extension of paralysis is unlikely

to occur 5 to 6 days after the onset of paralysis. Atrophy develops over several weeks. Rarely, a transverse myelitis with paraparesis, urinary retention, sensory complaints and signs and autonomic dysfunction including hyperhidrosis or hypohidrosis, and decreased limb temperature may occur (31,32).

Bulbar or brainstem poliomyelitis occurs in 10 to 15% of paralytic cases (30). It can involve any of the cranial nerves and the medullary reticular formation. Affected adults usually have bulbospinal poliomyelitis, whereas children are more likely to have isolated bulbar involvement. The most frequently involved cranial nerves are the VIIth, IXth, and Xth, resulting in facial weakness and difficulty with swallowing and phonation. Reticular formation involvement can result in respiratory problems with ataxic breathing, lethargy and obtundation, and cardiovascular dysfunction including hypotension, hypertension, and cardiac arrhythmias (33).

Chronic or persistent poliovirus infection occurs infrequently in children with immunodeficiency who receive the live oral vaccine (34,35). The immunodeficiency is usually agammaglobulinemia, but infection also rarely occurs in those with cellular immunodeficiency usually several months after vaccination (34–36). The affected individual may present with lower motor neuron (LMN) paralysis and progressive cerebral and intellectual dysfunction, with death in several months. Similar chronic infections have been caused by other enteroviruses (37).

Epidemiology

Incidence

The incidence of paralytic poliomyelitis peaked in the United States in 1952 with more than 20,000 cases (38). Because of the introduction of the killed IPV, or Salk vaccine, in 1954 and the live attenuated OPV, or Sabin vaccine, in 1961, the incidence has decreased to less than 10 cases per year in the United States (Fig. 2) (1,8,9,39). There is still a relatively high occurrence of the disease in Asia and Africa (40,41).

Transmission

Poliovirus is primarily spread by fecal-hand-oral transmission from one host to another. The virus is shed in oral secretions for several weeks and in the feces for several months (22,42). It is often introduced into the household by small children who are not toilet trained (43) and spreads in a family very rapidly, infecting most members in 4 to 5 days (42,44). Household spread depends on prior immunity, household size, and sanitary hygiene conditions (45). Transmission is related also to environmental factors such as sanitation, level of hygiene, crowded conditions, geography, the season, and host characteristics.

Endemic Versus Epidemic Activity

The geographic location and the accompanying temperature changes are factors that result in endemic or epidemic poliovirus activity. In tropical and semitropical areas, poliovirus circulates year around, the so-called endemic pattern, whereas in temperate zones, epidemics peak in the summer and early fall (45,46). From ancient times until the late 1800s, poliovirus activity was primarily endemic due to crowding, poor personal hygiene, and poor public sanitation (47,48). By early childhood, most individuals had been infected by all three types of poliovirus (49), and infrequently sporadic cases of paralytic poliomyelitis or true "infantile paralysis" were seen (50). This endemic pattern still occurs in semitropical and tropical underdeveloped areas of the world.

In the late 1800s, in developed temperate areas of the world, epidemic activity began to occur probably due to improved personal hygiene and public sanitation (2,51); accordingly, infants and small children were not previously exposed to poliovirus, creating a large pool of susceptible older children, adolescents, and adults. Because the latter are more likely to develop severe disease (3), when poliovirus infection sweeps through this virgin population, a high rate of paralysis can occur (22).

Predisposing Factors

There are other predisposing factors for paralytic poliomyelitis (3). Age is one factor; older children, adolescents, and adults have more severe and extensive paralysis and a higher incidence of death than infants and young children (52–54). Men and boys have a greater susceptibility to poliomyelitis (52,54). Tonsillectomy before or at the time of infection is associated with a higher incidence of bulbar involvement. Traumatic and injected extremities are more likely to become paralyzed,

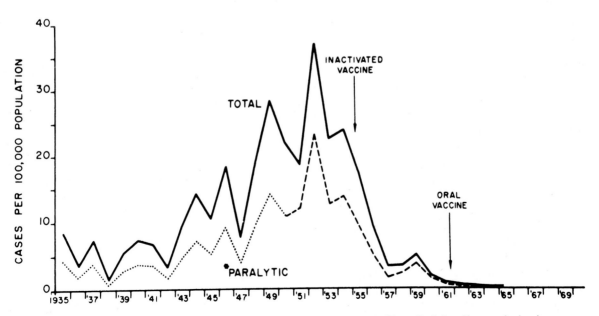

FIG. 2. Incidence of poliomyelitis in the United States, 1935–1964. (From Ref. 1, with permission.)

the so-called provoking effect (55). Physical exertion predisposes to more severe paralysis, whereas pregnancy increases the incidence of paralytic disease by about threefold (56).

Pathology and Pathogenesis

As previously noted, polioviruses and other enteroviruses are spread by fecal-hand-oral transmission. After replication in the oropharynx and intestinal mucosae, the virus replicates in the submucosal lymphatic tissue (57), leading to a primary viremia, followed by replication in nonneural target tissues, and secondary viremia and CNS invasion. The exact route the poliovirus takes to enter the CNS is unclear, but viremia is required for CNS invasion (58,59). There is evidence to suggest that poliovirus enters the neuraxis at areas where the blood–brain barrier is defective, such as the area postrema (60). Another possibility is that the virus reaches the neuromuscular junction during the viremia, entering the distal axon and transported by retrograde axonal transport to the CNS (61–63). Poliovirus dissemination in the CNS occurs along nerve fiber pathways, probably by fast axonal transport (57,63,64).

Pathologic changes are seen several days after poliovirus infection of anterior horn cells. Initially, the Nissl substance shrinks and dissolves, leading to diffuse chromatolysis and loss of basophilic staining (6). If infection does not resolve at this point (65), nuclear shrinkage, eosinophilic type B inclusions, and cellular membrane disintegration occur. The inflammatory response consists of meningeal, perivascular, and parenchymal infiltrates, initially composed of polymorphonuclear leukocytes over the first 24 to 48 hours, followed by mononuclear and microglial cell responses with neuronophagia (25,66).

Laboratory Studies

General laboratory tests are uninformative. The complete blood count may reveal a peripheral leukocytosis. Cerebrospinal fluid (CSF) abnormalities are similar to those seen with many other CNS viral infections. The CSF cell count is increased, which initially may be a polymorphonuclear leukocytosis followed by a shift to mononuclear cells in 12 to 48 hours (3). At times it may be important to repeat the lumbar puncture to exclude bacterial infection. The cell count often reaches several hundred cells per mm³ but can be as high as several thousand. It usually declines precipitously within 2 weeks. Initially, the CSF protein is normal or mildly elevated but may rise to 100 to 300 mg/dL over several weeks and may remain high for months. Hypoglycorrhachia is rarely seen (3). Newer generation magnetic resonance imaging studies may show localization of inflammation to the spinal cord anterior horns (67). Virus isolation and serologic studies are needed to confirm the diagnosis.

Poliovirus can be isolated from the oropharynx for several weeks and from the stool for several months (22,68). It is almost never isolated from the CSF (69). Because several enteroviruses may be isolated from the stool, serologic testing is needed to confirm the responsible virus type. A fourfold or greater rise in serum antibody titer between the acute and convalescent specimens is considered diagnostic. It is important to obtain the acute phase specimen as soon as possible to detect the fourfold rise. The convalescent phase sample should be obtained at least 2 weeks, and preferably 4 weeks, after the acute phase specimen is obtained. A CSF/serum antibody ratio of greater than 1:150 may also be diagnostic (70), as well as CSF IgM antipoliovirus antibody (71).

Differential Diagnosis

The combination of fever, headache, stiff neck, and asymmetric flaccid paralysis without sensory loss, and a CSF profile consistent with viral infection make paralytic poliomyelitis likely. The diagnosis may be difficult if these major manifestations are lacking or if unusual manifestations, such as urinary retention or sensory loss, occur. Nonpolio enteroviruses can also cause polio-like paralysis, although it is usually not as severe as that seen with poliovirus (3,72). Several other viruses can occasionally cause acute LMN paralysis, especially rabies (73) and herpes zoster (74). Other disease processes in the differential include transverse myelitis, acute spinal cord compression from epidermal abscess, Guillain-Barré syndrome, acute intermittent porphyria, toxic neuropathies, and botulism (69,72,75).

Management

Treatment

Treatment for paralytic poliomyelitis initially relies on supportive care followed by passive and then active physical therapy and orthopedic measures. Bedrest is recommended during the preparalytic stage because physical exercise can increase the severity of paralysis (3). Treatment of sore muscles with hot packs, fever with analgesics, and anxiety with anxiolytics may be calming. In addition, acute paralysis should be treated with hospitalization, appropriate positioning with splints to prevent contractures, foot boards to prevent foot drop, and frequent turning to prevent decubiti (69). Patients with bulbar involvement generally require fluid and electrolytes and, at times, cardiovascular, autonomic, and respiratory support (76). During the convalescent period, active physical therapy with nonfatiguing muscle-strengthening exercises and hydrotherapy may be beneficial. Braces and other orthoses may be needed for weak muscles or severe extremity paralysis. Arthrodesis, tendon transfers, leg-shortening procedures, and other orthopedic surgical interventions should be deferred for 1.5 to 2 years after maximum recovery has occurred (77,78).

Prevention

Vaccination is the mainstay of prevention. The *injectable* killed IPV and the live attenuated *OPV* have been very effective in decreasing the incidence of poliomyelitis (1,38). The advantages and disadvantages of each vaccine have been extensively debated (3,45). The killed vaccine results in relative short-term immunity of 5 to 10 years, necessitating frequent revaccinations, but it does not cause paralysis. A very high level of vaccination of the population is required with the killed vaccine to prevent the spread of wild-type virulent viruses in the community. In contrast, the live vaccine is effective in producing long-term immunity, possibly lifelong, producing immunity by exposure to vaccine strains circulating in the population (secondary spread) (79) and eliminating the circulation of wild-type virulent strains. However, the live vaccine rarely causes paralysis (55,80). Recently in the United States, the recommendations for vaccination have been changed to a sequential vaccination schedule of two doses each of the IPV followed by the OPV (81). Prevention can also occur by stopping the spread of infection through the use of good personal, family, and public hygiene. Handwashing and the use of clean utensils can decrease person-to-person fecal-hand-oral transmission (43). Adequate water and sewage treatment can decrease the spread of poliovirus (82).

Prognosis and Complications

With good supportive care, especially for respiratory insufficiency, death from paralytic poliomyelitis occurs in only 7 to 8% of patients (69). Death is usually the result of bulbar involvement with respiratory and cardiovascular impairment. Patients who survive an acute attack of paralytic poliomyelitis usually have significant recovery of motor function, although permanent and severe residual paralysis of one or two extremities is not uncommon. Motor improvement usually starts within weeks after onset, although in rare cases, extension of localized paralysis can be seen as late as the third or fourth week of illness (83). About a 50% recovery occurs in 3 months, and 75% in 6 months. Minimal further improvement occurs slowly over the next 2 years (84).

Acute and subacute complications include those related to immobility, such as decubiti, contractures, foot and wrist drop, and urinary tract infections. Pneumonia can result from bulbar muscle dysfunction and respiratory insufficiency. More chronic complications include osteoporosis, skeletal deformities such as scoliosis, reduced extremity growth, and PPS, discussed in the following section, which generally occurs 30 to 40 years after acute polio.

POST-POLIO SYNDROME

History

New muscle weakness as a late sequela of poliomyelitis was initially recognized by Charcot and others in 1875 (85–87). Between 1875 and 1975, about 200 cases were reported in the world's literature (23,88). Since 1975, a large "epidemic" of several thousand cases has occurred (23,89,90). They relate to the large epidemics of poliomyelitis that occurred during the first half of this century (reviewed in Ref. 91). Since our last in-depth review of this topic (91), recent advances have centered on the pathophysiology, etiology, and treatment of the muscle weakness. The generalized nonspecific manifestations and sympathetic and UMN involvement in poliomyelitis and PPS, including the epidemiology, muscle biopsy findings, etiologic hypotheses, symptomatic treatment, and management, have been previously reviewed by Jubelt and colleagues (23,91).

Clinical Manifestations

Definition of the Syndrome

PPS is a neurologic disorder that produces a cluster of symptoms in individuals who had acute paralytic poliomyelitis usually 30 to 50 years earlier. They commonly include progressive weakness, fatigue, and pain of muscles and/or joints and less commonly muscle atrophy, breathing and swallowing difficulties, sleep disorders, and cold intolerance. Some symptoms such as weakness, muscle fatigue, atrophy, and maybe generalized fatigue appear to be caused by a progressive degeneration or dysfunction of motor units and eventually motor neurons. Other symptoms such as joint pain are more likely the result of excessive wear and tear on different parts of the musculoskeletal system.

Because some of the manifestations, especially fatigue, are nonspecific, the syndrome itself can be hard to diagnose unless other musculoskeletal or neurologic components are present. *Fatigue* is the most common manifestation overall (89,91,92), but *new weakness*, sometimes accompanied by atrophy, is the signature for the neurologic disorder termed "post-polio progressive muscular atrophy" (23,89). The criteria for PPS now used by most investigators and clinicians in the field were first described by Mulder et al. (93): documentation of paralytic polio, partial recovery of function followed by a period of stabilization, and progressive neurologic deterioration (Table 1). The *musculoskeletal manifestations*, mainly joint and muscle pain, result from the combination of long-term residual weakness and the stress in joints, ligaments, and tendons.

Neurologic Manifestations

Fatigue is clearly the most prominent manifestation, occurring in up to 80% of patients (23,89,90,92) (Table 2).

TABLE 1. *Diagnostic criteria for post-polio syndrome*[a]

1. A prior episode of paralytic poliomyelitis with residual motor neuron loss (which can be confirmed through a typical patient history, a neurologic examination, and, if needed, an electrodiagnostic exam).
2. A period of neurologic recovery followed by an interval (usually 15 years or more) of neurologic and functional stability.
3. A gradual or abrupt onset of new weakness or abnormal muscle fatigue (decreased endurance), muscle atrophy, or generalized fatigue.
4. Exclusion of medical, orthopedic, and neurologic conditions that may be causing the symptoms mentioned in 3.

[a]Consensus of the Post-Polio Task Force.

It is generally described as a disabling generalized exhaustion, the "polio wall," that follows even minimal physical activity (94). Their fatigue also has been described by patients as "increasing physical weakness," "tiredness," "lack of energy," and "increasing loss of strength during exercise" (95); thus, it can either be perceived as generalized or muscular in origin (94,96). The fatigue can also affect mental as well as physical functioning, as for example when it is severe patients find it difficult to concentrate or collect their thoughts and appear confused (95). It may be improved by decreasing physical activity, pacing daily activities, and taking frequent rest periods and naps (96,97). PPS fatigue appears to respond better to sleep than that of the chronic fatigue syndrome, although frequent rest periods are also helpful.

The pathophysiology of fatigue is not clear. Bruno et al. (98) hypothesized that the age-related attrition of neurons in the substantia nigra and possible degeneration of reticular formation neurons, combined with the already decreased number of these neurons resulting from poliomyelitis, might cause impairment of the brain activating system. Others have related the fatigue to diffuse deterioration of the motor unit at the neuromuscular junction (97,99). Some PPS patients, 10 to 20%, have muscle fatigability reminiscent of myasthenia gravis (100), as similarly reported in amyotrophic lateral sclerosis (101). A number of medications can be used to treat the generalized fatigue as indicated below. One study found that neuromuscular junction transmission, as measured by jitter on single-fiber electromyography (SFEMG), improved with anticholinesterase treatment in up to 50% of PPS patients so studied, and 50% also experienced decreased general fatigue and muscle fatigability (102). A recently completed controlled double-blind trial of pyridostigmine in PPS was, however, negative (personal communication).

New slowly progressive muscle weakness is the most important neurologic problem, occurring in most affected patients (90,91,103) (Table 2). It appears to be related to a disintegration of the LMN unit (104,105) and can occur in muscles previously affected and partially or fully recovered or in unaffected muscles (90,91) (Table 2). Human electromyography (EMG) (106) and animal studies (107,108) indicate that some clinically unaffected muscles were involved subclinically during the acute poliomyelitis, but previously affected muscles were more likely than unaffected muscles to later become weak (90,91) (Table 2). The distribution of the new weakness, which is usually asymmetric, proximal, distal, or patchy, appears to correlate with the severity of paralysis at the time of the acute poliomyelitis and with the amount of recovery and thus with the number of surviving motor

TABLE 2. *Most common new late manifestations of poliomyelitis in patients referred to post-polio clinics*[a]

Symptom	Houston[b] (n=132)	Madison[c] (n=79)	Syracuse[d] (n=100) 1991–1993	Syracuse[d] (n=100) 1993–1997
Fatigue	89%	86%	83%	86%
Joint pain	71%	77%	72%	73%
Muscle pain	71%	86%	74%	73%
Weakness				
Previously affected muscles	69%	80%	88%	88%
Previously unaffected muscles	50%	53%	61%	59%
Total[e]	—	87%	95%	90%
Atrophy	28%	39%	59%	52%
Cold intolerance	29%	56%	49%	53%
Respiratory insufficiency	—	39%	42%	36%
Dysphagia	—	30%	27%	36%

[a]Modified from Ref. 91.
[b]Adapted from Ref. 90. All patients met criteria for PPS.
[c]Adapted from Ref. 92. All patients had histories and examinations compatible with diagnosis of previous poliomyelitis.
[d]First 200 patients with histories and examinations compatible with diagnosis of previous poliomyelitis.
[e]Total percent of patients with new weakness.

neurons (6,104,109). New atrophy does not occur as an isolated manifestation and is seen in fewer than half of patients with new weakness (90,110). In addition to the weakness and atrophy caused by the disintegration of the motor unit, rarely UMN signs can occur (23). They include hyperreflexia, Babinski signs, and occasionally spasticity. Of 180 PPS patients so studied, we found UMN signs in 15 (8.3%), 7 of whom underwent myelography or magnetic resonance imaging of the spinal cord to exclude compression (23). This percentage is very similar to the frequency of UMN signs found during acute poliomyelitis (23). *Muscle pain* or *myalgia*, which also occurs in most patients (90,91,103) (Table 2), appears to be due to overuse of weak muscles. Similar symptoms occur in overused weakened muscles in other neuromuscular diseases (23). The pain is a soreness or aching feeling that occurs with minimal exercise. A small number of patients can have muscle tenderness on palpation. Rest, braces, splints, and anti-inflammatory medications may be beneficial.

New muscle weakness may also involve specific muscles groups, causing respiratory insufficiency, bulbar muscle weakness, and sleep apnea. *Respiratory insufficiency* primarily occurs in patients with severe residual respiratory impairment with minimal reserve (111,112). Similar to limb weakness, respiratory failure is more likely to occur in patients who required respiratory support during the acute disease and hence had more severe disease and in those that contracted polio at an age older than 10 years (111). Patients with PPS and chronic respiratory failure lose an average of 1.9% of their vital capacity per year (113). It usually is due to respiratory muscle weakness but also to central hypoventilation because of the residual damage from earlier bulbar poliomyelitis (33). Other factors such as pulmonary or cardiac disease or scoliosis may contribute to the problem. Initially, respiratory failure begins with nocturnal alveolar hypoventilation, and patients may require only nighttime respiratory support (114). If already on nighttime respiratory support, they may eventually require total ventilator support (115). Bach (116) studied 145 post-poliomyelitis individuals who were managed by noninvasive alternatives to tracheostomy. Mouthpiece intermittent positive pressure ventilation, nasal intermittent positive pressure ventilation, manually and mechanically assisted coughing, and noninvasive blood gas monitoring in the home were the main techniques used for optimizing quality of life and for avoiding complications. With the use of these measures, acute respiratory failure and tracheal intubation were generally avoided.

Bulbar muscle weakness is now also a recognized component of PPS (117), of which *dysphagia* is the most common problem. Residual dysphagia occurs in 10 to 20% of polio survivors (118). It is primarily due to pharyngeal and laryngeal muscle weakness; however, local pharyngeal or esophageal problems should also be excluded. Some patients complain of food sticking, making swallowing slow or difficult, often with coughing and choking (118). Videofluoroscopic studies may reveal impaired tongue movements, delayed pharyngeal constriction, pooling in the valleculae or pyriform sinuses, and rarely aspiration, which is usually mild (117). Infrequently, other bulbar muscles, such as the facial muscles and vocal cords, may become weaker in PPS (119); dysarthria has also been reported (23).

Sleep apnea is not an uncommon problem in post-polio patients. It may be central, obstructive, or mixed (120,121). Most patients with central sleep apnea have a history of bulbar polio, and some required ventilatory support (120). It is probable that residual damage to the brainstem reticular formation predisposes to central sleep apnea. In comparison, obstructive sleep apnea appears to be related to pharyngeal muscle weakness, obesity, and musculoskeletal deformities (121). Respiratory muscle weakness may also contribute to sleep apnea (122).

Fasciculation and cramps without weakness, muscle pseudohypertrophy, and tingling paresthesias are other neuromuscular problems that may occur in post-polio patients, with or without new weakness (23).

Musculoskeletal Manifestations

Pain from joint instability is the major musculoskeletal problem and can occur without new weakness. The long-term overstress of joints because of residual weakness eventually results in joint deterioration. Progressive scoliosis, poor posture, unusual mechanics because of deformed joints, uneven limb size, failing tendon transfers, and failing joint fusions can all contribute to joint pain. It can also arise from overstressed tendons due to joint deformities or because of long-standing muscle weakness. These joint problems frequently lead to loss of mobility and a return to using old assistive devices (123). Compressive radiculopathies and mononeuropathies may occur as secondary musculoskeletal complications (23,124).

Other Manifestations

Other symptoms much less frequently reported include increased sleep requirements, cold intolerance, and psychologic stresses (23,90). Increased sleep requirements probably relate to severe fatigue. Many PPS patients complain of cold intolerance (90) (Table 2). They report worsening symptoms, including increasing generalized fatigue and weakness when exposed to cold temperatures (125). Patients may also develop coolness and color changes such as cyanosis and blanching of the affected extremity that relate to sympathetic intermediolateral column damage during prior acute poliomyelitis (126). Psychological symptoms, related to the reemergence of a supposedly old resolved problem and to the stresses of the required major changes in lifestyle, can be overwhelming at times (127,128).

Epidemiology

Prevalence

Data regarding the incidence and prevalence of PPS is quite variable. Codd et al. (103) found a prevalence of PPS of 22.4% in those with previous poliomyelitis, but a repeat study from the same institution found a prevalence of 64% (129). The 1987 National Health Interview Survey estimated that about half of the 1.63 million people in the United States who survived acute poliomyelitis had new late effects (PPS) (130). Another study from 1987 found a frequency of 42% (131). Ramlow et al. (132) detected a prevalence of 28.5% among all cases of paralytic poliomyelitis. The variation in prevalence appears to relate to the definition of PPS. About 50 to 64% of patients have new problems, but only about 20 to 30% have new progressive weakness. A large number of cases are seen because of the large epidemics of poliomyelitis that occurred in the United States in the 1940s and 1950s (23).

Delay in Onset of Post-Polio Syndrome

The delay in onset between acute poliomyelitis and PPS ranges from 8 to 71 years in various series (23). The more severe the acute polio, the earlier new symptoms are likely to occur (94). In various series the average interval is about 35 years (23,94,132,133).

Risk Factors

Several risk factors predispose to the development of PPS. One is the severity of the polio and resulting paralysis (94,129,134,135); another is the age at onset of the poliomyelitis. Acute poliomyelitis in adolescents and adults is more severe than in infants and small children (23), and the former patients are more likely to develop PPS (94,109). Another risk factor is the amount of recovery; the greater the recovery, the more likely PPS will occur (109), suggesting that reinnervation is unable to be maintained 30 to 40 years later. In those who do recover totally or partially, excessive exercise or overuse appears to predispose them to PPS (109,135).

Course of Post-Polio Progressive Muscular Atrophy

It is difficult to measure the course of many PPS manifestations; however, weakness lends itself to objective analysis. Mulder et al. (93) reported continuous progression of weakness during the 12 years of follow-up. Dalakas et al. (136) used Medical Research Council grading and noted stepwise or steady progression of weakness at an average rate of only 1% per year over a mean follow-up period of 12.2 years. Some studies with shorter follow-up periods of 2 (137), 2.5 (138), and 5 years (139) did not demonstrate progression of the weakness; however, two other studies (140,141), each with 4-year follow-up periods, found a rate of progression of 2% per year. Many patients have a stepwise course with plateaus, and progression may be difficult to demonstrate unless the follow-up period is of adequate duration, generally greater than 5 or even 10 years. Significant objective clinical weakening was noted by others (142), including weakness of bulbar musculature (117).

Laboratory Studies

Routine blood tests, including erythrocyte sedimentation rate, are normal except for the creatine kinase (CK), which may be mildly elevated (23,129,143,144). In one study, an increased creatine kinase level was more likely to occur in those with progressive weakness (129), and markedly elevated values probably indicate muscle overuse (145). In most studies, CSF parameters have been normal, although a mildly elevated protein content has been seen (23).

Electromyography

In 1987 (23), we analyzed EMG studies in 26 patients with old poliomyelitis. Concentric needle EMG of patients with old polio showed chronic denervation and reinnervation including abnormally increased motor unit potential amplitude, duration, and polyphasia and decreased interference patterns both in patients and in muscles with or without new weakness, tested years after acute polio, and in muscles that were clinically uninvolved during the acute disease. Active new denervation including fibrillation and positive sharp wave activity was usually of a mild degree (Table 3) and seen in some PPS patients with new weakness (range, 0 to 45%) but also in those without new weakness. Fasciculation was seen more frequently than acute denervation. Nerve conduction velocities were also generally normal. SFEMG revealed increased fiber density and the neuromuscular transmission defects of increased jitter and blocking (Table 3). The number of motor units with abnormal jitter and neuromuscular blocking correlated with the number of years since acute poliomyelitis (146). EMG and SFEMG studies, however, did not discriminate PPS from the asymptomatic cases (104). Wiechers (147) has been the only one to analyze macro-EMG and showed that large reinnervated motor units decreased with time from recovery of the acute disease, suggesting a loss of terminal sprouts.

It now appears that the enlarged motor units that develop by collateral sprouting after acute poliomyelitis never fully stabilize (148). There may be continuous denervation and reinnervation, with denervation becoming more prominent later in life as reinnervation becomes

TABLE 3. *Electromyography (EMG) in post-polio patients*

Standard (concentric needle) EMG
    Evidence of old, remote, or chronic denervation in >90% of patients, with increased duration or amplitude of MUP (often >10 mV) and decreased interference pattern
    Evidence of new or ongoing denervation—0–45% in various series, with spontaneous activity (fasciculations, fibrillations, positive waves) at a low level (1+).
    Does not discriminate symptomatic from asymptomatic post-polio patients
SFEMG
    Increased fiber density (very high) in 90% of patients
    Increasing % with abnormal jitter with increasing years since polio
    Neuromuscular blocking
    Does not discriminate symptomatic from asymptomatic post-polio patients
Macro-EMG
    Increased amplitude
    Amplitude may drop with progressive weakness

Modified from Ref. 91. See text for references.

less efficient. Progressive weakness appears to be the "end of the spectrum of all post-poliomyelitis patients" (149). Similar to clinical studies suggesting that good recovery is a major risk factor for PPS (109), SFEMG studies reveal a positive correlation between increased jitter and fiber density. They also suggest that muscles with enlarged motor units due to sprouting or recovery are more likely to become unstable later in life (110,150). Spontaneous activity, like jitter and blocking, appear to be more frequent in symptomatic muscles (151,152). Macro-EMG motor unit potential amplitudes are increased in post-polio muscles (141,153). In some muscles, the macro-EMG amplitudes may decrease in size as motor neurons die (154), whereas in others, it may increase as other motor neurons compensate (141). Despite the fact that EMG studies cannot be used to diagnose PPS because symptomatic and asymptomatic muscles have the same findings, the aforementioned studies have contributed greatly to our understanding of the pathophysiology of neuromuscular junction dysfunction after acute poliomyelitis. EMG studies can also exclude other diagnoses and determine the extent of the old acute poliomyelitis (155).

Muscle Biopsy

The biopsy findings of patients with old poliomyelitis reveal evidence of chronic denervation, reinnervation, and active denervation (23). The primary sign of chronic denervation and reinnervation is fiber type grouping. A sign of active denervation is the presence of small angulated fibers that arise with terminal sprout denervation; group atrophy, sometimes seen in amyotrophic lateral

sclerosis, is an infrequent finding in PPS. The expression of neural-cell adhesion molecules on the surface of muscle fibers is another finding that suggests active denervation (104,105). Unfortunately, chronic denervation and reinnervation and acute denervation have been seen in both symptomatic and asymptomatic post-polio patients, and muscle biopsies cannot clearly distinguish between them. Dalakas (156) found that originally affected muscles that had partially recovered had a variable degree of chronic and acute neurogenic atrophy or fiber-type grouping, with variable group atrophy and angulated fibers in some, combined with secondary myopathic features. Muscles originally affected that had fully recovered also showed signs of both chronic fiber-type grouping and recent denervation or angulated fibers, with few secondary myopathic features. Muscles originally spared clinically but newly symptomatic had signs of chronic denervation and reinnervation and recent denervation, but secondary myopathic features were minimal or absent. Asymptomatic post-polio patients had signs of chronic denervation and reinnervation but no signs of acute denervation or myopathy. These findings need to be confirmed in a larger sampling. The significance of the occasional findings of classic myopathic features (156,157) and lymphocytic infiltrates (156) remains unclear.

Etiology

Jubelt and Cashman (23) outlined nine possible mechanisms for the development of PPS (Table 4). Over the last 10 years, enough information has accumulated that the possibilities can now probably be narrowed even more. Normal aging alone cannot explain the development of PPS. The loss of anterior horn cells and motor

TABLE 4. *Possible etiology of the post-polio syndrome*

Death of remaining motor neurons with normal aging, coupled with the previous loss from poliomyelitis
Premature aging of cells permanently damaged by poliovirus
Premature aging of remaining normal motor neurons due to an increased metabolic demand (increased motor unit size after poliomyelitis)
Premature exhaustion of new terminal sprouts with advancing age in the large reinnervated motor units that developed after polio (possibly also excessive metabolic demand)
Chronic poliovirus infection
Predisposition to motor neuron degeneration because of the glial, vascular, and lymphatic changes caused by poliovirus
Poliomyelitis-induced vulnerability of motor neurons to secondary insults
Genetic predisposition of motor neurons to both poliomyelitis and premature degeneration
An immune-mediated syndrome

Modified from Ref. 23.

units with normal aging does not become prominent until after the age of 60 years (see Ref. 23). In other mammals, terminal sprouting also becomes impaired with aging, and sprouting is no longer able to keep up with the normal loss of terminal fibers that occurs throughout life as part of the constant remodeling at the neuromuscular junction (23). The age at which this occurs in humans is unknown. Muscle biopsy studies do not reveal a significant increase in small angulated fibers until after age 70 years (105). More important than chronologic age is the interval from the acute polio to the onset of symptoms, an interval that averages 30 to 40 years (23). A discussion of more likely possibilities follows.

Premature Exhaustion of New Sprouts Developing after Acute Poliomyelitis and of Their Motor Neurons due to Excessive Metabolic Demand

EMG and muscle biopsy studies have helped clarify this possible mechanism. Enlarged motor units that develop via sprouting after the acute polio may never fully stabilize (148). Findings from SFEMG studies reveal that the largest motor units are more likely to become unstable later in life (104,152), and with increasing time from the acute polio, neuromuscular transmission becomes more unstable, as increased jitter and blocking occur (146). Several studies have shown that spontaneous activity, jitter, and blocking occurred more frequently in symptomatic muscles (150,151). These findings are supported by muscle biopsy studies that describe an increasing number of angulated fibers accumulating over time with the eventual emergence of group atrophy (105). In fact, 30 to 40 years after the acute poliomyelitis, there is disintegration of the new terminal sprouts that form after the acute infection as demonstrated by the appearance of angulated fibers (156). A contributing factor in some is the reinnervation of fibers that may not result in effective synapses (150). This is followed by degeneration of axonal branches as shown by small group atrophy (104,157). It has been frequently hypothesized that the increased metabolic demand of an increased motor unit territory results in premature exhaustion and death of the motor neuron (23). Even though there are no definitive studies examining the cell soma to prove this, electrophysiologic and muscle biopsy data appear to be supportive. The overuse of muscles resulting in excessive muscular fatigue (158–160) may also contribute to the excessive metabolic demand on motor neurons, and premature exhaustion might also be enhanced by the prior poliovirus infection of motor neurons with residual damage (23).

Chronic Persistent Poliovirus Infection

Poliovirus and other picornaviruses can persist in the CNS of animals and cause delayed or chronic disease (23,161). Poliovirus and other enteroviruses can also persist in the CNS and systemically in immunodeficient children (23). Studies in tissue culture have found that poliovirus mutants can persist without killing the host cell (162,163) and can also persist in neurons (164). Support for the persistent poliovirus hypothesis was enhanced by the findings of Sharief et al. (165), who demonstrated poliovirus antibodies and poliovirus-sensitized cells in the CSF of post-polio patients. My collaborators and I have been unable to find poliovirus antibodies in the CSF of post-polio patients using isoelectric focusing and ELISA techniques (166,167), similar to others (136,168,169). Conclusive viral isolation and histochemical or hybridization studies have not as yet been reported using spinal cord tissues. However, CSF specimens have been examined for the presence of poliovirus RNA by polymerase chain reaction, and most studies have been negative or inconclusive (169–172).

An Immune-Mediated Disease

The strongest support for an inflammatory or immune-mediated mechanism for PPS stems from the study of Pezeshkpour and Dalakas (173) in which inflammation in the spinal cords of seven post-polio patients was found. It consisted of both perivascular and parenchymal lymphocytic infiltrates and neuronal degeneration and active gliosis. All changes were more prominent in the three patients with new weakness. Other findings that support this hypothesis are the finding oligoclonal bands in the CSF (136) and activated T cells in the peripheral blood (174). My collaborators and I have not found oligoclonal bands in these patients (104,166); however, other histologic studies suggest an immune-mediated or viral-induced pathogenesis or at least an inflammatory mechanism. Miller (175) examined the spinal cord from a post-polio patient and found perivascular intraparenchymal chronic inflammatory infiltrates primarily composed of B lymphocytes with rare macrophages and no T cells. Kaminski et al. (176) found inflammation in the spinal cords of eight of nine PPS patients so studied.

Management

The manifestations of PPS, such as fatigue, pain, and weakness, can be caused by other diseases; accordingly, the differential diagnosis and the exclusion of other diseases are important aspects in the evaluation of PPS patients, reviewed previously by Jubelt and Cashman (23).

Symptomatic Treatment and Supportive Care

The management of PPS has been primarily symptomatic and supportive (23) and based primarily on empirical observations and subjective reports, not objective analyses (Table 5) (177,178). However, objective treat-

TABLE 5. *Treatment of the post-polio syndrome*

Medical problems
  Respiratory insufficiency or failure: administer pneumovax and influenza vaccines, eliminate smoking, treat obstructive disease, assist ventilation
  Treat secondary cardiac failure
  Treat other complicating medical problems: anemia, thyroid disease, obesity, and others
Excessive fatigue
  Institute energy conservation measures
  Provide pharmacologic treatment: amantadine, pyridostigmine, amitriptyline, pemoline
Sleep disturbances
  Support respiratory insufficiency
  Treat sleep apnea
Musculoskeletal pain and joint instabilities
  Decrease mechanical stress on joints and muscles with lifestyle changes: weight loss, decrease activities causing overwork, return to using assistive devices (including orthoses, wheelchairs, adaptive equipment)
  Prescribe anti-inflammatory medications, heat, massage
  Evaluate and, infrequently, surgically repair orthopedic problems
Muscle weakness—stable or progressive
  Avoid overwork of weakened muscle
  Follow creatine kinase?
  As per above, decrease stress on muscles and joints
  Institute stretching exercises
  Prescribe nonfatiguing (submaximal, short duration) strengthening exercises
  Institute cardiopulmonary conditioning
Supportive psychological care
  Aid adjustment to second disability
  Encourage adjustment to required lifestyle changes

Modified from Ref. 91. See text for specific references.

ment studies are beginning to emerge. Respiratory insufficiency is increasingly being managed with noninvasive respiratory support with intermittent positive pressure ventilation using nasal masks and mouthpieces (113,116). Excessive generalized fatigue has been treated with energy conservation measures. Agre and Rodriquez (96) demonstrated that pacing of physical activities with work–rest programs decreased local muscle fatigue, increased work capacity, and resulted in recovery of strength in symptomatic post-polio patients. Generalized fatigue has also been treated pharmacologically with amantadine, amitriptyline, pyridostigmine, and pemoline. Amantadine lacked benefit in a small controlled study but may be helpful in selected cases (179). Amitriptyline has not been studied in a controlled trial but may help fatigue in a small percentage of cases, possibly by controlling pain. Pyridostigmine was beneficial in an open trial (180) but not in a recently completed controlled trial (personal communication). Pemoline has not been evaluated in a controlled study.

Essential to the treatment of sleep disorders in PPS patients is to first determine whether the cause is central, obstructive, or mixed and if there is respiratory insufficiency (121,122). Dysphagia can be improved by learning swallowing techniques (178). Musculoskeletal pain, muscle pain, and joint instabilities can be treated by pacing activities, decreasing mechanical stress by bracing and wheelchairs, and by the judicious use of anti-inflammatory medications (23,181). In a controlled study, Jones et al. (182) demonstrated that aerobic exercise could be tailored to post-polio patients to obtain positive cardiorespiratory training without the untoward effects on limb function.

Muscle-strengthening Exercises

Many recent experimental treatment studies have addressed the role of exercise in altering the progression of the new weakness, and a number suggest that exhaustive strengthening exercises of partially denervated muscles can result in overwork and progressive weakness (23,91). Excessive exercise along with too few motor neurons may result in progressive weakness (183). These findings are supported by similar results in animal studies (23).

Others have demonstrated that a nonfatiguing exercise program improves strength in post-polio patients. Feldman and Soskoine (184) analyzed the effect of nonfatiguing exercises in six post-polio patients over a 3-month period: 14 muscles improved in strength, 17 were unchanged, and in 1 strength decreased. Einarsson and Grimby (185) and Einarsson (186) analyzed the effects of a 6-week, isometric-isokinetic, nonfatiguing strengthening program at 6 and 12 months after training in 12 post-polio patients. These patients had Medical Research Council grade 4 strength in quadriceps muscle that subsequently increased 29% isokinetically with exercise. Fillyaw et al. (187) studied the effect of nonfatiguing resistance exercises in 17 PPS patients for up to 2 years. Their strength increased significantly in exercised compared with contralateral unexercised muscles. Agre et al. (188) evaluated the effect of a low-intensity, alternate-day, 12-week quadriceps muscle-strengthening resistance exercise program. Strength significantly improved without changes in motor units by EMG or in serum creatine kinase levels. Spector et al. (189) evaluated changes in the dynamic and isometric strength in newly weakened quadriceps muscles and in asymptomatic triceps muscles of six PPS patients after 10 weeks of progressive resistance muscle training. They found that the training led to significant gains in dynamic strength in both symptomatic and asymptomatic muscles, without histologic or serologic evidence of muscular damage. These studies suggest that significant short-term improvement in muscle strength occurs with nonfatiguing submaximal strength, short duration, repetitive exercises. The effects of long-term continuous exercise remains to be determined.

SUMMARY

Poliomyelitis is now a rare occurrence in the United States although still a significant problem in underdeveloped areas of the world. The large epidemics of poliomyelitis in the 1940s and 1950s are now reflected by the large number of polio survivors who are developing new late manifestations, referred to as the post-polio syndrome, or PPS. It is now a well-recognized entity that occurs on average about 35 years after the acute poliomyelitis. Common manifestations include generalized fatigue, joint deteriorations with pain, cold intolerance, and prominent neurologic problems. Neurologic problems include new weakness, muscle fatigue, muscle pain, muscle atrophy, respiratory insufficiency, dysphagia, sleep apnea, and possibly generalized fatigue. It is estimated that there are 1.63 million polio survivors in the United States and that half will develop PPS. It is a very slowly progressive syndrome. Older age at the onset of the acute poliomyelitis, the severity of the poliomyelitis, the amount of recovery, and overexercise or overuse of muscles are risk factors for early development. The etiology is unclear, although premature exhaustion of the new sprouts that develop after acute poliomyelitis and of their motor neurons appear to be important factors. Other possible causative factors include persistent poliovirus infection and an underlying immune-mediated process. Treatment is primarily supportive; however, nonfatiguing strengthening exercises can clearly improve strength over the short term.

REFERENCES

1. Paul JR. *History of poliomyelitis.* New Haven: Yale University Press, 1971.
2. Nathanson N, Martin JR. The epidemiology of poliomyelitis: enigmas surrounding its appearance, epidemicity and disappearance. *Am J Epidemiol* 1979;110:672–692.
3. Jubelt B, Lipton HL. Enterovirus infections. In: Vinken PF, Bruyn GW, Klawans HL, eds. *Handbook of clinical neurology. Vol. 12. Viral diseases.* Amsterdam: Elsevier Science Publishers, 1989:307–347.
4. Landsteiner K, Popper E. Übertragung der poliomyelitis acuta auf affen. *Z Immunitätsforsch* 1909;2:377–390.
5. Enders JF, Weller TH, Robbins FC. Cultivation of Lansing strain of poliomyelitis virus in cultures of various human embryonic tissues. *Science* 1949;109:85–87.
6. Bodian D. Poliomyelitis: pathologic anatomy. In: International Poliomyelitis Congress, ed. *Poliomyelitis: papers and discussions presented at the First International Poliomyelitis Conference.* Philadelphia: J.B. Lippincott, 1949:62–84.
7. Kessel JF, Pait CF. Differentiation of three groups of poliomyelitis virus. *Proc Soc Exp Biol Med* 1949;70:315–316.
8. Centers for Disease Control and Prevention. Summary of notifiable diseases, United States, 1993. MMWR Morb Mortal Wkly Rep 1993; 42:1–73.
9. Weibel RE, Benor DE. Reporting vaccine-associated paralytic poliomyelitis: concordance between the CDC and the National Vaccine Injury Compensation Program. *Am J Pub Hlth* 1996;86:734–737.
10. Racaniello VR, Baltimore D. Molecular cloning of poliovirus cDNA and determination of the complete nucleotide sequence of the viral genome. *Proc Natl Acad Sci USA* 1981;78:4887–4891.
11. Nomoto A, Omata T, Toyoda H, et al. Complete nucleotide sequence of the attenuated poliovirus Sabin 1 strain genome. *Proc Natl Acad Sci USA* 1982;79:5793–5797.
12. Stanway G, Hughes PJ, Mountford RC, et al. Comparison of the complete nucleotide sequences of the genomes of the neurovirulent poliovirus P3/Leon/37 and its attenuated Sabin vaccine derivation P3/Leon 12a, b. *Proc Natl Acad Sci USA* 1984;81:1539–1543.
13. Toyoda H, Kohara M, Karaoka Y, et al. Complete nucleotide sequences of all three poliovirus serotype genomes. Implication for genetic relationship, gene function and antigenic determinants. *J Mol Biol* 1984;172:561–585.
14. Kitamura N, Semler B, Rothberg PG, et al. Primary structure, gene organization and polypeptide expression of poliovirus RNA. *Nature* 1981;291:547–553.
15. LaMonica N, Meriam C, Racaniello VR. Mapping of sequences required for mouse neurovirulence of poliovirus type 2 Lansing. *J Virol* 1986;56:515–525.
16. Palmenberg AC. Sequence alignments of picornaviral capsid proteins. In: Semler BL, Ehrenfeld E, eds. *Molecular aspects of picornavirus infection and detection.* Washington, DC: American Society for Microbiology, 1989:211–241.
17. Pevear DC, Oh CK, Cunningham LL, Calenoff M, Jubelt B. Localization of genomic regions specific for the attenuated, mouse-adapted poliovirus type 2 strain W-2. *J Gen Virol* 1990;71:43–52.
18. Hogle JM, Cho M, Filman DJ. Three-dimensional structure of poliovirus at 2.9 Å resolution. *Science* 1985;229:1358–1365.
19. Wiegers K, Dernick R. Molecular basis of antigenic structures of poliovirus: implications for their evolution during morphogenesis. *J Virol* 1992;66:4597–4600.
20. Rossman MG, Palmenberg AC. Conservation of the putative receptor attachment site in picornaviruses. *Virology* 1988;164:373–382.
21. Mendelsohn CL, Wimmer E, Racaniello VR. Cellular receptor for poliovirus: molecular cloning nucleotide sequence, and expression of a new member of the immunoglobulin superfamily. *Cell* 1989;56: 855–865.
22. Horstmann DM. Epidemiology of poliomyelitis and allied diseases—1963. *Yale J Biol Med* 1963;36:5–26.
23. Jubelt B, Cashman NR. Neurological manifestations of the post-polio syndrome. *Crit Rev Neurobiol* 1987;3:199–220.
24. Bodian D. Poliomyelitis. In: Minckler J, ed. *Pathology of the nervous system.* New York: McGraw-Hill, 1972:2323–2394.
25. Jubelt B, Gallez-Hawkins G, Narayan O, Johnson RT. Pathogenesis of human poliovirus infection in mice. I. Clinical and pathological studies. *J Neuropathol Exp Neurol* 1980;39:1138–1148.
26. Hashimoto I, Hagiwara A, Komatsu T. Ultrastructural studies on the pathogenesis of poliomyelitis in monkeys infected with poliovirus. *Acta Neuropathol* 1984;64:53–60.
27. Dal Canto MC, Barbano RL, Jubelt B. Ultrastructural immunohistochemical localization of poliovirus during virulent infection of mice. *J Neuropathol Exp Neurol* 1986;45:613–617.
28. Moore M, Morens DM. Enteroviruses, including polioviruses. In: Belshe RM, ed. *Textbook of human virology.* Littleton: PSG Publishing, 1984:407–483.
29. Melnick JL, Ledinko N. Development of neutralizing antibodies against the three types of poliomyelitis virus during an epidemic period: the ratio of inapparent infections to clinical poliomyelitis. *Am J Hyg* 1953;58:207–222.
30. Howe HA, Wilson JL. Poliomyelitis. In: Rivers TM, Horsfall FL, eds. *Viral and rickettsial infections of man,* 3rd ed. Philadelphia: Lippincott, 1957:432–478.
31. Plum F. Sensory loss with poliomyelitis. *Neurology* 1956;6:166–172.
32. Foley KM, Beresford RH. Acute poliomyelitis beginning as transverse myelopathy. *Arch Neurol* 1974;30:182–183.
33. Plum F, Swanson AG. Central neurogenic hyperventilation in man. *Arch Neurol Psych* 1959;81:531–549.
34. Wyatt HV. Poliomyelitis in hypogammaglobulinemics. *J Infect Dis* 1973;128:802–806.
35. Wright PF, Hatch MH, Kasselberg AG, Lowry SP, Wadlington WB, Karzon DT. Vaccine-associated poliomyelitis in a child with sex-linked agammaglobulinemia. *J Pediatr* 1977;91:408–412.
36. Riker JB, Brandt CD, Chandra R, Arobio JO, Nakano JH. Vaccine-associated poliomyelitis in a child with thymic abnormality. *Pediatrics* 1971;48:923–929.
37. McKinney RE, Katz SL, Wilfert CM. Chronic enteroviral meningoencephalitis in agammaglobulinemic patients. *Rev Infect Dis* 1987;9: 334–356.
38. Centers for Disease Control. Poliomyelitis surveillance summary 1980–1981. 1982.

39. Strebel PM, Sutter RW, Cochi SL, et al. Epidemiology of poliomyelitis in the United States one decade after the last reported case of indigenous wild virus-associated disease. *Clin Infect Dis* 1992; 14:568–579.

40. Ramia S, Bakir TM, Al-Frayh AR, Bahakim H. Paralytic poliomyelitis and non-polio enteroviruses in Saudi Arabia. *J Trop Pediatr* 1987; 33:166–167.

41. Centers for Disease Control and Prevention. Recommendations of the International Task Force for Disease Eradication. *MMWR Morb Mortal Wkly Rep* 1993;42:1–38.

42. Kroon FP, Weiland HT, van Loon AM, van Furth R. Abortive and subclinical poliomyelitis in a family during the 1992 epidemic in the Netherlands. *Clin Infect Dis* 1995;20:454–456.

43. Fox JP, Gelfand HM, LeBlanc DR, Potash L, Clemmer DI, LaPenta D. The spread of vaccine strains of poliovirus in the household and in the community in southern Louisiana. In: International Poliomyelitis Congress, ed. *Poliomyelitis: papers and discussions presented at the Fifth International Poliomyelitis Conference.* Philadelphia: Lippincott, 1961:368–383.

44. Paul JR, Horstmann DM, Riordan JT, et al. An oral poliovirus vaccine trial in Costa Rica. *BulL WHO* 1962;26:311–329.

45. Melnick JR. Enteroviruses: polioviruses, coxsackieviruses, and new enteroviruses. In: Fields BN, ed. *Virology.* New York: Raven Press, 1990:549–605.

46. Meyer HM, Johnson RT, Crawford IP, Dascomb HE, Rogers NG. Central nervous system syndromes of "viral" etiology: a study of 713 cases. *Am J Med* 1960;29:334–347.

47. Melnick JL, Paul JK, Walton M. Serologic epidemiology of poliomyelitis. *Am J Public Health* 1955;45:429–437.

48. Honig EI, Melnick JL, Isacson P, Parr R, Myers IL, Walton M. An endemiological study of enteric virus infections: poliomyelitis, coxsackie, and orphan (ECHO) viruses isolated from normal children in two socioeconomic groups. *J Exp Med* 1956;103:247–262.

49. Paul JR, Melnick JL, Barnett VH, Colbblum N. A survey of neutralizing antibodies to poliomyelitis virus in Cairo, Egypt. *Am J Hyg* 1952;55:402–413.

50. Paul JR. Epidemiology of poliomyelitis. In: World Health Organization, ed. *Poliomyelitis.* Geneva: WHO Monograph Series, 1955:26.

51. Nolan JP, Wilmer BJ, Melnick JL. Poliomyelitis: its highly invasive nature and narrow stream of infection in a community of high socioeconomic level. *N Engl J Med* 1955;253:945–954.

52. Peart AFW. An outbreak of poliomyelitis in Canadian Eskimos in wintertime. *Can J Public Health* 1949;10:405–417.

53. Horstmann DM, Poliomyelitis: severity and type of disease in different age groups. *Ann NY Acad Sci* 1955;61:956–967.

54. Weinstein L. Influence of age and sex on susceptibility and clinical manifestations in poliomyelitis. *N Engl J Med* 1957;257:47–52.

55. Strebel PM, Ion-Nedelcu N, Baughman AL, Sutter RW, Cochi SL. Intramuscular injection within 30 days of immunization with oral poliovirus vaccine—a risk factor for vaccine-associated paralytic poliomyelitis. *N Engl J Med* 1995;332:500–506.

56. Rindge ME. Poliomyelitis in pregnancy: a report of 79 cases in Connecticut. *N Engl J Med* 1957;256:281–285.

57. Bodian D. Emerging concepts of poliomyelitis infection. *Science* 1955;122:105–108.

58. Nathanson N, Bodian D. Experimental poliomyelitis following intramuscular virus injection. II. Viremia and the effect of antibody. *Bull Johns Hopkins Hosp* 1961;108:320–333.

59. Nathanson N, Bodian D. Experimental poliomyelitis following intramuscular virus injection. III. The effect of passive antibody on paralysis and viremia. *Bull Johns Hopkins Hosp III* 1962;198–220.

60. Bodian D. Viremia in experimental poliomyelitis. I. General aspects of infection after intravascular inoculation with strains of high and low invasiveness. *Am J Hyg* 1954;60:339–357.

61. Nathanson N, Bodian D. Experimental poliomyelitis following intramuscular virus injection. I. The effect of neural block of a neurotropic and pantropic strain. *Bull Johns Hopkins Hosp* 1961;108:308–319.

62. Blitzinger K, Anzil AP. Neural route of infection in viral diseases of the central nervous system. *Lancet* 1974;2:1033–1035.

63. Jubelt B, Goldfarb SJ, Paradise MJ, Close MG. Fast axonal transport of human poliovirus (HPV) [abstract]. *Neurology* 1986;36[Suppl 1]:204.

64. Jubelt B, Narayan O, Johnson RT. Pathogenesis of human poliovirus infection in mice. II. Age dependency of paralysis. *J Neuropathol Exp Neurol* 1980;39:149–159.

65. Bodian D. The virus, the nerve cell, and paralysis. A study of experimental poliomyelitis in the spinal cord. *Bull Johns Hopkins Hosp* 1948;83:1–106.

66. Wolinsky JS, Jubelt B, Burke S, Narayan O. Hematogenous origin of the inflammatory response in acute poliomyelitis. *Ann Neurol* 1982; 11:59–68.

67. Kornreich L, Dagan O, Grunebaum M. MRI in acute poliomyelitis. *Neuroradiology* 1996;38:371–372.

68. Lipton L, Jubelt B. Enterovirus infections of the central nervous system. In: Tyler KL, Martin JB, eds. *Infectious diseases of the central nervous system.* Philadelphia: F.A. Davis, 1993:103–130.

69. Price RW, Plum F. Poliomyelitis. In: Vinken PJ, Bruyn GW, Klawans HL, eds. *Handbook of clinical neurology. Vol. 34. Infections of the nervous system. Part II.* Amsterdam: North-Holland Publishing Co., 1978:93–132.

70. Hovi TM, Stenvik M, Kinnunen E. Diagnosis of poliomyelitis by demonstration of intrathecal synthesis of neutralizing antibodies. *J Infect Dis* 1986;153:998–999.

71. Roivainen M, Agboatwalla M, Stenvik M, Rysa T, Akram DS, Hovi T. Intrathecal immune response and virus-specific immunoglobulin M antibodies in laboratory diagnosis of acute poliomyelitis. *J Clin Micro* 1993;31:2427–2432.

72. Gear JH. Nonpolio causes of polio-like paralytic syndromes. *Rev Infect Dis* 1984;6[Suppl 2]:S379–S384.

73. Chopra JS, Banerjee AK, Murthy JMK, Pal SR. Paralytic rabies: a clinico-pathological study. *Brain* 1980;103:789–802.

74. Thomas JE, Howard FM. Segmental zoster paresis, a disease profile. *Neurology* 1972;22:459–466.

75. Asbury AK. Diagnostic considerations in Guillain-Barré syndrome. *Ann Neurol* 1981;9[Suppl]:1–5.

76. Vogel E. Recognition, treatment and control of poliomyelitis. *Med Prog* 1950;242:899–908.

77. Raney RB, Brashear HR, Shands AR. *Shands' handbook of orthopaedic surgery.* St. Louis: C.V. Mosby, 1971:180–185.

78. James JIP. *Poliomyelitis: Essentials of surgical management.* London: Edward Arnold Ltd, 1987.

79. Chen RT, Hausinger S, Dajani AS. Seroprevalence of antibody against poliovirus in inner-city preschool children. Implications for vaccination policy in the United States. *JAMA* 1996;275:1639–1645.

80. Centers for Disease Control and Prevention. Monthly immunization table. *MMWR Morb Mortal Wkly Rep* 1994;43:743.

81. Centers for Disease Control and Prevention. Poliomyelitis prevention in the United States: introduction of a sequential vaccination schedule of inactivated poliovirus vaccine followed by oral poliovirus vaccine. Recommendations of the Advisory Committee on Immunization Practices (ACIP). *MMWR Morb Mortal Wkly Rep* 1997;46:1–25.

82. Tambini G, Andrus JK, Marques E, et al. Direct detection of wild poliovirus circulation by stool surveys of healthy children and analysis of community wastewater. *J Infect Dis* 1993;168:1510–1514.

83. Watkins AL. Progressive disabilities in poliomyelitis. In: International Poliomyelitis Congress, ed. *Poliomyelitis: papers and discussions presented at the Second International Poliomyelitis Conference.* Philadelphia: Lippincott, 1949:142–147.

84. Green WR. The management of poliomyelitis: the convalescent state. In: *Poliomyelitis: papers and discussions presented at the First International Poliomyelitis Conference.* Philadelphia: Lippincott, 1949: 165–185.

85. Carriere M. Amyotrophies secondaires. These de Montpelier, 1875. Cited in Potts, CS. A case of progressive muscular atrophy occurring in a man who had acute poliomyelitis nineteen years previously. With a review of the literature bearing upon the relations of infantile spinal paralysis to the spinal disease of later life. *Univ Pa Med Bull* 1903; 16:31–37.

86. Cornil Lepine. Sur un cas de paralysie generale spinale anterieure subaigue, suive d'autopsie. *Gax Med (Paris)* 1875;4:127–129.

87. Raymond M (clinical presentation with discussion by Charcot JM). Paralysie essentiele de l'enfance. Atrophie musculaire consecutive. *Gax Med (Paris)* 1875;4:225–226.

88. Wiechers DO. Late effects of polio: historical perspectives. *Birth Defects* 1987;23:1–11.

89. Dalakas MC, Sever JL, Madden DL, et al. Late post-poliomyelitis muscular atrophy: clinical, virologic and immunologic studies. *Rev Infect Dis* 1984;6[Suppl 2]:S562–S567.

90. Halstead LS, Rossi D. Post-polio syndrome: clinical experience with 132 consecutive outpatients. *Birth Defects* 1987;23:13–26.

91. Jubelt B, Drucker J. Post-polio syndrome: an update. *Semin Neurol* 1993;13:3:283–290.

92. Agre JC, Rodriquez AA, Sperling KB. Symptoms and clinical impressions of patients seen in a postpolio clinic. *Arch Phys Med Rehabil* 1989;70:367–370.

93. Mulder DW, Rosenbaum RA, Layton DD. Late progression of poliomyelitis or forme fruste amyotrophic lateral sclerosis? *Mayo Clin Proc* 1972;47:756–761.

94. Halstead LS, Wiechers DO, Rossi CD. Late effects of poliomyelitis: a national survey. In: Halstead LS, Wiechers DO, eds. *Late effects of poliomyelitis*. Miami: Symposia Foundation, 1985:11–31.

95. Berlly MH, Strauser WW, Hall KM. Fatigue in postpolio syndrome. *Arch Phys Med Rehab* 1991;72:115–118.

96. Agre JC, Rodriquez AA. Intermittent isometric activity: its effect on muscle fatigue in postpolio subjects. *Arch Phys Med Rehab* 1991;72:971–977.

97. Packer TL, Martins I, Krefting L, Brouwer B. Post-polio sequelae: activity and post-polio fatigue. *Orthopedics* 1991;14:1223–1226.

98. Bruno RL, Sapolsky R, Zimmerman JR, Frick NM. Pathophysiology of a central cause of post-polio fatigue. *Ann NY Acad Sci* 1995;753:257–275.

99. Baker PCH. Neuromuscular symptoms in patients with previous poliomyelitis: a New Zealand study. *NZ Med J* 1989;102:132–134.

100. Norris FH, Denys EH, Ü KS. Differential diagnosis of adult motor neuron disease. In: Mulder DW, ed. *The diagnosis and treatment of amyotrophic lateral sclerosis*. Boston: Houghton Mifflin, 1980:53–78.

101. Mulder DW, Lambert EH, Eaton LM. Myasthenic syndrome in patients with amyotrophic lateral sclerosis. *Neurology* 1959;9:627–631.

102. Trojan DA, Cashman NR. Anticholinesterases in post-poliomyelitis syndrome. *Ann NY Acad Sci* 1995;753:285–295.

103. Codd MB, Mulder DW, Kurland LT, Beard CM, O'Fallon WM. Poliomyelitis in Rochester, Minnesota, 1935–1955: epidemiology and long-term sequelae. A preliminary report. In: Halstead LS, Wiechers DO, eds. *Late effects of poliomyelitis*. Miami: Symposia Foundation, 1985:121–134.

104. Cashman NR, Maselli R, Wollman RL, Roos R, Simon R, Antel JP. Late denervation in patients with antecedent paralytic poliomyelitis. *N Engl J Med* 1987;317:7–12.

105. Dalakas M, Illa I. Post-polio syndrome: concepts in clinical diagnosis, pathogenesis, and etiology. *Adv Neurol* 1991;56:495–511.

106. Hayward M, Seaton D. Late sequelae of paralytic poliomyelitis: a clinical and electromyographic study. *J Neurol Neurosurg Psychiatry* 1979;42:117–122.

107. Bodian D, Howe HA. The pathology of early averted and nonparalytic poliomyelitis. *Bull Johns Hopkins Hosp* 1941;69:135–147.

108. Sabin AB, Ward R. Nature of non-paralytic and transitory paralytic poliomyelitis in Rhesus monkeys inoculated with human virus. *J Exp Med* 1941;73:757–770.

109. Klingman J, Chui H, Corgiat M, Perry J. Functional recovery: a major risk factor for the development of postpoliomyelitis muscular atrophy. *Arch Neurol* 1988;45:645–647.

110. Cashman NR, Maselli R, Wollmann R, Simon R, Heidkamp P, Antel JP. New muscle atrophy as a late symptom of the post-poliomyelitis syndrome. *Clin Ecol* 1987;5:11–13.

111. Dean E, Ross J, Read JD, Courtenay L, Madill KJ. Pulmonary function in individuals with a history of poliomyelitis. *Chest* 1991;100:118–123.

112. Blomstrand A, Baker B. Post-polio lung function. *Scand J Rehab Med* 1991;24:43–49.

113. Bach JR, Alba AS, Bohatiuk G, Saporitol Lee M. Mouth intermittent positive pressure ventilation in the management of postpolio respiratory insufficiency. *Chest* 1987;91:859–864.

114. Howard RS, Wiles CM, Spencer GT. The late sequelae of poliomyelitis. *J Med* 1988;66:219–232.

115. Bach JR, Alba AS, Bodofsky E, Curran FJ, Schultheiss M. Post-polio respiratory insufficiency. *Birth Defects* 1987;23:99–113.

116. Bach JR. Management of post-polio respiratory sequelae. *Ann NY Acad Sci* 1995;753:96–102.

117. Sonies BC, Dalakas MC. Progression of oral-motor and swallowing symptoms in the post-polio syndrome. *Ann NY Acad Sci* 1995;753:87–95.

118. Buchholz DW, Jones B. Post-polio dysphagia: alarm or caution? *Orthopedics* 1991;14:1303–1305.

119. Cannon S, Ritter FN. Vocal cord paralysis in postpoliomyelitis syndrome. *Laryngoscope* 1987;97:981–983.

120. Guilleminault C, Motta J. Sleep apnea syndrome as a long-term sequela of poliomyelitis. In: Guilleminault C, ed. *Sleep apnea syndromes*. New York: Alan R. Liss, 1978:309–315.

121. Steljes DG, Kryger MH, Kirk BW, Millar TW. Sleep in postpolio syndrome. *Chest* 1990;98:133–140.

122. Bach JR, Alba AS. Pulmonary dysfunction and sleep disordered breathing as post-polio sequelae: evaluation and management. *Orthopedics* 1992;14:1329–1337.

123. Anderson AD, Levine SA, Gellert H. Loss of ambulatory ability in patients with old anterior poliomyelitis. *Lancet* 1972;2:1061–1063.

124. Werner R, Waring W, Davidoff G. Risk factors for median mononeuropathy of the wrist in postpoliomyelitis patients. *Arch Phys Med Rehabil* 1989;70:464–467.

125. Bruno RL, Johnson JC, Berman WS. Motor and sensory functioning with changing ambient temperature in post-polio subjects: autonomic and electrophysiological correlates. In: Halstead LS, Wiechers DO, eds. *Late effects of poliomyelitis*. Miami: Symposia Foundation, 1985:95–108.

126. Smith E, Rosenblatt P, Limauro A. The role of the sympathetic nervous system in acute poliomyelitis. *J Pediatr* 1949;34:1–11.

127. Kohl SJ. Emotional response of patients with late effects of poliomyelitis. *Birth Defects* 1987;23:135–142.

128. Bruno RL, Frick NM. The psychology of polio as prelude to post-polio sequelae: behavior modification and psychotherapy. *Orthopedics* 1991;14:1185–1189.

129. Windebank AJ, Litchy WJ, Daube JR, Kurland LT, Codd MB, Iverson R. Late effects of paralytic poliomyelitis in Olmsted County, Minnesota. *Neurology* 1991;41:501–507.

130. Bruno RL. Post-polio sequelae: research and treatment in the second decade. *Orthopedics* 1991;14:1169–1170.

131. Speir JL, Owen RR, Knapp M, Canine JK. Occurrence of post-polio sequelae in an epidemic population. In: Halstead LS, Wiechers DO, eds. *Research and clinical aspects of the late effects of poliomyelitis*. White Plains, NY: March of Dimes Birth Defects Foundation, 1987:39–48.

132. Ramlow J, Alexander M, LaPorte R, Kaufmann C, Kuller L. Epidemiology of the post-polio syndrome. *Am Epidemiol* 1992;136:769–786.

133. Kidd D, Howard RS, Williams AJ, Heatley FW, Panayiotopoulos CP, Spencer GT. Late functional deterioration following paralytic poliomyelitis. *Q J Med* 1997;90:189–196.

134. Agre C, Rodriquez AA. Neuromuscular function: comparison of symptomatic and asymptomatic polio subjects to control subjects. *Arch Phys Med Rehabil* 1990;71:545–551.

135. Trojan DA, Cashman NR, Shapiro S, Tansey CM, Esdaile JM. Predictive factors for post-poliomyelitis syndrome. *Arch Phys Med Rehabil* 1994;75:770–777.

136. Dalakas MC, Elder G, Hallett M, et al. A long-term follow-up study of patients with post-poliomyelitis neuromuscular symptoms. *N Engl J Med* 1986;314:959–963.

137. Ivanyi B, Nelemans PJ, de Jonghe R, Ongerboer de Visser BW, DeVisser M. Muscle strength in post-polio patients: a prospective follow-up study. *Muscle Nerve* 1996;19:738–742.

138. Allen GM, Gandevia AS, Middleton J. Quantitative assessments of elbow flexor muscle performance using twitch interpolation in post-polio patients: no evidence for deterioration. *Brain* 1997;120:663–672.

139. Windebank AJ, Litchy WJ, Daube JR, Iverson RA. Lack of progression of neurologic deficit in survivors of paralytic polio: a 50 year prospective population-based study. *Neurology* 1996;46:80–84.

140. Agre JC, Grimby G, Rodriquez AA, Einarsson G, Swiggum ER, Franke TM. A comparison of symptoms between Swedish and American post-polio individuals and assessment of lower limb strength—a four-year cohort study. *Scand J Rehab Med* 1995;27:183–192.

141. Stalberg E, Grimby G. Dynamic electromyography and muscle biopsy changes in a 4-year follow-up: study of patients with a history of polio. *Muscle Nerve* 1995;18:699–707.

142. Munsat TL, ed. *Post-polio syndrome*. Boston: Butterworth Heinemann, 1991.

143. Nelson KR. Creatine kinase and fibrillation potentials in patients with late sequelae of polio. *Muscle Nerve* 1990;13:722–725.

144. Waring WP, McLaurin TM. Correlation of creatine kinase and gail measurement in the postpolio population. *Arch Phys Med Rehab* 1992;73:37–39.

145. Peach PE. Overwork weakness with evidence of muscle damage in a patient with residual paralysis from polio. *Arch Phys Med Rehab* 1990;71:248–250.

146. Wiechers DO, Hubbell SL. Late changes in the motor unit after acute poliomyelitis. *Muscle Nerve* 1981;4:524–528.

147. Wiechers DO. Pathophysiology and late changes of the motor unit after poliomyelitis. In: Halstead LS, Wiechers DO, eds. *Late effects of poliomyelitis*. Miami: Symposia Foundation, 1985:91–94.

148. Wiechers DO. New concepts of the reinnervated motor unit revealed by vaccine-associated poliomyelitis. *Muscle Nerve* 1988;11:356–364.

149. Ravits J, Hallett M, Baker M, Nilsson J, Dalakas M. Clinical and electromyographic studies of postpoliomyelitis muscular atrophy. *Muscle Nerve* 1990;13:667–674.

150. Maselli RA, Cashman NR, Wollman RL, Salazar-Grueso EF, Roos R. Neuromuscular transmission as a function of motor unit size in patients with prior poliomyelitis. *Muscle Nerve* 1992;15:648–655.

151. Ryniewicz G, Rowinska-Marcinska K, Emeryk B, Hausmanowa-Petrusewicz I. Disintegration of the motor unit in post-polio syndrome. Part I. Electrophysiological findings in patients after poliomyelitis. *Electromyogr Clin Neurophysiol* 1990;30:423–427.

152. Emeryk B, Rowinska-Marcinska K. Ryniewicz B, Hausmanowa-Petrusewicz I. Disintegration of the motor unit in post-polio syndrome. Part II. Electrophysiological findings in patients with post-polio syndrome. *Electromyogr Clin Neurophysiol* 1990;30:451–458.

153. Rodriquez AA, Agre JC, Harmon RL, Franke TM, Swiggus ER, Curt JT. Electromyographic and neuromuscular variables in post-polio subjects. *Arch Phys Med Rehab* 1995;76:989–993.

154. Lange DJ, Smith T, Lovelace RE. Postpolio muscular atrophy: diagnostic utility of macroelectromyography. *Arch Neurol* 1989;46:502–506.

155. Gawne AC, Pham BT, Halstead LS. Electrodiagnostic findings in 108 consecutive patients referred to a post-polio clinic: the value of routine electrodiagnostic studies. *Ann NY Acad Sci* 1995;753:383–385.

156. Dalakas MC. Morphological changes in the muscles of patients with post-poliomyelitis neuromuscular symptoms. *Neurology* 1988;38:99–104.

157. Drachman DB, Murphy SR, Nigam MP, Hills JR. "Myopathic" changes in chronically denervated muscle. *Arch Neurol* 1967;16:14–24.

158. Sharma KR, Braun-Kent J, Mynhier MA, Weiner MW, Miller RG. Excessive muscular fatigue in the postpoliomyelitis syndrome. *Neurology* 1994;44:642–646.

159. Sivakumar K, Sinnwell T, Yildiz E, McLaughlin A, Dalakas MC. Study of fatigue in muscles of patients with post-polio syndrome by *in vivo* [^{31}P] magnetic resonance spectroscopy: a metabolic cause for fatigue. *Ann NY Acad Sci* 1995;753:397–401.

160. Grimby L, Tollback A, Muller U, Larsson L. Fatigue of chronically overused motor units in prior polio patients. *Muscle Nerve* 1996;19:728–737.

161. Destombes J, Couderc T, Thiesson D, Girard S, Wilt SG, Blondel B. Persistent poliovirus infection in mouse motor neurons. *J Virol* 1997;71:1621–1628.

162. Colbere-Garapin F, Christodoulou C, Crainic R, Pelletier I. Persistent poliovirus infection of human neuroblastoma cells. *Proc Natl Acad Sci USA* 1989;86:7590–7594.

163. Borzakian S, Couderc T, Barbier Y, Attal G, Pelletier I, Colbere-Garapin F. Persistent poliovirus infection: Establishment and maintenance involve distinct mechanisms. *Virology* 1992;186:398–408.

164. Pavio N, Buc-Caron NH, Colbere-Garapin F. Persistent poliovirus infection of human fetal brain cells. *J Virol* 1996;70:6395–6401.

165. Sharief MK, Hentages R, Ciaidi M. Intrathecal immune response in patients with the post-polio syndrome. *N Engl J Med* 1991;325:749–755.

166. Salazar-Grueso EF, Grimaldi LM, Roos RP, Variakojis R, Jubelt B, Cashman NR. Isoelectric focusing studies of serum and cerebrospinal fluid in patients with antecedent poliomyelitis. *Ann Neurol* 1989;26:709–713.

167. Jubelt B, Salazar-Grueso EF, Roos RP, Cashman NR. Antibody titer to poliovirus in blood and cerebrospinal of patients with post-polio syndrome. *Ann NY Acad Sci* 1995;753:201–207.

168. Kurent JE, Brooks BR, Madden DL, Sever JL, Engel WK. CSF viral antibodies. Evaluation in amyotrophic lateral sclerosis and late-onset postpoliomyelitis progressive muscular atrophy. *Arch Neurol* 1979;36:269–273.

169. Melchers W, de Visser M, Jongen P, et al. The postpolio syndrome: no evidence for poliovirus persistence. *Ann Neurol* 1992;32:728–732.

170. Leon-Monzon ME, Dalakas MC. Detection of poliovirus antibodies and poliovirus genome in patients with the post-polio syndrome. *Ann NY Acad Sci* 1995;753:208–218.

171. Muir P, Nicholson F, Spencer GT, et al. Enterovirus infection of the central nervous system of humans: lack of association with chronic neurological disease. *J Gen Virol* 1996;77:1469–1476.

172. Leparc I, LeParc-Goffart I, Julien J, et al. Evidence of presence of poliovirus genomic sequences in cerebrospinal fluid from patients with postpolio syndrome. *J Clin Microbiol* 1996;34:2023–2026.

173. Pezeshkpour GH, Dalakas MC. Long-term changes in the spinal cords of patients with old poliomyelitis: signs of continuous disease activity. *Arch Neurol* 1988;45:505–508.

174. Ginsberg AH, Gale MJ Jr, Rose LM, Clark EA. T-cell alterations in late poliomyelitis. *Arch Neurol* 1989;46:497–501.

175. Miller DC. Post-polio syndrome spinal cord pathology. *Ann NY Acad Sci* 1995;753:185–193.

176. Kaminski JH, Tresser N. Hogan RE, Martin E. Pathological analysis of spinal cords from survivors of poliomyelitis. *Ann NY Acad Sci* 1995;753:390–393.

177. Young GR. Post-polio sequelae: energy conservation, occupational therapy, and the treatment of post-polio sequelae. *Orthopedics* 1991;14:1233–1239.

178. Silbergleit AK, Waring WP, Sullivan MJ, Maynard FM. Evaluation, treatment, and follow-up results of post polio patients with dysphagia. *Otolaryngol Head Neck Surg* 1991;104:333–338.

179. Stein DP, Dambrosia JM, Dalakas MC. A double-blind, placebo-controlled trial of amantadine for the treatment of fatigue in patients with the post-polio syndrome. *Ann NY Acad Sci* 1995;753:296–302.

180. Trojan DA, Cashman NR. An open trial of pyridostigmine in post-poliomyelitis syndrome. *Can J Neurol Sci* 1995;22:223–227.

181. Perry J, Fontaine JD, Mulroy S. Findings in post-poliomyelitis syndrome. *J Bone Joint Surg [Am]* 1995;77:1148–1153.

182. Jones DR, Speier J, Canine K, Owen R, Stull A. Cardiorespiratory responses to aerobic training by patients with postpoliomyelitis sequelae. *JAMA* 1989;261:3255–3258.

183. Herbison GJ, Jaweed MM, Ditunno JF Jr. Exercise therapies in peripheral neuropathies. *Arch Phys Med Rehab* 1983;64:201–205.

184. Feidman RM, Soskoine CL. The use of nonfatiguing strengthening exercises in post-polio syndrome. *Birth Defects* 1987;23:335–341.

185. Einarsson G, Grimby G. Strengthening exercise program in post-polio subjects. *Birth Defects* 1987;23:275–283.

186. Einarsson G. Muscle conditioning in late poliomyelitis. *Arch Phys Med Rehab* 1991;72:11–14.

187. Fillyaw MJ, Badger GJ, Goodwin GD, Bradley WG, Fries TJ, Skukla A. Post-polio sequelae: the effects of long term non-fatiguing resistance exercises in subjects with post-polio syndrome. *Orthopedics* 1991;14:1253–1256.

188. Agre JC, Rodriquez AA, Franke TM, Swiggum ER, Harmon RL, Curt JT. Low-intensity, alternate-day exercise improves muscle performance without apparent adverse effect in postpolio patients. *Am J Phys Med Rehab* 1996;75:50–58.

189. Spector SA, Gordon PL, Feurerstein IM, Sivakumar K, Hurley BF, Dalakas MC. Strength gains without muscle injury after strength training in patients with postpolio muscular atrophy. *Muscle Nerve* 1996;19:1282–1290.

Motor Disorders,
edited by David S. Younger.
Lippincott Williams & Wilkins, Philadelphia © 1999.

CHAPTER 35

Paraneoplastic Syndromes and Motor Dysfunction

Myrna R. Rosenfeld and Josep Dalmau

Paraneoplastic neurologic syndromes are disorders of nervous system function that occur in association with cancer but cannot be ascribed to metastases or direct infiltration of the nervous system by the tumor. They are important for two reasons. First, in two thirds of patients, neurologic symptoms precede the diagnosis of the tumor, and the correct identification of the disorder directs the search for an occult and potentially curable cancer. Second, these syndromes provide a model to study the relationship between cancer and the nervous system at the molecular level (1).

Paraneoplastic neurologic syndromes can affect any portion of the nervous system and can mimic many disorders. Furthermore, the fact that paraneoplastic disorders frequently develop before the presence of a cancer is known and that similar disorders may occur without cancer creates important diagnostic problems. The diagnosis of paraneoplastic syndromes relies on the index of suspicion by the clinician, which in turn depends on the type of syndrome and the detection of markers of paraneoplasia. The discovery that some antineuronal antibodies were highly associated with a specific paraneoplastic neurologic disorder and tumor type represented an important advance in early tumor diagnosis (2).

This chapter focuses on the paraneoplastic central and peripheral nervous system syndromes most commonly associated with motor dysfunction (Table 1).

M. R. Rosenfeld: Department of Neurology and Neuroscience, New York Hospital–Cornell Medical Center and Memorial Sloan-Kettering Cancer Center, New York, New York 10021.

J. Dalmau: Department of Neurology, Memorial Sloan-Kettering Cancer Center, New York, New York 10021.

PARANEOPLASTIC SYNDROMES OF THE CENTRAL NERVOUS SYSTEM

Paraneoplastic Encephalomyelitis and Sensory Neuronopathy

Paraneoplastic encephalomyelitis and sensory neuronopathy (PEM-SN) describes patients with cancer who develop clinical signs of dysfunction of various parts of the nervous system and postmortem signs of inflammation within the hippocampus, brainstem, cerebellum, spinal cord, dorsal root ganglia, and nerve roots (3). It may be associated with virtually all types of tumors; how-

TABLE 1. *Paraneoplastic syndromes associated with progressive motor dysfunction*

Paraneoplastic syndromes of the central nervous system
Paraneoplastic encephalomyelitis
Paraneoplastic cerebellar degeneration
(for subtypes see Table 2)
Motor neuron syndromes (for subtypes see Table 3)
Stiff-(man) person
Necrotizing myelopathy
Paraneoplastic syndromes of the peripheral nervous system
Guillain-Barré syndrome
Chronic sensorimotor neuropathy
Polyneuropathy associated with plasma cell dyscrasia and M-proteins
Paraneoplastic vasculitis of the nerve and muscle
Neuromyotonia
Paraneoplastic syndromes of the neuromuscular junction
Myasthenia gravis
Lambert-Eaton myasthenic syndrome (LEMS)
Polymyositis/dermatomyositis
Acute necrotizing myopathy
Carcinomatous neuromyopathy
Cachectic myopathy

ever, in more than 75% of patients, the underlying tumor is a small cell lung cancer (SCLC) (1,2). Those patients with SCLC usually have in their serum and cerebrospinal fluid (CSF) high titers of anti-Hu antibodies (4,5). The intrathecal synthesis of the antibody and the presence of inflammatory infiltrates in the nervous system and tumor suggest an immune origin of the disorder (6,7).

Most patients with PEM-SN develop signs and symptoms of multifocal involvement of the nervous system (8). Sensory symptoms secondary to dorsal root ganglia involvement are present in 75% of patients with PEM. The sensory loss may be severe, resulting in ataxia, pseudoathetotic movements, and difficulty walking with relative preservation of motor strength and cerebellar function.

Motor neuron dysfunction is a predominant symptom in 20% of affected patients. Although in some motor weakness is the presenting symptom, virtually all eventually develop signs referable to other areas of the nervous system. Only one patient with pure motor neuron dysfunction has been reported (9). In general, symptoms start with proximal loss of strength in the arms sometimes in an asymmetric pattern. Weakness of neck extensor muscles was the presenting finding in two patients at Memorial Sloan-Kettering Cancer Center. Muscle wasting and fasciculation are common. Reflexes may be hyperactive or abolished depending on other areas of the nervous system involved. Autonomic and respiratory failure, either of central or peripheral origin, are frequent causes of death. The main pathologic findings are perivascular inflammatory infiltrates, neuronal cell loss, and "neuronophagic" microglial nodules, which in the group of patients with motor neuron involvement, predominate in spinal cord gray matter, including the ventral horns and medulla (8,10).

CSF analysis shows increased protein concentration and pleocytosis in 80% of patients. The detection of the anti-Hu antibody in the serum and CSF confirms the paraneoplastic origin of the disorder and, in the case of undiagnosed tumor, directs the search for an SCLC. Treatment of the tumor or immune suppression does not usually improve the neurologic deficits (8,10–12).

When symptoms of PSN and motor weakness develop together and subacutely, they can mimic the Guillain-Barré syndrome (GBS). In these patients, the pathologic changes include inflammation and neuronal loss in the gray matter of the spinal cord and dorsal root ganglia (13).

Paraneoplastic Cerebellar Degeneration

This disorder is characterized by the subacute development of cerebellar dysfunction, which usually stabilizes in a few weeks or months and leaves the patient incapacitated with a pancerebellar syndrome. Initial symptoms include dizziness, nausea, vomiting, dysarthria, blurry vision, oscillopsia, and diplopia (1,14). The intensity and course of the symptoms and the association with other neurologic deficits can vary in individual patients, but these differences are less noticeable in those with a similar tumor or antineuronal antibody (Table 2).

The neoplasms most often involved in paraneoplastic cerebellar degeneration (PCD) include cancer of the lung, particularly SCLC; ovary and breast; and lymphoma. Postmortem studies in affected cases demonstrate near or total loss of Purkinje cells with relative preservation of other cerebellar neurons and Bergmann astrogliosis (Fig. 1). Inflammatory infiltrates, when present, usually involve the deep cerebellar nuclei. Focal demyelination may be present in the cerebellum, dorsal spinocerebellar, and posterior columns of the spinal cord (15).

The diagnosis of PCD should be suspected in any patient older than 50 years with subacute symptoms of cerebellar dysfunction. In the early stages, examination of the CSF usually demonstrates pleocytosis, increased protein, IgG content, and oligoclonal bands. The discovery that some patients harbor antineuronal antibodies (Fig. 2) and that some of these antibodies are associated with specific histologic types of tumors suggest that PCD is a syndrome rather than a disease and that different pathogenic mechanisms may result in similar symptoms (16,17). The detection of a well-characterized paraneoplastic antibody (Table 2) establishes the diagnosis and directs the search for the neoplasm. Other tests, such as

TABLE 2. Paraneoplastic cerebellar degeneration and antineuronal antibodies

Antibody	Antigens	Tumor	Sex	Symptoms	Prognosis/Death
Anti-Hu	HuD, HuC, Hel-N1,	SCLC Neuroblastoma	F > M	Pancerebellar, sensory neuropathy, PEM	Paraneoplasia > tumor
Anti-Yo	CDR62, CDR34	Ovary Breast	F >> M	Pancerebellar	Tumor > paraneoplasia
Anti-Ri	Nova	Breast, Gyn SCLC	F >> M	Ataxia, opsoclonus oculomotor dysfunction muscle spasms, rigidity	Tumor > paraneoplasia
Anti-Tr	Unknown	Hodgkin's	M > F	Pancerebellar	May respond to treatment
Anti-VGCC	P/Q-type, N-type VGCC	SCLC	M > F	Pancerebellar LEMS	Tumor > paraneoplasia

SCLC, small-cell lung cancer; Gyn, gynecologic; VGCC, voltage-gated calcium channel; LEMS, Lambert-Eaton myasthenic syndrome; PEM, paraneoplastic encephalomyelitis.

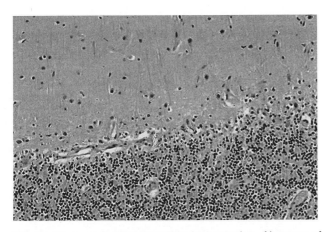

FIG. 1. Paraneoplastic cerebellar degeneration. Absence of Purkinje cells in a patient with small cell lung cancer and cerebellar degeneration associated with paraneoplastic encephalomyelitis and anti-Hu antibodies.

magnetic resonance imaging of the head, do not usually demonstrate changes in the acute phase of the disease, but atrophy of the cerebellum is usually seen several months after the development of neurologic symptoms.

Several antibodies have been identified in association with PCD (Table 2) as follows.

Anti-Yo

Patients with this antibody are typically postmenopausal women without a history of cancer (two thirds of patients) or with a recent diagnosis of cancer (one third of patients) (18). About 75% of patients have cancer of the ovary and 20% cancer of the breast. Rare exceptions include lung cancer and salivary gland cancer. The neurologic symptoms associated with anti-Yo antibodies include pancerebellar dysfunction with minor

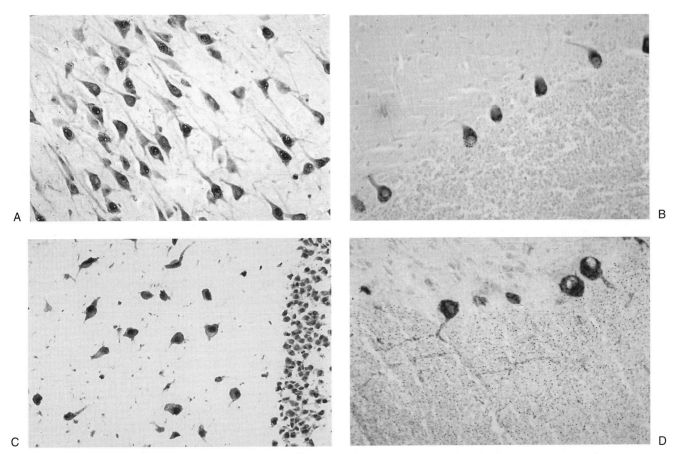

FIG. 2. Antineuronal antibodies in paraneoplastic disorders of the central nervous system. **A:** Anti-Hu antibodies. These antibodies react with 35- to 40-kDa proteins expressed in the nuclei and, to a minor degree, the cytoplasm of neurons of the central and peripheral nervous system. The Hu antigens are also expressed by the associated tumor, usually a small cell lung cancer. **B:** Anti-Yo antibodies. These antibodies react with 34- and 62-kDa proteins expressed in the cytoplasm of Purkinje cells and to a minor degree in the cytoplasm of neurons of the brainstem and the molecular layer of the cerebellum and by the associated tumor. The tumors more commonly involved are ovarian and breast cancer. **C:** Anti-Ri antibodies. These antibodies react with 55- and 80-kDa proteins expressed in the nuclei and, to a minor degree, the cytoplasm of neurons of the central nervous system. The same antigens are also expressed by the associated tumor, usually a breast cancer. **D:** Anti-Tr antibodies. These antibodies react with the cytoplasm of Purkinje cells and other neurons. Characteristically, the antibody reactivity has a dotlike pattern of staining in the molecular layer of the cerebellum. The tumor most frequently associated is Hodgkin lymphoma.

involvement, if any, of other areas of the nervous system including hyperactive reflexes, extensor plantar responses, and sensorimotor neuropathy. Treatment of the tumor with plasmapheresis and intravenous immunoglobulin (IVIg) does not usually affect the course of this disorder (11,12); however, there is a report of two patients who improved with cyclophosphamide (19).

Anti-Tr

Patients with this antibody are usually young men with Hodgkin lymphoma or rarely non-Hodgkin lymphoma (20,21). The neurologic disorder is a pancerebellar dysfunction, which usually develops after the diagnosis of the lymphoma or when the tumor is in remission. Treatment of the tumor results in a rapid and marked decrease of antibody titers. The cerebellar dysfunction of these patients may improve spontaneously, after treatment of the tumor, or symptomatic treatment with clonazepam. Most patients, however, have residual neurologic deficits.

Anti-Ri

Patients with this antibody usually have breast cancer (22). Other associated cancers include gynecologic tumors, carcinoma of the lung, and carcinoma of the bladder. In some patients, no tumor is found. Different from other paraneoplastic cerebellar disorders in which symptoms are pancerebellar, in anti-Ri patients the motor incoordination mainly affects the trunk and gait; 75% of patients have opsoclonus. Opsoclonus may improve spontaneously or with clonazepam, triazolam, or prednisone, leaving the patient with ocular flutter or dysmetria. Other symptoms include vertigo, nausea, dysphagia, ocular paresis, axial rigidity, muscle spasms, and confusion. Clinical response have been noted with cyclophosphamide and effective treatment of the tumor (23). One patient who developed episodes of muscle spasms, axial rigidity, and hyperventilation improved with baclofen (24).

Other

Paraneoplastic cerebellar dysfunction may occur in the absence of an antineuronal antibody, most often with SCLC and non-Hodgkin lymphoma (25).

The presence or absence of anti-Hu antibodies has clinical and prognostic implications. A study of 57 SCLC patients with PCD compared the clinical findings of patients with (44%) and without (56%) anti-Hu antibodies. Those with anti-Hu antibodies were likely to be women, to develop PEM-SN, to have tumor limited to chest, and to die as a result of the neurologic disease. In the same study, 17% of patients had Lambert-Eaton myasthenic syndrome (LEMS) irrespective of the anti-Hu

serology. Furthermore, a third of the anti-Hu seronegative SCLC patients with PCD had P/Q type voltage-gated calcium channel (VGCC) antibodies, suggesting that in these patients, LEMS was overlooked or that the antibodies were involved in the pathogenesis of the cerebellar dysfunction. Treatment with plasma exchange or IVIg improved LEMS but did not improve the cerebellar disorder (25).

In addition, several antineuronal antibodies directed against uncharacterized antigens have been reported (16,26), but their association with a specific paraneoplastic neurologic disorder, tumor type, or prognosis remains unknown.

Paraneoplastic Motor Neuron Disease

The association of systemic cancer with motor neuron disease (MND) (Table 3 is usually coincidental, but there are two situations in which the two disorders occur together, suggesting a paraneoplastic pathogenesis of the MND. The first is when symptoms of MND improve with treatment of the tumor, especially lung and renal cell carcinoma, thymoma, lymphoma, and Waldenström macroglobulinemia (27,28). The neuropathologic picture in these consists of anterior horn cell loss and variable lateral and dorsal column degeneration, without inflammatory cell infiltrates. The second is when a well-characterized paraneoplastic autoantibody is detected (8,10). For example, 20% of patients with anti-Hu–associated PEM-SN develop clinical or pathologic signs of MND during the course of the disease (Fig. 3). Some patients with Hodgkin and non-Hodgkin lymphoma develop a pure lower motor neuron (LMN) syndrome that may have a remitting course. This disorder was initially described in two young women with Hodgkin disease who developed quadriparesis with depressed or absent reflexes and normal sensation (29). In one, symptoms improved spontaneously before the Hodgkin disease was diagnosed; the other died of respiratory failure 14 months after the onset of the neurologic disorder. Later termed "subacute motor neuronopathy" (30), it classically affects patients with Hodgkin and non-Hodgkin lymphoma and leads to progressive, painless, asymmetric LMN weakness with little or no sensory involvement. The course of the neurologic disorder is generally independent of the course of the cancer. In some patients, there is spontaneous improvement with normalization of the neurologic examination. Neuropathologic findings include severe anterior horn cell degeneration, with mild or no inflammatory cell infiltrates, and variable demyelination and axonal loss in the posterior columns. A similar syndrome with poliomyelitis-like inflammatory infiltrates was also reported (31).

A prospective study (32) of patients with MND that underwent marrow biopsy showed an incidence of lymphoproliferative disorders of about 5%. The relationship

TABLE 3. *Paraneoplastic motor neuron syndromes*

Syndrome	Tumor	Pathology	Marker	Outcome
Lower motor neuron and elements of PEM/SN	SCLC	Moderate to severe inflammation; loss of lower motor neurons (spinal cord and brainstem)[a]	Anti-Hu	Progressive; no response to treatment of cancer or immune suppression
Amyotrophic lateral sclerosis	Lymphoma, CLL, plasma cell dyscrasia	No inflammation; lower and upper motor neuron, corticospinal tracts	NI	Progressive; no response to treatment of cancer or immune suppression
Lower motor neuron "subacute motor neuronopathy"	Hodgkin's and non-Hodgkin's lymphoma	Neuronal loss in anterior horns; mild inflammation. Variable demyelination and axonal loss in posterior columns	NI	Progressive; some patients improve spontaneously
Upper motor neuron (primary lateral sclerosis-like syndrome)	Breast cancer	No pathologic studies	NI	Progressive; no response to treatment of cancer or immune suppression

[a]Variable amounts of inflammation, gliosis, and neuronal loss in other areas of the nervous system (hippocampus, cerebellum, dorsal root ganglia, myenteric plexus, or autonomic ganglia).
SCLC, small-cell lung cancer; PEM/SN, paraneoplastic encephalomyelitis and sensory neuronopathy; CLL, chronic lymphocytic leukemia; NI, not identified.

of MND and lymphoproliferative disorders was recently reported among 26 new patients and 56 literature cases with either Hodgkin disease, follicular lymphoma, chronic lymphocytic leukemia, or malignant plasma cell dyscrasia (33). Overall, 55% had upper motor neuron signs clinically, including 56% of the postmortem cases in which pyramidal tracts showed degeneration (32–34).

In contrast to the predominant LMN involvement observed in the patients with anti-Hu associated PEM or lymphoproliferative disorders, a recent study identified a group of patients that developed a predominant upper motor neuron disorder, mimicking primary lateral sclerosis (10). These patients developed upper motor neuron disease in association with breast cancer by the time of

tumor diagnosis or recurrence. Treatment of the tumor did not modify the course of the disease in the five patients so studied, three of whom developed LMN involvement years later consistent with amyotrophic lateral sclerosis and two others that remained primary lateral sclerosis.

In summary, there are three specific settings in which a careful search for cancer is warranted: patients in whom the MND is part of the syndrome of PEM suggested by anti-Hu seropositivity and therein suspected of harboring an occult SCLC or another tumor; patients suspected of harboring a lymphoproliferative cancer so suggested by one or more of the following: an M-protein on immunofixation electrophoresis, elevation of the CSF protein content above 75 mg/dL, adenopathy, abnormal chest film, high erythrocyte sedimentation rate, anemia, leukocytosis, or the atypical clinical presentation of a pure LMN disorder or amyotrophic lateral sclerosis (33); and women with primary lateral sclerosis clinically that have abnormal mammography.

Necrotizing Myelopathy

Paraneoplastic necrotizing myelopathy has been reported in association with a variety of tumors, including lung and renal cancer, leukemia, and Hodgkin disease. Symptoms develop acutely or subacutely, including an ascending flaccid paralysis with sphincter dysfunction and involvement of all modalities of sensation (35,36). The CSF is usually acellular with an increased protein content. Myelography is normal or may show nonspecific spinal cord edema. Most reported patients have not been examined by magnetic resonance imaging, but increased T2 signal and patchy contrast enhancement in the cervical and thoracic spinal cord were identified in two

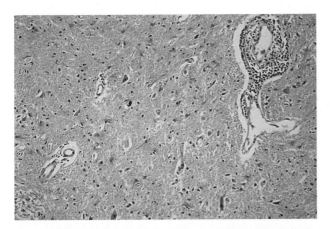

FIG. 3. Paraneoplastic motor neuron dysfunction. Anterior horn of the spinal cord of a patient with anti-Hu–associated encephalomyelitis and predominant lower motor neuron dysfunction. Note the absence of motor neurons and the presence of perivascular inflammatory infiltrates.

patients (37,38). The disorder results from a multiseg-
mental necrosis of both the gray and white matter with
few, if any, perivascular inflammatory infiltrates (39).

An identical syndrome results from intramedullary
metastases, viral infections (40) particularly of the herpes
group, toxic effects of radiation therapy and intrathecal
chemotherapy, septic infarction, and intramedullary granulomas.

PARANEOPLASTIC SYNDROMES OF THE PERIPHERAL NERVOUS SYSTEM

Signs and symptoms of peripheral neuropathy are often
found in cancer patients, particularly those with advanced
disease and significant weight loss. Most patients will
have an identifiable cause such as a nutritional deficit,
hepatic or renal failure, treatment with chemotherapeutic
agents, or leptomeningeal disease (1,2,14). Mononeuropathies in cancer patients are most often secondary to
compression of nerve by tumor or hemorrhage and infarction secondary to leukemic infiltration.

Guillain-Barré Syndrome

Patients with Hodgkin disease can present with rapidly
progressive motor neuropathy indistinguishable from
GBS (41–43). A few patients with solid tumors were
reported with concurrent GBS, but the small number of
cases precluded distinguishing a paraneoplastic pathogenesis. Neurologic symptoms have been reported during
active disease, in remission, and in some before relapse.
The course of the neuropathy is usually independent of the
lymphoma. These patients have the same response to
plasma exchange as those with idiopathic GBS.

Chronic Sensorimotor Neuropathy

This form of neuropathy occurs with any malignancy
but is most commonly associated with lung cancer. The
onset of the neuropathy usually follows the diagnosis of
the cancer but may precede it by several years. Patients
present with a distal symmetric polyneuropathy characterized by distal weakness, wasting, sensory loss, pain,
and decreased reflexes that slowly advances proximally
over the course of the disease, rarely with cranial nerve
involvement. The disease rarely stabilizes or shows a
remitting or relapsing course (1,44,45).

Routine laboratory studies are often unhelpful in distinguishing a paraneoplastic pathogenesis. Most patients
have normal CSF studies. Electrophysiologic studies
show evidence of axonopathy and occasionally slow conduction velocities indicative of concurrent demyelination.
Nerve biopsy can show axonal degeneration, segmental
demyelination, or a combination of the two. There have
been reports of responses with treatment of the cancer
and corticosteroids.

Approximately 10% of patients with a peripheral sensorimotor neuropathy of unknown etiology have a monoclonal gammopathy. These neuropathies are discussed in
a separate chapter.

Paraneoplastic Muscle Rigidity and Stiffness

Paraneoplastic muscle rigidity and stiffness results
from several disorders of the central nervous system and
peripheral nervous system, including neuromyotonia,
encephalomyelitis, and stiff-person syndrome. The small
number of patients reported and the lack of rigorous electrophysiologic and antineuronal antibody studies in some
cases make it difficult to compare and identify physio-
pathologic mechanisms that may be shared by these disorders.

Paraneoplastic neuromyotonia is characterized by continuous muscle fiber activity, associated with progressive
aching, stiffness, muscle cramps, myokymia, and hyperhidrosis (46). Some patients develop sensorimotor neuropathy. Electrophysiologic studies show bursts of high-
frequency atypical motor unit discharges that persist after
stopping a voluntary muscle contraction. These motor
discharges occur during sleep, general anesthesia, and
proximal nerve block but disappear by blocking the neuromuscular junction (46). Thymomas and SCLC are the
most frequently associated tumors (47,48). The autoimmune basis of this disorder is suggested by the demonstration of autoantibodies that interfere with the function
of K+ channels in patients with nonparaneoplastic neuromyotonia (49,50). Passive transfer of IgG from patients
with neuromyotonia to mice results in increased resistance to D-tubocurarine at the neuromuscular junction. A
similar mechanism has been suggested for paraneoplastic
neuromyotonia. These patients may improve with plasma
exchange.

Paraneoplastic rigidity and "spinal myoclonus" has
been called "progressive encephalomyelitis with rigidity"
(51,52) and results in rigidity involving trunk and limbs,
sometimes with mild distal sensory impairment. Painful
spasms can occur spontaneously or can be triggered by
various stimuli, including light touch, passive and active
limb movement, and sudden sounds. Most patients have
normal or absent tendon reflexes. Pathologic studies
show perivascular inflammatory infiltrates and neuronal
degeneration mainly involving the cervical portion of the
spinal cord and brainstem. Corticospinal tracts are usually preserved. The tumor most commonly involved is
SCLC. A woman with breast cancer, paraneoplastic opso-
clonus-myoclonus, ataxia, and anti-Ri antibodies developed a similar syndrome, including rigidity and muscle
spasms, but pathologic studies were not available.

Stiff-person syndrome is characterized by progressive
muscle stiffness, achiness, spasms, and rigidity involving
axial and proximal limb muscles. Muscle spasms are triggered by sensory or emotional stimuli and lead to limb

deformities and fractures. The rigidity consists of a boardlike contraction of affected muscles, which improves during sleep and with benzodiazepines. Electrophysiologic studies show continuous motor unit discharges. The tumors more commonly involved are SCLC, thymomas, and breast cancer (53,54). An autoimmune basis of this disorder was initially suggested by the identification of antibodies against glutamic acid decarboxylase in patients who had nonparaneoplastic stiff-person syndrome (55). More recently, a subset of patients with paraneoplastic stiff-person syndrome and breast cancer were found to harbor antibodies that react with amphiphysin, a 128-kDa synaptic protein (54–57). Antibodies against 125- to 130-kDa proteins have also been identified in one patient with colon carcinoma and one with Hodgkin disease (58). In patients with breast cancer and anti-amphiphysin antibodies, treatment of the tumor and use of steroids may result in neurologic improvement (54).

PARANEOPLASTIC SYNDROMES OF THE NEUROMUSCULAR JUNCTION AND MUSCLE

Lambert-Eaton Myasthenic Syndrome

Patients with this disorder develop antibodies that react with the presynaptic site of cholinergic synapses, blocking the entry of calcium necessary for the release of acetylcholine (59). Sixty percent of patients harbor an SCLC, which is usually detected 2 years after onset of neurologic symptoms. Tumors other than SCLC are rare, but lymphomas were reported in some patients (60). No tumor is identified in approximately 30% of patients (61).

In 60% of patients, the first symptom is lower extremity weakness. Less frequently, the presenting symptoms include generalized weakness, aching and stiffness of muscles, and autonomic dysfunction. Arm and leg weakness develops gradually, affecting proximal muscles. Autonomic dysfunction eventually affects 80% of the patients and includes dry mouth, impotence, constipation, and blurred vision. Cranial nerve involvement as manifested by diplopia, ptosis, slurred speech, and dysphagia is commonly mild or transient (61). Neurophysiologic studies demonstrate low-amplitude compound muscle action potentials at rest, with a decremental response at 3 Hz stimulation, and an incremental response of 100% or more at 50 Hz or after maximal voluntary contraction for 20 to 30 seconds.

The antigens recognized by LEMS antibodies are contained in the P/Q-type VGCC of the presynaptic cholinergic synapse. Similar channels are expressed in cerebellum, and extracts of cerebellum labeled with ω-conotoxin MVIIC, a toxin that specifically binds to P/Q type VGCC, are used in the immunoprecipation assay to detect antibodies in patients with LEMS (62). The specific epitopes of the VGCC complex recognized by these

antibodies are unknown. Antibodies against the β-subunit of the calcium channel (63) and against synaptotagmin (64) have been identified in the serum of LEMS patients. Recent studies have indicated two new putative epitopes located in the extracellular region of the α1A-subunit of the P/Q-type VGCC (65). In addition, 34% of patients with LEMS or their family members may harbor other organ-specific antibodies, suggesting a genetic predisposition to immunologic disorders (66).

Passive transfer of serum or IgG from patients with LEMS to animals reproduces the disease clinically, electrophysiologically, and morphologically (67,68). In patients with paraneoplastic LEMS, treatment of the tumor usually results in improvement of the neurologic disorder (69). Removal of antibodies by plasma exchange and treatment with IVIg or 3,4-diaminopyridine, alone or in conjunction with other therapies, are generally useful therapies (70–72).

Acute Necrotizing Myopathy

This rare disorder was described in patients with lung, gastric, breast, colon, and bladder tumors (73,74). Neurologic symptoms usually precede the diagnosis of the neoplasm. Presenting symptoms include muscle pain and symmetric limb weakness that rapidly progresses to involve respiratory, pharyngeal, and truncal muscles. Tendon reflexes are preserved. The course is usually fatal in 12 weeks. Serum creatine kinase levels are elevated and electrophysiologic studies show myopathic changes. Treatment with steroids and adrenocorticotropic hormone are generally ineffective; however, one patient improved after removal of a breast carcinoma.

Pathologic studies generally show widespread necrosis of skeletal muscle with little or no inflammation; however, one patient had polymyositis and another had peripheral neuropathy pathologically. It has been suggested that acute necrotizing myopathy represents a severe form of polymyositis with a more rapid course, more extensive muscle necrosis, and only rare evidence of inflammation. In one patient with acute necrotizing myopathy and bladder cancer, muscle biopsy demonstrated thickened capillaries with deposits of complement membrane attack complex, suggesting immune-mediated microangiopathy as a contributing factor (75). A resemblance to chemotherapy or cytokine- (interleukin-2, interferon-α) induced rhabdomyolysis has been noted (76).

Carcinomatous Neuromyopathy

This disorder presents clinically with proximal muscle weakness, decreased reflexes, and mild serum creatine kinase elevation. Electrophysiologic and pathologic studies show both myopathy and neuropathy. Electron microscopy demonstrated degeneration of intramuscular motor nerves in one case (77). Unlike patients with cachectic myopathy, these patients are generally well nourished, and symptoms precede the diagnosis of the tumor, usually a cancer of the lung.

Cachectic Myopathy

Paraneoplastic cachexia is common in patients with cancer and is characterized by anorexia, anemia, weakness, and weight loss. Affected patients develop a myopathy that is clinically and pathologically identical to myopathy found in patients with other chronic debilitating diseases. Despite diffuse muscle wasting, strength is often preserved until late in the course of the neoplastic disease. Myoedema or mounding phenomenon, an electrically silent focal contracture of skeletal muscle in response to muscle tapping, is often present. Pathologic studies show small fiber group atrophy that later progresses to show proliferation of myonuclei and fragmentation of muscle fibers. There is eventually muscle fiber necrosis with hyaline, granular, and vacuolar degeneration, without evidence of inflammation or nerve degeneration. Epidermal growth factor, tumor necrosis factor, and interleukin-6 may contribute to the pathogenesis of paraneoplastic cachexia (78–80).

Carcinoid Myopathy

Patients with carcinoid tumor develop progressive myopathy years after diagnosis (81–83). Symptoms include proximal muscle weakness, cramps, and tenderness of shoulder girdle muscles. Pathologic studies show nonspecific type II fiber atrophy, with absent or minimal inflammatory cell infiltrates. Cyproheptadine, a serotonin antagonist, improves both the myopathy and the carcinoid syndrome (82,84).

REFERENCES

1. Posner JB. *Neurologic complications of cancer.* Philadelphia: F.A. Davis, 1995.
2. Dalmau J, Posner JB. Paraneoplastic syndromes affecting the nervous system. *Semin Oncol* 1997;24:1–12.
3. Henson RA, Hoffman HL, Urich H. Encephalomyelitis with carcinoma. *Brain* 1965;88:449–464.
4. Dalmau J, Furneaux HM, Gralla RJ, Kris MG, Posner JB. Detection of the anti-Hu antibody in the serum of patients with small cell lung cancer—a quantitative Western blot analysis. *Ann Neurol* 1990;27:544–552.
5. Graus F, Elkon KB, Cordon-Cardo C, Posner JB. Sensory neuronopathy and small cell lung cancer: antineuronal antibody that also reacts with the tumor. *Am J Med* 1986;80:45–52.
6. Graus F, Segurado OG, Tolosa E. Selective concentration of anti-Purkinje cell antibody in the CSF of two patients with paraneoplastic cerebellar degeneration. *Acta Neurol Scand* 1988;78:210–213.
7. Jean WC, Dalmau J, Ho A, Posner JB. Analysis of the IgG subclass distribution and inflammatory infiltrates in patients with anti-Hu associated paraneoplastic encephalomyelitis. *Neurology* 1994;44:140–147.
8. Dalmau J, Graus F, Rosenblum MK, Posner JB. Anti-Hu associated paraneoplastic encephalomyelitis/sensory neuronopathy: a clinical study of 71 patients. *Medicine* 1992;71:59–72.
9. Verma A, Berger JR, Snodgrass S, Petito C. Motor neuron disease: a paraneoplastic process associated with anti-Hu antibody and small cell lung carcinoma. *Ann Neurol* 1996;40:112–116.
10. Forsyth PA, Dalmau J, Graus F, Cwik V, Rosenblum MK, Posner JB. Motor neuron syndromes in cancer patients. *Ann Neurol* 1997;41:722–730.
11. Graus F, Vega F, Delattre JY, et al. Plasmapheresis and antineoplastic treatment in CNS paraneoplastic syndromes with antineuronal autoantibodies. *Neurology* 1992;42:536–540.
12. Uchuya M, Graus F, Vega F, René R, Delattre J-Y. Intravenous immunoglobulin therapy in paraneoplastic neurologic syndromes with antineuronal autoantibodies. *J Neurol Neurosurg Psychiatry* 1996;60:388–392.
13. Graus F, Elkon KB, Lloberes P. Neuronal antinuclear antibody (anti-Hu) in paraneoplastic encephalomyelitis simulating acute polyneuritis. *Acta Neurol Scand* 1987;75:249–252.
14. Dalmau J, Graus F. Paraneoplastic syndromes. In: Loeffler JS, Black PMCL, eds. *Cancer of the nervous system.* Boston, MA: Blackwell Science 1997;674–700.
15. Henson RA, Urich H. *Cancer and the nervous system.* Oxford: Blackwell Science, 1982.
16. Voltz RD, Graus F, Posner JB, Dalmau J. Paraneoplastic encephalomyelitis: an update of the effects of the anti-Hu immune response on the nervous system and tumor. *J Neurol Neurosurg Psychiatry* 1997;63:133–136.
17. Mason WP, Graus F, Lang B, et al. Small-cell lung cancer, paraneoplastic cerebellar degeneration and the Lambert-Eaton myasthenic syndrome. *Brain* 1997;120:1279–1300.
18. Peterson K, Rosenblum MK, Kotanides H, Posner JB. Paraneoplastic cerebellar degeneration. I. A clinical analysis of 55 anti-Yo antibody-positive patients. *Neurology* 1992;42:1931–1937.
19. Stark E, Wurster U, Patzold U, Sailer M, Haas J. Immunological and clinical response to immunosuppressive treatment in paraneoplastic cerebellar degeneration. *Arch Neurol* 1995;52:814–818.
20. Hammack JE, Kotanides H, Rosenblum MK, Posner JB. Paraneoplastic cerebellar degeneration. II. Clinical and immunologic findings in 21 patients with Hodgkin's disease. *Neurology* 1992;42:1938–1943.
21. Graus F, Dalmau J, Valldeoriola F, et al. Immunological characterization of a neuronal antibody (anti-Tr) associated with paraneoplastic cerebellar degeneration and Hodgkin's disease. *J Neuroimmunol* 1997;74:55–61.
22. Luque FA, Furneaux HM, Ferziger R. et al. Anti-Ri: an antibody associated with paraneoplastic opsoclonus and breast cancer. *Ann Neurol* 1991;29:241–251.
23. Dropcho EJ, Kline LB, Riser J. Antineuronal (anti-Ri) autoantibodies in a patient with steroid-responsive opsoclonus myoclonus. *Neurology* 1993;43:207–211.
24. Casado JL, Gil-Peralta A, Graus F, Arenas C, Lopez JM, Alberca R. Anti-Ri antibodies associated with opsoclonus and progressive encephalomyelitis with rigidity. *Neurology* 1994;44:1521–1522.
25. Blumenfeld AM, Recht LD, Chad DA, DeGirolami U, Griffin T, Jaeckle KA. Coexistence of Lambert-Eaton myasthenic syndrome and subacute cerebellar degeneration: differential effects of treatment. *Neurology* 1991;41:1682–1685.
26. Dalmau J, Posner JB. Neurologic paraneoplastic antibodies (anti-Yo; anti-Hu; anti-Ri): the case for a nomenclature based on antibody and antigen specificity. *Neurology* 1994;44:2241–2246.
27. Rosenfeld MR, Posner JB. Paraneoplastic motor neuron disease. *Adv Neurol* 1991;56:445–459.
28. Evans BK, Fagan C, Arnold T, Dropcho EJ, Oh SJ. Paraneoplastic motor neuron disease and renal carcinoma. Improvement after nephrectomy. *Neurology* 1990;40:960–962.
29. Rowland LP, Schneck SA. Neuromuscular disorders associated with malignant neoplastic disorders. *J Chronic Dis* 1963;16:777–795.
30. Schold SC, Cho ES, Sonasundaram M, Posner JP. Subacute motor neuronopathy: a remote effect of lymphoma. *Ann Neurol* 1979;5:271–287.
31. Walton JN, Tomlinson BE, Pedru GW. Subacute "poliomyelitis" and Hodgkin's disease. *J Neurol Sci* 1968;6:435–445.
32. Rowland LP, Sherman WH, Latov N, et al. Amyotrophic lateral sclerosis and lymphoma: bone marrow examination and other diagnostic tests. *Neurology* 1992;42:1101–1102.
33. Gordon PH, Rowland LP, Younger DS, et al. Lymphoproliferative disorders and motor neuron disease: an update. *Neurology* 1997;48:1671–1678.

34. Younger DS, Rowland LP, Latov N, et al. Lymphoma, motor neuron diseases, and amyotrophic lateral sclerosis. *Ann Neurol* 1991;29:78–86.

35. Mancall EL, Rosales RK. Necrotizing myelopathy associated with visceral carcinoma. *Brain* 1964;87:639–659.

36. Ojeda VJ. Necrotizing myelopathy associated with malignancy. A clinicopathologic study of two cases and literature review. *Cancer* 1984; 53:1115–1123.

37. Glantz MJ, Biran H, Myers ME, Gockerman JP, Friedberg MH. The radiographic diagnosis and treatment of paraneoplastic central nervous system disease. *Cancer* 1994;73:168–175.

38. Gieron MA, Margraf LR, Korthals JK, Gonzalvo AA, Murtagh RF, Hvizdala EV. Progressive necrotizing myelopathy associated with leukemia: clinical, pathologic, and MRI correlation. *J Child Neurol* 1987; 2:44–49.

39. Gray F, Hauw JJ, Escourolle R, Castaigne P. Myelopathies necrosantes et pathologie neoplasique. *Rev Neurol* 1980;136:235–246.

40. Iwamasa T, Utsumi Y, Sakuda H, et al. Two cases of necrotizing myelopathy associated with malignancy caused by herpes simplex virus type 2. *Acta Neuropathol* 1989;78:252–257.

41. Lisak RP, Mitchell M, Zweiman B, Orrechio E, Asbury AK. Guillain-Barré syndrome and Hodgkin's disease: three cases with immunological studies. *Ann Neurol* 1977;1:72–78.

42. Klingon GH. The Guillain-Barré syndrome associated with cancer. *Cancer* 1965;18:163.

43. Croft PB, Urich H, Wilkinson M. Peripheral neuropathy of sensorimotor type associated with malignant disease. *Brain* 1967;90:31–36.

44. Trojaborg W, Frantzen E, Andersen I. Peripheral neuropathy and myopathy associated with carcinoma of the lung. *Brain* 1969;92:71–82.

45. Gomm SA, Thatcher N, Barber PV, Cumming WJK. A clinicopathological study of the paraneoplastic neuromuscular syndromes associated with lung cancer. *Q J Med* 1990;75:577–595.

46. Newsom-Davis J, Mills KR. Immunological associations of acquired neuromyotonia (Isaacs' syndrome). *Brain* 1993;116:453–469.

47. Waerness E. Neuromyotonia and bronchial carcinoma. *Electromyogr Clin Neurophysiol* 1974;14:527–535.

48. Garcia-Merino A, Cabello A, Mora JS, Liaño H. Continuous muscle fiber activity, peripheral neuropathy, and thymoma. *Ann Neurol* 1991; 29:215–218.

49. Sinha S, Newsom-Davis J, Mills K, Byrne N, Lang B, Vincent A. Autoimmune etiology for acquired neuromyotonia (Isaacs' syndrome). *Lancet* 1991;338:75–77.

50. Shillito P, Molenaar PC, Vincent A, et al. Acquired neuromyotonia: evidence for autoantibodies directed against K+ channels of peripheral nerves. *Ann Neurol* 1995;38:714–722.

51. Whiteley AM, Swash M, Urich H. Progressive encephalomyelitis with rigidity. *Brain* 1976;99:27–42.

52. Roobol TH, Kazzaz BA, Vecht CHJ. Segmental rigidity and spinal myoclonus as a paraneoplastic syndrome. *J Neurol Neurosurg Psychiatry* 1987;50:628–631.

53. Bateman DE, Weller RO, Kennedy P. Stiffman syndrome: a rare paraneoplastic disorder? *J Neurol Neurosurg Psychiatry* 1990;53:695–696.

54. Folli F, Solimena M, Cofiell R, et al. Autoantibodies to a 128-kd synaptic protein in three women with the stiff-man syndrome and breast cancer. *N Eng J Med* 1993;328:546–551.

55. Solimena M, Folli F, Aparisi R, Pozza G, De Camilli P. Autoantibodies to GABA-ergic neurons and pancreatic beta cells in stiff-man syndrome. *N Engl J Med* 1990;322:1555–1560.

56. De Camilli P, Thomas A, Cofiell R, et al. The synaptic vesicle-associated protein amphiphysin is the 128-kD autoantigen of stiff-man syndrome with breast cancer. *J Exp Med* 1993;178:2219–2223.

57. David C, Solimena M, De Camilli P. Autoimmunity in stiff-man syndrome with breast cancer is targeted to the C-terminal region of human amphiphysin, a protein similar to the yeast proteins, Rvs167 and Rvs161. *FEBS Lett* 1994;351:73–79.

58. Grimaldi LM, Martino G, Braghi S, et al. Heterogeneity of autoantibodies in stiff-man syndrome. *Ann Neurol* 1993;34:57–64.

59. Lang B, Newsom-Davis J, Wray D, Vincent A, Murray N. Autoimmune aetiology for myasthenic (Eaton-Lambert) syndrome. *Lancet* 1981;2: 224–226.

60. Goldstein JM, Waxman SG, Vollmer TL, Lang B, Johnston I, Newsom-Davis J. Subacute cerebellar degeneration and Lambert-Eaton myasthenic syndrome associated with antibodies to voltage-gated calcium channels: differential effect of immunosuppressive therapy on central

and peripheral defects. *J Neurol Neurosurg Psychiatry* 1994;57: 1138–1139.

61. O'Neill JH, Murray NM, Newsom-Davis J. The Lambert-Eaton myasthenic syndrome. A review of 50 cases. *Brain* 1988;111:577–596.

62. Motomura M, Johnston I, Lang B, Vincent A, Newsom-Davis J. An improved diagnostic assay for Lambert-Eaton myasthenic syndrome. *J Neurol Neurosurg Psychiatry* 1995;58:85–87.

63. Rosenfeld MR, Wong E, Dalmau J, et al. Serum from patients with Lambert-Eaton myasthenic syndrome recognize antigens homologous to the beta subunit of the Ca++ channel complex. *Ann Neurol* 1993;33:113–120.

64. Leveque C, Hoshino T, David P, et al. The synaptic vesicle protein synaptotagmin associates with calcium channels and is a putative Lambert-Eaton myasthenic syndrome antigen. *Proc Natl Acad Sci USA* 1992;89:3625–3629.

65. Takamori M, Iwasa K, Komai K. Antibodies to synthetic peptides of the α1A subunit of the voltage-gated calcium channel in Lambert-Eaton myasthenic syndrome. *Neurology* 1997;48:1261–1265.

66. Lennon VA, Kryzer TJ, Griesmann GE, et al. Calcium-channel antibodies in the Lambert-Eaton syndrome and other paraneoplastic syndromes. *N Engl J Med* 1995;332:1467–1474.

67. Kim YI. Passive transfer of Lambert-Eaton myasthenic syndrome: neuromuscular transmission in mice injected with plasma. *Muscle Nerve* 1985;8:162–172.

68. Kim YI, Neher E. IgG from patients with Lambert-Eaton syndrome blocks voltage-dependent calcium channels. *Science* 1988;239:405–408.

69. Chalk CH, Murray NM, Newsom-Davis J, O'Neill JH, Spiro SG. Response of the Lambert-Eaton myasthenic syndrome to treatment of associated small-cell lung carcinoma. *Neurology* 1990;40:1552–1556.

70. Newsom-Davis J, Murray NM. Plasma exchange and immunosuppressive drug treatment in the Lambert-Eaton myasthenic syndrome. *Neurology* 1984;34:480–485.

71. Bain PG, Motomura M, Newsom-Davis J, et al. Effects of intravenous immunoglobulin on muscle weakness and calcium-channel autoantibodies in the Lambert-Eaton myasthenic syndrome. *Neurology* 1996; 47:678–683.

72. Mcevoy KM, Windebank AJ, Daube JR, Low PA. 3,4-Diaminopyridine in the treatment of the Lambert-Eaton myasthenic syndrome. *N Engl J Med* 1989;321:1567–1571.

73. Brownell B, Hughes JT. Degeneration of muscle in association with carcinoma of the bronchus. *J Neurol Neurosurg Psychiatry* 1975;38: 363–370.

74. Vosskamper M, Korf B, Franke F, Schachenmayer W. Paraneoplastic necrotizing myopathy: a rare disorder to be differentiated from polymyositis. *J Neurol* 1989;236:489–492.

75. Emslie AM, Engel AG. Necrotizing myopathy with pipestem capillaries, microvascular deposits of the complement membrane attack complex (MAC) and minimal cellular infiltration. *Neurology* 1991;41:936–939.

76. Anderlini P, Buzaid AC, Legha SS. Acute rhabdomyolysis after concurrent administration of interleukin-2, interferon-alfa, and chemotherapy for metastatic melanoma. *Cancer* 1995;76:678–679.

77. Barron SA, Heffner RR. Weakness in malignancy: evidence for a remote effect of tumor on distal axons. *Ann Neurol* 1978;4:268–274.

78. Black K, Garrett IR, Mundy GR. Chinese hamster ovarian cells transfected with the murine interleukin-6 gene cause hypercalcemia as well as cachexia, leukocytosis and thrombocytosis in tumor-bearing nude mice. *Endocrinology* 1991;128:2657–2659.

79. Yoneda Y, Alsina MM, Watatani K, Bellot F, Schlessinger J, Mundy GR. Dependence of a human squamous carcinoma and associated paraneoplastic syndromes on the epidermal growth factor receptor pathway in nude mice. *Cancer Res* 1991;51:2438–2443.

80. Strassmann G, Jacob CO, Fong M, Bertolini DR. Mechanisms of paraneoplastic syndromes of colon-26: involvement of interleukin 6 in hypercalcemia. *Cytokine* 1993;5:463–468.

81. Berry EM, Maunder C, Wilson M. Carcinoid myopathy and treatment with cyproheptadine (Periactin). *Gut* 1974;15:34–38.

82. Swash M, Fox KP, Davidson AR. Carcinoid myopathy: serotonin-induced muscle weakness in man? *Arch Neurol* 1975;32:572–574.

83. Lederman RJ, Bukowski RM, Nickerson P. Carcinoid myopathy. *Cleve Clin J Med* 1987;54:299–303.

84. Moertel CG, Kvols LK, Rubin J. A study of cyproheptadine in the treatment of metastatic carcinoid tumor and the malignant carcinoid syndrome. *Cancer* 1991;67:33–36.

Motor Disorders,
edited by David S. Younger.
Lippincott Williams & Wilkins, Philadelphia © 1999.

CHAPTER 36

Motor Disorders Associated with Human Immunodeficiency Virus Infection

Daniel J. L. MacGowan and David M. Simpson

Since the beginning of the acquired immunodeficiency syndrome (AIDS) epidemic, an estimated 4.5 million persons have developed AIDS worldwide and 1 in 250 people of age 15 to 49 years are now infected with human immunodeficiency virus (HIV) type 1 (1). By December 1996, in the United States, 581,429 cases of AIDS in adults and adolescents were reported to the Centers for Disease Control and Prevention (CDC) (2). In 1993, the CDC revised its classification of AIDS to an absolute CD4+ lymphocyte count of less than 200 cells/μL (3). There are three categories of clinical infection: asymptomatic acute infection or primary generalized lympadenopathy, symptomatic, and AIDS indicator conditions, as previously described in 1987 (4). The degree of immunodeficiency is graded from 1 to 3 according to the CD4+ count, as follows: 1, at least 500 cells/μL; 2, 200 to 499 cells/μL; and 3, less than 200 cells/μL. Thus, the disease is now staged clinically and by the degree of immune deficiency. These classifications may be soon adapted to include serum HIV viral RNA load, which has been shown to predict outcome (5).

AIDS-associated neurologic conditions affect 40 to 60% of AIDS patients and are identified pathologically in over 90% (6–11). The incidence of neurologic disorders may be increasing despite improved antiretroviral and opportunistic infection treatments because patients now have a longer survival at more immunodeficient states, the time when the nervous system is most vulnerable (12). The scale of neurologic disease complicating HIV infection has been recently compared (13) with neuro-logic disorders in both the infected and uninfected community using CDC data (2) and statistics from San Francisco in the 1980s (14). The current annual incidence of primary central nervous system (CNS) lymphoma exceeds low-grade glioma. AIDS-associated progressive multifocal leukoencephalopathy (PML) is similar to that of Huntington's disease and myasthenia gravis combined, and HIV-related encephalopathy (HIVE) is equivalent to that of multiple sclerosis. Thus, the HIV pandemic is exerting profound effects on the prevalence and incidence of neurologic diseases overall. It remains unclear what effect highly active antiviral therapy with protease inhibitors or other novel agents (15) will have on the incidence of neurologic complications of HIV infection. Disorders of the motor system due to CNS and peripheral nervous system involvement, the topic of this chapter, can be a major or minor feature of the neurologic syndromes complicating HIV infection (Table 1).

CENTRAL NERVOUS SYSTEM MANIFESTATIONS

These may be divided into those of a *generalized* or *focal* types. The former group includes primarily HIV encephalopathy and HIV-associated cerebellar disease and myelopathy; the latter includes predominantly HIV-associated toxoplasmosis, primary CNS lymphoma, PML, and other focal proximate causes.

CENTRAL NERVOUS SYSTEM DISORDERS

Human Immunodeficiency Virus Encephalopathy

Clinical Features

HIVE, also known as AIDS-dementia complex (16) and HIV-1–associated cognitive motor complex (17), is the most frequent cause of dementia with signs of gener-

D. J. L. MacGowan: Neuro-AIDS Research Program and Departments of Neurology and Clinical Neurophysiology, Mount Sinai Medical Center, New York, New York 10029.

D. M. Simpson: Department of Neurology, Clinical Neurophysiology Laboratories and Neuro-AIDS Research Program, Mount Sinai Medical Center, New York, New York 10029.

TABLE 1. *Major HIV neurologic syndromes with motor system dysfunction*

Diagnosis	CD 4 count	Symptoms	Signs	Diagnostic studies	Therapy
HIV encephalopathy	<200 cells/mm³	Memory loss, gait disorder, behavioral change	Dementia, extrapyramidal and pyramidal signs, neuropsychiatric changes	MRI—periventricular white matter hyperintensities, lateral ventriculomegaly, +/– cortical atrophy CSF—⇑ β_2-microglobulin	High-dose AZT plus ddI, ddC, or d4T with a protease inhibitor Consider a clinical trial
Toxoplasma sulfadiazine, encephalitis	<200 cells/mm³	Headache, fever, confusion, lethargy, seizures, focal weakness	Focal hemiparesis, ataxia, sensory, visual field, or language deficits	Positive serum toxoplasma IgG MRI—single or multiple enhancing masses with edema	Pyrimethamine, clindamycin
Primary CNS lymphoma	<100 cells/mm³	Headache, confusion, lethargy, seizures, focal weakness	Focal hemiparesis, sensory, visual field, or language deficits	MRI—single or multifocal enhancing masses with edema CSF—Positive pcr for EBV DNA	Whole brain radiotherapy
Progressive multifocal leukoencephalopathy	<200 cells/mm³	Lethargy, confusion, focal weakness, speech disturbances	Focal hemiparesis, ataxia, sensory, visual field, or language deficits	MRI—nonenhancing subcortical white matter lesions without edema CSF—Positive pcr for JCV DNA	High-dose AZT plus ddI, d4T, or d4T with a protease inhibitor Consider a clinical trial
Cytomegalovirus encephalitis	<50 cells/mm³	Rapidly progressive confusion, apathy, weakness	Dementia, cranial neuropathies, pyramidal and extra-pyramidal signs	MRI—Peri-ependymal and meningeal enhancement CSF—Positive pcr for CMV-DNA	Ganciclovir +/– foscarnet
Cerebral infarction	<200 cells/mm³	Focal weakness, speech disturbance, vertigo, diplopia	Focal hemiparesis, ataxia, sensory, visual field, or language deficits	Echo—Merantic endocarditis CSF—VDRL, Cryptococcal antigen, Tb culture or pcr Urine—Pos. toxicology Serum—anticardiolipin abs, ⇑ ESR	Anticoagulation Antimicrobial therapy
Vacuolar myelopathy	<200 cells/mm³	Gait, urinary and erectile dysfunction. Lower extremity weakness	Spastic paraparesis, posterior column dysfunction, no sensory level	MRI/CSF—Normal or nonspecific SSEP's— Lower extremity Prolonged central conduction time	Symptomatic Clinical trial—? methionine replacement
Distal symmetric polyneuropathy	<200 cells/mm³	Distal numbness, paresthesias, pain	Stocking-glove sensory loss, decreased or absent ankle reflexes	NCV/EMG—Chronic, distal, predominantly sensory, sensorimotor axonopathy	ddI, ddC, or d4T withdrawal Tricyclic antidepressants Clinical trial
Mononeuritis multiplex Prednisone	>400 cells/mm³	Foot drop, wrist drop, facial weakness	Multifocal peripheral and/or cranial neuropathies	EMG/NCV—Multifocal axonal neuropathy. Nerve biopsy—CMV inclusions, vasculitis, inflammation	Early—None +/– Late—Ganciclovir
Inflammatory demyelinating polyneuropathy	>400 cells/mm³	Progressive generalized weakness and paresthesias	Generalized weakness, areflexia, mild sensory loss	NCV/EMG—Demyelination	Plasmapheresis, steroids
Progressive polyradiculopathy	<50 cells/mm³	Flaccid lower extremity weakness, paresthesias, urinary retention	Flaccid paraparesis, saddle anesthesia, decreased reflexes, urinary retention	CSF—Pos. pcr or culture for CMV DNA, ⇑ protein, neutrophilia MRI—Radicular enhancement	Ganciclovir +/– foscarnet
Myopathy	Any	Muscle weakness, myalgia, and weight loss	Proximal muscle weakness	⇑ CK, EMG—Irritative myopathy Muscle biopsy—Myofiber degeneration, inflammation, inclusions	AZT withdrawal Prednisone

HIV, human immunodeficiency virus; CNS, central nervous system; MRI, magnetic resonance imaging; CSF, cerebrospinal fluid; EBV, Epstein-Barr virus; JCV, JC virus; CMV, cytomegalovirus; VDRL, Venereal Disease Research Laboratory (test); ESR, erythrocyte sedimentation rate; SSEP's, somatosensory evoked potentials; NCV, nerve conduction velocity; CK, creatine kinase; EMG, electromyography.

alized pyramidal and extrapyramidal dysfunction. It resembles a parkinsonian state complicated by a subcortical type of dementia. Diagnostic criteria were defined by an American Academy of Neurology (AAN) Consortium to differentiate major and minor forms (18). HIVE is marked by poor concentration and psychomotor slowing rather than focal cortical brain abnormalities. Signs of extrapyramidal dysfunction, in particular bradykinesia, and frontal release increase over time in proportion to the level of immunodeficiency as measured by the CD4+ cell count (19,20). Snout and palmomental reflexes increase in frequency in HIV-infected Tanzanians according to the clinical stage of disease and are present in 23 to 39% of asymptomatic and in 69 to 87% of terminal AIDS cases, respectively (21). Pyramidal signs include spasticity, jaw jerk, hyperreflexia, and extensor plantar responses (16).

Radiologic Features

Brain magnetic resonance imaging (MRI) shows prominent, symmetric, periventricular, nonenhancing white matter hyperintensities that spare subcortical U-fibers, with secondary lateral ventriculomegaly ex vacuo (22). There is mild to moderate neocortical and caudate atrophy, with the latter correlating with cognitive impairment (23,24). Figure 1 shows the typical MRI appearance of HIVE.

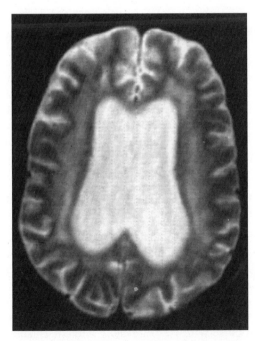

FIG. 1. T2-weighted magnetic resonance image of the brain of a 34-year-old HIV-infected man with dementia. There is diffuse enlargement of the lateral ventricles and hyperintense signal throughout the periventricular white matter, consistent with leukoencephalopathy. (From Simpson D, Tagliati M. Neurologic manifestations of HIV infection. *Ann Intern Med* 1994;121:771, with permission.)

Pathologic Features

The pathologic hallmark of HIVE is encephalitis marked by microglial nodules and multinucleated giant cells (25,26). The dominant areas affected are the periventricular white matter and basal ganglia, in particular the globus pallidus (27). Neocortical atrophy is less prominent (28), although an association has been shown between synaptic markers of neurologic damage and intra-CNS HIV burden, reflecting a reduction in cortical neuronal synaptic density and arborization (29). Figure 2 illustrates the histologic abnormalities. There is a correlation between cognitive decline and extent of periventricular white matter disease and neocortical atrophy. However, the extent of atrophy noted by MRI frequently does not correlate with autopsy findings, possibly due to fixation artifact and the absence of a consistent imaging finding for HIV multinucleated giant cell encephalitis (30). The neuropathology of the white matter lesions is heterogeneous, consisting of vacuolar leukoencephalopathy, angiocentric foci of hemosiderin laden macrophages, and multinucleated giant cell encephalitis with microglial nodules (30,31).

Pathophysiology

Pathologic mapping of HIV infection in the brain by immunohistochemistry for p24 core protein (27) shows the burden of infection to be in subcortical white matter and basal ganglia, with infection limited to macrophages and microglia. Productive infection of neurons using in situ polymerase chain reaction (PCR) hybridization techniques has been shown in only some studies (32). The degree of CNS HIV infection is surprisingly limited and

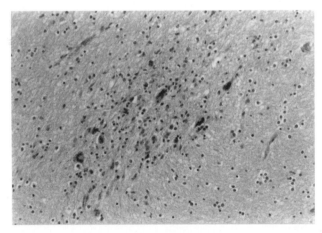

FIG. 2. HIV dementia. Photomicrograph showing a microglial nodule with multinucleated giant cells within the centrum semiovale. Hematoxylin-eosin, original magnification x25. (From Simpson D, Tagliati M. Neurologic manifestations of HIV infection. *Ann Intern Med* 1994;121:772, with permission.)

does not strongly correlate with either the degree of histopathology or the clinical severity of dementia (33). Similarly, there is a poor correlation of quantitative measurement, by PCR, of HIV-1 DNA in the fixed brain and HIV-1 RNA in cerebrospinal fluid (CSF) with clinical staging of HIVE (34–36). An annual prospective analysis showed a trend of rising CSF HIV-RNA levels in those patients who developed incident dementia (37). This suggests possible mechanisms of neuronal dysfunction that are secondarily related to the effects of HIV-infected macrophage infiltration. There may be multiple mechanisms including gp120, an HIV envelope glycoprotein, mediated glutamate excitotoxicity (38–40), increased release of cytokines, predominantly tumor necrosis factor alpha (TNF-α) (41–43), quinolinate (44), and eicosanoids (45). These hypotheses are supported by a series of studies showing correlation of neurologic deterioration with CSF levels of β_2-microglobulin (46,47), neopterin (48), and quinolinate (49). In addition, levels of intracerebral TNF-α and interleukin (IL)-1β mRNA measured by reverse transcriptase PCR correlate proportionally and inversely, respectively, with the presence of dementia (41).

Differential Diagnosis

Parkinsonism in AIDS may be precipitated by the use of neuroleptics, to which AIDS patients are particularly sensitive, especially with HIVE (50). It is important to consider the diagnosis of cytomegalovirus (CMV) encephalitis in patients with HIVE, because the clinical features may be very similar. Those that favor CMV encephalitis include rapid onset and progression; brainstem and cerebellar signs; evidence of systemic CMV disease, including retinitis and adrenalitis with signs of hypoadrenalism; and suggestive radiologic features such as periventricular or ependymal enhancement (51). The CSF in CMV encephalitis often contains an elevated protein content, with polymorphonuclear pleocytosis and hypoglcorrhachia, but it is most often nondiagnostic (51,52). However, PCR analysis for CMV DNA has a sensitivity of more than 80% and a specificity of more than 98% and is the diagnostic test of choice in the CSF (53,54). Neurosyphilis and cryptococcal meningitis should be routinely excluded by measurement of CSF Venereal Disease Research Laboratory (VDRL) test and cryptococcal latex antigen in AIDS patients with CNS dysfunction.

Figures 3 and 4 show the radiologic and pathologic typical of CMV encephalitis. The diagnosis of PML is considered in the radiologic diagnoses of HIV leukoencephalopathy. It can have a rapid onset and progression of focal signs such as hemiparesis, cerebellar and brainstem abnormalities, aphasia, visual field deficits, hemisensory deficits, and rarely focal extrapyramidal signs (55–57). Rarely, PML may present with nonfocal encephalopathy,

similar to HIV-associated dementia. The white matter abnormalities in PML are more focal, involve subcortical U-fibers, and can rarely show minor enhancement (58). These clinical and radiologic parameters assist in the differential diagnosis. Figures 5 and 6 show pathologic and MRI abnormalities observed in PML. However, as with all neurologic complications of HIV, multiple conditions may overlap in the same patient. The diagnostic approach to PML is discussed in more detail later.

Treatment

Zidovudine (AZT) in doses of 1,000 mg or more is the recommended treatment for HIV-associated dementia (59). There is also evidence of efficacy at doses of 600 mg (60); at this dose, there is a lower incidence of pathologic HIV encephalitis at autopsy (61). Penetration of AZT into the CSF has been shown to be independent of dose and may explain this possible efficacy at lower doses (62). The effects of new generation antiretroviral agents, including the protease inhibitors, are unknown. The currently available protease inhibitors Saquinavir, Ritonavir, and Norvir have poor CNS penetration. Despite this, the standard management of HIV dementia currently includes high-dose AZT; an additional nucleoside analogue inhibitor such as dideoxyinosine (ddI), dideoxycytidine (ddC), or stavudine (d4T); and a protease inhibitor.

Current experimental approaches have led to therapies that inhibit the indirect toxic effects of HIV-infected macrophages. A placebo-controlled trial of nimodipine, the AIDS Clinical Trials Group (ACTG) protocol 162, to inhibit calcium mediated excitotoxicity revealed trends in neuropsychological improvement that did not reach statistical significance (62a). A novel nucleoside analogue inhibitor, 1592 U89, which has good CNS penetration, is also under trial, as are NMDA glutamate receptor antagonists, including Memantine (63), and TNF-α inhibitors such as thalidomide and pentoxifylline.

Human Immunodeficiency Virus-related Cerebellar Disease

Cerebellar involvement is not a recognized sign of HIVE (16,18) and usually suggests a secondary or opportunistic cause. AIDS-related causes of cerebellar disease include PML (64,65) and CMV infection (66–68). Both can also be associated with brainstem signs and oculomotor disturbances. MRI shows diffuse white matter disease in those with HIVE, usually without enhancement, whereas those associated with opportunistic infection show meningeal, cortical, and ependymal enhancement (66,67). A rare cause of an acute pancerebellar syndrome in the drug-abusing population is a severe leukoencephalopathy caused by inhaled heroin, or "chasing the dragon" (69). It is a devastating white matter disorder of

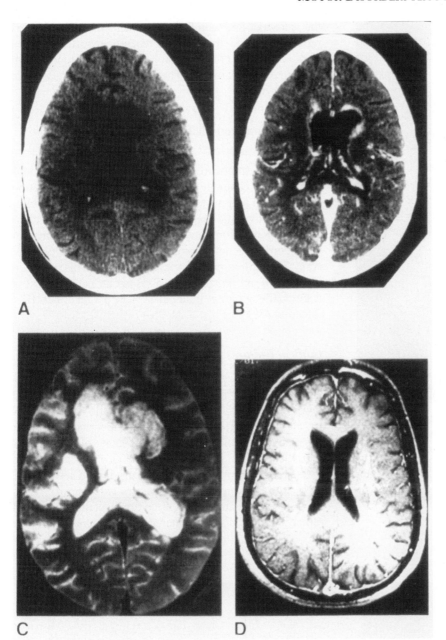

FIG. 3. Biopsy-proven cytomegalovirus encephalitis in advanced AIDS. **A:** Computed tomography (CT) and periventricular hypointensity. **B:** CT with contrast shows periventricular enhancement extending beyond the periventricular region. **C:** T2-weighted magnetic resonance image (MRI) shows periventricular hyperintensity with a right parenchymal lesion. **D:** Contrast-enhanced MRI in another patient with AIDS shows meningeal enhancement. (From Holland NR, Powers C, Matthews VP, et al. Cytomegalovirus encephalitis in AIDS. *Neurology* 1994;44:512, with permission.)

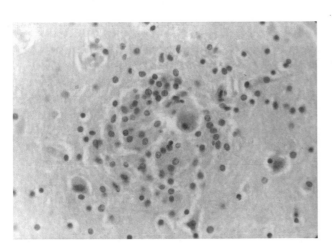

FIG. 4. Cytomegalovirus encephalitis. High power photomicrograph showing a microglial nodule with associated CMV inclusion. Hematoxylin and eosin, original magnification x250. (From Simpson D, Tagliati M. Neurologic manifestations of HIV infection. *Ann Intern Med* 1994;121:777, with permission.)

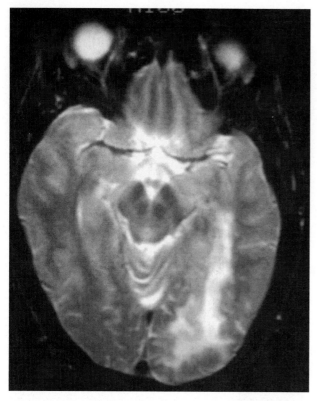

FIG. 5. Biopsy-proven progressive multifocal leukoencephalopathy. T2-weighted magnetic resonance scan shows a large confluent area of increased signal within the white matter of the right cerebral hemisphere. (From Simpson D, Tagliati M. Neurologic manifestations of HIV infection. *Ann Intern Med* 1994;121:776, with permission.)

the cerebral and cerebellar hemispheres that appears monophasic and irreversible, recently reported in New York (70), Oslo (71), as well as the original report from 1982 in Amsterdam (69). The contaminating causal agent is unknown.

Human Immunodeficiency Virus-associated Myelopathy

The most frequently encountered spinal cord pathology in AIDS is slowly progressive vacuolar degeneration of the lateral and posterior white matter tracts, with clinical and pathologic features similar to the subacute combined degeneration caused by B$_{12}$ deficiency. The thoracic cord is generally more affected than the cervical cord. This clinicopathologic entity, known as vacuolar myelopathy, presents in 20 to 55% of cases at autopsy but is clinically apparent in about 27% of patients with HIV infection (72).

Clinical Features and Diagnosis

The clinical features of vacuolar myelopathy are progressive spastic paraparesis, with prominent proximal lower limb weakness, frequent sensory and spinocerebellar ataxia, erectile dysfunction, and detrusor sphincter dyssynergia (72). Vacuolar myelopathy often coexists with distal sensory polyneuropathy (DSP) because ankle jerks are absent with stocking sensory loss, whereas knee jerks are brisk and plantar responses extensor (72). This does not necessarily imply a common pathogenesis but rather that both disorders increase in frequency with pro-

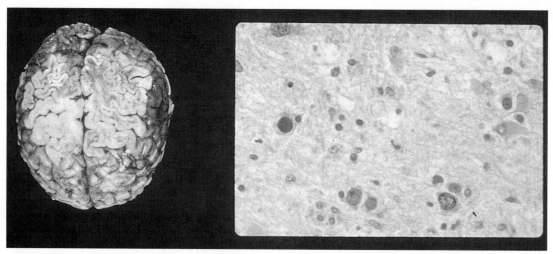

FIG. 6. Progressive multifocal leukoencephalopathy (PML) showing confluent demyelinated foci in the left hemisphere on ultrastructural horizontal sections and a histopathologic photomicrograph of the same lesion containing atypical astrocytes and oligodendroglia with intranuclear inclusions characteristic of JC virus, the etiologic agent of PML. (From Hair LS, Symmans F, Powers JM, et al. Progressive multifocal leukoencephalopathy in patients with human immunodeficiency virus. *Hum Pathol* 1992;23:663–667, with permission.)

gressive immune suppression. Features against the diagnosis of vacuolar myelopathy are acute onset, spinal sensory level, and evidence of focal cord involvement such as a Brown-Sequard syndrome (72), suggesting instead a secondary intra- or extramedullary opportunistic infection or neoplasm. Spinal MRI excludes structural spinal lesions. MRI findings in vacuolar myelopathy are usually normal or show nonspecific atrophy with subtle T2 posterolateral white matter hyperintensities (73,74). Peroneal and posterior tibial somatosensory evoked potentials show prolonged central conduction time (75). Additional use of popliteal fossa stimulation recordings help to differentiate peripheral from central conduction slowing (75). There is conflicting evidence for subclinical myelopathy by somatosensory evoked potential analysis in asymptomatic HIV-infected patients with CD4+ cell counts less than 200/mm^3 (76,77). Routine CSF analysis at this stage of infection is usually normal or shows mild abnormalities (72,78,79).

Pathology

This consists of early macrophage infiltration followed by increasing demyelination and vacuolation of the posterolateral white matter tracts of the thoracic cord (72,80–82). There is little or no axonal degeneration (80). Clinical severity correlates closely with the degree of pathologic involvement (72). A typical autopsy spinal cord specimen is shown in Fig. 7.

Pathophysiology

There is no evidence of direct HIV infection of the cord in vacuolar myelopathy (72,80,81). HIV-infected macrophages are present in the gray matter of the cord in the typical form of multinucleated giant cells and microglial nodules. They have not been demonstrated in the regions of vacuolar change (81,83–85). HIV myelitis affects the spinal cord gray matter (81). Vacuolar myelopathy does not correlate clinically with HIVE (72). Because vacuolar myelopathy does not seem to result from primary HIV infection, there have been alternative explanations for its development. Tyor et al. (82) found large numbers of major histocompatibilty (MHC) class I and II macrophages expressing TNF-α and IL-1 in regions of vacuolation. As with HIVE, there was also an increased level of neopterin, β2-microglobulin, and TNF-α in the CSF (82). The authors suggest a unifying hypothesis of HIV neuropathogenesis that is explained by cytokine-induced injury to neurons, oligodendrocytes, and Schwann cells by infiltrating HIV-infected macrophages, the so-called Trojan horses of HIV infection (86).

Other authors have proposed a metabolic theory on the basis of the underlying pathology, one that is similar to that of vitamin B$_{12}$ deficiency. Such deficiency was demonstrated in one study of AIDS patients with vacuolar myelopathy and neuropathy (87), although others have not confirmed this finding. Altered methionine metabolism as measured by a reduced serum and CSF S-adenosylmethionine/S-adenosylhomocysteine ratio was shown in two studies of HIV-infected patients with a range of central neurologic complications (88,89). S-adenosylmethionine deficiency leads to impaired transmethylation reactions and glutathione generation in the CNS. Hereditary disorders of methionine metabolism and nitrous oxide poisoning both lead to these metabolic abnormalities and cause vacuolar myelopathy (90,91). The pathogenesis of AIDS myelopathy may involve persistent immune activation in the CNS, leading to significant local production of cytokines, toxins, or oxygen radicals that cause membrane and myelin damage in the setting of secondary methyl group deficiency (80). There is no currently available treatment for vacuolar myelopathy, and antiretroviral agents do not appear to benefit, although controlled studies have not been done. Trials are underway using methionine or S-adenosylmethionine replacement in AIDS vacuolar myelopathy.

Differential Diagnosis

The presence of a sensory level, cervical cord involvement, and acute onset (72) suggests an alternative secondary cause, including primary CNS lymphoma (92), varicella zoster virus, CMV and herpes simplex virus transverse myelitis (93–97), neurosyphilis (98), abscess due to toxoplasma (99), mycobacterium tuberculosis (100,101), and aspergillus (102). Herpes zoster myelitis may occur without a rash (103). Contrast-enhanced MRI and CSF examination, including PCR for herpes viruses, are required to exclude these lesions.

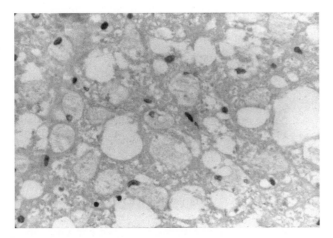

FIG. 7. Vacuolar myelopathy in AIDS. High power photomicrograph from the white matter of the spinal cord, showing large vacuoles. Macrophages are evident within the vacuoles. Hematoxylin-eosin, original magnification x250. (From Simpson D, Tagliati M. Neurologic manifestations of HIV infection. *Ann Intern Med* 1994;121:777, with permission.)

Coinfection with human T-cell lymphotropic viruses (HTLV) types I and II is being increasingly demonstrated in HIV-infected patients with and without myelopathy. Coinfection with HTLV-I dramatically increased the risk of myelopathy in HIV infection from 16 to 73% in a prospective case-control Brazilian study (104,110). HTLV-II is most commonly found in American Indians and intravenous drug users (105). The prevalence of myelopathy in a cohort of HTLV-I– and HTLV-II–infected potential blood donors was 2.4 and 0.25%, respectively (106). HTLV-II has now been well described as a cause of myelopathy (107). HTLV-II seropositivity was demonstrated in 25% of HIV-positive intravenous drug users in northern Manhattan and was associated with excess neurologic morbidity rather than specific myelopathy (108). The relation between these viruses and HIV with regard to neuropathogenesis is unknown. Serum HTLV-I and -II antibodies should be checked in HIV-infected patients with myelopathy.

FOCAL CENTRAL NERVOUS SYSTEM DISORDERS

Focal motor disorders, including hemiparesis, hemi-ataxia, dysmetria, rigidity, cogwheeling, chorea, and hemiballismus, suggest a focal infiltrating or mass lesion caused by an opportunistic infection or neoplasm. The differential diagnoses include protozoal, bacterial, or fungal abscesses; tumor; PML; cerebral infarct; CMV; herpes zoster virus or herpes simplex virus encephalitis; further separable by the presence or absence of mass effect and contrast enhancement on neuroimaging studies. Although toxoplasma encephalitis and primary CNS lymphoma are the most common causes of contrast enhancement on brain neuroimaging studies, PML is the most likely explanation when the lesions do not enhance. These disorders are discussed first, and the rarer causes of focal brain lesions in AIDS are described later.

Lesions with Mass Effect and Contrast Enhancement

Toxoplasma Encephalitis and Primary Central Nervous System Lymphoma

The most common cause of acute hemiparesis in AIDS is toxoplasma encephalitis; it is also the most frequent CNS mass lesion in patients with AIDS (2,6). Nearly 70% of patients present with hemiparesis and other focal signs such as ataxia, cranial nerve palsies, and secondary generalized seizures (67,109); however, nonfocal signs of headache, fever, confusion, and lethargy are almost equally as common. Toxoplasma mass lesions of the basal ganglia can produce hemidystonia (111), hemichorea (112), and unilateral akathisia (113).

The incidence of toxoplasma encephalitis is expected to fall with increasing use of sulfamethoxazole-trimethoprim prophylaxis (114–116). However, primary CNS lymphoma is increasing in incidence and may supersede toxoplasma as the most common cause of a focal brain lesion in AIDS (12). The two conditions cannot be easily distinguished clinically or radiologically; both cause single or multifocal enhancing mass lesions (117–119). However, fever, headache, seizures, and acute strokelike presentation are more common with toxoplasma encephalitis (120). Toxoplasma predilicts the basal ganglia and corticomedullary junction, whereas primary CNS lymphoma is most commonly seen in the periventricular regions and corpus callosum (11,118,119). Thallium-201 single-photon emission computed tomography of the brain demonstrates increased uptake with tumor but not infection. The demonstration of increased uptake was 100% sensitive and specific for CNS lymphoma when first reported (121), but lesions less than 6 to 8 mm often go undetected (122). Positron emission tomography and MR spectroscopy are useful in distinguishing these lesions. In patients with single or multiple focal enhancing brain lesions, empiric therapy with pyrimethamine and sulfadiazine is recommended if the patient is seropositive for toxoplasma IgG. Brain biopsy should be performed if improvement is not seen after 2 weeks of therapy because 91% of toxoplasma cases will then show clinical and radiologic improvement (109). This approach has been hampered by a 40% rate of allergic reactions, including the Stevens-Johnson syndrome and pancytopenia (122).

Toxoplasma-seronegative patients should undergo early biopsy (123). In two recent studies of AIDS patients with focal brain lesions (120,124), the use of routine antiprotozoal prophylaxis with sulfamethoxazole-trimethoprim significantly reduced the probability of toxoplasma encephalitis in seropositive patients from 0.78 to 0.59 (124). A negative patient has a diagnostic probability of 0.06 for toxoplasma encephalitis, making this diagnosis very unlikely (124). PCR for Epstein-Barr virus (EBV) DNA in the CSF has a sensitivity and specificity for primary CNS lymphoma that approaches 100% (53,54,125). Use of this test has been proposed in those patients on prophylaxis, provided lumbar puncture is determined to be safe, although it is still under research and not routinely available or standard clinical practice (124). A positive result should lead to early brain biopsy and antimicrobial therapy. It has been suggested that a positive thallium single-photon emission computed tomography and CSF PCR for EBV DNA replace the need for a brain biopsy and specific tissue diagnosis (124). The PCR test for toxoplasma DNA in the CSF has a similar specificity to that for EBV but a sensitivity of 50% (54,124). CSF for EBV DNA PCR may be very useful in a seronegative patient with a focal brain lesion. If lumbar puncture is contraindicated or unavailable, then a brain biopsy is necessary, which has a diagnostic sensitivity of 93 to 95% but a mortality of 1 to 2% and a morbidity of 4 to 12% due to hemorrhage (124,126–128). Steroids are recommended in patients with lesions that show significant mass effect on neuroimaging studies.

Toxoplasma encephalitis is treated with 50 to 75 mg of pyrimethamine, 4 to 6 g of sulfadiazine, and 10 to 20 mg of folinic acid daily for 3 to 6 weeks, and a clinical and radiologic response is seen in 68 to 95% of patients respectively (109,110,129). However, treatment has been complicated by a high rate of allergic reactions, an early mortality of up to 20% (130,131), residual neurologic deficits (132), inactivity against the tissue cyst, and unpredictable pharmacokinetics of pyrimethamine, usually prompt a loading dose of 100 to 200 mg (133). Sulfonamide-intolerant patients can be treated with the alternative regimen of clindamycin, pyrimethamine, and folinic acid, which has comparable efficacy (109,134), where pseudomembraneous colitis and neutropenia are the most important side effects. Atovaquone, azithromycin, and clarithromycin are alternatives (135,136). The standard treatment of primary CNS lymphoma is 3,000 to 4,000 cGy of whole brain radiation for 2 to 3 weeks, which improves survival from 1 to 4 months (137). A recent study showed no difference in outcome between empiric radiotherapy without biopsy compared with that preceded by stereotactic biopsy (138). The response rate of 77%, with a median survival of 42.5 months in the non-AIDS population with systemic and intrathecal methotrexate followed by combined radiotherapy and intravenous cytosine arabinoside (139), has been limited in patients with AIDS by disease-related mortality (140).

Focal Cerebral Lesion in Acquired Immunodeficiency Syndrome Without Mass Effect or Contrast Enhancement on Brain Neuroimaging Studies

When neuroimaging studies show a focal lesion without mass effect or ring enhancement, the most likely diagnosis is PML and the less likely diagnosis primary CNS lymphoma, with calculated probabilities of 0.6 and 0.12, respectively (124). The lesions in PML are usually multifocal and bilateral but may initially be single and unilateral (141). They are usually subcortical and restricted to the white matter of the supratentorial and infratentorial structures. Although the gray matter may be involved microscopically, the spinal cord is rarely involved. The frequency of enhancement on neuroimaging studies is less than 5% and faint and peripheral, if at all (141). The clinical and radiologic features of PML and its differentiation from primary HIV leukoencephalopathy has been described. In 80 to 90% of adults affected with PML, the proximate cause is believed to be a reactivation of latent JC virus infection (142). Cellular immunodeficiency results in productive infection of oligodendrocytes with hyperchromatic nuclear enlargement, bizarrely enlarged astrocytes, and extensive demyelination. JC virus can be demonstrated by electron microscopy, immunohistochemistry, and in situ hybridization PCR in oligodendrocytic nuclei. The diagnosis of PML has been altered by the use of PCR for JC viral DNA in CSF and has reduced the need for brain biopsy. The finding of JC viral DNA in CSF is almost 100% specific for PML, especially with the appropriate radiologic and clinical presentation (53,54,143). Its sensitivity of 70 to 80% is inferior to brain biopsy (124), but the latter is still the gold standard for the diagnosis of PML, especially with in situ hybridization PCR techniques.

Treatment of Progressive Multifocal Leukoencephalopathy

Intravenous and intraventricular cytarabine (ARA-C) had early reported success in uncontrolled series of patients with AIDS-associated PML (144,145,146); however, a recently completed randomized controlled therapeutic trial failed to show efficacy (146a). The prognosis of PML is generally poor with a mean survival of 4 months (147). The outcome of PML with newer generation combination antiretroviral therapies with protease inhibitors and nucleoside analogues is still unknown. It is possible that these drugs may improve the natural course of PML because the downregulation of HIV *tat* protein by these therapies decreases the transactivation of JC virus (148). Future therapeutic trials should take into account the case reports of unexplained spontaneous regression (149) and a survival beyond 1 year in 7% of cases so studied (150). However, these patients did not have cerebellar or brainstem involvement, frequently exhibited faint enhancement on MRI, and had inflammatory infiltrates in brain biopsy tissues.

Other Causes of Focal Cerebral Lesions in Acquired Immunodeficiency Virus

These include cerebral infarction; cryptococcus; tuberculoma; syphilitic gumma; metastatic systemic non-Hodgkin's lymphoma and Kaposi's sarcoma; CMV, varicella zoster virus, and herpes simplex virus; viral encephalitis; and abscess due to nocardia, candida, aspergillus, and histoplasma infection.

Cerebral Infarction

It is unclear if HIV itself is a stroke risk factor beyond that caused by cocaine, meningovascular syphilis (151,152), intravenous drug use, and endocarditis (153). In one review, cerebral infarction was explained by the comorbid factors of nonbacterial thrombotic (merantic) endocarditis; vasculitis due to concomitant herpes zoster virus, mycobacterium tuberculosis, and cryptococcus; thrombocytopenic hemorrhage; and hemorrhage into an abscess or tumor (153). HIV is also associated with antiphospholipid antibodies, although these are usually of the nonpathogenic IgM variety (154).

Recently, their role as a putative stroke risk factor has been questioned by the lack of association with an increased of stroke recurrence (155). Vasculitic cerebral infarction can be a complication of ipsilateral oph-thalmic herpes zoster virus infection (93).

Cryptococcoma

These are dilated perivascular spaces filled with viable cryptococci, a granulomatous reaction, and gelatinous material usually found in the basal ganglia (156). They usually do not enhance on neuroimaging studies and only cause mild mass effect. Smaller multiple cortical enhancing nodules can also occur (157), but neither are usually associated with focal symptoms or signs (156,157).

Tuberculoma and Tuberculous Meningitis

Tuberculomas are focal granulomatous abscesses due to hematogenous dissemination or local spread of tuberculosis from the subarachnoid space. They can occur with or without meningeal involvement and are seen in some patients with tuberculous meningitis (159). They occur at the corticomedullary junction but may be multiple in up to 34% of patients (160) and are more common in the supratentorial fossa (161). The resulting lesions ring enhance on neuroimaging studies with a central area of calcification, giving rise to the target sign (162). Full resolution of a cerebral tuberculoma requires months to years of antituberculous therapy and is most related to its size (160). Expansion of the mass can occur with initial treatment and may be accompanied by neurologic deterioration (163), which when present can sometimes be treated with adjunctive corticosteroids. Tuberculous meningitis in AIDS is associated with more frequent cerebral infarction and parenchymal tuberculomata (164). The former occur in 27% of HIV-infected patients and in 6% of uninfected cases (164). Diagnosis is aided in the HIV-infected population by a higher rate of a positive CSF culture detected in 50 to 64% of affected patients with HIV infection and in 10 to 30% of immunocompetent patients (165). This yield can be increased to a reported sensitivity of 48 to 100% and a specificity of greater than 94% (166) by PCR analysis in the CSF for mycobacterium tuberculosis DNA.

Syphilitic Gumma

Neurosyphilis may be complicated by localized granulomatous mass formation termed gumma (165). They are ring enhancing and can be associated with significant mass effect (168). Meningovascular syphilis typically presents with multifocal cerebral infarction (167). A positive serum VDRL or fluorescent treponemal antibody absorption test suggests the diagnosis, which is then confirmed by a positive CSF VDRL. However, the sensitivity of CSF-VDRL is only 30 to 70% (169), and the speci-ficity is altered by potential contamination of the CSF with blood. Thus, most authors recommend treating for neurosyphilis if the CSF shows an elevated protein content or pleocytosis, even with a negative VDRL (170). Absence of the CSF fluorescent treponemal antibody absorption may be used to exclude the diagnosis of neurosyphilis (170). It is treated with 12 to 14 million units of aequous penicillin G daily for 10 days (170). The goal is a negative serum and CSF VDRL, although some HIV-infected patients have a low positive titer after treatment.

Nocardia Asteroides

This opportunistic bacterial infection is increasingly more common in patients with AIDS and intravenous drug use (171). Pulmonary involvement, the most common presentation, is seen in 81% of patients (172). The next most frequent site of involvement is the CNS due to meningitis and secondary abscesses as a result of hematogenous spread from the lungs (173), although frank pulmonary involvement may be absent in up to 5% of cases (174). Nocardia abscesses present as ring-enhancing mass lesions on neuroimaging studies and may be multiple and multiloculated (175). The clinical presentation of nocardia is similar to toxoplasma encephalitis, although the presence of a cavitary lung infiltrate suggests the diagnosis (175). The 80% mortality rate may be partially explained by the 2- to 4-week period required for culture. It is treated with trimethoprim-sulfamethoxazole for a minimum of 6 months (175). Other focal cortical and subcortical enhancing mass lesions can be due to concomitant CMV (158), herpes zoster virus infection (98), and cerebral metastases from systemic non-Hodgkin's lymphoma and Kaposi's sarcoma (6,176).

PERIPHERAL NERVOUS SYSTEM MANIFESTATIONS

Peripheral Neuropathy

The clinically significant forms of neuropathy associated with HIV infection include DSP, mononeuritis multiplex, cranial neuropathy, and acute or chronic inflammatory demyelinating polyneuropathy, or Guillain-Barré syndrome and chronic inflammatory demyelinating polyneuropathy, respectively.

Distal Sensory Polyneuropathy

DSP occurs in the late immune-suppressed stages of HIV infection and is the most common neurologic complication of AIDS, present in 30% or more of patients after other causes of neuropathy have been excluded (10,185,204). The frequency of DSP increases with advancing immunosuppression, as reflected by falling CD4+ counts (205,206). Autopsy reveals pathologic evidence of DSP in nearly all patients with AIDS (207).

Clinical and Electrodiagnostic Features

The clinical features of DSP are symmetric distal numbness, paresthesias, and dysesthesias beginning in the legs, with later progression to the arms. Weakness is mild and generally confined to ankle dorsiflexor and evertor and intrinsic foot muscles (204,205,207,209). Neurologic examination reveals hypoactive or absent ankle reflexes with relative sparing of knee reflexes. The sensory deficit involves pinprick, temperature, and vibration in a stocking-and-glove pattern. Electrodiagnostic studies are generally consistent with a symmetric sensorimotor axonal polyneuropathy. The sural sensory nerve action potential is small or unobtainable and needle electromyography (EMG) generally shows mild to moderate changes and chronic denervation in distal muscles (206,210).

Pathophysiology

The electrophysiologic findings do not support the hypothesis that DSP is a dorsal root ganglionitis caused by CMV infection (209,211) or the excitotoxic effect of the HIV protein gp120 on sensory neurons (212). In addition, dorsal root ganglia show equal degrees of infiltration by macrophages and T cells in patients with and without DSP (213). There is evidence that the primary pathology in DSP is at the level of peripheral nerve rather than a dying back neuropathy from a ganglionitis or amyotrophic process. Nerve biopsies in two series have shown endoneurial infiltration by HIV-infected macrophages (213,214), and increased TNF-α mRNA levels have been demonstrated in peripheral nerve of patients with DSP when compared with those without DSP and in HIV-negative patients with axonal polyneuropathy (215). Consequently, DSP is similar to vacuolar myelopathy and HIV encephalopathy and may be another neurologic manifestation of the effects of infiltrating activated HIV-infected macrophages (86).

Differential Diagnosis

Several factors can contribute to the development of DSP in patients with AIDS, including diabetes, alcohol, thiamine, pyridoxine and B$_{12}$ deficiency, isoniazid, and, most frequently, the antiretroviral nucleoside analogue agents ddI, ddC, and d4T. Patients with underlying neuropathy from HIV-associated DSP and other causes of neuropathy have increased frequency of complications from nucleoside analogue therapy (218). They display an axonal polyneuropathy after 2 to 6 months of treatment that is clinically and electrophysiologically similar to HIV-associated DSP (216,217). The neurotoxic effects are dose dependent and are generally reversible on discontinuation of the drug (216,217). Clinical recovery occurs within 2 to 3 months after discontinuation but may be preceded by several weeks of intensified symptoms, termed the "coasting period" (216,217). Thus, discontinuation of the drug is the only useful means of differentiating this toxic neuropathy from DSP. However, some patients may tolerate rechallenge with lower doses of the antiretroviral agents.

Pathophysiology of Nucleoside Analogue-Induced Toxic Neuropathy

The mechanism for the toxic neuropathy complicating these therapies is unknown, but Famularo et al. (219) described several patients with a neuropathy that developed after treatment with ddI, ddC, and d4T and lower serum levels of acetyl-carnitine compared with those on ddI and AZT without neuropathy. The reduced levels of acetyl-carnitine may reflect drug-induced inhibition of mitochondrial τ-DNA polymerase (220), resulting in impaired transport of free fatty acids across the mitochondrial membrane and subsequent β-oxidation. It is unclear why AZT, a nucleoside analogue with similar effects on DNA polymerase, does not cause neuropathy (216). The drug is not associated with an increased risk of neuropathy in patients with CD4 counts of less than 200/mm^3 (221) and an otherwise high prevalence of neuropathy without treatment, so that a significant association with AZT therapy is not apparent.

Treatment of Distal Sensory Polyneuropathy

The primary treatment of DSP is symptomatic and includes analgesics, tricyclic antidepressants, anticonvulsants, mexilitine, and topical capsaicin (222); however, none have been effective in controlled studies. ACTG 242 was recently compared with amitriptyline and mexilitine, and both showed no more effectiveness than placebo (personal communication). Intranasal peptide-T appears to inhibit the excitotoxicity of gp120 on neurons in vitro (223) but was ineffective in a controlled trial (224). A large placebo-controlled study of subcutaneous recombinant human nerve growth factor, ACTG 291, is ongoing. The effect of the protease inhibitors and other novel antiretroviral agents on DSP is unknown.

Mononeuritis Multiplex

Mononeuritis multiplex presents with acute painful asymmetric sensorimotor deficits in the distribution of individual peripheral and cranial nerves (190,208,209, 225), often in association with fever, weight loss, and lymphadenopathy (225). Electrophysiologic studies show evidence of an asymmetric sensorimotor axonopathy neuropathy with frequent overlying symmetric DSP (208,225,228). Patients with CD4+/cell counts less than 100 cells/mm^3 can have evidence of systemic or intraneural invasion of CMV (228,229). Roullet et al. (228) described 15 patients with mononeuritis multiplex due to CMV infection present in nerve biopsy alone, in 2 by CSF culture, and inferred by clinical improvement, often ganciclovir, in the remaining 11 patients (228). Thirteen of 14 patients so studied had a positive CSF PCR analysis for CMV DNA. Nerve and muscle biopsies were performed in seven cases: three showed mild neurogenic atrophy and decreased numbers of myelinated fibers and two had perivascular polymorphonuclear inflammatory cell infiltrates with endoneurial cytomegalic cells characteristic of CMV. Of the remaining two, one had mixed perivascular infiltrates without cytomegalic cells and the other had necrotizing arteritis. The treatment response in their patients was short lived and most were prone to relapse, similar to CMV polyradiculitis. It is still unclear how specific CSF PCR analysis for CMV DNA is in this disease and whether serum PCR studies are more reliable.

Primary vasculitic neuropathy occurs in patients with early HIV disease, presumably due to immune-complex deposition similar to that caused by hepatitis B and C virus (192–195). The clinical presentation is generally asymmetric (193) but is occasionally symmetric late in the disease when distal lesions overlap and become confluent (196). Bradley and Verma (192) described two patients with a predominantly sensory neuropathy that improved with corticosteroids, and other cases had associated cryoglobulinemia (197). Neuropathy may be the singular presentation of vasculitis (193), although it is more commonly associated with an elevated erythrocyte sedimentation rate and other findings of polyarteritis nodosa (194). In both, nerve biopsy reveals necrotizing arteritis with intimal thickening and vascular stenosis or occlusion of epineurial vessels. Productive HIV infection was demonstrated in the perivascular inflammatory infiltrate of vascular endothelium in two cases (196). Steroid therapy has been associated with clinical improvement in many patients (192,227). There are rare cases of vasculitic neuropathy in patients with AIDS and advanced stages of immune suppression but not due to CMV infection (196,198).

Inflammatory Demyelinating Polyneuropathy

This is the least common form of peripheral neuropathy overall; it occurs early in the course of HIV infection, in the absence of frank immune suppression (186). The clinical presentation can be as Guillain-Barré syndrome or as chronic inflammatory demyelinating polyneuropathy, similar to the illness of uninfected patients. The presenting clinical features include generalized weakness, areflexia, and minor sensory loss. The diagnosis of HIV is suggested by the presence of minor CSF pleocytosis and a protein content greater than 100 mg/dL (186). In one series, the mean white blood cell count was 14 cells/mm³ as opposed to 1 cell/mm³ in patients without HIV-1 infection (187). Cranial neuropathies can occur, especially of the facial and trigeminal nerves (186,188). Nerve biopsy reveals macrophage-mediated demyelination and intense inflammatory cell infiltrates that do not stain for HIV RNA by in situ hybridization (186). Nerve conduction studies fulfill

criteria for demyelination (189). The prognosis of inflammatory demyelinating polyneuropathy in HIV infection, as reported in small series, is similar to patients without HIV infection. Treatment generally includes prednisone, plasma exchange, and intravenous immunoglobulin alone or in combination (186,190,191).

Cranial Neuropathy

Cranial involvement is frequent in HIV infection alone and with AIDS. In immunocompetent patients with high CD4+/cell counts, cranial neuropathies are often self-limited and resolve spontaneously. They presumably arise by immune mechanisms. Isolated cranial neuropathy, particularly of the facial nerve, may be the presenting manifestation of HIV infection. Facial nerve palsy in HIV-infected patients is indistinguishable clinically from Bell's palsy, although there is frequently CSF pleocytosis (199–201). The prognosis for facial motor recovery is excellent (202,203). It is prudent to check HIV status in patients with facial palsy, when factors or atypical features suggest immunodeficiency. Cranial neuropathies in AIDS are most commonly caused by cryptococcal, tuberculous, syphilitic meningitis, and leptomeningeal lymphoma (202). The facial nerve is the most commonly affected, followed by the abducens, oculomotor, hypoglossal, trigeminal, vestibulocochlear, optic, trochlear, glossopharyngeal, and vagal nerves (202). Hoarseness due to recurrent laryngeal nerve involvement has been reported (226). Intraaxial causes of cranial neuropathy in AIDS occur in association with PML, primary CNS lymphoma, brainstem infarction, and CMV encephalitis. Detailed MRI with contrast and repeated lumbar punctures are generally necessary to elucidate the proximate cause and exact diagnosis, especially in leptomeningeal lymphoma (230).

Polyradiculopathy

Clinical Features

Progressive polyradiculopathy is a well-described complication of AIDS. It presents with complaints of acute or subacute leg pain, paresthesia, weakness, and urinary retention (177–179). Associated flaccid leg weakness, areflexia, and sphincter incontinence may be mistaken for the cauda equina syndrome.

Laboratory Investigations

Electrophysiologic studies show evidence of acute axonopathy with unelicitable sensory nerve action potentials consistent with a predominant presentation in most cases (185). Contrast MRI of the lumbosacral spine may show enhanced clumped roots but may also be normal (178,179). The CSF in CMV-infected cases typically shows a polymorphonuclear pleocytosis, reduced glucose content, and raised protein content, although these typical features are more often absent (179) and should not be used as strict criteria in decisions to commence ganciclovir or foscarnet therapy. Culture for CMV is positive in up to 50% of cases (178,179). Previous or current systemic CMV disease, especially retinitis, supports an association with active infection. The study of choice is the demonstration of CMV-DNA in CSF by PCR, which has a sensitivity and specificity of about 100% in this disease (57,58,172).

Differential Diagnosis

The predominance of mononuclear CSF pleocytosis and a subacute presentation suggests an associated lymphoma, which usually implies a mean survival of 5 weeks or less and an association with cranial neuropathy (184). One series described four patients with a predominantly mononuclear cell pleocytosis who spontaneously recovered (178), although similar findings have not been reported in other series. Neurosyphilis is another cause of progressive polyradiculopathy (180).

Treatment

Ganciclovir or foscarnet therapy should be started early for this clinical syndrome while awaiting the CSF PCR result for CMV-DNA. Delay in treatment can result in irreversible axonal degeneration and a lack of subsequent response to treatment. There have been no controlled studies of antiviral therapy in CMV polyradiculopathy, although case reports have indicated a good outcome with early treatment. Occasional patients can relapse without maintenance treatment (179,181), and some may also develop viral resistance (182). A prospective study of ganciclovir and foscarnet alone and in combination using CSF PCR CMV-DNA to monitor the response is currently underway; similar laboratory monitoring was described in a small series of patients with CMV encephalitis (183).

Myopathy

The several syndromes of muscle involvement in HIV-infected patients include primary myopathy, a wasting syndrome, AZT-associated myopathy, and myopathy due to opportunistic infection (231,232) or neoplastic infiltration (233).

Primary Human Immunodeficiency Virus-associated Myopathy

Clinical Features

HIV-associated myopathy resembles sporadic polymyositis in uninfected patients (234) and shares similar clinical and laboratory criteria for diagnosis: progressive proximal weakness, elevation of the serum creatine kinase

(CK) level, a myopathic EMG, and supportive muscle biopsy (235). All four features make the diagnosis definite, whereas three make it probable. If two features are present and a biopsy is not performed, then the diagnosis is possible (236). The disorder occurs at any stage of infection but is most commonly seen in the early stages of HIV infection (234,236). Its prevalence is unknown, but autopsy data (238) show a frequency of nearly 25%, which contrasts with the reported rarity (237).

Laboratory Investigations

CK levels are moderately elevated, usually up to several-fold normal (226). Elevation of the CK level alone is not atypical in HIV infection, but such patients rarely have demonstrable weakness (237). EMG reveals fibrillation and positive sharp wave activity in up to 79% of affected patients (236) with a grossly myopathic recruitment pattern, typically in an affected proximal muscle such as the iliopsoas.

Pathology

The muscle biopsy in HIV-associated myopathy (Fig. 8) typically shows scattered myofiber degeneration and necrosis with phagocytosis and occasional inflammatory infiltration, although the latter less often than in HIV-seronegative polymyositis (234,236,238). Immunohistochemical studies show endomysial T-cell infiltrates of the CD8 phenotype, with MHC class 1 expression consistent with a primary T-cell–mediated cytotoxic process, similar to their seronegative counterparts (234). Evidence for direct HIV infection of myofibers was cited in one report (239), but it is unlikely to be an important pathogenetic

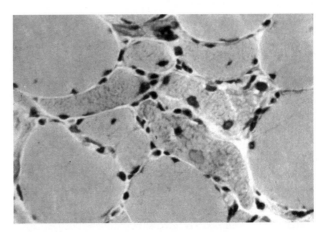

FIG. 8. HIV-associated myopathy. Photomicrograph of a quadriceps muscle biopsy reveals basophilic degenerating fibers without significant inflammatory cell infiltration. Hematoxylin-eosin, original magnification x100. (From Simpson D. Neuromuscular complications of human immunodeficiency virus infection. *Semin Neurol* 1992;12:39, with permission.)

mechanism overall. Most studies using in situ hybridization and PCR techniques have failed to demonstrate HIV in the myofibers but instead found HIV nucleic acid in the infiltrating endomysial macrophages and lymphocytes (240). These cells stained positive for TNF-α and IL-1 (241), suggesting a pathogenesis similar to those proposed for HIV encephalopathy, vacuolar myelopathy, and DSP (86).

Treatment

Improvement of HIV-associated myopathy has been reported with prednisone, usually beginning at 60 mg daily (236,255,259–261), but only one controlled study has been performed (258). The risk of a corticosteroid-related opportunistic infection should be weighed against the possible benefits of therapy, although in pneumocystis pneumonia, corticosteroids have had few adverse effects (262).

Rhabdomyolysis

Rhabdomyolysis with very high CK levels has been reported in all stages of HIV infection (248); similarly, HIV should be considered in affected patients. There is frequently fever, local muscle swelling, and sometimes compartment syndromes and renal failure. Three patients with acute rhabdomyolysis had HIV seropositivity but did not undergo muscle biopsy (249–251). In other cases muscle tissues showed isolated necrotic fibers without inflammation (248,252), but studies for HIV antigens were not performed. Concomitant systemic infections, malignancy, limb compression, local pyomyosits, neuroleptic and sulfonamide drugs, and didanosine can precipitate rhabdomyolysis (248). Its management usually includes adequate hydration, alkalinization, and careful monitoring of renal function.

Pathologic Variants of Primary Human Immunodeficiency Virus Myopathy

These include nemaline rod myopathy (242,243) and cases of skeletal muscle microvasculitis (193). Nemaline rod variants were described without evidence of inflammation or necrosis in a muscle biopsy in patients with clinical syndromes similar to those of primary HIV-associated myopathy. By electron microscopy the rods appear as electron-dense filamentous bodies with crystalline periodicity characteristic of nemaline rods. Similar findings were subsequently reported with equal frequency in primary HIV and AZT-related myopathy; accordingly, its existence as a separate entity is still unclear (234,236).

Coinfection with HTLV-I may be a proximate or contributing cause of HIV-related polymyositis (245). The pathology of HTLV-I– and HIV-associated myopathies are similar except for the predominance of infiltrating

CD4+, not CD8+ cells, in the former, some of which show productive infection with HTLV-I (244). Dickoff et al. (246) reported primary HTLV-I infection of myocytes by in situ hybridization techniques. Three biopsy-proven cases of inclusion body myositis were described (247), including two with HIV-1 and one with HTLV-I seropositivity. Their presentations were clinically and pathologically identical to other cases of sporadic inclusion body myositis due to the presence of rimmed vacuoles, MHC type 1 sarcolemmal expression, and infiltrating CD8+ lymphocytes along with retroviral-infected macrophages.

Human Immunodeficiency Virus Wasting Syndrome

This syndrome is characterized by unexplained weight loss of at least 10% of premorbid weight and 30 days or more of diarrhea. Frank weakness, when present, is progressive, proximal, and painless with marked muscular atrophy (254,255). This syndrome encompasses nearly 25% of AIDS events, similar to that seen in conjunction with CMV disease, bacterial pneumonia, and mycobacterium avium intracellulare sepsis (253). The pathologic features in skeletal muscle are nonspecific and show scattered myofiber degeneration and neurogenic atrophy, sometimes with associated inflammatory cells (256,257). Ragged red fibers were absent, and cytochrome *c* oxidase staining was normal in the biopsies of six patients with wasting syndrome so studied (256). The cause of the wasting syndrome is probably multifactorial, due to underlying anorexia and nutritional, endocrinologic, and gastrointestinal disorders with unexplained catabolic effects (255,256). The management includes correction of contributing systemic abnormalities. If the CK is elevated and the patient has a myopathy clinically and electrically, a muscle biopsy should be performed. A trial of the corticosteroid oxandrolone showed significant weight gain without hepatic or prothrombotic complications but no change in muscular strength (263).

Zidovudine Myopathy

AZT myopathy was first described by Dalakas et al. (260) among 15 patients and was compared with 5 cases of HIV-associated myopathy naive to AZT (260). The doses of AZT, 1,000 to 1,200 mg, was twice that commonly used in clinical practice. The clinical features of progressive proximal weakness and elevation of the CK were the same in both groups; however, the AZT-related cases also had myalgia. Muscle biopsies showed 5 to 50% of myofibers with ragged red changes on the modified Gomori Trichrome stain, similar to those seen in primary mitochondrial myopathy, but differed in a smaller more ragged appearance and a more marked myofibrillar disruption, leading to the term AZT fibers. In addition, all showed inflammatory myopathy with increased sarcolemmal MHC type 1 expression, cytoplasmic bodies, and nemaline rods. Electron microscopy in 13 cases showed abnormal swollen mitochondria with paracrystalline inclusions. The authors proposed that the mechanism of muscle toxicity with AZT was due to inhibition of mitochondrial DNA polymerase, leading to mitochondrial DNA depletion, reduced respiratory cycle enzymes, and subsequent energy failure (264). None of the five patients with HIV-associated myopathy naive to AZT showed ragged red fibers or electron micrographic evidence of mitochondrial abnormalities. AZT withdrawal resulted in improvement in clinical weakness preceded by a fall in the CK level in eight patients; no change or deterioration was seen in four others. Three of four cases of AZT myopathy also improved with prednisone. An overlapping HIV myopathy was proposed to explain the lack of response to AZT withdrawal.

Pathogenesis

Dalakas and colleagues (265–269) subsequently showed further evidence for a primary mitochondrial disorder by the demonstration of skeletal muscular carnitine deficiency, increased glycogen and lipid deposition, cytochrome oxidase deficiency, mitochondrial DNA depletion, and reduced phosphocreatine levels with delayed recovery postexercise as measured by magnetic resonance spectroscopy of the gastrocnemius. These authors also showed that the clinical and pathologic severity correlated significantly with the cumulative dose of AZT (270). Muscle biopsies of patients with myalgia and elevated CK, without weakness, showed electronmicrographic mitochondrial abnormalities and increased lipid but no ragged red fibers (266). Cumulative dose-related mitochondrial injury has been proposed, citing a spectrum of electron micrographic and ultrastructural abnormalities (266). Casademont et al. (272) detected mitochondrial DNA depletion in skeletal muscle biopsies and correlated the findings with weakness, myalgia, CK elevation, and proportion of red ragged fibers but not the cumulative AZT dose, suggesting an additional etiologic factor in this disorder. Other studies have not demonstrated the diagnostic specificity of ultrastructural and electronmicrographic features of mitochondrial abnormalities for AZT myopathy. Ragged red fibers may rarely be present or absent (236,261,273,274) in AZT-naive and normal patients (272), and muscle biopsies of affected patients may be normal, despite weakness and CK elevation (261). Some investigators were unable to distinguish HIV and AZT myopathy pathologically (236,273,274). Miller et al. (275) were unable to confirm MR spectroscopic abnormalities in affected patients (275), and the 100% specificity of cytochrome oxidase-deficient fibers could not be reproduced (276). The response to AZT withdrawal was inconsistent, demonstrating partial or complete improvement in 47 to 83% so studied (236,260,261,267,271); it is often limited to myalgia more than in weakness, whereas atrophy appears irreversible (271). Several inferential lines of evidence suggest a primary role for HIV infection in the myopathic process: the finding of inflammation in the muscle biopsies of patients with AZT myopathy, the occasional response to prednisone and the increased staining of AZT fibers for IL-1 and IL-1 mRNA (241), and the rarity of the disorder in animal models without HIV infection (277,278). Cupler et al. (279) found that patients with biopsy-proven AZT myopathy could continue treatment for greater than 6 months without further clinical deterioration. The urgency for discontinuation of AZT is therefore debatable.

Clinical Management and Treatment of Zidovudine Myopathy

The conflicting data on AZT myopathy has led to confusion as to the practical management of patients taking AZT who complain of muscular symptoms and/or have an elevated blood CK. A survey of the frequency of documented weakness, myalgias, and elevated CK was taken as part of the ACTG 016 trial comparing 1,000 mg AZT vs. placebo for 711 patients with CD4 counts between 200 and 800 (237). Myalgias and elevated CK were reported in 20 to 40% of both groups of patients. Actual weakness was seen in less than 2%, all on AZT, with improvement of weakness and a fall in the CK upon cessation of AZT. We would not recommend cessation of AZT for isolated myalgias or elevated CK in the absence of documented weakness or myopathic EMG. Similarly, we recommend a muscle biopsy only in those patients with demonstrable weakness or myopathic EMG. The significance of mitochondrial-type pattern abnormalities on biopsy in the absence of weakness is unclear because continued AZT use may not be associated with the development of weakness (279).

Motor Neuron Disease

There is yet no proven association between motor neuron disease and HIV infection. Nonetheless, there have been isolated case reports of motor neuron disease in HIV-infected patients (280–282), including one patient in whom motor neuron disease was associated with increased anti-asialo GM1 antibodies and a transient response to immune globulin (282).

Myasthenia Gravis

There are seven case reports of the association of myasthenia gravis with HIV infection (283). In two, myasthenia gravis was the presenting manifestation of HIV infection (283,284) and was unassociated with circulating acetylcholine receptor antibodies. Three had generalized myasthenia gravis with positive acetylcholine receptor antibodies. Myasthenia gravis improved in six with falling CD4 counts and progressive HIV disease-related immunodeficiency.

REFERENCES

1. World Health Organization. *The current global situation of the HIV/AIDS pandemic.* Geneva: World Health Organization Global Programme on AIDS, July 1994:1–11.
2. Centers for Disease Control and Prevention. U.S. HIV and AIDS cases reported through December 1996. *HIV/AIDS Surveillance Report* 1997;8.
3. Centers for Disease Control and Prevention. 1993 Revised classification system for HIV infection and expanded surveillance case definition for AIDS among adults and adolescents. *MMWR Morb Mortal Wkly Rep* 1992;41:(RR-17):1–4.
4. Centers for Disease Control and Prevention. Revision of the CDC surveillance case definition for acquired immunodeficiency syndrome. *MMWR Morb Mortal Wkly Rep* 1987;36[Suppl 1S]:1–15.
5. Mellors JW, Rinaldo CR, Gupta P, White RM, Todd JA, Kingsley LA. Prognosis in HIV-1 infection predicted by the quantity of virus in the plasma. *Science* 1996;272:1167–1170.
6. Levy RM, Bredesen DE, Rosenblum ML. Neurologic manifestations of the acquired immunodeficiency syndrome (AIDS): experience at UCSF and review of the literature. *J Neurosurg* 1985;62:475–495.
7. Petito CK. Review of central nervous system pathology in human immunodeficiency virus infection. *Ann Neurol* 1988;23:s54–s57.
8. Gray F, Gherardi R, Scaravilli F. The neuropathology of the acquired immunodeficiency syndrome (AIDS). *Brain* 1988;111:245–266.
9. Kure K, Llena JF, Lyman WD, et al. Human immunodeficiency virus-1 infection of the nervous system: an autopsy study of 268 adult, pediatric and fetal brains. *Hum Pathol* 1991;22:700–710.
10. de la Monte SM, Gabuzda DH, Ho DD, et al. Peripheral neuropathy in the acquired immunodeficiency syndrome. *Ann Neurol* 1988;23:485–492.
11. Snider WD, Simpson DM, Nielsen S, et al. Neurological complications of acquired immune deficiency syndrome: analysis of 50 patients. *Ann Neurol* 1983;14:403–418.
12. Bacellar H, Munoz A, Miller EN, et al. Temporal trends in the incidence of HIV-1 related neurologic diseases: Multicenter AIDS Cohort Study, 1985–1992. *Neurology* 1994;44:1892–1900.
13. Bendok B, Berger JR, Levy RM. *Acquired immunodeficiency syndrome and the nervous system: fifteen years of progress. AIDS and the Nervous System,* 2nd ed. Philadelphia, PA: Lippincott-Raven, 1997:1–11.
14. Rosenblum ML, Levy RM, Bredesen DE. Neurosurgical implications of the acquired immunodeficiency syndrome (AIDS). *Clin Neurosurg* 1988;34:419–445.
15. Carpenter CC, Fischl MA, Hammer SM, et al. Antiretroviral therapy for HIV infection in 1996: recommendations of an international panel. *JAMA* 1996;276:146–154.
16. Price RW, Brew BJ. The AIDS dementia complex. *J Infect Dis* 1988;158:1079–1083.
17. McArthur JC, Hoover DR, Bacellar H, et al. Nomenclature and research case definitions for neurological manifestations of human immunodeficiency virus type-1 (HIV-1) infection: report of a Working Group of the American Academy of Neurology AIDS Task Force. *Neurology* 1991;41:778–785.
18. The Dana Consortium on Therapy for HIV Dementia and Related Cognitive Disorders. Clinical confirmation of the American Academy of Neurology alogarithm for HIV-1 associated cognitive/motor disorder. *Neurology* 1996;47:1247–1253.
19. Marder K, Liu X, Stern Y, et al. Neurological signs and symptoms in a cohort of homosexual men followed for 4.5 years. *Neurology* 1995;45:261–267.
20. Marder K, Liu X, Stern Y, et al. Risk of human immunodeficiency virus type 1 related neurological disease in a cohort of intravenous drug users. *Arch Neurol* 1995;52:1174–1182.
21. Howlett WP, Nyka WM, Kvale G, Nilssen S. The snout and palmomental reflexes in HIV disease in Tanzania. *Acta Neurol Scand* 1995;91:470–476.
22. Portegies P, Enting RH, de Gans J, et al. Presentation and course of AIDS dementia complex: ten years of follow up in Amsterdam, the Netherlands. *AIDS* 1993;7:669–675.
23. Kieburtz K, Ketonen L, Cox C, et al. Cognitive performance and regional volume in human immunodeficiency virus type 1 infection. *Arch Neurol* 1996;53:155–158.
24. Dal Pan GJ, McArthur JC, Aylward E, et al. Patterns of cerebral atrophy in HIV-1 infected individuals: results of a quantitative MRI analysis. *Neurology* 1992;42:2125–2130.
25. Wiley CA, Achim C. Human immunodeficiency virus encephalitis is the pathological correlate of dementia in acquired immunodeficiency syndrome. *Ann Neurol* 1994;36:673–676.
26. Dickson DW, Lee SC, Hatch W, Mattiace LA, Brosnan CF, Lyman WD. Macrophages and microglia in HIV-1 related CNS neuropathology. *Assoc Res Nerv Ment Dis Res Publ* 1994;72:99–118.
27. Brew BJ, Rosenblum M, Cronin K, Price RW. AIDS dementia complex and HIV-1 brain infection: clinical-virological correlations. *Ann Neurol* 1995;38:563–570.
28. Seilhean D, Duyckaerts C, Vazeux R, et al. HIV-1 associated cognitive-motor complex: absence of neuronal loss in the cerebral neocortex. *Neurology* 1993;43:1492–1499.
29. Wiley CA, Masliah E, Morey M, et al. Neocortical damage during HIV infection. *Ann Neurol* 1991;29:651–657.
30. Everall IP, Chong WK, Wilkinson ID, et al. Correlation of MRI and neuropathology in AIDS. *J Neurol Neurosurg Psychiatry* 1997;62:92–95.
31. Schmidbauer M, Huemer M, Cristina S, Trabattoni GR, Budka H. Morphological spectrum, distribution and clinical correlation of white matter lesions in AIDS brains. *Neuropathol Appl Neurobiol* 1992;18:489–501.
32. Bagasra O, Lavi E, Boboroski L, et al. Cellular reservoirs of HIV-1 in the central nervous system of infected individuals: identification by the combination of in situ polymerase chain reaction and immunohistochemistry. *AIDS* 1996;10:573–585.
33. Glass JD, Wesselingh SL, Selnes OA, McArthur JC. Clinical-neuropathological correlation in HIV-associated dementia. *Neurology* 1993;43:2230–2237.
34. Shu F, Giometto G, Scaravilli F. HIV-1 DNA in brains in AIDS and pre-AIDS: correlation with the stage of disease. *Ann Neurol* 1996;40:611–617.
35. Conrad AJ, Schmid P, Syndulko K, et al. Quantifying HIV-1 RNA using the polymerase chain reaction on cerebrospinal fluid and serum of seropositive individuals with and without neurologic abnormalities. *J Acq Immun Def Syndr Hum Retrovirol* 1995;10:425–435.
36. Lubetzki C, Dubard T, Suarez S, Katlama C, Turell E, Calvez V. Cerebrospinal fluid HIV load and AIDS dementia. *Neurology* 1997;48:A387.
37. McArthur JC, Nance-Sproson T, Selnes OA, McLernon D, St Clair M, Lanier R. CSF HIV RNA: relationship to HIV-associated neurological disease. *Neurology* 1997;48:A388.
38. Toggas SM, Masliah E, Rockenstein EM, Rall GF, Abraham CR, Mucke L. Central nervous system damage produced by expression of the HIV-1 coat protein gp120 in transgenic mice. *Nature* 1994;367:188–193.
39. Lipton SA. Human immunodeficiency virus infected macrophages, gp120 and N-methyl-D-aspartate neurotoxicity. *Ann Neurol* 1993;33:227–228.
40. Epstein L, Gendelman HE. Human immunodeficiency virus type 1 infection of the nervous system: pathogenetic systems. *Ann Neurol* 1993;33:429–436.
41. Wesselingh SL, Power C, Glass JD, et al. Intracerebral cytokine messenger RNA expression in acquired immunodeficiency syndrome dementia. *Ann Neurol* 1993;33:576–582.
42. Tyor WR, Glass JD, Griffin JW, et al. Cytokine expression in the brain during the acquired immunodeficiency syndrome. *Ann Neurol* 1992;31:349–360.
43. Wilt SG, Milward E, Min Zhou J, et al. In vitro evidence for a dual role of tumour necrosis factor-α in human immunodeficiency virus type 1 encephalopathy. *Ann Neurol* 1995;37:381–394.
44. Heyes MP, Saito K, Major EO, Milstein S, Markey SP, Vickers JH. A mechanism of quinolinic acid formation by brain in inflammatory neurological disease: attenuation of synthesis of L-tryptophan by 6-chlorotryptophan and 4-chloro-3-hydroxyanthraniliate. *Brain* 1993;116:1425–1450.
45. Genis P, Jett M, Bernton EW, et al. Cytokines and arachidonic metabolites produced during human immunodeficiency virus (HIV)-infected macrophage-astroglia interactions: implications for the neuropathogenesis of HIV disease. *J Exp Med* 1992;176:1703–1718.
46. Brew BJ, Bhalla RB, Fleisher M, et al. Cerebrospinal fluid β2-microglobulin in patients infected with human immunodeficiency virus. *Neurology* 1989;39:830–834.

47. Brew BJ, Bhalla RB, Paul M, et al. Cerebrospinal fluid β2-microglobulin in patients with AIDS dementia complex: an expanded series including response to zidovudine treatment. *AIDS* 1992;6:461–465.

48. Brew BJ, Bhalla RB, Paul M, et al. Cerebrospinal fluid neopterin in human immunodeficiency virus type 1 infection. *Ann Neurol* 1990; 28:556–560.

49. Heyes MP, Brew BJ, Martin A, et al. Quinolinic acid in cerebrospinal fluid and serum in HIV-1 infection: relationship to clinical and neurological status. *Ann Neurol* 1991;29:202–209.

50. Hriso E, Kuhn T, Masdeu JC, Grundman M. Extrapyramidal symptoms due to dopamine-blocking agents with AIDS encephalopathy. *Am J Psychiatry* 1991;148:1558–1561.

51. Holland NR, Power C, Mathews VP, Glass JD, Forman M, McArthur JC. Cytomegalovirus encephalitis in acquired immunodeficiency syndrome (AIDS). *Neurology* 1994;44:507–514.

52. Kalayjian RC, Cohen ML, Bonomo RA, Flanigan TP. Cytomegalovirus ventriculoencephalitis in AIDS. *Medicine* 1993;72:67–77.

53. Cinque P, Scarpellini P, Vago L, Linde A, Lazzarin A. Diagnosis of central nervous system complications in HIV-infected patients: cerebrospinal fluid analysis by the polymerase chain reaction. *AIDS* 1997; 11:1–17.

54. Cinque P, Vago L, Dahl H, et al. Polymerase chain reaction on cerebrospinal fluid for diagnosis of virus-associated opportunistic diseases of the central nervous system in HIV-infected patients. *AIDS* 1996;10:951–958.

55. Berger JR, Kaszovitz B, Post MJ, Dickinson G. Progressive multifocal leukoencephalopathy associated with human immunodeficiency virus infection. A review of the literature with a report of sixteen cases. *Ann Intern Med* 1987;107:78–87.

56. Brooks BR, Walker DL. Progressive multifocal leukoencephalopathy. *Neurol Clin* 1984;2:299–313.

57. Von Einsiedel RW, Fife TD, Aksamit AJ, et al. Progressive multifocal leukoencephalopathy in AIDS: a clinicopathological study and review of the literature. *J Neurol* 1993;240:391–406.

58. Whiteman M, Post MJD, Berger JR, Limone L, Tate LG, Bell M. Progressive multifocal leukoencephalopathy in 47 patients. *Radiology* 1993;187:233–240.

59. Sidtis JJ, Gatsonis C, Price RW, et al. Zidovudine treatment of the AIDS dementia complex: results of a placebo controlled trial. *Ann Neurol* 1993;33:343–349.

60. Brouwers P, Hendricks M, Lietzau JA, et al. Effect of combination therapy with zidovudine and didanosine on neuropsychological functioning in patients with symptomatic HIV disease: a comparison of simultaneous and alternating regimens. *AIDS* 1997;11:59–66.

61. Maehlen J, Dunlop O, Liestol K, Dobloug JH, Goplen AK, Torvik A. Changing incidence of HIV-induced brain lesions in Oslo, 1983–1994: effects of zidovudine treatment. *AIDS* 1995;9:1165–1169.

62. Burger DM, Kraaijeveld CL, Meenhorst PL, et al. Penetration of zidovudine into the cerebrospinal fluid of patients infected with HIV. *AIDS* 1993;7:1581–1587.

62a. Navia BA, Dafni U, Simpson D, et al. A phase I/II trial of nimodipine for HIV-related neurologic complications. *Neurology* 1998;51:221–228.

63. Pellegrini JW, Lipton SA. Delayed administration of memantine prevents N-methyl-D-aspartate receptor mediated neurotoxicity. *Ann Neurol* 1993;33:403–407.

64. Parr J, Horoupian DS, Winkelman C. Cerebellar form of progressive multifocal leukoencephalopathy (PML). *Can J Neurosci* 1979;6: 123–128.

65. Jones HR, Hedley-Whyte T, Friedberg SR, et al. Primary cerebellopontine progressive multifocal leukoencephalopathy diagnosed premortem by cerebellar biopsy. *Ann Neurol* 1982;11:199–202.

66. Pierelli F, Tilia G, Damiani A, et al. Brainstem CMV encephalitis in AIDS: clinical case and MRI features. *Neurology* 1997;48:529–530.

67. Masdeu JC, Small CB, Weiss L, et al. Multifocal cytomegalovirus encephalitis in AIDS. *Ann Neurol* 1988;23:97–99.

68. Fuller GN, Guiloff RJ, Scaravilli F, Harcourt-Webster JN. Combined HIV-CMV encephalitis presenting with brain stem signs. *J Neurol Neurosurg Psychiatry* 1989;52:975–979.

69. Wolters EC, Van Wijngaarden GK, Stam FC, et al. Leucoencephalopathy after inhaling heroin pyrosylate. *Lancet* 1982;2:1233–1237.

70. Krigstein A, Armitage B, Kim PY. Heroin inhalation and progressive spongiform leukoencephalopathy. *N Engl J Med* 1997;336:589–590.

71. Celius EG, Andersson S. Leucoencephalopathy after inhalation of heroin: a case report. *J Neurol Neurosurg Psychiatry* 1996;60:694–695.

72. Dal Pan GJ, Glass JD, McArthur JC. Clincopathologic correlations of HIV-1 associated vacuolar myelopathy. An autopsy-based case-control study. *Neurology* 1994;44:2159–2164.

73. Dal Pan GJ, Berger JR. Spinal cord disease in human immunodeficiency virus infection. In: Berger JR, Levy RM, eds. *AIDS and the nervous system*, 2nd ed. Philadelphia: Lippincott-Raven, 1997:173–187.

74. Barakos JA, Mark AS, Dillon WP, Norman D. MR imaging of acute transverse myelitis and AIDS myelopathy. *J Comput Assist Tomogr* 1990;14:45–50.

75. Danisi F, Tagliati M, Di Rocco A, Mylin L, Simpson DM. Somatosensory evoked potentials in patients with evoked potentials in patients with HIV-1 associated myelopathy. *Neurology* 1997;48:A93.

76. Connolly S, Manji H, McAllister RH, et al. Neurophysiological assessment of peripheral nerve and spinal cord function in asymptomatic HIV-1 infection: results from the UCMSM/ medical research Council neurology cohort. *J Neurol* 1995;242:406–414.

77. Jabbari B, Coats M, Salazar A, Martin A, Scherokman B, Laws WA. Longitudinal study of EEG and evoked potentials in neurologically asymptomatic HIV infected patients. *Electroencephalogr Clin Neurophys* 1993;86:145–151.

78. Marshall DW, Brey RL, Cahill WT. Cerebrospinal fluid (CSF) findings in asymptomatic (AS) individuals infected by human immunodeficiency (HIV) virus. *Neurology* 1988;38:167–168.

79. Singer EJ, Syndulko K, Fahy-Chandon B, et al. Intrathecal IgG synthesis and albumin leakage are increased in subjects with HIV-1 neurological disease. *AIDS* 1994;7:265–271.

80. Tan SV, Guiloff RJ, Scaravilli F. AIDS-associated vacuolar myelopathy. A morphometric study. *Brain* 1995;118:1247–1261.

81. Petito CK, Vecchio D, Chen Y-T. HIV antigen and DNA in AIDS spinal cords correlate with macrophage infiltration but not with vacuolar myelopathy. *J Neuropathol Exp Neurol* 1994;53:86–94.

82. Tyor WR, Glass JD, Baumrind N, et al. Cytokine expression of macrophages in HIV-1 associated vacuolar myelopathy. *Neurology* 1993;43:1002–1009.

83. Rosenblum M, Scheck AC, Cronin K, et al. Disassociation of AIDS related vacuolar myelopathy and productive HIV infection of the spinal cord. *Neurology* 1989;39:892–896.

84. Henin D, Smith TW, DeGirolami U, Sughayer M, Hauw J-J. Neuropathology of the spinal cord in the acquired immunodeficiency syndrome. *Hum Pathol* 1992;23:1106–1114.

85. Kure K, Llena JF, Lyman WD, et al. Human immunodeficiency virus-1 infection of the nervous system. *Hum Pathol* 1991;22:700–710.

86. Tyor WR, Wesselingh SL, Griffin JW, McArthur JC, Griffin DE. Unifying hypothesis for the pathogenesis of HIV-associated dementia complex, vacuolar myelopathy, and sensory neuropathy. *J Acq Immun Def Syndr Hum Retrovirol* 1995;9:379–388.

87. Kieburtx KD, Giang DW, Schiffer RB, Vakil M. Abnormal vitamin B12 metabolism in human immunodeficiency infection. Association with neurological dysfunction. *Arch Neurol* 1991;48:312–314.

88. Keating JN, Trimble KC, Mulcahy F, Scott JM, Weir DG. Evidence of brain methyltransferase inhibition and early brain involvement in HIV-positive patients. *Lancet* 1991;337:935–939.

89. Castagna A, Le Grazie C, Accordini A, et al. Cerebrospinal fluid S-adenosylmethionine (SAMe) and glutathione concentrations in HIV infection: Effect of parenteral treatment with SAMe. *Neurology* 1995; 45:1678–1683.

90. Lazer RB, Fishman RA, Schaler JA. Neuropathy following abuse of nitrous oxide. *Neurology* 1978;28:504–506.

91. Surtees R, Leonard J, Austin S. Association of demyelination with deficiency of cerebrospinal fluid S-adenosylmethionine in inborn errors of metabolism of methyl transferase pathway. *Lancet* 1991;338:1550–1554.

92. Klein P, Zientek G, Vandenberg SR, Lothman E. Primary CNS lymphoma: lymphomatous meningitis presenting as a cauda equina lesion in an AIDS patient. *Can J Neurol Sci* 1990;17:329–331.

93. Gray F, Belec L, Lescs MC, et al. Varicella-zoster virus infection of the central nervous system in the acquired immune deficiency syndrome. *Brain* 1994;117:987–999.

94. Grant AD, Fox JD, Brink NS, Miller RF. Detection of varicella-zoster virus DNA using the polymerase chain reaction in an immunocompromised patient with transverse myelitis secondary to herpes zoster. *Genitourinary Med* 1993;69:273–275.

95. Mahieux F, Gray F, Fenelon G, et al. Acute myeloradiculitis due to cytomegalovirus as the initial manifestation of AIDS. *J Neurol Neurosurg Psychiatry* 1989;52:270–274.

96. Tucker T, Dix RD, Katzen C, Davis RL, Schmidley JW. Cytomegalovirus and herpes simplex virus ascending myelitis in a patient with acquired immunodeficiency syndrome. *Ann Neurol* 1985;18:74–79.

97. Britton CB, Mesa-Tejada R, Fenoglio CM, Hays AP, Garvey GG, Miller JR. A new complication of AIDS: thoracic myelitis caused by herpes simplex virus. *Neurology* 1985;35:1071–1074.

98. Berger JR. Spinal cord syphilis associated with human immunodeficiency virus infection: a treatable myelopathy. *Am J Med* 1992;92:101–103.

99. Resnieck DK, Comey CH, Welch WC, Martinez AJ, Hoover WW, Jacobs GB. Isolated toxoplasmosis of the thoracic spinal cord in a patient with acquired immunodeficiency syndrome. *J Neurosurg* 1995;82:493–496.

100. Woolsey RM, Chambers TJ, Chung HD, McGarry JD. Mycobacterial meningomyelitis associated with human immunodeficiency virus infection. *Arch Neurol* 1988;45:691–693.

101. Leibert E, Schluger NW, Bonk S, Rom WN. Spinal tuberculosis in patients with human immunodeficiency virus infection: clinical presentation, therapy and outcome. *Tubercle Lung Dis* 1996;77:329–334.

102. Woods GL, Goldsmith JC. Aspergillus infection of the central nervous system in patients with acquired immunodeficiency syndrome. *Arch Neurol* 1990;47:181–184.

103. Manian FA, Kindred M, Fulling KH. Chronic varicella-zoster virus myelitis without cutaneous eruption in a patient with AIDS: report of a fatal case. *Clin Infect Dis* 1995;21:986–988.

104. Harrison LH, Vaz B, Taveira DM, et al. Myelopathy among Brazilians coinfected with human T-cell lymphotropic virus type 1 and HIV. *Neurology* 1997;48:13–18.

105. Lee H, Swanson P, Rosenblatt J, et al. Relative prevalence and risk factors of HTLV-1 and HTLV-II infection in US blood donors. *Lancet* 1991;337:1435–1439.

106. Murphy EL, Fridey J, Smith J, et al. HTLV-associated myelopathy in a cohort of HTLV-1 and HTLV-II infected blood donors. *Neurology* 1997;48:315–320.

107. Lehky T, Flerlage ZN, Katz D, et al. Human T-cell lymphotropic virus type II associated myelopathy: clinical and immunologic profiles. *Ann Neurol* 1996;40:714–723.

108. Dooneief G, Marlink R, Bell K, et al. Neurologic consequences of HTLV-II infection in injection drug users. *Neurology* 1996;46:1556–1560.

109. Luft BJ, Hafner R, Korzun AH, et al. Toxoplasmic encephalitis in patients with the acquired immunodeficiency syndrome. *N Engl J Med* 1993;329:995–1000.

110. Porter SB, Sande M. Toxoplasmosis of the central nervous system in the acquired immunodeficiency syndrome. *N Engl J Med* 1992;327:1643–1648.

111. Nath A, Jankovic J, Pettigrew LC. Movement disorders and AIDS. *Neurology* 1987;37:37–41.

112. Navia BA, Petito CK, Gold JW, Cho ES, Jordan BD, Price RW. Cerebral toxoplasmosis complicating the acquired immune deficiency syndrome: clinical and neuropathological findings in 27 patients. *Ann Neurol* 1986;19:224–238.

113. Carrazone EJ, Rossitch E, Martinez J. Unilateral akathisia in a patient with AIDS and a toxoplasma suthalamic abscess. *Neurology* 1989;39:449–450.

114. Ammassari A, Murri R, Cingolani A, De Luca A, Antinori A. AIDS-associated cerebral toxoplasmosis: an update on diagnosis and treatment. *Curr Top Microbiol Immunol* 1996;219:201–214.

115. Oksenhendler E, Charreau I, Tournerie C, Azihary M, Carbon C, Aboulker JP. Toxoplasma gondii infection in advanced HIV infection. *AIDS* 1994;8:483–487.

116. Girard PM, Landman R, Gaudebout C, et al. Dapsone-pyrimethamine compared with aerosolized pentamidine as primary prophylaxis against *Pneumocystis carinii* pneumonia and toxoplasmosis in HIV infection. *N Engl J Med* 1993;328:1514–1520.

117. Ciricillo SF, Rosenblum ML. Use of CT and MR imaging to distinguish intracranial lesions and to define the need for biopsy in AIDS patients. *J Neurosurg* 1990;73:720–724.

118. Levy R, Mills C, Posin J, Moore S, Rosenblum M, Bredesen D. The efficacy and clinical impact of brain imaging in neurologically symptomatic AIDS patients: a prospective CT/MRI study. *J AIDS* 1990;3:461–471.

119. Dina TS. Primary central nervous system lymphoma versus toxoplasmosis in AIDS. *Radiology* 1991;179:823–828.

120. Raffi F, Aboulker J-P, Michelet C, et al. Prospective study criteria for the diagnosis of toxoplasmic encephalitis in 186 AIDS patients. *AIDS* 1997;11:177–184.

121. Ruiz A, Ganz W, Donovan Post J, et al. Use of Thallium-201 brain SPECT to differentiate cerebral lymphoma from toxoplasma encephalitis in AIDS patients. *Am J Neuroradiol* 1994;15:1885–1894.

122. Renold C, Sugar A, Chave JP, et al. Toxoplasma encephalitis in patients with the acquired immunodeficiency syndrome. *Medicine* 1992;71:224–239.

123. Mathews C, Barba D, Fullerton SC. Early biopsy versus empiric treatment with delayed biosy of non-responders in suspected HIV-associated cerebral toxoplasmosis: a decision analysis. *AIDS* 1995;9:1243–1250.

124. Antinori A, Ammassari A, De Luca A, et al. Diagnosis of AIDS-related focal brain lesions: A decision making analysis based on clinical and neuroradiological characteristics combined with polymerase chain reaction assays in CSF. *Neurology* 1997;48:687–694.

125. De Luca A, Antinori A, Cingolani A, et al. Evaluation of cerebrospinal fluid EBV-DNA and IL-10 as markers for in vivo diagnosis of AIDS-related primary central nervous system lymphoma. *Br J Haematol* 1995;90:844–849.

126. Luzzati R, Ferrari S, Nicolato A, et al. Stereotactic brain biopsy in human immunodeficiency virus-infected patients. *Arch Intern Med* 1996;5:565–568.

127. Levy Rm, Russell E, Yungbluth M, Hidvegi DF, Brody BA, DalCanto MC. the efficacy of image-guided stereotactic brain biopsy in neurologically symptomatic acquired immunodeficiency syndrome patients. *Neurosurgery* 1992;30:186–190.

128. Chappell ET, Guthrie BL, Orenstein J. The role of stereotactic biopsy in the management of HIV-related focal brain lesions. *Neurosurgery* 1992;30:825–829.

129. Haverkos HW. Assessment of therapy for toxoplasmic encephalitis. The TE study group. *Am J Med* 1987;82:907–914.

130. Luft BJ, Remington JS. Toxoplasmic encephalitis in AIDS. *Clin Infect Dis* 1992;15:211–222.

131. Pedrol E, Gonzalez-Clementz JM, Gatell JM, et al. Central nervous toxoplasmosis In AIDS patients: efficacy of an intermittent maintenance therapy. *AIDS* 1990;4:511–517.

132. Luft BJ, Hafner R. Toxoplasmic encephalitis [editorial]. *AIDS* 1990;4:593–595.

133. Mariuz P, Luft BJ. New therapeutic approaches to toxoplasmic encephalitis. *Curr Opin Infect Dis* 1991;826–833.

134. Danneman B, McCutchan JA, Israelski D, et al. Treatment of toxoplasmic encephalitis in patients with AIDS, a randomized trial comparing pyrimethamine plus clindamycin to pyrimethamine plus sulfadiazine. *Ann Intern Med* 1992;116:33–43.

135. Kovacs JA. Efficacy of atovaquone in treatment of toxoplasmosis in patients with AIDS. *Lancet* 1992;340:637–638.

136. Fernandez-Martin J, Leport C, Morlat P, et al. Pyrimethamine/clarithromycin combination therapy of acute toxoplasma in patients with AIDS. *Antimicrob Agents Chemother* 1991;35:2049–2052.

137. Baumgartner JE, Rachlin JR, Beckstead JH, et al. Primary central nervous system lymphoma: natural history and response to radiation therapy in 55 patients with acquired immunodeficiency syndrome. *J Neurosurg* 1990;73:206–211.

138. Donahue BR, Sullivan JW, Cooper JS. Additional experience with empiric radiotherapy for presumed human immunodeficiency virus-associayed primary central nervous system lymphoma. *Cancer* 1995;76:328–332.

139. DeAngelis LM, Yahalom J, Thaler HT, Kher U. Combined modality therapy for primary CNS lymphoma. *J Clin Oncol* 1992;10:635–643.

140. Forsyth PA, Yahalom J, DeAngelis L. Combined modality therapy in the treatment of primary central nervous system lymphoma in AIDS. *Neurology* 1994;44:1473–1479.

141. Whiteman MLH, Dandapani BK, Shebert RP, Post MJD. Progressive multifocal leukoencephalopathy in 47 HIV seropositive patients: neuroimaging with clinical and pathological correlation. *Radiology* 1993;187:233–240.

142. Walker DL, Padgett BL. The epidemiology of human polyomaviruses. In: Sever JL, Madden D, eds. *Polyomaviruses and human neurological disease*. New York: Alan R. Liss, 1983:99–106.

143. McGuire D, Barhite S, Hollander H, Miles M. JC virus DNA in cerebrospinal fluid of human immunodeficiency virus-infected patients: predictive value for progressive multifocal leukoencephalopathy. *Ann Neurol* 1995;37:395–399.

144. Portegies P, Algra PR, Hollar CM, et al. Response to cytarabine in progressive multifocal leukoencephalopathy in AIDS. *Lancet* 1991;337:680–681.

145. O'Riordan T, Daly PA, Hutchinson, Shattock AG, Gardner SD. Progressive multifocal leukoencephalopathy—remission with cytarabine. *J Infect* 1990;20:51–54.

146. Guarino M, DAlessandro R, Rinaldi R, et al. Progressive multifocal leukoencephalopathy in AIDS: treatment with cytosine arabinoside. *AIDS* 1995;9:819–820.

146a. Hall CD, Dafni U, Simpson D, et al. Failure of cytarabine in progressive multifocal leukoencephalopathy associated with human immunodeficiency virus infection. AIDS Clinical Trials Group 243 Team. *N Engl J Med* 1998;338:1345–1351.

147. Fong IW, Toma E, and The Canadian PML study group. The natural history of progressive multifocal leukoencephalopathy in patients with AIDS. *Clin Infect Dis* 1995;20:1305–1310.

148. Gendelman H, Phelps W, Feigenbaum L, et al. Transactivation of the human immunodeficiency virus long terminal repeat by DNA viruses. *Proc Natl Acad Sci USA* 1986;83:9759–9763.

149. Price RW, Nielsen S, Horten B, Rubina M, Padgett B, Walker D. Progressive multifocal leukoencephalopathy: a burnt out case. *Ann Neurol* 1983;13:485–490.

150. Berger JR, Mucke L. Prolonged survival and partial recovery in AIDS-associated progressive multifocal leukoencephalopathy. *Neurology* 1988;38:1060–1065.

151. Katz DA, Berger JR. Neurosyphilis in acquired immunodeficiency syndrome. *Arch Neurol* 1989;46:895–898.

152. Tyler KN, Sandberg E, Baum KF. Medial medullary syndrome and meningovascular syndrome: a case report in an HIV-infected man and a review of the literature. *Neurology* 1994;44:2231–2235.

153. Pinto AN. AIDS and cerebrovascular disease. *Stroke* 1996;27:538–543.

154. MacLean C, Flegg PJ, Kilpatrick DC. Anti-cardiolipin antibodies and HIV infection. *Clin Exp Immunol* 1990;81:262–266.

155. The Antiphospholipid Antibodies and Stroke Study Group (APASS). Anticardiolipin antibodies and the risk of recurrent thrombo-occlusive events and death. *Neurology* 1997;48:91–94.

156. Mathews VP, Alo PL, Glass JD, Kumar AJ, McArthur JC. AIDS-related CNS cryptococcosis: radiological-pathological correlation. *Am J Neuroradiol* 1992;13:1477–1486.

157. Tien RD, Chu PK, Hesselink JR, et al. Intracranial cryptococcosis in immunocompromised patients: CT and MRI findings in 29 cases. *Am J Neuroradiol* 1991;12:283–289.

158. Dyer JR, French MAH, Mallal SA. Cerebral mass lesions due to cytomegalovirus in patients with AIDS: report of two cases. *J Infect* 1995;30:147–151.

159. Dube MP, Holtom PD, Larsen RA. Tuberculous meningitis in patients with and without human immunodeficiency virus infection. *Am J Med* 1992;93:520–524.

160. Jinkins JR. Computed tomography of intracranial tuberculosis. *Neuroradiology* 1991;33:126–135.

161. Villoria MF, de la Torre J, Munoz L, et al. Intracranial tuberculosis in AIDS: CT and MRI findings. *Neuroradiology* 1992;34:11–14.

162. Van Dyk A. CT of intracranial tuberculosis with specific reference to the target sign. *Neuroradiology* 1988;30:329–336.

163. Afghani B, Liberman JM. Paradoxical enlargement or development of intracranial tuberculomas during therapy: case report and review. *Clin Infect Dis* 1994;19:1092–1099.

164. Berenguer J, Moreno S, Laguna F, Vicente T, et al. Tuberculous meningitis in patients infected with the human immunodeficiency virus. *N Engl J Med* 1992;326:668–672.

165. Kaplan JG, Sterman AB, Horoupian D, et al. Luetic meningitis with gumma: clinical, radiographic, and neuropathologic features. *Neurology* 1981;31:464–467.

166. Kox LKK, Sjoukje S, Kolk AHJ, et al. Early diagnosis of tuberculous meningitis by polymerase chain reaction. *Neurology* 1995;45:2228–2232.

167. Holland BA, Perrett LV, Mills CM. Meningovascular syphilis: CT and MR findings. *Radiology* 1986;158:439–442.

168. Berger JR, Waskin H, Pall L, Hensley G, Ihmedian I, Post MJD. Syphilitic cerebral gumma with HIV infection. *Neurology* 1992;42:1282–1287.

169. Hart G. Syphilis tests in diagnostic and therapeutic decision making. *Ann Intern Med* 1986;104:368–376.

170. Centers for Disease Control and Prevention. 1993 Sexually transmitted diseases treatment guidelines. *MMWR Morb Mortal Wkly Rep* 1993;42:27–46.

171. Uttamchandani RB, Daikos GL, Reyes RR, et al. Nocardiosis in 30 patients with advanced human immunodefciency virus infection. Clinical features and outcome. *Clin Infect Dis* 1994;18:348–353.

172. Palmer DL, Harvey RL, Wheeler JK. Diagnostic and therapeutic decisions in Nocardia asteroides infection. *Medicine* 1974;53:391–401.

173. Javaly K, Horowitz HW, Wormser GP. Nocardiosis in patients with human immunodeficiency virus infection. Report of two cases and review of the literature. *Medicine* 1992;71:128–138.

174. Beaman B, Burnside J, Edwards B, Causey W. Nocardial infection in the United States. 1972–1974. *J Infect Dis* 1976;134:286–289.

175. LeBlang SD, Whiteman MLH, Post MJD, et al. CNS Nocardia in AIDS patients: CT and MRI with pathologic correlation. *J Comput Assist Tomogr* 1995;19:15–22.

176. Gorin FA, Bale JF, Hacks-Miller M, Schwartz RA. Kaposi's sarcoma metastatic to the CNS. *Arch Neurol* 1985;42:162–165.

177. Eidelberg D, Sotrel A, Vogel H, et al. Progressive polyradiculopathy in the acquired immunodeficiency syndrome. *Neurology* 1986;36:912–916.

178. So YT, Olney RK. Acute lumbosacral polyradiculopathy in acquired immunodefciency syndrome: experience in 23 patients. *Ann Neurol* 1994;35:53–58.

179. Miller RF, Fox JD, Thomas P, et al. Acute lumbosacral polyradiculopathy due to cytomegalovirus in advanced HIV disease: CSF findings in 17 patients. *J Neurol Neurosurg Psychiatry* 1996;61:456–460.

180. Lanska MJ, Lanska DJ, Schmidley JW. Syphilitic polyradiculopathy in an HIV-positive man. *Neurology* 1988;38:1297–1301.

181. Kim YS, Hollander H. Polyradiculopathy due to cytomegalovirus: report of two cases in which improvement occurred after prolonged therapy and review of the literature. *Clin Infect Dis* 1993;17:32–37.

182. Tokumoto JIN, Hollander H. Cytomegalovirus polyradiculopathy caused by a ganciclovir-resistant strain. *Clin Infect Dis* 1993;17:854–856.

183. Cohen BA. Prognosis and response to therapy of cytomegalovirus encephalitis and meningomyelitis in AIDS. *Neurology* 1996;46:444–450.

184. Enting RH, Esselink RA, Portegies P. Lymphomatous meningitis in AIDS-related systemic non-Hodgkins lymphoma: a report of eight cases. *J Neurol Neurosurg Psychiatry* 1994;57:150–153.

185. So YT, Holtzman DM, Abrams DJ, et al. Peripheral neuropathy associated with acquired immunodeficiency syndrome: prevalence and clinical features from a population-based survey. *Arch Neurol* 1988;45:945–948.

186. Cornblath DR, McArthur JC, Kennedy PGE, Witte AS, Griffin JW. Inflammatory demyelinating peripheral neuropathies associated with human T-cell lymphotropic virus type III infection. *Ann Neurol* 1987;21:32–40.

187. Thornton CA, Latif AS, Emmanuel JC. Guillain-Barré syndrome associated with human immunodeficiency virus infection in Zimbabwe. *Neurology* 1991;41:812–815.

188. Paton P, Poly H, Gonnaud P-M, et al. Acute meningoradiculitis concomitant with seroconversion to human immunodeficiency virus type 1. *Res Virol* 1990;141:427–433.

189. Cornblath DR, Asbury AK, Albers JW, et al. Research criteria for diagnosis of chronic inflammatory demyelinating polyneuropathy (CIDP). *Neurology* 1991;41:617–618.

190. Miller RG, Parry CJ, Pfae MW, et al. The spectrum of peripheral neuropathy associated with ARC and AIDS. *Muscle Nerve* 1988;11:857–863.

191. Berger JR, Difini JA, Swerdloff MA, Ayyar RD. HIV seropositivity in Guillain-Barré syndrome. *Ann Neurol* 1987;22:393–394.

192. Bradley WG, Verma A. Painful vasculitic neuropathy in HIV-1 infection: relief of pain with prednisone therapy. *Neurology* 1996;47:1446–1451.

193. Gherardi R, Belec L, Mhiri C, et al. The spectrum of vasculitis in human immunodeficiency virus infected patients. *Arthritis Rheum* 1993;8:1164–1174.

194. Libman BS, Quismorio FP Jr, Stimmler MM. Polyarteritis nodosa-like vasculitis in human immunodeficiency virus infection. *J Rheumatol* 1995;22:351–355.

195. Said G, Lacroix-Ciaudo C, Fujimura H, Blas C, Faux N. The peripheral neuropathy of necrotising arteritis: a clinicopathological study. *Ann Neurol* 1988;23:461–465.

196. Gherardi R, Lebargy F, Gaulard P, Mhiri C, Bernaudin JF, Gray F. Necrotizing vasculitis and HIV replication in peripheral nerves. *N Engl J Med* 1989;321:685–686.

197. Stricker RB, Sanders KA, Owen WF, Kiprov DD, Miller RG. Mononeuritis multiplex associated with cryoglobulinemia in HIV infection. *Neurology* 1992;42:2103–2105.

198. Calabrese LH, Estes M, Yen-Lieberman B, et al. Systemic vasculitis in association with human immunodeficiency virus infection. *Arthritis Rheum* 1989;32:569–576.

199. Anonymous. Needlestick transmission of HTLV-III from a patient infected in Africa. *Lancet* 1984;2:1376–1377.

200. Piette AM, Tusseau F, Vignon D, et al. Acute neuropathy coincident with seroconversion for anti-LAV/HTLV-III. *Lancet* 1986;I:852.

201. Wiselka MJ, Nicholson KG, Ward SC, Flower AJE. Acute infection with human immunodeficiency virus associated with facial nerve palsy and neuralgia. *J Infect* 1987;15:189–194.

202. Lewis EM, Mahawar S, Wesley AM, Bredesen DE. Cranial neuropathies in AIDS patients. International conference on AIDS. 1989; 5:450.

203. Brown MM, Thompson A, Goh BT, Forster GE, Swash M. Bells palsy and HIV infection. *J Neurol Neurosurg Psychiatry* 1988;51:425–426.

204. Janssen R, Saykin A, Kaplan J, et al. Neurological complications of human immunodeficiency virus infection in patients with lymphadenopathy syndrome. *Ann Neurol* 1988;23:49–55.

205. Barohn RJ, Gronseth GS, LeForce BR, et al. Peripheral nervous system involvement in a large cohort of human immunodeficiency virus-infected individuals. *Arch Neurol* 1993;50:167–171.

206. Simpson DM, Tagliati M, Grinnell J, Godbold J. Electrophysiological findings in HIV infection: association with distal symmetrical polyneuropathy and CD4 level [abstract]. *Muscle Nerve* 1994;17: 1113–1114.

207. Griffin JW, Crawford TO, Tyor WR, et al. Predominantly sensory neuropathy in AIDS: distal axonal degeneration and unmyelinated fiber loss. *Neurology* 1991;41[Suppl 1]:374.

208. Lange DJ, Britton CB, Younger DS, et al. The neuromuscular manifestations of human immunodeficiency virus infections. *Arch Neurol* 1988;45:1084–1088.

209. Fuller GN, Jacobs JM, Guiloff RJ. Nature and incidence of peripheral nerve syndromes in HIV infection. *J Neurol Neurosurg Psychiatry* 1993;56:372–381.

210. Cornblath DR, McArthur JC. Predominantly sensory neuropathy in patients with AIDS and AIDS-related complex. *Neurology* 1988;38: 794–796.

211. Grafe MR, Wiley CA. Spinal cord and peripheral nerve pathology in AIDS: the role of cytomegalovirus and human immunodeficiency virus. *Ann Neurol* 1989;25:561–566.

212. Apostolski S, McAlarney T, Quattrini A, et al. The gp120 glycoprotein of human immunodeficiency virus type 1 binds to sensory ganglion neurons. *Ann Neurol* 1993;34:855–863.

213. Rizzuto N, Cavallaro T, Monaco S, et al. Role of HIV in the pathogenesis of distal symmetric peripheral polyneuropathy. *Acta Neuropathol* 1995;90:244–250.

214. Vital A, Beylot M, Vital C, Dleors B, Bloch B, Julien J. Morphological findings on peripheral nerve biopsies in 15 patients with human immunodeficiency virus infection. *Acta Neuropathol* 1992;83: 618–623.

215. Wesselingh SL, Power C, Fox R, et al. Cytokine messenger RNA expression in HIC-associated neurological disease. *J Cell Biochem* 1993;117D[Suppl]:78.

216. Simpson DM, Tagliati M. Nucleoside analogue-associated peripheral neuropathy in human immunodeficiency virus infection. *J Acq Immun Def Syndr Hum Retrovirol* 1995;9:153–161.

217. Berger AR, Arezzo JC, Schaumburg HH, et al. 2,3-Dideoxycytidine (ddC) toxic neuropathy. *Neurology* 1993;43:358–362.

218. Fichtenbaum CJ, Clifford DB, Powderly WG. Risk factors for dideoxynucleoside-induced toxic neuropathy in patients with the human immunodeficiency virus infection. *J Acq Immun Def Syndr Hum Retrovirol* 1995;10:169–174.

219. Famularo G, Moretti S, Marcellini S, et al. Acetyl-carnitine deficiency in AIDS patients with neurotoxicity on treatment with antiretroviral nucleoside analogues. *AIDS* 1997;11:185–190.

220. Lewis W, Dalakas MC. Mitochondrial toxicity of antiviral drugs. *Nat Med* 1995;1:417–422.

221. Bozzette SA, Santangelo J, Villasana D, et al. Peripheral nerve function in persons with asymptomatic or minimally symptomatic HIV disease: absence of zidovudine neurotoxicity. *J AIDS* 1991;4: 851–855.

222. Simpson DM, Wolfe DE. Neuromuscular complications of HIV infection and its treatment. *AIDS* 1991;5:917–926.

223. Brenneman DE, Buzy JM, Ruff MR, Pert CB. Peptide T sequences prevent neuronal cell death produced by the envelope glycoprotein (gp120) of the HIV virus. *Drug Dev Res* 1988;15:361–369.

224. Simpson DM, Dorfman D, Olney RK, et al. Peptide T in the treatment of painful distal neuropathy associated with AIDS: results of a placebo-controlled trial. *Neurology* 1996;47:1254–1259.

225. Lipkin WI, Parry G, Kiprov D, Abrams D. Inflammatory neuropathy in homosexual men with lymphadenopathy. *Neurology* 1985;35: 1479–1483.

226. Small PM, McPhaul LW, Sooy CD, Wofsy CB, Jacobson MA. Cytomegalovirus infection of the laryngeal nerve presenting as hoarseness in patients with acquired immunodeficiency syndrome. *Am J Med* 1989;86:108–110.

227. So YT, Olney RK. The natural history of mononeuritis multiplex and simplex in HIV infection. *Neurology* 1991;41[Suppl 1]:375.

228. Roullet E, Asseurus V, Gozlan J, et al. Cytomegalovirus multifocal neuropathy in AIDS: analysis of 15 cases. *Neurology* 1994;44: 2174–2182.

229. Said G, Lacroix C, Chemoulli P, et al. Cytomegalovirus neuropathy in acquired immunodeficiency syndrome: a clinical and pathological study. *Ann Neurol* 1991;29:139–146.

230. Berger JR, Flaster M, Schatz N, et al. Cranial neuropathy heralding otherwise occult AIDS-related large cell lymphoma. *J Clin Neurophthalmol* 1993;13:113–118.

231. Gherardi RK, Baudrimont M, Lionnet Fet al. Skeletal muscle toxoplasmosis in patients with acquired immunodeficiency syndrome: a clinical and pathological study. *Ann Neurol* 1992;32:535–542.

232. Belec L, Costanzo B, Georges AJ, Gherardi RK. HIV infection in African patients with tropical myositis. *AIDS* 1991;5:234.

233. Chevalier X, Amoura Z, Viard JP, Souissi P, Sobel A, Gherardi RK. Muscle lymphoma in patients with AIDS: a diagnostic problem with pyomyositis. *Arthritis Rheum* 1993;36:426–427.

234. Illa I, Nath A, Dalakas M. Immunocytochemical and virological characterisitics of HIV-associated inflammatory myopathies: similarities with seronegative polymyositis. *Ann Neurol* 1991;29:474–481.

235. Bohan A, Peter JB. Polymyositis and dermatomyositis. *N Engl J Med* 1975;292:344–347, 403–407.

236. Simpson DM, Citak KA, Godfrey E, Godbold J, Wolfe DE. Myopathies associated with human immunodeficiency virus and zidovudine. Can their effects be distinguished? *Neurology* 1993;43: 971–976.

237. Simpson DM, Slasor P, Dafni U, Berger J, Fischl MA, Hall C. Analysis of myopathy in a placebo-controlled zidovudine trial. *Muscle Nerve* 1997;20:382–385.

238. Wrzolek MA, Sher JH, Kozlowski PB, Rao C. Skeletal muscle pathology in AIDS: an autopsy study. *Muscle Nerve* 1990;13:508–515.

239. Seidman R, Peress N, Nuovo GJ. In situ detection of polymerase chain reaction-amplified HIV-1 nucleic acids in skeletal muscle in patients with myopathy. *Mod Pathol* 1994;7:369–375.

240. Leon-Monzon M, Lamperth L, Dalakas M. Search for HIV proviral DAN and amplified sequences in the muscle biopsies of patients with polymyositis. *Muscle Nerve* 1993;16:408–413.

241. Gherardi RK, Florea-Strat A, Fromont G, Poron F, Sabourin J-C, Authier J. Cytokine expression in the muscle of HIV infected patients: evidence for interleukin-1α accumulation in mitochondria of AZT fibers. *Ann Neurol* 1994;36:752–758.

242. Dalakas MC, Pezeshkpour GH, Flaherty M. Progressive nemaline (rod) myopathy associated with HIV infection. *N Engl J Med* 1987;317:1602–1603.

243. Dwyer BA, Mayer RF, Lee SC. Progressive nemaline rod myopathy as a presentation of human immunodeficiency virus infection. *Arch Neurol* 1992;49:440.

244. Higuchi I, Hashimoto K, Kashio N, et al. Detection of HTLV-1 provirus by in situ polymerase chain reaction in mononuclear inflammatory cells in skeletal muscle of viral carriers with polymyositis. *Muscle Nerve* 1995;18:854–858.

245. Wiley CA, Nerenberg M, Cros D, Soto-Aguilar M. HTLV-1 polymyositis in a patient also infected with the human immunodeficiency virus. *N Engl J Med* 1989;320:992–995.

246. Dickoff D, Simpson DM, Wiley CA, Mendelson SG, Farraye J, Wolfe DE, Wachsman W. HTLV-1 in acquired adult myopathy. *Muscle Nerve* 1993;16:162–165.

247. Cupler EJ, Leon-Monzon M, Semino-Mora C, Anderson TL, Dalakas MC. Inclusion body myositis in HIV-1 and HTLV-1 infected patients. *Brain* 1996;119:1887–1893.

248. Chariot P, Ruet E, Authier FJ, Levy Y, Gherardi RK. Acute rhabdomyolysis in patients infected by human immunodeficiency virus. *Neurology* 1994;44:1692–1696.

249. Mahe A, Bruet A, Chabin E, Fendler JP. Acute rhabdomyolysis coincident with primary HIV-1 infection [letter]. *Lancet* 1989;2:1454–1455.

250. Del Rio C, Soffer O, Widell JL, Judd RL, Slade BA. Acute human immunodeficiency virus infection temporally associated with rhabdomyolysis, acute renal failure, and nephrosis. *Rev Infect Dis* 1990; 12:282–285.

251. Lozano de Leon F, Gomez-Mateos JM, Iriarte LM, Garcia-Bragado F. Rhabdomyolysis in acute human immunodeficiency virus infection [letter]. *Med Clin* 1991;96:36–37.

252. Younger DS, Hays AP, Uncini A, Lange DJ, Lovelace RE, DiMauro S. Recurrent myoglobinuria and HIV seropositivity: incidental or pathogenic association? *Muscle Nerve* 1989;12:842–843.

253. Chan ISF, Neaton JD, Saravolatz LD, Crane LR, Osterberger J, for the Community Programs for Clinical Research on AIDS. Frequencies of opportunistic diseases prior to death among HIV-infected patients. *AIDS* 1995;9:1145–1151.

254. Berger JR, Pall L, Winfield D. Effect of anabolic steroids on HIV related wasting myopathy. *South Med J* 1993;86:865–866.

255. Simpson DM, Bender AN, Farraye J, et al. Human immunodeficiency virus wasting syndrome may represent a treatable myopathy. *Neurology* 1990;40:535–538.

256. Belec L, Mhiri C, Di Costanzo B, Gherardi RK. The HIV wasting syndrome. *Muscle Nerve* 1992;15:856–857.

257. Gherardi RK. Skeletal muscle involvement in HIV-infected patients. *Neuropathol Appl Neurobiol* 1994;20:232–237.

258. Hasset J, Tagliati M, Godbold J, et al. A placebo controlled study of prednisone in HIV-associated myopathy. *Neurology* 1994;44[Suppl]:A250.

259. Chalmers AC, Greco CM, Miller RG. Prognosis in AZT myopathy. *Neurology* 1991;41:1181–1184.

260. Dalakas MC, Illa I, Pezeshkpour GH, Laukaitis JP, Cohen B, Griffin JL. Mitochondrial myopathy caused by long-term zidovudine therapy. *N Engl J Med* 1990;322:1098–1105.

261. Manji H, Harrison MJG, Round JM, et al. Muscle disease, HIV and zidovudine: the spectrum of muscle disease in HIV-infected individuals treated with zidovudine. *J Neurol* 1993;240:479–488.

262. Consensus statement on the use of corticosteroids as adjunctive therapy for pneumocystis pneumonia in the acquired immunodeficiency syndrome. *N Engl J Med* 1990;323:1500–1504.

263. Berger JR, Pall L, Hall CD, Simpson DM, Berry PS, Dudley R. Oxandrolone in AIDS-wasting myopathy. *AIDS* 1996;10:1657–1662.

264. Simpson MV, Chin CD, Keilbough SA, Lin T-S, Prusoff WH. Studies on the inhibition of mitochondrial DNA replication of 3-azido-3-deoxythymidine and other dideoxynucleoside analogues which inhibit HIV replication. *Biochem Pharmacol* 1989;38:1033–1036.

265. Dalakas MC, Leon-Monzon ME, Bernardini I, Gahl WA, Jay CA. Zidovudine-induced mitochondrial myopathy is associated with muscle carnitine deficiency and lipid storage. *Ann Neurol* 1994;35:482–487.

266. Cupler EJ, Danon MJ, Jay C, Hench K, Ropka M, Dalakas MC. Early features of zidovudine-associated myopathy: histopathological findings and clinical correlations. *Acta Neuropathol* 1995;90:1–6.

267. Chariot P, Monnet I, Gherardi RK. Cytochrome c oxidase reaction improves histopathological assessment of zidovudine myopathy. *Ann Neurol* 1993;34:561–565.

268. Arnaudo E, Dalakas MC, Shanske S, Moraes CT, DiMauro S, Scon EA. Depeletion of muscle mitochondrial DNA in AIDS patients with zidovudine-induced myopathy. *Lancet* 1991;337:508–510.

269. Sinnwell TM, Sivakumar K, Soueidan S, et al. Metabolic abnormalities in skeletal muscle of patients receiving zidovudine therapy observed by 31-P in vivo magnetic resonance spectroscopy. *J Clin Invest* 1995;96:126–131.

270. Grau JM, Masanes F, Pedrol E, Caseademont J, Fernandez-Sola J, Urbano-Marquez A. Human immunodeficiency virus type 1 infection and myopathy: Clinical relevance of zidovudine therapy. *Ann Neurol* 1993;34:206–211.

271. Peters BS, Winer J, Landon DN, Stotter A, Pinching AJ. Mitochondrial myopathy associated with chronic zidovudine therapy in AIDS. *Q J Med* 1993;86:5–15.

272. Casademont J, Barrientos A, Grau JM, et al. The effect of zidovudine on skeletal muscle mtDNA in HIV-1 infected patients with mild or no muscle dysfunction. *Brain* 1996;119:1357–1364.

273. Morgello S, Wolfe DE, Godfrey E, Feinstein R, Tagliati M, Simpson DM. Mitochondrial abnormalities in human immunodeficiency virus-associated myopathy. *Acta Neuropathol* 1995;90:366–374.

274. Lane RJM, McLean KA, Moss J, Woodrow DF. Myopathy in HIV infection: the role of zidovudine and the significance of tubuloreticular inclusions. *Neuropathol Applied Neurobiol* 1993;19:406–413.

275. Miller RG, Carson PJ, Moussavi RS, et al. Fatigue and myalgia in AIDS patients. *Neurology* 1991;41:1603–1607.

276. Herzberg NH, Zorn I, Zwart R, Portegies P, Bolhuis PA. Major growth reduction and minor decrease in mitochondrial enzyme activity in cultured human muscle cells after exposure to zidovudine. *Muscle Nerve* 1992;15:706–710.

277. Lamperth L, Dalakas MC, Dagani F, Anderson J, Ferrari R. Abnormal skeletal and cardiac muscle mitochondria induced by zidovudine (AZT) in human muscle in vitro and in an animal model. *Lab Invest* 1991;65:742–751.

278. Reyes MG, Casanova J, Varricchio F, et al. Zidovudine myopathy [letter]. *Neurology* 1992;42:1252.

279. Cupler EJ, Hench K, Jay CA, et al. The natural history of zidovudine (AZT)-induced mitochondrial myopathy. *Neurology* 1994;44[Suppl 2]:A132.

280. Hoffman PM, Festaff BW, Giron CT, et al. Isolation of LAV/HTLV-3 from a patient with amyotrophic lateral sclerosis [letter]. *N Engl J Med* 1985;313:324–325.

281. Verma RK, Ziegler DK, Kepes JJ. HIV-related neuromuscular syndrome simulating motor neuron disease. *Neurology* 1990;40:544–546.

282. Simpson DM, Morgello S, Citak K, Corbo M, Latov N. Motor neuron disease associated with HIV and anti-asialo GM1 antibody. *Muscle Nerve* 1994;17:A1091.

283. Authier FJ, De Grissac N, Degos JD, Gherardi RK. Transient myasthenia gravis during HIV infection. *Muscle Nerve* 1995;18:914–916.

284. Wessel HB, Zitelli BJ. Myasthenia gravis associated with human T-cell lymphotropic virus type III infection. *Pediatr Neurol* 1987;3:238–239.

Motor Disorders,
edited by David S. Younger.
Lippincott Williams & Wilkins, Philadelphia © 1999.

CHAPTER 37

Neurotrophins and Nonneurotrophin Growth Factors: Impact on Motor and Other Systems

Douglas W. Zochodne

Recognition of the central and peripheral nervous systems as plastic and dynamic has led to hope that specific growth factors might yet protect the nervous system from disease, resurrect impaired connections, or support alternative pathways providing similar function. Recent advances in the understanding of these growth factors have identified several exciting concepts. First is the realization that motor systems, previously thought of as static in adults, have surprising responsiveness to certain growth factors after injury. Second is that a number of growth factors are elaborated by targets, sometimes in the periphery, and use retrograde transport to reach the cell body. Third is that growth factors can be synthesized by neurons and act on themselves in an autocrine fashion or on their neighbors in a paracrine fashion. Fourth is the understanding that growth factors have had tremendous redundancy in their actions. Although the absence of a given factor or its receptor may lead to severe developmental deficits, their deficiency appears to be compensated by the actions of other growth factors on shared receptors.

This chapter summarizes recent knowledge of growth factors that influence the peripheral and central nervous systems (CNS). These include the neurotrophin family of factors (Table 1). The first nerve growth factor (NGF) was identified over 40 years ago. Nonneurotrophin growth factors include ciliary neurotrophic factor (CNTF), insulin-like growth factors (IGFs), and glial-derived neurotrophic factor (GDNF). Specific animal models of disease that have used these growth factors are discussed. Finally, results of early clinical trials with these agents as available are presented.

D. W. Zochodne: Department of Clinical Neurosciences and The Neuroscience Research Group, University of Calgary and Department of Clinical Neurosciences, Foothills Hospital, Calgary, Alberta T2N 4N1, Canada.

NEUROTROPHINS

Neurotrophins are endogenous soluble proteins that regulate survival, growth, morphologic plasticity, and synthesis of proteins for the differentiated function of neurons (1). An important requirement is that the factor is retrogradely transported to the cells it putatively supports. NGF was described in 1953 by Levi-Montalcini and Hamburger (2) as a soluble factor isolated from mouse sarcoma tumors capable of inducing hyperplasia in sympathetic ganglia by stimulating neurite outgrowth. Five members of this family have now been described, each acting on a related tyrosine kinase (Trk) receptor: NGF, brain-derived neurotrophic factor (BDNF) (3,4), neurotrophin-3 (NT-3) (5,6), NT-4/5 (7), and NT-6 (8). NGF, NT-3, and BDNF are all transported retrogradely into sensory neurons of the dorsal root ganglia (DRG) of adult rats (9–11). BDNF is also retrogradely transported by motor neurons (11). Although there is overlap in receptor specificity, the primary receptors for these proteins have been labeled Trk A for NGF, Trk B for BDNF and NT-4/5, and Trk C for NT-3. Trk receptors mediate differentiation, survival, and loss of the proliferative capacity of subpopulations of neuronal cells through a number of intracellular second messengers. The survival benefit is conferred by blocking apoptotic cell death. Curiously, however, BDNF, NT-3, and NT-4/5 had the opposite effect of actually enhancing necrotic cell death (12). An additional low affinity receptor, p75, originally described in relationship to NGF, is probably responsive to all members of the neurotrophin family. p75 also appears to be required for retrograde transport of BDNF and NT-4/5 (13).

The interaction of a neurotrophin with its Trk receptor has been described in some detail. Neurotrophin dimers bind to Trk receptors to cause Trk dimerization and tyrosine autophosphorylation of Trk (14). Autophosphoryla-

TABLE 1. *Neurotrophins and other growth factors*

	Receptor	Target tissue (PNS)
Classic neurotrophins and their peripheral nerve targets		
Nerve growth factor (NGF)	TrkA, p75	Small fiber sensory neurons
		Sympathetic neurons
Brain-derived neurotrophic factor (BDNF)	TrkB, p75	Motor neurons
		Sensory neurons
Neurotrophin-3(NT-3)	TrkC, p75	Large sensory neurons
		Sympathetic neurons
		Motor neurons
Neurotrophin-4/5 (NT-4/5)	TrkB, p75	Motor neurons
		Sensory neurons
		Sympathetic neurons
Neurotrophin-6 (NT-6)	?	?
Other growth factors		
Factors that act on the gp 130 receptor complex		
Ciliary neurotrophic factor (CNTF)		
Leukemia inhibitory factor (LIF)		
Cardiotrophin-1 (CT-1)		
Growth factors discovered in other tissues with actions on the nervous system		
Basic fibroblast growth factor (bFGF)		
Acidic fibroblast growth factor (aFGF)		
Epidermal growth factor (EGF)		
Transforming growth factors alpha and beta (TGF beta, TGF alpha)		
Insulin-related growth factors		
Insulin		
Insulin-like growth factor I and II (IGFI and IGFII)		
Cytokines		
Interleukin-1		
Interleukin-6		
?Interleukin-11		
Other		
Glial-derived neurotrophic factor (GDNF)		

tion, in turn, activates several intracellular pathways (15). Neuron populations appear to support themselves and perhaps their neighboring cells in an autocrine (self-supporting) or paracrine (locally supporting) fashion using neurotrophin–Trk interactions (Fig. 1). This has been described in DRG where both Trk C and NT-3 transcripts are produced, that is, the factor and the receptor produced by the same population of cells (16). Evidence of the importance of this autocrine loop has been illustrated by Acheson et al. (17). They demonstrated that adult sensory ganglia cells in culture had a reduced survival when exposed to BDNF antisense oligonucleotides. The autocrine actions of neurotrophins have been suggested as a mechanism used by adult neurons to compensate for variations in target tissue support of neurons. In neonates, target support is critical for neuronal survival, whereas it is not in adults, perhaps because of autocrine support (18).

The role of the p75 receptor is still being sorted out, but it may act together with Trk receptors to enhance neurotrophin actions or as an influence of retrograde transport (13,19). Surprisingly, p75 may also mediate apoptosis, in contrast to the usual action of neurotrophins on Trk receptors (20).

There are complex interactions of the classic neurotrophins with other nonneurotrophin growth factors. For example, CNTF and leukemia inhibitory factor (LIF) (see below) may antagonize NGF actions on DRG neurons (21). Another example is the modulation of chick embryonic sensory neuron NT-3– and NT-4–mediated survival by transforming growth factor beta and LIF (22).

Nerve Growth Factor

NGF and its high affinity receptor, Trk A, have trophic actions that appear to be largely, but not exclusively, confined to small sensory and sympathetic neurons. Trk A receptors are required for survival of developing sympathetic neurons (23). Because Trk A receptors are particularly expressed in sensory and sympathetic cell populations, the influence of NGF directly on motor systems may be limited. Mice with Trk A knockout have severe neuronal loss in sensory and sympathetic ganglia and loss in the cholinergic forebrain, all incompatible with prolonged survival (24). There is evidence, however, that NGF may stimulate BDNF transcription (25,26). The roles of NGF and Trk A in counteracting axotomy-

Possible actions of neurotrophins and other growth factors on neurons

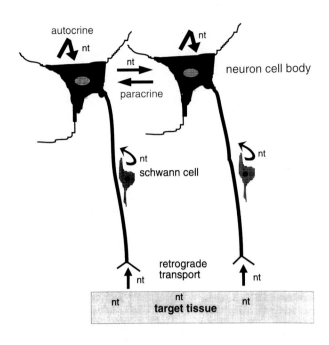

nt-neurotrophin or other growth factor

FIG. 1. Simplified scheme of routes of neurotrophin actions on neurons.

induced changes in DRG neurons have been reviewed in detail by Verge et al. (27). NGF is capable of reversing both the decline in peptide and protein expression after axotomy (substance P, alpha and beta calcitonine gene-related peptide [CGRP], neurofilament M subunit, Trk A, p75, fluoride-resistant acid phosphatase) and neuronal atrophy. In addition, NGF prevents increases in other cellular constituents after axotomy (galanin, NPY, VIP, and CCK) (27).

NGF administered in supraphysiologic doses may have hyperplastic actions. Intraventricular administration of high doses of NGF induced sprouting of sensory fibers, sympathetic fibers, and Schwann cell hyperplasia in a curious subpial distribution in rats (28). Intraventricular administration of NGF into the rat CNS prompted sprouting of cerebrovascular perivascular catecholamine sympathetic fibers (29).

Brain-derived Nerve Factor

BDNF was first identified in conditioned media of glioma cell lines and was subsequently isolated as a small basic protein from porcine CNS tissue (3,30,31). BDNF supports the survival of and neurite outgrowth from neural placode-derived sensory ganglia but, unlike NGF, not sympathetic neurons (32). BDNF is a potent motor neuron survival factor, rescuing neonatal spinal and cra-

nial motor neurons from death after axotomy (33,34). At least some survival mediating properties of BDNF would appear to act by enhancing the action of the antiapoptotic factor Bcl-2 (35). Targeted disruption of the BDNF gene (BDNF knockout) is associated with only a few weeks of animal survival and loss of vestibular and DRG neurons but not of facial motor neurons (36). In contrast, knock-out of the BDNF receptor gene, Trk B, is associated with yet earlier animal death after birth and loss of both spinal and cranial motor and DRG neurons (37). This discrepancy indicates that BDNF alone is not required to support motor neuron survival, whereas other neurotrophins, perhaps NT-4/5, are needed to activate the Trk B neurotrophin receptor.

In axotomized hypoglossal motor axons, loss of cholinergic immunoreactivity was prevented by central infusions of BDNF or NT-4/5 but not NGF or NT-3 (38,39). Interestingly, the injured motoneurons expressed Trk B receptors, known to bind BDNF and NT-4/5, and p75 but not Trk A or Trk C, which bind NGF and NT-3, respectively. BDNF is retrogradely transported to motor neurons after nerve section, Trk B has increased synthesis in motor neurons after section, and skeletal muscle has increased synthesis of BDNF after denervation (11, 40,41). BDNF production is also upregulated in Schwann cells after denervation (42), and it has been argued that its apparent upregulation in skeletal muscle after denervation may in fact be a result of Schwann cell proliferation in denervated intramuscular nerve stumps (43). Like other neurotrophins, it is not certain whether intraventricular infusion of BDNF might be of benefit because there are truncated nonfunctional Trk B receptors on ependymal cells (44,45). BDNF action is modulated by the inhibitory effects of abnormal truncated (lacking the Trk component) Trk B receptors because they form heterodimers with full-length receptors and inactivate them (46). BDNF acting through Trk B enhances synaptic efficacy in the hippocampus (47), enhances NMDA receptor maturation of cultured mouse cerebellar granule cells (48), and may play a role in the development of neuromuscular junctions (49,50). BDNF, NT-3, and NT-4/5, but not NGF, each increase the innervation of human muscle fibers cocultured with rat spinal cord explants (51). BDNF transcript is increased in rat brain after experimental cortical impact injuries (52). As discussed above, other trophic agents may influence BDNF. For example, NGF acting through Trk A regulates the BDNF transcription in DRG cells (25,26).

Neurotrophin 3

NT-3 is a 119 amino acid basic protein that exerts its actions as a dimer (6,53,54). Although NT-3 primarily binds to Trk C and p75, there is also weak binding to Trk B (55). Like Trk B, Trk C also exists in truncated nonfunctional forms (56). Like NGF, NT-3 may be thought of as a chiefly sensory neurotrophin, with supporting actions on large cell afferents that relay such information as muscle spindle activity and proprioception. NT-3 is retrogradely transported, particularly to large sensory neurons in DRG (11,33), and is expressed in muscle spindles (57). After axotomy in rats, NT-3 supports a population of larger sensory neurons not supported by NGF: NT-3 reverses axotomy-related changes in neurofilament subunit expression, p75 expression, and Trk C (27). In culture, NT-3 supports muscle sensory neurons (5). NT-3 supports the survival and differentiation of motor neurons and potentiates neuromuscular synapses in culture (58–60) but has no influence on adult sympathetic neurons (61). Although the actions of NT-3 are mediated through Trk C, there is evidence that cooperative activation of Trk B and C, perhaps in part through NT-3, is important in promoting survival of other cell types such as hippocampal neurons and cerebellar granule neurons (62). In addition, Trk B and Trk C transcripts appear in developing nigrostriatal neurons, indicating important development regulation of BDNF and NT-3 on this system (63). During development, NT-3 appears critical in the development of proprioceptive, nodose and auditory sensory neurons, and sympathetic neurons (64). NT-3–deficient transgenic mice have severe loss of sensory neurons, particularly spinal proprioceptive afferents and peripheral sensory organs (65). Trk C-deficient mice have loss of muscle sensory spindle afferents (66). In addition to its production by DRG neurons, spinal motor neurons appear to produce NT-3 during development (16). Like BDNF, NT-3 may also play a role in the development of neuromuscular junctions (50). NT-3 also enhances sprouting of corticospinal tracts during development and after lesions and rescues adult central noradrenergic cells (67,68).

Other Neurotrophins

NT-4/5 is another member of the neurotrophin family and supports the survival of developing sensory and sympathetic neurons (7). NT-4/5 differs from other neurotrophins in that it has more widespread distribution, suggesting its expression is less prone to environmental signals. Also, efficient signaling and retrograde transport both appear to depend particularly on the presence of the p75 receptor (69). NT-4/5 derived from muscle acts as an activity-dependent trophic signal for adult rat motor neurons (70). Like BDNF, NT-4/5 prevents axotomy-related facial motor neuron loss in newborn rats and changes in adult motor neuron choline acetyltransferase (71,72).

NONNEUROTROPHIN GROWTH FACTORS

Ciliary Neurotrophic Factors and Family

CNTF, initially described to support the survival of sympathetic neurons in the embryonic chick ciliary gan-

glion, is a 200 amino acid protein. CNTF is classified as a member of the alpha helical cytokine superfamily that includes LIF, interleukin 6, granulocyte colony-stimulating factor, and oncostatin M (73,74). CNTF, LIF, and a new growth factor, cardiotrophin-1, have receptor properties that are related, attributed to a signaling transducer known as gp130. In peripheral nerve, CNTF mRNA is detectable in Schwann cells but appears to require axonal contact to maintain its level (75). CNTF can be retrogradely transported by motor and sensory axons, and this transport is accelerated after a nerve lesion (76). CNTF protects developing motor neurons from cell death (77,78). In the adult, CNTF prevents neuronal degeneration of axotomized medial septal neurons (79) and of axotomized substantia nigra dopaminergic neurons (80). Systemic injections appear to induce sprouting by adult motor neurons (81,82). LIF rescued neonatal motor and sensory neurons after axotomy (83,84).

Insulin and Insulin-like Growth Factors

An important nonneurotrophin family of growth factors are the IGFs that are structurally related to insulin and were previously identified as somatomedins. IGF-I and IGF-II are single-chain polypeptides with A and B domains resembling those of insulin, a connecting C domain found in proinsulin but not in insulin, and a D domain (85). IGF-1, -2, and insulin all interact with the IGF-1 transmembrane Trk receptor that resembles the insulin receptor (86,87). IGF-2 also interacts with its own receptor, but the function of this receptor is less well understood (88). The actions of IGF are modulated by the presence of six IGF-binding proteins in the circulation and in tissues (89). IGF-1, IGF-1 receptor, and IGF-binding protein type 5 all appear to be locally elaborated in the microenvironment of injured peripheral nerves through Schwann cells (90). The influence of IGFs and insulin on the nervous system have only been recently examined. These actions may be quite diverse. For example, IGF-1 blocked toxin-induced apoptosis in cerebellar neurons in culture (91). The autocrine-paracrine promotion of hippocampal neuron survival involves interesting collaborative actions of IGF-1 and BDNF (92).

Glial-derived Neurotrophic Factor

GDNF belongs to the transforming growth factor beta family and supports midbrain dopaminergic neurons, Purkinje cells, and spinal motor neurons (93,94). GDNF also supported survival of GABAergic embryonic neurons transplanted intraocularly into adult rats (95). GDNF enhanced survival of motor neurons in culture and prevented axotomy related loss of newborn rat facial motor neurons (96). Indeed, the actions of GDNF were more potent than those of BDNF, CNTF, or LIF. In adults,

GDNF is expressed in skeletal muscle and transported retrogradely by motor nerves. It prevents axotomy-induced changes in choline acetyltransferase (ChAT) immunoreactivity in the facial nucleus (96,97). GDNF has demonstrated potential usefulness in experimental parkinsonism by supporting dopaminergic nigral cells (see below).

Growth Factors of Other Tissues

The fibroblast growth factor (FGF) family (98) includes acidic FGF and basic FGF (bFGF). FGFs exists in multiple molecular weight forms and appear to be liberated from the extracellular matrix by heparin (99). Both acidic FGF and bFGF have supporting actions in cell culture systems, where they prevent neuronal apoptotic cell death during development. bFGF may influence cholinergic differentiation (98). One difficulty in studying the FGFs is the possibility that some of their apparent neuronal trophic actions may be indirect because they come from glial or supporting cells (98). Some studies have evaluated FGF in models of neurologic disease. For example, unilateral cortical infarction in rats treated with acidic FGF increased the concentration of NGF and NGF transcript ipsilateral to the lesion (100). bFGF potentiated motor neuron sprouting by CNTF (82). bFGF rescued adult DRG cells in rats after a sciatic nerve section (101).

Additional growth factors not dealt with here but that have actions on the nervous system include epidermal growth factor (102) and the transforming growth factors alpha and beta (103).

Cytokines

Brain trauma appears to activate expression of NGF through interleukin-1β (104). Interleukin-1 from macrophages stimulates NGF production in peripheral nerves by nonneuronal cells (105). Interleukin-6 may be a directly acting growth factor (106). Inflammation may generate several growth factors that have actions on neurons beyond those of the interleukins (107).

Novel Growth Factors

A number of substances have been described as potential trophins in the nervous system but are not discussed in further detail: extracellular nucleotides and nucleosides (108), arachidonic acid (109), and CGRP are indirect promoters of nerve regeneration by their action as a mitogen for Schwann cells (110). Cysteine-rich neurotrophic factor is a newly identified non-neurotrophin growth factor isolated from the mollusk Lymnae stagnalis. Cysteine-rich neurotrophic factor promotes neurite outgrowth and influences motor neuron electrophysiologic properties apparently by acting on the p75 receptor (111).

NEUROTROPHINS, OTHER GROWTH FACTORS, AND HUMAN DISEASE

Motor Disorders

Retrograde changes in motor neurons after axotomy may have relevance in the ability of human motor neurons to restore function after injury. Changes in lower motor neurons have already been discussed. BDNF and NT-3 prevented axotomy-induced death of adult rat corticospinal neurons (112). Motor neuron degeneration in the wobbler mouse, a model of human motor neuron disease (MND), is slowed by BDNF (113). In this condition, an autosomal recessive disease, there is muscle wasting and limb paralysis leading to difficulty with walking (114). Treatment of the wobbler mice was yet more efficacious if BDNF was combined with CNTF (115). Treatment of progressive motor neuronopathy (pmn) in mice, another autosomal recessive model of human MND, was more successful with CNTF than GDNF (116,117).

Experimental Parkinsonism

The impact of growth factors on the substantia nigra, of relevance to human Parkinson disease, has been studied in a number of ways. Striatal neurons in culture have interesting but differential trophic support from several growth factors including IGF-1, NT-3, and bFGF (118). Neurotrophins provide protection against experimental parkinsonism induced by the toxin MPP+ in the striatum of neonatal rats. Kirschner et al. (119) reported that NGF, BDNF, bFGF, and NT-5 but not NT-3 were protective. NGF-producing neural stem cells transplanted into the striatum provided substantial protection against an excitotoxic lesion (120). Infusion of NT-4/5 but not NT-3 enhanced the function of nigral grafts in the rat model of parkinsonism induced by 6-hydroxydopamine (121). Fibroblast grafts producing BDNF protected against 6-hydroxydopamine loss of substantial nigra pars compacta domaminergic neurons in adult rat (122). BDNF and NT-4/5 also reversed alterations in neurotransmitter message induced by 6-hydroxydopamine (OHDA) (123,124). GDNF has demonstrated benefit in 6-OHDA, axotomy, and MPTP models of nigral injury in experimental parkinsonism (123–126).

Nerve Regeneration

The impact of growth factors on regenerating nerves has been mixed. Because neurotrophins turn off features of the cell body regeneration program, their potential impact on fiber regeneration is uncertain. He et al. (127) have suggested that NGF improves motor nerve regeneration. In another study, CNTF, delivered locally by a miniosmotic pump, improved regeneration of the rat sciatic nerve after transection, whereas NGF was not effective

(128). IGF-II has also been reported to increase the rate of sensory axon regeneration in sciatic nerves (129).

Peripheral Neuropathies

Peripheral neuropathies with involvement of motor fibers, sensory fibers, or both may be treatable by neurotrophins and other growth factors. The axotomy model has provided a great deal of information about target tissue influences on motor and sensory neurons. It has relevance for understanding neuropathy because retrograde changes in perikaryal properties and peptide expression, both of which are regulated by neurotrophins after a distal axonal insult, might have considerable bearing on their later ability to regenerate. Most experimental neuropathies have concentrated on sensory deficits. For example, Tomlinson et al. (130) suggested that NGF and NT-3 were of benefit in experimental diabetic neuropathy by reversing DRG changes in peptide expression and axonal conduction velocity deficits, respectively. The possible role of neurotrophins in diabetes has been reviewed in greater depth elsewhere (131). IGFs have been suggested as treatment for diabetic neuropathy because their levels are reduced in diabetes and because they may ameliorate the neural changes observed in experimental models of diabetes (132). Insulin itself, either by its actions on insulin receptors or by cross-occupying IGF-1 receptors, is capable of reversing conduction abnormalities in experimental diabetes independently of glycemic control, suggesting a possible trophic action (133). Anand (134) noted decreased skin NGF levels in diabetic patients and patients with leprosy. Because the axonal damage in leprosy is secondary to mycobacterium infection rather than NGF deficiency, the findings present the interesting possibility that skin denervation results in secondary NGF loss.

An important mechanism of recovery in any neuropathy is collateral sprouting. Collateral sprouting of motor and sensory fibers helps to reinnervate targets denervated from proximal lesions to nerves that are not likely to repair by regeneration. Diamond et al. (135) demonstrated that NGF supports collateral but not regenerative sensory sprouting. NT-3 was of benefit in the large fiber sensory neuropathy caused by high doses of pyridoxine (136), and NGF repaired the loss of DRG peptides in experimental taxol neuropathy (137). NGF has also been reported to be of benefit in cisplatin neuropathy (138).

Other

Trk B and Trk C mRNA transcripts decline in the spinal motor neurons of rats with aging, suggesting that loss of trophic support could account for motor deficits observed in elderly patients (139). Kokaia et al. (140) noted transient rises in BDNF, NGF, and Trk B expression in experimental cerebral infarcts of rats due to middle cerebral artery occlusion, suggesting that endogenous BDNF and NGF could play a role in recovery from human cerebral infarcts. Growth factors may also play a role in the repair from spinal cord injury. Nakahara et al. (141) implanted grafts of fibroblasts genetically modified to secrete NGF, NT-3, or bFGF into the central canal region of adult rat spinal cords. Sensory and noradrenergic dorsal root fibers were attracted into the graft, although BDNF grafts had no influence. Human chronic infusion of NT-3 and BDNF promoted CNS axonal regeneration through bridged semipermeable guidance channels in transected rat thoracic spinal cords (142).

One other interesting possible use of neurotrophins is to enhance activity or survival of fetal neuronal grafts in adults. Sinson et al. (143) used this strategy in rats with fluid percussion brain injuries. NGF did not enhance transplant survival but apparently improved memory.

EARLY CLINICAL TRIALS

An important criterion for the use of neurotrophins in human CNS and peripheral nervous system disorders is whether they penetrate the blood–brain and blood–nerve barriers. Poduslo and Curran (144) provided information on the permeability surface area of the trophins noting the following order of permeability: BDNF $\approx$ NT-3 > CNTF >> NGF for both the blood–nerve and blood–brain barriers.

Motor Neuron Disease

There has been particular interest in the use of neurotrophins or other growth factors in the treatment of MND. At the time of this writing, multicenter phase III trials of subcutaneously injected CNTF and BDNF have unfortunately been negative (145; Amgen Inc., personal communication). CNTF was associated with injection site reactions, cough, asthenia, nausea, anorexia, weight loss, and unexpected increased salivation, and there was an increased mortality rate with higher doses (145). A current trial studying intraventricular infusion of GDNF in patients with MND is underway (Amgen Inc., personal communication). Phase II trials of IGF-1 in MND are underway, but specific results have not yet been published (146,147). Some problems with subcutaneous IGF-1 in other clinical trials have included tachycardia, dyspnea, hypoglycemia, hypotension, and microvascular proliferation (148). Potential future trials of trophic agents might include combinations to provide some synergy of action.

Polyneuropathy

Phase II clinical trials of NT-3 and NGF in diabetic polyneuropathy have been completed, but details are not yet published (25,149). In phase I safety studies of healthy human volunteers, recombinant human NGF caused localized tenderness at the injection site, local pressure allodynia, and a lowering of heat pain thresholds (150). Some of these changes occurred at early times, indicating a local rather than central action. Petty et al. (151) noted myalgia at higher doses. A phase II trial of BDNF in Guillain-Barré syndrome with axonal degeneration was initiated but was prematurely terminated. It may be that a combination of NGF and NT-3 to support sensory neurons and BDNF to support motor neurons would be a rational approach to the treatment of mixed motor and sensory polyneuropathies that have axonal degeneration.

Other

Some benefits from IGF-1 have been reported in myotonic dystrophy in phase II studies (152) . NGF has been considered a potential treatment for disease of cholinergic neurons in Alzheimer disease, whereas BDNF, NT-3, and GDNF have been considered to be possible treatments for Parkinson disease (153). Perhaps one potential route to treatment of these conditions would be a stereotactic implantation of cells genetically engineered to secrete growth factors into the brains of patients with Alzheimer or Parkinson disease. This and other novel and interesting approaches toward trophin delivery are likely to be explored over the next few years.

ACKNOWLEDGMENTS

Brenda Boake provided expert secretarial assistance. Barbara Proksa reviewed the manuscript. The author was supported by the Alberta Heritage Foundation for Medical Research as a Medical Scholar and has received grant support from the Muscular Dystrophy Association of Canada and the Medical Research Council of Canada.

REFERENCES

1. Hefti F, Dento TL, Knusel B, Lapchak PA. Neurotrophic factors: what are they and what are they doing? In: Loughlin SE, Fallon JH, eds. *Neurotrophic factors*. Toronto: Academic Press, 1993:25–49.
2. Levi-Montalcini R, Hamburger V. A diffusible agent of mouse sarcoma, producing hyperplasia of sympathetic ganglia and hyperneurotization of viscera in the chick embryo. *J Exp Zool* 1953;123:233–287.
3. Barde Y-A, Edgar D, Thoenen H. Purification of a new neurotrophic factor from mammalian brain. *EMBO J* 1982;1:549–553.
4. Leibrock J, Lottspeich F, Hohn A, et al. Molecular cloning and expression of brain-derived neurotrophic factor. *Nature* 1989;341:149–152.
5. Hory-Lee F, Russell M, Lindsay RM, Frank E. Neurotrophin 3 supports the survival of developing muscle sensory neurons in culture. *Proc Natl Acad Sci USA* 1993;90:2613–2617.
6. Maisonpierre PC, Belluscio L, Squinto S, et al. Neurotrophin-3: a neurotrophic factor related to NGF and BDNF. *Science* 1990;247:1446–1451.
7. Berkemeier LR, Winslow JW, Kaplan DR, Nikolics K, Goeddel DV, Rosenthal A. Neurotrophin-5: a novel neurotrophic factor that activates trk and trkB. *Neuron* 1991;7:857–866.
8. Gotz R, Koster R, Winkler C, et al. Neurotrophin-6 is a new member of the nerve growth factor family. Nature 1994;372:266–269.
9. Hendry IA, Stockel K, Thoenen H, Iversen LL. The retrograde axonal transport of nerve growth factor. *Brain Res* 1974;68(1):103–121.
10. Schmidt RE, Yip HK. Retrograde axonal transport in rat ileal mesenteric nerves. Characterization using intravenously administered 125I-nerve growth factor and effect of chemical sympathectomy. *Diabetes* 1985;34:1222–1229.
11. DiStefano PS, Friedman B, Radziejewski C, et al. The neurotrophins BDNF, NT-3, and NGF display distinct patterns of retrograde axonal transport in peripheral and central neurons. *Neuron* 1992;8(5):983–993.
12. Koh JY, Gwag BJ, Lobner D, Choi DW. Potentiated necrosis of cultured cortical neurons by neurotrophins. *Science* 1995;268:573–575.
13. Curtis R, Adryan KM, Stark JL, et al. Differential role of the low affinity neurotrophin receptor (p75) in retrograde axonal transport of the neurotrophins. *Neuron* 1995;14:1201–1211.
14. Jing S, Tapley P, Barbacid M. Nerve growth factor mediates signal transduction through trk homodimer receptors. *Neuron* 1992;9:1067–1079.
15. Glass DJ, Yancopoulos GD. The neurotrophins and their receptors. *Trends Cell Biol* 1993;3:262–268.
16. Tojo H, Takami K, Kaisho Y, et al. Analysis of neurotrophin-3 expression using the lacZ reporter gene suggests its local mode of neurotrophic activity. *Neuroscience* 1996;71:221–230.
17. Acheson A, Conover JC, Fandl JP, et al. A BDNF autocrine loop in adult sensory neurons prevents cell death. *Nature* 1995;374:450–453.
18. Lindsay RM. Role of neurotrophins and trk receptors in the development and maintenance of sensory neurons: an overview. *Philos Trans R Soc Lond B Biol Sci* 1996;351:365–373.
19. Chao MV, Hempstead BL. p75 and Trk: a two receptor system. *Trends Neurosci* 1995;18:321–326.
20. Rabizadeh S, Oh J, Zhong L-T, et al. Induction of apoptosis by the low-affinity NGF receptor. *Science* 1993;261:345–348.
21. Mulderry PK. Neuropeptide expression by newborn and adult rat sensory neurons in culture: effects of nerve growth factor and other neurotrophic factors. *Neuroscience* 1994;59:673–688.
22. Krieglstein K, Unsicker K. Distinct modulatory actions of TGF-beta and LIF on neurotrophin-mediated survival of developing sensory neurons. *Neurochem Res* 1996;21:843–850.
23. Fagan AM, Zhang H, Landis S, Smeyne RJ, Silos-Santiago I, Barbacid M. Trk A, but not Trk C, receptors are essential for survival of sympathetic neurons in vivo. *J Neurosci* 1996;16:6208–6218.
24. Smeyne RJ, Klein R, Schnapp A, et al. Severe sensory and sympathetic neuropathies in mice carrying a disrupted Trk/NGF receptor gene. *Nature* 1994;368:246–249.
25. Apfel SC, Wright D, Dromia C, et al. Nerve growth factor stimulates BDNF mRNA expression in the peripheral nervous system. *Soc Neursci Abstr* 1995;21:196.
26. Apfel SC, Wright DE, Wiideman AM, Dormia C, Snider WD, Kessler JA. Nerve growth factor regulates the expression of brain-derived neurotrophic factor mRNA in the peripheral nervous system. *Mol Cell Neurosci* 1996;7:134–142.
27. Verge VM, Gratto KA, Karchewski LA, Richardson PM. Neurotrophins and nerve injury in the adult. *Philos Trans R Soc Lond B Biol Sci* 1996;351:423–430.
28. Winkler J, Ramirez GA, Kuhn HG, et al. Reversible Schwann cell hyperplasia and sprouting of sensory and sympathetic neurites after intraventricular administration of nerve growth factor. *Ann Neurol* 1997;41:82–93.
29. Isaacson LG, Billieu SG. Increased perivascular norepinephrine following intracerebroventricular infusion of NGF into adult rats. *Exp Neurol* 1996;139:54–60.
30. Monard D, Solomon F, Rentsch M, Gysin R. Glia-induced morphological differentiation in neuroblastoma cells. *Proc Natl Acad Sci USA* 1973;70:1894–1897.
31. Monard D, Stockel K, Goodman R, Thoenen H. Distinction between nerve growth factor and glial factor. *Nature* 1975;258:444–445.
32. Lindsay RM, Rohrer H. Placodal sensory neurons in culture: nodose ganglion neurons are unresponsive to NGF, lack NGF receptors but are supported by a liver-derived neurotrophic factor. *Dev Biol* 1985;112:30–48.
33. Yan Q, Elliott JL, Matheson C, et al. Influences of neurotrophins on mammalian motoneurons in vivo. *J Neurobiol* 1993;24:1555–1577.
34. Oppenheim RW, Yin QW, Prevette D, Yan Q. Brain-derived neurotrophic factor rescues developing avian motoneurons from cell death. *Nature* 1992;360:755–757.

35. Allsopp TE, Kiselev S, Wyatt S, Davies AM. Role of Bcl-2 in the brain-derived neurotrophic factor survival response. *Eur J Neurosci* 1995;7:1266–1272.

36. Jones KR, Farinas L, Backus C, Reichardt LF. Targeted disruption of the BDNF gene perturbs brain and sensory neuron development but not motor neuron development. *Cell* 1994;76:989–999.

37. Klein R, Smeyne RJ, Wurst W, et al. Targeted disruption of the trkB neurotrophin receptor gene results in nervous system lesions and neonatal death. *Cell* 1993;75:113–122.

38. Tuszynski MH, Mafong E, Meyer S. Central infusions of brain-derived neurotrophic factor and neurotrophin-4/5, but not nerve growth factor and neurotrophin-3, prevent loss of the cholinergic phenotype in injured adult motor neurons. *Neuroscience* 1996;71:761–771.

39. Yan Q, Matheson C, Lopez OT, Miller JA. The biological responses of axotomized adult motoneurons to brain-derived neurotrophic factor. *J Neurosci* 1994;14:5281–5291.

40. Koliatsos VE, Clatterbuck RE, Winslow JW, Cayouette MH, Price DL. Evidence that brain-derived neurotrophic factor is a trophic factor for motor neurons in vivo. *Neuron* 1993;10:359–367.

41. Piehl F, Frisen J, Risling M, Hokfelt T, Cullheim S. Increased trkB mRNA expression by axotomized motoneurones. *NeuroReport* 1994; 5:697–700.

42. Meyer M, Matsuoka I, Wetmore C, Olson L, Thoenen H. Enhanced synthesis of brain-derived neurotrophic factor in the lesioned peripheral nerve: different mechanisms are responsible for the regulation of BDNF and NGF mRNA. *J Cell Biol* 1992;119:45–54.

43. Griesbeck O, Parsadanian AS, Sendtner M, Thoenen H. Expression of neurotrophins in skeletal muscle: quantitative comparison and significance for motoneuron survival and maintenance of function. *J Neurosci Res* 1995;42:21–33.

44. Yan Q, Matheson C, Sun J, Radeke MJ, Feinstein SC, Miller JA. Distribution of intracerebral ventricularly administered neurotrophins in rat brain and its correlation with trk receptor expression. *Exp Neurol* 1994;127:23–36.

45. Anderson KD, Alderson RF, Altar CA, et al. Differential distribution of exogenous BDNF, NGF, and NT-3 in the brain corresponds to the relative abundance and distribution of high-affinity and low-affinity neurotrophin receptors. *J Comp Neurol* 1995;357:296–317.

46. Eide FF, Vining ER, Eide BL, Zang K, Wang XY, Reichardt LF. Naturally occurring truncated trkB receptors have dominant inhibitory effects on brain-derived neurotrophic factor signaling. *J Neurosci* 1996;16:3123–3129.

47. Levine ES, Dreyfus CF, Black IB, Plummer MR. Selective role for trkB neurotrophin receptors in rapid modulation of hippocampal synaptic transmission. *Brain Res Mol Brain Res* 1996;38:300–303.

48. Muzet M, Dupont JL. Enhancement of NMDA receptor maturation by BDNF in cultured mouse cerebellar granule cells. *NeuroReport* 1996;7:548–552.

49. Kwon YW, Gurney ME. Brain-derived neurotrophic factor transiently stabilizes silent synapses on developing neuromuscular junctions. *J Neurobiol* 1996;29:503–516.

50. Wang T, Xie K, Lu B. Neurotrophins promote maturation of developing neuromuscular synapses. *J Neurosci* 1995;15:4796–4805.

51. Braun S, Croizat B, Lagrange MC, Warter JM, Poindron P. Neurotrophins increase motoneurons' ability to innervate skeletal muscle fibers in rat spinal cord-human muscle cocultures. *J Neurol Sci* 1996;136:17–23.

52. Yang K, Perez-Polo JR, Mu XS, et al. Increased expression of brain-derived neurotrophic factor but not neurotrophin-3 mRNA in rat brain after cortical impact injury. *J Neurosci Res* 1996;44:157–164.

53. Hohn A, Leibrock J, Bailey K, Barde YA. Identification and characterization of a novel member of the nerve growth factor/brain-derived neurotrophic factor family. *Nature* 1990;344:339–341.

54. Radziejewski C, Robinson RC, DiStefano PS, Taylor JW. Dimeric structure and conformational stability of brain-derived neurotrophic factor and neurotrophin-3. *Biochemistry* 1992;31:4431–4436.

55. Chao MV. Neurotrophin receptors: a window into neuronal differentiation. *Neuron* 1992;9:583–593.

56. Valenzuela DM, Maisonpierre PC, Glass DJ, et al. Alternative forms of rat Trk C with different functional capabilities. *Neuron* 1993;10: 963–974.

57. Copray JC, Brouwer N. Selective expression of neurotrophin-3 messenger RNA in muscle spindles of the rat. *Neuroscience* 1994;63: 1125–1135.

58. Wong V, Arriaga R, Ip NY, Lindsay RM. The neurotrophins BDNF, NT-3 and NT-4/5, but not NGF, up-regulate the cholinergic phenotype of developing motor neurons. *Eur J Neurosci* 1993;5:466–474.

59. Henderson CE, Camu W, Mettling C, et al. Neurotrophins promote motor neuron survival and are present in embryonic limb bud. *Nature* 1993;363:266–270.

60. Lohof AM, Ip NY, Poo M-M. Potentiation of developing neuromuscular synapses by the neurotrophins NT-3 and BDNF. *Nature* 1993; 363:350–353.

61. Birren SJ, Lo L, Anderson DJ. Sympathetic neuroblasts undergo a developmental switch in trophic dependence. *Development* 1993;119: 597–610.

62. Minichiello L, Klein R. Trk B and Trk C neurotrophin receptors cooperate in promoting survival of hippocampal and cerebellar granule neurons. *Genes Dev* 1996;10:2849–2858.

63. Jung AB, Bennett JP Jr. Development of striatal dopaminergic function. III. Pre-and postnatal development of striatal and cortical mRNAs for the neurotrophin receptors Trk BTK+ and Trk C and their regulation by synaptic dopamine. *Brain Res* 1996;94:133–143.

64. Chalazonitis A. Neurotrophin-3 as an essential signal for the developing nervous system. *Mol Neurobiol* 1996;12:39–53.

65. Farinas I, Jones KR, Backus C, Wang XY, Reichardt LF. Severe sensory and sympathetic deficits in mice lacking neurotrophin-3. *Nature* 1994;369:658–661.

66. Klein R, Silos-Santiago I, Smeyne RJ, et al. Disruption of the neurotrophin-3 receptor gene trkC eliminates Ia muscle afferents and results in abnormal movements. *Nature* 1994;368:249–251.

67. Schnell L, Schneider R, Kolbeck R, Barde YA, Schwab ME. Neurotrophin-3 enhances sprouting of corticospinal tract during development and after adult spinal cord lesion. *Nature* 1994;367:170–173.

68. Arenas E, Persson H. Neurotrophin-3 prevents the death of adult central noradrenergic neurons in vivo. *Nature* 1994;367:368–371.

69. Ibanez CF. Neurotrophin-4: the odd one out in the neurotrophin family. *Neurochem Res* 1996;21:787–793.

70. Funakoshi H, Belluardo N, Arenas E, et al. Muscle-derived neurotrophin-4 as an activity-dependent trophic signal for adult motor neurons. *Science* 1995;268:1495–1499.

71. Koliatsos VE, Cayouette MH, Berkemeier LR, Clatterbuck RE, Price DL, Rosenthal A. Neurotrophin 4/5 is a trophic factor for mammalian facial motor neurons. *Proc Natl Acad Sci USA* 1994;91: 3304–3308.

72. Friedman B, Kleinfeld D, Ip NY, et al. BDNF and NT-4/5 exert neurotrophic influences on injured adult spinal motor neurons. *J Neurosci* 1995;15:1044–1056.

73. Bazan JF. Neuropoietic cytokines in the hematopoietic fold. *Neuron* 1991;7:197–208.

74. Hall AK, Rao MS. Cytokines and neurokines: related ligands and related receptors. *Trends Neurosci* 1992;15:35–37.

75. Sendtner M, Stöckli KA, Thoenen H. Synthesis and localization of ciliary neurotrophic factor in the sciatic nerve of the adult rat after lesion and during regeneration. *J Cell Biol* 1992;118:139–148.

76. Curtis R, Adryan KM, Zhu Y, Harkness PJ, Lindsay RM, DiStefano PS. Retrograde axonal transport of ciliary neurotrophic factor is increased by peripheral nerve injury. *Nature* 1993;365:253–255.

77. Arakawa Y, Sendtner M, Thoenen H. Survival effect of ciliary neurotrophic factor (CNTF) on chick embryonic motoneurons in culture: comparison with other neurotrophic factors and cytokines. *J Neurosci* 1990;10:3507–3515.

78. Sendtner M, Kreutzberg GW, Thoenen H. Ciliary neurotrophic factor prevents the degeneration of motor neurons after axotomy. *Nature* 1990;345:440–441.

79. Hagg T, Quon D, Higaki J, Varon S. Ciliary neurotrophic factor prevents neuronal degeneration and promotes low affinity NGF receptor expression in the adult rat CNS. *Neuron* 1992;8:145–158.

80. Hagg T, Varon S. Ciliary neurotrophic factor prevents degeneration of adult rat substantia nigra dopaminergic neurons in vivo. *Proc Natl Acad Sci USA* 1993;90:6315–6319.

81. Kwon YW, Gurney ME. Systemic injections of ciliary neurotrophic factor induce sprouting by adult motor neurons. *NeuroReport* 1994;5: 789–792.

82. Gurney ME, Yamamoto H, Kwon Y. Induction of motor neuron sprouting in vivo by ciliary neurotrophic factor and basic fibroblast growth factor. *J Neurosci* 1992;12:3241–3247.

83. Cheema SS, Richards L, Murphy M, Bartlett PF. Leukemia inhibitory

factor prevents the death of axotomised sensory neurons in the dorsal root ganglia of the neonatal rat. *J Neurosci Res* 1994;37:213–218.

84. Cheema SS, Richards LJ, Murphy M, Bartlett PF. Leukaemia inhibitory factor rescues motoneurones from axotomy-induced cell death. *NeuroReport* 1994;5:989–992.

85. LeRoith D, Roberts CT, Jr. Insulin-like growth factors. *Ann NY Acad Sci* 1993;692:1–9.

86. Ullrich A, Gray A, Tam AW, et al. Insulin-like growth factor I receptor primary structure: comparison with insulin receptor suggests structural determinants that define functional specificity. *EMBO J* 1986;5:2503–2512.

87. Steele-Perkins G, Turner J, Edman JC, et al. Expression and characterization of a functional human insulin-like growth factor I receptor. *J Biol Chem* 1988;263:11486–11492.

88. Morgan DO, Edman JC, Standring DN, et al. Insulin-like growth factor II receptor as a multifunctional binding protein. *Nature* 1987;329:301–307.

89. Baxter RC, Martin JL. Binding proteins for the insulin-like growth factors: structure, regulation and function. *Prog Growth Factor Res* 1989;1:49–68.

90. Cheng HL, Randolph A, Yee D, Delafontaine P, Tennekoon G, Feldman EL. Characterization of insulin-like growth factor-I and its receptor and binding proteins in transected nerves and cultured Schwann cells. *J Neurochem* 1996;66:525–536.

91. Fernandez-Sanchez MT, Garcia-Rodriguez A, Diaz-Trelles R, Novelli A. Inhibition of protein phosphatases induces IGF-1-blocked neurotrophin-insensitive neuronal apoptosis. *FEBS Lett* 1996;398:106–112.

92. Lindholm D, Carroll P, Tzimagiogis G, Thoenen H. Autocrine-paracrine regulation of hippocampal neuron survival by IGF-1 and the neurotrophins BDNF, NT-3 and NT-4. *Eur J Neurosci* 1996;8:1452–1460.

93. Lin LF, Doherty DH, Lile JD, Bektesh S, Collins F. GDNF: a glial cell line-derived neurotrophic factor for midbrain dopaminergic neurons. *Science* 1993;260:1130–1132.

94. Mount HT, Dean DO, Alberch J, Dreyfus CF, Black IB. Glial cell line-derived neurotrophic factor promotes the survival and morphologic differentiation of Purkinje cells. *Proc Natl Acad Sci USA* 1995;92:9092–9096.

95. Price ML, Hoffer BJ, Granholm AC. Effects of GDNF on fetal septal forebrain transplants in oculo. *Exp Neurol* 1996;141(2):181–189.

96. Henderson CE, Phillips HS, Pollock RA, et al. GDNF: a potent survival factor for motoneurons present in peripheral nerve and muscle. *Science* 1994;266:1062–1064.

97. Yan Q, Matheson C, Lopez OT. In vivo neurotrophic effects of GDNF on neonatal and adult facial motor neurons. *Nature* 1995;373:341–344.

98. Unsicker K, Grothe C, Ludecke G, et al. Fibroblast growth factors: their roles in the central and peripheral nervous system. In: Louglin SE, Fallon JH, eds. *Neurotrophic factors.* Toronto: Academic Press, 1993:313–338.

99. Lobb RR. Clinical applications of heparin-binding growth factors. *Eur J Clin Invest* 1988;18:321–336.

100. Figueiredo BC, Pluss K, Skup M, Otten U, Cuello AC. Acidic FGF induces NGF and its mRNA in the injured neocortex of adult animals. *Brain Res Mol Brain Res* 1995;33:1–6.

101. Otto D, Unsicker K, Grothe C. Pharmacological effects of nerve growth factor and fibroblast growth factor applied to the transectioned sciatic nerve on neuron death in adult rat dorsal root ganglia. *Neurosci Lett* 1987;83:156–160.

102. Morrison R. Epidermal growth factor: structure, expression and functions in the central nervous system. In: Louglin SE, Fallon JH, eds. *Neurotrophic factors.* Toronto: Academic Press, 1993:339–357.

103. Puolakkainen P, Twardzik DR. Transforming growth factors alpha and beta. In: Loughlin SE, Fallon JH, eds. *Neurotrophic factors.* Toronto: Academic Press, 1993:359–389.

104. DeKosky ST, Styren SD, O'Malley ME, et al. Interleukin-1 receptor antagonist suppresses neurotrophin response in injured rat brain. *Ann Neurol* 1996;39:123–127.

105. Lindholm D, Heumann R, Meyer M, Thoenen H. Interleukin 1 regulates synthesis of nerve growth factor in non neuronal cells of rat sciatic nerve. *Nature* 1987;330:658–659.

106. Otten UH, Gradient RA. Post natal expression of interleukin-6 (IL-6) and 1L-6 receptor transcripts in the peripheral nervous system. *Soc Neurosci Abstr* 1995;21:35.

107. Richardson PM, Lu X. Inflammation and axonal regeneration. *J Neurol* 1994;242[Suppl 1]:S57–S60.

108. Neary JT, Rathbone MP, Cattabeni F, Abbracchio MP, Burnstock G. Trophic actions of extracellular nucleotides and nucleosides on glial and neuronal cells. *Trends Neurosci* 1996;19:13–18.

109. Katsuki H, Okuda S. Arachidonic acid as a neurotoxic and neurotrophic substance. *Prog Neurobiol* 1995;46:607–636.

110. Cheng L, Khan M, Mudge AW. Calcitonin gene-related peptide promotes Schwann cell proliferation. *J Cell Biol* 1995;129:789–796.

111. Fainzilber M, Smit AB, Syed NI, et al. CRNF, a molluscan neurotrophic factor that interacts with the p75 neurotrophin receptor. *Science* 1996;274:1540–1543.

112. Giehl KM, Tetzlaff W. BDNF and NT-3, but not NGF, prevent axotomy-induced death of rat corticospinal neurons in vivo. *Eur J Neurosci* 1996;8:1167–1175.

113. Ikeda K, Klikosz B, Green T, et al. Effects of brain-derived neurotrophic factor (BDNF) on motor dysfunction in wobbler mouse motor neuron disease. *Ann Neurol* 1995;37:505–511.

114. Mitsumoto H, Bradley WG. Murine motor neuron disease (the wobbler mouse): degeneration and regeneration of the lower motor neuron. *Brain* 1982;105(Pt 4):811–834.

115. Mitsumoto H, Ikeda K, Klinkosz B, Cedarbaum JM, Wong V, Lindsay RM. Arrest of motor neuron disease in wobbler mice cotreated with CNTF and BDNF. *Science* 1994;265:1107–1110.

116. Sagot Y, Tan SA, Baetge E, Schmalbruch H, Kato AC, Aebischer P. Polymer encapsulated cell lines genetically engineered to release ciliary neurotrophic factor can slow down progressive motor neuronopathy in the mouse. *Eur J Neurosci* 1995;7(6):1313–1322.

117. Sagot Y, Tan SA, Hammang JP, Aebischer P, Kato AC. GDNF slows loss of motoneurons but not axonal degeneration or premature death of pmn/pmn mice. *J Neurosci* 1996;16:2335–2341.

118. Nakao N, Odin P, Lindvall O, Brundin P. Differential trophic effects of basic fibroblast growth factor, insulin-like growth factor-1, and neurotrophin-3 on striatal neurons in culture. *Exp Neurol* 1996;138:144–157.

119. Kirschner PB, Jenkins BG, Schulz JB, et al. NGF, BDNF and NT-5, but not NT-3 protect against MPP+ toxicity and oxidative stress in neonatal animals. *Brain Res* 1996;713:178–185.

120. Martinez-Serrano A, Bjorklund A. Protection of the neostriatum against excitotoxic damage by neurotrophin-producing, genetically modified neural stem cells. *J Neurosci* 1996;16:4604–4616.

121. Haque NS, Hlavin ML, Fawcett JW, Dunnett SB. The neurotrophin NT4/5, but not NT3, enhances the efficacy of nigral grafts in a rat model of Parkinson's disease. *Brain Res* 1996;712:45–52.

122. Levivier M, Przedborski S, Bencsics C, Kang UJ. Intrastriatal implantation of fibroblasts genetically engineered to produce brain-derived neurotrophic factor prevents degeneration of dopaminergic neurons in a rat model of Parkinson's disease. *J Neurosci* 1995;15:7810–7820.

123. Sauer H, Wong V, Bjorklund A. Brain-derived neurotrophic factor and neurotrophin-4/5 modify neurotransmitter-related gene expression in the 6-hydroxydopamine-lesioned rat striatum. *Neuroscience* 1995;65:927–933.

124. Sauer H, Rosenblad C, Bjorklund A. Glial cell line-derived neurotrophic factor but not transforming growth factor beta 3 prevents delayed degeneration of nigral dopaminergic neurons following striatal 6-hydroxydopamine lesion. *Proc Natl Acad Sci USA* 1995;92:8935–8939.

125. Beck KD, Valverde J, Alexi T, et al. Mesencephalic dopaminergic neurons protected by GDNF from axotomy-induced degeneration in the adult brain. *Nature* 1995;373:339–341.

126. Tomac A, Lindqvist E, Lin LF, et al. Protection and repair of the nigrostriatal dopaminergic system by GDNF in vivo. *Nature* 1995;373:335–339.

127. He C, Chen Z, Chen Z. Enhancement of motor nerve regeneration by nerve growth factor. *Microsurgery* 1992;13:151–154.

128. Newman JP, Verity AN, Hawatmeh S, Fee WE Jr, Terris DJ. Ciliary neurotrophic factor enhances peripheral nerve regeneration. *Arch Otolaryngol Head Neck Surg* 1996;122:399–403.

129. Glazner GW, Lupien S, Miller JA, Ishii DN. Insulin-like growth factor II increases the rate of sciatic nerve regeneration in rats. *Neuroscience* 1993;54:791–797.

130. Tomlinson DR, Fernyhough P, Diemel LT. Neurotrophins and peripheral neuropathy. *Philos Trans R Soc Lond B Biol Sci* 1996;351:455–462.

131. Zochodne DW. Neurotrophins and other growth factors in diabetic neuropathy. *Semin Neurol* 1996;16:153–161.

132. Ishii DN. Implication of insulin-like growth factors in the pathogenesis of diabetic neuropathy. *Brain Res Brain Res Rev* 1995;20:47–67.

133. Singhal A, Cheng C, Sun H, Zochodne DW. Near nerve local insulin prevents conduction slowing in experimental diabetes. *Brain Res* 1997;763:209–214.

134. Anand P. Neurotrophins and peripheral neuropathy. *Philos Trans R Soc Lond B Biol Sci* 1996;351:449–454.

135. Diamond J, Holmes M, Coughlin M. Endogenous NGF and nerve impulses regulate the collateral sprouting of sensory axons in the skin of the adult rat. *J Neurosci* 1992;12:1454–1466.

136. Helgren ME, Torrento K, DiStefano PS, et al. NT-3 attenuates proprioceptive deficits in the adult rat with a large fiber neuropathy. *Soc Neurosci Abstr* 1994;20:455.

137. Schmidt Y, Unger JW, Bartke I, Reiter R. Effect of nerve growth factor on peptide neurons in dorsal root ganglia after taxol or cisplatin treatment and in diabetic (db/db) mice. *Exp Neurol* 1995;132:16–23.

138. Apfel SC, Lipton RB, Arezzo JC, Kessler JA. Nerve growth factor prevents toxic neuropathy in mice. *Ann Neurol* 1991;29:87–90.

139. Johnson H, Hokfelt T, Ulfhake B. Decreased expression of Trk B and Trk C mRNAs in spinal motoneurons of aged rats. *Eur J Neurosci* 1996;8:494–499.

140. Kokaia Z, Zhao Q, Kokaia M, et al. Regulation of brain-derived neurotrophic factor gene expression after transient middle cerebral artery occlusion with and without brain damage. *Exp Neurol* 1995;136:73–88.

141. Nakahara Y, Gage FH, Tuszynski MH. Grafts of fibroblasts genetically modified to secrete NGF, BDNF, NT-3, or basic FGF elicit differential responses in the adult spinal cord. *Cell Transplant* 1996;5:191–204.

142. Xu XM, Guenard V, Kleitman N, Aebischer P, Bunge MB. A combination of BDNF and NT-3 promotes supraspinal axonal regeneration into Schwann cell grafts in adult rat thoracic spinal cord. *Exp Neurol* 1995;134:261–272.

143. Sinson G, Voddi M, McIntosh TK. Combined fetal neural transplantation and nerve growth factor infusion: effects on neurological outcome following fluid-percussion brain injury in the rat. *J Neurosurg* 1996;84:655–662.

144. Poduslo JF, Curran GL. Permeability at the blood-brain and blood-nerve barriers of the neurotrophic factors: NGF, CNTF, NT-3, BDNF. *Brain Res Mol Brain Res* 1996;36:280–286.

145. Miller RG, Petajan JH, Bryan WW, et al. A placebo-controlled trial of recombinant human ciliary neurotrophic (rhCNTF) factor in amyotrophic lateral sclerosis. *Ann Neurol* 1996;39:256–260.

146. Murphy M, Reid K, Hilton DJ, Bartlett PF. Generation of sensory neurons is stimulated by leukemia inhibitory factor. *Proc Natl Acad Sci USA* 1991;88:3498–3501.

147. Murphy MF, Felice K, Gawel M, et al. A double-blind, placebo-controlled study of myotrophin (CEP-151) in the treatment of amyotrophic lateral sclerosis. *Ann Neurol* 1995;38:335.

148. Le Roith D. Seminars in medicine of the Beth Israel Deaconess Medical Center. Insulin-like growth factors. *N Engl J Med* 1997;336:633–640.

149. Apfel S, Adornato B, Cornblath D, et al. Clinical trial of recombinant human nerve growth factor (rhNGF) in peripheral neuropathy. *Neurology* 1995;45[Suppl 4]:A278.

150. Dyck PJ, Peroutka S, Rask C, et al. Intradermal recombinant human nerve growth factor induces pressure allodynia and lowered heat-pain threshold in humans. *Neurology* 1997;48:501–505.

151. Petty BG, Cornblath DR, Adornato BT, et al. The effect of systemically administered recombinant human nerve growth factor in healthy human subjects. *Ann Neurol* 1994;36:244–246.

152. Slonim AE, Rosenthal H, Manzione D, Goldberg T. Clinical trial of recombinant human insulin-like growth factor-1 in myotonic dystrophy. *Ann Neurol* 1995;38:334.

153. Ebendal T, Lonnerberg P, Pei G, et al. Engineering cells to secrete growth factors. *J Neurol* 1994;242[Suppl 1]:S5–S7.

PART V

Neurorehabilitation

Motor Disorders,
edited by David S. Younger.
Lippincott Williams & Wilkins, Philadelphia © 1999.

CHAPTER 38

Principles of Neuromuscular Rehabilitation

John R. Bach and Heakyung Kim

Once the diagnosis of a progressive neuromuscular disease is made, there is a tendency to inform the patient or family that there is no effective intervention. This is done despite the availability of physical medicine interventions that can in many instances prolong life without hospitalization or tracheostomy and, in virtually all instances, temporarily restore considerable function to the patient. The worst case scenario is advanced amyotrophic lateral sclerosis (ALS), in which 88 (1) to 97% (2) of lives are prolonged and function maximized by physical medicine interventions. In 1991, the Honorable Justice Sam Filer, stricken with advanced ALS and essentially no functional movement other than that of his eyelids for over 3 years, communicated the following by computer-driven voice synthesizer:

> Throughout the process of amyotrophic lateral sclerosis, I have learned many things. I have learned that having ALS does not necessarily mean a death sentence, that I am not living with a life-threatening disease, but rather with a life-enhancing condition. I have learned, moreover, that it is possible to continue to live a life of quality... I have learned that I have much to offer (3).

The judge is not at all unique. Other 24-hour ventilator users with advanced ALS or other severe neuromuscular conditions continue gainful employment and have a positive attitude about their lives (2). Optimism can be encouraged in similarly affected patients by making aspects of neuromuscular rehabilitation available in a multidisciplinary care program to optimize the patient's options.

J. R. Bach: Department of Physical Medicine and Rehabilitation, UMDNJ-The New Jersey Medical School, Newark, New Jersey 07103.

H. Kim: Department of Physical Medicine and Rehabilitation, UMDNJ-The New Jersey Medical School and Department of Rehabilitation Medicine, University Hospital, Newark, New Jersey 07103.

DEFINITIONS

A *disease* is a pathologic condition with a set of symptoms and signs. An *impairment* results from the loss or abnormality of psychologic, physical, or anatomic structures or function or disease therein (4). When an impairment prohibits the accomplishment of a task required for personal independence or physical well-being, then a *disability* is created. The World Health Organization defines disability as any restriction or lack resulting from an impairment of ability to perform an activity in the manner or within the range considered normal for a human being (4). For example, impairment of either respiratory muscle function, airway obstruction, or anatomic destruction of the lungs can lead to a disabled cough mechanism. To assess the status of the general abilities of patients, rehabilitation specialists evaluate activities that are normally performed on a daily basis to maintain personal independence, such as the ability to breathe, eat, bathe, groom, toilet, move about, and communicate, all of which have an impact on our capacity to live independently. When deficiencies are evident, then it is necessary to assist or substitute the abnormal body function with physical medicine aids.

According to the World Health Organization, a *handicap* is the disadvantage of a given individual that results from an impairment or a disability that limits or prevents the fulfillment of a role that is normal for that individual (4). Some patients with acquired immunodeficiency syndrome may be handicapped socially without being physically disabled. A child receiving full ventilatory support by an indwelling tracheostomy tube may be banned from attending school or even from returning home because, according to state regulations, the presence of an "open wound" necessitates continual family or nursing attention. The same patient using physical medicine aids for noninvasive ventilatory support might be permitted to return to the community (5,6).

Patients with neuromuscular impairments, can have resulting disability may be due to breathing dysfunction, skeletal muscle dysfunction, musculotendinous contractures, primary skeletal or cardiopulmonary pathology, poor endurance, other associated disease pathology, or some combination of impairments. The patient can be further handicapped by architectural barriers, public policies, inadequate finances, family support, or education. Clinicians should identify and differentiate the disease process, impairments, disabilities, and handicaps faced by the patient so that physical medicine interventions and psychosocial support can be instituted and the person returned to the fullest possible physical, mental, social, and economic independence. Physical medicine interventions pertain to the use of equipment or activities that may include noninvasive methods of ventilatory support and cough facilitation, exercises, range-of-motion, and surgical interventions based on pathokinesiologic principles to maximize breathing, coughing, nutrition, and physical functioning.

MANAGEMENT STAGES

It is useful to consider the example of the three clinical stages of Duchenne muscular dystrophy (DMD) (Table 1). The clinician who understands the management principles for DMD can apply them to patients with other neuromuscular conditions.

Ambulatory Stage

In this stage, the diagnosis of DMD is established and the patient and family are told about possible treatment interventions, and the major options in each subsequent management stage are discussed. This is particularly important for optimizing compliance for later surgical therapies to maintain leg function, prevent scoliosis, avoid later hospitalizations for pulmonary morbidity and tracheostomy, and to prolong survival without invasive measures. Psychological support is important to prevent feelings of guilt or sympathy from disrupted family psychodynamics, alienated family members, and to avert overprotection to the point of delaying the patient's emotional maturity and the assumption of self-directed activities and decision making.

Musculotendinous Contracture Management

The pathokinesiology of progressive gait difficulty has been described for DMD (7,8), but it applies equally well to other myopathies, childhood polymyositis, and spinal muscular atrophy (SMA). Asymmetric hip extensor weakness leads to anterior and lateral pelvic tilt, asymmetric hip flexor contractures, and accentuated lumbar lordosis. Tensor fascia lata and iliotibial band contractures lead to a wide-based gait with internal rotation and flexion at the knees. With increasing quadriceps weakness, the patient stabilizes the knee by keeping the weight line anterior to the knee, but it must also be kept behind the hips because of weak hip extensors. Intact plantar flexors encourage toe walking and lead to equinus deformity that initially stabilizes the knees. Iliotibial tract tightness increases the torque on the femur and flexes the knee until the center of gravity shifts from behind the hip to the front of the knees. Strong foot evertor and tibialis posterior muscles destabilize the subtalar joint and lead to falls on uneven surfaces and later on level surfaces. Unless aggressively treated, the average age of wheel-

---

TABLE 1. *Management principles for neuromuscular disease*

Ambulatory stage
1. Genetic counseling
2. Early counseling regarding future physical medicine options
3. Psychological support to prevent counterproductive family psychodynamics, to encourage goal oriented activities, and to prepare the patient to be a self-directed individual
4. Early prevention or reduction of musculotendinous and chest wall and lung contractures
5. Supportive physical and occupational therapy and possibly splinting and therapeutic exercise
6. Pathokinesiologically justified surgical and bracing interventions
7. Prevention of cardiac complications

Wheelchair-dependent stage
8. Maintenance of proper nutrition
9. Facilitation of activities of daily living
10. Early surgical prevention or correction of back deformity
11. Prevention of cardiac complications
12. Maintenance of pulmonary compliance and normal alveolar ventilation

Stage of prolonged survival
13. Facilitation of independence with assistive devices and methods
14. Prevention of cardiac complications
15. Use of physical medicine respiratory muscle aids to assist alveolar ventilatory and clear airway secretions
16. Augmentative communication
17. Quality of life considerations

chair dependence in DMD is 8.6 to 9.5 years (range, 6 to 15 years) (9–12).

Although leg weakness plays a major role in the eventual loss of walking, musculotendinous contractures destabilize the gait prematurely as seen by its prevention or early correction with bracing until walking ceases (13). An early prophylactic approach to preventing contractures depends on careful monitoring of the patient's muscle strength, articular range-of-motion, and ability to walk and rise from the floor (14). Surgically lengthening the Achilles tendon and hamstrings resection of the iliotibial bands, lengthening of hip flexor muscles, and transferring the tibialis posterior tendon to the dorsum of the foot to improve ankle dorsiflexors equalize strength in each joint. These are generally performed between ages 4 and 7 (Fig. 1) (14). These procedures are safer and better tolerated when performed early in the disease and require less postoperative physical therapy and stabilization gait. They also break the vicious cycle of weakness that leads to imbalance and contractures. Early surgical rehabilitation also reverses and prevents leg contractures during the ambulatory stage without long-term physical therapy, burdensome splinting, or bracing (13,14). Similar principles have been applied to patients with milder myopathies, but those with better proximal strength require only certain elements of the surgical intervention such as tendo-Achilles lengthening or tibialis posterior tendon transfer. Other approaches to the management of leg contractures include daily muscle stretching with or without concomitant bracing, stretching, and physical therapy (13,14). By comparison, in the 1950s, Paul (15) found a third of patients with DMD stopped walking before age 6 years. When contractures are prevented by early surgery and a short course of postoperative physical therapy, ongoing physical therapy and splinting are unnecessary.

The nighttime use of plaster casting in combination with physical therapy is another approach; however, they should be redone every 6 months, are extremely uncomfortable and therefore poorly tolerated, and effective programs place considerable long-term burden on patients and their families. It has been suggested that this approach maintains ambulation to age 10.3 years (16,17).

Early conservative management, then musculotendinous releases, resection of iliotibial bands, and long-leg bracing when the patient is approaching wheelchair dependence prolongs ambulation or at least the ability to stand (18,19), but this late intervention is less well tolerated and requires intensive postoperative physical therapy and the use of cumbersome, expensive, and often poorly tolerated long-leg braces.

Simple ankle–foot orthoses are not indicated for assisted ambulation in patients with neuromuscular disease unless the muscle weakness is limited to the ankles and knees. They can sometimes be used along with Lofstrand crutches after late surgical contracture releases. They slow the speed of walking and make rising from a chair or going up steps more difficult because of reduced knee flexion and ankle extension. In patients with Charcot-Marie-Tooth neuropathy and other conditions with primarily distal involvement, polypropylene ankle–foot orthoses relieve toe dragging and support pes cavus supinated feet. A plastic or metal ankle–foot orthosis with an adjustable locked ankle also provides knee and ankle control by improving tibial stability in these cases.

Maintaining Pulmonary Compliance

Just as frequent passive range-of-motion is necessary to maintain the integrity and mobility of peripheral extremity articulations, deep insufflations are important in patients with diminished vital capacity (VC) to maintain pulmonary compliance and adequate volumes for an effective cough (20). There are no published guidelines in the use of daily deep insufflations, but they are useful in patients with a VC of 50% or less of predicted normal, especially those in the stage of wheelchair dependence.

Exercise

Increased functional demands can be damaging to immature muscles, and dystrophic muscles are likewise more susceptible to overuse atrophy (21). Greater weakness was found in the preferred upper (22) and lower (23) extremities of dystrophic individuals than in the opposite nonpreferred limbs. Serum creatine kinase levels increase more so after exercise in dystrophic patients than in normal subjects. In patients with advanced weakness, even routine activities can cause overuse atrophy.

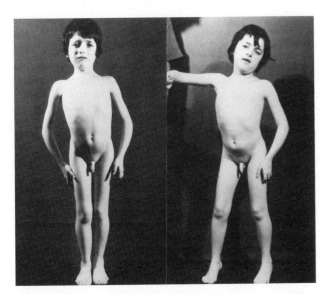

FIG. 1. Boy with Duchenne muscular dystrophy unable to stand without assistance before (right) and able to walk without assistance or bracing after (left) extensive release of lower extremity contractures and transfer of tibialis posterior muscles. (Photo courtesy of Dr. Yves Rideau.)

deLateur and Giaconi (24) found that strengthening and endurance training improved strength and slowed progression of weakness early in the course of DMD (24). Vignos and Watkins (25) noted a 50% increase in strength over 4 months, with gains usually maintained for a year after resistance exercise training of antigravity muscles. Milner-Brown and Miller (26) reported similarly increased strength and work tolerance and decreased fatigue in 20- to 53-year-old patients with facioscapulohumeral, myotonic, Becker, and limb-girdle muscular dystrophies; SMA; and assorted polyneuropathies. However, the initial strength had to be greater than 15 to 20% of normal. Fowler (27) suggested that dynamic high-resistance exercise training was potentially beneficial and resulted in gains in strength if the degree of weakness was not severe or if the rate of clinical progression and the intensity of the exercise program was relatively slow. However, the period of daily exercise was limited and took into account the individual's daily physical activity level. Unfortunately, exercise programs do not benefit the patients that need help the most. There is little evidence that they result in prolonged functional abilities. Fowler and Goodgold (28) recommended starting an exercise program early in the course of the disease, restricted to individuals with slowly progressive disorders, and the use of only submaximal resistance or high-repetition aerobic exercise. Similarly, Vignos and Watkins (25) recommended 2 to 3 hours of standing, walking, or swimming per day, as long as the patient felt rested after a night's sleep. All patients should be encouraged to stay active with activities they enjoy while avoiding muscle strain.

Cardiac Considerations

Although cardiac arrhythmias are rarely a problem in young neuromuscular patients, they can be life-threatening in those with Emery-Dreifuss muscular dystrophy who require close monitoring and possibly chemical treatment even during the ambulatory stage. Cardiac monitoring can usually be empirically delayed until the stage of wheelchair dependence.

Nutritional Considerations

Undernutrition results from the inability to feed oneself, swallowing impairments, shortness of breath, aspiration of food, the presence of an indwelling tracheostomy tube, decreased appetite due to bowel disturbances, restrictions of food textures and flavors, and impairment in taste, especially in those receiving tracheostomy and intermittent positive pressure ventilation (IPPV) (29).

Patients should be weighed regularly and weight changes considered in the context of their diseases. As little as a 10% loss of ideal weight can be associated with loss of physiologic adaptability and increased morbidity (30). This is particularly true in patients with impaired

pulmonary defense mechanisms. Food deprivation impairs respiratory muscle function by reducing available energy substrates. Diaphragm isometric strength (31,32), endurance, maximum static inspiratory and expiratory pressures (31,32), and maximum voluntary ventilation decrease during a fast (32), as does hypoxic (33,34) and hypercapnic (35) ventilatory drive. Ventilatory failure can also occur with chronic starvation. Rats restricted to a third of their normal caloric intake for 6 weeks developed emphysema-like lung changes (36), similar to the lesions found in starved individuals from Warsaw ghettos (37). Malnutrition impairs cell-mediated and humoral immunity (38,39) and alveolar macrophage phagocytic activity (40,41) and increases bacterial adherence to the lower airways in patients with tracheostomy tubes (42). In addition, deficiencies in specific nutrients can affect respiratory function.

Obesity may be a complicating factor and can compromise ventilatory dynamics. However, by the time a patient requires a ventilator, severe weight loss and undernutrition often supervene. The average weight of a DMD patient at the time of ventilator use was 70 pounds (43). The serum albumin and transferrin levels reflect the protein synthetic ability of the liver. Both have half-lives of just under 2 weeks; therefore, the serum levels reflect long-term, not short-term, changes in protein status. Retinol-binding protein and prealbumin are more useful for assessing short-term nutritional status because of the shorter half-life of 12 hours and 2 days, respectively (29). Other useful tests include total iron-binding capacity and serum vitamin A, C, and E levels.

Food intake can be assessed by use of a diet diary to compare calorie and nutrient intake with ideal quantities. However, the ideal intake levels of inactive patients differ from those in the general population. The following equation calculates the daily recommended caloric intake of children with DMD: Kcal = 2,000 - age (years) × 50 (44). For advanced DMD and other patients with neuromuscular disease, caloric needs may not exceed normal resting energy expenditure, estimated to be 110% of the basal metabolic rate. Patients commonly go from being able to eat foods of all consistencies to soft or pureed foods and later to high-calorie thick liquid nutritional supplements. Patients should be referred for gastrostomy when they can no longer be fed without aspiration, especially when there are signs of chronic undernutrition and arterial oxyhemoglobin desaturation due to aspiration of upper airway secretions.

Stage of Wheelchair Dependence

Scoliosis Prevention

Severe scoliosis develops in virtually all patients with SMA type I and II, in up to 90% of patients with DMD (45), and in many other childhood-onset neuromuscular disorders. The higher the plateau VC, that is, the highest

VC ever attained by the patient, the less likely is the development of scoliosis and the longer one can wait before intervening (46).

The usual indication for scoliosis-reduction surgery is a curvature of 40° or more in a patient who has failed thoracolumbar bracing and in whom cardiopulmonary function is adequate enough for reasonably safe intervention. Although this is appropriate for many patients with idiopathic and other nonneuromuscular forms of scoliosis, it is often inappropriate in patients with neuromuscular diseases. Wheelchair seating modifications and thoracolumbar bracing are useful in delaying surgical intervention in those with infantile SMA but should be avoided in patients with DMD because they do not affect the ultimate degree of curvature (47). In DMD, the delay in intervention until a curvature of 40° is obtained is usually associated with inadequate pulmonary function (Fig. 2) (48). In a third of patients with DMD and a relatively low plateau VC, waiting until the scoliotic curve attains 40° results in diminution of the VC to under 30% of predicted normal levels and virtually precluded surgical intervention (48).

Scoliosis develops early in childhood in patients with SMA. The most common approach to limit progression of their irreversible curvature is by total contact plastic thoracolumbar bracing to allow normal early vertebral growth, followed by spinal instrumentation and fusion after age 6 (49–51). Failure to prevent scoliosis results in a variety of sequelae: loss of the ability to sit because of the protrusion of the ribs into the abdominal wall, loss of balance and comfort when seated, the need for complicated and expensive seating modifications and custom seating systems, low back pain, compressive lumbar radiculopathies, ischial discomfort and skin breakdown, inability to use an intermittent abdominal pressure ventilator for ventilatory assistance (52), and hindrances in the use of mobile arm supports for self-feeding (53).

During the stage of wheelchair dependence, the presence of an excessive spinal curvature and the vital capacity should be monitored at 6-month intervals and surgical intervention recommended (48,54–57). Some investigators recommend prophylactic intervention in all patients (57). We recommend that DMD patients with a plateau VC below 1,500 mL undergo surgical intervention as soon as they are wheelchair dependent and have any pelvic obliquity. A plateau VC of 1,500 to 2,000 mL and a curvature of 20 to 40° are also indications for intervention. Patients with a plateau VC of more than 2,000 mL can safely delay intervention until the curve reaches 40°.

Of the surgical approaches to reduce scoliotic curves, some, but not all, include spinal fusion. Perhaps the ideal

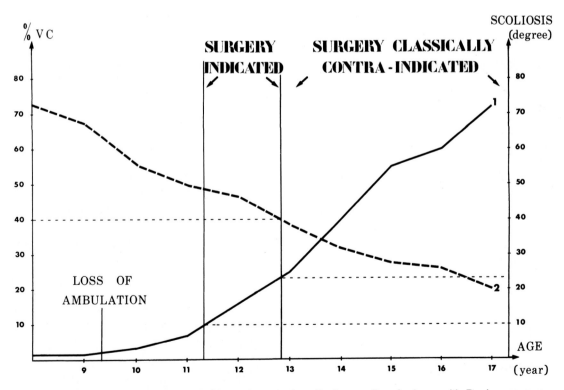

FIG. 2. This plot of vital capacity (VC) vs. degree of scoliosis over time for boys with Duchenne muscular dystrophy with low plateau VCs (about one third of Duchenne patients' VCs plateau below 1,600 mL before 14 years of age) shows that by the time scoliosis reaches 23°, the VC has decreased to 40% of predicted normal, thereby increasing the risk of general anesthesia and perioperative pulmonary complications. The safe surgical window is presented (between the solid lines).

method is not yet in general practice (46). Spinal fusion methods should be used for definitive interventions in all patients with DMD and nonfusion methods reserved for interventions deemed temporary as for SMA children under age 6.

Prevention of Cardiac Complications

Holter monitoring should be performed on a regular basis in conjunction with other standard studies of cardiac function such as chest radiographs, electrocardiography, and either echocardiography and radioscintigraphy scanning in patients with Emery-Dreifuss muscular dystrophy because they can have life-threatening cardiac arrhythmias, even in the presence of normal cardiac ejection. There is little, if any, evidence that cardiac arrhythmias pose a serious risk in patients with other dystrophies or myopathies, except of course when the ejection fraction is severely diminished, indicative of advanced cardiomyopathy.

Neuroendocrine activation is triggered by congestive heart failure (58). Measurements of plasma atrial natriuretic peptide (59–63) and norepinephrine are useful for estimating the severity of dilated cardiomyopathy and congestive heart failure (64,65). Norepinephrine concentrations have been shown to be an independent predictor of prognosis for patients with congestive heart failure (64,65). Atrial natriuretic peptide levels, normally about 10 pg/mL in young adults, increase as a function of cardiothoracic ratio and with the ratio of the preejection period to left ventricular ejection time. Atrial natriuretic peptide concentrations increase in DMD patients once left ventricular ejection fractions decrease to under 25% (66). Most such patients have a poor prognosis despite effective use of respiratory muscle aids. Thus, norepinephrine and atrial natriuretic peptide concentrations are useful for evaluating heart failure and monitoring treatment. Trials of the use of the angiotensin-converting enzyme inhibitor captopril, and hydralazine in the treatment of patients with severely decreased ventricular function, with or without congestive heart failure, demonstrated significant improvements in left ventricular ejection fraction and neuroendocrine levels (67). Patients with severe left ventricular dysfunction are at risk for developing mural thrombi and embolic complications that should be managed by anticoagulation. The correction of chronic hypercapnia with the use of inspiratory muscle aids is useful in reversing cor pulmonale and right ventricular failure.

Facilitation of Activities of Daily Living

Arm Function

Arm weakness parallels leg and diaphragm weakness in patients with neuromuscular disease. For example, by age 13 the strength of arm muscle groups in patients with DMD was only 4% of normal (68). Affected patients lose the ability to feed themselves by late adolescence when substitute movements, like flexing the trunk to meet the hand, balancing the forearm on the tip of the elbow, using objects as levers for the forearm, and using the fingers to crawl up the opposite arm, no longer work. A variety of mechanical systems can be useful for self-feeding, including an overhead sling counterweight and motorized system of arm suspension (68) and a ball-bearing forearm orthosis or mobile arm support (69); however, the latter requires adequate elbow flexor strength (69). When these are no longer adequate because of progressive weakness, finger-operated robotic arms mounted on a wheelchair (Fig. 3) (70,71), finger-controlled motorized wheelchairs, and environmental control systems permit patients to continue to feed themselves and perform many other upper extremity activities.

Other useful adaptive aids include long-handled combs, brushes, sponges, toilet paper holders, and shoe horns; flexible shower hoses; shower–tub transfer seats; grab bars; elevated toilet seats; bedside commode chairs; hospital beds; dressing and kitchen aids; and lifts (72). The latter can be useful for transfers and to facilitate bowel evacuation. For example, the patient is placed onto a lift with a seat that has a central cutout area, as is the case with many lift seats. The buttocks are slowly lowered almost to the commode, and with the feet on the floor, the legs are placed into an abdomen–bowel evacuation position, and time is greatly reduced. Condom drainage systems can increase independence. The need for the frequent turning of severely disabled patients in bed at night can be eliminated by use of a bed that slowly turns the patient from side to side (Motion Bed, J.H. Emerson Co.,

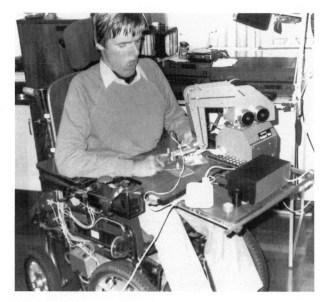

FIG. 3. Duchenne muscular dystrophy patient using a robot manipulator to perform electronic work.

Cambridge, MA). The home visit of an occupational therapist can aid the physician in prescribing the devices and home modifications that are most useful. With the use of assistive devices, many neuromuscular patients have gone on to achieve professional educations and gainful employment (73).

Communication

The selection of an appropriate communication system depends on the disease and its stage of evolution. Nonelectronic communication systems, including the use of paper and pencil, letter and phrase boards, and direct selection techniques using eye movements, are easily accessible to many patients and often adequate enough for most situations. Some patients with SMA type I and ALS who become aphonic can learn to use a personal computer with keyboard emulator software to drive a voice synthesizer and possibly a printer (74). Simple blinking operates an eye switch activated by infrared limbus–pupil reflection; electro-ocular switches may also be used (75). The Eye Gaze System (LC Technologies, Inc., Fairfax, VA) (Fig. 4) is an integrated system that provides access to the electronic devices in the patient's environment but requires careful positioning for accurate use.

Bach et al. (73) reported the experience of 22 patients with aphonia and ALS who were dependent on 24-hour ventilatory support for an average of 2.8 years while communicating with personal computer/voice synthesizer systems. Five patients used the system for over 5 years. One patient who used the technologic aids for 10 years earned a living by writing prose and poetry for a greeting card manufacturer. The ability to communicate had a positive effect on psychological outlook and longevity. In another study of patients with ALS managed by tracheostomy IPPV without mention of augmentative communication, mean longevity was only 11 months (76).

Patients with functional forearm musculature who have severe shoulder weakness, such as those with facioscapulohumeral muscular dystrophy, benefit from scapular stabilization to the rib cage and scapula-fixing orthoses to prevent winging. These can permit arm abduction, and flexion to greater than 90°.

Mobility

Patients with good trunk stability and function, particularly those with poor endurance, benefit from a motorized scooter, with elevated seats to facilitate transfers, attached baskets for carrying objects, and ventilator trays. They can be readily disassembled into three or four pieces of maximal weight 40 pounds and placed into the trunk or back seat of an automobile. Adapted strollers are available for children who are unable or too young to propel a wheelchair and require positioning support; however, their complexity varies. Like wheelchairs, the bases can have an option that allows the parent to recline a child as necessary, and with some, the base can be quickly reversed to permit parents to conveniently reposition a child with seizures or who requires ventilatory support.

For maximal efficiency, wheelchairs should be of proper size and have accessories to increase the function and quality of life of the user. The value of the wheelchair to the physically challenged individual cannot be overstated. Wheelchair prescription is appropriate for long-distance travel, through shopping malls, and along areas of uneven terrain and at outdoor events for patients with poor endurance or standing balance but who can other-

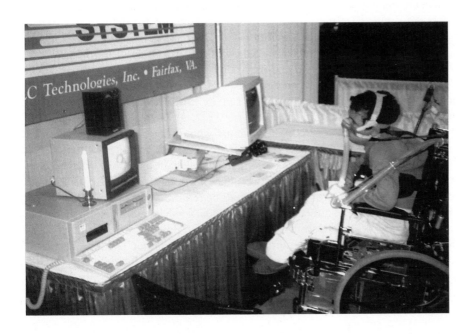

FIG. 4. Duchenne muscular dystrophy ventilator consumer using the Eye Gaze Electronic Communication and Environmental Control System. The gaze of the user's eye on the computer screen (right monitor) is monitored (left monitor) and triggers the computer.

wise walk with a cane, a walker, or orthosis. The ideal wheelchair is a light folding type for ease of transfer in an automobile. A more substantial manual or a power wheelchair is indicated for patients with greater walking difficulties. The patient must be measured for proper fit, and coat and orthotic use must be considered when applicable. Most wheelchairs have an overall width of 24 to 28 inches. Wider, more heavily constructed chairs can be made for obese individuals. A seat belt should be used for those with poor sitting balance or weak trunk musculature.

Two types of lightweight wheelchairs are available, those with rigid and those with nonrigid frames. A rigid-framed chair has a solid immovable base and an axis that connects one wheel to the other. They are suited for the active individuals who will use the chair on a variety of uneven terrains. Because of the solid axis, these frames provide more stability, a smoother ride, and are more durable. Such wheelchairs support more weight and accessories like ventilators and robot arms. A disadvantage of the rigid-frame wheelchair is that it cannot be folded and put into a car. However, the pin and lock configuration of "quick release" wheels permits rapid wheel removal to decrease the diameter of the chair in half for storage in the trunk of an automobile. Wheelchairs with a non-rigid frame have a cross-bar connecting one side of the wheelchair to the other. They fold to decrease their width in half. The cross-frame, however, wears out with use, compromising the integrity and stability of the wheelchair. Nevertheless, wheelchair users may prefer a cross-frame wheelchair because of its convenience. Both options should be tried to determine the one most appropriate for the user's lifestyle and environmental restrictions.

Most individuals with neuromuscular conditions require adjustable removable leg rests with heel straps. Offset foot plates and heel loops are used for individuals with severe ankle and foot deformities. The feet are maintained flat on the plates to discourage further deformity. Elevating foot rests increase the turning radius of the wheelchair and are generally used in conjunction with a reclining back in the presence of lower extremity edema, postural hypotension, and pressure sores that cannot be managed effectively in other ways. Individuals with poor endurance may also require a reclining seat. The ability to recline with extended knees reduces the tendency to develop flexion contractures of the knees and hips and allows the user to rest more comfortably. A neck or head support may be necessary for individuals with advanced ALS, infantile SMA, and/or DMD. Neck rests with a forehead strap provide both lateral and anterior-posterior support.

The user has the option of having full-length wheelchair arms or desk arms. Desk arms are preferable because they permit the user to approach and use tables. Full-length arms may be useful to support a lap board to facilitate the performance of school work, gainful employment, and recreational activities. Elevating arms are an option but are rarely required by users with neuromuscular weakness. However, the wheelchair arms must be removable to facilitate transfers.

Special seating modifications are required for individuals with weakness, instability, and deformity of the trunk, pelvis, or spine. The individual must be positioned and aligned properly to discourage pelvic obliquity. When bony prominences or pelvic obliquity are severe, a proper seating system can provide a stable surface while accommodating the deformities. The pelvis can be supported by a firm seat cushion supporting both ischia to keep the pelvis level and balanced. Several seating systems should be tried for comfort and function before one is prescribed. Commercially available seating systems include the Roho (Roho Inc., Belleville, IL), Jay (Jay Medical Ltd., Boulder, CO), and Avanti (Invacare, Inc., Elyria, OH) systems. Wedges, padded inserts, and lateral trunk supports are added as needed to maximize comfort and support. Seats can also be fully contoured for patients with severe deformity (77). Some seating systems permit users to vary their sitting positions by adjusting the upright sitting posture to increase head and upper extremity control and to reduce skin pressure and pressure ulcers. The "Tilt-in-Space" system (La Bac Systems, Inc., Denver, CO) shifts the user and the wheelchair seat and back simultaneously to change the seating orientation and shift skin pressures. Users can operate the tilt themselves via a switch.

Motorized wheelchairs are essential for the independent mobility of many severely disabled individuals. The same considerations for standard wheelchairs apply to motorized wheelchairs. In addition, motorized wheelchairs have drive trains and operation systems that must be chosen to satisfy the needs of the particular patient. A front-wheel-drive wheelchair is more maneuverable in the confined spaces of the home. A rear-wheel drive grips the ground better and is superior for outdoor use. When finger function is present, power wheelchairs can be operated by joy-stick controls. Otherwise, tongue, chin, and sip-and-puff controls are usually used. When neck, finger, and lip musculature are inadequate, any volitional muscle activity can be adapted to operate the chair (Fig. 5).

Although patients who are able to drive standard wheelchairs are infrequently dependent on daytime ventilator use, motorized wheelchair operators often require daytime support. When it is estimated that daytime ventilatory assistance will be required within 3 years, any prescribed power or standard wheelchair should have the capability of carrying a ventilator tray and holding additional batteries and possibly a charger. Daytime ventilator support is conveniently provided by the delivery of IPPV via a mouthpiece fixed onto wheelchair controls or, for joy-stick control users, fixed by a metal gooseneck clamp adjacent to the mouth (Fig. 6).

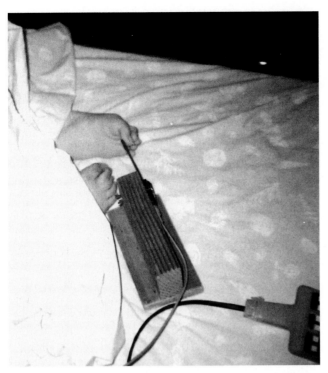

FIG. 5. A patient with Duchenne muscular dystrophy using a ventilator whose best functional movement is with his big toe. He uses his toe to trigger his computer.

Other considerations when prescribing a motorized wheelchair include its style for personal preference; adjustability of the control box for sensitivity of operation; programming chair speed, acceleration, and turning radius; noise; brake efficiency; tire treads and suspension

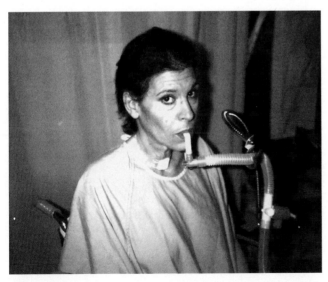

FIG. 6. Patient with muscular dystrophy whose tracheostomy tube was removed after 5 months of failed ventilator weaning attempts. She uses 24-hour mouthpiece intermittent positive pressure ventilation delivered during daytime hours via a mouthpiece held adjacent to the mouth by a metal gooseneck clamp.

system for smoothness of ride on flat unlevel surfaces or on grass; curb-jumping ability; battery recharger; durability; warranty; and price. Some motorized wheelchairs can stand the patient and can be operated while standing. Patients and care providers must be trained to properly and safely operate the wheelchair to prevent accidents and injuries for both the user and pedestrians. Training includes lifting and lowering the wheelchair onto and off of curbs, steps, and ramps.

CONCLUSION

The impact of progressive musculoskeletal impairment can become increasingly intrusive on the physical, emotional, and social functioning of affected patients. However, interventions in each stage of disability can optimize function and maintain continued community living despite severe physical disability. Physical medicine interventions therefore increase patient management options and optimize quality of life for patients with neuromuscular diseases. The stage of prolonged survival will be considered in Chapter 40.

REFERENCES

1. Moss AH, Oppenheimer EA, Casey P, et al. Patients with amyotrophic lateral sclerosis receiving long-term mechanical ventilation: advance care planning and outcomes. *Chest* 1996;110:249–255.
2. Bach JR. Amyotrophic lateral sclerosis: communication status and survival with ventilatory support. *Am J Phys Med Rehabil* 1993;72: 343–349.
3. Bach JR. Perspectives, indications, and the ethics of prolonging "meaningful life" for individuals with progressive neuromuscular disease. *J Neuro Rehab* 1992;6:61–66.
4. World Health Organization (WHO). *International classification of impairments, disabilities, and handicaps: a manual of classification relating to the consequences of disease.* Geneva: World Health Organization, 1980.
5. Bach JR, Intintola P, Alba AS, Holland I. The ventilator-assisted individual: cost analysis of institutionalization versus rehabilitation and in-home management. *Chest* 1992;101:26–30.
6. Bach JR. Case studies of respiratory management. In: Bach JR, ed. *Pulmonary rehabilitation: the obstructive and paralytic conditions.* Philadelphia: Hanley & Belfus, 1996:331–346.
7. Johnson EW. Pathokinesiology of Duchenne muscular dystrophy: implications for management. *Arch Phys Med Rehabil* 1977;58:4–7.
8. Sutherland DH, Olshen R, Cooper L, et al. The pathomechanics of gait in Duchenne muscular dystrophy. *Dev Med Child Neurol* 1981;23: 3–22.
9. Demos J. Early diagnosis and treatment of rapidly developing Duchenne de Boulogne type myopathy. *Am J Phys Med* 1971;50:271–284.
10. Roland LP, Laycer RB. The X-linked muscular dystrophies. In: Vinken PJ, Bruyn GW, eds. *Handbook of clinical neurology.* New York: North Holland Publishing, 1979:349–414.
11. Glorion B, Burgot D, Bonnard C. Myopathie Duchenne de Boulogne et chirurgie des membres inferieurs: 60 cas operes. *Readapt Revalid* 1987;3:8–13.
12. Gardner-Medwin D. Clinical features and classification of the muscular dystrophies. *Br Med Bull* 1980;36:109–115.
13. Bach JR, McKeon J. Orthopedic surgery and rehabilitation for the prolongation of brace-free ambulation of patients with Duchenne muscular dystrophy. *Am J Phys Med Rehabil* 1991;70:323–331.
14. Rideau Y, Duport G, Delaubier A, Guillou C, Renardel-Irani A, Bach JR. Early treatment to preserve quality of locomotion for children with Duchenne muscular dystrophy. *Semin Neurol* 1995;15:9–17.
15. Paul WD. Medical management of contractures in muscular dystrophy.

In: *Proceedings of the Third Medical Conference of Muscular Dystrophy Associations of America*, New York, 1954.

16. Scott OM, Hyde SA, Goddard C, Dubowitz V. Prevention of deformity in Duchenne muscular dystrophy. A prospective study of passive stretching and splintage. *Physiotherapy* 1981;67:177–180.

17. Rideau Y, Bach J. Efficacit therapeutique dans la dystrophie musculaire de Duchenne. *J Readapt Med* 1982;2:96–100.

18. Harris SE, Cherry DB. Childhood progressive muscular dystrophy and the role of physical therapy. *Phys Ther* 1974;54:4–12.

19. Seeger BR, Caudrey DJ, Little JD. Progression of equinus deformity in Duchenne muscular dystrophy. *Arch Phys Med Rehabil* 1985;66: 286–288.

20. Bach JR. Pulmonary rehabilitation and respiratory muscle aids. In Younger DS (ed): *Motor Disorders.* Philadelphia: Lippincott Williams & Wilkins, 1999: (*in press*).

21. Dangain J, Vrbova G. Response of normal and dystrophic muscles to increased function demand. *Exp Neurol* 1986;94:796–801.

22. Johnson EW, Braddom R. Over-work weakness in facioscapulohumeral muscular dystrophy. *Arch Phys Med Rehabil* 1971;52:333–336.

23. Blanger AY, Nol G, Ct C. A comparison of contractile properties in the preferred and non-preferred leg in a mixed sample of dystrophic patients. *Am J Phys Med Rehabil* (*in press*).

24. deLateur BJ, Giaconi RM. Effect on maximal strength of submaximal exercise in Duchenne muscular dystrophy. *Am J Phys Med* 1979;58: 26–36.

25. Vignos PJ, Watkins MP. The effect of exercise in muscular dystrophy. *JAMA* 1966;197:843–848.

26. Milner-Brown HS, Miller RG. Muscle strengthening through high-resistance weight training in patients with neuromuscular disorders. *Arch Phys Med Rehabil* 1988;69:14–19.

27. Fowler WM Jr. Management of musculoskeletal complications in neuromuscular diseases: weakness and the role of exercise. *Phys Med Rehabil* 1988;489–507.

28. Fowler WM, Goodgold J. Rehabilitation management of neuromuscular diseases. In: Goodgold J, ed. *Rehabilitation medicine*. Washington: C.V. Mosby, 1988:298–316.

29. Axen KV. Nutrition in chronic obstructive pulmonary disease. In: Haas F, Axen K, eds. *Pulmonary therapy and rehabilitation principles and practice*, 2nd ed. Baltimore: Williams & Wilkins, 1991:95–105.

30. Blackburn GL, Bistrian BR, Maini BS, Schlamm HT, Smith MF. Nutritional and metabolic assessment of the hospitalized patient. *JPEN* 1977;1:11–22.

31. Kelsen SG, Ference M, Kaoor S. Effects of prolonged undernutrition on structure and function of the diaphragm. *J Appl Physiol* 1985;58: 1354–1359.

32. Arora NS, Rochester DF. Respiratory muscle strength and maximal voluntary ventilation in undernourished patients. *Am Rev Respir Dis* 1982;126:5–8.

33. Baier H, Somani P. Ventilatory drive in normal man during semi-starvation. *Chest* 1984;85:222–225.

34. Doekel RC Jr, Zwillich CW, Scoggin CH, Kryger M, Weil JV. Clinical semistarvation: depression of hypoxic ventilatory response. *N Engl J Med* 1976;295:358–361.

35. Askanazi J, Rosembaum SH, Hyman AI, Rosenbaum L, Milie-Emili J, Kinney JM. Effects of parenteral nutrition on ventilatory drive. *Anesthesiology* 1980;53[Suppl]:185(abst).

36. Kerr JS, Riley DJ, Lanza-Jacoby S, et al. Nutritional emphysema in the rat: influence of protein depletion and impaired lung growth. *Am Rev Respir Dis* 1985;131:644–660.

37. Laaban JP, Rabba A, Kouchakyi B. Nutrition et insuffisance respiratoire. *Medecine et Hygiene* 1995;53:833.

38. McMurray DN, Loomis SA, Casazza LJ, Rey H, Miranda R. Development of impaired cell mediated immunity in mild and moderate malnutrition. *Am J Clin Nutr* 1981;34:68–77.

39. Good RA. Nutrition and immunity. *J Clin Immunol* 1981;1:3–11.

40. Moriguchi S, Sonc S, Kishino Y. Changes of alveolar macrophages in protein deficient rats. *J Nutr* 1983;113:40–46.

41. Martin TR, Altman LC, Alvares OF. The effects of severe protein-calorie malnutrition on antibacterial defense mechanisms in the rat lung. *Am Rev Respir Dis* 1983;128:1013–1019.

42. Niederman MS, Merrill WW, Ferranti RD, Pagano KM, Palmer LB, Reynolds HY. Nutritional status and bacterial binding in the lower respiratory tract in patients with chronic tracheostomies. *Ann Intern Med* 1984;100:795–800.

43. Bach JR, Tippett DC, McCrary MM. Bulbar dysfunction and associated cardiopulmonary considerations in polio and neuromuscular disease. *J Neuro Rehab* 1992;6:121–128.

44. Griffiths RD. Controlling weight in muscle disease to reduce the burden. *Physiotherapy* 1989;75:190–192.

45. Heckmatt J, Rodillo E, Dubowitz V. Management of children: pharmacological and physical. *Br Med Bull* 1989;45:788–801.

46. Duport G, Gayet E, Pries P, et al. Spinal deformities and wheelchair seating in Duchenne muscular dystrophy: twenty years of research and clinical experience. *Semin Neurol* 1995;15:29–37.

47. Emery AEH. Duchenne muscular dystrophy: genetic aspects, carrier detection and antenatal diagnosis. *Br Med Bull* 1980;36:117–122.

48. Rideau Y, Glorion B, Delaubier A, Tarle O, Bach J. Treatment of scoliosis in Duchenne muscular dystrophy. *Muscle Nerve* 1984;7:281–286.

49. Brown JC, Zeller JL, Swank SM, Furumasu J, Warath SL. Surgical and functional results of spine fusion in spinal muscular atrophy. *Spine* 1989;14:763–770.

50. Merlini L, Granata C, Bonfiglioli S, Marini ML, Cervellati S, Savini R. Scoliosis in spinal muscular atrophy: natural history and management. *Dev Med Child Neurol* 1989;31:501–508.

51. Phillips DP, Roye DP, Farcy JC, Leet A, Shelton YA. Surgical treatment of scoliosis in a spinal muscular atrophy population. *Spine* 1990; 15:942–945.

52. Bach JR, Alba AS. Total ventilatory support by the intermittent abdominal pressure ventilator. *Chest* 1991;99:630–636.

53. Yasuda YL, Bowman K, Hsu JD. Mobile arm supports: criteria for successful use in muscle disease patients. *Arch Phys Med Rehabil* 1986; 67:253–256.

54. Jenkins JG, Bohn D, Edmonds JF, Levison H, Barker GA. Evaluation of pulmonary function in muscular dystrophy patients requiring spinal surgery. *Crit Care Med* 1982;10:645–649.

55. Kumano K, Tsuyama N. Pulmonary function before and surgical correction of scoliosis. *J Bone Joint Surg [Am]* 1982;64A:242–248.

56. Cambridge W, Drennan JL. Scoliosis associated with Duchenne muscular dystrophy. *J Pediatr Orthop* 1987;7:436–440.

57. Smith AD, Koreska J, Moseley CF. Progression of scoliosis in Duchenne muscular dystrophy. *J Bone Joint Surg [Am]* 1989;71A: 1066–1074.

58. Floras JS. Clinical aspects of sympathetic activation and parasympathetic withdrawal in heart failure. *J Am Coll Cardiol* 1993;22:72A–84A.

59. Burnett JC, Kao PC, Hu DC, et al. Atrial natriuretic peptide elevation in congestive heart failure in humans. *Science* 1968;231:1145–1147.

60. Gottlieb SS, Kukin ML, Ahern D, Packer M. Prognostic importance of atrial natriuretic peptide in patients with chronic heart failure. *J Am Coll Cardiol* 1989;13:1534–1539.

61. Yanagisawa A, Yokata N, Miyagawa M, et al. Plasma levels of atrial natriuretic peptide in patients with Duchenne's muscular dystrophy. *Am Heart J* 1990;120:1154–1158.

62. Kawai H, Adachi K, Kimura C, et al. Secretion and clinical significance of atrial natriuretic peptide in patients with muscular dystrophy. *Arch Neurol* 1990;47:900–904.

63. Kameda K. Clinical significance of the relationship between cardiac insufficiency and atrial natriuretic peptide and dystrophin in patients with Duchenne muscular dystrophy. *Sapporo Med J* 1991;60: 535–543.

64. Cohn JN, Levine B, Olivari MT, et al. Plasma norepinephrine as a guide to prognosis in patients with chronic congestive heart failure. *N Engl J Med* 1984;311:819–823.

65. Francis GS, Cohn JN, Johnson G, Rector TS, Goldman S, Simon A. Plasma norepinephrine, plasma renin activity, and congestive heart failure: relations to survival and the effects of therapy in V-HeFT. *Circulation* 1993;87:40–48.

66. Kameda K. Clinical significance of the relationship between cardiac insufficiency and atrial natriuretic polypeptide and dystrophin in patients with Duchenne muscular dystrophy. *Sapporo Med J* 1991;60:535–546.

67. Ishikawa Y, Bach JR, Sarma RJ, et al. Cardiovascular considerations in the management of neuromuscular disease. *Semin Neurol* 1995;15: 93–108.

68. James WV, Orr JF. Upper limb weakness in children with Duchenne muscular dystrophy—a neglected problem. *Prosthet Orthot Int* 1984;8: 111–113.

69. Yasuda YL, Bowman K, Hsu JD. Mobile arm supports: criteria for successful use in muscle disease patients. *Arch Phys Med Rehabil* 1986; 67:253–256.

70. Bach JR, Zeelenberg A, Winter C. Wheelchair mounted robot manipulators: long term use by patients with Duchenne muscular dystrophy. *Am J Phys Med Rehabil* 1990;69:59–69.

71. Valenza J, Guzzardo SL, Bach JR. Functional interventions for individuals with neuromuscular disease. In: Bach JR, ed. *Pulmonary rehabilitation: the obstructive and paralytic conditions.* Philadelphia: Hanley & Belfus, 1996:371–394.

72. Brammell CA. Assistive devices for patients with neuromuscular diseases: the role of the occupational therapy. In: Maloney FP, Burks JS, Ringel SP, eds. *Interdisciplinary rehabilitation of multiple sclerosis and neuromuscular disorders.* New York: J.B. Lippincott, 1985: 259–276.

73. Bach JR, O'Brien J, Krotenberg R, Alba A. Management of end stage respiratory failure in Duchenne muscular dystrophy. *Muscle Nerve* 1987;10:177–182.

74. Brody H. The great equalizer: PCs empower the disabled. *PC/Computing,* Ziff-Davis Pub. Co., 1989:83–93.

75. van der Meer KJH. An electro-ocular switch for communication of the speechless. *Med Prog Technol* 1983/1984:10:135–141.

76. Goulon M, Goulon-Goeau C. Sclerose Latrale amyotrophique et assistance respiratoire. *Rev Neurol* 1989;145:293–298.

77. Gibson DA, Albisser AM, Koreska J. Role of the wheelchair in the management of the muscular dystrophy patient. *Can Med Assn J* 1975; 113:964–967.

Motor Disorders,
edited by David S. Younger.
Lippincott Williams & Wilkins, Philadelphia © 1999.

CHAPTER 39

Orthoses and Adaptive Equipment in Neuromuscular Disorders

Barry Rodstein and Dennis D. J. Kim

An orthosis is a device, such as a brace or splint, that is applied externally to the body. It modifies the functional and structural characteristics of the neuromuscular and musculoskeletal systems. The term orthotic is a term that refers to the study and practice of bracing, not to the actual device. Adaptive devices are external appliances, including orthoses, canes, crutches, walkers, reachers, and wheelchairs, that are used to improve function.

The management of neuromuscular disorders changes continuously because of significant medical and technologic advances, including those in molecular biology, genetics, and immunology. This has resulted in more precise diagnoses, superior care, and increased lengths of survival. Thus, there are more patients with neuromuscular diseases, some elderly, requiring adaptive equipment and orthoses, and it is prudent for physicians involved in their care to be familiar with these. This chapter reviews the basic approach to bracing in neuromuscular disease.

An orthosis is named for the joint that the brace crosses, beginning proximally, followed by the word orthosis. The general term "foot" is used for joints distal to the ankle. Thus, a brace that begins at the leg, crosses the ankle, and ends at the foot is referred to as an ankle–foot orthosis (AFO). If the brace begins at the thigh, crosses the knee and ankle, and ends at the foot, it is called a knee–ankle–foot orthosis (KAFO). Many specific braces are referred to by nonstandard names based on their function, design, or where they were developed: reciprocating gait orthosis, patella tendon-bearing AFO (PTB AFO), and University of California at Berkeley Laboratories Foot Orthosis are such examples.

B. Rodstein and D. J. Kim: Department of Rehabilitation Medicine, Albert Einstein College of Medicine and Montefiore Medical Center, Bronx, New York 10467.

GENERAL PRINCIPLES FOR ORTHOSES IN MOTOR DISORDERS

The exact purpose of a brace and its goal should be obvious to a patient; otherwise, it will not be used. A common pitfall in our zeal to fix the patient and normalize gait is to overbrace, resulting in orthoses that are unnecessarily awkward or too heavy to use. A useful approach is to begin with the simplest brace that is likely to result in safe and functional ambulation and use a more cumbersome one only when necessary. This is particularly true for KAFOs and longer braces, in which the weight of the brace is an important consideration.

Often, control is achieved at one joint by moving or controlling adjacent ones. This usually requires that the adjacent joints are either functional or able to be braced. The most common example is control of the knee with an AFO, which requires intact hip musculature, particularly extensor muscles. Knee buckling can be prevented by the combination of a dorsiflexion stop at the ankle and active hip extension, so that a KAFO is not needed.

An essential concept in bracing is that forces are applied to at least three points. Two of them, applied to one side of the limb or body part, stabilizes it, whereas the third exerts the necessary counterforce in between them. The magnitude of the counterforce equals the sum of the opposing forces (1).

For orthoses that involve the foot, such as the KAFO or AFO, the shoe is an integral part of the system even if it is not an actual part of the orthosis because the throat or the portion anterior to the tongue is a necessary point to the three point system and the one that exerts the most force. Other areas along which forces are applied are the metatarsal heads through the sole of the shoe or a footplate and the upper calf by means of a proximal band. As a rule, a shoe without a wide padded area and firm closures, such as penny loafers and pumps and those with elastic laces, should not be used with a brace. An orthosis with a footplate inside the shoe can be used with standard shoes, ideally with removable insoles that can be taken out to accommodate the orthosis. If this is not possible, a shoe one-half size longer or wider may suffice. Patients unable to tie standard laces should have looped Velcro closures with a D-ring. Footwear can have an impact on the dynamic response of the orthosis because even minor changes in heel design and height, sole material, or angle of the toe spring can affect the biomechanics of walking. Decisions and instructions regarding footwear should be made with the orthosis in mind.

Orthoses of the leg can exert significant pressure on the skin. When the primary function of an orthosis is to control movement of a joint, pressure and shear forces will be inversely proportional to the length of the lever arm and the area over which force is applied. To minimize undue pressure on the skin, force should be applied as far as possible from the fulcrum using the longest possible lever arm, and the area of contact should be maximized. The type of orthosis and the materials used should be carefully chosen for insensate or obese patients and in those with significant edema along the area to be braced. Whenever possible, forces should be applied by a tubular or closed structure producing the equivalent of a thin-walled pressure vessel, in which the resulting hydrostatic forces provide considerably greater resistance to torsional stress, allowing the use of thinner materials as compared with an open design (2,3). Examples are the circumferential designs of the thigh enclosure in a KAFO and most spinal orthoses.

Patients with useful motion in a joint should have braces designed to allow this motion. For example, allowing useful dorsiflexion will improve gait, especially at late stance phase. This approach aids in preserving and improving range of movement, particularly in the triceps surae because weight bearing in the lengthened position provides useful muscle stretching. Standing by means of a tilt table or a standing frame is one of the best ways to improve range of motion (ROM) at the ankles in patients unable to ambulate (2). Resting night splints assist in preventing contractures; however, the knee should be in extension to stretch the gastrocnemii and soleus muscles. ROM maintenance should be instituted early and aggressively because correction of contractures is much more difficult than prevention, if not impossible.

Whenever possible, it is important to design braces to accommodate the anticipated changes that occur as a result of progressive neuromuscular disease. For example, when choosing an AFO, an articulating ankle with adjustable dorsiflexion and plantar flexion is better than one with a fixed ankle. Any patient, but particularly those with waxing and waning diseases such as multiple sclerosis, are prone to discard braces that are no longer used and should be reminded not to do so.

Materials

Orthoses were first made of leather, fabric, and metal and attached directly to shoes. Polypropylene and other modern plastics are now preferred by patients because they offer better control through closer fit and decrease energy expenditure due to lighter weight. In addition, they are more cosmetically appealing. They are of two types: thermoplastic and thermosetting plastic. Thermoplastic orthoses can be repeatedly remolded by reheating. Thermosetting plastics are liquid resins at room temperature and harden when set. They are applied to mesh laminates under vacuum pressure to form the composite material. Although they are more durable, high-temperature thermoplastics such as polypropylene are suitable for many bracing needs and are sometimes chosen because of their lower cost and ease of modification. Thermoplastic orthoses can be reinforced with composite inserts, but they do not become an integral part of the brace and are thus not as strong as the laminated ones (4). Thermosetting plastics are superior in cases of high stress, such as in weight transfer, PTB AFO, and obesity. Laminated braces are lighter, stronger, and more versatile. Because lower forces are required for upper extremity and temporary lower extremity bracing, lower temperature thermoplastics such as polyethylene are generally acceptable; they are also easier to modify. For short-term use on sensate patients, prefabricated braces are often appropriate but should not be considered in cases of significant sensory impairment, edema, foot deformity, or obesity.

Pediatric Bracing

The prime goal of pediatric orthotics is to prevent deformity; however, when one already exists, efforts should be aimed at correcting it. When that is not possible, the orthosis should be designed to accommodate the deformity. Children should be seen for frequent brace adjustments during growth spurts because of changes in girth and height and contours of the ankle and calf portions.

Several factors are important to increase acceptance of braces in children. First, the brace should be comfortable. This usually requires use of a soft lining or padding. Second, there should be parental acceptance of the brace. Parents should be educated in its use and purpose and in differentiating pain due to poor fit from annoyance due to the confinement imposed by the brace. The ease of donning and doffing also increases patient use and parental acceptance of the brace. Bright colors, patterns, buttons, buckles, and cartoon characters can make the brace more cosmetically appealing.

COMMON LOWER EXTREMITY ORTHOSES

Ankle–Foot Orthoses

AFOs are versatile, relatively inexpensive, and cosmetically inoffensive. They are the most commonly used lower extremity orthoses. Table 1 lists the major types of AFOs, their biomechanical functions, conditions in which they are deemed appropriate, and particular advantages and disadvantages.

Double Upright Ankle–Foot Orthoses with Shoe

This prototypical AFO (Fig. 1) consists of hinge joints connected proximally to steel, aluminum, or titanium uprights. A posterior calf band with an anterior strap fixes the uprights to the leg, and a stirrup fixes the brace distally to the shoe. A split stirrup can be removed to allow for its use in different shoes, which must be modified by attaching a caliper box to accept the stirrup. A light, thin, and durable solid stirrup can be riveted directly to the shoe and should be used in patients with severe spasticity; in weight transfer AFOs (5), as for example, a PTB AFO; in those who tamper with their braces. A variation on the double-upright AFO is a custom-made footplate, which is placed inside the shoe, which should have adequate room to accommodate it, such as extra depth shoes and sturdy sneakers with removable insoles.

As with other AFOs, the upper margin of the calf band must end at least 2 to 3 cm below the fibular head to avoid injury of the peroneal nerve. The ankle should be aligned with the lateral orthotic joint slightly anterior to the lateral malleolus, and the medial joint should be slightly posterior to the medial malleolus. The joints can have a single posterior channel or both posterior and anterior channels. Pins or springs can be placed in these channels and adjusted to limit or assist motion as necessary. Commonly used configurations include a single long-length posterior channel that provides a dorsiflexion assist with a spring or a plantar flexion stop with a pin, or dual channels that in addition provide a dorsiflexion stop. These joints are easily adjusted by turning a screw to vary the allowable motion or amount of assist. The Klenzak joint is widely used and has a particularly long posterior channel to accommodate a long spring that enables effective dorsiflexion assist. A brace can be configured to provide plantar flexion assist, but there are few clinical applications for this, and the dorsal aspect of the foot does not tolerate any substantial pressure.

Modifications can be made to this type of brace to address a wide variety of conditions. A T- or Y-strap can be used to control pronation or supination. For excessive pronation, the strap is attached to the medial side of the shoe and buckled around the lateral upright to produce a force directing the subtalar joint inward; the opposite configuration can be used to control supination.

Although extremely versatile and effective, traditional double-upright AFOs are used much less because of the advancement of modern synthetic thermoplastics and composite materials. The double-upright AFO is still the ideal choice for patients with severe spasticity, an insensate foot, fluctuating edema, or a severe foot deformity requiring a custom-molded shoe. In addition, patients who have been using this type of brace for many years may not wish to change. In developing countries, the technology for plastic braces may not be available, making the double-upright brace the default choice.

Spring-wire (Piano-wire) Ankle–Foot Orthoses

The spring-wire AFO (Fig. 2) is a variation on the double-upright AFO in which the heavy uprights are replaced with stainless steel wires coiled at the ankle to provide a spring action that assists dorsiflexion. Like the double-upright AFO, the distal end is attached directly to an orthopedic shoe, which can accommodate edema and allow shoe modifications. It has the advantages of being lighter in weight, less conspicuous, and providing better dorsiflexion assistance. However, neither varus-valgus control nor plantar-dorsiflexion stops are possible, and, like the double-upright AFO, replacement of the shoe requires an orthotist. This brace is used primarily for isolated dorsiflexion weakness when a plantar leaf spring ankle–foot orthosis (PLSO) cannot be used due to edema, loss of sensation, ulcers, or advanced deformity of the foot requiring shoe modifications.

Single Upright Ankle–Foot Orthoses

One modification that makes this brace lighter is a single upright and joint on the AFO instead of two. This provides control and assist in the sagittal plane but does not prevent internal or external rotation of the leg. The single joint is subject to significant torsional stress and is less durable unless an extra-heavy joint is used, negating the decrease in weight. Thus, single upright AFO are usually not indicated and infrequently prescribed.

Veterans Administration Prosthetic Center Ankle–Foot Orthoses

This simple lightweight metal brace clips onto the back of a shoe and provides dorsiflexion assist. Although inexpensive, it requires a sturdy orthopedic shoe to be effective and shifting of the posterior upright on the calf can be problematic for some patients. The PLSO has largely superseded the Veterans Administration Prosthetic Center brace, which is now primarily used as a trial dorsiflexion-assist brace in the clinic setting.

Plastic Ankle–Foot Orthoses

These are the most common AFOs today. They provide an intimate fit and are lightweight, washable, cost-

TABLE 1. *Characteristics and application of various AFOs*

AFO design	Functions provided	Functions not provided	Better choice for	Advantages	Disadvantages
Double upright	DF stop DF assist PF stop Knee control Medial-lateral control		CVA Changing conditions Fluctuating edema Patient prefers this type of brace	Versatile Adjustable Accommodates edema and foot deformities Safer with insensate skin	Heavy Less cosmetic than plastic AFO Requires shoe modification
Springwire	DF assist	DF stop PF stop Knee control Medial-lateral control	Foot drop (especially when PLSO contraindicated) Low motor neuron disease with stable ankle Conditions where PLSO would be useful, but is contraindicated due to edema or foot deformity (see PLSO)	Accommodates edema and foot deformities Safer with insensate skin	Less cosmetic than plastic AFO Requires shoe modification Heavier than PLSO due to increased weight of footwear
Articulated plastic	DF stop DF Assist (mild) PF stop Knee control Medial-lateral control	Strong DF assist	CVA Changing conditions Tight heel cords (stabilizes the subtalar joint so that stretching occurs at the crural joint)	Versatile Adjustable Lightweight Cosmetic No special shoes required	Cannot be used with fluctuating edema or severe foot deformity Requires caution with insensate foot Less durable than solid AFO Expensive
PLS	DF assist	PF stop DF stop Medial-lateral control Knee control	Foot drop Low motor neuron disease with stable ankle Anterior compartment syndrome Myotonic dystrophy Post-polio syndrome ALS (with mild or no spasticity)	Lightweight Cosmetic Durable Inexpensive Washable No special shoes required	Ineffective for equinus deformity Unable to resist spasticity Minimal mediolateral control Cannot be used with fluctuating edema Requires caution with insensate foot Does not stabilize the ankle
Semisolid	PF stop Medial-lateral control Mild DF assist	DF stop DF assist Knee control	CVA with mild-moderate spasticity ALS with moderate spasticity	Lightweight Cosmetic Durable Washable No special shoes required Tolerated better than solid AFO	Cannot be used with fluctuating edema Requires caution with insensate foot May prevent useful ankle motion Not ideal for bilateral use (although may be better than solid AFO)
Solid	DF stop PF stop Knee control Medial-lateral control	DF assist	CVA with severe spasticity Conditions requiring immobilization of the ankle	Lightweight Cosmetic Durable Washable No special shoes required	Cannot be used with fluctuating edema Requires caution with insensate foot May prevent useful ankle motion Not good for bilateral use

AFO, ankle foot orthosis; PLS, posterior leaf spring; DF, dorsiflexion; PF, plantar flexion; CVA, cerebrovascular accident; PLSO, posterior leaf spring orthosis; ALS, amyotrophic lateral sclerosis.

effective, and relatively cosmetic. A one-piece plastic AFO does not have a true joint, but the amount of ankle motion can be controlled by modifying the ankle trim line, thickness, and properties of the plastic. The footplate usually ends just proximal to the metatarsal heads and are

sometimes referred to as ¾ footplates. Although a full footplate improves push off, is more difficult to don and doff, and increases the risk of breakdown, they are indicated in conditions associated with excessive toe flexor tone or flexion contractures of the toes but are infre-

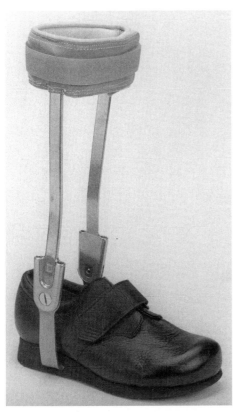

FIG. 1. Double-upright ankle–foot orthosis with dual-channel joints.

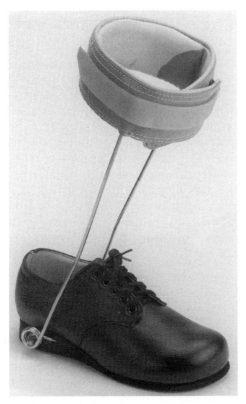

FIG. 2. Spring-wire ankle–foot orthosis.

quently used in adults. A hybrid can be made combining a plastic shoe insert and hinged joint with either a plastic calf shell or a metal upright attached to a calf band.

Plantar Leaf Spring Ankle–Foot Orthoses

This widely used lightweight plastic AFO is made of high-temperature thermoplastic polypropylene (Fig. 3). It is lightweight, inexpensive, relatively easy to fabricate, washable, cosmetically benign, and allows for ease in exchange of footwear. The degree of trimming and thickness of the material determines the amount of spring action and thus dorsiflexion assist and the amount of mediolateral control. It can be used for almost all conditions involving flaccid dorsiflexor weakness but is less well suited for resisting plantar flexion as, for example, in upper motor neuron (UMN) disorders with excessive spasticity or if there is substantial mediolateral ankle instability. In those situations, an articulated or less flexible brace is preferable. Dorsiflexion can be easily restored by a PLSO for complete foot drop due to peroneal palsy, lumbosacral root or plexus lesion, or compartment syndrome. The primary function of this brace is control of the swing phase of walking and therefore needs only to support the weight of the foot and shoe, approximately 2 pounds (6). When a patient has dorsiflexion and plantar flexion weakness, such as in a sciatic nerve injury, a dorsiflexion-assist AFO can satisfy the needs for daily walking activities, particularly in geriatric patients, whose gait pattern may not demand strong push off.

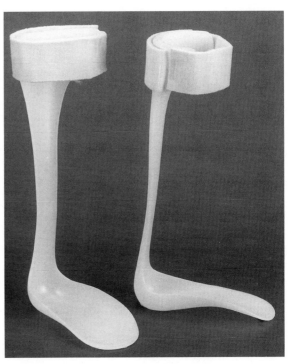

FIG. 3. Plantar leaf spring ankle–foot orthosis, made with polypropylene.

458 / CHAPTER 39

Semisolid and Solid Ankle–Foot Orthoses

In this AFO, the trim lines of the calf shell are brought somewhat more anterior than in the PLSO. This results in increased resistance to plantar flexion and dorsiflexion and increased control of mediolateral motion. If the trim lines are brought further anterior to surround the ankle, there is minimal ankle motion and the brace is then referred to as a solid AFO (Fig. 4). Solid and semisolid AFOs are more durable than articulated AFOs. Gait difficulties may arise with these braces or in other circumstances that result in further diminished ankle ROM. Although not yet in common use, designs are beginning to appear in which polyethylene is added to allow more flexibility, and a horizontal slit is made posteriorly to allow sagittal motion. Such a design may allow for a very lightweight dorsiflexion-assist brace, functionally similar to a PLSO but providing better medial-lateral control.

Articulating Plastic Ankle–Foot Orthoses

These braces use hinged joints attached to plastic proximal and distal components (Fig. 5). In many ways, they combine the advantages of both double-upright and solid AFOs and are the second most common type of lower extremity orthoses. They are probably the most commonly prescribed AFO in patients with spasticity. Like double-upright AFOs, various configurations allow for combinations of plantar and dorsiflexion stops and mild dorsiflexion assist. They are lightweight, relatively cosmetic, and quite versatile. Because of the solid footplate and mediolateral stability they provide, they can control

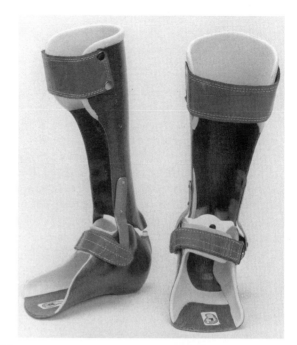

FIG. 5. Articulating ankle–foot orthosis with instep strap, made with laminated plastic.

the subtalar joint and thus facilitate appropriate stretching of the triceps surae and Achilles tendon.

However, compared with nonarticulating AFOs, they are considerably more expensive and less durable, and their joints and attachments are under higher stress and therefore more prone to excessive wear and early failure. Thus, when very high forces are expected, as for example with obesity or very high tone, a solid AFO is still preferable.

Spiral and Hemispiral Ankle–Foot Orthoses

The spiral and hemispiral AFOs were designed to permit the natural internal and external rotation of the leg with respect to the foot while controlling ankle and subtalar motion. This theoretic advantage over other AFO is offset by material fatigue and difficulty initially and subsequently maintaining proper fit. The hypothetical advantage of allowing physiologic tibial rotation and subtalar motion may not actually occur due to the footplate of the brace that restricts subtalar motion. These AFO are not in widespread use (7).

Patellar Tendon-bearing Ankle–Foot Orthoses

This particular solid AFO is designed with a snug-fitting bivalved calf portion to partially relieve distal weight bearing by distributing weight to the medial tibial condyle, patellar tendon, and the soft tissues of the leg. They are useful in patients with foot ulcers, tibial fractures, painful heel conditions, avascular necrosis of the ankle or foot, and Charcot joints. It should usually be

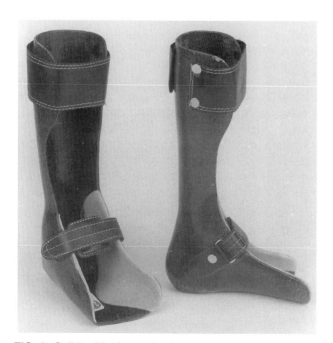

FIG. 4. Solid ankle–foot orthosis with instep strap, made with laminated plastic.

custom-made to optimize weight distribution. A rocker-bottom and ankle reinforcements are often incorporated to minimize ankle movement and active push off (8). The PTB AFO is usually contraindicated in patients with vascular insufficiency because of the high forces distributed along the popliteal artery (9). In this instance, a solid ankle-anterior shell AFOs, with rocker-bottom sole to prevent significant motion from the ankle to the midfoot and Plastazote lining, should be used instead.

Knee–Ankle–Foot Orthoses

These should be prescribed with discretion, such as when it is necessary to control the knee directly, when an AFO or another indirect intervention is not adequate, or when the ankle or foot must be suspended or controlled. Impaired proprioception at the knee may necessitate bracing proximal to the calf; however, if only knee control alone is necessary, a knee orthosis (KO) may be the better choice. KAFO are used in rheumatoid and other generalized arthritides to stabilize the joints, especially since weakness is usually not the main problem and the weight of the braces is less important. They are also used in patients with poliomyelitis and the post-polio syndrome (PPS) wherein the nature of the paralysis is spotty, there is no spasticity, and sensation is intact. Many patients with poliomyelitis have been successfully managed with KAFO for several decades. Bracing for UMN conditions is usually more complex and difficult to achieve than in flaccid conditions because of poor trunk balance and central motor control and the frequent presence of ataxia, apraxia, involuntary movements, and spasticity (10). While obstacles can often be overcome by an AFO, the problems are compounded with KAFO, and thus their use in UMN conditions is rarely beneficial.

Alternatives to Knee–Ankle–Foot Orthoses

Less-cumbersome solutions should be considered before prescribing a KAFO. Knee buckling, for example, can be addressed by using an AFO with the ankle fixed in 5 to 10° of plantar flexion, thereby increasing the knee extension moment and assisting the weakened quadriceps. This may reduce the risk of falling and obviate or delay the need for KAFO. One problem with this approach is that genu recurvatum may result in excessive strain on the knee capsule and ligaments. In addition, as with patients using KAFO to ambulate, weak proximal lower extremity or trunk muscles may limit lifting of the limbs or trunk sufficiently to clear the feet for swing-to or swing-through gait. When further control of the knee is necessary, an AFO can be used with a temporary KO in anticipation of partial quadriceps recovery or while the patient is being trained in a more secure gait pattern. Diabetic plexopathy truncal radiculopathy, diabetic amyotrophy, and acute inflammatory demyelinating polyneuropathy are diseases wherein ultimate improvement can occur and in which an AFO and temporary KO may be appropriate.

Design Considerations

Distally, the design of a KAFO is essentially the same as an AFO and uses the various types of plastic or metal designs described in the previous section. To this is added a thigh band or plastic shell with intervening hinges that can limit or lock motion. In some designs, the joint is offset so that in early stance it is posterior to the ground reaction force, thereby creating an extension moment that increases knee stability. The proximal thigh band should end about 1 to 2 cm below the ischial tuberosity with the patient standing (6). When knee flexion is particularly difficult to control, an anterior prepatellar band can be added. If a significant change in condition is expected, an adjustable joint should be used. When locking knee joints are used, the patient has to unlock the knee to sit.

With the changing axis of rotation of an anatomic knee joint, the fixed-axis mechanical joint will not move completely in unison with the knee resulting in shifting of the orthosis with knee flexion and extension and discomfort. Polycentric knees are designed to minimize this discrepancy but are only needed when a significant amount of knee motion will occur during ambulation. Because patients requiring KAFO will generally not ambulate with a great amount of knee motion, polycentric joints are usually not necessary and are more commonly used in athletic KOs.

Ambulation with Bilateral Knee–Ankle–Foot Orthoses

Most patients with bilateral weakness who require KAFO to ambulate find that the effort of donning and doffing them, the weight of the braces, and the energy expenditure of walking with both knees locked all preclude functional ambulation; in fact, it would be difficult for many healthy individuals without impairments. Patients with paraplegia resulting from complete spinal cord injuries were reported to consume 500% more oxygen per meter when ambulating with bilateral KAFO and crutches than normal subjects. Furthermore, their speed of walking is 29 m/min compared with 80 m/min in normal subjects (6). Patients will often plead fervently for KAFO and are quite genuine in their belief that they will use them to ambulate; however, functional or even regular therapeutic ambulation is rare. The exception is in patients with poliomyelitis or young, vigorous, and highly motivated patients who choose to ambulate despite the fact that wheelchair mobility is faster and more efficient. Bilateral KAFO should not be prescribed, particularly when one considers their cost, unless there is a strong indication that they will be used in daily activities.

Scott-Craig Knee–Ankle–Foot Orthoses

This orthosis was specifically designed to enable patients with cord injury to stand and walk. The ankle joint is fixed in approximately 10° of dorsiflexion and the knee joints are locked, placing the center of gravity anterior to the ankle and knee. The patient is able to hyperextend the hips and passively hang on the Y-ligaments, so that the center of gravity is behind the hip and balance is achieved. The knee joints are designed to allow easy unlocking for sitting. This KAFO is not of great use in other neuromuscular disorders with weakness.

Reciprocating Gait Orthoses

This is a particular type of hip–knee–ankle–foot orthosis in which flexion of one hip is mechanically linked to extension of the other. This type of brace, which is rarely indicated in adults due to the high energy cost of ambulation, is well-tolerated in children and often enables patients with spinal cord injury or myelodysplasia to ambulate.

Knee Orthosis

The KO is primarily used for musculoskeletal conditions; however, it is also used in patients with isolated quadriceps weakness resulting in recurvatum; nevertheless, when sufficient, a cane is often the best orthosis. The prototypical KO for recurvatum is the articulated Swedish knee cage, which uses a three-point design to create a flexion force at the knee. One or two anterior bands above and one below the knee are connected by lateral uprights to a hinge joint at the knee, where a posterior band is placed. A major problem with most KO is the cylindrical shape of the leg that makes it difficult to avoid significant longitudinal and rotational movement of the brace, often making other bracing strategies such as AFO preferable.

Quadriceps-Assist Orthosis

In patients with DMD without plantar flexion contractures, knee buckling may be a significant factor limiting ambulation. Gluteus maximus weakness precludes the use of hip extension to substitute for quadriceps weakness, and the quadriceps assist orthosis may be useful (2). This brace consists of a neoprene knee sleeve with anterior spring steel stays that are wound to assist knee extension.

Functional Electrical Stimulation

The use of functional electrical stimulation (FES) in paralysis dates back to the 1960s (12). An intact motor unit is required. Electrical stimulation of the common peroneal nerve can be used to improve gait and obviate the need for bracing in UMN lesions causing foot drop. The device consists of electrodes placed behind or below the fibular head, a battery-operated stimulator, and a switch placed between the heel and the shoe. When the heel is off the ground, the circuit is activated, resulting in dorsiflexion and thus clearance of the foot in the swing phase. At heel strike, the circuit is broken, allowing the foot to land flat (11). More complex FES packages are available and are in limited use for patients with paraplegia. New interest and promise have arisen in this field with the recent advances in electronics and biotechnology. Nevertheless, FES is still in the research phase. Major barriers include failure of electrodes, nonphysiologic recruitment pattern, early fatigability, technical limitations of sensors, and, in paraplegics, the high energy cost of ambulation. FES can be used when there is minimal or no spasticity. Furthermore, because bracing provides a far simpler, more reliable, and cost-effective approach to paralysis, FES may never become a widespread alternative.

PATIENT EVALUATION

Team Approach

This time-consuming approach is advantageous in the long run because inappropriate prescription of adaptive equipment or orthoses is ineffective, costly, and can delay the patient's functional recovery. This can be a significant source of frustration for the patient, sometimes straining the relationship with their physician, therapists, family, and caretakers. Furthermore, if the wrong brace is ordered, it can be difficult to obtain funding for a replacement. The physician is best trained to advise on prognosis, contraindications, or other disease-specific issues. Physiatrists are ideal in this role because they are knowledgeable in gait and bracing, neuromuscular and musculoskeletal function, and the long-term effects of disease. Neurologists, primary care providers, and orthopedists may also assume this role. A physical or occupational therapist trained in many of these areas will spend a significant amount of time with the patients and therefore have insight into their physical and cognitive abilities. The orthotist will fabricate the orthosis and is able to advise on bracing strategies and the biomechanical characteristics and limitations of a given design. The patient will often go directly to the orthotist for minor adjustment, repair, or modification of the brace. It is imperative to have communication and accessibility between the patient and the orthotist. Social services may be required at times to assist in resolving issues such as funding for equipment and orthotist services. Involvement of family members in the initial evaluation may improve patient compliance, particularly in children. When bracing needs are straightforward, the full team approach is not always necessary.

Preprescription Evaluation

A preprescription evaluation is crucial in determining the appropriate brace for the patient and in establishing the ROM, strength, tone, and stability. ROM testing for two-joint muscles, as for example in the gastrocnemii, hamstrings, tensor fascia lata, and rectus femoris, should include a notation of the position in which testing was done, as for example, dorsiflexion tested with knee flexed or extended, particularly given the tendency of two-joint muscles to become tight. For normal gait, 5° of ankle dorsiflexion is necessary and 10° is ideal. Plantar flexion contractures of more than 5° interfere with ambulation and if possible should be stretched before bracing. If a plantar flexion contracture is not correctable, the brace will have to accommodate it. ROM at the hip must be considered when prescribing AFO or KAFO because hip flexion contractures increase lumbar lordosis and reduce stride length, thereby reducing the speed and efficiency of ambulation. Assessment of tone is extremely important because the presence of spasticity or clonus can limit bracing options. Severe spasticity and clonus of the gastrocsoleus may preclude the use of certain AFO. Treatments include stretching and antispasticity medications and, in selected cases, nerve or muscle blocks with phenol or botulinum toxin.

Conditions involving weakness or ligamentous laxity can affect stability of the joint with an increased risk of injury requiring orthotic intervention. Anteroposterior and mediolateral stability should be assessed in the knee and ankle; mediolateral instability of the ankle, for example, may indicate that a solid or hinged AFO is more appropriate than a PLSO.

It is next necessary to observe the patient walking. The knees should be visible to assess for buckling or recurvatum. Often, problems will not be apparent for a few minutes until muscle imbalance and fatigue lead to the emergence of a foot slap, spastic foot dragging, knee buckling, or genu recurvatum, especially when observations are made on more demanding conditions such as on different terrains and at various speeds of walking. When it is unclear exactly what type of brace is necessary, a trial of one or the other may be appropriate either in a brace clinic or for more extended periods with a physical therapist. A stock PLSO or Veterans Administration Prosthetic Center clip-on AFO may be used to determine whether a simple dorsiflexion assist brace will suffice. More complex bracing may require an adjustable double-upright trial AFO strapped to the patient's shoe.

The prescription should be as detailed and specific as possible, and a copy should be kept in the patient's record. Communication between the patient and orthotist should be open so that frequent adjustments can be made and financial problems can be quickly resolved.

Checkup and Gait Analysis After Delivery

Upon delivery of the brace, the physician should compare it with the written prescription, noting any discrepancies. The brace is put on the patient, observing any undue pressure areas and checking the location of the orthotic joints and fit of the shoes. The patient should walk for several minutes while the team observes for unexpected gait deviations. It is best to take a systematic approach, observing the patient along proximal to distal points, or vice versa, to avoid missing subtle gait deviations. After the brace has been worn for at least 15 minutes, it is removed and the skin is examined. If any redness is observed, the brace should be modified to reduce pressure on affected areas. Any complaints or questions should be addressed at this time (11).

PITFALLS AND COMPLICATIONS ENCOUNTERED WITH USE OF ORTHOSES

Unnecessary Bracing and the Importance of Follow-up

The importance of avoiding unnecessary bracing or overbracing has already been reviewed. After bracing, the patient should be followed by the physician for an extended period to assess any changes in bracing needs, especially for conditions that are not static. A patient who develops foot drop due to radiculopathy or peroneal palsy, for example, may recover enough dorsiflexion to obviate the need for the orthosis. It is not uncommon for patients to use heavy braces for several years until a physician or other health-care provider discovers that it is no longer needed. By avoiding unnecessary bracing and providing frequent follow-up, such occurrences can be prevented. Of course, it may also be discovered that more aggressive bracing is needed, particularly with progressive conditions.

Skin Breakdown

Patients with severely impaired sensation, significant edema, spasticity, deformity, or contractures are at particular risk for skin breakdown and require extra attention in the design of the brace and subsequent follow-up. The navicular tubercle, the malleoli, and the area of the trim lines of the orthosis are particularly likely problem points. Extra-soft lining, extra-depth footwear, use of more accommodating materials, and patient education reduce the incidence of breakdown, although the extra lining will increase the bulk of the brace.

When discomfort, erythema, or actual skin breakdown occurs, a particularly useful technique is to mark the affected area with a transferable medium such as lipstick and to have the patient don the brace. Areas of higher pressure will have more of a mark, and this information can be used to determine exactly how to modify the brace and where to relieve pressure. It is important to realize, however, that breakdown is not always an indication that the brace is too tight but may result from dynamic biomechanical gait abnormalities. For example, if the

Achilles tendon is too tight, the patient may pronate in the brace, substituting subtalar motion for ankle motion and resulting in pressure and friction in the navicular area. In such a case, the solution may be a heel lift to accommodate the deformity rather than flaring of the brace.

Problems Resulting from Limitation of Ankle Range of Motion

Certain problems may arise when ROM at the ankle is severely limited either by disease or by a solid, semi-solid, or metal upright AFO. In normal gait, the foot rapidly plantar flexes upon heel strike, controlled by eccentric contraction of the anterior compartment musculature to stabilize the knee. A fixed ankle will prevent this response, and the tibia will continue forward abruptly to achieve foot flat, forcing the knee and hip into excessive flexion. The quadriceps, which may already be weak due to underlying neuromuscular disease, are thus under an increased demand to prevent buckling of the knee. One solution is to cushion or bevel the heel of the shoe so as to move the ground reaction force further anterior and thus diminish the flexion moment at the knee. Because this moves the ground reaction force anterior to the ankle as well, it aids weak ankle dorsiflexor muscles by decreasing the plantar flexor moment. Derived from prosthetics jargon, the cushion heel is often referred to as the SACH, or the solid ankle cushion heel. Patients with mild hyperextension of the knee or genu recurvatum can be treated with a small heel lift placed under the AFO or external to the shoe. A heel lift places the ankle in plantar flexion and may result in an increased extension moment at the knee.

A rocker sole added to an orthopedic shoe mimics the action of the ankle and metatarsophalangeal (MTP) joints and aids in roll off, push off, and unweighting of the metatarsal heads, simulating ankle dorsiflexion. Use of a rocker sole requires a stiff sole and an additional elevation of one-quarter to one-half inch to the heel on the rocker side and to the heel and sole on the contralateral side to avoid a resulting leg length discrepancy. The combined use of a SACH heel and rocker sole in the shoe simulates dorsiflexion and plantar flexion in the gait cycle, even though the ankle is relatively fixed. This SACH plus rocker combination can be used whenever there is minimal or no motion at the ankle, as for example because of fusion, fracture, cast immobilization, orthosis design, pain, or arthritis.

Bilateral bracing poses a particular challenge. When rigid ankle AFO are used bilaterally, the contralateral limb is prevented from compensating, thus compounding the difficulties. Consequently, patients seldom tolerate bilateral solid AFO, and hinged or flexible joints should be used.

A solid ankle affects the patient during transitional movements. Normally, when rising from a chair, for example, the ankle is dorsiflexed to move the center of gravity anteriorly; thus, with a solid ankle, alternative strategies must be used. This is also true for movements such as bending or climbing up stairs. Because the ankle is locked, balance adjustments must be made at the hip or by stepping, which can be awkward.

Cane and Crutch Palsy

Those who depend heavily on their canes, such as poliomyelitis patients, should be informed of the possibility of developing secondary compression neuropathies in the hand. This is particularly true for elderly patients as they become more reliant on assistive devices for ambulation or for those who prematurely abandon their AFO or KAFO, causing them to lean on their canes excessively.

The syndrome of cane palsy is due to a lesion at the palm of the hand distal to the carpal and ulnar tunnels. It results in ulnar and median intrinsic muscle weakness and wasting with minimal sensory loss due to involvement of the terminal motor branches of the deep palmar branch of the ulnar and recurrent branch of the median nerves. There are treatment options to reduce pressure on these nerves, including use of a KAFO contralateral to the affected hand, weight control, or use of platform crutches, a walker, or a wheelchair.

Crutch palsy results from compression of the radial nerve at the fascial edge of the latissimus dorsi muscle by axillary crutches. Unlike the Saturday night radial nerve palsy or posterior interosseous nerve entrapment syndrome, there is weakness of the triceps muscle. As with cane palsy, therapy is aimed at reducing pressure on the nerve with the temporary use of platform crutches instead. The lesion is usually a neurapraxic one, and the prognosis for full recovery is good. Axillary artery thrombosis can rarely follow prolonged use of axillary crutches (13).

Other Compression Neuropathies

Carpal tunnel syndrome occurs in patients who use canes and crutches, whereas ulnar neuropathy at the elbow occurs in those who use wheelchairs. Better padding of the handle and armrest of the wheelchair reduces the latter complication.

Unauthorized Alteration

Braces that are altered by patients, often beyond repair, necessitate the fabrication of a new one. Those patients likely to engage in this activity should be educated as to the importance of leaving modifications to the appropriate professionals. It is particularly helpful to provide good communication and access to the orthotist so that patients can resolve problems before becoming frustrated and attempting to solve them themselves.

MANAGEMENT OF SPECIFIC ISSUES

Upper Motor Neuron Disorders

The spasticity and clonus of a UMN disorder may be exacerbated by a solid AFO. Even patients with moderate ankle clonus, however, can do well with a dorsiflexion assist brace, sometimes even a PLSO, without aggravating the clonus. When spasticity is severe, a solid AFO is indeed appropriate. If ataxia is present, bracing can be detrimental; in some cases, however, weighting of the extremity can improve gait, and in these patients bracing may be beneficial.

Dropped Head Syndrome

This syndrome is due to focal weakness of extensor neck muscles in association with inflammatory myopathy, myasthenia gravis, or motor neuron disease (14–16). A lightweight cervical orthosis that assists extension while providing firm support may be more beneficial than traditional restrictive cervical orthoses. Two such braces are pictured in Fig. 6 and are designed to allow for tracheostomy care.

Amyotrophic Lateral Sclerosis

The braces of a patient with amyotrophic lateral sclerosis should be supportive, minimally restrictive, and lightweight. For dorsiflexion weakness at the ankle, a PLSO is preferable to a heavier brace. A lightweight cervical orthosis should be considered if significant extensor neck weakness is present.

Loss of Sensation and Balance

Although it is commonly stated that patients with diminished sensation tolerate plastic braces poorly due to decreased proprioceptive input, however, when an AFO bridges the affected areas, as for example in stocking-and-glove neuropathies, the orthosis may actually transmit vibratory and position stimuli proximally to less affected areas. This can provide important feedback, allowing more physiologic and therefore more functional ambulation (11). Whenever orthoses are used in patients with decreased pain and light touch sensation, there should be frequent inspection of the insensate skin, particularly with plastic orthoses because they make intimate contact with the skin.

Charcot-Marie-Tooth Disease

Charcot-Marie-Tooth disease patients do well with plastic AFO because of their lighter weight. In general, a custom-made brace is appropriate due to diminished sensation and significant foot deformities. Patients with

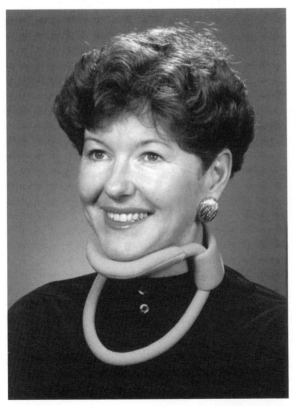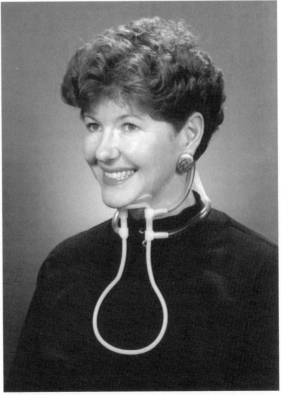

FIG. 6. A: Headmaster collar. **B:** Canadian collar.

distal sensory and proprioceptive loss may shift their weight at the ankle or knees in an attempt to sense the supporting surface at more proximally placed joints where proprioception is intact. Similarly, with severe sensory loss, a cane augments balance by transmitting proprioceptive input to the upper extremity.

The development of a cavus deformity is probably hastened by substitution of toe extensors for weak dorsiflexor muscles and thus may be delayed by early bracing. Dorsiflexion weakness is best managed with a lightweight spring-loaded dorsiflexion-assist orthosis such as a custom-made PLSO with accommodative footwear. When the deformity is severe, posterior tibial transfer, osteotomy, or tarsal arthrodeses may be necessary.

Polio and the Post-Polio Syndrome

Bracing in poliomyelitis and the PPS is often successful because of the spotty nature of the weakness, lack of spasticity, and intact sensation. The continued use of orthoses and adaptive devices is often indicated in these patients despite their ability to get by without them. Frequently, patients with poliomyelitis will have spent decades with minimal or no bracing, and with advancing age and possibly weakness due to PPS, more aggressive means are often needed for safe ambulation to prevent degenerative changes, improve stability, and prevent malalignment of affected joints. Assistive devices such as canes, crutches, wheelchairs, and scooters are often useful as well. Cane palsy may occur in PPS due to increased reliance on assistive devices.

Acute Inflammatory Demyelinating Polyneuropathy or the Guillain-Barré Syndrome

Most patients with Guillain-Barré syndrome recover significant motor function. Nonetheless, an important consideration is to prevent contractures and to reduce overuse fatigue during recuperation. If contractures develop, they will usually be more detrimental to overall function than the residual neuropathy, and heavy bracing should be avoided.

Neuropathic Foot Drop due to a Compartment Syndrome

The anterior tibial compartment syndrome is frequently caused by trauma or fracture and complicated vascular surgery and often results in ischemic peroneal neuropathy. Early weight bearing and ambulation are necessary to prevent plantar flexion contracture. In addition to standing and stretching in the tilt table, early application of a dorsiflexion-assist AFO should be contemplated. An open fasciotomy wound does not preclude bracing, because an effective dorsiflexion-assist AFO can be designed to minimize pressure on the wound. The surgeon should be informed of the extreme importance of preventing contractures even if this interferes with closure of the wound.

Myopathies

The use of orthoses in myopathies is limited. These diseases typically affect proximal muscles more than distal, and orthotic control of proximal joints such as hips, trunk, and shoulders is highly unsatisfactory. Myotonic muscular dystrophy, inclusion body myositis, and facioscapulohumeral dystrophy can present with quadriceps weakness and foot drop, requiring bracing.

ADAPTIVE EQUIPMENT

Ambulation aids such as canes, crutches, and walkers are technically upper extremity orthoses that provide increased stability and safety. They can reduce the load on one or both lower extremities and improve sensory feedback by transmitting information to the upper extremity. They also alert the public that the user needs special consideration. The use of these devices requires functional upper extremities and adequate strength.

Canes

A cane is the most basic adaptive device and supports up to 25% of body weight (17). In unilateral conditions, it is used on the opposite side of the impairment to reduce the load on the affected lower extremity, but they can also be used bilaterally. Wide-based canes are most stable and consist of a platform with three or four legs connected to a shaft and handle, with variable base widths. Although heavier and clumsier than a standard cane, they stand by themselves so that it is not necessary to lean or hook them when not in use. When a cane is used for a prolonged period of time, a functional grip cane, as opposed to the standard C-cane, improves comfort and minimizes the risk of developing problems from excessive pressure to the palm. When fitting a patient for a cane, the top should come up to the level of the greater trochanter, resulting in 20 to 30° of elbow flexion.

Crutches

Crutches are indicated when the impairment is more severe and requires greater support. Whereas a cane conveys balance and sensory feedback, crutches allow the transfer of a significant amount of weight to the upper extremities. This may be problematic, however, in neuromuscular diseases when there is accompanying upper extremity weakness. Bilateral axillary crutches transfer 80% of body weight away from the lower extremities. Although they are commonly padded, this should be avoided because it may encourage increased axillary weight bearing and lead to compression neuropathy of the radial nerve in the axilla. The crutch handle should measure similar to a standard cane, and because it is oriented obliquely to the floor, the total length of the crutch should be about 3 to 5 cm longer than the distance from the anterior axillary fold to the bottom of the heel.

Nonaxillary crutches are less cumbersome and can transfer 40 to 50% of body weight. The most common of these, Lofstrand crutches, consists of an adjustable aluminum shaft with a molded hand piece and an adjustable forearm piece with an open cuff. This design allows the user to release the hand piece while retaining the crutch, thus freeing the hands for other activities. The wooden forearm orthosis, or Kenny Stick, is basically an axillary crutch with shortened proximal end at the level of the forearm and a closed forearm cuff. For patients with distal weakness, they are even easier to retain than Lofstrand crutches (18). Canadian crutches are similar to Lofstrands with longer uprights and a second half cuff that extends above the elbow. The crutch tips for patients with triceps weakness should be checked routinely for wear. Special tips are available for use in the rain, ice, and snow. Patients that cannot bear weight along the forearm or those with wrist or hand weakness due to arthritis, fractures, and neuromuscular diseases should consider platform crutches.

Walkers

A walker should be used when maximum stability is needed, particularly in disorders of balance and coordination. They require good bilateral grasp and arm strength and result in a slowed and more awkward gait. As with crutches, a platform can be added when weight bearing through the forearm is problematic. Although they provide less stability, rolling walkers allow for a more natural gait pattern and require less upper extremity coordination. They are particularly useful in patients with Parkinson disease because they minimize starts and stops. These ambulatory aids may be unsafe if the user is unable to keep themselves within the base of support of the walker. Newer lightweight walkers are more efficient for patients with neuromuscular disease.

Wheelchairs

A wheelchair is indicated when walking becomes unsafe, impossible, or impractical, even with the use of the above devices. Quite commonly, the patient and their family see the failure to ambulate as a defeat. The physician must emphasize that their wheelchair allows safer and more efficient mobility. Some patients are able to ambulate indoors or even limited distances outdoors but require a wheelchair for longer distances to improve their safety and level of independence. A standard wheelchair is inappropriate for patients who spend most of the day in them. A great variety of lightweight designs and different

cushions, seat backs, headrests, armrests, and other components are available. Complex wheelchairs should be prescribed with the input of a multidisciplinary team, including the physiatrist, other physicians, therapists, and the equipment vendor. Concomitant with the cessation of ambulating, complications due to underlying disease and increased immobility, including scoliosis, pressure ulcers, deconditioning, and contractures, can rapidly arise, requiring additional attention.

A manually powered wheelchair is preferable to a motorized chair because they are more durable, lighter in weight and therefore easier to transport, less expensive, and allow greater access in confined spaces. They are often the only significant exercise that a patient may receive. A motorized wheelchair or scooter should only be considered when a patient is unable to propel themselves independently, when greater mobility is required for independence at work or school, and to avoid undue strain upon already weakened limbs. Prescription considerations are similar to those for manual chairs; numerous control devices are available to accommodate various impairments.

UPPER EXTREMITY ORTHOSES

Upper extremity orthoses are primarily used to prevent or minimize contractures and to improve function in patients with neuromuscular diseases. There are two basic types, static and dynamic, with the former being a fixed or rigid device and the latter allowing some movement. The term functional is sometimes applied to a splint designed to directly increase function, as opposed to resting splints, which are designed to prevent or stretch contractures.

As with lower extremity bracing, it is important to keep in mind the purpose of the orthosis and whether it is likely to be used. In functional bracing, patients are only likely to continue to use orthoses if this enables them to do things that they otherwise could not. A patient with bilateral deficits is more likely to use a functional orthosis because the other hand may not be able to compensate. With resting splints, comfort and ease of donning and doffing are paramount. Cosmesis is much more of an issue with upper extremity orthoses given the visibility of the hand and another reason why an upper extremity orthosis may be rejected. Orthoses that cover the volar aspect of the hand can be problematic because they interfere with sensation, which is a primary function of the hand. Sometimes, this can be alleviated by a dorsal design, minimizing the impact on sensory feedback. Orthoses that hinder sensation can be used at rest, whereas a less cumbersome one can be used during activities.

Wrist–Hand Orthoses

These are the most common types of upper extremity orthoses and usually consist of a volar support with dorsal forearm straps. When indicated, variations are available with the support applied to the dorsal surface and ventral straps.

Resting Hand Splint

This widely used volar splint is designed to prevent contractures by maintaining the hand in a functional position, preserving the balance between extrinsic and intrinsic muscles. It also provides joint protection and is applicable to UMN conditions that result in increased tone.

Tenodesis Splints

The fingers normally flex somewhat with wrist extension and extend with wrist flexion. So-called tenodesis is enhanced by orthoses that use a hinged parallelogram design to approximate the thumb and fingers when the wrist is extended. The patient should be prepared and trained before the brace is ordered, and the finger flexors should be left to develop mild contractures so that with passive wrist extension, the distal and proximal interphalangeal joints flex, aiding in tenodesis. The classic indication for these is a C6 tetraplegia, although they can also be used in other conditions in which hand weakness is significant.

Wrist Cock-up Splint

This static splint supports the wrist in a functional position of about 20 to 30° of extension and improves grip by placing a slight stretch on the finger flexors (tenodesis) providing protection and functional improvement when there is weakness of wrist extension and grip. For good leverage, it should begin about two thirds the way up the forearm and should extend no further than the distal palmar crease. This splint is often used in carpal tunnel syndrome, in which case a more neutral wrist position of 0 to 20° of extension is preferable.

Balanced Forearm Orthosis

This orthosis can be attached to a supporting structure such as a wheelchair or pelvic band and consists of a ball-bearing hinge joint at the elbow with a forearm trough. It is configured to support the forearm and allow for flexion and extension at the elbow along the horizontal plane, essentially eliminating the effect of gravity. In cases of proximal weakness, including the shoulder with relative sparing of the hand, it can increase independence in the activities of daily living, but elbow strength should be grade 2 or more. An overhead sling arrangement can also be used for trial purposes. When shoulder strength is adequate but elbow weakness is a problem, a dynamic flexion-assist orthosis can be made by using arm and forearm cuffs connected by a spring joint. Elbow exten-

sion can usually be substituted by gravity (19). In cases of complete paralysis, tendon transfer may be beneficial.

Shoulder Slings

The basic shoulder sling is known to virtually everyone. It positions the arm in adduction and internal rotation with the elbow flexed. By limiting motion at the shoulder, it contributes to contractures, and minimizes opportunities for the patient to reincorporate use of the extremity into the activities of daily living; it and should therefore only be used acutely or for protection during transfers. A sling with a humeral cuff and chest straps that support the humerus and reduce subluxation while interfering much less with shoulder motion should be used for shoulder subluxation resulting from paralysis.

SUMMARY

The judicious use of orthoses and adaptive equipment can greatly benefit the patient with a neuromuscular disease. A thorough knowledge of the biomechanics of ambulation and upper extremity function and the capabilities and limitations of bracing are necessary to prescribe orthoses correctly. The physician should focus on function, maintenance of ROM, and joint preservation, although the patient will often be more concerned about cosmesis, comfort, and ease of donning and doffing them. If the patient agrees with a chosen orthosis or brace, compliance will be best when the goals of both the patient and physician are suitably addressed.

ACKNOWLEDGMENT

Lynn Nichols, CO, J-V-Prosthetics & Orthotics Inc. for providing information and samples of orthoses.

REFERENCES

1. Stillwell GK, Thorsteinsson G. Rehabilitation procedures. In: Dyck T, Thomas PK, Lambert E, Bunge R, eds. *Peripheral neuropathy,* 3rd ed. Philadelphia: W.B. Saunders, 1992:1692–1708.
2. Siegel IM. *Muscle and its diseases: an outline primer of basic science and clinical method.* Chicago: Year Book Medical Publishers, 1986.
3. Redford JB. Orthotics: general principles. *Phys Med Rehabil* 1987;1: 1–10.
4. Cinque AA. Laminated versus polypropylene: what's best for patients? *O & P Business News* 1997;June 15:8–12.
5. *Lower-limb orthotics.* New York: Prosthetic Orthotic Publications, 1986.
6. Zablotny CM. Use of orthoses for the adult with neurologic involvement. In: Nawoczenski DA, Epler, ME, eds. *Orthotics in functional rehabilitation of the lower limb.* Philadelphia: W.B. Saunders, 1997:207–243.
7. Rubin GR, Staros AS. Orthotic and prosthetic management of foot disorders. In: Jhass MJ, ed. *Disorders of the foot and ankle: medical and surgical management,* 2nd ed. Philadelphia: W.B. Saunders, 1991: 2808–2833.
8. Hennessey WJ, Johnson EW. Lower limb orthoses. In: Braddom RL, ed. *Physical medicine and rehabilitation.* Philadelphia: W.B. Saunders, 1996:333–358.

9. Chambers RB, Elftman N. Orthotic management of the dysvascular patient. In: Goldberg B, ed. *Atlas of orthoses and assistive devices,* 3rd ed. St. Louis: Mosby, 1997.

10. Merritt JL. Knee-ankle-foot orthotics: long leg braces and their practical applications. *Phys Med Rehabil* 1987;1:67–82.

11. Halar E, Cardenas D. Ankle-foot orthoses: clinical implications. *Phys Med Rehabil* 1987;1:45–66.

12. Weber RJ. Functional neuromuscular stimulation. In: DeLisa JA, Gans BM, eds. *Rehabilitation medicine principles and practice*, 2nd ed. Philadelphia: J.B. Lippincott, 1993:463–476.

13. Brooks AL, Fouler SB. *J Bone Joint Surg* 1964;46:863–864.

14. Suarez GA, Kelly JJ. The dropped head syndrome. *Neurology* 1992;42: 1625–1627.

15. Hoffman D, Gutmann L. The dropped head syndrome with chronic inflammatory demyelinating polyneuropathy. *Muscle Nerve* 1994;17: 808–810.

16. Katz JS, Wolfe GI, Burns DK, Bryan WW, Fleckenstein JL, Barohn RJ. Isolated neck extensor myopathy: a common cause of the dropped head syndrome. *Neurology* 1996;46:917–921.

17. Scheinberg L, Smith CR. Rehabilitation of patients with multiple sclerosis. *Neurol Clin* 1987;5:585–600.

18. Ragnarsson KT. Lower extremity orthotics, shoes, and gait aids. In: DeLisa JA, Gans BM, eds. *Rehabilitation medicine principles and practice*, 2nd ed. Philadelphia: J.B. Lippincott, 1993:492–506.

19. Irani KD. Upper limb orthoses. In: Braddom RL, ed. *Physical medicine and rehabilitation*. Philadelphia: W.B. Saunders, 1996:321–332.

Motor Disorders,
edited by David S. Younger.
Lippincott Williams & Wilkins, Philadelphia © 1999.

CHAPTER 40

Respiratory Muscle Aids

John R. Bach

Inspiratory and expiratory muscle aids are manual or mechanical devices that assist in inspiratory or expiratory muscle function by applying forces on the body or intermittent pressure changes to the airway. Those that act on the body include the negative pressure body ventilators (NPBV) that create atmospheric pressure changes around the thorax and abdomen, body ventilators and exsufflation devices that apply forces directly to the body to mechanically displace respiratory muscles; and others that apply intermittent pressure changes directly to the airway. Positive pressure blowers deliver a continuous flow of positive airway pressure (CPAP). These act like a pneumatic splint to maintain airway and alveolar patency and to increase functional residual capacity but do not directly assist respiratory muscle function or substitute for respiratory muscle assistance.

In a 1992 report of a survey of 273 Jerry Lewis Muscular Dystrophy Association clinic directors and 167 clinics, most discouraged ventilator use (Fig. 1); the most common reason, 56% overall, was the anticipated poor patient quality of life. Accordingly, 62 clinics (37%) were not managing patients using ventilators. The preponderance of ventilator use was tracheostomied patients (Fig. 2). In only 43 clinics, ventilators were used electively. Only two physicians who discouraged use of mechanical ventilation indicated familiarity with methods of noninvasive ventilatory aid assistance. Respiratory muscle aids that postpone or eliminate the otherwise inevitable development of acute respiratory failure and hospitalization are an alternative to endotracheal intubation, tracheostomy, or death (1). Noninvasive respiratory muscle aids are preferred by most who later switch from tracheostomy to noninvasive intermittent positive pressure ventilation (IPPV). They are preferred

for swallowing, sleep, speech comfort, appearance, comfort, convenience, and security (Fig. 3) (2).

No medications are effective in increasing spontaneous alveolar ventilation and respiratory muscle strength (3). Inspiratory muscle training does not reduce the incidence of respiratory complications or hospitalization rates (3). Respiratory muscle aids have been used in selected patients by pulmonary, physical medicine, and rehabilitation specialists to avert respiratory complications, acute respiratory failure (4,5), and tracheostomy. This chapter reviews the assessment of patients, the available respiratory aid modalities, and the use in patients with motor disorders and respiratory insufficiency.

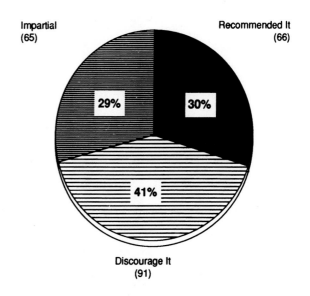

FIG. 1. Muscular Dystrophy Association directors' attitudes toward ventilatory aid (n = 222). (From Ref. 1, with permission.)

J.R. Bach: Departments of Physical Medicine and Rehabilitation and of Neurosciences, UMDNJ-The New Jersey Medical School, Newark, New Jersey 07103.

Ventilator Systems of DMD Patients Currently Followed by MDA Directors (n=105 clinics)

Ventilator Systems of Non-DMD Patients Currently Followed by MDA Directors (n=105 clinics)

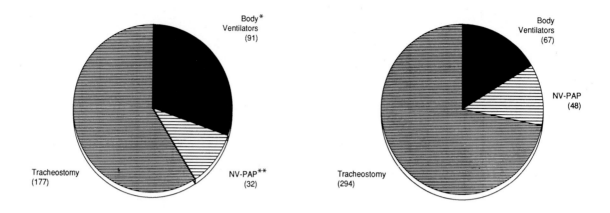

Body* Ventilators (91)

Tracheostomy (177)

NV-PAP** (32)

Body Ventilators (67)

NV-PAP (48)

Tracheostomy (294)

*Body Ventilators = iron lung, chest shell, pulmowrap
**NV-PAP = assisted ventilation via the nose and/or mouth

FIG. 2. Noninvasive ventilatory support systems used by Muscular Dystrophy Association clinic patients (n = 167 clinics). Body ventilators include iron lung, chest shell, and wrap style ventilators. Positive pressure methods include ventilation via the nose or mouth. (From Ref. 2, with permission.)

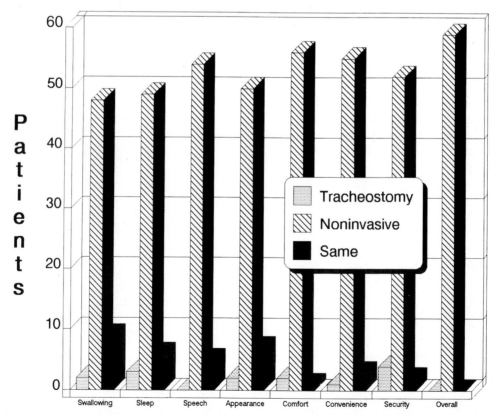

FIG. 3. The preferences of 59 patients switched from tracheostomy to noninvasive aids, including 8 who switched to body ventilators, 18 to noninvasive intermittent positive pressure ventilation (IPPV) methods, and 33 to a combination of body ventilators and noninvasive IPPV methods. (From Ref. 2, with permission.)

GOALS OF INTERVENTION

Respiratory failure is the inevitable outcome for conventionally managed patients with progressive neuromuscular disorders. Three goals in the pulmonary management of patients at risk for respiratory failure can avert respiratory failure: improvement of pulmonary compliance by chest wall and lung "range-of-motion exercises," maintenance at all times of normal alveolar ventilation, and monitoring of cough flow.

The lungs and chest wall should be fully mobilized several times a day. This prevents chronic atelectasis, contractures, loss of elasticity, and inadequate insufflation to generate an effective cough or raise the voice. Patients with a vital capacity (VC) below 50% of the predicted normal mean can be taught to stack air by receiving consecutive breaths without exhalation from a manual resuscitator, volume ventilator, or mechanical insufflator-exsufflator (In-Exsufflator, J. H. Emerson Co., Cambridge, MA).

Full insufflations are most conveniently delivered by a mouthpiece. If, however, the oral and buccal musculature is weak or there is difficulty in grasping a mouthpiece and greater volumes can be insufflated by a nose piece, then the latter method should be used. A mouthpiece can be used with mild hand pressure applied to a lipseal phalange. Patients who have mastered glossopharyngeal breathing (GPB) can also use this method for maximal insufflation. The ultimate goal is to approach the predicted inspiratory capacity or maximum insufflation capacity, the maximum volume of air that can be held.

Air stacking improves alveolar ventilation and the distribution of air to underventilated areas, (6), decreases microscopic atelectasis, and may not only help maintain static lung compliance, but also may temporarily improve dynamic pulmonary compliance (7). The higher resulting volumes increase unassisted and assisted peak cough flows (PCF). The ability to stack air indicates the potential to receive IPPV by a mouthpiece or nasal interface. Those patients undergoing extubation or decanulation of a tracheostomy tube who are still unable to breathe independently can be switched to IPPV. Hyperinflation two to four times per day delivers a gradually increased volume of air until the predicted inspiratory capacity is reached or further increases can not be tolerated. Regular deep insufflations via anesthesia masks, and later via mouth or nasal interfaces, was studied in over 100 children age 18 months or older with spinal muscular atrophy (8,9).

Maximizing Cough Flows: Expiratory Muscle Aids

Patients with restrictive pulmonary syndromes often cannot generate a sufficient PCF to expel airway debris, and accordingly, episodes of acute respiratory failure most often occur during otherwise benign upper respiratory tract infections (10). A flow rate of 160 L/min is necessary to expel airway secretions (11). The inability to take or receive a 2L volume of air, hold it with a closed glottis, generate sufficient thoracoabdominal pressure using intercostal and abdominal muscles, and create an explosive decompression upon glottic opening all contribute to a decreased PCF. Thus oropharyngeal muscle function and airway patency are important determinants of PCF. Debris that occurs during respiratory infections or that results from aspiration of saliva or food can precipitate life-threatening plugging of the airways and acute respiratory failure. This is also true for intubated or tracheotomized patients who necessarily have increased airway secretion and are unable to close the glottis to generate the pressures needed for an effective cough.

Airway suctioning via the mouth or nose is ineffective and poorly tolerated. Suctioning via an endotracheal tube does not mobilize deep secretions and has many potential complications. Suction catheters will usually fail to enter the left main stem bronchus (12). Repeated suctioning irritate airway membranes, exacerbating secretions and causing inflammatory changes, edema, and wheezing. This necessitates further bronchial sunctioning. Over time, granulation formation can narrow the airway. Mucous plugs that adhere to the cuff or the wall of a tube can not be removed and may eventually plug a bronchus, causing atelectasis and airway collapse. Tracheal intubation and tracheostomy tubes incapacitate mucociliary and alveolar macrophage activity, which can be further impaired by chronic bacterial colonization and malnutrition (13). Swallowing and communication are hampered or precluded by the presence of indwelling tubes (14). Chest percussion and postural drainage is performed while positioned in as many as nine different positions to maximally clear bronchopulmonary segments (15), but its effect on morbidity and mortality is debatable (16–21) and has not been shown more effective than an effective cough alone (22).

Chest percussion also causes hypoxia and oxyhemoglobin desaturation (20), increases sputum volume, and is ineffective in patients who produce less than 30 ml of sputum per day. It may be beneficial for patients with chronic bronchitis and atelectasis, but appears to be of no benefit in treating pneumonia or viral bronchitis, or as a postoperative therapy (21).

Various techniques of a manually assisted cough are effective but underused (23). To be optimally effective for patients with a VC less than 1,500 mL, it must be preceded by a deep assisted insufflation (24) and followed by anterior chest compression and an abdominal thrust to generate 3 L/sec or more of PCF. Manually assisted coughing may be inadequate during severe respiratory tract infections or in patients with an MIC that is not significantly greater than the VC. These patients can benefit from the use of mechanically assisted coughing.

Mechanical insufflator-exsufflator (In-Exsufflator, J. H. Emerson Inc.) may be useful in selected patients with neuromuscular disorders. It delivers an adjustable positive pressure insufflation followed by an adjustable negative pressure exsufflation via anesthetic mask or an indwelling tube. About 10 L/sec of delivered expiratory flow carries airway debris up into the mouth or indwelling tube, where it can then be easily suctioned. An abdominal thrust can be manually applied during the exsufflation cycle to further increase flows. Mechanical insufflation-exsufflation can increase VC and normalize oxygen saturation (SaO$_2$) as secretions and mucous plugs are cleared. The optimal use of mechanical exsufflation can be instrumental in allowing continued ventilatory support without a tracheostomy (5,25–28). Few if any complications have been reported in over 40 years and in thousands of applications (26–29). It facilitates ventilator weaning and benefits patients with neuromuscular weakness who aspirate food or who have periodic difficulties in managing profuse upper airway secretions.

Inspiratory Muscle Aids

Body Ventilators

The iron lung is the best known NPBV. It induces alveolar ventilation by cyclically creating subatmospheric pressure in a chamber that covers at least the chest and abdomen. They are still the mainstay of intensive care unit ventilatory support in some European centers (30) and continue to be used by some adults, although more practical and effective noninvasive IPPV methods are now available (31,32). The iron lungs are really only practical in small children, such as those with spinal muscular atrophy, who prefer them to noninvasive IPPV methods because of difficulty with use of a mouthpiece. The Portalung is a small light iron lung that achieves equivalent negative pressures and ventilatory volumes. The negative chamber pressure is created by the action of a pressure generator or ventilator that is separate from the chamber itself. The cuirass or chest shell ventilator firmly covers the anterior chest and upper abdomen and creates negative or subatmospheric pressure under the shell. Although less effective than the iron lung, it is adequate for most patients without significant back deformity, intrinsic lung disease, or impaired pulmonary compliance. Unlike other NPBV, the chest shell can be used in the daytime and in the seated position. It is the ventilator of choice for assistance during tracheostomy site closure and during extubation for those being converted from IPPV via endotracheal intubation to mouthpiece or nasal IPPV (33). It may also be an alternative to continuous nasal IPPV or iron lung use by infants with spinal muscular atrophy who otherwise lack ventilator-free breathing ability.

Wrap ventilators provide greater volumes than the chest shell ventilator using similar principles. Properly and carefully placed, a firm plastic grid covers the thorax and abdomen and may be applied to a rigid backplate to optimize effectiveness. The grid and the body underneath can be covered by a variety of wraps of various composition and in several forms. One popular design is windproof nylon or Gortex (W.C. Gore & Assoc. Inc., Elkton,

MD) in the style of a poncho or one-piece suit. The Gortex makes a cooler more flexible wrap than plastic or cloth, and it increases comfort and expense. The wrap is sealed around the patient's wrists, neck, and abdomen or lower extremities, depending on the intended style.

Rocking bed ventilators rock the patient from 15 to 30° above and below the horizontal line, shifting abdominal contents against the diaphragm to assist ventilation. It is the least effective but easiest of body ventilators (34) to use. The weight-shifting effect protects the skin against breakdown and improves bowel motility. The majority of patients using NPBVs have obstructive apneas and oxyhemoglobin desaturations during sleep. This can cause fatigue and other symptoms of chronic alveolar hypoventilation, high blood pressure and recurrent aspirations. Apart from small children, patients with respiratory infection or during tracheostomy closure (35–39), there is little current need for NPBV.

The intermittent abdominal pressure ventilator (IAPV) is the method of choice for daytime ventilatory support in wheelchair-dependent patients with less than 1 hour of ventilator-free breathing ability (40). It is only effective when the patient is in a seated position and may not be effective for those with scoliosis or the extremes of body weight. About 250 (40) to 1,200 mL (5) of tidal volumes can be provided by its action and can be supplemented by autonomous breathing effort when possible, as well as by GPB. IAPV has been used for nocturnal ventilatory support of individuals that sleep in a seated upright position. Daytime use of IAPV can complement nocturnal mouthpiece or nasal IPPV.

NONINVASIVE INTERMITTENT POSITIVE PRESSURE VENTILATION

These methods provide ventilatory assistance via the mouth (5,25,32,33,40–42), nose (36,41,43–47), or both together (42,43,48,49) in either portable volume-cycled (PLV-100, Lifecare International Inc., Westminster, CO; LP 10, Aquetron Inc., Minneapolis, MN) or pressure-cycled ventilators (BiPAP, Respironics Inc., Monroeville, PA). BiPAP should not be used for adolescents or adults unless the VC is greater than 2,000 mL because it cannot provide high enough volumes for assisted coughing when airway secretions are present. An assist-control mode present on the volume-cycled ventilator enables the patient to trigger the machine. Volume-cycled ventilator volumes of less than 900 mL are useful for introducing mouthpiece or nasal IPPV, but these are gradually increased to 1,500 mL or more to permit the patient to control the depth of the assisted breath. The improvement in SaO$_2$ and carbon dioxide levels equals or exceeds those obtained by body ventilator use (36). There appears to be less hypercapnia and fewer rapid eye movement-associated desaturations, sleep disturbances, or arousals with noninvasive IPPV (50). Patients for whom normal ventilation is maintained

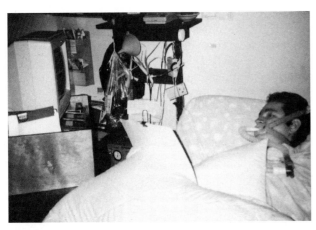

FIG. 4. Patient with Duchenne muscular dystrophy who has used 24-hour mouthpiece intermittent positive pressure ventilation (IPPV) for 12 years, now with less than 5 minutes of ventilator-free breathing ability. He uses mouthpiece IPPV with lipseal retention for sleep.

during daytime hours and who do not have depressed ventilatory drive mechanisms or receive supplemental oxygen can maintain normal SaO_2 and $PaCO_2$ during sleep by use of these methods despite little or no measurable VC (36).

Intermittent Positive Pressure Ventilation Mouthpiece

The mouthpiece for IPPV is either kept in the patient's mouth or, more often, fixed onto the motorized wheelchair controls adjacent to the patient for assisted breaths as needed (51). It has the advantage of simplicity, low expense, and different available styles. The rate, rhythm, and volume of speech are more normal for mouthpiece IPPV users and swallowing is less compromised than for those using tracheostomy or nasal IPPV. Mouth-stick activities are unhindered by mouthpiece IPPV unless the patient has little or no significant ventilator-free breathing ability, in which case the IAPV or nasal IPPV is usually preferred for daytime aid when using a mouthstick.

It can also be used for nocturnal ventilatory support with lipseal retention (Fig. 4) to avoid potentially severe oxyhemoglobin desaturation (Fig. 5) and loss of the mouthpiece (39). A soft flexible scuba mouthpiece or a bite mouthpiece may be substituted for additional comfort and relief of orthodontic pressure. Cotton pledgets can be placed into the nostrils and sealed in place by adhesive tape, or nose clips can be used for an airtight oronasal seal (39) for relief of any nasal leakage. For patients who require pressures over 40 to 45 cm H_2O, a custom-molded acrylic nasal interface (Fig. 6) or a custom acrylic mouthpiece with bite plate retention and acrylic lipseal can be constructed (43). Patients without reliable attendant care to aid in placement of a strap retention system can use a custom-made acrylic interface with bite plate retention (43). This can be put on independently without needing to put one's hands behind the head to affix retention straps. This interface can also be easily removed by a tongue thrust. Mouthpiece IPPV safely and effectively ventilates patients both day and night and is associated with few difficulties (33). It is of paramount importance in the conversion of patients from tracheostomy to noninvasive aid (11) and can also be used in ventilator weaning (52).

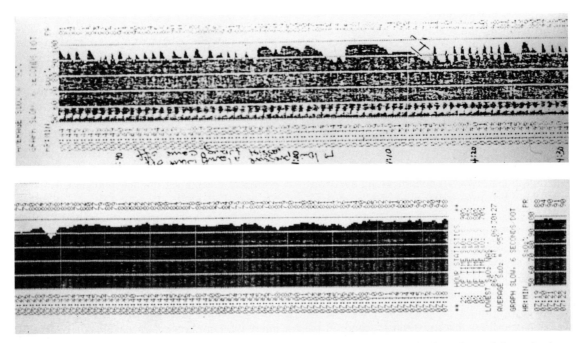

FIG. 5. Normalization of oxyhemoglobin saturation with reduction of leakage of ventilator-delivered volumes by switching from nocturnal nasal intermittent positive pressure ventilation (IPPV) (top) to mouthpiece IPPV with lipseal retention (bottom).

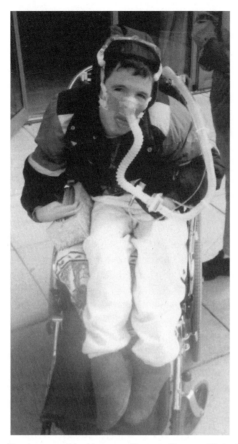

FIG. 6. Custom-molded low-profile acrylic nasal interface for nasal intermittent positive pressure ventilation (IPPV) being used here for daytime ventilatory support for a Duchenne muscular dystrophy ventilator user with no ventilator-free breathing ability and insufficient lip strength to grab a mouthpiece for mouthpiece IPPV.

Nasal Intermittent Positive Pressure Ventilation

First described in 1981 (53) and used for 24-hour ventilatory support in 1987 (54), nasal IPPV has become the preferred method of ventilatory support during sleep (36). Commercially available CPAP masks are most often used as nasal interfaces for nasal IPPV. CPAP masks were initially designed to provide a leakage-free patient–ventilator hose interface for CPAP pressures less than 15 cm H_2O; however, they can be used for nasal IPPV at pressures exceeding 20 cm H_2O. All commercially available CPAP masks are held in place by a headgear or strap assembly. When generic nasal CPAP masks are uncomfortable or not airtight, custom-molded interfaces can be made (36). SEFAM assembly kits can be used to make several styles of custom nasal interfaces (Lifecare Inc.) (41). They contain elastic strap sets, a small plastic housing, and sufficient silicone putty to make three to six interfaces. The putty is mixed and molded by the patient or caregiver into interfaces that are strap retained. Firm durable custom acrylic nasal interfaces can also be fabricated (Fig. 6) (43). Nasal IPPV can also be used for daytime aid when the patient's lips or neck are too weak to grab a mouthpiece and IAPV is ineffective.

During sleep, the open systems of mouthpiece and nasal IPPV are apparently effective because of central nervous system-mediated reflex muscle activity that cuts off excessive air leakage and reverses leakage-associated oxyhemoglobin desaturations (55). Closed systems of noninvasive IPPV are possible by using lipseal retention with the nose plugged or an oral–nasal interface.

Oral–Nasal Intermittent Positive Pressure Ventilation

Covering both the nose and the mouth with an oral–nasal interface is rarely necessary because simple mouthpiece, lipseal, and nasal IPPV are generally effective for most patients. Nonetheless, comfortable available strap-retained oral–nasal interfaces are commercially available (Respironics, Murrysville, PA). A custom-molded strapless oral–nasal interface is often used by patients unable to place strap-retention systems (43). One consists of an acrylic bite plate with metal clasps for retention to the teeth that is affixed to an extraoral shell and connected to a respirator hose. It can be open to both the nose and mouth, allowing concurrent nasal and mouthpiece IPPV, and provides an essentially closed system. It can be thrust out by tongue movement alone. It should not be used for children who necessarily have rapidly changing dentition.

GLOSSOPHARYNGEAL BREATHING

Self-administered GPB indirectly assists expiratory muscles and supports ventilation by providing large volumes of air and increasing PCF (56); it also expands the lungs to maintain elasticity and raises the volume of one's voice. Patients who master GPB can awaken from sleep using it, only to discover that their ventilators are no longer functioning. The patient is instructed to take as deep a breath as possible and then augment it by GPB. The glottis captures boluses of air and projects them into the lungs. The vocal cords close with each "gulp." One breath usually consists of six to eight gulps of 60 to 200 mL each. During the training period, the efficiency of GPB is monitored spirometrically by measuring the number of milliliters of air per gulp and the gulps per breath and breaths per minute; an excellent training manual and video is also available (57). A GPB rate of 12 to 14 per minute can provide patients with normal tidal volumes, minute ventilation, and hours of ventilator free time (Fig. 7) even in those with little or unmeasurable VC (51). The maximum depth of a GPB should be equal to that of the maximum insufflation capacity.

Baydur et al. (38) reported two ventilator-assisted patients with Duchenne muscular dystrophy who successfully used GPB for ventilator-free breathing. We worked with five Duchenne patients, others with polio and other neuromuscular diseases, and patients with spinal cord injury who similarly mastered GPB for hours of ventilator-free breathing. The presence of a tracheostomy tube virtually precludes successful use of GPB, because even with the tube plugged, gulped air leaked around the tube and out the tracheostomy site. Therefore, its use justifies removal

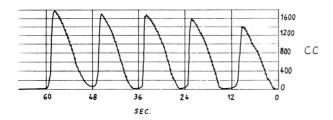

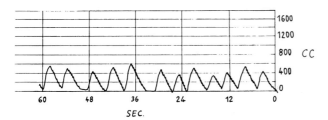

FIG. 7. Top: Glossopharyngeal breathing (GPB) minute ventilation 8.39 L/min with GPB breaths averaging 1.67 L, 20 gulps, and 84 mL/gulp for each breath in a patient with a vital capacity of 0 mL. Bottom: Same patient using GPB at usual tidal volumes with minute ventilation 4.76 L/min, 12.5 breaths, average eight gulps per breath, and 47.5 mL/gulp performed over a 1-minute period. (From Ref. 51, with permission.)

of air indwelling tracheostomy tubes when standard extubation criteria are satisfied (11).

OXIMETRY MONITORING AND BIOFEEDBACK

Hypercapnic patients not using ventilatory support and those being converted from tracheostomy to noninvasive IPPV can use oximetry as feedback to guide the need for mouthpiece and nasal IPPV. The SaO_2 alarm is set from 93% to 94%, and the patient is instructed to take a slightly deeper breath to normalize the SaO_2 and to take mouthpiece assisted breaths when tired. Over time, patients with progressive muscular weakness spend longer periods of time on IPPV maintaining adequate ventilation, even up to 24 hours without the need of hospitalization. In this manner, oximetry feedback can also be used to reset central ventilatory drive. Oximetry biofeedback can be particularly useful in the management of upper respiratory tract infections. In patients that use nasal IPPV during sleep, decreases in SaO_2 can be caused by obstruction to flow by nasal congestion and secretions. Oral nasal decongestant may be helpful. Patients can switch to lipseal IPPV or other noninvasive aids guided by nocturnal SaO_2 monitoring (11,58). Patients with a VC of less than 1,000 mL or an assisted PCF of less than 5 L/sec should undergo continuous daytime SaO_2 monitoring during respiratory tract infections. When the SaO_2 decreases below 95%, either noninvasive IPPV or mechanical or manual coughs are used as needed to maintain normal alveolar ventilation and SaO_2. Oximetry is used to prevent any prolonged decrease in SaO_2 and prevent respiratory insufficiency. Oximetry screens for hypoventilation, mucus plugging, atelectasis, pneumonia, and other intrinsic lung conditions. Dehydra-

tion or decreases in SaO_2 baseline below 95% can indicate the need for chest x-ray and possible hospitalization.

MAINTENANCE OF RESPIRATORY MUSCLE STRENGTH AND ENDURANCE

Inspiratory resistive exercise training improves respiratory muscle endurance (59,60,62) but has not been shown to increase VC, maximum inspiratory, or expiratory pressures (59–61). The degree of improvement in endurance correlated with the level of VC and maximum inspiratory pressure at the outset of training, but no patient with less than 30% of predicted VC improved (59). This is the level of VC at which patients are at high risk for mucous plug-associated respiratory failure and at which they often require nocturnal ventilatory assistance (36). Unfortunately, the improvement in endurance does not delay deterioration in respiratory muscle function or the need for ventilator use. To the contrary, the training itself may be hazardous for certain patients such as those with amyotrophic lateral sclerosis in whom decreases in VC and inspiratory pressures proceed rapidly despite training (63).

COUNSELING

Early and effective use of physical medicine respiratory muscle aids is essential if hospitalizations and episodes of acute respiratory failure are to be avoided. Likewise, physical interventions to facilitate rehabilitation are important to optimize quality of life. Counseling is needed to explain the various options. The patient should also be cautioned to avoid obesity, heavy meals, extremes of temperature, high humidity, excessive fatigue, home oxygen use, crowded areas or exposure to respiratory tract pathogens, and sedatives. Early and appropriate attention during intercurrent respiratory tract infections with the oximetry-noninvasive IPPV-assisted coughing protocol should also be reinforced. The need for influenza and bacterial vaccinations and even antiviral agents such as amantadine should be considered. Because patients with progressive neuromuscular diseases can now have greatly increased survival, goal-oriented activities and plans for the future should also be entertained.

REFERENCES

1. Bach JR. Ventilator use by muscular dystrophy association patients: an update. *Arch Phys Med Rehabil* 1992;73:179–183.
2. Bach JR. A comparison of long-term ventilatory support alternatives from the perspective of the patient and care giver. *Chest* 1993;104:1702–1706.
3. Bach JR. Pulmonary rehabilitation. In: DeLisa JD, ed. *Rehabilitation medicine: principles and practice.* Philadelphia: J.B. Lippincott, 1993:952–972.
4. Bach JR. Update and perspectives on noninvasive respiratory muscle aids. Part 1. The inspiratory muscle aids. *Chest* 1994;105:1230–1240.
5. Bach JR, Alba AS. Noninvasive options for ventilatory support of the traumatic high level quadriplegic. *Chest* 1990;98:613–619.
6. Alvarez SE, Peterson M, Lunsford BR. Respiratory treatment of the adult patient with spinal cord injury. *Phys Ther* 1981;61:1737–1745.
7. Miller WF: Rehabilitation of patients with chronic obstructive lung disease. *Med Clin North Am* 1967;51:349–361.
8. Barois A, Bataille J, Estournet B. La ventilation a domicile par voie buccale chez l'enfant dans les maladies neuromusculaires. *Agressologie* 1985;26:645–649.

9. Barois A, Estournet B, Duval-Beaupere G, Bataille J, Leclair-Richard D. Amyotrophie spinale infantile. *Rev Neurol (Paris)* 1989;145:299–304.

10. Bach JR, Rajalaman R, Ballanger F, Kulessa R. Neuromuscular ventilatory insufficiency: the effect of home mechanical ventilator use vs. oxygen therapy on pneumonia and hospitalization rates. *Am Phys Med Rehabil* 1998;77:8–19.

11. Bach JR, Saporito LR. Criteria for extubation and tracheostomy tube removal for patients with ventilatory failure: a different approach to weaning. *Chest*

12. Fishburn MJ, Marino RJ, Ditunno JF Jr. Atelectasis and pneumonia in acute spinal cord injury. *Arch Phys Med Rehabil* 1990;71:197–200.

13. Mohsenin V, Ferranti R, Loke JS. Nutrition for the respiratory insufficient patient. *Eur Respir J* 1989;2:663s–665s.

14. Leonard C, Criner GJ. Swallowing function in patients with tracheostomy receiving prolonged mechanical ventilation. *International Conference on Pulmonary Rehabilitation and Home Ventilation.* Abstracts. 1991:58.

15. Pineda HD. Rehabilitation management of pulmonary/respiratory diseases. In: Goodgold J, ed. *Rehabilitation medicine.* St. Louis: C.V. Mosby, 1988:374–383.

16. Graham WGB, Bradley DA. Efficacy of chest physiotherapy and intermittent positive-pressure breathing in the resolution of pneumonia. *N Engl J Med* 1978;299:624–627.

17. Kirilloff LH, Owens GR, Rogers RM, Mazzocco MC. Does chest physical therapy work. *Chest* 1985;88:436–444.

18. Make B. Pulmonary rehabilitation: myth or reality? *Clin Chest Med* 1986;7:519–540.

19. van der Schans CP, Piers DA, Postma DS. Effect of manual percussion on tracheobronchial clearance in patients with chronic airflow obstruction and excessive tracheobronchial secretions. *Thorax* 1986;41:448–452.

20. Connors AF, Hammon WE, Martin RJ, Rogers RM. Chest physical therapy: the immediate effect on oxygenation in acutely ill patients. *Chest* 1980;78:559–564.

21. Eid N, Buchheit J, Neuling M, Phelps H. Chest physiotherapy in review. *Respir Care* 1991;36:270–282.

22. De Boeck C, Zinman R. Cough versus chest physiotherapy: a comparison of the acute effects on pulmonary function in patients with cystic fibrosis. *Am Rev Respir Dis* 1984;129:182–184.

23. Massery M. Manual breathing and coughing aids. *Phys Med Rehabil Clin North Am* 1996;2:407–422.

24. Bach JR. Mechanical insufflation-exsufflation: comparison of peak expiratory flows with manually assisted and unassisted coughing techniques. *Chest* 1993;104:1553–1562.

25. Bach JR, O'Brien J, Krotenberg R, Alba A. Management of end stage respiratory failure in Duchenne muscular dystrophy. *Muscle Nerve* 1987;10:177–182.

26. Barach AL, Beck GJ, Bickerman HA, Seanor HE. Physical methods simulating cough mechanisms. *JAMA* 1952;150:1380–1385.

27. Barach AL, Beck GJ, Smith RH. Mechanical production of expiratory flow rates surpassing the capacity of human coughing. *Am J Med Sci* 1953;226:241–248.

28. Barach AL, Beck GJ. Exsufflation with negative pressure: physiological studies in poliomyelitis, bronchial asthma, pulmonary emphysema, and bronchiectasis. *Arch Intern Med* 1954;93:825–841.

29. Bach JR. Update and perspectives on noninvasive respiratory muscle aids. Part 2. The expiratory muscle aids. *Chest* 1994;105:1538–1544.

30. Corrado A, Gorini M, De Paola E: Alternative techniques for managing acute neuromuscular respiratory failure. *Semin Neurol* 1995;15:84–89.

31. Splaingard ML, Frates RC, Jefferson LS, Rosen CL, Harrison GM. Home negative pressure ventilation: report of 20 years of experience in patients with neuromuscular disease. *Arch Phys Med Rehabil* 1985;66:239–242.

32. Curran FJ, Colbert AP. Ventilator management in Duchenne muscular dystrophy and postpoliomyelitis syndrome: twelve years' experience. *Arch Phys Med Rehabil* 1989:70;180–185.

33. Bach JR, Alba AS, Saporito LR. Intermittent positive pressure ventilation via the mouth as an alternative to tracheostomy for 257 ventilator users. *Chest* 1993;103:174–182.

34. Goldstein RS, Molotiu N, Skrastins R, Long S, Contreras M. Assisting ventilation in respiratory failure by negative pressure ventilation and by rocking bed. *Chest* 1987;92:470–474.

35. Bach JR, Penek J. Obstructive sleep apnea complicating negative pressure ventilatory support in patients with chronic paralytic/restrictive ventilatory dysfunction. *Chest* 1991;99:1386–1393.

36. Bach JR, Alba AS. Management of chronic alveolar hypoventilation by nasal ventilation. *Chest* 1990;97:52–57.

37. Bach JR, Alba AS, Bohatiuk G, Saporito L, Lee M. Mouth intermittent

38. Baydur A, Gilgoff I, Prentice W, Carlson M, Fischer A. Decline in respiratory function and experience with long-term assisted ventilation in advanced Duchenne's muscular dystrophy. *Chest* 1990;97:884–889.

39. Bach JR. Prevention of morbidity and mortality with the use of physical medicine aids. In: Bach JR, ed. *Pulmonary rehabilitation: the obstructive and paralytic conditions.* Philadelphia: Hanley & Belfus, 1996:303–329.

40. Bach JR, Alba AS. Total ventilatory support by the intermittent abdominal pressure ventilator. *Chest* 1991;99:630–636.

41. Leger P, Jennequin J, Gerard M, Robert D. Home positive pressure ventilation via nasal mask for patients with neuromuscular weakness or restrictive lung or chest-wall disease. *Respir Care* 1989;34:73–79.

42. Viroslav J, Rosenblatt R, Morris-Tomazevic S. Respiratory management, survival, and quality of life for high level traumatic tetraplegics. *Respir Care Clin North Am* 1996;2:313–322.

43. McDermott I, Bach JR, Parker C, Sortor S. Custom-fabricated interfaces for intermittent positive pressure ventilation. *Int J Prosthodont* 1989;2:224–233.

44. Bach JR, Alba AS. Noninvasive options for ventilatory support of the traumatic high level quadriplegic. *Chest* 1990;98:613–619.

45. Carroll N, Branthwaite MA. Control of nocturnal hypoventilation by nasal intermittent positive pressure ventilation. *Thorax* 1988;43:349–353.

46. Ellis ER, Bye PTP, Bruderer JW, Sullivan CE. Treatment of respiratory failure during sleep in patients with neuromuscular disease, positive-pressure ventilation through a nose mask. *Am Rev Respir Dis* 1987;135:148–152.

47. Kerby GR, Mayer LS, Pingleton SK. Nocturnal positive pressure ventilation via nasal mask. *Am Rev Respir Dis* 1987;135:738–740.

48. Bach JR, McDermott I. Strapless oral-nasal interfaces for positive pressure ventilation. *Arch Phys Med Rehabil* 1990;71:908–911.

49. Ratzka A. Uberdruckbeatmung durch Mundstuck. In: Frehse U, ed. *Spatfolgen nach Poliomyelitis: Chronische Unterbeatmung und Moglichkeiten selbstbestimmter Lebensfuhrung Schwerbehinderter.* Munchen, West Germany: Pfennigparade eV, 1989:149.

50. Goldstein RS, Avendano MA. Long-term mechanical ventilation as elective therapy: clinical status and future prospects. *Respir Care* 1991;36:297–304.

51. Bach JR, Alba AS, Bodofsky E, Curran FJ, Schultheiss M. Glossopharyngeal breathing and non-invasive aids in the management of post-polio respiratory insufficiency. *Birth Defects* 1987;23:99–113.

52. Bach JR. Alternative methods of ventilatory support for the patient with ventilatory failure due to spinal cord injury. *J Am Paraplegia Soc* 1991;14:158–174.

53. Delaubier A. Traitement de l'insuffisance respiratoire chronique dans les dystrophies musculaires. In: Ridean Y, ed. *Memoires de certificat d'etudes superieures de reeducation et readaptation fonctionnelles.* Paris: Universite R Descarte, 1984:1–124.

54. Bach JR, Alba AS, Mosher R, Delaubier A. Intermittent positive pressure ventilation via nasal access in the management of respiratory insufficiency. *Chest* 1987;92:168–170.

55. Bach JR, Robert D, Leger P, Langevin B. Sleep fragmentation in kyphoscoliotic individuals with alveolar hypoventilation treated by nasal IPPV. *Chest* 1995;107:1552–1558.

56. Sortor S, McKenzie M. *Toward independence: assisted cough* (video). Dallas, TX: BioScience Communications of Dallas, 1986.

57. Dail CW, Affeldt JE. *Glossopharyngeal Breathing* (video). Los Angeles, CA: Los Angeles Department of Visual Education, College of Medical Evangelists, 1954.

58. Bach JR. Pulmonary rehabilitation considerations for Duchenne muscular dystrophy: the prolongation of life by respiratory muscle aids. *Crit Rev Phys Rehabil Med* 1992;3:239–269.

59. DiMarco AF, Kelling JS, DiMarco MS, Jacobs I, Shields R, Altose MD. The effects of inspiratory resistive training on respiratory muscle function in patients with muscular dystrophy. *Muscle Nerve* 1985:8:284–290.

60. Martin AJ, Stern L, Yeates J, Lepp D, Little J. Respiratory muscle training in Duchenne muscular dystrophy. *Dev Med Child Neurol* 1986;28:314–318.

61. Rodillo E, Noble-Jamieson CM, Aber V, Heckmatt JZ, Muntoni F, Dubowitz V. Respiratory muscle training in Duchenne muscular dystrophy. *Arch Dis Child* 1989;64:736–738.

62. Smith PEM, Coakley JH, Edwards RHT. Respiratory muscle training in Duchenne muscular dystrophy [letter]. *Muscle Nerve* 1988;11:784–785.

63. Schiffman PL, Belsh JM. Effect of inspiratory resistance and theophylline on respiratory muscle strength in patients with amyotrophic lateral sclerosis. *Am Rev Respir Dis* 1989;139:1418–1423.

positive pressure ventilation in the management of post-polio respiratory insufficiency. *Chest* 1987;91:859–864.

Motor Disorders,
edited by David S. Younger.
Lippincott Williams & Wilkins, Philadelphia © 1999.

CHAPTER 41

Evaluation and Management of Swallowing and Voice Disorders

Celia F. Stewart, Andrew Blitzer, and Mitchell F. Brin

New technology, better understanding of the phenomena, and new treatments have all led to improvement in the diagnosis and care of motor disorders. Until recently, swallowing and voice symptoms were frequently overlooked because it was believed that little could be done to enhance these functions. However, new treatments for patients with paralysis and paresis, Parkinson's disease (PD), and hyperkinetic movement disorders have changed this outlook. These new treatments have helped patients experience not only improved swallowing and voice functions but also improved quality of life.

When rehabilitation is planned by an interdisciplinary team, more comprehensive and effective treatment is provided. At a minimum, the team should include a speech–language pathologist, otolaryngologist, and neurologist. Team members evaluate those aspects of rehabilitation that relate to their area of specialization and work together to form an integrated treatment plan. These combined efforts result in comprehensive management of swallowing and voice disorders.

This chapter focuses on current evaluations and treatments of swallowing and speech disorders for patients with movement disorders including specific criteria and methods of laboratory diagnosis, treatment, and outcome. The chapter is divided into two major sections: swallowing and voice. The first section particularly highlights new methods for the assessment and management of dysphagia. The second part reviews in particular new treatments for flaccid, hypokinetic, and hyperkinetic voice disorders.

SWALLOWING DISORDERS

Aspiration of food, liquids, or secretions into the tracheobronchial tree can produce life-threatening pulmonary disease. Aspiration is usually caused by a dysfunction of the oral, pharyngeal, or esophageal phases of swallowing and can result from a variety of disorders. Intermittent or persistent aspiration can lead to cough, intermittent fever, recurrent tracheobronchitis, atelectasis, pneumonia, and empyema. In addition, aspiration can be associated with weight loss, cachexia, and dehydration.

A normal swallow is a synchronized coordinated program of muscle contractions and relaxations that move the bolus of food posteriorly in the oral cavity, through the laryngeal inlet, and then into the esophagus (1). It is very rapid, and many actions occur simultaneously or in a rapid sequence. If the swallowing events are not coordinated, aspiration, choking, nasal reflux, or regurgitation can occur.

The physiology of swallowing is divided into four parts: the oral preparatory, oral proper, pharyngeal, and esophageal phases (1). During the *oral preparatory phase,* the food is taken into the mouth and an oral seal is maintained anteriorly by closing the lips and posteriorly by lowering the soft palate. This keeps food from spilling out of the mouth before the initiation of the swallow. The tongue and teeth prepare the bolus for swallowing by identifying and crushing big particles of food and by mixing the food with saliva. The food is then collected by the tongue and compressed against the palate, shaped, and coated with mucous. The time food remains in the mouth is highly variable and is a matter of individual preference.

C. F. Stewart: Department of Speech-Language Pathology and Audiology, New York University and Movement Disorders Center, Department of Neurology, Mount Sinai School of Medicine and the Mount Sinai Hospital, New York, New York 10029.

A. Blitzer: New York Center for Voice and Swallowing Disorders at St. Luke's/Roosevelt Hospital Center, Head and Neck Surgical Group, New York, New York 10019.

M. F. Brin: Movement Disorders Program, Department of Neurology, Mount Sinai Medical Center, New York, New York 10029.

The *oral phase* begins at the end of the oral preparatory phase when the bolus is squeezed toward the oropharynx (1). The bolus is held between the palate and the tongue and pushed posteriorly. The soft palate elevates so that the food can enter the pharynx and then separates the nasopharynx from the oropharynx, creating pressure in the swallowing system and making a nasal seal and preventing nasal reflux. When the bolus reaches the faucial pillars, the larynx is elevated and tucked under the tongue (2), and a swallow is then triggered. Aspiration can occur if the bolus spills posteriorly before the larynx is elevated, if the bolus is not cohesive, if the bolus is not a proper size, or if food particles remain in the mouth after the swallow.

The *pharyngeal phase* of swallowing begins when the bolus passes the faucial pillars and enters the pharynx (1). Respiration is interrupted during this phase of swallowing. The tongue base first moves posteriorly as the epiglottis is tipped posterior and inferior and the larynx is raised by the supraglottic musculature. The bolus is diverted posterolateral, away from the airway by the epiglottis. The bolus then descends into the hypopharynx, whereas the airway is protected by the epiglottis, by collapse of the aryepiglottic folds and false folds, and by the adduction of the vocal folds (2–5). If the swallow is not triggered, the bolus can catch in the valleculae or pyriform sinuses and can spill into the airway if not adequately protected.

The final stage of the swallow, the *esophageal phase*, begins as the esophagus is pulled open, creating a negative pressure that sucks the bolus through the upper esophageal sphincter (1). Problems can occur if the upper esophageal sphincter fails to relax and open or if the esophagus fails to contract in a peristaltic action to move the food through the esophagus. The esophageal phase ends when the food enters the stomach.

Assessment

The diagnosis and evaluation of swallowing disorders requires a careful history, physical examination, and often video fluoroscopic-modified barium swallow and fiberoptic evaluation. The patient and family can be helpful in identifying the specific swallowing problems. A quick assessment of the severity of the disorder can be suggested by the amount of body weight lost due to the swallowing disorder (6). Different types of medical problems lead to distinctive patterns of swallowing disorders. In general, the onset and course of the swallowing disorder differs depending on the proximate cause and whether dysphagia is a result of a neurogenic disorder or another problem. For example, oral difficulty can result from a variety of factors, including ill-fitting dentures, xerostomia, or poor neurologic control. The patient can frequently identify which types of foods are easily tolerated and ones that cause difficulty. This information helps with assessment because different types of foods cause different challenges to the swallowing system. For instance, solids are usually more difficult to swallow when there is a structural blockage or narrowing and liquids are usually more difficult when the movement of the tongue and pharynx is limited (6).

Physical assessment requires visual examination of swallowing structures and functions. Patients can be observed while swallowing their secretions, drinking liquids, and eating a variety of foods. Although the physical assessment is limited, it can reveal the patient's normal eating routine and obvious oral and pharyngeal disorders (6). Physical assessment is not adequate for identification of aspiration, and so further examination is necessary with video fluoroscopy, manometry, or nasal endoscopy. In addition, speech and language, neurologic, and otolaryngologic assessments can increase knowledge of the disorder and identify patients who may benefit from behavioral therapy.

One way to assess for aspiration and to identify subtle changes within the phases of the swallow is by use of a modified barium swallow or "cookie swallow." The patient is kept in the natural upright position and eats small amounts of food of different consistencies coated with barium to assess the oral, pharyngeal, and esophageal phases of the swallow. The radiographic examination is videotaped so it can be replayed later. The swallowing effort can be analyzed for adynamic areas, relative or true obstructions, and asynchronous movements. The dynamic movements of laryngeal elevation, tongue base motion, and degree of upper esophageal sphincter or cricopharyngeus muscle opening can be assessed. In addition, laryngeal penetration and aspiration of barium can be observed. Valuable information can be obtained by analysis of the consistency of the bolus, the position of the patient, and any other associated dysfunction (1,7); and by compensatory strategies such as changing the patient's position and the consistency of the bolus to facilitate swallowing.

Manometry combined with video fluoroscopy can measure pressures in the pharynx, cricopharyngeus, and esophagus and identify subtle failures of pressure generation or hyperfunction of the sphincter, but it does not yield information about aspiration itself. Therefore, the two are used together to accurately evaluate dysphagia and aspiration (8).

Fiberoptic endoscopic evaluation of swallowing can directly observe phenomena in the larynx and pharynx, including, first, pooling of secretions, immobility of the vocal folds, and frank aspiration of secretions. If there is no risk to further testing, the patient can be fed a soft material, usually applesauce colored with green food dye, to improve the observation of swallowing and to then detect the propulsion of the food by the tongue base, the efficacy of the oropharyngeal contraction, the clearance of the vallecula, hypopharyngeal contraction, clearance of the material from the pyriform sinuses, and whether laryngeal penetration ever occurs. It is also an adjunctive technique to the barium swallow for intervention or modification of diet in the course of routine follow-up (9,10).

Fiberoptic endoscopic evaluation of swallowing and sensory testing (FEESST) quantifies supraglottic and pharyngeal sensory discrimination thresholds. It is performed while the patient is awake. A pressure- and duration-controlled puff of air is delivered to the anterior wall of the pyriform sinus via an internal port within a flexible fiberoptic laryngoscope. The patient indicates when the puff of air is felt. It begins with a suprathreshold stream of air for 5 seconds to orient the patient to the expected sensation. During the test, the puff of air is sustained for 50 ms while the pressure is varied according to standard psychophysical testing methods. After a minute rest, the patient is given six repeated stimuli. Each one lasts about 10 seconds with a 10-second rest. The subjects are instructed to raise their hand within 2 seconds of feeling the air pulse. Both the right and left side of the supraglottic are compared. Previous studies have shown a progressive diminution of sensory capacity in the laryngopharynx with increasing age (11–14). From age 20 to 40 years, the mean pressure threshold was 2.07 ± 0.2 mm Hg; from 41 to 60 years, the mean pressure threshold was 2.22 ± 0.34 mm Hg; and at 61+ years, the normal mean threshold was 2.68 ± 0.63 mm Hg (11–14). These studies suggest that sensory deficits play a role in the development of dysphagia and aspiration in the elderly. In addition, one study (15) found a significantly reduced number of small myelinated fibers in the superior laryngeal nerve in patients 60 years or older. In the study by Kidd et al. (16) on stroke victims, impaired pharyngeal sensation and the severity of the stroke were both related to the development of aspiration pneumonia. In that analysis, sensory assessment was done with the touch of an orange stick in the hypopharynx. More precise techniques can reveal silent sensory deficits in stroke victims. Although patients may not complain of dysphagia, sensory deficits may nonetheless contribute to aspiration and even pneumonia.

Treatment

Swallowing therapy should be based on behavioral observation during the swallowing effort and other phenomena identified on a video-modified barium swallow or other procedures. Patients can have a swallowing disorder of one phase of the swallow due to dystonia or flaccid paralysis of the oral cavity and pharynx. Generalized mechanical failure leading to severe impairment of all phases of swallowing occurs in patients with amyotrophic lateral sclerosis, brainstem strokes, generalized myopathies, and in those with traumatic injuries. The type and location of the impairment dictate the types of treatment that will be effective.

Treatment should be directed at correcting or compensating the underlying defect. Behavioral therapies are most beneficial when patients have mild to moderate dysphagia and can maintain oral feedings rather than alternate feeding routes. The consistency of the food, head position, and quantity of food can be assessed and modified for each patient to allow the maximum swallowing situation for that patient.

Patients with oral preparatory and oral phase disorders due to unilateral hypoglossal nerve paralysis may be asymptomatic, but bilateral hypoglossal paralysis is generally devastating. Swallowing therapy can be of benefit in some patients. For example, rotation of the head toward the weaker side mechanically blocks the vulnerable vallecula and pyriform sinus. Gravity can be used to pull the food toward the stronger side by having the patient lay with the weakened side facing upward. The viscosity of a meal can be reduced so that food moves through the oral cavity with less resistance. In patients who cannot swallow, the oral phase can be bypassed by using gavage feeding.

Patients with pharyngeal phase dysphagia can have velopharyngeal insufficiency and laryngeal incompetence. The former causes rhinolalia, decreased pressure during swallowing, and nasal reflux. Symptomatic treatment ranges from behavioral techniques of thermal stimulation to prosthetic appliances that elevate the soft palate. There are surgical procedures to augment the soft palate and posterior pharyngeal wall and pharyngeal flaps.

Patients with true cricopharyngeal or relative achalasia may be helped by cricopharyngeal myotomy to correct the associated dysphagia and aspiration. However, it is not indicated for dysphagia due to a variety of neurologic conditions such as dystonia. Patients who have difficulty in all phases of swallowing from generalized mechanical failure related to amyotrophic lateral sclerosis, brainstem stroke, and myopathy have limited or no benefit from cricopharyngeal myotomy.

Patients with mild pharyngeal phase disorders who aspirate food and liquids can benefit from behavioral changes that slow the movement of the food or strengthen the musculature. The speed with which the food travels can be altered by manipulating the consistency of the food and changing head postures. The muscles may be strengthened by thermal stimulation and supraglottic swallow procedures. These techniques help the patient to eat even when they have mild to moderate aspiration. Patients with more severe pharyngeal phase disorders chronically aspirate copious amounts of their secretions and can benefit from separation of the airway and food passages. Tracheotomy is the most common method of providing this separation. The airway can be protected from secretions or food substances with a cuffed tube, which can also provide direct access for good pulmonary toilet. It is not, however, the best way to manage glottic incompetence. An open glottic chink may be due to anatomic deficiency, mechanical impairment, or neuromuscular disability, and when incompetent and symptomatic due to lack of compensation by the contralateral fold, correction should be considered by one of several methods, including augmentation by injection of various substances, thyroplasty, and laryngeal framework surgery.

Vocal fold injection was first performed using paraffin, but that caused granulomas. Glycerine, cartilage, bone dust, and Tantalum were later used with varying success. Arnold (17) used Teflon and glycerine with good results. Teflon paste injection is currently used, generally in an awake patient via the oral route. Its advantages are permanence and relative ease of injection. The disadvantages are local fibrosis, granuloma formation, and scarring at the site of the injection with later voice dysfunction. Collagen and fat injection can be used to augment and support paralyzed and incompetent vocal folds. They are not permanent and resorb with time but have the advantage of producing good glottic waves on phonation.

Surgical medialization of the vocal folds by thyroplasty or laryngeal framework surgery with placement of an implant, is the treatment of choice for patients with a glottal gap or paralysis and incompetence. It is performed under local anesthesia so that the patient can phonate, swallow, and breathe while sizing and positioning for maximum effectiveness. An external incision is made through the skin of the neck overlying the larynx. After the thyroid cartilage is exposed, a window of about 1 cm in length is created in the cartilage at the level of the vocal fold and a pocket is made in the inner perichondrium. The cartilage, Silastic, or hydroxylapatite implant is positioned to provide maximum voice quality. The larynx can be examined with a fiberoptic instrument during the surgery to observe the position of the vocal fold and the degree of closure of the glottal gap. Almost immediately, the patient has a louder voice, stronger cough, and improved swallowing without aspiration of liquids.

Another approach to pharyngeal phase disorders is the use of nerve–muscle pedicle grafts along the paralyzed muscles to allow partial reinnervation of the vocal fold. The grafts are made from the nerve–muscle pedicle of the anterior belly of the omohyoid muscle. Motion is often not restored, but increased muscle tone allows adequate glottic closure, with an improved voice and decreased aspiration.

Patients with more severe pharyngeal phase disorders and intractable aspiration and pneumonia require more drastic measures. One temporary measure is a glottic prosthesis to block the upper airway and prevent soiling of the lower airway; however, a tracheostomy is required for breathing. A new type of stent made of silicone and inserted through the tracheostomy site allows phonation while sealing the glottic opening (18).

Several surgical procedures provide airway protection by closing the larynx or diverting the pathway. The treatment requires a tracheostomy for breathing and pulmonary toilet. Laryngeal closure is temporary and is accomplished via sewing, which causes scarring to occlude the airway, but the patient can eat without soiling the airway. Another temporary approach to severe aspiration is laryngotracheal diversion, in which the trachea is separated with the lower end coming out to the skin and the upper end sewn end-to-side to the esophagus. As a result, material that penetrates the larynx goes back to the food passage; therefore, aspiration is impossible. When all else fails, simple laryngectomy with externalization of the lower airway prevents aspiration but eliminates the possibility of a normal voice; however, this operation, unlike the others already discussed, is irreversible.

Treatment of combined oral and pharyngeal phase defect in swallowing includes nonoral and nasogastric tube feedings, both of which are effective but must be monitored closely. Patients with nasogastric tubes that have erosion of the esophagus due to friction of the tube on the esophagus continue to aspirate due to reflux of material around the tube. These patients may need a gastrostomy, tracheostomy, or other laryngeal and pharyngeal procedures to prevent life-threatening aspiration.

The care of patients with swallowing disorders is most effective when a team of professionals assesses the patient's needs and cooperatively plans a course of treatment. The team should consist of an otolaryngologist, speech–language pathologist, and nutritionist. Other professionals such as a pulmonary specialist and gastroenterologist are needed in selected patients. Some patients with degenerative diseases require ongoing evaluation and management of their dysphagia to maintain the least restrictive method for consuming the food and adequate nutrition.

VOICE DISORDERS

Neurologic voice disorders are the result of weakness, lack of coordination, and/or involuntary movements or postures of the vocal folds; current therapy focuses on restoring appropriate alignment, support, and vibratory pattern of the vocal folds (19–22). The movements of the vocal folds are controlled by specific muscle groups. During quiet respiration, the vocal folds are moved to the intermediate position by the posterior cricoarytenoid muscles. Conversely, during phonation the vocal folds are stiffened and adducted by the thyroarytenoid, lateral cricoarytenoid, and interarytenoid muscles.

During optimal phonation, the movements of the vocal folds follow a predictable pattern. After inhalation, exhalation is initiated and the vocal folds are simultaneously stiffened and adducted to phonation neutral position (the vocal folds are adducted close enough to vibrate but not to touch) (23). The ventricular vocal folds are not adducted during speech. As a puff of air passes between the vocal folds, a slight negative pressure is generated by the air flowing through the narrow opening and the vocal folds are sucked together. The medial movement of the membranous portion of the vocal folds close the glottis and blocks the flow of air. Therefore, air pressure builds up below the vocal folds and eventually blows the vocal folds apart. The elastic qualities of the vocal folds and the suction created by the air moving between the vocal folds brings the vocal folds back to midline (23,24). The oscillation or vibration of the vocal folds results in phonation, but deviations from this alignment or pattern of vibration can lead to voice disorders.

The movements of the muscles can be identified by needle electromyography (EMG). EMG is most useful in determining whether vocal fold immobility results from mechanical fixation or paralysis. Acute spontaneous activity, including fibrillations and positive sharp waves, are much more clearly identified in limb muscles where complete relaxation and electrical silence can be achieved. Quiet baseline data of laryngeal muscles may be difficult to collect because they are continuously active during respiration, breath holding, and phonation. Consequently, these studies are performed while a patient is engaged in breathing, phonating, sniffing, holding their breath, or changing pitch. Motor unit potentials in the larynx are optimally studied with monopolar or concentric needle electrodes because they offer increased accuracy; surface electrode recordings are less accurate because of the comparatively longer distance from the motor end-plate specificity between muscles. Monopolar and concentric needles can be placed perorally or percutaneously. Those placed perorally are either via direct laryngoscopy or by indirect viewing of the larynx. The percutaneous technique is used most frequently for placing monopolar, concentric, or hooked-wire electrodes with the patient in the recumbent position and the neck slightly extended. The procedure is relatively painless and does not require local anesthesia. A ground electrode is generally placed over the sternum, and a reference lead is placed over the cheek. The thyroid and cricoid cartilages are palpated and used as landmarks. After the thyroarytenoid-vocalis muscle complex is identified, the needle electrode is passed through the skin in the midline of the neck, through cricothyroid membrane, and advanced superiorly and laterally until it pierces the muscle and insertional activity is identified. The thyroarytenoid-vocalis muscle usually has continuous motor activity during phonation. The needle should be advanced in several different directions within the muscle.

If there are questions about vocal fold abduction, especially in patients with stridor and breathy dysphonia, the posterior cricoarytenoid muscle should be examined because it is the only abductor muscle of the larynx. There are two methods for locating the muscle. In the first, the larynx is rotated away from the examiner and the needle is passed through the strap muscles behind the posterior cricoarytenoid muscle. The second, is by passing the needle through the skin in the midline, through the cricothyroid membrane, and angling it slightly laterally. The needle transverses the airway and passes

through the rostrum of the cricoid cartilage until it impales the posterior cricoarytenoid muscle (25).

Voice Disorders and New Treatments Associated with Flaccid Vocal Folds

Various conditions can produce a weak and breathy voice resulting from vocal fold immobility; the latter is generally caused by fixed or flaccid vocal folds. The conditions that produce joint fixation include rheumatoid arthritis, Lyme disease, lupus erythematosus, and other collagen vascular disorders that result in an open glottic chink and a breathy voice. Mechanical trauma to the cricoarytenoid joint with scarring can produce a fixed vocal fold. Immobile vocal folds occur in patients with invasive laryngeal carcinoma and secondary fixation. It can be neurogenic in origin, resulting from damage to the vagus nerve alone or in association with chest trauma and in malignant lesions of the thyroid, esophagus, or lung that invade the recurrent nerve. Patients who undergo cardiac, pulmonary, esophageal, mediastinal, laryngeal and skull base, or brainstem surgery can sustain vagal lesions, causing a vocal fold paralysis with sensory loss and pharyngeal paralysis. Damage to the vagus nerve can result from central nervous system disease, including multiple sclerosis, stroke, and head trauma. Finally, vocal fold paralysis can be caused by a lesion of the recurrent laryngeal nerve, particularly in association with neurotropic virus infection.

Assessment

A fixed vocal fold should be distinguished from a paralyzed one in order to provide proper treatment. In mechanical vocal fold fixation, immobility can be improved by repairing the mechanical problem, removing the cancer, or treating the underlying medical condition. Alternatively, the therapy of flaccid vocal folds can focus on compensatory processes. However, both disorders lack movement of the affected side and result in absence of vocal fold adduction at rest. The diagnosis generally can be reached with laryngeal EMG and direct palpation, observing for passive mobility. With mechanical lesions, the laryngeal joint does not move when well or at all. When manipulated by an outside source, EMG signals show normal activity with vocal fold paralysis; the joint moves when touched and EMG shows denervation. Vocal fold paralysis or paresis can be unilateral or bilateral. The voice is usually breathy and diplophonic and cannot generate a strong glottal croup. Patients frequently complain of running out of breath when talking because of the lack of glottal closure. The paralyzed vocal fold usually rests in the paramedian position but can rest at midline or at any position of abduction. Over time, some patients with unilateral vocal fold paralysis can compensate for the paralyzed vocal fold by adducting the opposite vocal fold beyond the midline and attaining glottal closure.

Treatment

Appropriate therapy of vocal fold paralysis depends on the permanency of the lesion and includes supportive injections and surgical therapy. Neuropathic flaccid vocal fold paralysis resolves spontaneously in many cases, usually within a year of onset if the nerve is intact and if the EMG shows reinnervation process. Surgical intervention should be considered after 6 months, especially if there is no evidence of reinnervation, because spontaneous recovery is unlikely. Surgical medialization of the flaccid vocal folds is performed by thyroplasty or laryngeal framework surgery with an implant. It is monitored fiberoptically and done while the patient is awake, able to phonate, and placement and size of the implant can be monitored, ultimately for better voice production. The procedure results in a louder voice, a stronger cough, and an improved ability to swallow without aspiration of liquids. The recovery period is brief, and patients can resume a normal routine shortly after surgery. Some patients report awareness of the implants shortly after surgery, but that disappears within a few days.

Behavioral voice therapy benefits some patients with flaccid vocal folds. It focuses on maximizing vocal folds adduction while reducing activity in other muscles. The expiratory drive is decreased so that effort matches the decreased medial compression of the vocal folds. A more appropriate relationship is established by matching these two forces, and the vocal folds then vibrate rather than blow along the stream of breath. It also helps those who have undergone surgical medialization of the flaccid vocal folds. One other technique effective in optimizing voice production is rotation of the head toward the flaccid vocal fold because it changes the position of the vocal folds and improves the loudness and quality of the voice.

Voice Disorders Associated with Parkinson's Disease

Communicative defects, including hypokinetic dysarthria, occur in approximately 89% of patients in all stages of idiopathic PD (26). Mild dysphonia is an early finding (27), and a change in voice can be an early sign that improves with successful treatment of PD (28).

Assessment

In the early stages of PD, dysphonia can be so mild and intermittent as to escape awareness. Awareness of voice symptoms develops slowly as patients notice that they are asked to frequently repeat themselves. As PD worsens, the ability to communicate degenerates and hypokinetic dysarthria develops, which frequently involves impairment in voice, articulation, and fluency. The progression may be random or may occur in association with fluctuations in medications and fatigue. When the symptoms are unpredictable, the patient cannot rely on the quality of speech and cannot effectively predict when he or she can properly communicate. The most common voice symptoms associated with hypokinetic dysarthria include decreased voice loudness with a monopitch and monoloud inflection and prosodic insufficiency (19,29). Among 200 patients with PD so studied (26), 15% had breathiness, 45% had hoarseness, and 29% had roughness of the voice. Using a pneumotachometer, sustained phonation was shorter, and the total amount of air used during the phonation was less in the PD group than in normal control subjects (30). One group (31) found that shimmer and jitter were twice that of the patients with PD. This was thought to be related to a large cycle-to-cycle variation in the amplitude of acoustic output pressure. The measurement of the harmonic-to-noise ration was half of normal, perhaps related to the vocal fold elasticity. They also described a tremor of 4 to 7 Hz with a probable thalamic or cerebellar source.

Some patients with PD have articulatory and fluency impairment, including imprecise consonants; inappropriate silences; short rushes of speech; variable speech rates; and repetition of words, phrases, and sentences (29,32). Imprecise articulation is related to improper tongue elevation to achieve complete closure on stops and inadequate constriction for fricatives (33). These abnormalities were corroborated by cinefluorography and EMG that showed low amplitude and short duration motor unit potentials. A few patients so studied exhibited progressive acceleration of words toward the end of a sentence similar to the festination of gait (32). As these symptoms increase, the patterns of inflection for expression of humor, sarcasm, concern, and emphasis can disappear (32). Talking can be laborious and frustrating for the patients, and over time they may talk less and become restricted at home, socially, and at work.

Communication can also be impaired due to loss of spontaneous facial, hand, and body gestures. Nonverbal communication through gestures and facial expression reinforces communicative messages and cues comprehension of speech. When nonverbal communication is restricted, it may be easier for the patient to sit passively and listen rather than to participate by gesturing or speaking. If a patient does not smile and nod when he or she talks with an old friend, the friend may misunderstand the intention and meaning of the speech and believe the patient is angry, bored, or disinterested. Friends may stop initiating greetings or conversations with the patient, and the patient can become isolated.

Some patients with PD can have word finding and fluency difficulty, resulting in excessive speech pauses, hesitations, and gaps; the decline in verbal fluency can also be related to aging (34–36). Despite the origin of the anomia, difficulty retrieving words can interfere with communication by causing vague speech, difficulty interjecting speech into a conversation, and breaks in conversation.

Direct observations of the motor speech mechanism reveal decreased muscle strength, speed, range of motion, accuracy, steadiness, and increased tone of the facial, oral, and respiratory structures. Diadochokinesis is often imprecise and slow, whereas articulation for speech can be very fast. Evaluation of respiration reveals decreased vital capacity, irregular cycles, shallow breathing, inflexibility in breathing patterns, and poor synchronization of respiration with phonation and articulation. The respiratory deficits are associated with decreased voice loudness and short phrases with illogical breath groups.

Fiberoptic laryngeal examination can reveal a normal larynx, bowing of the membranous portion of the vocal folds, incomplete adduction of the arytenoid cartilages, asymmetry of the position of the arytenoid from lack of coordinated posterior cricoarytenoid muscle activity, asymmetry of the cricothyroid muscle contraction, and tremor (37). Glottographic evaluation of the larynx can show bowing of the vocal folds during speaking and coincide with a breathy voice and short phrasing (37). The cough is often weak with reduced pitch and loudness. Patients use increased effort when talking and have decreased loudness of their voices. If patients increase the loudness and projection of their voices, the vibratory pattern usually improves.

Treatment

Over the last few years, behavioral and surgical therapies have been developed to increase voice quality for patients with PD. The former is most beneficial for those with mild to moderate PD; however, the choices are limited in the most advanced stages. Patients may need to rely on assistive or alternate communicative devices and surgical therapies to bring the vocal folds to a medial position to compensate for incomplete adduction and bowing.

Behavioral Therapies

Behavioral treatment focuses on several parts of speech production, including increasing loudness of the voice, improving precision of articulation, and hastening word retrieval. Choosing the area of emphasis by identifying areas of maximal deficit is important to achieve maximum gains and to select a therapy that truly helps the disorder.

Voice loudness is problematic in early PD and responds well to speech therapy (22,27,38). It is normally determined by habit, intent, expiratory drive, and posture. Behavioral modification of loudness and voice projection requires coordination of respiratory excursions, phonation, and articulation. The former is amenable to therapy, and the gains are often maintained long after therapy ends (22,38,39). Tape recording the voice can be useful because it allows comparisons of the voice of the patient and therapist; in addition, most patients are unaware of a weakened voice until heard for themselves (40). Speech loud-

ness can be affected by the expiratory drive, posture, and levels of activity. During normal respiration, the chest wall expands and the diaphragm descends and flattens. If the expiratory drive is reduced, the loudness of speech, length of phrases, and precision of articulation is reduced. Furthermore, if the patient's posture is slumped forward, chest wall expansion and diaphragm movement is reduced. If loudness is not improved with direct therapy, breathing exercises can be used to improve the speed and excursion of the muscles of respiration, and modifications in posture can be used to create better movement of the muscle of respiration. In addition, respiration can be improved indirectly by increasing the patient's level of activity and by having the patient work in physical therapy (41).

Stamina for maintaining the louder voice can be enhanced by gradually lengthening utterances and increasing the complexity of the utterances. Patients begin by repeating short and then long spontaneous utterances. Gradually increasing the length and propositionality of speech can lead to projection of a loud clearer voice. A patient that can sustain a loud clear voice during everyday speaking tasks can be discharged from therapy confident that the gains will be sustained for at least 3 to 6 months (22,38,39) and perhaps longer if periodically reinforced.

An electronic device can provide amplification and the solution to the problem of decreased voice loudness, but most patients with PD have a combination of decreased loudness and imprecise articulation. If the speech is unintelligible because of a combination of the two, little benefit will likely be gained from amplification (42).

Articulation may be imprecise because of oral and facial muscle bradykinesia, decreased motor coordination, and increased pharyngeal secretions (43–47). Consonants and vowels are produced when the articulators make specific sequences of movements. If the movements of the articulators are slow or imprecise, the lips, tongue, jaw, and soft palate will not reach their target positions and the resulting speech sounds will be distorted. There are exercises to increase the range, speed, and accuracy of the articulatory movements, improve articulation and overall speech intelligibility. Saliva that accumulates when swallowing can affect articulation. Behavioral therapy, directed at increasing the frequency of volitional swallows, also improves articulation.

Improvement in word retrieval is another potential focus of behavioral therapy. One way to improve recall is to practice retrieval of words by categories and word associations. When words are recalled more easily, the patient is better able to focus on the motor aspects of loud, clear, and more fluent speech.

Surgical Therapies

Several different surgical procedures can be used in patients with vocal fold bowing and breathy dysphonia. Augmentation with Teflon, collagen, or fat in carefully selected patients can improve speech loudness and maximum phonation time; however, low pitch, dysarthria, and slowness of speech may persist. Each material has potential benefits and shortcomings. Teflon causes stiffness along the vocal fold edge, increases harshness, and decreases intelligibility (48). Collagen is usually reabsorbed. Autologous fat must be overinjected to correct the deformity that follows later reabsorption. Type I thyroplasty or laryngeal framework surgery with medialization using an implant reversibly corrects bowing of the vocal folds (49–51).

The comparative effectiveness of type 1 thyroplasty and Teflon injection to bring the vocal folds to a medial position was evaluated in 24 patients with PD and in 6 patients with Shy-Drager syndrome (SDS) at Columbia-Presbyterian Medical Center. All but one patient with SDS had mild to moderate dysphonia related to asymmetric and disorganized laryngeal motion, and 20 PD patients had short maximum phonation time. All underwent direct laryngeal examination by fiberoptic laryngoscopy or stroboscopy. Of the 30 so studied, 10 had bowed vocal folds and 20 had slow vocal cord motion, asymmetry, or tremor alone or in combination. Twenty patients, in addition, had mild to moderate dysarthria, related to a slow or ineffectual tongue motion, and imprecise articulation (Fig. 1). Six of eight patients with bowed vocal folds treated with Teflon augmentation of the middle third of the vocal fold or type I thyroplasty had improved loudness but continued to have a slowed speech pattern. Harshness persisted in all but two patients who had a near normal phonatory ability, and there were no complications.

When there are respiratory symptoms, other steps should be undertaken. Sleep studies should be performed because life-threatening apnea and respiratory dysrhythmia can occur that is preventable by tracheostomy. Pulmonary function tests to measure airflow during speaking in severe PD and SDS may reveal an inadequate flow of air across to the larynx during speaking for effective speech. Augmentation of the vocal folds in these patients will not improve the hypophonia; rather, it may make respiratory efforts worse. Speech and pharmacotherapy (19) are still the mainstays of therapy in difficult therapeutic problems (19,52).

Botulinum Toxin Therapy for Hyperkinetic Voice Disorders

General Considerations

Type A botulinum toxin (BTX-A) is effective in voice disturbances associated with dystonia, Tourette syndrome, and certain other vocal tremors. Micromolar doses of BTX-A injected into selected muscles causes chemical denervation. BTX-A was initially used in the treatment of strabismus and blepharospasm (53). It is a

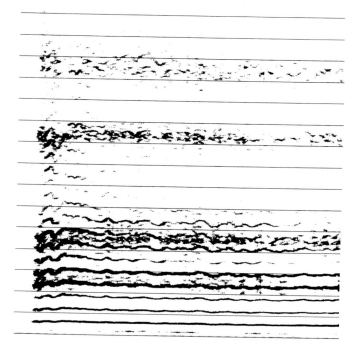

FIG. 1. Narrow band spectrogram /a/: A 65-year-old male patient with Parkinson disease has dysphonia characterized by hypophonia and a rough, breathy, and monopitch voice quality. His voice fades at the end of breath groups and his articulation is mildly imprecise. His voice production is consistent with speech compromise due to poor presentation of air to the vocal folds. This narrow-band spectrogram was made on the DSP Sona-Graph 5500 during steady-state phonation of sustained /a/ at a moderate pitch and loudness. Periodic and quasi-periodic frictional noise is observed between the spectral bands and in the high frequencies. In addition, his higher harmonics are weak. Acoustic analysis yielded an average fundamental frequency of 130 Hz; jitter of 28.147%; shimmer of 0.75dB; and a signal-to-noise ratio of 5.723 dB. The jitter is high and the signal-to-noise ratio is low.

potent neurotoxin that presynaptically blocks the release of acetylcholine from nerve endings (53,54). It specifically cleaves the SNAP-25 target protein, causing inhibition of synaptic acetylcholine vesicle exocytosis along nerve endings.

The treatment is performed with the patient awake via a special hollow monopolar Teflon-coated needle under EMG guidance to add precision to the site of injection. The injection of the thyroarytenoid muscle blocks adductor movements and is identified by having the patient utter sustained vowel sounds. Injection of the posterior cricoarytenoid muscle decreases vocal fold abduction and is activated with sniffing sounds. The effects of injection are temporary and need to be repeated every 3 to 5 months or when symptoms recur. The strength of the response can be controlled by adjusting the dose or by repeating the injection. Transient adverse side effects vary with the muscle injected. There may be mild temporary choking on thin liquids, a weak breathy voice quality, and weakness when coughing, laughing, and yelling with thyroarytenoid muscle injection (55). The transient adverse effects of posterior cricoarytenoid injection include mild stasis of solid food in the pharynx and short-term inhalatory stridor. Patients at risk for aspiration are poor candidates for BTX therapy.

Treatment of Focal Laryngeal Dystonia (Spasmodic Dysphonia)

Dystonia is an action-induced hyperkinetic motor disorder due to abnormal involuntary muscle contraction; at rest, the body part appears normal (19,56–58). Spasmodic dysphonia or focal laryngeal dystonia is a rare voice disorder that starts in early adulthood and responds well to BTX (19,59). It occurs alone or in association with blepharospasm and oromandibular dystonia (60). In spasmodic dysphonia, the act of speaking elicits dystonic movements. The vocal folds appear normal at rest and during sustained vowels, but when speech is initiated, the laryngeal muscles contract inappropriately, causing abnormal movements and muscle spasms (19,56,57). Movements of the vocal folds in spasmodic dysphonia are optimal during sustained vowels but deviate with connected speech.

Fiberoptic studies of the vocal folds during connected speech usually shows adductor and abductor movements (61) and either compensatory abductor, adductor dystonic breathing pattern, or both. About 90% of all patients have adductor spasmodic dysphonia with adductor spasms of four possible types (62): type I, adduction with excess force; type II, hyperadducted vocal folds and ventricular folds; type III, forceful adduction and anterior movement of the arytenoid cartilages; type IV, the arytenoid cartilages are pulled far forward, touching the pedicle of the epiglottis and causing sphincteric closure of the glottis (62).

In patients with an abductor spasmodic dysphonia, the vocal folds start in the appropriate position when phonation is initiated but are pulled open into an abducted posture during speech. At times, the vocal folds remain abducted or the position of the vocal folds involuntarily oscillates between abduction and adduction.

In mixed spasmodic dysphonia, a combination of adductor and abductor spasmodic dysphonia occurs with a mixture of a strained–strangled, rough, breathy quality and frequent voice breaks (63). The symptoms of the mixed type form a continuum, with some patients having predominantly adductor characteristics and others mainly abductor spasms.

Two variations of vocal fold movement have been observed in patients with spasmodic dysphonia: compensatory abductor spasmodic dysphonia and adductor spasmodic dysphonia. The former is found in patients with adductor spasmodic dysphonia who volitionally produce a breathy voice by whispering and do not fully contract their vocal folds to prevent the adductor spasms of strained–strangled voice production and voice breaks. Compensatory adductor spasmodic dysphonia occurs in patients with abductor spasmodic dysphonia that attempt to prevent breathiness by hypercontracting the vocal folds (19,56,57). Both patterns are rare, but the latter is the most common.

Adductor breathing dystonia is a variant of laryngeal dystonia. It occurs during respiration and results in vocal stridor and air hunger (19,64). These patients do not become hypoxic and the stridor abates during sleep. Two of 12 patients reported lacked coordination between movements of the vocal folds, diaphragm, and chest wall muscles with paradoxical diaphragmatic and chest wall movements (65).

Assessment of Voice and Speech Symptoms

Both forms of spasmodic dysphonia cause interrupted, rough, breathy speech with frequent voice arrests and decreased loudness, especially with connected speech. In addition, the symptoms of adductor spasmodic dysphoria are increased with expiratory effort. Some patients with abductor spasmodic dysphonia hyperventilate when they talk and speak on both inhalation and exhalation. Patients with true mixed adductor–abductor spasmodic dysphonia have both breathy and strained–strangled symptoms. The characteristics of mixed spasmodic dysphonia lie along a continuum with some patients having a predominately adductor type and others, a predominately abductor type.

A pattern of fluctuation is observed in the voice during a day, or over several days. They seem random, but the severity of the voice symptoms usually worsens in stressful speaking situations such as on the telephone or when talking to groups (66). Symptoms may also worsen when the person is ill, tense, or fatigued. Some individuals experience improved phonation when they wake up in the morning, feel strong emotions, and speak to their physician (66–68). Voice production frequently improves when patients make one-word responses such as "hi" or "no." Voice production is generally normal when patients do nonspeech acts such as laughing, shouting, whispering, singing, yawning, sighing, belching, coughing, clearing their throats, sustaining vowels, producing falsetto, and hiccuping (59,69–73). This pattern of fluctuation is not observed with other types of voice disorders.

Another speech symptom associated with adductor spasmodic dysphonia is increased effort. Patients report feeling effort in their throats, chests, stomachs, and articulators during speech. Effortful speech may improve with laughing, shouting, whispering, singing, yawning, sighing, belching, coughing, clearing their throats, sustaining vowels, producing falsetto, and hiccuping (59). It can be so severe that patients will smile and nod rather than talking so that they do not trigger the effort.

Onset, Medical History, and Symptoms

As with other types of focal cranial dystonia, most symptoms begin in adulthood (56). The average age at onset for spasmodic dysphonia is 38 years with a range of 3 to 85 years (19,56). Spasmodic dysphonia occurs more frequently in women (58%) than in men (56). The cause of spasmodic dysphonia is unknown, but the onset has been associated with trauma, exposure to phenothiazine drugs, head colds, flu, laryngitis, upper respiratory infections, and a genetic predisposition (19,74,75). In addition, no geographic, environmental, or occupational patterns have been associated with the onset of spasmodic dysphonia.

The onset may be gradual or abrupt, but it commonly begins as a mild intermittent voice disorder that gradually worsens over 1 to 3 years. The disorder typically reaches a plateau. In those with abrupt onset, a chronic voice disorder can develop that worsens, remains the same, or improves over time (59,66,76,77); however, it rarely resolves.

Although spasmodic dysphonia typically occurs in isolation as a focal dystonia, other dystonic symptoms can accompany it, including Meige syndrome (78), blepharospasm (19,79), idiopathic torsion dystonia (80), torticollis (59), oromandibular, and writers' cramp (79), overall in up to 16% of patients (60,81,82).

Up to 12% of patients with spasmodic dysphonia have a family history of dystonia (19). Our understanding of the genetics of the disorder has improved, and family and linkage studies have identified several genetic locations. A marker for some cases of childhood-onset dystonia has been found on chromosome 9 (83), an autosomal dominant dopa-responsive dystonia on chromosome 14q, X-linked Filipino torsion dystonia, and an autosomal dominate non-dopa–responsive idiopathic torsion dystonia (ITD) related to *DTY1* gene mapped to chromosome 9q34 (83–90). Identification of the genes and understanding their function may eventually lead to a better treatment or cure for dystonia.

Treatment

BTX-A is the treatment of choice for adductor spasmodic dysphonia (54,91,92); it has also been used for the abductor form (19–21,55,56,60,93). Since 1984, our group alone has treated 901 affected patients, including 747 with adductor and 154 with abductor spasmodic dysphonia.

The average starting dose of BTX-A for adductor spasmodic dysphonia is the injection of 1 unit in each side with a dose range of 0.005 to 30 units. After the first dose, the strength of the dose is modified according to the patient's response. Most patients continue at this dose, some have staggered doses a few weeks apart, whereas others receive small unilateral doses. Some receive frequent minidoses bilaterally, and still other patients receive larger doses. These different treatment patterns allow us to individualize the treatment and maximize the patient's voice production while reducing side effects. By decreasing the size of the dose, the breathiness associated with adductor injections can be reduced, but the length of benefit also decreases.

Most patients have a good response to the injections and suffer few side effects. The average time to effect of the BTX was 2.4 days, with a peak effect at 9.0 days, and an average duration of benefit of 15.1 weeks. Rated on a scale of increasingly normal status from 0 to 100% normal function, the rating before treatment was 52.4% and afterward 89.7% for best speaking, representing an improvement of 37.33%. Transient side effects include mild breathiness in a third of the patients; mild choking on liquids in 15%; and less than 1% had local pain or sore throat, slight blood-tinged sputum, or dermal itchiness with or without a rash after the injection. In the patients so studied, there was a functional pretreatment rating of 81% at the time of mobile vocal fold injection and 60% when an immobile vocal fold was treated.

In abductor spasmodic dysphonia, the posterior cricoarytenoid muscle of the most mobile vocal fold is injected with an initial dose of 3.75 units. After the unilateral injection, up to 20% of patients with abductor spasmodic dysphonia so treated develop a good voice without breathy breaks. The others received additional doses of BTX into the contralateral posterior cricoarytenoid muscle in doses ranging from 0.625 to 2.5 units based on vocal quality, the presence of noisy breathing, the amount of vocal fold adduction during speech, and the glottal size during quiet respiration and during speech. Patients initially rated themselves as functioning at 54.8% of normal and improved to an average of 66.7%.

Some patients have required injections into other muscles or surgical procedures to improve their voices. Nine of 154 patients continued to have breathy voice or tremor after treatment and were injected with BTX into the cricothyroid muscle. Five of nine had improved voice, and one worsened. Ten patients received unilateral type I thyroplasty to medialize the vocal fold mechanically. The patients with surgical treatment along with BTX injections raised the mean improved function of 82%.

Short periods of behavioral voice therapy can be beneficial when combined with BTX treatment. Voice therapy can help decrease breathiness after adductor injections and maximize vocal quality and length of benefit from injections for both adductor and abductor spasmodic dysphonia. Some patients with adductor spasmodic dysphonia have excessive breathiness after BTX injection. They have a history of using increased expiratory drive to compensate for the hyperadduction of the vocal folds. By increasing their expiratory drive, they could balance the increased medial compression and force the vocal folds to vibrate. If they continue to use this expiratory pattern when the vocal folds are weakened, they will blow the vocal folds out of phonation neutral position and vibration will not occur. In addition, if they continue to use increased expiratory drive, the vocal folds will fatigue. These patients respond well to a short period of therapy directed at decreasing expiratory drive.

A second group of patients that benefit from behavioral therapy are those who wish to maximize the benefit they receive from BTX. Therapy for both adductor and abductor patients focuses on decreasing expiratory drive, decreasing the effort at the level of the vocal folds, coordinating the expiratory drive and the effort levels, and decreasing extraneous muscle activity (62) and decreasing extraneous muscle activity in the head and neck areas (62,94). In addition, an amplifier can be used to increase the loudness of the voice on the telephone and in small or large groups (95).

Voice Symptoms and Treatment for Tourette Syndrome

A second hyperkinetic disorder that responds to BTX is Tourette syndrome. It is characterized by rapid ticlike movements and peculiar vocalizations. These can be accompanied by facial grimacing and sudden movements of the head, neck, shoulders, arms, trunk, and legs (96–98). Involuntary contractions of the respiratory, phonatory, and articulatory system result in simple and complex phonic tics. Simple motor tics involve only one group of muscles, causing brief isolated ticlike movements. Simple phonic tics consist of inarticulate noises such as sniffing, throat clearing, grunting, squeaking, screaming, coughing, blowing, and sucking. Complex motor tics are coordinated sequenced movements resembling motor acts or gestures that are inappropriately intense and timed. Complex tics are usually linguistically meaningful such as coprolalia, echolalia, and palilalia. When phonic tics are loud, they can cause irritation to the vocal folds that often lead to dysphonia (96–98).

Assessment

When phonic tics are loud, they can result in the vocal folds having increased lateral excursions of the membranous portion of the vocal folds and increased medial compression resulting in excess force. If this occurs, the vocal folds can become irritated, swollen, and hyperemic, and nodules or polyps can form. These changes in the structure of the vocal folds can result in dysphonia in the speaking and singing voice, including roughness, breathiness, and stridency. One way to decrease the strength with which the vocal folds contract during vibration is to weaken them by injecting BTX into the thyroarytenoid muscle.

Treatment

The treatment of Tourette syndrome is exemplified in the following case report (99). A 28-year-old man experienced frequent, brief, loud, screaming vocal tics that were unresponsive to haloperidol benztropine mesylate because of sedation and only partial tic relief. As an adult, he had shoulder shrugging and eye blinking, but his most disabling symptoms were simple and complex phonic tics, including loud screams, grunting, saying vowels and words, coprolalia, and loud talking. He made approximately 100 to 180 loud screams per day, each lasting 3 to 7 seconds. His screaming could be heard from a considerable distance. He held a few jobs during that time but had to quit because of his phonic tics. He also had minimal social relationships. When his vocal tics were severe, he became very depressed, requiring inpatient psychiatric care. He was unable to work and was socially isolated. He required brief admissions to a psychiatric inpatient unit when tics were severe (99).

Examination of the movement of the vocal folds during loud phonic tics revealed hyperadduction of the cartilaginous portion of the vocal folds and increased excursions of the membranous portion during phonation (99). The increased excursions of the vocal folds resulted in increased medial compression of the membranous portion and increased friction. An empirical trial of BTX-A, using laryngeal dystonia protocol, was initiated to decrease the severity of tics. BTX-A was injected into the thyroarytenoid muscles using EMG guidance (99).

After injection of the thyroarytenoid muscle, the hyperadduction of the thyroid cartilages was reduced and the lateral excursions and medial compression of the membranous portion of the vocal folds decreased. The vocal tics decreased approximately 50% in volume and 10% in frequency, leading to an improvement in social functioning (99). His speaking voice improved from moderately to severely rough to only moderately rough. He had large laryngeal nodules before the injections that decreased in size by one third. The number of psychiatric hospitalizations decreased from 45 in 14 months to 23 in 14 months. The side effects from the BTX injection included a brief mild period of increased hoarseness and minimal trouble swallowing liquids (99).

Voice Symptoms and Treatment of Essential Tremor, Dystonia, and Myoclonus

The physiologic basis of the involuntary, rhythmic, oscillatory changes (100) in frequency and amplitude of the voice can be caused by tremor in the intrinsic and extrinsic laryngeal muscles, the pharyngeal muscles, the respiratory muscles, the articulators, and the extremities. Tremor of the lateral cricoarytenoid, interarytenoid, and posterior cricoarytenoid muscles result in rhythmic abduction and adduction of the vocal folds (101). Tremulous movements of the extrinsic laryngeal and pharyngeal muscles result in rhythmical vertical movement of the larynx (102). Vocal tremor occurs alone or in association with essential tremor, orthostatic tremor (103), PD (31,

104,105), cerebellar ataxia, dystonia (19,57), myoclonus (19,103), motor neuron disease (106,107), or developmental speech and language deficits (108). A vocal tremor can also result from changes in subglottal air pressure induced by tremor in the external and internal intercostal muscles (109–111). Vibrations in the tongue, soft palate, and jaw have been reported to contribute to a vocal tremor (101,110). In addition, gross tremors elsewhere in the body can be referred to the larynx as a secondary tremor (26,112).

Specific patterns in the speed, amplitude, and regularity of tremors have been identified for specific types of tremors. A normal physiologic vocal tremor is a fast rhythmical tremor in the 8- to 20-Hz range (113) with amplitudes of 25%. Tremors that accompany neurologic diseases are slower and have been reported to range from 4 to 8 Hz (102,109,110,114). The amplitude of the oscillations ranges widely (102,113,114). Neurologic tremors can be regular throughout sustained phonation, can crescendo in amplitude and slow in frequency toward the end of phonation (102), or can be too variable and irregular to analyze (113) (Fig. 2).

Essential Voice Tremor

An essential voice tremor occurs in 10 to 20% of the patients with essential tremor (110) and is a rhythmical oscillatory movement of 4 to 12 Hz (115–118). It can be the first or only symptom of the disease or it can accompany tremors in other parts of the body (102,109,111, 112). When it occurs with tremors in other parts of the body, it may parallel the onset of the other symptoms or may have a sudden independent onset (102,112).

The voice symptoms associated with essential tremor include rhythmic quavering in pitch and loudness, especially during sustained vowel prolongation and continuant consonants; pitch and phonating breaks; and degraded intelligibility (102). Pitch breaks occur when the pitch involuntarily and abruptly shifts to a lower or higher frequency and phonation breaks occur when phonation involuntarily ceases (110,119). These breaks have been identified with visible vertical oscillations of the vocal folds, larynx, hyolaryngeal complex, or a combination of these structures (29). A vocal tremor seems worse under emotional stress or fatigue (102,112). Essential tremor is typically absent at rest, maximal during maintenance of a posture, reduced during movement, and often accentuated at the termination of a movement (115,118,120).

Laryngeal Dystonic Tremor (Spasmodic Dysphonic)

Tremors associated with dystonia are usually slow, irregular, have a directional predominance, and increase when the patient assumes a posture opposed to the primary dystonic contractions (121). In addition, there is

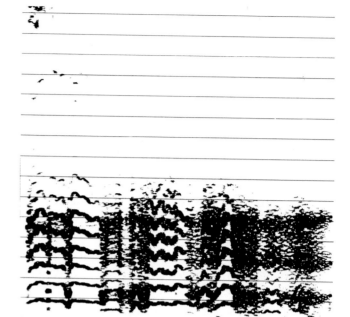

FIG. 2. Narrow-band spectrogram /a/: A 40-year-old female with a two-year history of spasmodic dysphonia and vocal tremor characterized by a moderate-to-severe rough, strain-strangled voice quality, moderate intermittent irregular vocal tremor and severely reduced voice loudness. This narrow-band spectrogram was made on the DSP Sona-Graph 5500 during steady state phonation of sustained /a/ at a moderate pitch and loudness. The spectrogram begins on the left with clearly defined harmonics. About one-fifth of the way into the spectrogram, we observe a pitch break where the harmonics split in two and a second tracing is observed between the original harmonics. When the pitch break resolves, a jagged harmonic associated with vocal tremor emerges. Then the harmonics deteriorate into quasi-random turbulent noise that represents an increase in the strain-strangled quality. In addition the higher harmonics are weak. Acoustic analysis yielded an average fundamental frequency of 188 Hz; jitter of 9.927%; shimmer of 0.789dB; and a signal-to-noise ratio of 13.176 dB.

generally a preferred position in which the tremor is less prominent. Many patients with spasmodic dysphonia have vocal tremor in addition to their other vocal symptoms of strain–strangled voice stoppages, monopitch, and an abnormally low pitch level (59,60,67,122).

Postural tremors caused by dystonia can be difficult to distinguish from essential tremors (123–125). Differentiating between tremulous voice due to essential tremor or dystonia is particularly difficult because all vocal folds are never fully at rest (one set of muscles or the other is always contracting) and they cannot twist or turn but can only adduct or abduct inappropriately (102,123).

A comparison between dystonic vocal tremor and essential vocal tremor suggests that approximately 30% of the patients with spasmodic dysphonia have vocal tremor (126). Essential tremor patients have greater regularity in vocal arrests and vocal tremor than spasmodic dysphonia patients (113,127,128). In essential tremor, frequency oscillations are more predominant that amplitude oscillations, whereas in spasmodic dysphonia patients, only amplitude oscillations were reported (113). Clinically, we have found that patients with spasmodic dysphonia have an improvement or elimination of their vocal tremor when they whisper.

Injections of BTX-A have been used with 21 adults, and dramatic results have been identified in our preliminary series. The BTX is injected into the cricothyroid muscle with the same technique used to treat patients with spasmodic dysphonia. Injections into the thyroarytenoid muscles resulted in improvement from a mean of 35.0% of normal function to a mean of 87.5% of normal function (123). Some patients had tremors in the sternohyoid and sternothyroid muscles, and injections into these muscles can be associated with an increased incidence of dysphagia.

Myoclonus

Myoclonic movements are brief, sudden, shocklike involuntary actions. They are caused by muscular contractions (positive myoclonus) or by inhibitions (negative myoclonus or "asterixis") originating in the central nervous system (129–131). Myoclonic symptoms affecting cranial structures are called "oculopalatal" or "brachial" myoclonus. Guillain et al. (132) proposed the term myoclonus for the syndrome affecting the brachial musculature because nystagmus was associated with physiologically and phenomenally different eye movements.

Pharyngeal and laryngeal myoclonic movements are observable as involuntary unconscious movements of the soft palate and pharynx of 1.5 to 3 Hz with a range of 0.3 to 100 Hz (133). Further exploration often documents synchronous jerks affecting the eyes, face, palate, larynx, diaphragm, neck, shoulders, and arm, giving rise to the syndrome "myoclonies velopharyngolaryngo-oculo-diaphragmatiques" (134). The pharyngeal movements can be unilateral (with the palate and uvula often drawn to one side) or bilateral and symmetric. The rhythmic myoclonic movements nearly always persist in sleep, can vary in rate with respiration (135), and can be suppressed by some patients. Once myoclonus begins, it rarely resolves (136).

Patients complain of clicking in their ears, broken speech patterns, and/or slow tremors. The clicking in their ears is thought to be due to movement of the tensor veli palatini muscle as it opens the eustachian tube (137). This clicking can often be heard on examination of the ears. The broken speech pattern produced by laryngeal, palatal, pharyngeal, or diaphragmatic myoclonus simulates the dysphonia heard in laryngeal dystonia or tremor (138). Examination of the vocal folds frequently reveals slow rhythmic adduction and abduction of the vocal folds with the same timing and frequency as the palatal, pharyngeal,

and possibly diaphragmatic contractions. Myoclonus is usually unresponsive to pharmacotherapy; nevertheless, some patients will respond to 5-hydroxytryptophan (139, 140), carbamazepine (141), clonazepam (142,143), tetrabenazine (143), and trihexyphenidyl (144,145). The clicking in the ears caused by focal palatal myoclonus is usually a minor annoyance but can become problematic when associated with spread of symptoms to other muscles. Treatment with tenotomy of the tensor veli palatini, stapedius, or tensor tympani muscles and myringotomy and BTX has had varying degrees of success (146).

SUMMARY

Neurologic disorders can impair speech and swallowing skills. Frequently, these impairments can be minimized and the patient's quality of life improved. Because each specialist offers a unique set of knowledge and experience, optimal treatment is provided when a team of professionals, including a speech–language pathologist, otolaryngologist, and neurologist, works together and plans the therapeutic approach.

REFERENCES

1. Logemann JE. *Evaluation and treatment of swallowing disorders.* San Diego: College Hill Press, 1983:214–227.
2. Didio LJ, Anderson MC. *The "sphincters" of the digestive system.* Baltimore: Williams & Wilkins, 1968.
3. Ardan GM, Kemp FH. The protection of laryngeal airway during swallowing. *Br J Radiol* 1952;25:406–416.
4. Atkinson M, Kramer P, Wyman SM, Ingelfinger FJ. The dynamics of swallowing. I. Normal pharyngeal mechanisms. *J Clin Invest* 1957;36:581–588.
5. Negus JE. The second stage of swallowing. *Acta Otol* 1949;78[Suppl]:78–82.
6. Baredes S, Blitzer A, Krespi YP, Logemann JA. Swallowing disorders and aspiration. In: Blitzer A, Brin MF, Sasaki CT, Fahn S, Harris K, eds. *Neurological disorders of the larynx.* New York: Thieme, 1992:201–213.
7. Ekberg O, Nylander G. Cineradiography of the pharyngeal stage of deglutition in 250 patients. *Br J Radiol* 1982;55:258–262.
8. McConnell FMS. Analysis of pressure generation and bolus transit during pharyngeal swallowing. *Laryngoscope* 1988;98:71–78.
9. Langmore SE, Schatz K, Olsen N. Endoscopic and video fluoroscopic evaluations of swallowing and aspiration. *Ann Otol Rhinol Laryngol* 1991;100:678–681.
10. Murray J, Langmore SE, Ginsberg S, Dostie A. The significance of accumulated oropharyngeal secretions and swallowing frequency in predicting aspiration. *Dysphagia* 1996;11:99–103.
11. Aviv JE, Martin JH, Jones ME, et al. Age related changes in pharyngeal and supraglottic sensation. *Ann Otol Rhinol Laryngol* 1994;103:749–752.
12. Aviv JE, Martin JH, Sacco RL, et al. Supraglottic and pharyngeal sensory abnormalities in stroke patients with dysphagia. *Ann Otol Rhinol Laryngol* 1996;105:92–97.
13. Aviv JE, Sacco RL, Thomson J, et al. Silent laryngopharyngeal sensory deficits after stroke. *Ann Otol Rhinol Laryngol* 1997;106:87–93.
14. Aviv JE, Martin JH, Keen MS, Debell M, Blitzer A. Air pulse quantification of supraglottic and pharyngeal sensation: a new technique. *Ann Otol Rhinol Laryngol* 1993;102:777–780.
15. Mortelliti AJ, Malmgren LT, Gacek RR. Ultrastructural changes with age in the human superior laryngeal nerve. *Arch Otolaryngol Head Neck Surg* 1990;116:1062–1069.
16. Kidd D, Lawson J, Macmahon J. Aspiration in acute stroke: a clinical study with video fluoroscopy. *Q J Med* 1993;86:825–829.

17. Arnold GE. Vocal rehabilitation of paralytic dysphonia. *Arch Otolaryngol* 1962;76:358–368.
18. Eliachar I, Roberts JK, Hayes JD, Tucker HM. A vented laryngeal stint with phonatory and pressure relief capability. *Laryngoscope* 1987;97:1264–1268.
19. Brin MF, Fahn S, Blitzer A, Ramig LO, Stewart C. Movement disorders of the larynx. In: Blitzer A, Brin MF, Sasaki CT, Fahn S, Harris K, eds. *Neurological disorders of the larynx.* New York: Thieme, 1992:240–248.
20. Ludlow CL. Treatment of speech and voice disorders with botulinum toxin. *JAMA* 1990;264:2671–2676.
21. Ludlow CD, Naunton RF, Sedory SE, Schulz GM, Hallett M. Effects of botulinum toxin injections on speech in adductor spasmodic dysphonia. *Neurology* 1988;38:1220–1225.
22. Ramig LO. Speech therapy for patients with Parkinson's disease. In: Koller W, Paulson G, eds. *Therapy of Parkinson's disease.* New York: Marcel Dekker, 1994.
23. Liebermann P. Direct comparison of subglottal and esophageal pressure during speech. *J Acoust Soc Am* 1968;48:1159–1164.
24. Zemlin WR. *Speech and hearing science: anatomy and physiology,* 3rd ed. Englewood Cliffs, NJ: Prentice Hall, 1988.
25. Blitzer A. Laryngeal electromyography. In: Gould W, Rubin RJ, Karovin G, Sataloff R, eds. *Diagnosis and treatment of voice disorders.* New York: Igaku Shoin, 1994.
26. Logemann J, Fisher H, Boshes B, Blondsky E. Frequency and cooccurrence of vocal tract dysfunctions in the speech of a large sample of parkinsonian patients. *J Speech Hear Dis* 1978;43:47–57.
27. Stewart CF, Winfield A, Hunt A, et al. Speech dysfunction in early Parkinson's disease. *Mov Disord* 1995;10:562–565.
28. Tetrud JW. Preclinical Parkinson's disease: detection of motor and nonmotor manifestations. *Neurology* 1991;41:69–72.
29. Darley FL, Aronson AE, Brown JR. *Motor speech disorders.* Philadelphia: W.B. Saunders, 1975.
30. Mueller PB. Parkinson's disease: motor speech behavior in a selected group of patients. *Folia Phoniatr* 1971;23:333–346.
31. Ramig LA, Scherer RC, Titze IR, Ringel SP. Acoustic analysis of voices of patients with neurologic disease: rationale and preliminary data. *Ann Otol Rhinol Laryngol* 1988;97:164–172.
32. Selby G. Parkinson's disease. In: Vinken PJ, Buryn GW, eds. *Handbook of clinical neurology.* Amsterdam: North-Holland Publishing Co., 1968:6.
33. Logemann JA, Fisher HB. Vocal tract control in Parkinson's disease: phonetic feature analysis of misarticulations. *J Speech Hear Dis* 1981; 46:348–352.
34. Gurd JM, Ward CD. Retrieval from semantic and letter-initial categories in patients with Parkinson's disease. *Neuropsychologia* 1989; 27:734–746.
35. Hanley JR, Dewick HC, Davis ADM. Playfer J, Turnbull C. Verbal fluency in Parkinson's disease. *Neuropsychologia* 1990;28, 7:737–741.
36. Scott SA, Caird FI. The response of the apparent receptive speech disorder of Parkinson's disease to speech therapy. *J Neurol Neurosurg Psychiatry* 1984;47:302–304.
37. Hanson DG, Gerbatt BR, Ward PH. Glottographic measurement of vocal dysfunction: a preliminary report. *Ann Otol Rhinol Laryngol* 1983;92:413–420.
38. Ramig LO. Therapy for patients with Parkinson's disease. *NCVS Status Progr Rep* 1993;5:83–90.
39. Ramig LO, Bonitati CM. The efficacy of voice therapy for patients with Parkinson's disease. *NCVS Status Progr Rep* 1991;1:61–86.
40. Hoberman SG. Speech techniques in aphasia and Parkinsonism. *J Mich State Med Soc* 1958;57:1720–1723.
41. Palmer SS, Mortimer JA, Webster DD, Bistevins R, Dickinson GL. Exercise therapy for Parkinson's disease. *Arch Phys Med Rehabil* 1986;67:741–745.
42. Greene CL, Watson BW. The value of speech amplification in Parkinson's disease patients. *Folia Phoniatr* 1968;20:250–257.
43. Caligiuri MP. Labial kinematics during speech in patients with Parkinsonian rigidity. *Brain* 1987;110:1033–1044.
44. Denny-Brown D. *The basal ganglia and their relation to disorders of movement.* London: Oxford University Press, 1962.
45. Gath I, Yair E. Analysis of vocal tract parameters in parkinsonian speech. *J Acoust Soc Am* 1988;84:1628–1634.
46. Hunker CJ, Abbs JH, Barlow SM. The relationship between parkinsonian rigidity and hypokinesia in the orofacial system: a quantitative analysis. *Neurology* 1982;32:749–754.

47. Connor NP, Abbs JH, Cole KJ, Gracco VL. Parkinsonian deficits in serial multiarticulate movements for speech. *Brain* 1989;112: 997–1009.
48. Ford CN. Laryngeal injection techniques. In: Ford CN, Bless DM, eds. *Phonosurgery: assessment and surgical management of voice disorders.* New York: Raven Press, 1991:123–141.
49. Blaugrund SM, Isshiki N, Taira T. Phonosurgery. In: Blitzer A, Brin MF, Sasaki CT, Fahn S, Harris K, eds. *Neurological disorders of the larynx.* New York: Thieme, 1992:190–201.
50. Isshiki N, Okamura H, Ishikawa T. Thyroplasty type I (lateral compression) for dysphonia due to vocal cord paralysis or atrophy. *Acta Otolaryngol* 1975;80:465–473.
51. Koufman JA. Laryngoplasty for vocal cord medialization: an alternative to Teflon. *Laryngoscope* 1986;96:726–731.
52. Ramig LO, Scherer RC. Speech therapy for neurologic disorders of the larynx. In: Blitzer A, Brin MF, Sasaki CT, Fahn S, Harris K, eds. *Neurological disorders of the larynx.* New York: Thieme, 1992:163–182.
53. AAO Statement. Botulinum toxin therapy of eye muscle disorders. Safety and effectiveness. American Academy of Ophthalmology. *Ophthalmology* 1989;(Pt 2.):37–41.
54. American Academy of Neurology. Assessment: the clinical usefulness of botulinum toxin-A in treating neurologic disorders. Report of the Therapeutics and Technology Assessment Subcommittee of the American Academy of Neurology. *Neurology* 1990;40:1332–1336.
55. Brin MF, Fahn S, Moskowitz C, et al. Localized injections of botulinum toxin for the treatment of focal dystonia and hemifacial spasm. *Adv Neurol* 1988;50:599–608.
56. Blitzer A, Brin MF. Laryngeal dystonia: a series with botulinum toxin therapy. *Ann Otolaryngol Rhinol Laryngol* 1991;100:85–89.
57. Blitzer A, Brin MF, Fahn S, Lovelace RE. Localized injections of botulinum toxin for the treatment of focal laryngeal dystonia (spastic dysphonia). *Laryngoscope* 1988;98:193–197.
58. Brin MF, Blitzer A, Fahn S, Gould W, Lovelace RE. Adductor laryngeal dystonia (spastic dysphonia): treatment with local injections of botulinum toxin (Botox). *Mov Disord* 1989;4:287–296.
59. Aronson AE, Brown JR, Litin EM, Pearson JS. Spastic dysphonia. I. Voice, neurologic, and psychiatric aspects. *J Speech Hear Disord* 1968; 33:203–218.
60. Blitzer A, Lovelace RE, Brin MF, Fahn S, Fink ME. Electromyographic findings in focal laryngeal dystonia (spasmodic dysphonia). *Ann Otol Rhinol Laryngol* 1985;94:591–594.
61. Aronson AE. *Clinical voice disorders.* New York: Thieme, 1985.
62. Stewart CF, Brin MF, Blitzer A. Spasmodic dysphonia. In: Ferrand CT, Bloom RL, eds. *Introduction to organic and neurogenic disorders of communication.* New York: Thieme Medical Publications Inc. 1997:301–318.
63. Cannito MP, Johnson JP. Spasmodic dysphonia: a continuum disorder. *J Communicat Dis* 1981;14:215–223.
64. Grillone O, Blitzer A, Brin M. Treatment of adductor breathy dysphonia with botulinum toxin. *Laryngoscope* 1994;104:30–33.
65. Braun N, Abd A, Baer J, Blitzer A, Stewart C, Brin M. Dyspnea in dystonia. *Chest* 1995;107:1309–1316.
66. Izdebski K, Dedo HH. Spastic dysphonia. In: Darby JK, ed. *Speech evaluation in medicine.* New York: Grune Stratton, 1981:105–127.
67. Aronson AE, Brown JR, Litin EM, Pearson JS. Spastic dysphonia. II. Comparison with essential (voice) tremor and other neurologic and psychogenic dysphonias. *J Speech Hear Disord* 1968;33:219–231.
68. Segre R. Spasmodic aphonia. *Folia Phoniatr* 1951;3:150–165.
69. Arnold GE. Spastic dysphonia. *Logos* 1959;2:3–14.
70. Bloch CS, Hirano M, Gould WJ. Symptom improvement of spastic dysphonia in response to phonatory tasks. *Ann Otol Rhinol Otolaryngol* 1985;94:51–54.
71. Finitzo T, Freeman F. Spasmodic dysphonia, whether and where: results of seven years of research. *J Speech Hear Res* 1989;32: 541–555.
72. Izdebski K, Dedo HH. Selecting the side of recurrent laryngeal nerve section for spastic dysphonia. *Otolaryngol Head Neck Surg* 1981;89: 423–426.
73. Ludlow CL, Connor NP. Dynamic aspects of phonatory control in spasmodic dysphonia. *J Speech Hear Res* 1987;30:197–206.
74. Gordon MF, Brin MF, Giladi N, Hunt A, Fahn S. Dystonia precipitated by peripheral trauma. *Mov Disord* 1990;5:236.
75. Robe E, Brumlik J, Moore P. A study of spastic dysphonia. *Laryngoscope* 1960;70:219–245.

76. Ludlow CL, Naunton RF, Bassich CJ. Procedures for the selection of spastic dysphonia patients for recurrent laryngeal nerve section. *Otolaryngol Head Neck Surg* 1984;92:24–31.

77. Wolfe VI, Ratusnik DL, Feldman H. Acoustic and perceptual comparison of chronic and incipient spastic dysphonia. *Laryngoscope* 1979; 9:1478–1486.

78. Jacome, DE, Yanez GY. Spastic dysphonia and Meige disease [letter]. *Neurology* 1980;30:349.

79. Aminoff MJ, Dedo HH, Izdebski K. Clinical aspects of spasmodic dysphonia. *J Neurol Neurosurg Psychiatry* 1978;41:361–365.

80. Marsden CD, Sheehy MP. Spastic dysphonia, Meige disease, and torsion dystonia [letter]. *Neurology* 1982;32:1202.

81. Blitzer A, Brin MF. Spasmodic dysphonia (laryngeal dystonia). In: Gates G, ed. *Current therapy in otolaryngology—head and neck surgery*, 4th ed. Toronto: B.C. Decker, 1990:346–348.

82. Blitzer A, Brin MF, Stewart C. Botulinum toxin management of spasmodic dysphonia (laryngeal dystonia): a 12 year experience in over 900 patients. *Laryngoscope* 1998;108:1435–1441.

83. Ozelius LJ, Kramer PL, deLeon D, et al. Strong allelic association between the torsion dystonia gene (DTY1) and loci on chromosome 9q34 in Ashkenazi Jews. *Am J Hum Genet* 1992;50:619–628.

84. Wilhelmsen KC, Weeks DE, Nygaard TG, et al. Genetic mapping of the Lubag (X-linked dystonia-parkinsonism) in Filipino kindred to the pericentromeric region of the X chromosome. *Ann Neurol* 1991;29: 124–131.

85. Fahn S, Moskowitz C. X-linked recessive dystonia and parkinsonism in Filipino males. *Ann Neurol* 1988;24:179(abstr).

86. Kupke KG, Lee LV, Muller U. Assignment of the X-linked torsion dystonia gene to Xq21 by linkage analysis. *Neurology* 1990;40: 1438–1442.

87. Nygaard TG, Marsden CD, Fahn S. Dopa-recessive dystonia: long term-treatment response and prognosis. *Neurology* 1991;41: 174–181.

88. Bressman SB, deLeon D, Kramer PL, et al. Dystonia in Ashkenazi Jews: clinical characterization of a founder mutation. *Ann Neurol* 1994;36:771–777.

89. Bressman SB, Heiman GA, Nygaard TG, et al. A study of idiopathic torsion dystonia in a non-Jewish family: evidence for genetic heterogeneity. *Neurology* 1994;44:283–287.

90. Ichinose H, Ohye T, Takahashi E. Hereditary progressive dystonia with marked diurnal fluctuation caused by mutations in the GPT cyclohydrolase I gene. *Nat Genet* 1994;8:236–242.

91. National Institutes of Health Consensus Development Conference. Clinical use of botulinum toxin. 1990;8:8.

92. American Academy of Otolaryngology—Head and Neck Surgery Policy Statement. Botox for spasmodic dysphonia. *AAO-HNS Bull* 1990; 9:8.

93. Blitzer A, Brin MF, Stewart C, Fahn S. Abductor laryngeal dystonia: a series treated with botulinum toxin. *Laryngoscope* 1992;102: 163–167.

94. Murry T, Woodson GE. Combined modality treatment of adductor spasmodic dysphonia with botulinum toxin and voice therapy. *J Voice* 1995;9:460–465.

95. Blitzer A, Stewart CF. Abductor spasmodic dysphonia. In: Stemple J, ed. *Voice therapy: clinical studies*. Chicago: Mosby Year Book, 1993: 147–153.

96. Pauls DK, Towbin KE, Lekman JF, Zahner GE, Cohen DJ. Gilles de la Tourette's syndrome and obsessive-compulsive disorder: evidence supporting a genetic relationship. *Arch Gen Psych* 1986;43: 1180–1182.

97. Kurlan R. Tourette's syndrome: current concepts. *Neurology* 1989;39: 1625–1630.

98. Shapiro AK, Shapiro ES, Young JG, Feinberg TE. Studies of treatment. In: Shapiro AK, Shapiro ES, Young JG, Feinberg TE, eds. *Guilles de la Tourette syndrome*, 2nd ed. New York: Raven Press, 1988:384–385.

99. Salloway S, Stewart C, Israeli L, et al. Botulinum toxin for refractory vocal tics. *Mov Disord* 1996;11:746–748.

100. Cohen AH, Rossingnol S, Grillner S. *Neural control of rhythmic movements in vertebrates*. New York: John Wiley & Sons, 1988.

101. Ardan G, Kinsbourne M, Rushworth G. Dysphonia due to tremor. *J Neurol Neurosurg Psychiatry* 1966;29:219–223.

102. Brown JR, Simonson J. Organic voice tremor: a tremor of phonation. *Neurology* 1963;13:520–525.

103. Yokota J, Imai H, Seki K, Ninomiya C, Mizuno Y. Orthostatic tremor associated with voice tremor. *Eur Neurol* 1992;32:354–358.

104. Aronson AE. *Clinical voice disorders: an interdisciplinary approach*, 3rd ed. New York: Thieme, 1990.

105. Seguier N, Spira A, Dordain M, Lasar P, Chevrie-Muller C. Relationship between speech disorders and other clinical manifestations of Parkinson's disease. *Folia Phoniatr* 1994;26:108–126.

106. Carrow E, Rivera V, Mauldin M, Shamblin L. Deviant speech characteristics in motor neuron disease. *Arch Otolaryngol* 1974;100: 212–218.

107. Aronson AE, Ramig LO, Winholtz WS, Silber SR. Rapid voice tremor, or flutter, in amyotrophic lateral sclerosis. *Ann Otol Rhinol Laryngol* 1992;101:511–518.

108. Amorosa H, von Benda U, Dames M, Schaferskupper P. Defects in fine motor coordination in children with unintelligible speech. *Eur Arch Psych Neurol Sci* 1986;236:26–30.

109. Hachinski VC, Thomsen IV, Buch NH. The nature of primary vocal tremor. *Can J Neurol Sci* 1975;2:195–197.

110. Lebrun Y, Devreux R, Rousseau JJ, Darimont P. Tremulous speech. *Folia Phoniatr* 1982;34:134–142.

111. Tomoda H, Shibasaki H, Huroda Y, Shin T. Voice tremor: dysregulation of voluntary expiratory muscles. *Neurology* 1987;37:117–122.

112. Findley LJ, Gresty M. Head facial and voice tremor. *Adv Neurol* 1988; 49:239–253.

113. Ludlow C, Bassich C, Connor N, Coulter D. Phonatory characteristics of vocal fold tremor. *J Phonet* 1986;14:509–515.

114. Ramig LA, Shipp T. Comparative measures of vocal tremor and vocal vibrato. *J Voice* 1987;2:162–167.

115. Critchley E. Clinical manifestation of essential tremor. *J Neurol Neurosurg Psychiatry* 1972;35:365–372.

116. Davis CH, Kunkle CE. Benign essential (heredofamilial) tremor. *Arch Intern Med* 1951;87:808–816.

117. Duvoisin RC. Benign essential tremor. In: Rowland LP, ed. *Merritt's textbook of neurology*. Philadelphia: Lea & Febiger, 1984:525–526.

118. Marshall J. Pathology of tremor. In: Findley LJ, Capildeo R, eds. *Movement disord: tremor*. New York: Oxford University Press, 1984: 95–123.

119. Meeuwis CA, Baarsma EA. Essential (voice) tremor. *Clin Otolaryngol* 1985;10:54.

120. Findley LJ. The pharmacology of essential tremor. In: Marsden CD, Fahn S, eds. *Movement disorders 2*. London: Butterworth, 1987: 438–458.

121. Elble RJ, Moody C, Higgins C. Primary writing tremor. A form of focal dystonia? *Mov Disord* 1990;5:118–126.

122. Rosenfield DB, Donovan DT, Sulek M, Viswanath NS, Inbody GP, Nudelman HB. Neurogenic aspects of spasmodic dysphonia. *J Otolaryngol* 1990;19:231–236.

123. Brin MB, Blitzer A, Stewart CF. Vocal tremor. In: Findley LJ, Koller WC, eds. *Handbook of tremor disorders*. New York: Marcel Dekker, 1995:495–520.

124. Lou JS, Jankovic J. Essential tremor: clinical correlates in 350 patients. *Neurology* 1991;41:234–238.

125. Lang A, Quinn N, Marsden CD. Essential termor [letter]. *Neurology* 1992;42:1432–1434.

126. Schaefer SD. Neuropathology of spasmodic dysphonia. *Laryngoscope* 1983;93:1183–1184.

127. Aronson AE, Hartman DE. Adductor spastic dysphonia as a sign of essential (voice) tremor. *J Speech Hear Disord* 1981;46:52–58.

128. Hartman DE, Abbs JH, Vishwanat B. Clinical investigations of adductor spastic dysphonia. *Ann Otol Rhinol Laryngol* 1988;97:247–252.

129. Fahn S, Marsden CD, Van Woert MH. Definition and classification of myoclonus. *Adv Neurol* 1986;43:1–5.

130. Marsden CD, Hallett M, Fahn S. The nosology and pathophysiology of myoclonus. In: Marsden CD, Fahn S, eds. *Movement disorders*. London: Butterworth Scientific, 1982:196–248.

131. Young RR, Shahani BT. Asterixix: one type of negative myoclonus. *Adv Neurol* 1986;43:137–156.

132. Guillain G, Nollaret P, Rees A, Mai Wand OH, Garland MH. Duex cas de myoclonies synchrones et rythmees velo-pharyngo-laryngo-oculo-diaphragmatiques. Le probleme anatomizue et physiopathologiqque de ce syndrome. *Rev Neurol* 1931;2:545–566.

133. Lapresle J, Ben Hamida M. The dentato-olivary pathway. Somatotopic relationship between the dentate nucleus and intralateral inferior olive. *Arch Neurol* 1970;22:135–143.

134. Guillain G. The syndrome of synchronous and rhythmic palato-pharyngo-laryngo-oculo-diaphragmatic myoclonus. *Proc R Soc Med* 1938;31:1031–1038.

135. Dubinsky RM, Hallet M. Palatal myoclonus and facial involvement in other types of myoclonus. *Adv Neurol* 1988;49:263–278.

136. Jacobs L, Newman RP, Bozian D. Disappearing palatal myoclonus. *Neurology* 1981;31:748–751.

137. Rondot P, Ben Hamida M. Myoclonus du voille et myoclonus squelit-tiques. Etude clinique et anatomique. *Rev Neurol* 1968;119:59–83.

138. Doody RS, Rosenfield DB. Spasmodic dysphonia associated with palatal myoclonus. *Ear Nose Throat J* 1990;69:829–832.

139. Magnussen I, Dupont E, Prange HA, et al. Palatal myoclonus treated with 5-hydroxy tryptophan and decarboxylase-inhibitor. *Acta Neurol Scand* 1977;55:251–253.

140. Williams A, Goodenberger D, Calne DB. Palatal myoclonus following herpes zoster ameliorated by 5-hydroxy tryptophan and carbidopa. *Neurology* 1978;28:358–359.

141. Sakai T, Murakami S. Palatal myoclonus responding to carbamazepine [letter]. *Ann Neurol* 1981;9:199–200.

142. Gauthier S, Young SN, Baxter DW. Palatal myoclonus associated with a decrease in 5-hydroxyindole acetic acid in cerebrospinal fluid and responding to clonazepam. *Can J Neurol Sci* 1981;8:51–54.

143. Jankovic J, Pardo R. Segmental myoclonus: clinical and pharmaco-logic study. *Ann Neurol* 1986;43:1025–1031.

144. Jabbari B, Rosenberg M, Scherokman B, Gunderson CH, McBurney JW, McClintock W. Effectiveness of trihexyphenidyl against pendular nystagmus and palatal myoclonus: evidence of cholinergic dysfunc-tion. *Mov Disord* 1987;2:93–98.

145. Jabbari B, Scherokman B, Gunderson CH, Rosenberg M, Miller J. Treatment of movement disorders with trihexyphenidyl. *Mov Disord* 1989;4:202–212.

146. Hanson B, Ficara A, McQuade M. Bilateral palatal myoclonus. Patho-physiology and report of a case. *Oral Surg Oral Med Oral Pathol* 1985;59:479–481.

Motor Disorders,
edited by David S. Younger.
Lippincott Williams & Wilkins, Philadelphia © 1999.

CHAPTER 42

Treatment of Bladder, Bowel, and Sexual Disorders

George D. Baquis

Disturbances of bladder and bowel continence and sexual function are common and can complicate the care of patients with central and peripheral nervous system motor disorders. Urinary incontinence affects approximately 13 million Americans, 15 to 35% of institutionalized persons older than 60 years of age, and more than 50% of nursing home residents. It is a major cause of institutionalization of the elderly (1). The prevalence of fecal incontinence ranges from 10 to 17% of nursing home residents (2). Approximately 7% of men experience impotence, and as many as 37% complain of unsatisfactory erectile function (3). As many as one in three married women rarely or never achieve orgasm (3).

These disorders have traditionally been considered together because the organs affected are physically proximate to each other and share a similar peripheral nerve innervation. Although disturbances of bladder, bowel, and sexual function may occur simultaneously as a result of a shared disease, they may also occur separately with a different pathophysiology and thus need to be considered separately. In the absence of a recognized underlying generalized nervous system disease, proper clinical assessment is generally directed to specific disorders unique to the bladder, bowel, and sexual organs. They require examination techniques and expertise that are not part of the traditional neurologic examination and may not be familiar to many neurologists.

This chapter reviews basic principles of clinical function; laboratory diagnosis; and treatment of bladder, bowel, and sexual disorders.

GENERAL CONSIDERATIONS

The storage and periodic elimination of urine are performed by the bladder, smooth muscle urethral sphincter, and striated muscle urethral sphincter (4). Efferent parasympathetic nerve supply to the bladder detrusor muscle is conveyed by pelvic nerves that originate in the intermediolateral cell column of the sacral spinal cord from S2 to S4. Sympathetic nerves supply the bladder via the inferior hypogastric nerves and originate in the intermediolateral nuclei of the thoracic spinal cord from T11 to L2. They activate beta receptors in the bladder dome, alpha receptors in the bladder base (trigone), and alpha receptors of urethral smooth muscle fibers (5). The striated muscle of the external urethral and external anal sphincters are supplied by pudendal nerve branches that originate in Onufrowicz nucleus in the anterior horn of sacral spinal cord segments S1 to S3 (6). The pelvic floor striated muscle, including the puborectalis and perivaginal striated muscle, is supplied directly by pelvic nerve branches (7). The ascending and proximal colon derives parasympathetic innervation from the vagus nerve, and the descending colon receives parasympathetic innervation via the pelvic nerves and sympathetic innervation via the lumbar splanchnic and hypogastric plexi (8). The internal anal smooth muscle sphincter possesses both alpha- and beta-adrenergic receptors (8). Penile erection is mediated via parasympathetic impulses that initiate the necessary penile vascular changes (3). In women, parasympathetic activity increases vaginal secretions in association with clitoral swelling (3). Sympathetic nerves supply the vas deferens, seminal vesicle, prostate, and bladder vesicle neck. These sympathetic efferents in men close the proximal bladder neck to retrograde flow and induce the emission of semen through rhythmic smooth muscle contraction and in women induces contraction of genital smooth muscle during orgasm (3). The complex

G. D. Baquis: Department of Neurology, Tufts University School of Medicine and Electromyography Laboratory, Division of Neurology, Baystate Medical Center, Springfield, Massachusetts 01199.

central nervous system integration of the peripheral somatic and autonomic systems is accomplished in neuronal centers within the spinal cord, pons, midbrain, and other subcortical and cortical structures (3–5).

CLASSIFICATION

The classification of neurogenic bladder and bowel dysfunction has been based on the anatomic localization of nervous system disease lesions, the associated neurologic and urologic findings, and pathophysiologic mechanisms when known (1,2,9,10). The classification of neurogenic fecal incontinence has generally been described based on associated neurologic diseases rather than by pathophysiologic mechanisms (2,10,11). Neurogenic sexual dysfunction is similarly generally categorized based on associated neurologic diseases. Neurogenic disturbances of male sexual function include both erectile and ejaculatory dysfunction (12); and in women, disturbances of vaginal lubrication and of orgasm (3).

CLINICAL ASSESSMENT

The clinical evaluation of bladder, bowel, and sexual disturbances should commence with a directed history and physical examination. Assessment of the abdomen; external genitalia; rectal sphincter muscle and puborectalis muscle tone and contraction; perianal and perineal sensation; and abdominal, cremasteric, bulbocavernosus, anal wink, and cutaneous reflexes should be performed. Pelvic examination of women and the definitive visualization of the bladder by cystoscopy and of the anorectum and colon by endoscopy require the assistance of subspecialists. The evaluation of bladder incontinence generally includes measurement of the postvoid residual, which is performed by catheterization or pelvic ultrasound, and a urinalysis to detect hematuria, pyuria, bacteriuria, glycosuria, and proteinuria (1). Cystometry is helpful when the diagnosis is uncertain, a known coexistent neurologic condition exists, or a therapeutic trial based on initial evaluation has been unsuccessful (1). There are techniques for the assessment of bladder sensation, capacity, and compliance and the presence and magnitude of both voluntary and involuntary bladder contractions. Neurophysiologic studies are helpful in detecting and elucidating the pathophysiology of an underlying neurogenic disease, including pudendal nerve conduction studies; urethral sphincter, anal sphincter, and pelvic floor striated muscle needle electromyography (EMG); bulbocavernosus reflex latency measurements; pudendal somatosensory evoked potentials; and cortical evoked potentials after direct bladder or urethral stimulation (13,14).

Studies for fecal incontinence include anal manometry, cinedefacography, conduction studies along the pudendal nerve, and needle EMG of the anal sphincter (2,10,11). At the least, these tests help establish the underlying neurogenic basis for fecal incontinence when the diagnosis is uncertain or a coexisting neurologic disease exists. However, anal manometry is not a well-standardized test (11) and in conjunction with cinedefacography measures the anorectal angle formed by contraction of the puborectalis muscle, but its significance in fecal continence is not well understood (11). Although the utility of these studies for the treatment of fecal incontinence remains a topic of discussion, their use often helps direct therapy (15).

Specialized tests for the neurologic evaluation of sexual dysfunction include studies of nocturnal penile tumescence and rigidity; vasoactive pharmacologic maneuvers to detect erectile capacity; and electrophysiologic studies of the pudendal nerve, bulbocavernosus reflex responses, pudendal somatosensory evoked potentials, and penile biothesiometry (12).

TREATMENT: GENERAL FEATURES

Urinary Incontinence

Urge incontinence may be associated with detrusor instability, detrusor hyperreflexia, detrusor sphincter dyssynergia, and urethral instability (16,17). Anticholinergic agents are effective in detrusor instability and hyperreflexia. Oxybutynin has direct smooth muscle relaxant and anticholinergic effects and is the agent of choice (17, 18). Propantheline is a second choice, and dycyclomine, which is a less well-studied anticholinergic agent with smooth muscle relaxant properties, is an alternative (1). Their effects include urinary retention, xerostomia, blurred vision, constipation, nausea, and mental changes. The tricyclic antidepressant imipramine decreases bladder contractility and increases sphincter resistance and may be helpful but has side effects that limit its use in elderly patients (1). Bladder training with emphasis on patient education and scheduled voiding, in conjunction with pelvic floor exercises to strengthen periurethral and perivaginal striated muscles, reduces urgency and urge incontinence in women (1). Biofeedback using multimeasurement feedback such as simultaneous measurement of pelvic, abdominal, and detrusor activity can reduce incontinence and is suggested for use in conjunction with pelvic muscle exercises and bladder training (1). Patients who participate in behavioral management programs derive maximal benefit when ongoing reinforcement and support are provided (1). Multiple studies describe the benefit of treatment with pelvic electrical stimulators. These devices produce contraction of the sphincter and pelvic floor muscles. Vaginal-, anal-, and surface skin-stimulating electrodes are described, and the parameters of use, such as electrode location and stimulation frequency, intensity, and duration, vary between studies. Adverse effects are minimal, and this treatment can be used with other therapies (1). Surgical treatment of detrusor instability includes bladder denervation, augmentation intestinoplasty, and urinary diversion procedures, but these are generally reserved for patients that are refractory to other treatments (1).

Stress incontinence may be associated with hypermobility of the bladder neck in women or with neurogenic sphincter deficiency (16). Pelvic floor exercises, biofeedback, and pelvic electrical stimulation improve stress urinary incontinence in older and younger patients (1,19). Pelvic exercises using vaginal weighted cones have been associated with reduction in incontinence episodes in premenopausal women (1,19,20). Patients with neurogenic sphincter deficiency may respond with a decreased number of incontinent episodes to phenylpropanolamine, an alpha receptor agonist, or to pseudoephedrine (1,19, 20). Oral or vaginal estrogen therapy may benefit some patients with stress or mixed stress and urgency incontinence. Although it is proposed that estrogens may restore urethral mucosal coaptation and increase responsiveness of alpha-adrenergic urethral sphincter smooth muscle receptors, their mechanism of action is not well understood (1,19,21). Imipramine benefits some women who fail to respond to the combination of estrogen and phenylpropanolamine (1). There are surgical therapies of bladder neck hypermobility that include retropubic suspension, needle bladder neck suspension, and anterior vaginal repair. Intrinsic sphincter deficiency may respond to sling procedures. Both men and women may respond to periurethral injection of materials such as polytetrafluoroethylene, collagen, or autologous fat (1).

Overflow incontinence can be caused by loss of bladder contractility or bladder outlet obstruction. Bladder hypocontractility in the absence of outlet obstruction may respond to bethanechol (18,19). Alternative therapy includes intermittent straight catheterization.

Detrusor external sphincter dyssynergia represents the contraction of the detrusor during simultaneous contraction of the external urethral sphincter. It interferes with bladder emptying and is usually seen in association with intrinsic spinal cord disease. Alpha-adrenergic blocking agents such as terazosin, baclofen, and benzodiazapines have been used, but none selectively relax sphincter striated muscle, and adverse side effects limit their usefulness (22). Other described therapies include anticholinergic medication with intermittent catheterization, intrathecal baclofen via an implantable pump, external sphincterotomy, sphincter stent prosthesis, and laser sphincterotomy (22).

Fecal Incontinence

There are medical, biofeedback, and surgical treatments for neurogenic fecal incontinence (2,11). Initial therapy generally includes institution of a high-fiber diet, stool-bulking agents, daily tap water enemas, or glycerin suppositories with a program of planned bowel evacuations (11). The antidiarrheal agent loperamide helps control diarrhea when no other therapy is available (2).

Biofeedback with intrarectal balloon distention and monitoring of anal external sphincter contraction reduces the frequency of incontinent episodes in patients who retain rectal sensation and voluntary sphincter contraction; success correlates more with improvement in rectal sensation than with sphincter strengthening (2). Pelvic electrical stimulation with surface electrodes or an anal plug electrode and pelvic exercises improves symptoms of mild incontinence (23,24). Surgical approaches include direct repair of the external anal sphincter; posterior anal repair with plication of the levator ani, puborectalis, and levator ani muscles; anal encirclement to mechanically tighten the anus; implantation of an artificial sphincter; anal encirclement with portions of adjacent skeletal muscle; and colostomy, especially in refractory incontinence (2).

Sexual Dysfunction

Disorders of male sexual dysfunction generally receive greater attention than female sexual dysfunction, about which there is relatively less published. Underlying and accompanying psychological disorders, including anxiety and depression, need to be addressed and coexistent medical diseases identified and treated (3).

Specific therapies for male erectile dysfunction include the use of vasoactive medications, application of vacuum-constriction devices, and implantation of penile prostheses. Oral sildenafil, an inhibitor of cyclic guanosine monophosphate, improves erectile function in men with erectile dysfunction of organic, psychogenic, and mixed causes (25). Adverse effects and complications include hypotension (can potentiate the hypotensive effect of nitrates), headache, flushing, dyspepsia, and transient visual disturbance (26). The intracavernosal injection of alprostadil is an effective therapy in patients with neurogenic, vasculogenic, and psychogenic erectile dysfunction. Side effects and complications include local pain, hematoma or ecchymosis formation, priapism, and penile fibrosis (27). The efficacy of alprostadil was demonstrated with a transurethral preparation without the side effects of the injected form of the medication (28). A variety of other drugs have been used, including the alpha-adrenergic blockers phenoxybenzamine, phentolamine, and yohimbine and the smooth muscle dilator papaverine (3). Vacuum devices consist of a canister tube connected to a vacuum pump. Negative pressure draws blood into the penis, and tumescence is maintained by a band placed at the base of the penis (3). Adverse effects include decreased penile sensation, impaired ejaculation, ecchymosis, and rare penile necrosis. Erectile function may also be restored by surgical placement of a semirigid or inflatable penile prosthesis; however, the possible complications include infection, erosion, penile gangrene, and malfunction of inflatable devices (3). Ejaculatory dysfunction may respond to local mechanical vibration or to electrical stimulation of sympathetic outflow via intrarectal electrodes (29). Little information exists regarding the treatment of local pain, pelvic muscle spasm, and diminished vaginal secretions that can result in sexual dysfunction in women with neurologic disease.

TREATMENT OF SPECIFIC DISEASES

Stroke

Urinary incontinence has an incidence of 57 to 83% early after stroke, with gradual improvement over 6 subsequent months (30,31). The causes of urinary incontinence include disruption of micturition pathways, stroke-related cognitive dysfunction, language deficits, concurrent neuropathy, and medication effects (32). Acute urinary retention may be the initial presenting feature, but over time, frequency, urgency, and urge incontinence may become the primary complaints (31). In a study of 639 first-time stroke patients, urinary incontinence at onset was the single best predictor of moderate or severe disability at 3 and 12 months (33); incontinence has been associated with prolonged hospital stay (34). In a sample of 532 patients seen within 7 days of an acute stroke, 53% of incontinent patients died within 6 months of their stroke (35). In a prospective study cohort of 492 stroke patients, urinary incontinence was an independent predictor of death at 1 year (36).

A variable pattern is present on urodynamic testing, which may reflect timing of the procedure after the stroke or the anatomic extent and location of the stroke (37). Cystometry of 39 patients revealed uninhibited detrusor contractions in 18 of 21 patients with frontal, putaminal, or internal capsule lesions on brain computed tomography when examined at a mean of 19 months after stroke. Uninhibited sphincter relaxation was associated with internal capsule but not with putaminal lesions (38). Other studies revealed detrusor hyperreflexia and uninhibited sphincter relaxation with cortical and internal capsule lesions in most patients with voiding disorders (39,40). In a group of 19 patients studied at a mean of 69.4 days after stroke, 21% had bladder hyporeflexia, but these patients were either taking anticholinergic medications or had diabetes mellitus (33). Incomplete bladder emptying may also be present in continent poststroke patients and may be associated with a higher rate of urinary tract infections (41).

Patients under consideration of prostatectomy for symptoms of bladder outlet obstruction should be approached cautiously because the incidence of unsatisfactory results has been reported as high as 50%, and those operated on within a year of their stroke seemed to do worse (42). Treatment of stroke-related urinary incontinence should be based on the underlying pattern of the incontinence, which is not always clinically apparent, and on the knowledge that this pattern may change with time.

Fecal incontinence can follow unilateral and bilateral frontal ischemic infarction (43,44). Bowel incontinence is closely associated with urinary incontinence (45) and impaired mobility (46). It tends to resolve during the first 2 months after the stroke (46). Patients with fecal incontinence on hospital admission or at discharge from the hospital had a less favorable outcome (47).

Strokes resulting in hemiplegia are associated with a decline in coital frequency in men and women (3). The most common sexual problems are erectile and ejaculatory dysfunction in men and vaginal lubrication and orgasm in women (3). The prevalence of sexual dysfunction in a study of 27 men with unilateral strokes was greater in association with right hemisphere lesions than with left hemisphere lesions (48). An increased percentage of both men and women reported diminished libido after stroke, although cases of increased sexual interest and activity have been described (3).

Dementia

Disturbances of micturition and defecation have been associated with lesions of the anteromedial frontal lobe, including the anterior cingulate gyrus and genu of the corpus callosum (43,49), and may also occur in patients who are socially aware but not demented. The presence of subcortical white matter lesions on magnetic resonance imaging in patients with Alzheimer's disease, so selected for absence of vascular disease risk factors, symptomatic cerebrovascular disease, or cardiovascular disease, were all associated with an increased frequency of urinary incontinence (50,51). Although bladder and bowel incontinence are frequent accompaniments of vascular dementia and Binswanger disease, and urinary incontinence may be an earlier feature in vascular dementia than in senile dementia of the Alzheimer type (50), careful clinical and urodynamic descriptions are lacking (52–54). Longitudinal data on the temporal relationship of cognitive decline in Alzheimer disease to the development of urinary and fecal incontinence demonstrates a significantly earlier onset of incontinence in patients with diffuse Lewy body disease and those with Alzheimer disease with vascular lesions or Lewy bodies compared with those with Alzheimer disease alone (55). The prevalence of urinary incontinence in patients with Alzheimer disease varies from 16 to 40% and is related to the severity of dementia (56). The development of urinary incontinence in patients with Alzheimer disease is predictive of institutionalization (57). Urinary incontinence is one of the symptoms of normal pressure hydrocephalus that can improve after ventricular shunting. Early symptoms consist of urgency and frequency, and late symptoms can include urgency incontinence accompanied by fecal incontinence (58). Cystometrograms show uninhibited bladder contractions at small volumes (58,59).

Side effects limit pharmacologic management in this patient group. Treatment options for urinary incontinence include prompt voiding with regularly scheduled toileting; simple alterations in environment, including addition of toileting or ambulation devices; strategies to improve ambulation; steps to eliminate bowel impaction; fluid restriction at night for nocturia; absorbent pads; external collection devices; and intermittent catheterization (1). Treatment of fecal incontinence in the elderly includes stool-bulking agents, antidiarrheal agents, and scheduled toileting at a fixed time each day. Biofeedback and behavioral measures may be limited by patient comprehension of instructions (60). Sexual disinhibition has been described in 7% of patients (56).

Parkinsonian Syndromes

Parkinson's disease (PD), multiple system atrophy (MSA), and Shy-Drager syndrome are all associated with urinary incontinence. The incidence of bladder dysfunction with PD ranges from 37 to 71% (61). Symptoms include frequency, urgency, urge incontinence, hesitancy, and retention (61,62). Detrusor hyperreflexia associated with sphincter relaxation is the most common urodynamic pattern (61). Sphincter bradykinesia or failure of perineal floor muscle relaxation during detrusor contraction and pseudo-dyssynergia or voluntary perineal floor muscle contraction in response to detrusor contraction have also been described (61,62). Urodynamic studies in patients receiving medication and repeated several hours after stopping medication are associated with both improvement and worsening of bladder hyperreflexia (63). However, the urodynamic pattern of a cohort of L-dopa treated and untreated men did not significantly differ (61).

Careful cystometry is indicated in patients with symptoms of obstruction being considered for prostatectomy, because normal preoperative voluntary sphincter control has been associated with a lower risk of postoperative incontinence (64). Although stress incontinence is the most common cause of incontinence in nonparkinsonian women, a urodynamic study revealed detrusor instability in 70.6% of women with PD who experience symptoms of urge and stress incontinence (65). Patients with MSA may experience urgency, frequency, and nocturia, and women may experience stress incontinence. Cystometry may reveal detrusor hyperreflexia, but detrusor atonia and urinary retention can also occur (66). Women undergoing surgery for stress incontinence may fail to improve (67). Treatment with intermittent catheterization, anticholinergic medication, and desmopressin spray may improve continence (68). Findings of denervation and reinervation by urethral and anal sphincter EMG are common in patients with MSA but are rarely seen with idiopathic PD (68).

Patients with Shy-Drager syndrome can initially have bladder hyperreflexia and later develop bladder atonia (69). An open bladder vesicle neck was present at rest in five patients undergoing cystometry (70), and evidence of external urethral sphincter denervation may be present by needle EMG (70). Urinary symptoms of urgency, urge incontinence, and obstruction may be present in patients with progressive supranuclear palsy, and urodynamic studies may reveal detrusor hyperreflexia, uninhibited striated sphincter relaxation, and detrusor sphincter dyssynergia (71). External sphincter needle EMG may reveal neurogenic abnormalities (71).

Constipation in PD may result from failure of sphincter muscle relaxation and paradoxical contraction during defecation (72). EMG of the anal sphincter in Shy-Drager syndrome reveals evidence of chronic reinervation (70, 73). Age, severity of illness, and depression are important predictors of sexual function in men with PD, and the frequency of sexual dysfunction may be similar to that with other chronic illnesses (74). In PD, L-dopa may improve libido out of proportion to motoric improvement, and men are more likely to notice this than women (3). Impotence is a common symptom of MSA and may be the presenting symptom (66,67).

Multiple Sclerosis

Bladder dysfunction in multiple sclerosis (MS) arises as a result of interruption of pathways from the pontine micturition center to the sacral spinal cord (75). Common symptoms include urgency, frequency, and urge incontinence. Hesitancy, poor or interrupted urinary stream, dribbling, and incomplete emptying also occur (75). Urodynamic abnormalities include detrusor hyperreflexia, incomplete bladder emptying, and detrusor sphincter dyssynergia (75,76). Up to one half of MS patients without urinary complaints may have abnormal urodynamic studies. The presence of urinary symptoms correlates with longer duration of disease, the severity of pyramidal or sensory lesions, and the total disability score (77,78). Bladder symptoms generally correlate poorly with any single urodynamic finding (79,80). For example, the presence of irritative bladder symptoms may not be associated with uninhibited detrusor contractions, and some patients with obstructive symptoms may not have bladder areflexia (79). Also, the pattern of urodynamic abnormality may change over time with development of new detrusor hyperreflexia or detrusor sphincter dyssynergia, the development of which is a urodynamic indicator of progressive MS (80). Sphincter dyssynergia in men may be associated with a higher risk of complications such as urosepsis and vesicoureteral reflux (81). Lack of response to treatment based on urodynamic assessment may be related to progression of MS (82). Patients with detrusor hyperreflexia may respond well to treatment with oxybutynin or propantheline (75,83). Refractory nocturia may respond to desmopressin (84). Bladder areflexia is treated with intermittent catheterization and is not usually responsive to bethanechol (75). Bladder hyperreflexia with dyssynergia is effectively managed with anticholinergic therapy in combination with intermittent catheterization (75). Detrusor sphincter dyssynergia has been reported to respond to intrathecal baclofen (85).

Constipation and fecal incontinence can occur alone or in combination with urinary incontinence (86–88). In women, fecal incontinence may reflect a combination of factors, including central nervous system disease, pelvic peripheral nervous system disease, and injury acquired with childbirth (87). Evaluation of radiopaque marker transit and anorectal manometry has revealed increased colonic transit time and spontaneous rectal contractions and fecal incontinence in MS patients (89). Defacography has shown evidence of rectal outlet obstruction with failure of the puborectalis and anal sphincter muscles to relax (90). Paradoxical contraction of the puborectalis muscle in constipated MS patients may be the anal equivalent of detrusor sphincter dyssynergia of the bladder (91). Patients with MS and fecal incontinence experience rectal sensation at a higher volume, increased thresholds of phasic external anal sphincter contraction, decreased maximal voluntary anal pressures, and require smaller volumes of rectal distention to inhibit internal sphincter tone than normal control subjects (92). Similar less severe findings may be present in continent MS patients (92). Treatment is empiric and includes a high-fiber diet, adequate fluid intake, a regular defecation schedule with use of glycerin suppositories or digital stimulation, loperamide for loose stools, and regular exercise (93).

Sexual dysfunction in men includes erectile dysfunction, decreased penile sensation, inability to ejaculate, and premature ejaculation (94). Female patients report decreased vaginal lubrication and decreased vaginal sensation (94). Both men and women may have trouble achieving orgasm, and the presence of sexual dysfunction is associated with depression, bladder dysfunction, and bowel dysfunction. Some patients have reported an improvement in sexual dysfunction after corticosteroid treatment of MS symptoms other than sexual dysfunction (94). Erectile dysfunction may respond to intracorporeal papaverine injections, and yohimbine therapy may improve ejaculatory ability (95).

Caudae Equina Syndrome

Injury to the caudae equina can cause dysfunction of both the bladder and pelvic floor musculature and can result from a variety of disorders including trauma, disc herniation, and tumor compression (96). Most disc herniations occur at the L4-5 level, and some patients may present with bladder and bowel incontinence (97). Postoperative improvement correlates with early emergent diagnosis and treatment (97–99). Early decompression improves the ability to retain or regain erectile function (97). Bladder areflexia is the predominant pattern of urodynamic dysfunction and can be associated with impaired electromyographic sphincter activity and denervation of pelvic floor

muscles (100–102). Bowel dysfunction consists of both constipation (103) and fecal incontinence (97) that improves after surgical decompression. Recovery of bladder function is a slow process that takes place over months to years (104). Conservative treatment consists of intermittent catheterization guided by urodynamic abnormalities (96,99,104).

Spinal Cord Injury

Spinal cord trauma initially results in a state of spinal shock that lasts 6 to 8 weeks and is associated with an acontractile bladder. External sphincter EMG activity returns before bladder activity. As reflexive bladder activity returns, the urodynamic pattern of function generally includes a hypercontractile bladder alone or with external sphincter dyssynergia. Treatment includes intermittent catheterization to maintain low bladder pressures and to prevent upper urologic tract disease (105). Selected patients may benefit from pharmacologic therapy tailored to urodynamic findings, sphincterotomy, or augmentation cystoplasty (105). Autonomic dysreflexia, an exaggerated sympathetic outflow response to an afferent spinal stimulation, which usually manifests as a rise in blood pressure with slowing of heart rate (106), should be avoided through careful bladder management (105).

Spinal cord transection results in bowel dysfunction that consists of intractable constipation, fecal impaction, overflow fecal incontinence, and distention-induced uncontrolled reflex defecation. Patients with lack of volitional control rely on reflexes to complete defecation (107). Continence may be preserved without fecal impaction through avoidance of dehydration, a diet high in fiber, and a regular toileting regimen (107).

Residual sexual function depends on the level of injury. Reflex sexual activity is absent during spinal shock (3). Thoracic and cervical level lesions are generally associated with retention of reflex penile erections and occasional ejaculation in males and with vaginal secretions as part of a genital reflex in females (108). Conus medullaris lesions are usually associated with absence of penile erections and vaginal secretions (108).

Peripheral Neuropathy

Bladder, bowel, and sexual dysfunction can result from peripheral nervous system injury affecting somatic motor, sensory, and the autonomic nervous system. Diabetic cystopathy is present in 26 to 87% of diabetic patients and correlates with the presence of a generalized polyneuropathy (109,110). The onset is usually insidious, with progressive urinary retention, hesitancy, weak urinary stream, dribbling, nocturia, and impaired sensation of bladder filling. Common cystometric findings include detrusor areflexia with impaired sensation of bladder filling; however, patients with diabetes not uncommonly manifest detrusor hyperreflexia on urodynamic study, and men may exhibit features of bladder outlet obstruction (111). In elderly diabetic patients, the presence of bladder hyperreflexia and occasional detrusor sphincter dyssynergia may reflect coexistent associated neurologic diseases such as stroke or prior spinal trauma (112). Treatment of patients with bladder areflexia includes scheduled voiding along with the crede maneuver, cholinergic medications such as bethanechol, and intermittent catheterization (113). Because the onset of polyneuropathy can be delayed and progression slowed by intensive therapy in patients with diabetes mellitus (114), it is possible that intensive therapy could also favorably affect diabetic bladder dysfunction. Other toxic and metabolic polyneuropathies may be the cause of urinary retention, including pernicious anemia, hypothyroidism, alcohol related, vitamin E deficiency, and porphyria (115). Urinary retention occurs in Guillain-Barré syndrome; urodynamic studies may reveal a flaccid bladder with external urethral denervation. Incontinence is rare and usually reflects urinary overflow (116).

Fecal incontinence occurs in up to 20% of diabetics, may be nocturnal, and can coincide with diarrhea (117). Sphincter tone may be diminished on examination, and incontinence may be related to abnormal internal or external anal sphincter function (118,119). An increased perceptive threshold to rectal balloon distention suggests the presence of sensory dysfunction, and this may contribute to incontinence by impaired perception of rectal fullness (92). Biofeedback therapy can improve fecal incontinence in some patients (119).

Sexual dysfunction in male diabetic patients includes retrograde ejaculation, which is believed to be caused by contractile failure of the internal vesicle sphincter of the bladder during ejaculation. This may respond to sympathomimetic medications (120). Erectile dysfunction affects more than a third of diabetic men and accounts for about 9% of evaluations in a medical clinic for impotence (121, 122). Abnormalities of the bulbocavernosus reflex latency time and the dorsal nerve of the penis conduction velocity support peripheral nervous system dysfunction as an etiology for impotence in diabetic men (122–124). Sexual dysfunction in diabetic women includes inadequate lubrication, anorgasmia, and dyspareunia (125). Both men and women can experience loss of libido, and psychological factors can play a role and need to be considered in the overall approach to treatment (3,126,127). Therapeutic options include penile prosthetic insertion, vacuum constriction devices, and local pharmacologic injection therapy (121,128).

Plexopathy and Mononeuropathy

Pelvic plexus or pudendal nerve injury may be a consequence of major pelvic surgery such as abdominoperineal resection or radical hysterectomy, as well as trauma and childbirth. Hysterectomy causes damage to the pelvic plexus and contributes to incontinence later in life (129). Features noticed in women undergoing radical hysterectomy and pelvic lymphadenectomy include decreased or altered awareness of bladder distention, stress incontinence, prolonged postoperative urinary retention, and hypertonic cystometry findings (130). The hypertonicity could reflect excessive unopposed parasympathetic tone or an intrinsic increase in bladder myogenic tone secondary to surgical dissection adjacent to the bladder and irritation from the indwelling bladder catheter (130,131). Tumor invasion of the pelvic plexus by destruction of the somatic, parasympathetic, and sympathetic nerves results in bladder areflexia with retention, constipation, and impotence (132, 133). Voiding dysfunction occurs after abdominoperineal resection of the rectum in up to 69% of patients, and symptoms usually subside in 3 to 6 months. Urodynamic findings are variable and include patients with areflexic bladders and some with hyperreflexic bladders and decreased proximal urethral pressure (134,135). Bladder areflexia may be replaced later by hyperreflexia (134). Bladder outlet obstruction, ascribed to the prostate, may be present in men (135). Removal of the cardinal ligaments or a long cuff of the upper vagina during hysterectomy may increase the likelihood of a plexus neuropathy. The posterior pelvic plexus and parasympathetic nerves may be damaged during mobilization of the rectum during abdominoperineal resection (136). Some women develop intractable constipation after hysterectomy associated with increased rectal compliance and volume, which may reflect incidental parasympathetic nerve injury (137). Functional obstruction of the colon may result from malignant tumor infiltration of the splanchnic nerves, celiac plexus, semilunar ganglia, and vagus nerves and is thought to reflect an imbalance of sympathetic and parasympathetic innervation or Ogilvie syndrome (138). If conservative management to decompress the colon fails, surgery may be indicated to prevent cecal rupture (138).

Sexual dysfunction may result from resection of the rectum and includes erectile and ejaculatory dysfunction in men and decreased vaginal secretions, dyspareunia, and diminished orgasm in women. The incidence is highest in abdominoperineal resection procedures and lower with anterior procedures, features which suggests that the extent of local surgical trauma is an etiologic factor (139). The incidence of impotence is about 11% in men with lumbosacral plexus neuropathy secondary to tumor invasion (133).

Stress urinary incontinence and genitourinary prolapse in women are associated with prolongation of the pudendal nerve terminal motor latency (PNTML) (140,141). Single-fiber EMG of the pubococcygeus and anal sphincter muscles with genitourinary prolapse, with or without stress urinary incontinence, shows increased fiber density, consistent with reinnervation (142–144). These findings are more common in women who experience prolonged labor and vaginal delivery and may reflect direct pressure effect or stretching of the pudendal nerve (143). Vaginal dissection may be associated with perineal motor nerve injury and can worsen preexisting perineal neuropathy in patients with stress incontinence (145). EMG of pelvic floor muscles reveals asymmetric and uncoordinated levator muscle activation patterns in parous stress-incontinent women (146). Constipation, in addition to obstetric history, may be associated with the development of pudendal nerve damage and stress urinary incontinence (147). Fecal incontinence is commonly present in women with stress urinary incontinence and is associated with weakness of the internal and external anal sphincters, the puborectalis, and other striated muscles of the pelvic floor (148–150) and with prolongation of the PNTML measured to the rectal sphincter (151). This may result from injury to the pudendal nerves or direct injury to the pelvic nerves during vaginal delivery and is associated with multiparity, forceps delivery, and high birth weight (152).

Occult lacerations and direct muscle injury of the external anal sphincter may accompany neurogenic injury and contribute to incontinence (153,154). PNTML measurement in patients with untreated fecal incontinence may progressively worsen but is not always associated with clinical worsening of incontinence (155). An association of PNTML with the extent of pelvic descent during straining has been suggested to represent the result of recurrent trauma to the pudendal nerves during perineal descent (156,157). However, other studies have not suggested this relationship. The flaccid and noncontractile muscle movement abnormalities present on videoproctography of patients with neuropathic fecal incontinence were not present in those with chronic constipation without fecal incontinence and control patients (158). A prospective study of 213 patients with disturbances of defecation did not demonstrate a correlation between perineal descent and PNTML (159). A sensory deficit of the rectum and anal canal may occur in isolation or accompany anorectal motor dysfunction and contribute to fecal incontinence (160,161).

Conservative management includes pelvic electrical stimulation, pelvic floor exercises, and biofeedback therapy (162). Treatment of refractory patients includes surgical repair of the sphincter. The identification of extensive external striated sphincter injury by EMG may be valuable in predicting response to surgical sphincter repair (163). Unilateral or bilateral pudendal neuropathy is associated with a reduced likelihood of an excellent result from repair of anterior anal sphincter defects after obstetric delivery (164,165). However, overlap does exist in preoperative PNTML values between patient groups achieving good versus poor long-term results (166).

Myopathy

Urinary and fecal incontinence are uncommon accompaniments of most myopathies. Fecal incontinence with myotonic dystrophy may be increased with diarrhea. EMG of the puborectalis and external anal sphincter muscle of patients with myotonic dystrophy revealed abnormalities consistent with both a myopathy and reinnervation (167). Exercise-induced urinary incontinence and muscle weakness were the presenting features of a 68-year-old man with acid maltase deficiency (168). Stress incontinence with pelvic floor muscle involvement may be an early feature of limb girdle muscular dystrophy (169). Urinary incontinence is occasionally present in Duchenne muscular dystrophy but most likely is a result of upper motor neuron abnormalities, perhaps associated with scoliosis or spinal fusion and not due to a myopathy of the detrusor or external sphincter muscle (170).

CONCLUSION

The symptoms of bladder incontinence, bowel incontinence, and sexual dysfunction can result from a large and diverse group of neurologic conditions. The laboratory assessment provides useful additional diagnostic information that can be used to guide rational therapy and predict outcome. Currently, treatment is primarily symptomatic. A carefully planned therapy program, which may involve healthcare professionals from many disciplines, can result in significant clinical improvement. Future therapy will require an improved understanding of the pathophysiologic mechanisms underlying the neurologic basis of these diseases.

REFERENCES

1. Fantl JA, Newman DK, Colling J, et al. Urinary incontinence in adults: acute and chronic management. Clinical Practice Guideline No. 2, 1996 update. Rockville, MD: U.S. Department of Health and Human Services, Agency for Health Care and Policy Research. AHPCR Publication No. 96-0682. March 1996.
2. Madoff RD, Williams JG, Caushaj PF. Fecal incontinence. *N Engl J Med* 1992;326:1002–1007.
3. Lechtenberg R, Ohl DA. *Sexual dysfunction*. Philadelphia: Lea & Febiger, 1994.
4. de Groat WC. Anatomy and physiology of the lower urinary tract. *Urol Clin North Am* 1993;20:383–401.
5. Chai TC, Steers WD. Neurophysiology of micturition and continence. *Urol Clin North Am* 1996;23:221–236.
6. Onufrowicz B. On the arrangements and function of the cell groups of the sacral region of the spinal cord in man. *Arch Neurol* 1901;3: 387–417.
7. Swash M. Pelvic floor incompetence. In: Rushton DN, ed. *Handbook of neuro-urology*. New York: Marcel Dekker, 1994:303–327.
8. Banwell JG, Creasey GH, Aggarwal AM, Mortimer JT. Management of the neurogenic bowel in patients with spinal cord injury. *Urol Clin North Am* 1993;20:517–527.
9. Blaivas JG, Chancellor MB. Classification of neurogenic bladder disease. In: Chancellor MB, Blaivas JG, eds. *Practical neuro-urology—genitourinary complications in neurological diseases*. Boston: Butterworth-Heinemann, 1995:25–32.
10. Henry MM. Pathogenesis and management of fecal incontinence in the adult. *Gastroenterol Clin North Am* 1987;16:35–45.
11. Jorge JMN, Wexner SD. Etiology and management of fecal incontinence. *Dis Colon Rectum* 1993;36:77–97.
12. Report of the Therapeutics and Technology Subcommittee of the American Academy of Neurology. Assessment: neurological evaluation of male sexual dysfunction. *Neurology* 1995;45:2287–2292.

13. Fowler CJ. Pelvic floor neurophysiology. *Methods Clin Neurophysiol* 1991;2:1–24.
14. Vodusek DB. Evoked potential testing. *Urol Clin North Am* 1996;23:427–446.
15. Wexner SD, Jorge JMN. Colorectal physiological tests: use or abuse of technology? *Eur J Surg* 1994;160:167–174.
16. Chancellor MB, Blaivas JG. Urinary incontinence and neurological implication. In: Chancellor MB, Blaivas JG, eds. *Practical neuro-urology—genitourinary complications in neurologic disease.* Boston: Butterworth-Heinemann, 1995:259–273.
17. Swami SK, Abrams P. Urge incontinence. *Urol Clin North Am* 1996;23:417–425.
18. Wein AJ, Van Arsdalen K, Levin RM. Pharmacologic therapy. In: Krane RJ, Siroky MB, eds. *Clinical neuro-urology.* Boston: Little, Brown, 1989:523–557.
19. Wise BG, Cardozo L. Urinary incontinence. In: Rushton DN, ed. *Handbook of neuro-urology.* New York: Marcel Dekker, 1994:181–207.
20. Bourcier A, Juras JC. Nonsurgical therapy for stress incontinence. *Urol Clin North Am* 1995;22:613–627.
21. Kultke JJ, Bergman A. Hormonal influence on the urinary tract. *Urol Clin North Am* 1995;22:629–639.
22. Chancellor MB, Rivas DA. Management of sphincter dyssynergia. In: Chancellor MB, Blaivas JG, eds. *Practical neuro-urology—genitourinary complications in neurological disease.* Boston: Butterworth-Heinemann, 1995:309–324.
23. Binnie NR, Kawimbe BM, Papachrysostomou M, Smith AN. Use of the pudendo-anal reflex in the treatment of neurogenic faecal incontinence. *Gut* 1990;31:1051–1055.
24. Keighley MRB. Management of faecal incontinence and results of surgical treatment. *Br J Surg* 1983;70:463–468.
25. Goldstein I, Lue TE, Padma-Nathan H, et al. Oral sildenafil in the treatment of erectile dysfunction. *N Engl J Med* 1998;338:1397–1404.
26. Sildenafil: an oral drug for impotence. *Med Lett* 1998;40:51–52.
27. Linet OI, Ogring FG, the Alprostadil Study Group. Efficacy and safety of intracavernosal alprostadil in men with erectile dysfunction. *N Engl J Med* 1996;334:873–877.
28. Padma Nathan H, Hellstrom WJ, et al. Treatment of men with erectile dysfunction with transurethral alprostadil. Medicated Urethral System for Erection (MUSE) study group. *N Engl J Med* 1997;336:1–7.
29. Brindley GS. Impotence and ejaculatory failure. In: Rushton DN, ed. *Handbook of neuro-urology.* New York: Marcel Dekker, 1994:329–348.
30. Currie CT. Urinary incontinence after stroke. *BMJ* 1986;293:1322–1323.
31. Burney TL, Senapati M, Desai S, Choudhary ST, Badlani GH. Effect of cerebrovascular accident on micturition. *Urol Clin North Am* 1996;23:483–490.
32. Gelber DA, Good DC, Laven LJ, Verhulst SJ. Causes of urinary incontinence after acute right hemisphere stroke. *Stroke* 1993;24:378–382.
33. Taub NA, Wolfe CDA, Richardson E, Burney PGJ. Predicting the disability of first-time stroke sufferers at 1 year. *Stroke* 1994;25:352–357.
34. Maguire PA, Taylor IC, Stout RW. Elderly patients in acute medical wards: factors predicting length of stay in hospital. *Br Med J* 1986;292:1251–1253.
35. Wade DT, Hewer RL. Outlook after an acute stroke: urinary incontinence and loss of consciousness compared in 532 patients. *Q J Med* 1985;56:601–608.
36. Anderson CS, Jamrozik KD, Broadhurst RJ, Stewart-Wynne EG. Predicting survival for 1 year among different subtypes of stroke. *Stroke* 1994;25:1935–1944.
37. Brittain KR, Peet SM, Castleden CM. Stroke and incontinence. *Stroke* 1998;29:524–528.
38. Tsuchida S, Noto H, Yamaguchi O, Itoh M. Urodynamics studies on hemiplegic patients after cerebrovascular accident. *Urology* 1983;21:315–318.
39. Khan Z, Starer P, Yang WC, Bhola A. Analysis of voiding disorders in patients with cerebrovascular accidents. *Urology* 1990;34:265–270.
40. Khan Z, Hertanu J, Yang WC, Melman A, Leis E. Predictive correlation of urodynamic dysfunction and brain injury after cerebrovascular accident. *J Urol* 1981;126:86–88.
41. Garrett VE, Scott JA, Costich J, Aubrey DL, Gross J. Bladder emptying assessment in stroke patients. *Arch Phys Med Rehabil* 1989;70:41–43.
42. Lum SK, Marshall VR. Results of prostatectomy in patients following a cerebrovascular accident. *Br J Urol* 1982;54:186–189.
43. Ishii N, Nishihara Y, Imamura T. Why do frontal lobe symptoms predominate in vascular dementia with lacunes? *Neurology* 1986;36:340–345.
44. Bogousslavsky J, Regli F. Anterior cerebral artery territory infarction in the Lausanne stroke registry—clinical and etiologic patterns. *Arch Neurol* 1990;47:144–150.
45. Ween JE, Alexander MP, D Esposito M, Roberts M. Incontinence after stroke in a rehabilitation setting: outcome associations and predictive factors. *Neurology* 1996;47:659–663.
46. Brocklehurst JC, Andrews K, Richards B, Laycock PJ. Incontinence in stroke patients. *J Am Geriatr Soc* 1985;33:540–542.
47. Jongbloed L. Prediction of function after stroke: a critical review. *Stroke* 1986;17:765–776.
48. Coslett HB, Heilman KM. Male sexual function. Impairment after right hemisphere stroke. *Arch Neurol* 1986;43:1036–1039.
49. Andrew J, Nathan PW. Lesions of the anterior frontal lobes and disturbances of micturition and defaecation. *Brain* 1964;87:233–265.
50. Thal LJ, Grundman M, Klauber MR. Dementia: characteristics of a referral population and factors associated with progression. *Neurology* 1988;38:1083–1090.
51. Bennett DA, Gilley DW, Wilson RS, Huckman MS, Fox JH. Clinical correlates of high signal lesions on magnetic resonance imaging in Alzheimer's disease. *J Neurol* 1992;239:186–190.
52. Roman GC. Senile dementiae of the Binswanger type. *Arch Neurol* 1987;258:1782–1788.
53. Tarvonen-Schroder S, Roytta M, Raiha I, Kurki T, Rajala T, Sourander L. Clinical features of leuko-araiosis. *J Neurol Neurosurg Psychiatry* 1996;60:431–436.
54. NINDS-AIREN International Workshop. Vascular dementia: diagnostic criteria for research studies. *Neurology* 1993;43:250–260.
55. Del-Ser T, Munoz DG, Hachinski V. Temporal pattern of cognitive decline and incontinence is different in Alzheimer's disease and diffuse Lewy body disease. *Neurology* 1996;46:682–686.
56. Burns A, Jacoby R, Levy R. Psychiatric phenomena in Alzheimer's disease. IV. Disorders of behavior. *Br J Psych* 1990;157:86–94.
57. Newmans AJ, Forsler DP, Kay DWK. Dependency and community care in presenile Alzheimer's disease. *Br J Psych* 1995;166:777–782.
58. Fisher CM. Hydrocephalus as a cause of disturbances of gait in the elderly. *Neurology* 1982;32:1358–1363.
59. Jonas S, Brown J. Neurogenic bladder in normal pressure hydrocephalus. *Urology* 1975;5:44–50.
60. Romero Y, Evans JM, Fleming KC Phillips SF. Constipation and fecal incontinence in the elderly population. *Mayo Clin Proc* 1996;71:81–92.
61. Pavlakis AJ, Siroky MB, Goldstein I, Krane R. Neurologic findings in Parkinson's disease. *J Urol* 1983;129:80–83.
62. Berger Y, Blaivas JG, DeLarocha ER, Salinas JM. Urodynamic findings in Parkinson's disease. *J Urol* 1987;138:836–839.
63. Fitzmaurice H, Fowler CJ, Rickards D, et al. Micturition disturbance in Parkinson's disease. *Br J Urol* 1985;57:652–656.
64. Staskin DS, Vardi Y, Siroky MB. Post-prostatectomy continence in the parkinsonian patient: the significance of poor voluntary sphincter contraction. *J Urol* 1988;140:117–118.
65. Khan Z, Starer P, Bhola A. Urinary incontinence in female Parkinson disease patients. Pitfalls of diagnosis. *Urology* 1989;33:486–489.
66. Wenning GK, Shlomo YB, Magalhaes M, Daniel SE, Quinn NP. Clinical features and natural history of multiple system atrophy. *Brain* 1994;117:835–845.
67. Beck RO, Betts CD, Fowler CJ. Genitourinary dysfunction in multiple system atrophy: clinical features and treatment in 62 cases. *J Urol* 1994;151:1336–1341.
68. Eardley I, Quinn NP, Fowler CJ, et al. The value of urethral sphincter electromyography in the differential diagnosis of parkinsonism. *Br J Urol* 1989;64:360–362.
69. Sakakibara R, Hattori T, Tojo M, Yamanishi T, Yasuda K, Hirayama K. Micturitional disturbance in multiple system atrophy. *Jpn J Psychiatr Neurol* 1993;47:591–598.
70. Salinas JM, Berger Y, De La Rocha RE, Blaivas JG. Urological evaluation in the Shy Drager syndrome. *J Urol* 1986;135:741–743.
71. Sakakibara R, Hattori T, Tojo M, Yamanishi T, Yasuda K, Hirayama K. Micturitional disturbance in progressive supranuclear palsy. *J Autonomic Nerv Syst* 1993;45:101–106.
72. Christmas TJ, Kempster PA, Chapple CR, et al. Role of subcutaneous apomorphine in parkinsonian voiding dysfunction. *Lancet* 1988;2:1451–1453.
73. Sakuta M, Nakanishi T, Toyokura Y. Anal muscle electromyograms

differ in amyotrophic lateral sclerosis and Shy-Drager syndrome. *Neurology* 1978;29:1289–1293.

74. Lipe H, Longstreth WT Jr, Bird TD, Linde M. Sexual function in married men with Parkinson's disease compared to married men with arthritis. *Neurology* 1990;40:1347–1349.

75. Fowler CJ, Kerrebroeck PEV, Nordenbo A, Van Poppel H. Treatment of lower urinary trct dysfunction in patients with multiple sclerosis. *J Neurol Neurosurg Psychiatry* 1992;55:986–989.

76. Hinson JL, Boone TB. Urodynamics and multiple sclerosis. *Urol Clin North Am* 1996;23:475–481.

77. Bemelmans BLH, Hommes OR, Van Kerrebroeck PEV, et al. Evidence for early lower urinary tract dysfunction in clinically silent multiple sclerosis. *J Urol* 1991;145:1219–1224.

78. Awad SA, Gajewski JB, Sogbein K, Murray JT, Field CA. Relationship between neurological and urological status in patients with multiple sclerosis. *J Urol* 1984;132:499–502.

79. Blaivas JG, Bhimani G, Labib KB. Vesicourethral dysfunction in multiple sclerosis. *J Urol* 1979;122:342–347.

80. Goldstein I, Siroky MB, Sax DS, Krane RJ. Neurologic abnormalities in multiple sclerosis. *J Urol* 1982;128:541–545.

81. Blaivas JG, Barbalias GA. Detrusor-external sphincter dyssynergia in men with multiple sclerosis: an ominous urologic condition. *J Urol* 1984;131:91–94.

82. McGuire EJ, Savastano JA. Urodynamic findings and long term outcome management of patients with multiple sclerosis induced lower urinary tract dysfunction. *J Urol* 1984;132:713–715.

83. Gajewski JB, Awad SA. Oxybutynin versus propantheline in patients with multiple sclerosis and detrusor hyperreflexia. *J Urol* 1986;135:966–968.

84. Kinn AC, Larsson PO. Desmopressin: a new principle for symptomatic treatment of urgency and incontinence in patients with multiple sclerosis. *Scand J Urol Nephrol* 1990;24:109–112.

85. Nanninga JB, Frost F, Penn R. Effect of intrathecal baclofen on bladder and sphincter function. *J Urol* 1989;142:101–105.

86. Chia YW, Fowler CJ, Kamm MA, Henry MM, Lemieux MC, Swash M. Prevalence of bowel dysfunction in patients with multiple sclerosis and bladder function. *J Neurol* 1995;242:105–108.

87. Swash M, Snooks SJ, Chalmers DHK. Parity as a factor in incontinence in multiple sclerosis. *Arch Neurol* 1987;44:504–508.

88. Hinds JP, Eidelman BH, Wald A. Prevalence of bowel dysfunction in multiple sclerosis. A population survey. *Gastroenterology* 1990;98:1538–1542.

89. Weber J, Grise P, Roquebert M, et al. Radiopaque markers transit and anorectal manometry in 16 patients with multiple sclerosis and urinary bladder dysfunction. *Dis Colon Rectum* 1987;30:95–100.

90. Gill KP, Chia YW, Henry MM, Shorvon PJ. Defecography in multiple sclerosis patients with severe constipation. *Radiology* 1994;191:553–556.

91. Chia YW, Gill KP, Jameson JS. Paradoxical puborectalis contraction is a feature of constipation in patients with multiple sclerosis. *J Neurol Neurosurg Psychiatry* 1996;60:31–35.

92. Caruana BJ, Wald A, Hinds JP, Eidelman BH. Anorectal sensory and motor function in neurogenic fecal incontinence—comparison between multiple sclerosis and diabetes mellitus. *Gastroenterology* 1991;100:465–470.

93. Hinds JP, Wald A. Colonic and anorectal dysfunction associated with multiple sclerosis. *Am J Gastroenterol* 1989;84:587–595.

94. Mattson D, Petrie M, Srivastava DK, McDermott M. Multiple sclerosis—sexual dysfunction and its response to medications. *Arch Neurol* 1995;52:862–868.

95. Betts CD, Jones SH, Fowler CG. Fowler CJ. Erectile dysfunction in multiple sclerosis. *Brain* 1994;117:1303–1310.

96. Appell RA. Voiding dysfunction and lumbar disc disorders. *Probl Urol* 1993;7:35–40.

97. Shapiro S. Caudae equina syndrome secondary to lumbar disc herniation. *Neurosurg* 1993;32:743–747.

98. O'Flynn KJ, Murphy R, Thomas DG. Neurogenic bladder dysfunction in lumbar intervertebral disc prolapse. *Br J Urol* 1992;69:38–40.

99. O'Laoire SA, Crockard NA, Thomas DG. Prognosis for sphincter recovery after operation for caudae equina compression owing to lumbar disc prolapse. *BMJ* 1981;282:1852–1854.

100. Bradley WE, Andersen JT. Neuromuscular dysfunction of the lower urinary tract in patients with lesions of the caudae equina and conus medullaris. *J Urol* 1976;116:620–621.

101. Sandri SD, Fanciullacci F, Politi P, Zanollo A. Urinary disorders in intervertebral disc prolapse. *Neurourol Urodyn* 1987;6:11–19.

102. Pavlakis AJ, Siroky MB, Goldstein I, Krane RJ. Neurologic findings in conus medullaris and caudae equina injury. *Arch Neurol* 1983;40:570–573.

103. Emmett JL, Love JG. Urinary retention in women caused by asymptomatic protruded lumbar disk: report of 5 cases. *J Urol* 1968;99:597–606.

104. Hellstrom P, Kortelainen P, Kontturi M. Late urodynamic findings after surgery for cauda equina syndrome caused by a prolapsed lumbar intervertebral disk. *J Urol* 1986;135:308–312.

105. Wheeler IS, Walter JW. Acute urologic management of the patient with spinal cord injury. *Urol Clin North Am* 1993;20:403–411.

106. Perkash I. Long term urologic management of the patient with spinal cord injury. *Urol Clin North Am* 1993;20:423–434.

107. Banwell JG, Creasey GH, Aggarwal AM, Mortimer JT. Management of the neurogenic bowel in patients with spinal cord injury. *Urol Clin North Am* 1993;20:517–526.

108. Smith EM, Bodner DR. Sexual dysfunction after spinal cord injury. *Urol Clin North Am* 1993;20:535–542.

109. Frimodt-Moller C. Diabetic cystopathy: epidemiology and related disorders. *Ann Intern Med* 1980;92(Pt 2):318–321.

110. Ellenberg M. Development of urinary bladder dysfunction in diabetes mellitus. *Ann Intern Med* 1980;92(Pt 2):321–323.

111. Kaplan SA, Te AE, Blaivas JG. Urodynamic findings in patients with diabetic cystopathy. *J Urol* 1995;153:342–344.

112. Starer P, Libow L. Cystometric evaluation of bladder dysfunction in elderly diabetic patients. *Arch Intern Med* 1990;150:810–813.

113. Frimodt Moller C, Mortenson S. Treatment of diabetic cystopathy. *Ann Intern Med* 1980;92(Pt 2):327–328.

114. Diabetes control and complications trial research group. The effect of intensive treatment of diabetes on the development and progression of long-term complications in insulin-dependent diabetes mellitus. *N Engl J Med* 1993;329:977–986.

115. Nickell K, Boone TB. Peripheral neuropathy and peripheral nerve injury. *Urol Clin North Am* 1996;23:491–499.

116. Ropper AH, Wijdicks EFM, Truax BT. *Guillain-Barré syndrome.* Philadelphia: F.A. Davis, 1991.

117. Valdovinos MA, Camilleri M, Zimmerman BR. Chronic diarrhea in diabetes mellitus: mechanisms and an approach to diagnosis and treatment. *Mayo Clin Proc* 1993;68:691–702.

118. Schiller LR, Santa Ana CA, Schmulen AC, Hendler RS, Harford WV, Fordtran JS. Pathogenesis of fecal incontinence in diabetes mellitus. Evidence for internal-anal-sphincter dysfunction. *N Engl J Med* 1982;307:1666–1671.

119. Wald A, Tunuguntla AK. Anorectal sensorimotor dysfunction in fecal incontinence and diabetes mellitus. Modification with biofeedback therapy. *N Engl J Med* 1984;310:1282–1287.

120. Ellenberg M. Diabetes and sexual dysfunction. *NY St J Med* 1982;82:927–930.

121. Price DE. Managing impotence in diabetes. *BMJ* 1993;307:275–276.

122. Slag MF, Morley JE, Elson MK, et al. Impotence in medical clinic outpatients. *JAMA* 1983;249:1736–1740.

123. Kaneko S, Bradley WE. Penile electrodiagnosis. Value of bulbocavernosus reflex latency versus nerve conduction velocity of the dorsal nerve of the penis in diagnosis of diabetic impotence. *J Urol* 1987;137:933–935.

124. Daniels JS. Abnormal nerve conduction in impotent patients with diabetes mellitus. *Diabetes Care* 1989;12:449–454.

125. Campbell LV, Redelman MJ, Borkman M, et al. Factors in sexual dysfunction in diabetic female volunteer subjects. *Med J Aust* 1989;151:550–552.

126. Schiavi RC. Psychological treatment of erectile disorders in diabetic patients. *Ann Intern Med* 1980;92(Pt 2):337–339.

127. Lustman RJ, Clouse RE. Relationship of psychiatric illness to impotence in men with diabetes. *Diabetes Care* 1990;13:893–895.

128. Whitehead ED. Diabetes-related impotence and its treatment in the middle-aged and elderly. Part II. *Geriatrics* 1987;42:77–85.

129. Brown JS, Seeley DG, Fong J, Black DM, Ensrud KE, Grady D. Urinary incontinence in older women: who is at risk? *Obstet Gynecol* 1996;87:715–721.

130. Forney JP. The effect of radical hysterectomy on bladder physiology. *Am J Obstet Gynecol* 1980;138:374–382.

131. Seski JC, Diokno AC. Bladder dysfunction after radical abdominal hysterectomy. *Am J Obstet Gynecol* 1977;128:643–651.

132. Woodside JR, Crawford ED. Urodynamic features of pelvic plexus injury. *J Urol* 1980;124:657–658.

133. Jaeckle KA, Young DF, Foley KM. The natural history of lumbosacral plexopathy in cancer. *Neurology* 1985;35:8–15.

134. Blaivas JG, Barbalias GA. Characteristics of neural injury after abdomino-perineal resection. *J Urol* 1983;129:84–87.

135. Yalla SV, Andriole GL. Vesicourethral dysfunction following pelvic visceral ablative surgery. *J Urol* 1984;132:503–509.

136. Mundy AR. An anatomical explanation for bladder dysfunction following rectal and uterine surgery. *Br J Urol* 1982;54:501–504.

137. Varma JS. Autonomic influences on colorectal motility and pelvic surgery. *World J Surg* 1992;16:811–819.

138. Nanni G, Garbini A, Luchetti P, et al. Ogilvie's syndrome (acute colonic pseudo-obstruction): review of the literature (October 1948–March 1980) and report of four additional cases. *Dis Colon Rectum* 1982;25: 157–166.

139. Fegiz G, Trenti A, Bezzi M, et al. Sexual and bladder dysfunctions following surgery for rectal carcinoma. *Ital J Surg Sci* 1986;16:103–109.

140. Snooks SJ, Badenoch DF, Tiptaft RC, Swash M. Perineal nerve damage in genuine stress urinary incontinence. An electrophysiological study. *Br J Urol* 1985;57:422–426.

141. Smith ARB, Hosker GL, Warrell DW. The role of pudendal nerve damage in the aetiology of genuine stress incontinence in women. *Br J Obstet Gynaecol* 1989;96:29–32.

142. Smith ARB, Hosker GL, Warrell DW. The role of partial denervaton of the pelvic floor in the aetiology of genitourinary prolapse and stress incontinence of urine. A neurophysiologic study. *Br J Obstet Gynaecol* 1989;96:24–28.

143. Allen RE, Hosker GL, Smith ARB, Warrell DW. Pelvic floor damage and childbirth: a neurophysiologic study. *Br J Obstet Gynaecol* 1990; 97:770–779.

144. Anderson RS. A neurogenic element to urinary stress incontinence. *Br J Obstet Gynaecol* 1984;91:44–45.

145. Zivkovic F, Tamussino K, Ralph G, Schied G, Auer-Grumbach M. Long-term effects of vaginal dissection on the innervation of the striated urethral sphincter. *Obstet Gynecol* 1996;87:257–260.

146. Deindl FM, Vodusek DB, Hesse U Schussler B. Pelvic floor activity patterns: comparison of nulliparous continent and parous urinary stress incontinent women. A kinesiological study. *Br J Urol* 1994;73:413–417.

147. Spence-Jones C, Kamm MA, Henry MM, Hudson CN. Bowel dysfunction: a pathogenic factor in uterovaginal prolapse and urinary stress incontinence. *Br J Obstet Gynaecol* 1994;101:147–152.

148. Swash M. Anorectal incontinence: electrophysiological tests. *Br J Surg* 1985;72[Suppl]:S14–S22.

149. Lubowski DZ, Nicholls RJ, Burleigh DE, Swash M. Internal anal sphincter in neurogenic fecal incontinence. *Gastroenterology* 1988;95: 997–1002.

150. Snooks SJ, Henry MM, Swash M. Anorectal incontinence and rectal prolapse: differential assessment of the innervation to puborectalis and external anal sphincter muscles. *Gut* 1985;26:470–476.

151. Kiff ES, Swash M. Slowed conduction in the pudendal nerves in idiopathic (neurogenic) faecal incontinence. *Br J Surg* 1984;71:614–616.

152. Snooks SJ, Swash M, Henry MM, Setchell M. Risk factors in childbirth causing damage to the pelvic floor innervation. *Int J Colorectal Dis* 1986;1:20–24.

153. Sultan AH, Kamm MA, Hudson CN, Thomas JM, Bartram CI. Anal-sphincter disruption during vaginal delivery. *N Engl J Med* 1993;329: 1905–1911.

154. Snooks SJ, Henry MM, Swash M. Faecal incontinence due to external anal sphincter division in childbirth is associated with damage to the innervation of the pelvic floor musculature: a double pathology. *Br J Obstet Gynaecol* 1985;92:824–829.

155. Hill J, Mumtaz A, Kiff ES. Pudendal neuropathy in patients with idiopathic faecal incontinence progresses with time. *Br J Surg* 1994;81: 1494–1495.

156. Kiff ES, Barnes PRH, Swash M. Evidence of pudendal neuropathy in patients with perineal descent and chronic straining at stool. *Gut* 1984; 25:1279–1282.

157. Jones PN, Lubowski DZ, Swash M, Henry MM. Relation between perineal descent and pudendal nerve damage in idiopathic faecal incontinence. *Int J Colorectal Dis* 1987;2:93–95.

158. Pinho M, Yoshioka K, Keighley M. Are pelvic floor movements abnormal in disordered defecation? *Dis Colon Rectum* 1991;34: 1117–1119.

159. Jorge JMN, Wexner SD, Ehrenpries ED, et al. Does perineal descent correlate with pudendal neuropathy? *Dis Colon Rectum* 1993;36: 475–483.

160. Bielefeldt K, Enck P, Erckenbrecht JF. Sensory and motor function in the maintenance of anal continence. *Dis Colon Rectum* 1990;33: 674–678.

161. Rogers J, Henry MM, Misiewicz JJ. Combined sensory and motor deficit in primary neuropathic faecal incontinence. *Gut* 1988;29:5–9.

162. Richardson DA. Conservative management of urinary incontinence—a symposium. *J Reprod Med* 1993;38:659–661.

163. Cheong DMO, Vaccaro CA, Salanga VD, Wexner SD, Phillips RC, Hanson MR. Electrodiagnostic evaluation of fecal incontinence. *Muscle Nerve* 1995;18:612–619.

164. Sangwan YP, Coller JA, Barrett RC. Unilateral pudendal neuropathy. Impact on outcome of anal sphincter repair. *Dis Colon Rectum* 1996; 39:686–689.

165. Laurberg S. Swash M, Henry MM. Delayed external sphincter repair for obstetric tear. *Br J Surg* 1988;75:786–788.

166. Carrero PS, Kamm MA, Nicholls RJ. Long term results of post anal repair for neurogenic faecal incontinence. *Br J Surg* 1994;81:140–144.

167. Herbaut AG, Nogueira MC, Panzer JM, Zegers de Beyl D. Anorectal incontinence in myotonic dystrophy: a myopathic involvement of pelvic floor muscles [letter]. *Muscle Nerve* 1992;15:1210–1211.

168. Chancellor AM, Warlow CP, Webb JN, Lucas MG, Besley GT, Broadhead DM. Acid Maltase deficiency presenting with a myopathy and exercise induced urinary incontinence in a 68 year old male [letter]. *J Neurol Neurosurg Psychiatry* 1991;54:659–660.

169. Dixon PJ, Christmas J, Chapple CR. Stress Incontinence due to pelvic floor muscle involvement in limb-girdle muscular dystrophy. *Br J Urol* 1990;65:653–654.

170. Carress JB, Kothari MJ, Bauer SB, Shefner JM. Urinary incontinence in Duchenne muscular dystrophy. *Muscle Nerve* 1996;19:819–822.

Motor Disorders,
edited by David S. Younger.
Lippincott Williams & Wilkins, Philadelphia © 1999.

CHAPTER 43

Management of Spasticity

Andrew B. Lassman and Saud A. Sadiq

Spasticity is a common clinical feature of central nervous system motor disorders. Untreated, spasticity may compound disability and negatively impact on functional aspects of daily living. Current management of spasticity is based on an understanding of the pathophysiologic mechanisms underlying the disorder. This has led to more effective and safe treatments for most patients with spasticity. This chapter reviews aspects of the pathophysiology and treatment of spasticity, including intrathecal therapy.

DEFINITIONS AND KEY CLINICAL FEATURES

Spasticity results from upper motor neuron lesions and the disinhibition of velocity-dependent increase in muscle tone during stretch. With rapid stretching of an affected muscle, there is a brief tone-free period, followed by an abrupt catch with increasing muscular tone to a peak, after which resistance dissipates like opening a clasp knife. The associated positive clinical signs of the resulting disinhibition are hyperreflexia, Babinski signs, and extensor and painful flexor spasms. The negative signs of spasticity are upper motor neuron weakness, fatigability, and incoordination (1–6).

Rigidity, usually associated with extrapyramidal disorders, may be mistaken for spasticity; however, it leads to increased constant muscle tone throughout the range of the muscle stretch response, like bending a lead pipe. With few exceptions, such as in secondary dystonia in which signs of both rigidity and spasticity may coexist, rigidity is generally not associated with hyperreflexia or Babinski signs (5,6).

The most common causes of spasticity are traumatic brain injury and spinal cord injury (SCI); multiple sclerosis (MS); cerebral palsy (CP); stroke; compressive myelopathy, transverse myelitis or myelopathy due to human T-cell lymphotropic virus type I, human immunodeficiency virus, or Lyme infection; spinal cord tumors; and dystonia. Less common causes are familial spastic paraplegia, stiff-person syndrome, primary lateral sclerosis, postencephalitic conditions, and certain spastic paraplegia due to specific enzymatic or metabolic disorders. It is important to accurately determine the underlying condition resulting in spasticity to optimize treatment.

PATHOPHYSIOLOGY

Normal muscle tone reflects a balance or equilibrium between inhibitory and excitatory inputs to the alpha motor neuron (αMN). An alteration of this equilibrium results in spasticity, and current treatments are designed to correct this imbalance. To better understand the rationale of drug therapy for spasticity, we now consider the normal pathways involved in maintaining muscle tone.

Basic Circuitry: The Stretch Reflex

A reflex consists of an input to the αMN resulting in an output. The input pathway is relatively complex and is modulated by several excitatory and inhibitory signals reviewed below. Stretch reflex output is simple and occurs with the generation of an action potential and release of acetylcholine at the neuromuscular junction. This induces a muscle end-plate potential with release of calcium ions from the muscle sarcoplasmic reticulum. An energy-requiring release of calcium enables myosin and actin filaments to slide over one another, the final outcome of which is myofiber contraction (7).

There are several inputs to the αMN. In the simple stretch reflex, Ia spindle afferents from muscle spindle stretch receptors enter the dorsal horn of the spinal cord

A. B. Lassman: Columbia University College of Physicians and Surgeons and Department of Neurology, New York Presbyterian Hospital, New York, New York 10032.

S. A. Sadiq: Department of Neurology, Albert Einstein College of Medicine and St. Luke's–Roosevelt Hospital, New York, New York 10019.

and synapse with the αMN in the ventral horn, with the excitatory amino acids glutamate and aspartate as neurotransmitters. These afferents also synapse on the αMN of synergist muscles to enhance contraction and on inhibitory interneurons to inhibit contraction of antagonist muscles. The sensitivity of muscle spindle afferents is maintained by gamma motor neurons (γMN) that regulate fusimotor muscle spindle tone. When a muscle is stretched, fusimotor discharges increase regulating γMN activity and reflex muscle tone (8).

Increased Excitatory Input

On the basis of this simple circuitry, one could postulate several potential mechanisms for spasticity. For example, spasticity could result from hyperexcitability of the agonist αMN, perhaps from a change in membrane properties (2,9); however, disruptions of synaptic input to the αMN are more likely than intrinsic alterations (10). Excessive activity of the fusimotor system could yield a spindle that is overly sensitive to stretch, although evidence for this is lacking (4,6,11–14). At the level of the αMN, potential therapies could involve interrupting the afferent (anterior rhizotomy) or afferent (posterior rhizotomy) αMN pathways. A decrease in calcium ion release can be achieved with dantrolene. A reduction in acetylcholine release at the neuromuscular junction can be obtained with local injection of botulinum toxin (BTX), and there are also useful physical therapy modalities (Table 1).

Pathways Mediating Both Excitatory and Inhibitory Input

Several descending pathways may also contribute to spasticity. Some influence fusimotor tone by increasing excitatory synapses on αMNs; the latter synapse on αMN and transmit their signals by the excitatory amino acid glutamate. However, the circuitry is complex and is not completely delineated. Two major descending pathways,

the inhibitory norepinephrine-mediated dorsal reticulospinal tract and the excitatory serotonin-mediated medial reticulospinal tract, exert balancing influences on muscle tone. Other descending pathways, such as the corticospinal, rubrospinal, and vestibulospinal pathways, also exert a modulating influence. Spasticity could result from a lack of upper motor neuron influence on the inhibitory dorsal reticulospinal tract that shifts the balance toward the excitatory medial reticulospinal tract and vestibulospinal tract (2,3). Potential therapies at this level include enhancement of adrenergic inhibitory activity with the use of clonidine and tizanidine and reduction of serotonergic excitatory activity with cyproheptadine (Table 1).

Decreased Inhibitory Input

Many interneurons participate in the stretch reflex pathway, including Ia and Ib inhibitory interneurons and Renshaw neurons (15). Ia inhibitory interneurons receive excitatory afferent input from the Ia afferents and inhibit αMNs of antagonistic muscles, known as "reciprocal inhibition." Ib inhibitory interneurons are more complex. Golgi tendon organs transmit information about muscle tension via Ib afferents to interneurons, but the Ib interneurons also receive Ia afferent information and have a more integrative role. Hence, the term interneurons mediating group I nonreciprocal inhibition is probably more accurate (9). Renshaw cells, another type of interneuron, receive several types of input, including branches of αMNs, afferent inputs, descending pathways, and other interneurons. In turn, Renshaw cells synergistically inhibit αMNs, γMNs, Ia inhibitory interneurons, and other Renshaw cells. The latter have complex connections with many other cells via a feedback loop. They have a role in the firing of αMNs by integrating signals from both descending pathways and afferent input (9).

Presynaptic inhibition of Ia afferents reduces the excitatory impact of Ia afferents on αMNs; both afferent inputs and descending pathways induce such presynaptic inhibition (9). Inadequate presynaptic inhibition of muscle spindles contribute to spasticity. The transmitter γ-aminobutyric acid (GABA) is an important mediator of presynaptic inhibition. Enhancement of GABA or GABA-like transmission is one method of treatment (4). Medications such as baclofen, diazepam, clonazepam, and ivermectin exert much of their antispasticity effect by enhancement of GABA transmission (Table 1).

THERAPEUTIC MODALITIES

The goal of treatment is to prevent or reduce the undesirable consequences of spasticity that include decreased mobility, disabling pain, contractures, dependency for activities of daily living and hygiene, sexual dysfunction, and sleep disturbances. Untreated, they lead to low self-esteem and mood disorders. In all cases, treatment should

TABLE 1. *Pathophysiologic basis of treatment of spasticity*

Site of action	Neurotransmitter	Treatment
Muscle	Calcium	Dantrolene
Neuromuscular junction	Acetylcholine	Botulinum toxin
Inhibitory inputs to alpha motor neurons (segmental and diffuse central)	GABA	Baclofen, diazepam, clonazepam, ivermectin
Inhibitory reticulospinal	Norepinephrine	Tizanidine, clonidine
Excitatory reticulospinal	Serotonin	Cyproheptadine
Afferents to alpha motor neuron	NA	Dorsal rhizotomy

improve overall function and not just reduce spasticity. Indeed, in some cases, a certain degree of spasticity has functional value such as in the barely ambulatory patient with spastic paraparesis in whom overtreatment would render the patient nonambulatory.

The management of spasticity should ideally be based on ongoing clinical assessment, leading to an appropriate therapeutic plan that includes one or more of the following options listed in order of least to most aggressive: physical therapy, oral medications, BTX injections, intrathecal baclofen (ITB) therapy, and surgical ablative procedures.

Clinical Assessment

A thorough clinical assessment is crucial in formulating a logical management plan. It requires a team approach with the input of a variety of physician and non-physician specialists. A complete history and examination is performed to determine the severity of spasticity and its impact on function. The patient should be examined supine and erect and on more than one visit. Posture may have an effect on spasticity, and the severity varies to a certain extent from day to day. The Ashworth Scale (22, 23), in modified version shown in Table 2, is an objective bedside scale of spasticity that can be easily used. Rating scales are useful both in the initial assessment and in determining treatment benefit. Functional assessment of patient-performed tasks such as ambulation, dressing, transferring, and turning in bed are also useful.

The underlying neurologic condition causing spasticity and the associated complications such as urinary tract infections and decubitus ulcers, which can potentially exacerbate the spastic condition, should be stabilized and optimally treated (2,16–21). Acute worsening of spasticity is almost always a manifestation of an associated medical change such as a relapse in a patient with MS or unsuspected infection. A step-ladder management plan

with clearly defined and appropriate goals should be instituted. The physician, therapist, and, above all, the patient should agree on these goals. The patient should understand the limitations of treatment. For example, treatment may allow easier transfers or relieve associated pain but will not strengthen a weak limb or restore lost function (2).

Role of Physical Therapy

Physical therapy is effective without the side effects of medication, and may be all that is needed. Spasticity leads to muscle immobilization and changes in muscle fiber length and number. Physical therapy can interrupt this vicious cycle and improve active function and patient comfort. In addition, physical therapy may enhance the effects of some oral medications, such as baclofen (24), and is best initiated before the development of muscle shortening to maintain muscle length and elasticity. Thus, physical therapy should be initiated as soon as possible. It includes passive range of motion exercises, joint mobilization, positioning and stretching, bracing, strengthening, and serial casting (20,25).

Standard Antispasticity Agents

Baclofen

If physical therapy is not satisfactory as the only therapy, oral baclofen is usually the drug of choice for spasticity due to intrinsic spinal cord disease (20) and MS (18,26), although one might consider other treatments for patients with a history of hallucinations or seizures (21). Baclofen is a GABA analogue, and although its precise mechanism of action is not known, it probably acts as a GABA-β agonist to inhibit spinal reflexes by hyperpolarizing afferent inputs.

TABLE 2. *Modified Ashworth scales for assessment of muscle tone*

Muscle tone		Spasm score		Reflex scale	
Scale	Definition	Scale	Definition	Scale	Definition
1	No increase in tone	0	No spasm	0	None
2	Minimal increase in tone; movement of affected part gives a "catch"	1	Mild spasms only present upon stimulation	1	Hyporeflexia
3	Moderate increase in tone but affected part easily moved	2	Spontaneous spasms occurring at less than once per hour	2	Normal
4	Severe increase in tone and affected part moved with difficulty	3	Frequent spontaneous spasms occurring between 1 to 10 times an hour	3	Pathologically brisk but no clonus
5	Fixed and rigid muscle	4	Very frequent spasms occurring at more than 10 every hour	4	Unsustained clonus, less than four beats
				5	Unsustained clonus, more than four beats
				6	Sustained clonus

Where possible, the exact dose to be taken should be determined by both the patient and physician, and most patients can work out an individual schedule tailored to their needs. Physicians often give too little baclofen to patients who can tolerate higher doses (27). High doses are not associated with treatment discontinuation, as found in a study that showed about 20% of patients with MS had taken doses greater than 80 mg/day (28). When initiating treatment, it is usual to start with a 10-mg nighttime dose to determine effect. There is a wide variation in dose tolerance relative to adverse effects ranging from 10 to 200 mg; this is probably the single most important determinant of efficacy.

An early double-blind study of baclofen treatment in patients with MS showed a significant reduction in spasticity with concomitant relief of painful spasms and clonus and improved range of joint motion that helped maintain functional status (29). A similar study also found an improvement in spasticity, especially in reducing painful spasms (30). A more recent study of 30 patients with MS treated with medication and stretching showed a benefit of baclofen alone (24). Although baclofen is used less in other conditions associated with spasticity, a therapeutic trial is warranted in most cases. In one case of stiff-person syndrome, a patient bedridden for 3 years became ambulatory after 1 month of daily oral baclofen (31). A double-blind placebo-controlled trial of 20 children also demonstrated the efficacy of baclofen in reducing spasticity from CP (32). It also provides beneficial anxiolytic effects in some patients (33). However, not all spasticity-associated conditions respond to baclofen. A double-blind placebo-controlled study of patients with SCI showed no significant reduction of spasticity with baclofen (34). Oral baclofen penetrates the blood–brain barrier poorly. Therefore, to obtain therapeutic levels, many patients require high doses that induce unacceptable weakness, lethargy, somnolence, or other side effects (27). Perceived weakness as an adverse effect to baclofen is usually an unmasking effect and results from decreased resistance to muscular contraction (35). Toxicity generally indicates subclinical renal insufficiency (36), and overdose can be life threatening (37). When baclofen is discontinued after long-term use, it should be tapered gradually because rapid withdrawal has been associated with hallucinations, seizures, manic psychosis, dyskinesia, and hyperthermia (6,38–45).

Diazepam and Clonazepam

These medications are useful in the management of spasticity either as single agents or in combination due to synergistic actions (46). The benzodiazepines diazepam and clonazepam, facilitate the presynaptic inhibitory actions of GABA on GABA-β receptors but may have other antispasticity actions (4,6). Diazepam is effective in the treatment of spasticity associated with the stiff-person syndrome (6,47). A study of 13 affected patients followed at the Mayo Clinic for 30 years demonstrated the efficacy of diazepam in reducing spasms, especially when combined with rehabilitation (48). The efficacy of clonazepam in treating spasticity from CP was demonstrated by a double-blind, placebo-controlled, crossover study of 12 children (49). Another double-blind study of 22 children demonstrated that diazepam and dantrolene together were more effective than placebo, and the combination was more effective than either alone (50). However, benzodiazepines have undesirable sedative effects during waking hours and the potential for addiction and dangerous withdrawal symptoms when abruptly discontinued (6,18,51,52); they may also affect body weight (53). In fact, diazepam is often considered less preferable when compared with other medications (6,46). In a double-blind study of 105 patients comparing diazepam and tizanidine, fewer adverse effects related to treatment discontinuation occurred with tizanidine (54). Similarly, when the adverse effect profile of diazepam was compared with dantrolene (55) or baclofen (56), diazepam was tolerated less well than either of the other medications. In a study comparing clonazepam with baclofen, both were about equally effective, with clonazepam perhaps more beneficial in patients with mild cerebral causes of spasticity, whereas baclofen was more effective in severe spinal spasticity (57). In general, these agents are best used in small doses in combination therapy. The greatest efficacy is in patients with nocturnal spasms. Occasionally, in treatment-resistant cases of severe spasticity, as sometimes seen in spastic dystonia patients, high-dose diazepam (50 to 100 g/day) may be a last resort before consideration of intrathecal therapy.

Tizanidine and Clonidine

Tizanidine and clonidine are α_2-adrenergic agonists that inhibit the release of excitatory amino acids from both spinal interneurons and the dorsal reticulospinal tract (58,59). The effects of clonidine have been studied in chronic spinalized rats (60). It leads to reduced αMN excitability, decreased spontaneous electromyogram activity, less tonic activity, reduced amplitude of hindlimb muscles and respective reflexes, and an increase in the threshold for electronically induced reflexes (60).

Clonidine, alone or in combination with other agents, improved spasticity associated with SCI, brainstem infarction, MS, and traumatic brain injury (61–66), often in spite of an inadequate response to other medications. However, its use is limited because of adverse sympatholytic side effects, including bradycardia, and hypotension, sedation, dry mouth, and sexual dysfunction. Transdermal delivery of clonidine is also effective and may decrease side effects (65–70). The combination of intrathecal clonidine and baclofen effectively reduced complications from spasticity in a patient with SCI after ITB alone became ineffective (71).

In comparison, tizanidine, another α_2-adrenergic agonist, has the advantage of causing less hypotension. Initial studies showed that patients who did not adequately improve on baclofen, dantrolene, or diazepam found objective improvement with tizanidine (72,73). Several studies have compared the two agents. A double-blind trial of 12 patients with spasticity treated with baclofen or tizanidine effectively decreased passive stretch responses compared with placebo; however, tizanidine was more effective than baclofen (74). A double-blind comparative study of 21 patients with MS and spasticity similarly showed efficacy of both agents in reduction of spasms and clonus; however, tizanidine was more effective in improving strength, bladder function, and activities of daily living (75). Other studies have been less conclusive. Tizanidine and baclofen were minimally effective in improving spastic gait compared with placebo in one study (76). Four other studies that compared baclofen with tizanidine among 206 patients with spasticity due to MS, cerebrovascular lesions and other causes, reported improvement in many patients, but the differences between the two agents were not significant (44,77–79). Nonetheless, some patients favored tizanidine (77,79).

The subject of tizanidine efficacy was recently reviewed by Young (80). A randomized, placebo-controlled, double-blind clinical trial of spasticity due to MS showed that tizanidine was subjectively more effective than placebo in treating spasms and clonus. However, a reduction in muscle tone as measured objectively by the Ashworth Scale was not seen (81). Other studies of patients with MS (82) and SCI (83) showed an objective benefit in muscle tone by the Ashworth Scale but without functional improvement in activities of daily living. Despite a number of studies showing significant subjective or objective benefit with tizanidine, the efficacy of its use as a treatment for spasticity has still been challenged (84). An important side effect of tizanidine is sedation (85); others include hypotension, dizziness, asthenia, dry mouth, and, less frequently, hepatic damage and hallucinations (73,81–83,85,86). The conflicting efficacy data and the side effects render tizanidine a second-line medication. The starting dose is 2 mg at bedtime, gradually increasing to a maximum of 36 mg/day in three to four daily divided doses. In all patients, liver function tests should be monitored (83).

Dantrolene

Dantrolene inhibits calcium release from muscle sarcoplasmic reticulum, disrupting contraction and reducing tone in spastic muscles (4,27). The drug exerts its actions independent of neuronal circuitry. Early studies demonstrated improvement in some aspects of spasticity, although not without caveats. In 11 hemiplegic patients, dantrolene improved fine muscle control but did not significantly improve daily living functions (87). Among 23 patients with hemiplegia, clonus decreased and gait improved with treatment, although patients over age 50 responded less well (88). In a study involving 77 patients treated for up to 2 years with dantrolene, signs of muscle spasm, clonus, tone, and hyperreflexia improved, but functional improvement was less noticeable and side effects were common (89). In a double-blind placebo-controlled study, dantrolene was effective in about a third of patients suffering from spasticity of various causes, but all patients reported adverse effects, some of which led to discontinuation of treatment (90). Patients with spasticity after stroke showed improvement in activities of daily living with long-term administration (91).

It is argued that dantrolene is the drug of choice in spasticity of cerebral origin (20,66), especially childhood CP (92). However, a double-blind study of 20 children with CP showed that although dantrolene reduced muscle contraction force, little if any significant objective functional improvement was noted (93). Others found similar results and question the preference of dantrolene as the drug of choice in spasticity of cerebral origin (94). In those with spasticity of spinal origin, especially MS, dantrolene is generally not helpful (94,95).

The adverse effects of dantrolene include potentially severe liver toxicity, effusive pleural and pericardial disease, sedation, weakness, diarrhea, acne, and lymphoma. As with tizanidine, liver function studies should be performed before and during treatment with dantrolene, and the medication should be discontinued if abnormalities are found (6,18,27,55,95–102). In summary, dantrolene at doses of 25 to 400 mg/day is useful in spasticity of cerebral origin but should probably be reserved for patients that are unresponsive to other oral medications.

Cyproheptadine

Cyproheptadine, 5-hydroxytryptamine, is a serotonin antagonist that exerts its antispasticity actions via the medial reticulospinal tract (103), evidence for which comes from animal studies (104).

In one small study of patients with SCI or MS, oral cyproheptadine significantly decreased clonus and spasms (105). In a study of 25 patients with SCI, there was no essential difference between cyproheptadine-, clonidine-, and baclofen-related improvement of lower extremity tone by the Ashworth Scale or by other objective measures of spasticity (106). Studies have also demonstrated the ability of cyproheptadine to improve gait and function in addition to reducing spasms (107,108). When cyproheptadine was combined with clonidine and a locomotion training program, two patients, both wheelchair-bound by severe spasticity from SCI, became ambulatory with crutch assistance (109).

The adverse effects associated with cyproheptadine include sedation, dizziness, ataxia, tinnitus, blurred vision, hypotension, dry mouth, gastrointestinal upset, and fever. The anticholinergic effects occasionally lead to urinary retention in the occasional patient (110,111). In summary, cyproheptadine is most useful in patients with MS and SCI, usually in conjunction with other antispasticity medications. The usual dose is 4 to 20 mg/day.

Botulinum Toxin

The effects of overly active αMNs, whatever the cause, are treatable with injections of BTX into affected muscles. BTX impairs the release of acetylcholine at the neuromuscular junction (112). The use of BTX in the treatment of spasticity is briefly outlined below and described in Chapter 44. Both open-label and double-blind placebo-controlled studies demonstrated the clinical utility of BTX in the improvement of muscle tone and function in spasticity from many causes (113–124); however, bruising at the injection site, weakness, flulike symptoms, and antibody development can limit its use.

Ivermectin

Ivermectin is an antiparasitic agent with anti-onchocerciasis activity. Its mechanism of action in spasticity is due to the enhancement of GABA release and the postsynaptic binding of GABA at parasite receptors (125,126) and possible GABA agonist activity (127). In an open-label pilot study of 10 patients with SCI spasticity, the subcutaneous injection of an initial dose of 0.2 mg/kg, followed 2 weeks later by an injection of 0.4 mg/kg, and maintenance doses of 0.4 to 1.6 mg/kg thereafter for several weeks, resulted in improvement in objective measures of spasticity in all 10 patients and decreased Ashworth Scores in 7. There were no side effects; in fact, some described improvement in mood, sphincter function, and sleep (127).

Use of Intrathecal Baclofen in Treatment of Spasticity

ITB therapy delivered via a surgically implanted programmable pump has been one of the most significant advances in the treatment of spasticity. ITB was approved by the U.S. Food and Drug Administration for use in spasticity of spinal cord origin in 1992 and of cerebral origin in 1996. It is used most commonly in patients with MS, SCI, CP, and traumatic brain injury, but a beneficial response is seen in a variety of other disorders (Table 3).

As reviewed by McLean (128), 168 patients in nine independent studies demonstrated the effectiveness of ITB in spasticity. Spasticity was relieved in 164 (98%), abolished in 130 (98%), bladder function improved in 18 (78%), and overall function improved in 55 (71%). Other studies yielded similar results in spasticity from spinal trauma, MS, and cerebral and other diseases (129–132).

ITB has many advantages in the treatment of severe spasticity when compared with oral baclofen. Oral baclofen penetrates the blood–brain barrier poorly, and

TABLE 3. *Disorders responsive to intrathecal baclofen*

Spinal origin spasticity	Cerebral origin spasticity
Multiple sclerosis	Traumatic brain injury
Spinal cord injury	Cerebral palsy
Spinal cord infarction	Stroke
Transverse myelitis	Dystonia (usually secondary forms)
Spinal tumor	Multiple sclerosis
Compressive myelopathy	Anoxic brain injury
Primary lateral sclerosis	Postencephalitis
Stiff-person syndrome	Inherited metabolic and developmental disorders
Hereditary spastic paraparesis	Miscellaneous, e.g., arachnoid cyst, Laurence-Moon-Biedl syndrome, etc.

From ref. 128, with permission.

thus lumbar cerebrospinal fluid (CSF) concentrations are low, for example, 60 mg orally results in 24 μg/mL baclofen CSF concentration. By contrast, direct delivery of 60 μg baclofen resulted in a spinal CSF baclofen concentration of 1,240 μg/mL (27). Thus, to obtain an adequate therapeutic response, patients require such high and frequent oral doses of the medication that the dosing becomes inconvenient or the side effects become intolerable. Because the currently used device for delivery of ITB is a programmable pump, fine tuning of the clinical response is possible.

There are disadvantages to ITB. Its implementation requires surgery. Filling follow-ups may be frequent, and cosmetic issues arise. There is also a lack of awareness among the medical community about ITB, and patients may be referred for ITB inappropriately or not at all even when they might benefit from its use. When ITB is used with the appropriate precautions, it is safe, with most difficulties related to pump implantation, catheter blocking, accidental overdose, and problems generally associated with inexperience. The most common adverse effects from the medication include drowsiness, weakness, dizziness, and seizures in patients with a prior history of seizures or head trauma. Less frequently, there may be blurred vision, headaches, hypotension, numbness, constipation, slurred speech, lethargy, reversible coma, and respiratory depression with overdoses (27).

The following criteria should be fulfilled before proceeding to catheter placement to avoid unnecessary pump implantation (128):

1. Disabling spasticity of a moderate to severe degree or intolerable pain.
2. Spasticity that is not due to reversible neurologic disease or trauma and has been present and stable for more than 6 months.
3. Failure of oral therapy despite maximal doses or unacceptable adverse effects. Treatment with three to four oral agents is advised before consideration of ITB. In cerebral origin spasticity, particularly in CP,

oral treatment response is so poor that ITB may be indicated without a prolonged oral trial.

4. Patients or their caregivers that understand the risks and benefits involved with the intrathecal pump that can participate in the necessary follow-up care of refilling the medication reservoir.

At our institution, all patients that meet the above selection criteria for ITB therapy undergo a complete assessment and screening test. A detailed neurologic history and physical examination are performed with specific attention to grading of the spasticity and its associated features by the Ashworth and Spasm Scales (Table 2) (130). Eligible patients have a fall in their score by at least one point after the ITB screening test doses, given as follows: a lumbar puncture is performed, drawing out 2 to 3 mL of CSF in a sterile manner for later reintroduction; 150 μL of baclofen (75 μg at 500 μg/mL) is drawn into a tuberculin syringe and mixed with 500 μL of CSF in the same syringe via the lumbar catheter; the entire amount is injected back into the patient; and the baclofen dose is chased with 2 to 3 mL of CSF obtained earlier. The patient is monitored hourly for adverse effects with particular attention to drowsiness and respiratory difficulties and spasticity reassessed at 2, 4, and 6 hours for improvement of signs and symptoms related to spasticity. The object of the screening process is to assess spasticity relief and not to achieve functional goals. Some patients may encounter profound weakness with the test dose, but this effect may not occur after pump implantation when ITB is given by continuous infusion rather than as a bolus, and titration of dose and effect is possible.

Patients who respond to ITB without serious adverse affects may be referred to neurosurgical care for pump implantation. Positive responders usually have dramatic subjective improvement in spasticity as judged by the patient and experience significant objective improvement as judged by a unequivocal fall in post-trial Ashworth scores (133–135).

ITB therapy should generally be reserved for centers specializing in spasticity treatment because surgical implantation and postimplant maintenance complications are minimal when the appropriate expertise is available.

Selective Dorsal Rhizotomy

For patients who do not benefit satisfactorily from physical therapy or pharmacologic interventions, referral for therapeutic neurosurgical procedures may provide relief in selected patients. Many procedures are available and are reviewed elsewhere (136,137). The following discussion is limited to selective dorsal rhizotomy (SDR).

Physiologically, SDR most likely reduces spasticity by removing the stimulating afferent input of muscle stretch receptors on motor neurons. The term "selective" refers to attempted sectioning of only those inputs that are contributing to spastic signs and symptoms. However, SDR invariably leaves the patient with some undesirable sensory deficits. The history and details of the procedure are reviewed by Albright (138) and others (139). In the pediatric population, SDR can improve muscle tone, range of motion, and gait (140). In one study of 178 children with CP, early SDR at age 2 and 4 years decreased the need for some, although not all, orthopedic procedures to correct lower extremity deformities compared with SDR at ages 5 and 19 (141). A study of 16 children with spastic diplegia from CP had experienced statistically significant improvement in cognition 6 months after SDR compared with normal children and with those with CP who did not undergo SDR (142).

Although SDR certainly provides relief to many patients, we generally recommend referral for such neurosurgical procedures only after other management modalities have failed to effectively treat the signs and symptoms of spasticity. ITB is remarkably efficacious with few adverse effects in patients who are appropriately screened, and SDR is appropriate for patients who fail the screening test for ITB and are refractory to other therapies. However, in patients with CP there is still some controversy. In 1992, Albright (138) preferred SDR for mild spasticity in children with CP because the treatment was definitive. For children with more moderate spasticity that used the increase in tone to assist in ambulation, ITB was recommended because the dose could be optimized for each patient. For more severely affected children, there was no clear recommendation, weighing permanent benefit of SDR on lower extremity spasticity against the upper and lower extremity benefits of ITB on a case by case basis. Subsequent studies in children with cerebral spasticity treated by SDR or with ITB have not established either therapy as clearly superior to the other (143–145).

REFERENCES

1. Landau WM. Spasticity: what is it? What is it not? In: Feldman RG, Young RR, Koella WP, eds. *Spasticity: disordered motor control.* Chicago: Mosby-Year Book, 1980:17–24.
2. Young RR. Spasticity: a review. *Neurology* 1994;44[Suppl 9]:S12–S20.
3. Brown P. Pathophysiology of spasticity. *J Neurol Neurosurg Psychiatry* 1994;57:773–777.
4. Davidoff RA. Antispasticity drugs: mechanisms of action. *Ann Neurol* 1985;17:107–116.
5. Adams RD, Victor M, Ropper AH. *Principles of neurology.* New York: McGraw-Hill, 1997.
6. Young RR, Delwaide PJ. Drug therapy: spasticity. *N Engl J Med* 1981; 304:28–33, 96–99.
7. Ghez C. Muscles: effectors of the motor systems. In: Kandel ER, Schwartz JH, Jessell TM, eds. *Principles of neural science.* New York: Elsevier, 1991:548–563.
8. Gordon J, Ghez C. Muscle receptors and spinal reflexes: the stretch reflex. In: Kandel ER, Schwartz JH, Jessell TM, eds. *Principles of neural science.* New York: Elsevier, 1991:564–580.
9. Davidoff RA. Skeletal muscle tone and the misunderstood stretch reflex. *Neurology* 1992;42:951–963.
10. Heckman CJ. Alterations in synaptic input to motor neurons during partial spinal cord injury. *Med Sci Sports Exerc* 1994;26:1480–1490.
11. Hagbarth K-E, Wallin G, Löfstedt L. Muscle spindle responses to stretch in normal and spastic subjects. *Scand J Rehab Med* 1973;5: 156–159.
12. Hagbarth K-E, Wallin G, Löfstedt L, Aquilonius S-M. Muscle spindle

activity in alternating tremor of parkinsonism and in clonus. *J Neurol Neurosurg Psychiatry* 1975;38:636–641.

13. Burke D. A reassessment of the muscle spindle contribution to muscle tone in normal and spastic man. In: Feldman RG, Young RR, Koella WP, eds. *Spasticity: disordered motor control.* Chicago: Mosby-Year Book, 1980;261–278.

14. Burke D. Critical examination of the case for or against fusimotor involvement in disorders of muscle tone. *Adv Neurol* 1983;39:133–150.

15. Gordon J. Spinal mechanisms of motor coordination. In: Kandel ER, Schwartz JH, Jessell TM, eds. *Principles of neural science.* New York: Elsevier, 1991:581–595.

16. Young RR. Role of tizanidine in the treatment of spasticity. *Neurology* 1994;44[Suppl 9]:S4–S5.

17. Lindau WM. Spasticity: the fable of a neurological demon and the emperor's new therapy. *Arch Neurol* 1974;31:217–219.

18. DeLisa JA, Little J. Managing spasticity. *Am Fam Physician* 1982;26:117–122.

19. Ditunno JF, Formal CS. Chronic spinal cord injury. *N Engl J Med* 1994;330:550–556.

20. Katz RT. Management of spasticity. *Am J Phys Med Rehabil* 1988;67:108–116.

21. Merritt JL. Management of spasticity in spinal cord injury. *Mayo Clin Proc* 1981;56:614–622.

22. Ashworth B. Preliminary trial of carisoprodol in multiple sclerosis. *Practitioner* 1964;192:540–542.

23. Bohannon RW, Smith MB. Interrater reliability of a modified Ashworth scale of muscle spasticity. *Phys Ther* 1987;67:206–207.

24. Brar SP, Smith MB, Nelson LM, Franklin GM, Cobble ND. Evaluation of treatment protocols on minimal to moderate spasticity in multiple sclerosis. *Arch Phys Med Rehabil* 1991;72:186–189.

25. Perry J. Rehabilitation of spasticity. In: Feldman RG, Young RR, Koella WP, eds. *Spasticity: disordered motor control.* Chicago: Mosby-Year Book, 1980:87–100.

26. Giesser B. Multiple sclerosis. Current concepts in management. *Drugs* 1985;29:88–95.

27. Blanck TJ, Sadiq SA. General anesthetics and anesthesia-associated drugs. In: Rowland LP, Klein DF, eds. *Current neurologic drugs.* Philadelphia: Current Medicine, 1996:239–308.

28. Smith CR, LaRocca NG, Giesser BS, Scheinberg LC. High-dose oral baclofen: experience in patients with multiple sclerosis. *Neurology* 1991;41:1829–1831.

29. Feldman RG, Kelly-Hayes M, Conomy JP, Foley JM. Baclofen for spasticity in multiple sclerosis. Double-blind crossover and three-year study. *Neurology* 1978;28:1094–1098.

30. Sawa GM, Paty DW. The use of baclofen in treatment of spasticity in multiple sclerosis. *Can J Neurol Sci* 1979;6:351–354.

31. Miller F, Korsvik H. Baclofen in the treatment of stiff-man syndrome. *Ann Neurol* 1981;9:511–512.

32. Milla PJ, Jackson AD. A controlled trial of baclofen in children with cerebral palsy. *J Int Med Res* 1977;5:398–404.

33. Hinderer SR. The supraspinal anxiolytic effect of baclofen for spasticity reduction. *Am J Phys Med Rehabil* 1990;69:254–258.

34. Hinderer SR, Lehmann JF, Price R, White O, deLateur BJ, Deitz J. Spasticity in spinal cord injured persons: quantitative effects of baclofen and placebo treatments. *Am J Phys Med Rehabil* 1990;69:311–317.

35. Smith MB, Brar SP, Nelson LM, Franklin GM, Cobble ND. Baclofen effect on quadriceps strength in multiple sclerosis. *Arch Phys Med Rehabil* 1992;73:237–240.

36. Asien ML, Dietz M, McDowell F, Kutt H. Baclofen toxicity in a patient with subclinical renal insufficiency. *Arch Phys Med Rehabil* 1994;75:109–111.

37. Ghose K, Holmes KM, Matthewson K. Complications of baclofen overdose. *Postgrad Med J* 1980;56:865–867.

38. Lees AJ, Clarke CR, Harrison MJ. Hallucinations after withdrawal of baclofen. *Lancet* 1977;1:858.

39. Stien R. Hallucinations after sudden withdrawal of baclofen. *Lancet* 1977;2:44–45.

40. Arnold ES, Rudd SM, Kirshner H. Manic psychosis following rapid withdrawal from baclofen. *Am J Psychiatry* 1980;137:1466–1467.

41. Terrence CF, Fromm GH. Complications of baclofen withdrawal. *Arch Neurol* 1981;38:588–589.

42. Kirubakaran V, Mayfield D, Regachary S. Dyskinesia and psychosis in a patient following baclofen withdrawal. *Am J Psychiatry* 1984;141:692–693.

43. Garabedian-Ruffalo SM, Ruffalo RL. Adverse effects secondary to baclofen withdrawal. *Drug Intell Clin Pharm* 1985;19:304–306.

44. Stien R, Nordal HJ, Oftedal SI, Sletteb M. The treatment of spasticity in multiple sclerosis: a double-blind clinical trial of a new anti-spastic drug tizanidine compared with baclofen. *Acta Neurol Scand* 1987;75:190–194.

45. Mandac BR, Hurvitz EA, Nelson VS. Hyperthermia associated with baclofen withdrawal and increased spasticity. *Arch Phys Med Rehabil* 1993;74:96–97.

46. Lataste X, Emre M, Davis C, Groves L. Comparative profile of tizanidine in the management of spasticity. *Neurology* 1994;44[Suppl 9]:S53–S59.

47. Kuhn WF, Light PJ, Kuhn SC. Stiff-man syndrome: case report. *Acad Emerg Med* 1995;2:735–738.

48. Lorish TR, Thorsteinsson G, Howard FM Jr. Stiff-man syndrome updated. *Mayo Clin Proc* 1989;64:629–636.

49. Dahlin M, Knutsson E, Nergardh A. Treatment of spasticity in children with low dose benzodiazepine. *J Neurol Sci* 1993;117:54–60.

50. Nogen AG. Medical treatment of spasticity in children with cerebral palsy. *Childs Brain* 1976;2:304–308.

51. Rall TW. Hypnotics and sedatives; ethanol. In: Gilman AG, Rall TW, Nies AS, Taylor P, eds. *Goodman and Gilman's the pharmacological basis of therapeutics.* New York: McGraw-Hill, 1993:345–382.

52. Waldman HJ. Centrally acting skeletal muscle relaxants and associated drugs. *J Pain Symptom Manage* 1994;9:434–441.

53. Frisbie JH, Aguilera EJ. Diazepam and body weight in myelopathy patients. *J Spinal Cord Med* 1995;18:200–202.

54. Bes A, Eyssette M, Pierrot-Deseilligny E, Rohmer F, Warter JM. A multi-centre, double-blind trial of tizanidine, a new antispastic agent, in spasticity associated with hemiplegia. *Curr Med Res Opin* 1988;10:709–718.

55. Pinder RM, Brogden RN, Speight TM, Avery GS. Dantrolene sodium: a review of its pharmacological properties and therapeutic efficacy in spasticity. *Drugs* 1977;13:3–23.

56. Roussan M, Terrence C, Fromm G. Baclofen versus diazepam for the treatment of spasticity and long-term follow-up of baclofen therapy. *Pharmatherapeutica* 1985;4:278–284.

57. Cendrowski W, Sobczyk W. Clonazepam, baclofen and placebo in the treatment of spasticity. *Eur Neurol* 1977;16:257–262.

58. Coward DM. Tizanidine: neuropharmacology and mechanism of action. *Neurology* 1994;44[Suppl 9]:S6–S11.

59. Delwaide PJ, Pennisi G. Tizanidine and electrophysiologic analysis of spinal control mechanisms in humans with spasticity. *Neurology* 1994;44[Suppl 9]:S21–S28.

60. Tremblay LE, Bedard PJ. Effect of clonidine on motor neuron excitability in spinalized rats. *Neuropharmacology* 1986;25:41–46.

61. Nance PW, Shears AH, Nance DM. Reflex changes induced by clonidine in spinal cord injury patients. *Paraplegia* 1989;27:296–301.

62. Stewart JE, Barbeau H, Gauthier S. Modulation of locomotor patterns and spasticity with clonidine in spinal cord injured patients. *Can J Neurol Sci* 1991;18:321–332.

63. Maynard FM. Early experience with clonidine in spinal spasticity. *Paraplegia* 1986;24:175–182.

64. Sandford PR, Spengler SE, Sawasky KB. Clonidine in the treatment of brainstem spasticity. Case report. *Am J Phys Med Rehabil* 1992;71:301–303.

65. Khan OA, Olek MJ. Clonidine in the treatment of spasticity in patients with multiple sclerosis. *J Neurol* 1995;242:712–715.

66. Dall JT, Harmon RL, Quinn CM. Use of clonidine for treatment of spasticity arising from various forms of brain injury: a case series. *Brain Inj* 1996;10:453–458.

67. Hoffman BB, Lefkowitz RJ. Catecholamines and sympathomimetic drugs. In: Gilman AG, Rall TW, Nies AS, Taylor P, eds. *Goodman and Gilman's the pharmacological basis of therapeutics.* New York: McGraw-Hill, 1993:187–220.

68. Gerber JG, Nies AS. Antihypertensive agents and the drug therapy of hypotension. In: Gilman AG, Rall TW, Nies AS, Taylor P, eds. *Goodman and Gilman's the pharmacological basis of therapeutics.* New York: McGraw-Hill, 1993:784–813.

69. Yablon SA. Sipski ML. Effect of transdermal clonidine on spinal spasticity. A case series. *Am J Phys Med Rehabil* 1993;72:154–157.

70. Weingarden SI, Belen JG. Clonidine transdermal system for treatment of spasticity in spinal cord injury. *Arch Phys Med Rehabil* 1992;73:876–877.

71. Middleton JW, Siddall PJ, Walker S, Molloy AR, Rutkowski SB. Intrathecal clonidine and baclofen in the management of spasticity and neuropathic pain following spinal cord injury: a case study. *Arch Phys Med Rehabil* 1996;77:824–826.

72. Sie OG, Lakke JP. The spasmolytic properties of 5-chloro-4-(2-imidazolin-2-yl-amino)-2, 1,3-benzothiadiazole hydrochloride (DS 103-282): a pilot study. *Clin Neurol Neurosurg* 1980;82:273–279.

73. Lapierre Y, Bouchard S, Tansey C, Gendron D, Barkas WJ, Francis GS. Treatment of spasticity with tizanidine in multiple sclerosis. *Can J Neurol Sci* 1987;14:513–517.

74. Hassan N, McLellan DL. Double-blind comparison of single doses of DS103-282, baclofen and placebo for suppression of spasticity. *J Neurol Neurosurg Psychiatry* 1980;43:1132–1136.

75. Smolenski C, Muff S, Smolenski-Kautz S. A double-blind comparative trial of new muscle relaxant, tizanidine (DS 103-282), and baclofen in the treatment of chronic spasticity in multiple sclerosis. *Curr Med Res Opin* 1981;7:374–383.

76. Corston RN, Johnson F, Godwin-Austen RB. The assessment of drug treatment of spastic gait. *J Neurol Neurosurg Psychiatry* 1981;44:1035–1039.

77. Newman PM, Nogues M, Newman PK, Weightman D, Hudgson P. Tizanidine in the treatment of spasticity. *Eur J Clin Pharmacol* 1982;23:31–35.

78. Eyssette M, Rohmer F, Serratrice G, Warter JM, Boisson D. Multi-centre, double-blind trial of a novel antispastic agent, tizanidine, in spasticity associated with multiple sclerosis. *Curr Med Res Opin* 1988;10:699–708.

79. Medici M, Pebet M, Ciblis D. A double-blind, long-term study of tizanidine ("Sirdalud") in spasticity due to cerebrovascular lesions. *Curr Med Res Opin* 1989;11:398–407.

80. Young RR (supplement editor). Role of tizanidine in the treatment of spasticity. *Neurology* 1994;44[Suppl 9]:S1–S80.

81. Smith C, Birnbaum G, Carter JL, Greenstein J, Lublin FD, the US Tizanidine Study Group. Tizanidine treatment of spasticity caused by multiple sclerosis: results of a double-blind, placebo-controlled trial. *Neurology* 1994;44[Suppl 9]:S34–S43.

82. The United Kingdom Tizanidine Trial Group. A double-blind, placebo-controlled trial of tizanidine in the treatment of spasticity caused by multiple sclerosis. *Neurology* 1994;44[Suppl 9]:S70–S78.

83. Nance PW, Bugaresti J, Schellenberger K, Sheremata W, Martinez-Arizala A, the North American Tizanidine Study Group. Efficacy and safety of tizanidine in the treatment of spasticity in patients with spinal cord injury. *Neurology* 1994;44[Suppl 9]:S44–S52.

84. Lindau WM, Young RR. Tizanidine and spasticity. *Neurology* 1995;45:2295–2296.

85. Miettinen TJ, Kanto JH, Salonen MA, Scheinin M. The sedative and sympatholytic effects of oral tizanidine in helathy volunteers. *Anesth Analg* 1996;82:817–820.

86. Wallace JD. Summary of combined clinical analysis of controlled clinical trials with tizanidine. *Neurology* 1994;44[Suppl 9]:S60–S69.

87. Jonsson B, Ladd H, Afzelius-Frisk I, Lindberg-Broman AM. The effect of dantrium on spasticity of hemiplegic patients. *Acta Neurol Scand* 1975;51:385–392.

88. Steinberg FU, Ferguson KL. Effect of dantrolene sodium on spasticity associated with hemiplegia. *J Am Geriatr Soc* 1975;23:70–73.

89. Joynt RL. Dantrolene sodium: long-term effects in patients with muscle spasticity. *Arch Phys Med Rehabil* 1976;57:212–217.

90. Luisto M, Moller K, Nuutila A, Palo J. Dantrolene sodium in chronic spasticity of varying etiology. A double-blind study. *Acta Neurol Scand* 1982;65:355–362.

91. Ketel WB, Kolb ME. Long-term treatment with dantrolene sodium of stroke patients with spasticity limiting the return of function. *Curr Med Res Opin* 1984;9:161–169.

92. Molnar GE. Long-term treatment of spasticity in children with cerebral palsy. *Int Disabil Stud* 1987;9:170–172.

93. Joynt RL, Leonard JA Jr. Dantrolene sodium suspension in treatment of spastic cerebral palsy. *Dev Med Child Neurol* 1980;22:755–767.

94. Whyte J, Robinson KM. Pharmacologic management. In: Glenn MB, Whyte J, eds. *The practical management of spasticity in children and adults*. Philadelphia: Lea & Febiger, 1990:201–226.

95. Ward A, Chaffman MO, Sorkin EM. Dantrolene, a review of its pharmacodynamic and pharmacokinetic properties and therapeutic use in malignant hyperthermia, the neuroleptic malignant syndrome and an update of its use in muscle spasticity. *Drugs* 1986;32:130–168.

96. Mahoney JM, Bachtel MD. Pleural effusion associated with chronic dantrolene administration. *Ann Pharmacother* 1994;28:587–589.

97. Miller DH, Haas LF. Pneumonitis, pleural effusion and pericarditis following treatment with dantrolene. *J Neurol Neurosurg Psychiatry* 1984;47:553–554.

98. Petusevsky ML, Faling LJ, Rocklin RE, et al. Pleuropericardial reaction to treatment with dantrolene. *JAMA* 1979;242:2772–2774.

99. Knutsson E, Martensson A. Action of dantrolene sodium in spasticity with low dependence on fusimotor drive. *J Neurol Sci* 1976;29:195–212.

100. Meyler WJ, Bakker H, Kok JJ, Agoston S, Wesseling H. The effect of dantrolene sodium in relation to blood levels in spastic patients after prolonged administration. *J Neurol Neurosurg Psychiatry* 1981;44:334–339.

101. Pembroke AC, Saxena SR, Kataria M, Zilkha KD. Acne induced by dantrolene. *Br J Dermatol* 1981;104:465–468.

102. Wan HH, Tucker JS. Dantrolene and lymphocytic lymphoma. *Postgrad Med J* 1980;56:261–262.

103. Garrison JC. Histamine, bradykinin, 5-hydroxytryptamine, and their antagonists. In: Gilman AG, Rall TW, Nies AS, Taylor P, eds. *Goodman and Gilman's the pharmacological basis of therapeutics*. New York: McGraw-Hill, 1993:575–599.

104. Tremblay LE, Bedard PJ. Action of 5-hydroxytryptamine, substance P, thyrotropin releasing hormone and clonidine on spinal neuron excitability. *J Spinal Cord Med* 1995;18:42–46.

105. Barbeau H, Richards CL, Bedard PJ. Action of cyproheptadine in spastic parapertic patients. *J Neurol Neurosurg Psychiatry* 1982;45:923–926.

106. Nance PW. A comparison of clonidine, cyproheptadine and baclofen in spastic spinal cord injured patients. *J Am Paraplegia Soc* 1994;17:150–156.

107. Wainberg M, Barbeau H, Gauthier S. Quantitative assessment of the effect of cyproheptadine on spastic paretic gait: a preliminary study. *J Neurol* 1986;233:311–314.

108. Wainberg M, Barbeau H, Gauthier S. The effects of cyproheptadine on locomotion and on spasticity in patients with spinal cord injuries. *J Neurol Neurosurg Psychiatry* 1990;53:754–763.

109. Fung J, Stewart JE, Barbeau H. The combined effects of clonidine and cyproheptadine with interactive training on the modulation of locomotion in spinal cord injured patients. *J Neurol Sci* 1990;100:85–93.

110. Houang M, Leroy B, Forin V, Sinnassamy P, Bensman A. Acute urine retention: a rare mode of revelation of cervico-dorsal syringomyelia caused by cyproheptadine. *Arch Pediatr* 1994;1:260–263.

111. Silberstein SD. Agents for migraine and other headaches. In: Rowland LP, Klein DF, eds. *Current neurologic drugs*. Philadelphia: Current Medicine, 1996:20–73.

112. Ford B, Fahn S. Agents for treating Parkinson disease and other movement disorders. In: Rowland LP, Klein DF, eds. *Current neurologic drugs*. Philadelphia: Current Medicine, 1996:309–327.

113. Borg-Stein J, Pine ZM, Miller JR, Brin MF. Botulinum toxin for the treatment of spasticity in multiple sclerosis. New observations. *Am J Phys Med Rehabil* 1993;72:364–368.

114. Yablon SA Agana BT, Ivanhoe CB, Boake C. Botulinum toxin in severe upper extremity spasticity among patients with traumatic brain injury: an open-labeled trial. *Neurology* 1996;47:939–944.

115. Bhakta BB, Cozens JA, Bamford JM, Chamberlain MA. Use of botulinum toxin in stroke patients with severe upper limb spasticity. *J Neurol Neurosurg Psychiatry* 1996;61:30–35.

116. Simpson DM, Alexander DN, O'Brien CF, et al. Botulinum toxin type A in the treatment of upper extremity spasticity: a randomized, double blind, placebo-controlled trial. *Neurology* 1996;46:1306–1310.

117. Hesse S, Lucke D, Malezic M, et al. Botulinum toxin for lower limb extensor spasticity in chronic hemiparetic patients. *J Neurol Neurosurg Psychiatry* 1994;57:1321–1324.

118. Grazko MA, Polo KB, Jabbari B. Botulinum toxin A for spasticity, muscle spasms, and rigidity. *Neurology* 1995;45:712–717.

119. Pierson SH, Katz DI, Tarsy D. Botulinum toxin A in the treatment of spasticity: functional implications and patient selection. *Arch Phys Med Rehabil* 1996;77:717–721.

120. Burbaud P, Wiart L, Dubos JL, et al. A randomised, double blind, placebo controlled trial of botulinum toxin in the treatment of spastic foot in hemiparetic patients. *J Neurol Neurosurg Psychiatry* 1996;61:265–269.

121. Koman LA, Mooney JF, Smith BP, Goodman A, Mulvaney T. Man-

agement of spasticity in cerebral palsy with botulinum-A toxin: report of a preliminary, randomized, double-blind trial. *J Pediatr Orthop* 1994;14:299–303.

122. Gooch JL, Sandell TV. Botulinum toxin for spasticity and athetosis in children with cerebral palsy. *Arch Phys Med Rehabil* 1996;77:508–511.

123. Pullman SL, Greene P, Fahn S, Pedersen SF. Approach to the treatment of limb disorders with botulinum toxin A. Experience with 187 patients. *Arch Neurol* 1996;53:617–624.

124. Hesse S, Jahnke MT, Luecke D, Mauritz KH. Short-term electrical stimulation enhances the effectiveness of Botulinum toxin in the treatment of lower limb spasticity in hemiparetic patients. *Neurosci Lett* 1995;201:37–40.

125. Webster LT Jr. Drugs used in the chemotherapy of helminthiasis. In: Gilman AG, Rall TW, Nies AS, Taylor P, eds. *Goodman and Gilman's the pharmacological basis of therapeutics*. New York: McGraw-Hill, 1993:959–977.

126. Kanwar RS, Varshneya C. Neuropharmacological effects of ivermectin in mice. *Ind J Physiol Pharmacol* 1995;39:421–422.

127. Costa JL, Diazgranados JA. Ivermectin for spasticity in spinal-cord injury. *Lancet* 1994;343:739.

128. McLean BN. Intrathecal baclofen in severe spasticity. *Br J Hosp Med* 1993;49:262–267.

129. Penn RD. Intrathecal baclofen for spasticity of spinal origin: seven years of experience. *J Neurosurg* 1992;77:236–240.

130. Coffey RJ, Cahill D, Steers W, et al. Intrathecal baclofen for intractable spasticity of spinal origin: results of a long-term multicenter study. *J Neurosurg* 1993;78:226–232.

131. Abel NA, Smith RA. Intrathecal baclofen for treatment of intractable spinal spasticity. *Arch Phys Med Rehabil* 1994;75:54–58.

132. Albright AL, Barron WB, Fasick MP, Polinko P, Janosky J. Continuous intrathecal baclofen infusion for spasticity of cerebral origin. *JAMA* 1993;270:2475–2477.

133. Akman MN, Loubser PG, Donovan WH, O'Neill ME, Rossi CD. Intrathecal baclofen: does tolerance occur? *Paraplegia* 1993;31:516–520.

134. Gianino J. Intrathecal baclofen for spinal spasticity: implications for nursing practice. *J Neurosci Nurs* 1993;25:254–264.

135. Albright AL, Cervi A, Singletary J. Intrathecal baclofen for spasticity in cerebral palsy. *JAMA* 1991;265:1418–1422.

136. Barolat G. Surgical management of spasticity and spasms in spinal cord injury: an overview. *J Am Paraplegia Soc* 1988;11:9–13.

137. Kasdon DL, Abramovitz JN. Neurosurgical approaches. In: Glenn MB, Whyte J, eds. *The practical management of spasticity in children and adults*. Philadelphia: Lea & Febiger, 1990:259–267.

138. Albright AL. Neurosurgical treatment of spasticity: selective posterior rhizotomy and intrathecal baclofen. *Stereotact Funct Neurosurg* 1992;58:3–13.

139. McLaughlin JF, Bjornson KF, Astley SJ, et al. The role of selective dorsal rhizotomy in cerebral palsy: critical evaluation of a prospective clinical series. *Dev Med Child Neurol* 1994;36:755–769.

140. Thomas SS, Aiona MD, Pierce R, Piatt JH. Gait changes in children with spastic diplegia after selective dorsal rhizotomy. *J Pediatr Orthop* 1996;16:747–752.

141. Chicoine MR, Park TS, Kaufman BA. Selective dorsal rhizotomy and rates of orthopedic surgery in children with spastic cerebral palsy. *J Neurosurg* 1997;86:34–39.

142. Craft S, Park TS, White DA, Schatz J, Noetzel M, Arnold S. Changes in cognitive performance in children with spastic diplegic cerebral palsy following selective dorsal rhizotomy. *Pediatr Neurosurg* 1995;23:68–75.

143. Albright AL, Barry MJ, Fasick MP, Janosky J. Effects of continuous intrathecal baclofen infusion and selective posterior rhizotomy on upper extremity spasticity. *Pediatr Neurosurg* 1995;23:82–85.

144. Steinbok P, Daneshvar H, Evans D, Kestle JR. Cost analysis of continuous intrathecal baclofen versus selective functional posterior rhizotomy in the treatment of spastic quadriplegia associated with cerebral palsy. *Pediatr Neurosurg* 1995;22:255–264.

145. Nance P, Schryvers O, Schmidt B, Dubo H, Loveridge B, Fewer D. Intrathecal baclofen therapy for adults with spinal spasticity: therapeutic efficacy and effect on hospital admissions. *Can J Neurol Sci* 1995;22:22–29.

Motor Disorders,
edited by David S. Younger.
Lippincott Williams & Wilkins, Philadelphia © 1999.

CHAPTER 44

Botulinum Toxin for Motor Disorders

Mitchell F. Brin

Local injection of botulinum toxin type A (BTX-A) is effective and often primary therapy for blepharospasm, cervical dystonia, spasmodic dysphonia, jaw and limb dystonia with or without tremor, and spasticity (Table 1) (1–9).

BACKGROUND

The bacterium *Clostridium botulinum* produces seven serologically distinct toxins, designated A, B, C, D, E, F, and G (10). Partial amino acid sequences reveal regions of structural homology (11) for most serotypes, and although antigenically distinct, they possess similar molecular weights and have a common subunit structure (12). The toxins are synthesized as single polypeptide chains of approximate molecular weight of 150 kDa (13). In this form, the toxin molecules have relatively little potency as neuromuscular blocking agents. The single-chain toxin is cleaved by bacterial enzymes or by trypsin to yield a dichain molecule. In animals, an endogenous protease cleaves the protein. The result is a heavy chain of 100 kDa, linked by a disulfide bond to a light chain with a molecular weight of 50 kDa, and associated with a molecule of zinc (Zn^{2+}) (14,15). The cleaved form of the molecule paralyzes neuromuscular transmission. Reduction of the disulfide bonds that link the two chains causes complete loss of toxicity before internalization.

When botulinum neurotoxin is isolated from bacterial cultures, it is normally associated with nontoxic macromolecules such as proteins or nucleic acids (16). The protein hemagglutinin associates noncovalently with type A toxin. When administered parenterally for therapeutic use, the nontoxic proteins do not enhance the activity of the neurotoxin and may even interfere slightly. When administered orally, however, the nontoxic proteins enhance its activity, possibly by protecting the neurotoxin

from proteolytic enzymes in the gut (16). BTX exerts its effect at the neuromuscular junction by inhibiting the release of acetylcholine (ACh), causing paralysis. The three steps involved in toxin-mediated paralysis include binding, internalization, and inhibition of ACh neurotransmitter release. The toxin must enter the nerve ending to exert its poisoning effect (17). Both pharmacologic (12,13) and morphologic (18,19) data suggest that internalization occurs via the receptor-mediated endocytotic/lysosomal vesicle pathway. The binding of toxin to nerves is selective and saturable. In vitro studies with synaptosomal preparations suggest an interaction of both high and low affinity sites and some specificity for toxin type (18,19). The C-terminal half of the heavy chain determines cholinergic specificity and binding, whereas the light chain is the intracellular toxic moiety (20,21). The internalization process is independent of Ca^{2+} concentration and partially dependent on nerve stimulation (22,23) but entirely dependent on energy (20,21). In experimental systems, internalization is hastened in an acid medium and retarded in a cooled system (21).

After internalization, a segment of the toxin penetrates the endosomal membrane into the cytosol by an unknown mechanism. The toxin then causes lesions in the pathway of secretion of ACh (20,24,25). The N-terminal half of the heavy chain is responsible for the translocation of the inhibitory segment across the membrane. BTX does not affect the synthesis or storage of ACh (20,21,26). Nerve endings poisoned by BTX can still induce release of normal quanta of acetylcholine, although nonphysiologic techniques must be used.

BTX is an enzyme acting as a Zn^{2+} endopeptidase (21) that modifies the release of synaptosomes of the microtubular subsystem. The light chains of BTX-A, -B, and -E, in addition to tetanus toxin, are each associated with one molecule of Zn^{2+} (14). The binding is reversible, and histidines are involved in zinc coordination, as is characteristic of zinc endopeptidases. BTX-E has proteolytic activity that is expressed when the approximately 150-

M. F. Brin: Department of Neurology, Movement Disorders Program, Mount Sinai Medical Center, New York, New York 10029.

TABLE 1. *Botulinum toxin: conditions characterized by excessive muscle contraction: regions with proven efficacy*

Dystonic spasms
  Blepharospasm
  Cervical dystonia
  Laryngeal dystonia
  Oromandibular dystonia
  Occupational cramps
  Limb dystonia
  Dystonic tremor
Nondystonic excessive muscle contraction
  Back spasm
  Bladder: detrusor-sphincter dyssynergia
  Bruxism
  Cosmetic (hyperfunctional facial lines): "brow furrows," "frown lines," "crows' feet," platysma lines
  Gastrointestinal: achalasia, anismus (constipation), cricopharyngeal spasm, lower esophageal sphincter spasms, rectal spasms, rectal fissures
  Eyelid spasms: hemifacial spasm and synkinesis, benign eyelid fasciculation
  Headache (muscle contraction, migraine)
  Hyperhidrosis
  Myokymia
  Oscillopsia
  Presurgical stabilization
  Spasticity: stroke, cerebral palsy, head injury, paraplegia, multiple sclerosis, neurodegenerative disease
  Sports medicine injuries
  Stuttering
  Tics
  Temporomandibular joint associated muscle spasm
  Tremor: Parkinson disease, essential tremor, hereditary chin tremor
  Vaginismus

Modified from Brin MF. Treatment of dystonia. In: Jankovic J, Tolosa E, eds. *Parkinson's disease and movement disorders.* New York: Williams & Wilkins, 1998.

kDa neurotoxic protein is nicked into a dichain neurotoxin. Proteolytic activity is isolated to the N-terminal 50-kDa light chain. Intracellular proteins that are targets of the enzymatic effect of the clostridial neurotoxins are thought to be responsible for effective docking of a neurotransmitter vesicle onto the inner surface of the plasma membrane (25,27). Vesicular docking seems to be involved in the formation of a complex that includes proteins from the cytoplasm including gamma-SNAP, alpha-SNAP, NSF, and SNAP-25 and those that are inserted permanently in the vesicle such as VAMP/synaptobrevin and the target plasma membrane protein syntaxin. These proteins are responsible for the ATP-dependent translocation of an intact neurotransmitter-containing vesicle from the cytosol to the plasma membrane (15). Cleavage of any of these proteins interferes with the proper binding and fusion of a vesicle to the plasma membrane and therefore impedes exocytosis-mediated neurotransmitter release. BTX-D and BTX-F cleave VAMP/synaptobrevin but at a different site than BTX-B (28). BTX-A and BTX-E cleave another translocation protein, SNAP-25, and BTX-C acts

by cleaving syntaxin and SNAP-25 (29,30). It has therefore become clear that the primary action of BTX is the disruption of fusion proteins responsible for neurotransmitter vesicle release from the nerve terminal. The preparations of botulinum toxin, namely BOTOX, Dysport, and NeuroBloc, are each distinct (31,32) and each measured in units of biologic activity. Treating physicians should know which product they are using, especially in settings where multiple products and/or serotypes are available.

CLINICAL USE OF BOTULINUM TOXIN

The local intramuscular injection of minute doses of BTX-A was first used in the treatment of strabismus (2). The goal was to block cholinergic neuromuscular junctions and rebalance neural input to the extraocular rectus muscles; this realigned muscle forces, straightened the eyes, and enhanced convergence (33). Other similar drugs, including alpha-bungarotoxin, were considered but had limitations, including lack of selectivity, short duration of action, and substantial antigenicity. BTX had the advantage of being a potent neuromuscular blocking agent with few undesirable side effects. Alan Scott, who first developed the toxin, applied it to patients with blepharospasm (34,35). Subsequently, we and others began to use the toxin for additional disorders characterized by inappropriate muscle contraction. These are considered below.

Dystonia

The underlying pathophysiology of dystonia is unknown. It is a neurologic syndrome dominated by involuntary muscle contractions that may be sustained (tonic), spasmodic (rapid or clonic), patterned, or repetitive. The muscle movements frequently cause abnormal postures, including twisting (e.g., torticollis), flexing or extending (e.g., anterocollis, retrocollis, writer's cramp), and adducting or abducting (e.g., blepharospasm, spasmodic dysphonia) movements. It can be idiopathic or symptomatic of another disorder. It can involve any voluntary muscle. Because the movements and resulting postures are often unusual and the condition is rare, it is one of the most frequently misdiagnosed neurologic conditions (36). We estimate at least 150,000 cases of idiopathic dystonia in this country (37,38). About 1 in 3,000 people is diagnosed with dystonia, but the true prevalence is probably much higher. Cervical dystonia is likely the most commonly diagnosed form of focal dystonia, but graphospasm (writer's cramp) may be the most prevalent form. Despite advances in understanding the genetics of many forms of dystonia, gene-directed therapy is not yet available. Genetic studies support the assertion of pathology in the basal ganglia and its connections (39–41), but neurochemical (42–44), biochemical (45), anatomic (46–48), and neuroimaging (49–52) studies have not revealed a common neurochemical substrate. Although presumed for many years to be primarily a motor disorder, the motor signs of dystonia may be in part a reflection of aberrant sensory input (53–55). Specific pharmacotherapy is also not yet available for most cases of dystonia, and the mainstay of therapy is still supportive and symptomatic. Local injection of BTX is now primary therapy for many patients with dystonia and is secondary therapy for those that have failed other modalities.

The results of BTX-A therapy has been summarized elsewhere (6–8). Local injection of BTX-A benefits 90% of patients with blepharospasm, hemifacial spasm, and laryngeal dystonia and more than 75% of those with cervical dystonia and jaw-closing oromandibular dystonia. The treatment of upper limb dystonia is challenging because of the variety of postures and the potential consequences of hand weakness, although many patients obtain relief from therapy. The onset of drug effect occurs within 72 hours and peaks by 1 week. Relief of symptoms lasts 3 to 4 months, although some patients derive a longer period of benefit. Toxin-related side effects are typically reversible and related to excessive weakness in the injected or adjacent muscles. Occasionally there can be a rash or flulike syndrome; however, with rare exception, they are self-limited.

Spasticity

Spasticity is characterized by a velocity-dependent increase in tonic stretch reflexes or "muscle tone" due to hyperexcitability of stretch reflexes. It is the most discernable component of the upper motor neuron syndrome (56) in those with lesions of the corticospinal tracts. Some patients with both spasticity and rigidity will often prove to have only task or position-specific increased tone, as one might see in dystonia.

There are numerous case reports and double-blind studies (57–62) establishing the clinical utility of BTX-A in managing both pediatric and adult-acquired spasticity (Table 2). They show an improvement in the degree of spasticity and the quality of life. Adults with acquired spasticity that displayed a good range of motion early in the course of their disease fared better than those with fixed or nearly fixed contractures, so suggesting the value of early intervention with BTX before the onset of fixed contractures or severe limitation in range of motion.

The importance of early intervention in pediatric cerebral palsy to promote more normal limb growth and functionality has been suggested by the hereditary spastic mouse model (63). Mouse calf muscles that were 16% shorter than normal ultimately grew to within 2% of normal length after injections of BTX-A.

A more favorable cost-effectiveness ratio and degree of improvement in spasticity was demonstrated for BTX-A injections compared with baclofen in the management of spasticity after stroke (64). The average extent of improvement in spasticity with BTX-A plus physiotherapy was 3

TABLE 2. *Spasticity disorders that may respond to botulinum toxin therapy*

Cerebral palsy
Prevalence: 500,000–750,000 in the United States
36% hemiplegia
33% spastic diplegia
12% dyskinesia
Incidence: 1–3 infants per 1,000 live births (154)
Multiple sclerosis
Prevalence: 250,000 in the United States (155)
Incidence: 8,000 new cases/yr (156)
Spinal cord injury
Prevalence: 150,000–200,000 in United States
Incidence: 7,000–10,000 new cases/yr (157)
Stroke
Prevalence: 2 million survivors in United States
Incidence: 400,000–500,000 new cases per year
Initial mortality high: ~38% within first month
200,000 die from stroke-related causes
Incidence decreasing but prevalence increasing due to enhanced survival (158)
Traumatic brain injury (TBI)
Incidence: 500,000 new cases per year in United States
Of survivors after 1 year: 50% good recovery; 31% moderate disability; 16% severely disabled; 3% vegetative state
20/100,000 or 44,000 per year survive TBI with moderate to severe physical or neurobehavioral sequelae (159)

times greater than for baclofen plus physiotherapy and 10 times greater than physiotherapy alone without a difference in cost.

Laryngeal Disorders

BTX-A has been used to treat both inappropriately closed and open laryngeal muscles in patients with laryngeal dystonia (65–71). BTX-A combined with voice therapy produced improved air flow rates through the larynx for periods of 6 months or longer (72). Patients treated with BTX-A plus speech therapy had better outcomes than those who did not receive adjunctive therapy. Laryngeal injection of BTX-A has been used to treat patients with chronic aspiration and failure of normal laryngeal reflexes that close the larynx (73). BTX-A injection of the posterior cricoarytenoid muscles and aryepiglottic folds brings the vocal folds into apposition and protects the airway in preparation for surgical closure of the larynx, which may be complicated by persistent abduction of the vocal folds.

Dysphagia due to spasm of the cricopharyngeal component of the inferior constrictor of the pharynx and herniation of the posterior wall of the pharynx can be relaxed with BTX-A, resulting in improved swallowing (74–76).

Gastrointestinal Disorders

Achalasia results from failure of relaxation of the lower esophageal sphincter during swallowing. BTX-A injection of the lower esophageal sphincter using an endoscopically guided approach led to improved swallowing function with quantitative decreases in muscle sphincter pressures (77–85) after two treatments in up to 68% of patients (86). BTX-A has also been used to treat diffuse esophageal spasm in those with nonachalasic esophageal dysmotility (87). Spasm of the sphincter of Oddi leading to biliary obstruction was treated with BTX-A using a long sclerotherapy needle in two patients (88). In one, sphincteric pressure was reduced by 50%, and the other had a 50% improvement in bile flow. The usefulness of this technique is limited by the inaccessibility of the muscle to be injected, and it has not gained widespread use.

BTX has been used in both open and double-blind studies for the treatment of chronic constipation (89,90) and anal fissures (91–94) caused by rectal spasm that fails to heal in the setting of increased rectal tone with secondarily inadequate drainage of the rectal circulation. One hundred units of BTX-A was administered to a patient with Parkinson disease and chronic constipation due to failure of relaxation and excessive contraction of the puborectalis muscle (95). Improved defecation and a moderate reduction in resting pressures was later shown by anorectal manometry.

Genitourinary Disorders

BTX-A has been successfully used in the treatment of urinary sphincter spasm (91–93) and recently to relieve vaginismus (96). Routine therapy of vagismus includes sequentially using dilators of increasing size. We injected the perivaginal muscles of a patient with resistant vagismus. After treatment, she resumed sexual intercourse, with a resultant remission of over 30 months. We suspect that the initial treatments permitted her to have intercourse, which then resulted in adequate chronic vaginal dilation.

Hyperhidrosis

Early observations of decreased sweating in response to BTX-A occurred among patients treated for hemifacial spasm. Patients have been reported to have decreased sweating after injection into the face or axilla (97–104). One patient with palmar hyperhidrosis had no recurrence of sweating for 14 weeks (105). Injection of 1 unit of BTX-A into the forearm of another patient caused regional loss of thermoregulatory sweating for over a year (106). We treated a patient with familial hyperhidrosis, formerly treated by bilateral sympathectomy in which multiple small injections of BTX-A into the fingers and palm led to clinical improvement.

Acquired Nystagmus

Acquired nystagmus resistant to pharmacotherapy is treated with retrobulbar injection of large doses of BTX-

A to infiltrate the extraocular muscles, paralyzing and fixing the eyeball in a neutral position (101–103). By injecting one eye every 4 to 5 months and patching the other, the patient fixates with the injected eye while avoiding the jiggling associated with the nystagmoid eye.

Preoperative Use

Cervical disease may be associated with dystonia and motor tics. Preoperative treatment with BTX-A facilitated surgery in four patients, including two each with chronic motor tics or cervical dystonia and severe neck disease undergoing laminectomy and stabilization (107).

Chronic Muscular Pain

BTX may reduce pain independent of its effect on muscle spasm in our original studies of BTX-A in cervical dystonia patients (108) and even exceeded motor benefit. Subsequent reports documented a reduction in pain with BTX-A therapy in two patients with taut cervical bands and trigger points along the trapezius and splenius capitis muscles, although the benefit may have been due to the placement of needles alone (109). Improvement was also shown among patients with the fibromyalgia-myofacial pain syndrome when injected with BTX-A into trigger points (110), but some found conflicting results (111). Others (112,113) have had success in the treatment of headache with BTX-A in either orofacial pain or masseter hypertrophy and anecdotally in chronic tension headache in an open-treatment study (114).

Tics and Tremor

Three studies reported the use of BTX-A in the treatment of motor and vocal tics, including those associated with Tourette's syndrome (115–117). Tremor disorders have also been treated with BTX-A (118–128). One study (118) examined BTX-A treatment in patients with essential tremor alone and in those with tremor associated with torticollis; both groups showed improvements. Additional studies demonstrated benefit with injections of BTX-A into activated muscles associated with palatal tremor and ear clicks (122), parkinsonian tremors (124), vocal tremors (121,126,128), and the rare disorder of hereditary chin tremor (127).

Cosmetic Indications: Hyperfunctional Facial Lines

BTX-A has also been used for its beneficial cosmetic effects, particularly in the reduction of facial wrinkles and frown lines (129–135). Photographs of patients before and after treatment at rest and with activation of the wrinkle showed significant efficacy of BTX-A in improving facial appearance (134).

BTX-A has also been used to provide additional contralateral symmetry to patients with hemifacial spasm, therefore giving better cosmetic appearance (136).

ADDITIONAL CONSIDERATIONS

Antibodies to BTX-A have rarely been detected in patients exposed either by food poisoning (137) or for the management of dystonia (138–146). Some patients who have developed BTX-A antibodies benefited from injections by immunologically distinct preparations. The benefits of BTX-F appear to last only about 1 month (147–151). BTX-B is currently in clinical trial (152,153).

ACKNOWLEDGMENT

Supported in part by The Bachmann-Strauss Foundation.

REFERENCES

1. AAO Statement. Botulinum-A toxin for ocular muscle disorders. *Lancet* 1986;1:76–77.
2. AAO Statement. Botulinum toxin therapy of eye muscle disorders. Safety and effectiveness. American Academy of Ophthalmology. *Ophthalmology* 1989;(Pt 2):37–41.
3. American Academy of Neurology. Assessment: the clinical usefulness of botulinum toxin-A in treating neurologic disorders. Report of the Therapeutics and Technology Assessment Subcommittee of the American Academy of Neurology. *Neurology* 1990;40:1332–1336.
4. AAO-HNS. American Academy of Otolaryngology-Head and Neck Surgery Policy Statement: Botox for spasmodic dysphonia. *AAO-HNS Bull* 1990;9:8.
5. National Institutes of Health Consensus Development Conference. Clinical use of botulinum toxin. National Institutes of Health Consensus Development Statement, November 12–14, 1990. *Arch Neurol* 1991;48:1294–1298.
6. Jankovic J, Hallett M. *Therapy with botulinum toxin.* New York: Marcel Dekker, 1994.
7. Moore AP. *Handbook of botulinum toxin treatment.* Oxford: Blackwell Scientific, 1993.
8. AAN Assessment. The clinical usefulness of botulinum toxin-A in treating neurologic disorders. Report of the Therapeutics and Technology Subcommittee of the American Academy of Neurology. [review]. *Neurology* 1990;40:1332–1336.
9. Spasticity Study Group. Spasticity: etiology, evaluation, management and the role of botulinum toxin type A. *Muscle Nerve* 1997;20[Suppl 6]:S1–S231.
10. Simpson LL. The origin, structure, and pharmacological activity of botulinum toxin. *Pharmacol Rev* 1981;33:155–188.
11. Simpson LL. The binding fragment from tetanus toxin antagonizes the neuromuscular blocking actions of botulinum toxin. *J Pharmacol Exp Ther* 1984;229:182–187.
12. Simpson LL, DasGupta BR. Botulinum neurotoxin type E: studies on mechanism of action and on structure-activity relationships. *J Pharmacol Exp Ther* 1983;224:135–140.
13. DasGupta BR. Structure of botulinum neurotoxin. In: Jankovic J, Hallett M, eds. *Therapy with botulinum toxin.* New York: Marcel Dekker, 1994.
14. Schiavo G, Rossetto O, Santucci A, DasGupta BR, Montecucco C. Botulinum neurotoxins are zinc proteins. *J Biol Chem* 1992;267: 23479–23483.
15. Brin MF. Botulinum toxin: chemistry, pharmacology, toxicity, and immunology. *Muscle Nerve* 1997;20[Suppl 6]:S146–S168.
16. Schantz EJ, Johnson EA. Properties and use of botulinum toxin and other microbial neurotoxins in medicine. *Microbiol Rev* 1992;56:80–99.
17. Simpson LL. Kinetic studies on the interaction between botulinum toxin type A and the cholinergic neuromuscular junction. *J Pharmacol Exp Ther* 1980;212:16–21.
18. Black JD, Dolly JO. Interaction of ^{125}I-labeled botulinum neurotoxins with nerve terminals. II. Autoradiographic evidence for its uptake into motor nerves by acceptor-mediated endocytosis. *J Cell Biol* 1986;103: 535–544.
19. Black JD, Dolly JO. Interaction of ^{125}I-labeled botulinum neurotoxins with nerve terminals. I. Ultrastructural autoradiographic localization and quantitation of distinct membrane acceptors for types A and B on motor nerves. *J Cell Biol* 1986;103:521–534.
20. Simpson LL. Peripheral actions of the botulinum toxins. In: Simpson LL, ed. *Botulinum neurotoxin and tetanus toxin.* New York: Academic Press, 1989:153–178.
21. Dolly JO. General properties and cellular mechanisms of neurotoxins. In: Jankovic J, Hallett M, eds. *Therapy with botulinum toxin.* New York: Marcel Dekker, 1994.
22. Nathan P, Dimitrijevic MR, Sherwood AM. Reflex path length and clonus frequency [letter]. *J Neurol Neurosurg Psychiatry* 1985;48: 725.
23. Hughes R, Whaller BC. Influence of nerve ending activity and of drugs on the rate of paralysis of rat diaphragm preparations by clostridium botulinum type A toxin. *J Physiol* 1962;160:221–223.
24. Dolly JO, Ashton AC, McInnes C, et al. Clues to the multi-phasic inhibitory action of botulinum neurotoxins on release of transmitters. *J Physiol* 1990;84:237–246.
25. Martin TFJ. Stages of regulated exocytosis. *Trends Cell Biol* 1997;7: 271–276.
26. Gundersen CB. The effects of botulinum toxin on the synthesis, storage and release of acetylcholine. *Prog Neurobiol* 1980;14:99–119.
27. Barinaga M. Secrets of secretion revealed. *Science* 1993;260:487–489.
28. Huttner WB. Snappy exocytoxins. *Nature* 1993;365:104–105.
29. Blasi J, Chapman ER, Yamasaki S, Binz T, Niemann H, Jahn R. Botulinum neurotoxin-C1 blocks neurotransmitter release by means of cleaving HPC-1/syntaxin. *EMBO J* 1993;12:4821–4828.
30. Williamson LC, Halpern JL, Montecucco C, Brown JE, Neale EA. Clostridial neurotoxins and substrate proteolysis in intact neurons: botulinum neurotoxin c acts on synaptosomal-associated protein of 25 kda. *J Biol Chem* 1996;271:7694–7699.
31. Brin MF, Blitzer A. Botulinum toxin—dangerous terminology errors [letter]. *J R Soc Med* 1993;86:494.
32. Marsden CD. Botulinum toxin—dangerous terminology errors [reply]. *J R Soc Med* 1993;86:494.
33. Scott AB. Botulinum toxin injection of eye muscles to correct strabismus. *Trans Am Ophthalmol Soc* 1981;79:734–770.
34. Jacobs L, Bender MB. Palato-ocular synchrony during eyelid closure. *Arch Neurol* 1976;33:289–291.
35. Scott AB, Rosenbaum A, Collins CC. Pharmacologic weakening of extraocular muscles. *Invest Ophthalmol Vis Sci* 1973;12:924–927.
36. Fahn S. The varied clinical expressions of dystonia. *Neurol Clin* 1984; 2:541–554.
37. Spinella GM, Sheridan PH. Research opportunities in dystonia: National Institute of Neurological Disorders and Stroke workshop summary. *Neurology* 1994;44:1177–1179.
38. Nutt JG, Muenter MD, Aronson A, Kurland LT, Melton LJ III. Epidemiology of focal and generalized dystonia in Rochester, Minnesota. *Mov Disord* 1988;3:188–194.
39. Gasser T. Advances in the genetics of movement disorders: implications for molecular diagnosis. *J Neurol* 1997;244:341–348(abst).
40. Ichinose H, Nagatsu T. Molecular genetics of hereditary dystonia—mutations in the GTP cyclohydrolase I gene. *Brain Res Bull* 1997;43: 35–38(abst).
41. Nygaard TG. Dopa-responsive dystonia. *Curr Opin Neurol* 1995;8: 310–313.
42. Hornykiewicz O, Kish SJ, Becker LE, Farley I, Shannak K. Brain neurotransmitters in dystonia musculorum deformans. *N Engl J Med* 1986; 315:347–353.
43. Jankovic J, Svendsen CN, Bird ED. Brain neurotransmitters in dystonia. *N Engl J Med* 1987;316:278–279.
44. de Yebenes JG, Brin MF, Mena MA, et al. Neurochemical findings in neuroacanthocytosis. *Mov Disord* 1988;3:300–312.
45. Brin MF, Moskowitz C, Fahn S. Dystonia clinical research center tissue resource facility: investigations on collected tissue. *Adv Neurol* 1988; 50:215–222.
46. Obeso JA, Gimenez Roldan S. Clinicopathological correlation in symptomatic dystonia. *Adv Neurol* 1988;50:113–122.
47. Zweig RM, Hedreen JC, Jankel WR, Casanova MF, Whitehouse PJ,

Price DL. Pathology in brainstem regions of individuals with primary dystonia. *Neurology* 1988;38:702–706.

48. Zweig RM, Hedreen JC. Brain stem pathology in cranial dystonia. *Adv Neurol* 1988;49:395–407.

49. Ceballos-Baumann AO, Passingham RE, Warner T, Playford ED, Marsden CD, Brooks DJ. Overactive prefrontal and underactive motor cortical areas in idiopathic dystonia. *Ann Neurol* 1995;37:363–372.

50. Eidelberg D, Moeller JR, Ishikawa T, et al. The metabolic topography of idiopathic torsion dystonia. *Brain* 1995;118:1473–1484.

51. Brooks D. PET studies on dystonia. *Focus Dystonia* 1994;14–15 (abst).

52. Playford ED, Fletcher NA, Sawle GV, Marsden CD, Brooks DJ. Striatal [F-18]dopa uptake in familial idiopathic dystonia. *Brain* 1993; 116:1191–1199.

53. Hallett M, Toro C. Dystonia and the supplementary sensorimotor area. *Adv Neurol* 1996;70:471–476.

54. Hallett M. Is dystonia a sensory disorder [editorial]? *Ann Neurol* 1995; 38:139–140.

55. Kaji R, Rothwell JC, Katayama M, et al. Tonic vibration reflex and muscle afferent block in writer's cramp. *Ann Neurol* 1995;38:155–162.

56. Lance JW. Symposium synopsis. In: Feldman RG, Young RR, Koella WP, eds. *Spasticity: disordered motor control.* Chicago: Year Book Medical Publishers, 1980.

57. Snow BJ, Tsui JK, Bhatt MH, Varelas M, Hashimoto SA, Calne DB. Treatment of spasticity with botulinum toxin: a double-blind study. *Ann Neurol* 1990;28:512–515.

58. Dykstra DD, Sidi AA. Treatment of detrusor-sphincter dyssynergia with botulinum A toxin: a double-blind study. *Arch Phys Med Rehabil* 1990;71:24–26.

59. Koman LA, Mooney JF III, Smith BP, Goodman A, Mulvaney T. Management of spasticity in cerebral palsy with botulinum-A toxin: report of a preliminary, randomized, double-blind trial. *J Pediatr Orthop* 1994;14:299–303.

60. Corry IS, Cosgrove AP, Walsh EG, McClean D, Graham HK. Botulinum toxin A in the hemiplegic upper limb: a double-blind trial [see comments]. *Dev Med Child Neurol* 1997;39:185–193.

61. Jabbari B, Polo KB, Ford G, Grazko MA. Effectiveness of botulinum toxin A in patents with spasticity. *Mov Disord* 1995;10:379(abst).

62. Simpson DM, Alexander DN, O'Brien CF, et al. Botulinum toxin type a in the treatment of upper extremity spasticity: a randomized, double-blind, placebo-controlled trial. *Neurology* 1996;46:1306–1310.

63. Cosgrove AP, Graham HK. Botulinum toxin A prevents the development of contractures in the hereditary spastic mouse. *Dev Med Child Neurol* 1994;36:379–385.

64. Wallesch CW, Maes E, Lecomte P, Bartels C. Cost-effectiveness of botulinum toxin type A injection in patients with spasticity following stroke: a German perspective. *Eur J Neurol* 1997;4[Suppl 2]:S53–S58.

65. Brin MF, Blitzer A, Stewart C. Laryngeal dystonia (spasmodic dysphonia): observations of 901 patients and treatment with botulinum toxin. *Adv Neurol* 1998;78:237–252.

66. Blitzer A, Brin MF, Stewart C. Botulinum toxin management of spasmodic dysphonia (laryngeal dystonia): a 12 year experience in over 900 patients. *Laryngoscope* 1998;108:1435–1441.

67. Brin MF, Stewart C, Viswanath NS, Beardsley A, Blitzer A, Rosenfield D. Pilot study: laryngeal botulinum toxin (botox) injections for disabling stuttering in adults. *Neurology* 1992;42[Suppl 3]:376(abst).

68. Blitzer A, Brin MF. Laryngeal dystonia: a series with botulinum toxin therapy. *Ann Otol Rhinol Laryngol* 1991;100:85–90.

69. Brin MF, Blitzer A, Stewart C, Fahn S. Botulinum toxin: now for abductor laryngeal dystonia. *Neurology* 1990;40[Suppl 1]:381(abst).

70. Brin MF, Blitzer A, Fahn S, Gould W, Lovelace RE. Adductor laryngeal dystonia (spastic dysphonia): treatment with local injections of botulinum toxin (Botox). *Mov Disord* 1989;4:287–296.

71. Brin MF, Blitzer A, Fahn S, Lovelace RE. Laryngeal dystonia (LD) at the Dystonia Clinical Research Center (DCRC): clinical and electromyographic features in 110 cases. *Neurology* 1988;129(abst).

72. Murry T, Woodson GE. Combined-modality treatment of adductor spasmodic dysphonia with botulinum toxin and voice therapy. *J Voice* 1995;9:460–465.

73. Pototschnig CA, Schneider I, Eckel HE, Thumfart WF. Repeatedly successful closure of the larynx for the treatment of chronic aspiration with the use of botulinum toxin A. *Ann Otol Rhinol Laryngol* 1996; 105:521–524.

74. Blitzer A, Komisar A, Baredes S, Brin MF, Stewart C. Voice failure after tracheoesophageal puncture: management with botulinum toxin. *Otolaryngol Head Neck Surg* 1995;113:668–670.

75. Schneider I, Pototschnig C, Thumfart WF, Eckel HE. Treatment of dysfunction of the cricopharyngeal muscle with botulinum A toxin—introduction of a new, noninvasive method. *Ann Otol Rhinol Laryngol* 1994;103:31–35.

76. Blitzer A, Brin MF. Use of botulinum toxin for diagnosis and management of cricopharyngeal achalasia. *Otolaryngol Head Neck Surg* 1997; 116:328–330.

77. Pasricha PJ, Rai R, Ravich WJ, Hendrix TR, Kalloo AN. Botulinum toxin for achalasia: long-term outcome and predictors of response [see comments]. *Gastroenterology* 1996;110:1410–1415.

78. Pasricha PJ, Ravich WJ, Hendrix TR, Sostre S, Jones B, Kalloo AN. Treatment of achalasia with intrasphincteric injection of botulinum toxin—a pilot trial. *Ann Intern Med* 1994;121:590–591.

79. Pasricha PJ, Ravich WJ, Hendrix TR, Sostre S, Jones B, Kalloo AN. Intrasphincteric botulinum toxin for the treatment of achalasia. *N Engl J Med* 1995;332:774–778.

80. Pasricha PJ, Ravich WJ, Kalloo AN. Botulinum toxin for achalasia. *Lancet* 1993;341:244–245.

81. Pasricha PJ, Ravich WJ, Kalloo AN. Effects of intrasphincteric botulinum toxin on the lower esophageal sphincter in piglets. *Gastroenterology* 1993;105:1045–1049.

82. Eaker EY, Gordon JM, Vogel SB. Untoward effects of esophageal botulinum toxin injection in the treatment of achalasia. *Dig Dis Sci* 1997;42: 724–727(abst).

83. Cohen S, Parkman HP. Treatment of achalasia—from whalebone to botulinum toxin [editorial]. *N Engl J Med* 1995;332:815–816.

84. Ferrari AP, Siqueira ES, Brant CQ. Treatment of achalasia in Chaga's disease with botulinum toxin. *N Engl J Med* 1995;332:824–825.

85. Annese V, Basciani M, Lombardi G, et al. Perendoscopic injection of botulinum toxin is effective in achalasia after failure of myotomy or pneumatic dilation. *Gastrointest Endosc* 1996;44:461–465.

86. De Looze DA. Botulinum toxin in the treatment of achalasia. *Eur J Neurol* 1997;4[Suppl 2]:S85–S89.

87. Miller LS, Parkman HP, Schiano TD, et al. Treatment of symptomatic nonachalasia esophageal motor disorders with botulinum toxin injection at the lower esophageal sphincter. *Dig Dis Sci* 1996; 41:2025–2031.

88. Pasricha PJ, Miskovsky EP, Kalloo AN. Intrasphincteric injection of botulinum toxin for suspected sphincter of Oddi dysfunction. *Gut* 1994; 35:1319–1321.

89. Hallan RI, Williams NS, Melling J, Waldron DJ, Womack NR, Morrison JF. Treatment of anismus in intractable constipation with botulinum A toxin. *Lancet* 1988;2:714–717.

90. Joo JS, Agachan F, Wolff B, Nogueras JJ, Wexner SD. Initial North American experience with botulinum toxin type A for treatment of anismus. *Dis Colon Rectum* 1996;39:1107–1111.

91. Gui D, Cassetta E, Anastasio G, Bentivoglio AR, Maria G, Albanese A. Botulinum toxin for chronic anal fissure [see comments]. *Lancet* 1994;344:1127–1128.

92. Albanese A, Bentivoglio AR, Cassetta E, Viggiano A, Maria G, Gui D. The use of botulinum toxin in the alimentary tract [review]. *Aliment Pharmacol Ther* 1995;9:599–604.

93. Jost WH, Schimrigk K. Botulinum toxin in therapy of anal fissure [letter; comment]. *Lancet* 1995;345:188–189.

94. Mason PF, Watkins MJ, Hall HS, Hall AW. The management of chronic fissure in-ano with botulinum toxin. *J R Coll Surg Edinb* 1996;41: 235–238.

95. Albanese A, Maria G, Bentivoglio AR, Brisinda G, Cassetta E, Tonali P. Botulinum toxin in the treatment of chronic constipation in Parkinson's disease. *Eur J Neurol* 1997;4[Suppl 2]:S81–S84.

96. Brin MF, Vapnek JM. Treatment of vaginismus with botulinum toxin injections [letter]. *Lancet* 1997;349:252–253.

97. Schulze-Bonhage A, Schroder M, Ferbert A. Botulinum toxin in the therapy of gustatory sweating. *J Neurol* 1996;243:143–146.

98. Bushara KO, Park DM, Jones JC, Schutta HS. Botulinum toxin—a possible new treatment for axillary hyperhidrosis. *Clin Exp Dermatol* 1996;21:276–278.

99. Bushara KO, Park DM. Botulinum toxin and sweating. *J Neurol Neurosurg Psychiatry* 1994;57:1437–1438.

100. Shumway-Cook A. Role of the vestibular system in motor development: theoretical and clinical issues. In: Forssberg H, Hirschfeld H, eds. *Movement disorders in children.* Basel: Karger, 1992:209–216.

101. Helveston EM, Pogrebniak AE. Treatment of acquired nystagmus with botulinum A toxin. *Am J Ophthalmol* 1988;106:584–586.

102. Repka MX, Savino PJ, Reinecke RD. Treatment of acquired nystagmus with botulinum neurotoxin A. *Arch Ophthalmol* 1994;112:1320–1324.

103. Thomas R, Mathai A, Braganza A, Billson F. Periodic alternating nystagmus treated with retrobulbar botulinum toxin and large horizontal muscle recession. *Indian J Ophthalmol* 1996;44:170–172.

104. Naver H, Aquilonius SM. The treatment of focal hyperhidrosis with botulinum toxin. *Eur J Neurol* 1997;4[Suppl 2]:S75–S80.

105. Naumann M, Flachenecker P, Brocker EB, Toyka KV, Reiners K. Botulinum toxin for palmar hyperhidrosis [letter]. *Lancet* 1997;349:252.

106. Cheshire WP. Subcutaneous botulinum toxin type a inhibits regional sweating: an individual observation. *Clin Auton Res* 1996;6:123–124.

107. Adler CH, Zimmerman RS, Lyons MK, Simeone F, Brin MF. Perioperative use of botulinum toxin for movement disorder-induced cervical spine disease. *Mov Disord* 1996;11:79–81.

108. Brin MF, Fahn S, Moskowitz C, et al. Localized injections of botulinum toxin for the treatment of focal dystonia and hemifacial spasm. *Mov Disord* 1987;2:237–254.

109. Acquadro MA, Borodic GE. Treatment of myofascial pain with botulinum A toxin [letter]. *Anesthesiology* 1994;80:705–706.

110. Cheshire WP, Abashian SW, Mann JD. Botulinum toxin in the treatment of myofascial pain syndrome. *Pain* 1994;59:65–69.

111. Paulson GW, Gill W. Botulinum toxin is unsatisfactory therapy for fibromyalgia. *Mov Disord* 1996;11:459.

112. Clark GT, Koyano K, Browne PA. Oral motor disorders in humans. *J Calif Dent Assoc* 1993;21:19–30.

113. Doyle M, Jabbari B. Hypertrophic branchial myopathy treated with botulinum toxin type A. *Neurology* 1994;44:1765–1766.

114. Relja M. Treatment of tension-type headache by local injection of botulinum toxin. *Eur J Neurol* 1997;4[Suppl 2]:S71–S74.

115. Salloway S, Stewart CF, Israeli L, et al. Botulinum toxin for refractory vocal tics. *Mov Disord* 1996;11:746–748.

116. Scott BL, Jankovic J, Donovan DT. Botulinum toxin injection into vocal cord in the treatment of malignant coprolalia associated with tourette's syndrome. *Mov Disord* 1996;11:431–433.

117. Jankovic J. Botulinum toxin in the treatment of dystonic tics. *Mov Disord* 1994;9:347–349.

118. Jankovic J, Schwartz K. Botulinum toxin treatment of tremors. *Neurology* 1991;41:1185–1188.

119. Jankovic J, Schwartz K, Clemence W, Aswad A, Mordaunt J. A randomized, double-blind, placebo-controlled study to evaluate botulinum toxin type A in essential hand tremor. *Mov Disord* 1996;11:250–256.

120. Henderson JM, Ghika JA, Van Melle G, Haller E, Einstein R. Botulinum toxin A in non-dystonic tremors. *Eur Neurol* 1996;36:29–35.

121. Stager SV, Ludlow CL. Responses of stutterers and vocal tremor patients to treatment with botulinum toxin. In: Jankovic J, Hallett M, eds. *Therapy with botulinum toxin*. New York: Marcel Dekker, 1994:481–490.

122. Deuschl G, Lohle E, Toro C, Hallett M, Lebovics RS. Botulinum toxin treatment of palatal tremor (myoclonus). In: Jankovic J, Hallett M, eds. *Therapy with botulinum toxin*. New York: Marcel Dekker, 1994:567–576.

123. Jedynak CP, Vidailhet M, Sharshar T, Lubetzki C, Lyon-Caen O, Agid Y. Segmental analysis of multiple sclerosis midbrain tremor as a target of botulinum toxin type A injections: functional improvement and long term follow-up. *Mov Disord* 1995;10:402(abst).

124. Trosch RM, Pullman SL. Botulinum toxin A injections for the treatment of hand tremors. *Mov Disord* 1994;9:601–609.

125. Jedynak CP, Bonnet AM. Botulinum A toxin injections for the treatment of hand tremors. *Ann Neurol* 1992;32:250(abst).

126. Ludlow CL. Treating the spasmodic dysphonias with botulinum toxin: a comparison with adductor and abductor spasmodic dysphonia and vocal tremor. In: Tsui JKC, Calne DB, eds. *Handbook of dystonia*. New York: Marcel Dekker, 1995:431–446.

127. Gordon K, Cadera W, Hinton G. Successful treatment of hereditary trembling chin with botulinum toxin. *J Child Neurol* 1993;8:154–156.

128. Brin MF, Blitzer A, Stewart C. Vocal Tremor. In: Findley LJ, Koller WC, eds. *Handbook of tremor disorders*. New York: Marcel Dekker, 1995:495–520.

129. Carruthers JD, Carruthers JA. Treatment of glabellar frown lines with C. botulinum-A exotoxin. *J Dermatol Surg Oncol* 1992;18:17–21.

130. Blitzer A, Brin MF, Keen MS, Aviv JE. Botulinum toxin for the treatment of hyperfunctional lines of the face. *Arch Otolaryngol Head Neck Surg* 1993;119:1018–1022.

131. Blitzer A, Brin MF. Evaluation and management of hyperfunctional muscular disorders of the head and neck. *Adv Oto Head Neck Surg* 1994;7:1–28.

132. Keen M, Blitzer A, Aviv J, et al. Botulinum toxin for hyperkinetic facial lines: results of a double blind placebo controlled study. *Plast Reconstr Surg* 1994;94:94–99..

133. Carruthers A, Kiene K, Carruthers J. Botulinum A exotoxin use in clinical dermatology. *J Am Acad Dermatol* 1996;34:788–797.

134. Blitzer A, Binder WJ, Aviv JE, Keen MS, Brin MF. The management of hyperfunctional facial lines with botulinum toxin: a collaborative study of 210 injection sites in 162 patients. *Arch Otolaryngol Head Neck Surg* 1997;123:389–392.

135. Carruthers A, Carruthers J. Cosmetic uses of botulinum A exotoxin. *Adv Dermatol* 1997;12:325–348.

136. Armstrong MW, Mountain RE, Murray JA. Treatment of facial synkinesis and facial asymmetry with botulinum toxin type A following facial nerve palsy. *Clin Otolaryngol* 1996;21:15–20.

137. Paton JC, Lawrence AJ, Manson JI. Quantitation of *Clostridium botulinum* organisms and toxin in the feces of an infant with botulism. *J Clin Microbiol* 1982;15:1–4.

138. Biglan AW, Gonnering R, Lockhart LB, Rabin B, Fuerste FH. Absence of antibody production in patients treated with botulinum A toxin. *Am J Ophthalmol* 1986;101:232–235.

139. Gonnering RS. Negative antibody response to long-term treatment of facial spasm with botulinum toxin. *Am J Ophthalmol* 1988;105:313–315.

140. Hatheway CH, Snyder JD, Seals JE, Edell TA, Lewis GE. Antitoxin levels in botulism patients treated with trivalent equine botulism antitoxin to toxin types A, B, and E. *J Infect Dis* 1984;150:407–412.

141. Dezfulian M, Hatheway C, Yolken R, Bartlett J. Enzyme-linked immunosorbent assay for detection of *Clostridium botulinum* type A and type B toxins in stool samples of infants with botulism. *J Clin Microbiol* 1984;20:379–383.

142. Dezfulian M, Bitar R, Bartlett J. Kinetics study of immunological response to *Clostridium botulinum* toxin. *J Clin Microbiol* 1987;25:1336–1337.

143. Tsui JK, Wong NLM, Wong E, Calne DB. Production of circulating antibodies to botulinum-A toxin in patients receiving repeated injections for dystonia. *Ann Neurol* 1988;24:181(abst).

144. Doellgast GJ, Triscott MX, Beard GA, et al. Sensitive enzyme-linked immunosorbent assay for detection of *Clostridium botulinum* neurotoxins A, B, and E using signal amplification via enzyme-linked coagulation assay. *J Clin Microbiol* 1993;31:2402–2409.

145. Doellgast GJ, Beard GA, Bottoms JD, et al. Enzyme-linked immunosorbent assay and enzyme-linked coagulation assay for detection of *Clostridium botulinum* neurotoxin-A, neurotoxin-B, and neurotoxin-E and solution–or-phase complexes with dual-label antibodies. *J Clin Microbiol* 1994;32:105–111.

146. Siatkowski RM, Tyutyunikov A, Biglan AW, et al. Serum antibody production to botulinum-A toxin. *Ophthalmology* 1993;100:1861–1866.

147. Greene PE, Fahn S. Response to botulinum toxin F in seronegative botulinum toxin A-resistant patients. *Mov Disord* 1996;11:181–184.

148. Sheean GL, Lees AJ. Botulinum toxin F in the treatment of torticollis clinically resistant to botulinum toxin A. *J Neurol Neurosurg Psychiatry* 1995;59:601–607.

149. Ludlow CL, Hallett M, Rhew K, et al. Therapeutic use of type F botulinum toxin [letter]. *N Engl J Med* 1992;326:349–350.

150. Greene PE, Fahn S. Use of botulinum toxin type-F injections to treat torticollis in patients with immunity to botulinum toxin type-A. *Mov Disord* 1993;8:479–483.

151. Rhew K, Ludlow CL, Karp BI, Hallett M. Clinical experience with botulinum toxin F. In: Jankovic J, Hallett M, eds. *Therapy with botulinum toxin*. New York: Marcel Dekker, 1994:323–328.

152. Tsui JKC, Hayward M, Mak EKM, Schulzer M. Botulinum toxin type B in the treatment of cervical dystonia: a pilot study. *Neurology* 1995;45:2109–2110.

153. Lew MF, Adornato BT, Duane DD, et al. Botulinum toxin type B (BotB): a double-blind, placebo-controlled, safety and efficacy study in cervical dystonia. *Neurology* 1997;49:701–707.

154. Stanley F, Alberman E. *The epidemiology of the cerebral palsies*. Philadelphia: J.B. Lippincott, 1984.

155. Adams RD, Victor M. Multiple sclerosis and allied demyelinated diseases. In: *Principles of neurology*, 5th ed. New York: McGraw-Hill, 1993:776–798.

156. Cobble ND, Dietz MA, Grigsby J, Kennedy PM. Rehabilitation of the patient with multiple sclerosis. In: DeLisa JA, ed. *Rehabilitation medicine: principles and practice*, 2nd ed. Philadelphia: J.B. Lippincott, 1993:861–885.

157. Staas WE, Formal CS, Gershkoff AM, et al. Rehabilitation of the spinal cord-injured patient. In: DeLisa JA, ed. *Rehabilitation medicine: principles and practice*, 2nd ed. Philadelphia: J.B. Lippincott, 1993.

158. Garrison SJ, Rolak LA. Rehabilitation of the stroke patient. In: DeLisa JA, ed. *Rehabilitation medicine: principles and practice*, 2nd ed. Philadelphia: J.B. Lippincott, 1993:801–824.

159. Whyte J, Rosenthal M. Rehabilitation of the patient with traumatic brain injury. In: DeLisa JA, ed. *Rehabilitation medicine: principles and practice*, 2nd ed. Philadelphia: J.B. Lippincott, 1993:825–860.

Motor Disorders,
edited by David S. Younger.
Lippincott Williams & Wilkins, Philadelphia © 1999.

CHAPTER 45

Multidisciplinary Integrated Psychosocial and Palliative Care

Peregrine L. Murphy, Maura L. Del Bene, and Steven M. Albert

I ask knowledge what it can tell me of life. Knowledge replies that what it can tell me is little, yet immense. Whence this universe came, or whither it is bound, or how it happens to be at all, knowledge cannot tell me. Only this: that the will-to-live is everywhere present, even as in me. I do not need science to tell me this; but it cannot tell me anything more essential. Profound and marvelous as chemistry is, for example, it is like all science in the fact that it can lead me only to the mystery of life, which is essentially in me, however near or far away it may be observed.

Albert Schweitzer (1)

Life and death are intensely personal and social experiences. The way an individual faces life-threatening disease and obtains support from others reflects the shared beliefs and values of the particular culture, society, and treating physicians (2). Over the past several years, it has become clear that the optimal care of patients with progressive motor disorders includes attention to both psychosocial and medical needs. Regardless of the etiologic diagnosis, the goals of pyschosocial and palliative care are to enhance, or at least maintain, quality of life by keeping the disruptive features of the disease to a minimum. Such care reinforces independence and self-esteem and enhances useful coping strategies and treatment options while actively identifying and modifying maladaptive behaviors. In progressive and ultimately fatal disorders without known cure or effective therapy, such as amyotrophic lateral sclerosis (ALS), a psychosocial and

P.L. Murphy: Eleanor and Lou Gehrig Muscular Dystrophy Association/Amyotrophic Lateral Sclerosis Research Center, Neurologic Institute, New York Presbyterian Hospital, New York, New York 10032.

M. L. Del Bene: The Eleanor and Lou Gehrig Muscular Dystrophy Association/Amyotrophic Lateral Sclerosis Research Center, Neurological Institute and Department of Education Research and Standards, New York Presbyterian Hospital, New York, New York 10032.

S. M. Albert: Gertrude H. Sergievsky Center, Columbia University, New York, New York 10032.

palliative model of care can help the patient live and die in a desired manner.

This chapter focuses on the integrated palliative and psychosocial care of patients with ALS; however, the concepts are applicable to other progressive neuromuscular disorders. The essential aspects of the classification, diagnosis, laboratory evaluation, and pharmacotherapy of inherited and acquired ALS are reviewed in preceding chapters in this volume (1–5,31–32,38–40,41–43).

GENERAL CONSIDERATIONS

The psychological and social needs of a patient with progressive motor disorders should be ascertained as soon as possible after the diagnosis is made and discussed with the patient and family, because the emotional reaction to the perceived loss of bodily integrity commences right away. Denial, fear, and anxiety are early reactions, followed later by depression and anger, with an intensity and duration that depend on the severity and rate of progression of the illness, individual character, family variables, and envisioned changes in lifestyle. For several reasons there may be lingering doubts or disbelief of the diagnosis even after a lengthy evaluation. First, the diagnosis of ALS is a clinical one, substantiated by laboratory studies, in particular, electromyography and muscle biopsy, with an accuracy of about 95% in experienced hands. Second, the time to correct diagnosis may lag by weeks or months, with some patients given alternative diagnoses or inaccurate information about the disease. In one study, a third each of 33 patients and their families complained that the diagnosis of ALS was withheld too long or crudely relayed (3). At the time of diagnosis, the leading concern in one half of patients was the prospect of becoming disabled and dependent on others, followed by the uncertainly in the length, mode of progression, and nature of the terminal phases of the illness. Third, neurologists can have different styles of communication, with some transmitting their sense of helplessness about the disease and concentrating on the inevitable clinical decline and time to death and others proactively engaging the patient in useful dialogue. Experienced ALS clinicians recommend as many visits as necessary to address personal concerns, treatment expectations, and other questions, because information overload frequently occurs after the initial discussion of the diagnosis.

ALS presents particular challenges because the cause of the disease is not well understood; for the most part, the course of ALS is relentlessly progressive with few stable plateau periods, and approximately 50% of patients die within 3 to 5 years of diagnosis. Its predictable pattern of functional decline permits evaluation of the effects of psychological, social measures, and therapeutic interventions on prognosis and outcome. Measures of psychological well-being were related to outcome in a cohort of 144 patients with ALS in which depression, hopelessness, and perceived stress are more likely to occur in patients with advanced physical disability who are closer to death (4).

An integrated medical and psychosocial approach usually reveals potential medical problems earlier and provides a more effective utilization of resources, particularly in the present managed care environment. The multidisciplinary team includes a neurologist; advanced care or clinical research nurse; physiatrist; physical and occupational therapists; speech, swallowing, and otolaryngologic specialists; psychologist or psychiatrist; clergy; social worker; respiratory and vocational therapists; and nutritionist. Advanced-trained nurses can provide valuable leadership by virtue of their pivotal position as contact person for patients, their families, and other team specialists.

CHALLENGE OF PSYCHOSOCIAL CARE

It is in reverence for life that knowledge passes over into experience . . . My life bears its meaning in itself. And this meaning is to be found in living out the highest and most worthy idea which my will-to-live can furnish. . . .

Albert Schweitzer (5)

In this section we consider the psychosocial aspects of the relationships between the patient, family, and healthcare team and five specific suggestions to optimize them.

1. *Ensure that the relationship established with the patient and their family is professional, with clearly established boundaries and expectations.*

Healthcare professionals should strive to create as best as possible a warm, welcoming, hospitable environment. To offer hospitality, in the true sense of the word, is to offer an environment that restores the patient's spirit and their physical nature (6). Hospitality and hospital are of the same Latin root, *hospitis*, which means host, guest, or friend (7). Practically speaking, optimal relationships are based on mutual respect, resembling how one would like to be treated if diagnosed with the same condition. Some clinicians believe that an atmosphere of informality may best

help the patient feel at ease. One way to create such informality is to refer to both patients and team members by their first names. This degree of informality is appropriate in patient care if everybody on the team, including the physician, are called by first names. Realistically, it is quite rare for a patient to refer to the physician by his or her first name even when invited to do so. To refer to the patient by their first name conveys a paternalistic posture and lack of gender sensitivity even if it is not intended to do so (8). This style of communication infantilizes the patient and can be perceived as rude and threatening to the patient's dignity. In contrast to those clinicians wishing to promote informality in the clinician–patient relationship, others believe that excessive informality erodes boundaries and leads to confusion (9). With increasing awareness of the need to empower patients, effort has been toward fostering balanced gender-sensitive egalitarian models of team care (10) that convey mutual dignity and respect.

2. *Identify coping strategies and take into account interpersonal communication styles of the patient.*

There are perhaps as many styles of coping as there are individual personalities. It may be useful to elicit information about the ways in which the patient faced challenges that occurred in the past to plan treatment strategies for the present and certainly for the future. There may be underlying emotional, spiritual, intellectual, and cultural factors that interfere with adequate communication, understanding of the disease process, and the successful integration of coping strategies. The patient's reaction to a diagnosis that is terminal is akin to the reaction observed in individuals experiencing trauma. Denial may be observed, or patients may insist that they are coping well, when in fact they may not be. Although this defense mechanism is inordinately useful to the patient (it enables an individual to maintain a sense of competence in the face of actual incompetence [11]), the healthcare team would be wise to recognize that this coping strategy is frequently used. It also has been advised that the healthcare team should not force the acceptance of a frank or poor prognosis or confront denial directly (11). Instead, one should recognize that denial is a common reaction, understand its positive and negative effects, emphasize the patient and family's strengths, and encourage alignment with the medical team. An awareness and understanding of the patient's patterns of coping; current functioning; psychological status, including cognitive change and impairment; and spiritual and cultural orientation can help to facilitate that alignment. Reframing through the utilization of the positive aspects of denial and emphasizing of concerns of safety will orient the patient and family toward reality and help them view the diagnosis of ALS as a challenge and not a crisis situation (12).

3. *Identify coping mechanisms, strategies, and interpersonal communication styles of the patient's family.*

Relationships with the patient's primary caregivers should be actively pursued. This effort may lead to insight into the system of family interdependence (13) and identification of the members that will be the most influential in effecting change and supporting the use of certain assistive devices. Cultural factors may be important determinants of a successful relationship, as for example when the eldest son of an affected father holds the most influence in a family because of the cultural norms. Language barriers may hamper interpersonal communication, for example, when English is not the primary language spoken at home. In our experience, family members may not openly express helplessness, frustration, anger, fear, and concern about the patient in front of the patient or to all members of the interdisciplinary team. The technique of reframing (14) (again emphasizing the positive aspects of denial and concerns of safety always orienting toward reality) may be useful in ALS family support groups. Group facilitators are mindful that the emphasis is not what is happening to the family but how the family is relating to what is happening (12).

4. *Ensure that an analysis of interdisciplinary treatment goals has been conducted to ascertain how psychosocial support might complement the medical plan of care.*

The provision of psychosocial support can be facilitated or diminished by the behaviors and treatment goals of the interdisciplinary team. It is important for team members to share common goals and establish close communicative ties. Any tendency of the family to manipulate or split the team should be made apparent to all concerned and put into perspective.

5. *Ensure that the coping strategy and interpersonal communication of health professionals are continually self-assessed and open to outside counsel.*

Healthcare professionals should be aware of their own behaviors. Just as the patient and family are asked to meet the diagnosis of ALS as a continual challenge, so should the healthcare team. One manner of self-assessment is to ask a set of related questions. Have our behaviors promoted problem-solving and positive adaptation or dependency in patients with ALS and other progressive motor illness? Whose psychological needs are being met—the patient's or ours? Are we being realistic in our behavioral self-assessment? Have we been creative in our approach to alternative treatments? Do we need supportive guidance from a psychiatric nurse clinician, psychologist, or psychiatrist in responding to a patient and their family, particularly when psychological dysfunction is evident? Are we aware of our own psychological functioning, dysfunctioning and maladaptive patterns? Have we promoted collegiality and collaboration among all our team members?

INTEGRATED PALLIATIVE CARE

To act as one-caring, then, is to act with special regard for the particular person in a concrete situation. We act not to achieve for ourselves a commendation but to protect or enhance the welfare of the cared-for. Because we are inclined toward the cared-for, we want to act in a way that will please him. But we wish to please him for his sake and not for the promise of his grateful response to our generosity.

Nel Noddings (15)

Palliative therapy should be offered at all stages of ALS to promote confidence, encourage independence, reduce the burden of physical handicaps, and sustain relationships with family, friends, and colleagues.

The gradual loss of ambulation is a nearly universal feature of progressive motor disease that leads to consultation with physiatry and physical and occupational therapy. These professionals, as well as other members of the interdisciplinary team, will guide the patient in their increasing reliance on assistive devices to maintain independence. In ALS, leg weakness and spasticity are the causes of gait difficulty. Mild to moderately affected patients derive benefit from a cane or walker. Ankle–foot orthoses and other bracing maneuvers may improve balance, preserve energy, promote safety, and avert fatigue that might otherwise preclude the participation of some patients in social activities. When frequent falls occur, a wheelchair may be necessary. Contemporary lightweight chairs are easy to operate and are portable. Self-propelled larger units offer the potential for continued independence even in advanced disease, but they are more expensive and heavier than manually propelled ones.

Communication impairments resulting from dysarthria, anarthria, and dysphonia are challenges for patients with ALS and their healthcare providers. Speech difficulty leads to a sense of isolation, enhances preexisting dysfunctional communication styles, and may limit the ability to communicate basic needs, such as suctioning or repositioning. Consultation with an experienced speech pathologist is essential early in the diagnosis before problems in communication become overtly apparent. Under normal circumstances, speech is possible through the combined action of the lips, tongue, palate, and larynx. Bulbar weakness and spasticity lead to a mixed pattern of dysarthria. Hyperadduction of the vocal cords leads to elevated laryngeal resistance in exhalation and a raspy voice. Flaccid weakness of one or both vocal cords causes a breathy hypernasal voice due to escape of air into the nasal pharynx; in addition, there may be slow strained vocalization with poor pronunciation of consonants.

Management of bulbar symptoms in patients diagnosed with ALS begins with speech, language, and otolaryngologic assessments. It may be helpful to educate patients with bulbar ALS in oromotor exercises for mild impairments and to encourage early intervention for evaluation of augmentative aids. Verbal communication can be prolonged in tracheostomized patients as long as speech is intelligible, in spite of respiratory dependency, by cuffless tubes or intermittent positive pressure ventilation. Computer-assisted aids and electronic communication systems are useful for maintaining communication to family, friends, and the healthcare team and in allowing the patient to actively participate in the decision-making process even late in the illness.

Optimal management of dysphagia and nutritional requirements is important in the psychosocial and physical well-being of patients with ALS and other progressive neuromuscular disorders. Dysphagia precedes ventilatory difficulty in three fourths of patients with ALS and is present in virtually all others late in the illness (16). Normal swallowing requires the coordinated function of structures of the oral cavity, pharynx, larynx, and esophagus. Chewed food moves posteriorly in the oral cavity through constrictor muscles and other pharyngeal spaces to the esophagus where peristaltic movement carries it past the gastric sphincter and into the stomach. Alterations in smell, taste, and fear of aspiration and respiratory weakness can contribute to the occurrence of weight loss even before overt dysphagia is present. Weakness of lip, cheek, lingual, neck muscles, hyperactive pharyngeal gag and cough reflexes, dyspnea, spinal hyperlordosis, and balance difficulty due to axial weakness can all impair the early phase of swallowing; esophageal weakness and dismotility compromise lower esophageal function. The clinical evaluation includes a review of clinical symptoms and signs of dysphagia and inspection of the nasopharynx, larynx, and esophageal paths by fiberoptic and video fluoroscopic studies. Liquids are generally more difficult to swallow than solids. Pooling of liquids and secretions may be found along the vallecula and pyriform sinuses or in the laryngeal vestibule, increasing the likelihood for aspiration.

Even the treatment of mild dysphagia includes dietary counseling, oromotor exercises, and positioning devices for the head and trunk. With bulbar involvement, aspiration can be improved by the management of secretions, abnormal breathing patterns, assisted coughing or chest physical therapy, oropharyngeal suctioning, and percutaneous endoscopic gastrostomy (PEG) placement. Nasogastric tubes are typically not used due to local irritation and an offensive appearance. The PEG is the most used procedure for dysphagia management due to its appeal. The ease of implementation, low risk for individuals with a forced vital capacity of 50% of predicted or greater (16), and minimal anesthesia are factors that contribute to PEG utilization. PEG may prolong survival in ALS (17), particularly before weight loss becomes too great, but its impact on the quality of life is still unknown (18,19). Its routine use runs counter to the view that death due to starvation or malnutrition in ALS is a painless, final, merciful act and is one of many options to be considered for prolongation of life (20–23).

Respiratory symptoms inevitably occur in all patients with ALS, often in association with an ineffective cough, difficulty in clearing secretions, and in the aspiration of fluids or food. An astute clinician will recognize the signs of impending respiratory insufficiency, including agita-

tion, lethargy, orthopnea, poor cough, increased use of accessory muscles, diminution of the volume of speech, and disturbed sleep. Pulmonary consultation can provide helpful information regarding respiratory muscle function to the ALS clinician. Pulmonary muscle function tests are the most reliable and sensitive measures of respiratory strength capacity and life expectancy and are optimally performed every 3 to 6 months. As vital capacity approaches 50% of predicted capacity, noninvasive intermittent positive-pressure aids should be introduced. Some patients decided early in the course of their illness to pursue tracheostomy and are comfortable considering life assisted with ventilation, knowing that they may be unable to move and, at some point, unable to communicate.

The decision to proceed with endotracheal intubation or indwelling tracheostomy should be discussed as openly and supportively as possible with the patient and family members in advance of impending emergencies to remain in compliance with patient preferences for medical decision making. Similarly, documentation with respect to advance directives, healthcare proxy, or, in the case of some states, durable power of attorney, should be completed and placed in the patient's chart and copies distributed to appropriate team members. The optimal situation for home ventilatory support includes adequate financial resources and psychosocial and medical support systems, including proximity to a clinic or hospital for the treatment of complications or emergencies (24).

Drooling is a vexing problem in ALS that is associated with oropharyngeal and lower lip muscle weakness, faulty containment and overflow of secretions, but usually not hypersalivation. Early in the disease, patients report a small pool of saliva on the pillow case upon awakening or excessive secretions from the mouth requiring frequent dabbing of facial tissue. Beyond the embarrassment and social isolation it causes, drooling is associated with a heightened risk of aspiration. Medications such as tricyclic antidepressants and atropine-like drugs, with potent anticholinergic effects, reduce salivation by blocking parasympathetic outflow; however, they also have the potential for urinary retention, confusion, and hallucinations.

Care for the mental health of patients with ALS is a steady challenge (25,26). It includes recognition and treatment of clinically significant depression, anxiety, lability of mood, and dementia. The seemingly healthy adjustment to serious illness often includes the denial of depression and anxiety that may be helped through referrals to psychiatry, psychology, social work, or pastoral care and with pharmacotherapy. Observations suggest that treatment for depression has an impact on denial and facilitates adaptive coping mechanisms.

Anxiety disorders and obsessive thought disorders associated with ALS have been less well studied, but experience suggests that they might also be amenable to counseling and antianxiety drugs. Lability of mood, leading to extreme laughter or tearfulness, is especially common among patients with ALS and is probably related to pseudobulbar palsy and frontal lobe release mechanisms. Experience suggests a role for counseling to improve insight and pharmacotherapy for depression. There is increasing awareness of clinical and pathologic syndromes of dementia in association with ALS (26). Mental disturbances in ALS-associated dementia are often minor compared with those with frank Alzheimer's disease and can be easily overlooked by the busy clinician. Cognitive change is subtle and can include variable impairment in reasoning, abstraction, decision-making, goal-directed planning, and organizational ability. For example, these subtle cognitive changes may be seen in the reluctance to introduce formal mechanisms of healthcare planning, such as institution of advance care directives or a healthcare proxy.

Contact with friends and family and the satisfaction with that contact are two important elements in the psychosocial well-being of patients with ALS. Observations have found that the identification of a spiritual frame of reference or worshipping community also serves of benefit. In fact, social contact is central after ambulation ceases, ability to perform activities of daily living is reduced, and hopefulness and interest in the future are lost (9).

Attitudes about terminal or hospice care have varied over time, and such attitudes differ among individual physicians and patients. The term hospice has evolved from its medieval concept as a place of rest for the sick and weary on a long journey. Today's concept is seen more as when medical science cannot add further days to life (expectancy), at least more life will be added to each day (by hospice care). Hospice care offers medical and social services for terminally ill patients and their families, which includes guidance in coping with physical, emotional, spiritual, and psychological distress. This philosophy of care can take place in the home, hospital, or in other dedicated facilities. There has been increasing acceptance of the patient's right to allow a terminal disease to take its course in a hospice setting without treatment to prolong life, with the physician serving the patient's interest (27). Some have advocated legal and ethical standards to protect this right (20,25). Others have found these rights essential to living and leaving a life with dignity.

ACKNOWLEDGMENTS

This chapter is dedicated to the many patients that have received psychosocial care and palliative care from the Eleanor and Lou Gehrig MDA/ALS Center at Columbia-Presbyterian Medical Center (CPMC), New York; to the Muscular Dystrophy Association (MDA), which supports that care; to Dr. Elisabeth K. J. Koenig, The Rev. Dr. John Koenig, and The Rev. William A. Doubleday of General Theological Seminary, New York, who influenced our thoughts on the psychosocial care of patients; and to Lewis P. Rowland, M.D., for his leadership and support.

REFERENCES

1. Schweitzer A. The will to live. In: Joy CR, ed. *Albert Schweitzer: an anthology*. Boston: Beacon Press, 1947:251.
2. Starr P. *The social transformation of American medicine: the rise of a sovereign profession and the making of a vast industry*. New York: Basic Books, 1982.
3. Mayer RF. Living with amyotrophic lateral sclerosis. In: Charash LI, Lovelace RE, Leach CF, et al., eds. *Muscular dystrophy and other neuromuscular diseases: psychosocial issues*. New York: Haworth Press, 1991:23–30.
4. McDonald ER, Wiedenfeld SA, Hillel A, Carpenter CL, Walter RA. Survival in amyotrophic lateral sclerosis. The role of psychological factors. *Arch Neurol* 1994;51:17–23.
5. Schweitzer A. Reverence for life. In: Joy CR, ed. *Albert Schweitzer: an anthology*. Boston, Beacon Press, 1947:261.
6. Koenig J. *New Testament hospitality: partnership with strangers as promise and mission*. Philadelphia: Fortress Press, 1985.
7. Hendrick R. [Revised by Padol L.] *Latin made simple*. New York: Doubleday, 1992.
8. Campbell-Heider N, Hart C. Updating the nurse's bedside manner. *Image J Nurs Scholar* 1993;25:133–139.
9. Lawton MP, Moss M, Glicksman A. The quality of the last year of life of older persons. *Milbank Q* 1990;68:1–28.
10. Henson RH. Analysis of the concept of mutuality. *Image J Nurs Scholar* 1997;29:77–81.
11. Naugle RI. Denial in rehabilitation: its genesis, consequences, and clinical management. In: Marinelli RP, Dell Orto AE, eds. *The psychological & social impact of disability*. New York: Springer Publishing Company, 1991:139–151.
12. Hulnick MR, Hulnick HR. Life's challenges: curse or opportunity? Counseling families of persons with disabilities. In: Marinelli RP, Dell Orto AE, eds. *The psychological & social impact of disability*. New York: Springer Publishing Company, 1991:258–268.
13. Friedman EH. *Generation to generation: family process in church and synagogue*. New York: The Guilford Press, 1985.
14. Bandler R, Grinder J. *Frogs into princes*. Moab, UT: Real People Press, 1979.
15. Noddings N. *Caring: a feminine approach to ethics & moral education*. Berkeley: University of California Press, 1984:24.
16. Strand EA, Miller RM, Yorkston KM, Hillel AD. Management of oral-pharyngeal dysphasia symptoms in ALS. *Dysphasia* 1996;11:129–139.
17. Mazzini L, Corra T, Zaccala M, Mora G, Del Piano M, Galante M. Percutaneous endoscopic gastrostomy and enteral nutrition in amyotrophic lateral sclerosis. *Neurology* 1995;242:695–698.
18. Schmitz P. The process of dying with and without feeding and fluids by tube. *Law Med Health Care* 1991;19:23–26.
19. Gelinas DF, Miller RG. Optimizing PEG management in ALS. Presented at the 6th International Symposium on ALS/MND, Dublin, Ireland, 1995(abst).
20. American Academy of Neurology Ethics and Humanities Subcommittee. Position statement: certain aspects of the care and management of profoundly and irreversibly paralyzed patients with retained consciousness and cognition. *Neurology* 1993;43:222–223.
21. American Academy of Neurology Ethics and Humanities Subcommittee. Commentary: competent patients with advanced states of permanent paralysis have the right to forgo life-sustaining therapy. *Neurology* 1996;43:224–225.
22. Sullivan RJ. Accepting death without artificial nutrition or hydration. *J Gen Intern Med* 1993;8:220–224.
23. Bernat JL, Gert B, Mogielnicki RP. Patient refusal of hydration and nutrition: an alternative to physician-assisted suicide or voluntary active euthanasia. *Arch Intern Med* 1993;153:2723–2728.
24. Moss AH, Casey P, Stocking CB, Roos RP, Brooks BR, Siegler M. Home ventilation for amyotrophic lateral sclerosis patients: outcomes, costs, and patient, family, and physician attitudes. *Neurology* 1993;43:438–443.
25. American Academy of Neurology Ethics and Humanities Subcommittee. Special article: palliative care in neurology. *Neurology* 1996;46:870–872.
26. Massman PJ, Sims J, Cooke N, Haverkamp LJ, Appel V, Appel SH. Prevalence and correlates of neuropsychological deficits in amyotrophic lateral sclerosis. *J Neurol Neurosurg Psychiatry* 1996;61:450–455.
27. Miller RJ. Hospice as an alternative to euthanasia. *Law Med Health Care* 1992;20:127–132.

Subject Index

DATE DUE